## MY TWO SONS

I have two sons.
One was born in a mighty
fine Texas town.
The other died there.

My baby son was full of love.
He gave me great gifts of
laughter,
hugs and kisses.
He gave me the great gift
of sorrow.
When he died, I thought
I would die.
But then he taught me how to
live.

My living son now has a brother
who can teach him great lessons
in life.
He is blessed among children.
But he must grow, and seek
these difficult lessons.
He will be alone.
I cannot show him the way.

The force of his life will lead
him to understand and comprehend
meaning in sorrow,
the significance of human care,
a strength to carry him beyond
himself.

My living son is a good child.
He has a soul.
He will suffer more than his
dear dead brother.
His little brother's soul will
always be as it now stands.
God bless the soul of my dear
baby son.
He has gone to meet his morning
sun.
God bless the soul of my living
son.
His race in life has just begun.

**P. L. C.**

# CHILD HEALTH MAINTENANCE
## Concepts in family-centered care

# Child health maintenance

## Concepts in family-centered care

**PEGGY L. CHINN, R.N., Ph.D.**

Professor of Nursing,
School of Nursing,
Wright State University,
Dayton, Ohio

**SECOND EDITION**

with **377** illustrations

# The C. V. Mosby Company

ST. LOUIS • TORONTO • LONDON    1979

**SECOND EDITION**

**Copyright © 1979 by The C. V. Mosby Company**

All rights reserved. No part of this book may be reproduced
in any manner without written permission of the publisher.

Previous edition copyrighted 1974

Printed in the United States of America

The C. V. Mosby Company
11830 Westline Industrial Drive, St. Louis, Missouri 63141

**Library of Congress Cataloging in Publication Data**

Chinn, Peggy L        1941-
    Child health maintenance.

    Includes bibliographical references and index.
    1.  Pediatric nursing.  2.  Children—Care and
hygiene.  I.  Title. [DNLM:  1.  Child care.
2.  Pediatric nursing.  3.  Family.  4.  Child
development.   WY159 C5395ca]
RJ245.C49 1979        610.73′62        78-12101
ISBN 0-8016-0950-X

GW/VH/VH   9  8  7  6  5  4  3  2  1      03/B/355

# Preface

The second edition of *Child Health Maintenance: Concepts in Family-Centered Care* represents a major stage in the development of the text. During the writing, I was reminded of the first five years in the life of a child, when growth and development leads to major changes in the child's stature as well as to significant gains in maturity over the infantile state. Just as the milieu of the family shapes the development of the child, this book reflects changes in the milieu of the nursing profession over the past five years.

Of particular importance is the profession's development of the concepts of nursing diagnosis and of quality assurance in nursing practice. My own expanded concepts of health needs, health problems, and nursing diagnosis are presented in the text along with the significant work that has resulted in the Nursing Problem Classification for Children and Youth and the Standards of Maternal-Child Nursing Practice. These two major developments have occurred since the publication of the first edition, and I am pleased to include them as integral components of this edition.

The basic philosophy of child health nursing presented in the first edition remains in this revision. The child is viewed as a unique, holistic individual developing within the context of family and society. The conceptual frame of reference of physical, learning and thought, social, and inner competencies has been developed further. Several approaches for nursing assessment and intervention related to each competency area have been added for each stage of development. Application of the theoretical bases for development in each competency area has been more completely developed for nursing assessment and intervention. For example, the theoretical function of play is presented for each stage of development, and play approaches for assessment and for nursing intervention are described.

A primary aim of the first edition was to stimulate the problem-solving capacity of the student or practitioner. With the second edition, it is anticipated that critical thinking as well as problem-solving skills are stimulated. The text provides specific theory needed to stimulate critical examination of the nurse's basis for practice. Further, where evidence to support existing theory is lacking or where existing theories are inadequate to explain observed phenomena, the need for further development of understanding is discussed. The cases included in each unit present examples of comprehensive use of the nursing process, use of the problem-oriented record, and illustrative health needs and problems of children. Further, the cases serve as a point of reference for the use of the case audit guide (presented in the Appendix) for simulated experience in examining the quality of nursing practice.

Nursing management of major health problems for each stage of development has been more completely conceptualized and includes health maintenance and illness problems. In these sections, nursing is considered to have certain areas of independent responsibility for the child's attainment and maintenance of health, as well as certain areas of desired and necessary collaborative function with other health care workers. Although there has been a major expansion in the presentation of medical diagnoses of physical health problems, the emphasis remains on the conceptualization of nursing problems and responsible nursing intervention.

Appreciation is extended to the many agencies and individuals who granted permission to include their material and who cooperated in obtaining illustrations. In particular, I wish to thank the American Nurses' Association, who gave permission to include the Standards for Maternal and Child Health Practice, and Minnesota Systems Research, Inc., who gave permission to include the Nursing Problem Classification for Children and Youth. It is my hope that these valuable resources will stimulate the development of nursing diagnoses and facilitate the process of quality assurance in nursing practice.

Appreciation is extended to the Children's Medical Center of Dallas, Texas, the Dallas County Hospital District, Parkland Memorial Hospital, and St. Thomas Day Care Center for granting permission to take photographs that are included in this edition. Special acknowledgment is given to each of the parents and young people who willingly gave permission to have themselves or their children photographed.

A very special acknowledgment is extended to Tommie Wallace for providing the photographic illustrations that have been added to this edition and to Cheryl Hundley for designing the assessment tools and preparing the cases that are included in each unit. Appreciation is expressed to Jean Tillman for contributing the section on home deliveries.

I am grateful to all who have reviewed or used the first edition and offered valuable suggestions for the revision, many of whom I have never met. I am particularly grateful to Jo Ann Ashley for her insightful critique of subtle attitudes and values that were conveyed in the manuscript and who assisted in the revision of the section on the family and in the conceptualization of nursing practice that has been developed in this edition. Finally, I would like to express gratitude to the many individuals who knowingly or unknowingly made it possible for me to take the time and devote my energy to complete this edition and to those who gave needed support and encouragement throughout the period of preparation.

**Peggy L. Chinn**

# Contents

Contents

Contents

## 17 Death and dying during childhood and adolescence, 689

## 18 Children and youth with long-term physical problems, 703

## 19 The child with learning problems, 784

Co-authored with Philip C. Chinn, Ed.D.

## 20 The child with long-term social and inner problems, 802

Co-authored with Philip C. Chinn, Ed.D.

## Appendix, 865

# Child health maintenance

The major goal of health care is to promote the child's and the family's motivation to seek health and to use their own resources to attain, maintain, or regain optimal health and function. Whether the child is healthy or unhealthy, the health care system provides a major service in assisting the child and family to reach and maintain this ideal goal of health. The individual who assumes the responsibilities associated with professional membership on the health care delivery team in society must understand the child and the family and the many factors that contribute to the promotion and maintenance of health. When the child and family are burdened with stresses that interfere with the maintenance of health, these stresses become important factors in assisting the family to attain or return to a more satisfying state of health. The role of the nurse is to fulfill those functions sanctioned by society as within the realm of nursing care and that traditionally have focused on the promotion of the individual's ability to attain, maintain, or regain optimal health. In the chapters that follow, we will consider the child, the family, and society, and the health care services that are offered in today's society to children and families.

The purposes of Chapter 1, "The Challenge of the Child," are (1) to present an overview of the processes of growth and development, (2) to present a conceptual frame of reference that can be used by the nurse in understanding the child and in meeting the challenge of rendering meaningful, sound nursing care, which enhances the achievement of maximal life and health for each child, and (3) to consider basic facilitating factors that enhance the attainment of mature life competencies.

The purposes of Chapter 2, "Child Nursing Today . . . and Tomorrow," are (1) to portray briefly the history of child nursing, (2) to discuss

Child health
maintenance

implementation of health care for children specifically relating this to professional nursing, (3) to describe in general terms nursing assessment of the child, and (4) to describe generally nursing management of child health needs. The nursing process, comprised of nursing assessment and implementation of nursing care, is more specifically developed in the units that follow for each developmental period of childhood.

Chapter 3, "Understanding Family and Society," is aimed toward the purposes of (1) reviewing the essential features and problems of culture and environment, (2) discussion of the predominant features of the family unit as it has existed in the past and is beginning to emerge today, (3) discussion of the manner in which families as a unit influence competency development in children, and (4) consideration of the experience of crisis within the family unit and its implications for nursing care.

# The challenge of the child

In today's world the concept of growth and development during childhood has expanded in proportion with advances in all fields of science. Increased ability to observe physical and biochemical events scientifically during intrauterine life has led to increased awareness and knowledge of the effects of fetal events on the individual's later life. The behavioral sciences have contributed to significant changes in ways children of technologic societies are reared and taught. Discoveries in the physiologic and medical sciences have yielded the ability to alter the course of human life when deformity or debilitating disease occurs.

Nursing has long shared with many professions dealing with children and families the goal of improving the life and health of the child and enhancing the process of physical and emotional development of children. Thus nursing practice and research have been intimately concerned with improving and investigating effects of nursing intervention upon children and their families. Many related disciplines have contributed to this process, but a great gap exists between knowledge that can reliably serve to define the goal of care for children and applied practices that are sound and relevant to achieving optimal health.

## LIFE AS AN OPEN SYSTEM
### The concept of growth

Growth refers to changes in structure or size. During childhood the physical changes in weight, height, and body proportion are readily noticeable. In addition the child completes a uniform sequence of changes in body cell content. The child's fat and muscle tissues change in kind, distribution, and mass. Metabolic and biochemical processes change as life progresses toward maturity. The cells of the central nervous system change as maturity progresses. This process directly influences the process of development.[13,24]

### The concept of development

Development refers to changes in kind or quality. Development evolves from maturation of physical and mental capacities and learning. It is the progression of events that leads to maturity and integration. The child cannot achieve maturity until physical growth is complete, and yet developmental maturity cannot be pinpointed at a particular point in life. Emotional maturity has many interpretations; it is difficult to describe completely the close interrelationships of all aspects of life. Physical, emotional, and social factors have made the exact study of

**3**

human nature elusive and difficult. Philosophy and theology have long influenced the study of development and the thinking of those most earnestly seeking knowledge of the child. This is understandable, because children and adults are beings with the unique ability to think, feel, ponder, deliberate, and reason. The endless quest for understanding of development and life processes is enhanced through understanding of certain principles and characteristics that can describe but do not necessarily explain the developmental process.

## Principles of growth and development

### Openness and change

The person, incorporating body, mind, and spirit, may be thought of as a system that constantly receives from the environment and gives to the environment. This concept of the person as an open system is useful in understanding many problems of development during childhood, because at no other period during life is the process of physical and emotional change so apparent. In addition the child is seen as an individual with maximal potential for further change and development within the limitations of heritable factors.[42]

### Heredity and environment

Parents and those in science and service professions have long deliberated over the influences of heredity and environment in shaping personality and behavior. It is now generally acknowledged that both factors influence all behavior. The issue seems to recur in regard to the proportion of behavior that can be attributed to inherited traits and that portion that has been shaped by parents or other significant people, either knowingly or unknowingly. The issue becomes a very practical one, for example, when a child has begun to exhibit some undesirable behavioral trait, and society must decide the destiny, not only of the child, but also of the family and community. Will the child be left within the family unit, and can the behavior be therapeutically changed? Is the child destined to behave in such a manner because of a predetermined personality trait? Mothers have been identified as extremely significant "shapers" of their child's behavior, but a particular child's future can never be projected to determine precisely the influence a particular mother may have exerted. The great complexity of this issue has baffled behavioral and physical scientists for years.

Children are products of their heredity and past environment. The predetermined hereditary factors cannot be significantly altered. But the present complex environment, including the people in the child's life, the climate and condition of the external and internal environment, the child's nutrition, and society and culture, provides the immediate stimulus for current behavior. The interaction of heredity and environment may be described as a proportional contribution depending upon the extent of influence of each factor. For example, a child who possesses average analytical reasoning ability may be stimulated to achieve advanced academic standing through encouraging and enhancing family and school settings or may experience academic failure in the presence of a discouraging, stifling family and school environment.[2]

### Predictable patterns and stages

Development proceeds according to a predictable, continuous pattern for all children. Individual variations, discussed in the next section, occur in the rate and quality of attainment of these predictable patterns. Damage to the body structure or central nervous system can alter the pattern of development, and development that does not follow the usual sequence is indicative of damage or malfunction. Child nursing practice depends upon thorough familiarity with the expected patterns of development. Emotional development and social adjustment are predictably characterized by phases of equilibrium and disequilibrium. Children swing from periods when they are in focus and harmony with their families and peers to other points, when they are difficult to live with and seem unusually tense, indecisive, or insecure.

Development of the body proceeds in a cephalocaudal and proximodistal fashion (Fig. 1-1). Increases in size and maturation of the neuromuscular functions of the body begin first in the head and proceed toward the hands and

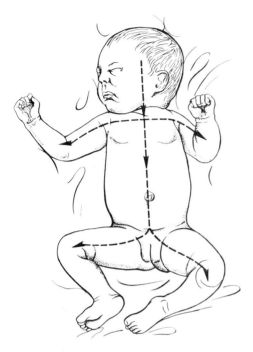

**Fig. 1-1.** Development of the body proceeds in a cephalocaudal and proximodistal fashion.

feet. Development also proceeds from the general to the specific; gross, large muscle functions are present before the finer abilities of the hands and fingers. The fetus reaches term with a relatively large head and small limbs, and the abilities for functioning are more advanced for the head than for the limbs.

Developmental patterns have been clearly identified through scientific observations in many areas of functioning. Motor development was one of the earliest developmental patterns described, and it is sometimes equated with the total concept of physical development.[19] Closely associated with motor development is the development of speech, and patterns in the acquisition of speech have been fully described.[5,31] Patterns and sequences in emotional and social behavior likewise have been described for various cultures and have been conceptualized from several different theoretic frameworks. There appear to be cross-cultural similarities, but the process of identifying universal traits is far from complete.[14,32]

The widely influential theories of Freud and others who followed him depend heavily upon the concept of sequential, predictable patterns of emotional and social development. The child has also been observed to follow well-described patterns in intellectual, analytical thinking and concept formation abilities.[37] These abilities may be further described for specific abstractions such as time, self, death, moral and religious beliefs, humor, beauty, and interests, and they are heavily influenced by the child's culture.[25,32,36]

The classic works of the Yale Clinic of Child Development[19,20,21,22] have described in detail many of the predictable features of development. Although many of these findings have been challenged, they have remained as a major foundation in developmental evaluation, and they continue to be a valuable resource for understanding salient features of a particular stage of childhood.

Throughout child development literature, stages of development are identified either by age groupings or in terms implying age groupings. Since all children do not develop at the same rate in all areas of functioning and because of variations in quality of development, there is some dissatisfaction with the use of defined "stages" in describing the developmental patterns. However, the conceptual formation of defined stages of development according to roughly approximate age groups aids in describing behavior and development. The six major developmental periods, which will be described in subsequent chapters, are:

1. *Prenatal period.* This period begins at some point before conception. It is considered to be one of the most important developmental periods because of the extremely rapid rate at which development proceeds. The nurse who is involved with the care of the child will inevitably need to understand the influences of the prenatal period in order to obtain a meaningful history and to associate relevant factors with the child's state of health at any current stage of development.

2. *Newborn and infancy periods.* A distinction is made between the overlapping periods termed "infancy" and "newborn." The *newborn* period extends through the critical first month of life and is considered in detail because of the importance of this period for the parents and

**5**

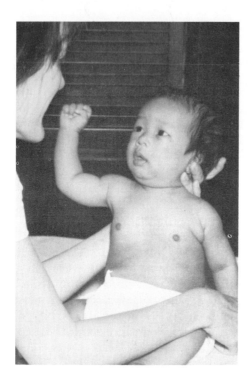

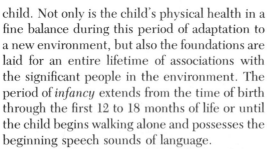

**Fig. 1-2.** The 6-week-old child has passed the newborn period and is now a more mature, stable infant who is beginning to become a more active participant in family life.

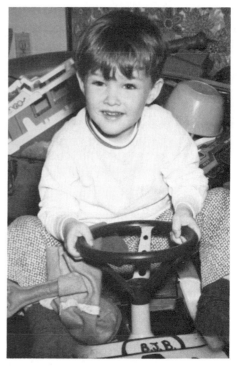

**Fig. 1-3.** Toddlerhood is a period of significant personality, mental, and physical development.

child. Not only is the child's physical health in a fine balance during this period of adaptation to a new environment, but also the foundations are laid for an entire lifetime of associations with the significant people in the environment. The period of *infancy* extends from the time of birth through the first 12 to 18 months of life or until the child begins walking alone and possesses the beginning speech sounds of language.

3. *Toddlerhood.* In Western societies the period of life from the time the child begins to walk and talk until about the age of 3 years marks a significant time of physical and emotional development. Motor development progresses significantly, and the child achieves a degree of physical and emotional autonomy while maintaining the close identity with the primary family unit. Of particular significance to nursing is the fact that characteristic health problems exist during the toddler years, which merit nursing assessment, prevention, and management. These health problems are re-

lated to physical characteristics of anatomy and cellular structure in the young child and to motor and cognitive features, which render the child relatively dependent, defenseless, and prone to illness and injury.

4. *Early childhood.* The period between about 3 years of age and the time the child enters the formal school setting is distinguished by the child's early entry into the world of peers. Most children in this age period experience early contacts with other children of their own age and reach a level of physical and emotional ability to begin interaction, to respond to their peers, and to begin social interactions with a variety of persons. Increased physical defenses against disease, the increased maturity in physical dexterity, and increasing cognitive ability give children a greater defense against health problems, but they still maintain greater risk than the older child. The meaning of this age period has great significance as a period of readiness to enter the larger social world beyond the

family and provides for a transition from family-oriented development to society- and peer-oriented development.

5. *Later childhood.* The childhood years begin when children begin to enter the world of their peers, which in Western culture is usually marked by entrance into school. For the purposes of this book the ages of 5 or 6 will be considered as the beginning of the later childhood years. At this point children gain a more advanced level of resistance to a number of the health problems of the earlier years and advance in cognitive abilities to a point that their interests turn away from the immediate family to the wider world of peers. They possess enough maturity to begin to relate to others as individuals in their own right and to practice advanced skills of socialization on their own. The end of this period is marked by the onset of puberty, at which time many developmental tasks continue but are cast against the background of adolescence.

6. *Adolescence.* The point of puberty, or sexual maturity, marks the beginning of adolescence. In all societies there is some significance associated with this point in life, but the nature of its interpretation varies greatly. In the United States adolescence is a period of transition, great stress and adjustment, of personal exploration and trial. In societies that are not technologically oriented, adolescence is more a period of entrance and acceptance into the adult world, and greater adult responsibilities are given to the adolescent at an earlier period. The end point of adolescence is reached when the individual demonstrates readiness to assume full adult responsibilities of financial, emotional, and social independence. Under usual circumstances in Western societies, this point is reached between the ages of 18 and 21, but wide variations exist.[6]

### Individual differences in development

Knowledge of the predictable characteristics of development at various points during the childhood years is a practical necessity in knowing and predicting realistic expectations for a child's behavior. Within this framework, however, any child may exhibit a wide range of behavior, which represents a unique set of physical and personality characteristics. The real challenge in working with a child is to determine in a nonjudgmental fashion whether the behavior and physical ability are within a normal, acceptable range for this particular child.

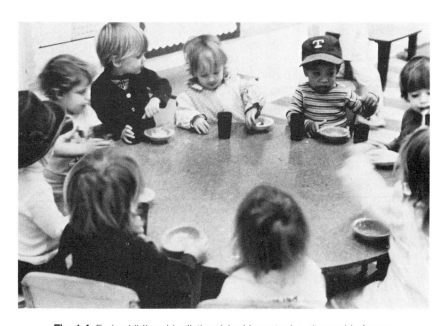

**Fig. 1-4.** Early childhood is distinguished by entry into the world of peers.

The guidelines for this decision arise from many sources: the child's society and culture, expectations determined through scientific observation, and factors arising from the child's genetic and environmental endowment. Usually a child functions at a clearly acceptable level in most areas of development. When deviations occur, there can be total deviation from normally expected development in all areas, or a child may function at expected levels in most areas with an unusually slow or unusually accelerated rate or different quality in one or two areas. Complete evaluation of developmental standing when differences occur is a multidisciplinary task. The nurse may detect differences but must rely upon educators, psychologists, speech and hearing specialists, physicians, and other appropriate persons for obtaining reliable and valid evaluation of the nature of the child's developmental standing.

### The importance of early development

When development is within normal limits, one period prepares the child for the next. Cultural expectations in regard to the attainments of each period in life enhance the sequential dependency of one stage upon the preceding one, but the fact remains that the child can most ef-

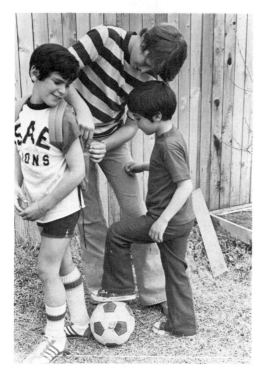

**Fig. 1-5.** Later childhood is a period when interests begin to center on the wider world of peers.

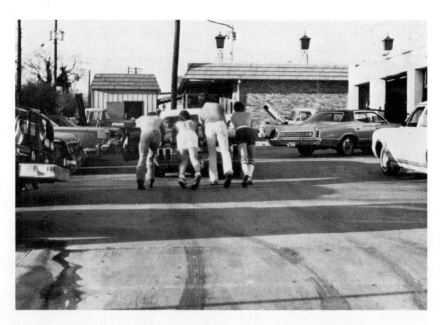

**Fig. 1-6.** The adolescent begins entrance into the adult world.

fectively move into the next period, either physically or emotionally, when successful completion of the tasks of the preceding period have been mastered.[35] In addition there is evidence supporting the notion that there are critical periods of development after which the task of the period cannot be mastered.[17,25,32,48] For example, if a child is not able to master the vocalizations of speech sounds during the first year of life, he or she is in jeopardy of never being able to function adequately in the area of verbal communication.[5,31] Unfavorable emotional experiences in early years exert a severe impact on the child's future, whereas an older child is more able to cope with adverse circumstances. Although environmental intervention for certain deficiencies in development has been demonstrated to be more effective for humans than for animals in cases of delayed development, there remains a significant handicap when intervention is delayed or when certain physical or mental limitations are present.

Early patterns of behavior persist throughout life within the range of normalcy expected. Various investigators and theorists identify the first two to five years of life as the critical period for formation of basic personality traits.[17,45] The many factors contributing to the formation of permanent characteristics and traits include the child's genetic inheritance, undetermined prenatal environmental factors, the family and society as an infant and young child, the relationship to the environment, the emotional milieu, and the degree of cognitive and learning stimulation in the environment. The significance of the early years of life arises from the rapidity of growth and development during this period. While some progress may be made in efforts to alter the effects of early development at a later point in life, there remains an overwhelming preference for intervention during the period of earliest development.

## A CONCEPTUAL FRAMEWORK FOR NURSING CARE OF THE CHILD

Development of the individual may be conceptualized as beginning at the point of conception and gradually progressing toward maturity (Fig. 1-7). The sphere of experience and interaction with the environment gradually widens,

and the unique individual acquires traits in four major areas: physical, learning and thought, social, and inner competencies.

Human development is an open system, with a multitude of influences operating upon the uniqueness of the individual; in turn the individual influences the environmental factors. The multiple factors that influence development of the individual are depicted in Fig. 1-8. The developmental process may be further depicted as a constant movement among the parts of the circle, illustrating the constant interaction and interdependence among the parts. The total impact of these multidimensional factors is constantly exerting influence on the child in all areas of development. The nursing focus becomes that of merging what is known about the influencing factors of the open system with the child's particular developmental competencies and needs for future development.

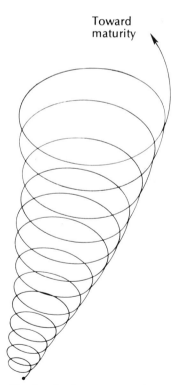

Toward
maturity

The beginning—conception

**Fig. 1-7.** The widening sphere of the individual's unique, progressive development throughout life toward physical, learning and thought, psychosocial, and inner competencies.

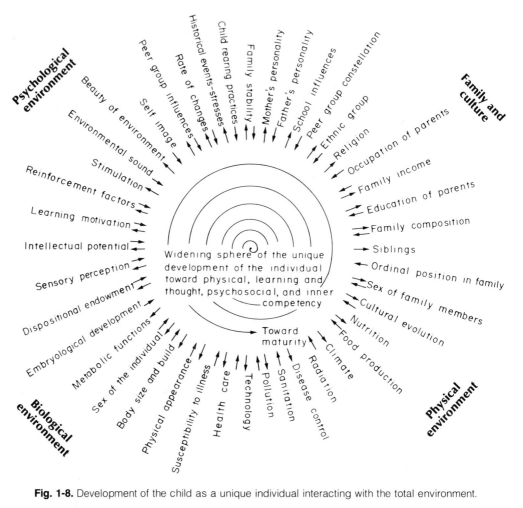

**Fig. 1-8.** Development of the child as a unique individual interacting with the total environment.

An in-depth study of specific personality and developmental theories is beyond the scope of this book, but reviews will provide a useful framework for the nurse in understanding the complexities and needs of the child. Regardless of theoretical position, the growth and development process may be conceptualized as being a gradual movement toward the attainment of adultlike competencies, fitness, and ability necessary for successful living.[46] These basic competencies may be further described as follows:

### Physical competency

*Physical competency* includes the ability of the individual to use various motor and neurologic capacities to attain mobility and manipulation capabilities. It also includes the ability to physically take care of one's own biologic and physiologic needs. The child begins helpless and relatively immobile and grows gradually to the point where he or she maintains personal responsibility for physical health and provides for physical performance and mobility. The concept of physical competency incorporates the physiologic functions of each body system. All assessment parameters that reflect the anatomy and physiology of the body are considered to be representative of the child's physical competency. Physical competency is interpreted in light of the child's developmental stage and in light of findings in relation to each of the other competency areas but can be objectively described in detail. The description of physical competency is one of the most highly developed and is an area of assessment in which nursing function overlaps significantly with assessment of the physician. However, the primary objectives of the nurse in describing physical competency are to identify and describe the objective findings, to identify all parameters of normal function, and to describe any deviations from that which is normally expected. Interpretation of physical competency in terms of the principles of growth and development is a major focus of the nursing assessment.

The concept of physical competency also includes all environmental factors that impinge upon the child's physical development, physical ability, and physical systems. In assessing physical competency the nurse describes such parameters as the child's nutritional intake, environmental pollutants, and factors in the environment that operate to protect the child from disease or to increase chances for developing health problems. Physical environmental factors may be conceptualized as influencing the developmental spiral shown in Fig. 1-7.

## Learning and thought competency

*Learning and thought competency* includes the development of language and thought process, cognitive maps and abstractions, perceptions, and communication capabilities. The child at birth is able to communicate crudely a few basic physiologic needs and begins to assimilate multiple stimuli, which eventually grow into conceptualizations and cognitive structures.

Learning and thought competency may be conceptualized as the child's ability to use complex mental powers to perform those operations deemed to be unique human cognitive traits. The advanced ability to reason, to solve increasingly complex problems, to give cognitive attention to affective dimensions of human existence, to idealize, fantasize, and project into the future are among the many learning and thought traits acquired during the years of growth and development. In addition the child acquires the ability to ponder, to meditate, to give deliberate thought to philosophic and religious ideas presented by the family and society.

Assessment tools for learning and thought competency are not yet well developed, and the major tools available to nurses are those that have been developed to fulfill the purposes of educators. Thus, language development, intellectual skill, and reading and mathematical skill may be tested and described. The major nursing goals in relation to the assessment of learning and thought are the interpretations of the child's ability in terms of the norms of growth and development and of the interrelationships between learning and thought competency and each of the other competency areas.

Factors in the environment that influence learning and thought competency are considered for each stage of development and depend upon the major cognitive tasks that are a focus of development at the time of the assessment. For example, during infancy and early childhood, stimulation and reinforcement factors provided by the family are of primary importance. During later childhood, factors in the school or other formal learning environments are of major significance, as are the influence of the peer group and the activities of the peer group that extend beyond school and that influence the child's learning and thought development.

## Social competency

*Social competency* includes the child's development of interpersonal relationships—affiliations with significant people and peers and sociocultural interactions with individuals and groups of people. The processes of separation and affiliation constantly interact until an ability is achieved during adulthood that allows the individual to attain security and comfort from a variety of interpersonal relationships.

Assessment of social competency includes a description of the nature and quality of the child's interactions with significant others as well as with strangers. The interpretation of social behavior is made in terms of the norms of growth and development, as well as the primary expectations for the child's developmental stage by the family and culture. During early childhood the interactions of the infant and the mother or other significant persons are of major importance. The behaviors observed during this period are those of eye contact, touch, and attentiveness of each individual to the other. As the child develops and grows, the range of so-

**11**

cial behaviors increases significantly. The child is expected to relate to an increasing wider circle of persons. Behavior is increasingly shaped by the social and cultural environment. Thus, assessment of the child's actual behavior, as well as the social and environmental factors that influence behavior, are of major importance in assessment and interpretation of social competency.

Nursing assessment tools for social competency are not yet well developed. Nursing function and the functions of the social work profession overlap in this area. Nursing interprets assessment of social competency with a major emphasis and focus on the perspective of the health and development of the individual child and family; the profession of social work observes, interprets, and acts with a major emphasis on the society and groups in society. As in other areas of professional overlap the complementary nature of the two professions is important in providing for the comprehensive health care of individuals and society.

### Inner competency

*Inner competency* includes the individual's developing awareness of self, the ability to cope as a separate person with the multitude of factors that influence the self, and acceptance and realization of self. The child at first experiences herself or himself as part of others and is not able to assume responsibility and accountability for thoughts, behavior, or being until a measure of maturity is achieved. An inner sense of security and well-being characterizes the healthy child at any stage of development, but the personality traits characteristic of each stage of life are identified through various theories of personality development.

Describing inner competency of the child is a major challenge for the nurse. This area of competency is intimately tied to the development of each of the other competency areas and exerts an influence on the child's state of health in every area of development. Likewise, each of the other competency areas exerts an influence on the development of inner competency. The interactions between social and inner competency, for example, are so closely interrelated that they often cannot be described as separate

areas of development. However, it is important to attempt to observe the behaviors that signify the child's inner sense of self as completely as possible and to make a deliberate effort to observe all cues that give an indication of the child's inner sense of esteem, security, confidence, self and body image, and well-being.

Tools for assessment of inner competency are limited, and for the profession of nursing, play, the interview, and self-report from the child are the major means of obtaining data related to inner competency. Other possible parameters of inner competency include body language, personal habits, daily patterns of living, drawings of the self, and expressions of the self through play. Because of limited knowledge of the meaning of these behaviors, it is difficult to make interpretations, but the behavior can be described to convey the nature of the child's inner competency. When there is an indication of the need for further assessment of inner competency, the nurse depends upon the skill of persons in psychology to provide more complete data related to inner competency.

These four major competencies develop simultaneously from some point after conception and constantly interact and influence one another. They may be enhanced or caused to deteriorate by the multiple factors influencing development and, in fact, each competency becomes a factor influencing the others. For example, a child's social competency will be severely limited if his or her self-realization is low.

### Integration of competencies

The child does not exist in four separate parts but as a whole, total individual. However, it is necessary to conceptualize development in the four major competency areas in order to take into account each of the parameters of self that contribute to the child's unique wholeness. Therefore, upon completing the assessment of each of the competency areas, the nurse has a comprehensive basis upon which to summarize and make a summary assessment of the child as a complete human being. The interpretation of the individual's level of development is made by taking into account each of the competency areas and weighing consideration of the ways in which each area of competency interacts with the others. In addition, the nurse can plan for ways in which nursing management is to be designed in order to provide maximal interaction of effects from one competency area to another. For example, the adolescent suffering from acne (physical competency interference) will also have an effect in each of the other competency areas. Learning and thought may be interfered with due to the physical and emotional discomfort of the acne. There is a major interference in the social competency of the individual, and the inner competency of the individual is influenced by altering the self-image or body image. Nursing interpretation of this problem must include each area of consideration, and intervention is planned to provide for maximal health in each competency. Simply helping the adolescent to minimize the acne condition will provide an effect in all competency areas, but maximal health in each competency area is achieved only through intervention aimed toward meeting the learning and thought, social, and inner needs of the person.

In considering nursing care of the child, the major competencies to be developed throughout life become the framework and focus. Rather than primary consideration of the disease or health state of the child or the medical diagnosis or prescription, the nurse considers primarily the child's individual needs in developing life competencies. The state of health or illness, medical diagnosis, or any of the other factors influencing development become essential parts of the nursing assessment. These influence to some extent the nursing diagnosis and plan of management, but the primary issue for the nurse is: *How does this factor* (physical trait, divorce, illness, social condition, etc.) *affect this individual child's ability to:*

1. Perform physically and biologically
2. Learn and think
3. Relate socially to others
4. Develop an adequate sense of self

The child is a unique totality representing a single human existence. What he or she is and what he or she becomes are dependent upon many problems that are beyond the scope and realm of nursing care. The nurse's challenge is to maintain the perspective of the whole child—the total essence, which is somehow different from the separate influences and parts of existence—and to serve as an advocate for factors that enhance the optimal development of the unique self. In so doing the nurse is able to provide a number of services and functions on behalf of the child. Other needs may be met through a wide range of resources available on the health care team or in the community, or from the significant people in the child's life.

## THEORY FOR CHILD NURSING

Interpretation of assessment data in each competency area depends upon a background of knowledge of major theories related to the nature and development of each competency. Theories provide descriptions of the developmental phenomena and explanation and understanding of the nature of these phenomena. They provide a means of establishing developmental norms or the expected behavior for a child of a given age and stage of development. Theoretical norms are viewed in light of family and cultural expectations but are useful guides in interpretation of observed behavior. The following section presents a brief overview and summary of the theories used in this text to describe and explain the meaning of developmental traits during childhood.

### Physical competency

Theories of physiologic development and of physical and motor behavior throughout life are based on the assumption that development in humans proceeds in a predictable, orderly fashion. This assumption implies that all human development is similar, and study of one human at a given age and stage provides knowledge of all other humans at that stage of life. Change in function is presumed to be dependent upon what preceded the change, and each successive change will influence successive changes. It is generally recognized that there are variations in developmental sequence in physical function, but alterations of the expected, predicted pattern are viewed as abnormalities.

Timiras, in *Developmental Physiology and Aging*,[43] presented a comprehensive review of theories of physiologic development from the prenatal period through adulthood and aging.

**13**

The embryonic and hereditary genesis of each body system is described as is the developmental nature of the system's function throughout life. Normal development is emphasized, but explanations of variations of normal development are included. The regulation of growth of each system is discussed, as well as means for measuring growth and development of each of the body systems at various stages of growth. Although these theories provide an important source for background knowledge, the nurse in child health needs to acquire understanding of the measurement approaches that are used in determining the development of a child's physiologic growth. Of particular importance are measurement and assessment approaches needed to differentiate normal versus abnormal development. For example, delayed growth during adolescence is difficult to define based on the relationship between age, body size, and development of secondary sexual characteristics. Rather, it is essential to take into account neurologic, endocrine, and environmental influences on the time of growth and development at puberty. Using knowledge of the theories and knowledge of the individual adolescent, the nurse guides and counsels the adolescent and family in regard to any concern. In summary, knowledge of physiologic theory such as that presented by Timiras is essential in conducting the nursing assessment and is used in counseling and teaching.

The physical development approach of Gesell and Amatruda[18] in their early studies of child development at Yale University has provided a frame of reference for most subsequent descriptions of child behavior. This theory described the physical and behavioral traits of infants and children at different ages. Since their early work, many researchers have sought to verify the adequacy of these descriptions and to describe and explain variations of normal development. Brazelton[8] described the first year of life in terms of three basic behavior types: average, quiet, and active. This approach recognizes the common traits of development that exist for all infants but also acknowledges the interaction of heredity and environment in shaping the development of physical motor traits. One of the most frequently expressed concerns of mothers

and families is that regarding the appearance of developmental landmarks, particularly in the first few years of life. The child health nurse needs a sound basis in theories of developmental landmarks and a knowledge of the variations that have been acknowledged to occur within normal limits.

Theories of abnormalities of physical development are presented in several medical resources and provide a background for pathophysiology and application of these principles in medical practice.[13,40,49] These resources are valuable for collaborative nursing practice and provide a theoretical background for nursing management of physiologic deviations from health. Application of these theories in nursing practice is primarily in the realm of family and child education and will be included in this text with emphasis on use of theory in nursing practice.

## Learning and thought competency

There exists a wide diversity of theory related to learning and thinking processes. One of the bases for the diversity is differences in assumptions on which theories are based. Many learning theories are based on the notion that the human mind is predetermined in function and that it develops according to predictable, orderly stages of development. Other learning theories are based on the alternate notion that the mind is largely subject to shaping by the environment and that learning ability can be altered. Research evidence supports each of these notions, depending on the kind of cognitive or mental ability studied. For example, it has been substantiated that the human mind responds to positive and negative stimuli in a predictable fashion, independent of age or stage of development. However, the kind of learning that occurs as a result of positive or negative reinforcement can be shaped and altered by selecting the stimuli and environmental conditions in accord with the age and stage of development of the child. Learning and thinking are complex human functions and have been the object of extensive study in Western society.

Piaget and Inhelder[37] provided a major contribution to the study and understanding of cognitive development. Their theory describes stages of cognitive development throughout the

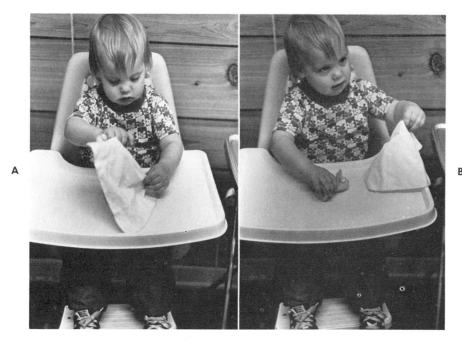

**Fig. 1-9.** This 13-month-old child demonstrates cognitive permanence of object. **A,** Child demonstrates awareness that toy continues to exist even though it is hidden. **B,** Child finds toy, and the event reinforces developing cognitive awareness of permanence of object.

developmental years. Through a natural unfolding of ability, the child acquires sequentially predictable cognitive abilities. Given adequate environmental stimuli and an intact neurologic system, the child gradually matures toward full ability to conceptualize. The theory of Piaget and other scientists in his tradition offers many implications for planning the learning process in nursing situations and for assessment of the child's ability to learn at a given stage of development.

Bruner[9,10] developed a theory of learning and education that offers a basis for understanding readiness to learn, intuitive and analytic thinking, and motivation. The importance of enactment of ideas in behavior as a component of learning is a concept of Bruner's that has particular relevance for nursing care of children and the learning activities in which nurses engage with children.

Chomsky's model[12] of the development of language provides an explanation of the acquisition of language, a critical component of learning and thought competency. The acquisition of meaning for words is critical to the acquisition of language and can be described in terms of the child's behavior. Children express words used in their own understanding of the term, and as others in their environment respond to this use of terms, they gradually refine their understanding of the meaning until they use the term in accord with those around them. Nursing assessment of the use of language by a child is possible by observing the appropriate use of words in the child's language; this observation gives valuable information about learning and thinking.

**Social competency**

Social competency is interpreted using the theories of Lewin,[27] Sullivan,[41] and Bowlby.[7] Each of these theorists views interpersonal interactions in a different dimension, but their theories are based on the premise that human behavior and personality arise from the nature and traits of human interaction. Lewin's field theory states that change depends upon the state of the psychologic field at any point in **15**

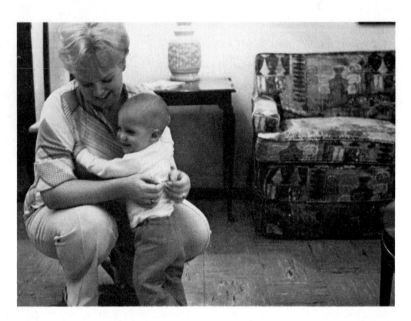

**Fig. 1-10.** This 10-month-old infant has just returned to mother after briefly wandering a few feet from her, demonstrating the process of exploring brief separation and returning to the attachment figure for reassurance.

time. Past events in life may affect the behavior, but the contemporary, here and now, situation has the greatest effect. For Lewin the person must be viewed in terms of the current life space or of all of the facts existing for the individual or group. All of the parts of the person's life space are interdependent and exert an influence on behavior.

Sullivan's interpersonal theory of psychiatry states that the individual personality is comprised of an enduring pattern of recurrent interpersonal relationships or situations.[41] Heredity and maturation are recognized as important factors in development, but social interactions are of primary importance in the development of distinctly human traits of personality. Interpersonal experiences are considered to have such a major impact on the person that they shape and alter all physiologic functions of the individual, as well as the psychologic traits. Dynamisms, or habits, personifications, or self-images, and cognitive processes are the major concepts of Sullivan's theory.

Bowlby[7] has made a major contribution in describing the nature of attachments and separations in human life. His theory provides a basis for understanding behaviors of infants and mothers and of the family group as the child grows and matures to adulthood. The behaviors contributing to the formation of an affectional bond are described in detail, as are the behaviors that signal inadequate bonding.

Theories of family structure are drawn from the work of Duvall,[15] who describes the structure and function of the family unit. Although the family unit is changing in structure and to some extent in function, it remains a vital and deep-rooted unit of Western society. The roles of various family members, the interactions between them, and the ways in which they serve to meet one another's needs are important dimensions of the nursing assessment and often provide the focus of nursing management.

### Inner competency

Theories of the self and development of the self are based on the assumption that humans possess a unique trait of a sense or knowledge of inner self or spirit. Some theories view this inner self as a natural unfolding and inherent trait common for all human individuals, which develops according to predictable patterns and stages. Others view the self as a trait of potential, the development of which depends upon factors in the environment and upon the will of the person to develop self. Erikson[16] described the development of identity of the self and the ego through successive stages that naturally unfold. Through the stages the child experiences challenges to accomplish identity tasks. Accomplishment of each successive task provides the foundation for a healthy self-identity. Each stage is dependent upon the other and must be successfully accomplished in order for the child to proceed to successful accomplishment of the next. The influence of the family and the environment is significant to the child, but the motivation to achieve the challenges of identity arises from within.

Maslow[29] and Rogers[38] have presented two theoretical views of the process of self-actualization or realization of the potential of the self. Each position views self-development as a lifelong process, involving gradual maturity and discovery of the inner meaning of the self. Relationships with others and the psychologic environment are important to the individual development, but the self existing within the individual must be fully expressed and experienced by the individual alone. The realization of inner potential leads to creativity, to making good life choices, to inner peace and congruency, to seeking and maintaining satisfying life relationships with others. There are no developmental stages described, but the behaviors of self-actualization can exist at all stages of the life cycle. Each of these theorists presents views of the therapeutic or healthy environment that facilitate the process of self-actualization. These descriptions are important in nursing practice and are useful in assessment of the child and family environment as well as in nursing management.

## Nursing theory

Throughout this text, these and other theories will be described in detail, along with indications of their application in nursing practice. Some theories or models have limited applicability, but others provide an underlying basis for nursing practice. No theory from another discipline is to be applied in practice without careful analysis of the potential of the theory for practice. However, without a theoretical basis and rationale for nursing practice, actions in

nursing hold little or no potential for the development of a science upon which practice can be built and which will yield understanding and prediction of the outcomes of nursing actions.

Statements have developed in recent years in the nursing literature that provide a beginning conceptualization of the process of nursing, and the conceptual meaning of nursing acts as well as the outcomes of those acts. In Chapter 2 a conceptualization of nursing practice for child health care is presented upon which this text is developed. This is a descriptive conceptual frame of reference, and the theories described above are useful in defining and implementing practice.

Other frameworks that have appeared in nursing literature in recent years have particular relevance for child nursing practice, such as those of Martha Rogers,[39] The Nursing Conference Development Group,[33,34] The Maternal-Child Nursing Department of the University of Maryland,[4] and Dorothy Johnson.[23] Rogers presents a conceptualization of the person as a unified whole—an open, developing human system. Life proceeds along a space-time continuum, a concept that holds potential value for the study of childhood health and states of wellbeing. Life pattern and organization are self-regulating, dynamic qualities that fulfill the potentialities of living. Life is also conceptualized as having an inherent rhythmic quality that is essential to the essence of living. There is constant exchange of energy and matter between the human field and the environment. Among the implications of these concepts for nursing practice is the basic premise that nursing actions are planned according to the uniqueness of the individual and to enable the individual to be in harmony with the environment rather than in conflict with it. The concept of movement has been substantiated to be relevant in infant growth and development, providing a stimulus for development during this period of life. Other applications are yet to be tested and the concepts have yet to be tested extensively. However, it has provided a stimulus for investigation and application of potentially important principles in practice.

The Nursing Development Conference Group formulated a description of nursing that **17** is based on Orem's general concept of nursing.[33,34] The system of nursing is based on the underlying premise that recipients of nursing care have the ability, right, and responsibility to assume a meaningful role in their own health care, in identification of the goals of care, and in the means of achieving these goals. Nursing is conceptualized as existing and having meaning within the context of society. There are three basic elements of the nursing system: therapeutic self-care demand, nursing agency, and self-care agency. Therapeutic self-care demand incorporates the action that needs to be taken, a standard against which the actions can be judged, and a standard for change in the actions. The nurse and client both participate in determining the therapeutic self-care demand elements. Nursing agency is the prime regulatory force for the system, in that the nurse has the ability to receive and judge signals from the environment and the client that serve to provide knowledge and a basis for judging and taking action. Self-care agency is also a regulatory mechanism that provides the primary input to determine therapeutic self-care demand and to regulate the nursing agency in the system. Use of this conceptualization of nursing practice provides for optimal participation by the child/adult client in the nursing situation. In addition, several propositions presented about self-care agency provide a stimulus for the study and further development of specific nursing approaches and management.

The faculty of the Maternal-Child Nursing Department of the University of Maryland has developed a conceptual basis for maternal-child nursing practice. The construct is based on four concept areas: motion, sensation, cognition, and affiliation. These concepts are viewed as interrelated and as integral to the growth and development of the child. Assessment techniques that provide data to support these concepts and their relationships have been developed. The intent of those working with this framework is to determine predictions of later physical, cognitive, and emotional development in order to design early prevention approaches in nursing practice.[4]

Johnson[23] presented a behavioral system upon which nursing care can be based, which consists of eight subsystems: achievement, affiliative, aggressive-protective, dependency, eliminative, ingestive, restorative, and sexual. There are four input modes (visual, auditory, olfactory, and tactile) and four output modes (verbal, motor, excretory, and physical). Each subsystem has its own input and output mechanisms. Behavior is goal-oriented. Nursing serves to assess each subsystem and its function in the behavioral system and to assist the client in making choices and taking actions that promote optimal health and growth of the system. Nursing also provides for the sustenal imperatives of the client, which are protection, nurturance, and stimulation. Incorporation of the framework into nursing practice provides a basis for assessment, diagnosis, management, and evaluation of care.

## FACILITATING GROWTH

Only in recent years has parenthood been regarded as a subject worthy of careful study and preparation. The normative crisis that occurs in our modern world as young adults become parents may be conceptualized as the assumption of a new role and, as such, conforming to societal expectations for behavior.[3,14,26] The nurse is inevitably involved in many of the dynamics of this role development. The issues range in kind and complexity from the initial stages of parenthood immediately postpartum to ongoing processes such as teaching and assisting parents to provide adequate nutrition for a growing family or helping a family to achieve effective discipline and emotional security. With a few regrettable exceptions, most parents enter parenthood with the noblest intentions to produce a healthy, well-adjusted member of society according to the demands and expectations of that society or subculture. Few parents deliberately begin with the intent of rearing a disturbed or handicapped child. In reality, there are many failures. In Western cultures parents are often blamed, and the child rarely bears personal responsibility for failure to fit the accepted norm. Even in the case of physical deformity at birth, parents in this society enter into grueling exploration and soul-searching for the cause or the antecedents of the child's deformity. Likewise, emotional or physical disasters are most often blamed on the inadequacies of parents.

## Factors that enhance competency development

What should parents do to furnish society with people who are more acceptable to it than unacceptable? The question often arouses concern that cripples the very effort given in the answer. A totally acceptable answer can never be given, and although there is an increasing number of sound theories, approaches, and ideas related to child-rearing, human beings are not subject to alteration in a predictable manner. Parents who are successful can be studied and analyzed. The complexities of the situation only become enhanced. The nurse may give advice, only to be frustrated by the parents' inability to do the very thing they wish to do. The chapters that follow will seek to explore many sound and applicable approaches that have evolved in recent years, but a formula for success cannot be offered.[28,48] Facilitating growth toward the attainment of adultlike competencies in living is the basic goal of healthy parenthood. The following five facilitating factors may be identified as essential for all children.

First, the child's basic physical and biologic needs must be met. Initially the infant is totally dependent upon other people for satisfaction of every physical need and slowly learns to communicate needs and then to assume some responsibility for satisfaction of these needs until total independence is achieve in adulthood. Efforts toward effective parenthood without consideration of the basic needs of nutrition, warmth, physical hygiene, and protection from infectious disease render efforts in other areas relatively ineffective.

Second, the child needs to feel the emotional security of being wanted and loved, without being required to conform or perform in exchange. Although a parent cannot convey such a feeling without possessing the actual emotion, there can be circumstances in the total situation that either enhance or detract the child's perception of the parent's true intent. Nursing assessment and intervention can effectively assist a family to achieve the maximal level of emotional functioning possible for the particular situation.

Third, the child should experience the opportunity for unhampered inner development. This implies an environment that is accepting of the child at a given stage of development, while providing restrictions imposed with reason and consistency and offering psychologic space to make mistakes and learn from them. The child needs freedom to explore, experiment, and discover the self within the confines of safe limitations that prohibit danger to or thoughtless disregard of himself or herself and others.[35]

Fourth, the child needs to experience success and happiness based on real experience and achievement. He or she needs to experience performance abilities as realistically as possible. The toddler must learn how far he or she can climb without falling. The child must learn how much effort it takes to learn to do something new. The adolescent must experience real responsibility to learn to assume independence. Thus the child gradually is able to assume the competencies needed for adequate adult living. Cultural definitions of success and happiness become increasingly important to the child in this respect, because these determine the experience available to the child. In a society that is extremely materialistic, the child who is deprived of material wealth may develop a self-concept that equates deprivation with unhappiness and lack of personal success. Few efforts to reverse this effect are successful in erasing the conceptions developed throughout childhood.

Finally, the child must be allowed to make the emotional shift from attachments centered on the parental family or its substitute to attachments to the peer group and members of the peer generation. This very demanding and often painful process begins during early childhood and is enhanced by emotional factors involved in meeting the preceding needs.

## Influence of historical "mood"

The modern characteristic of rapid change affects every aspect of a child's life. Fashionable theories of child-rearing are subject to change from year to year, undermining the very trait of consistency that parents strive to achieve. The form of the family in today's world is increasingly subject to change, as are other traditional institutions, in an effort to incorporate new ideas and new technology. Thus one major challenge in regard to child-rearing in today's world is to enhance the child's ability to cope with change, increasing technology, and complexity of the world to come.[11,44]

### Influence of life themes

Upon entering parenthood, each individual brings a personal history of childhood and the experiences that shaped physical development and personality. Most parents tend to rear their own children in much the same manner as they themselves were reared, even when they verbally state they wish to improve or change their own child-rearing techniques. When the moment comes to make an unexpected decision or take some sort of action in relation to the child, their own childhood experience becomes the most ready resource upon which to draw, and the action or the decision is often administered in a very similar manner to that of their own parents.

Families and individuals within families grow with certain life themes dominating all behavior. Some families are extremely materialistic; others are not. Some families center their interest and expectations for one another on intellectual or academic pursuits. Families establish expectation for all family members according to these themes. For example, loyalty to the members of the family is stressed in one family, while members of another family live highly separate, individualized lives that seldom touch one another in action, thought, or activity. Families teach their members habits of personal care; some maintain neat surroundings, others are cluttered. Some families place a high priority on physical appearance, while others do not. A life theme for some families is survival—the basic needs of the family are so difficult to meet that there is little time or energy left for other types of concerns. Some families place a high priority on seeking pleasure, others on religion, others on a family hobby or business. Children and youth most often continue the predominant themes of their own childhood family. There are areas of life that children deliberately break away from, or they may change in some respect to suit their own personal preference. A person may determine to forsake the religion of childhood and to rear his or her own children without religion or in a different religion. The parent often continues, however, to behave under the influence of many of the basic tenets of the childhood faith, maintaining some of its basic life themes such as honesty, humanitarianism, or other moral codes.

Conflicts in life themes grow as life's complexity increases. The child experiences conflicting values and expectations from each significant person in life. The child is encouraged to cooperate and help others but is also encouraged to compete and excel. Whichever theme dominates the individual colors all behavior and experience and shapes future parenting practices.[48]

### Children: a priority in health care

Maternal and child health has been a priority for programs of the World Health Organization since its inception. Representatives from all participating countries agree that there are several significant reasons for establishing adequate maternal and child health care for the well-being of their country and their country's future. These reasons are specifically important in considering the pervasive influence of health care services to children and so will be considered here.

1. Children are the future of a nation or community. They are essential for the survival of any group of people.

2. Mothers and children form a majority of the population. The proportion of children in a given population tends to rise in less developed areas where lifespan tends to be short. Mothers and children comprise as much as two thirds of the total population.

3. Children are particularly vulnerable to disease. The less well-developed an area, the greater the percentage of deaths occurring in children under 5 years, rising to 50%.

4. Most diseases that cause death or morbidity in children are preventable. One major problem has been communicable disease, which

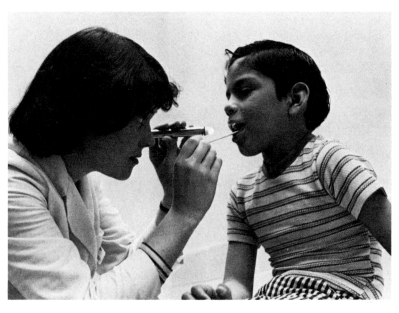

**Fig. 1-11.** The nurse provides important health care services in the areas of health screening, health guidance and counseling, and assisting families to attain and maintain optimal health.

is preventable through immunization programs and treatable through antibiotic treatment and supportive care. Malnutrition is another major health problem that is often related to lack of knowledge about the use of available foods for good health.

5. Maternal and child health services have been demonstrated to provide an appealing introduction to rational health care for the entire community. Families in most cultures value their children greatly, and they appreciate seeing them healed or helped through adequate health care efforts. The learning that is then applied for all members of the family benefits the entire community.

6. Decreased childhood disease leads to a decreased social burden from having to sustain individuals whose lives are damaged physically or mentally. The comparative cost to society of caring for a chronically ill or handicapped child is great when cast against the cost of prevention and early recognition and treatment programs.

7. Children are not able to articulate their own needs and health care problems. Traditionally, in most countries this problem is further accentuated by the fact that women, who are assigned the role of advocating the child's needs

and meeting them, have little or no role in the formation of political, administrative, or community policies. Thus children, who are not able to speak for themselves, have their traditional advocate placed in a relatively ineffectual role.[47]

The First National Congress on the Quality of Life in 1972 recognized that mothers and children must be the highest priority in health care to safeguard the future of the nation. The following Declaration of Interdependence* was adopted, expressing a commitment to protect the quality of life of children:

We Declare:

That the Nation's highest priority should be its children

That the destiny of each child should reflect his individual potential rather than the result of environmental or economic deprivation

That the opportunity to be born healthy should be accorded to each American

That social, educational, physical, mental, emotional, and environmental conditions that cause human blight affect children of all classes, all

*From American Medical Association: Quality of life: the early years, Acton, Mass., 1974, Publishing Sciences Group, Inc., pp. 39-40.

**21**

races, and all persuasions and therefore are a national problem

That human blight perpetuates the cycle of unhealthy mother–unhealthy child–unhealthy mother–and ultimately an unhealthy Nation

That prevention of human blight is more fruitful and more economical than the costs of individual, institutional, and social care

That the achievement of these goals demands an end to fragmentation and the beginning of a new interdependent relationship among all governmental, social, welfare, health, medical, educational, religious, and legal agencies. Having so declared:

We the Undersigned,

Commit ourselves to seek an end to human blight

Pledge ourselves to a new era of cooperation among each and all of us

Dedicate ourselves to an interdependent effort to achieve for each American child his basic inalienable right: A Life of Quality.

Reflecting on the problems of parenthood, we emphasize the very real possibilities in the future for society at large to become more involved in assuring optimal development for all children. The child must be given first priority if indeed the world of tomorrow is to be a better one. Although the basic responsibility for a child rests with the family, the future of society is at stake. Total dedication toward fulfillment of this basic responsibility can enhance the possibility of improving the lot of the young child within the family. Health and adjustment in later life have their roots in appropriate health care and experience in early childhood, and the nurse is challenged to join this effort of investment in the future.

## STUDY QUESTIONS

1. Discuss the principles of growth and development, illustrating each with examples from your own experience or that of children you know.
2. Identify a child who has an unusual characteristic in one of the four basic competencies. Discuss ways in which this unusual characteristic has affected development of each of the competencies.
3. Discuss your ideas of the challenges of parenthood in your own culture and community. What ideas can you propose that would enhance or help parents with problems of child-rearing?
4. Describe your own life themes. What conflicting themes can you identify? Which have been the most consistent throughout your development?

## REFERENCES

1. American Medical Association: Quality of life: the early years, Acton, Mass., 1974, Publishing Sciences Group, Inc.
2. Anastasi, A.: Heredity, environment, and the question "how?" Psychological Rev. **65:**197-208, 1958.
3. Anthony, E. J., and Benedek, T., editors: Parenthood; its psychology and psychopathology, Boston, 1970, Little, Brown and Co.
4. Barnard, K., and Neal, M. V.: Maternal-child nursing research; a review of the past and strategies for the future, Nurs. Res. **26:**193-200, May-June, 1977.
5. Bellugi, U., and Brown, R., editors: The acquisition of language, Chicago, 1970, University of Chicago Press.
6. Bernard, H. W.: Human development in Western culture, ed. 4, Boston, 1975, Allyn & Bacon, Inc., Publishers.
7. Bowlby, J.: Attachment and loss, vol. I, Attachment, New York, 1969, Basic Books, Inc.
8. Brazelton, T. B.: Infants and mothers; differences in development, New York, 1970, Delacorte Press.
9. Bruner, J. S.: The process of education, New York, 1963, Random House, Inc.
10. Bruner, J. S.: The relevance of education, New York, 1971, W. W. Norton & Co., Inc.
11. Buder, L., and others: Where we are: a hard look at family and society, New York, 1970, Child Study Association of America.
12. Chomsky, N.: Syntactic structures. The Hague, 1957, Mouton.
13. Cooke, R. E., editor: The biologic basis of pediatric practice, New York, 1968, McGraw-Hill Book Co.
14. Damon, W.: The social world of the child, San Francisco, 1977, Jossey-Bass, Inc., Publishers.
15. Duvall, E. M.: Family development, ed. 5, Philadelphia, 1977, J. B. Lippincott Co.
16. Erikson, E. H.: Identity; youth and crisis, New York, 1968, W. W. Norton & Co., Inc.
17. Escalona, S. K.: The roots of individuality, Chicago, 1968, Aldine Publishing Co.
18. Gesell, A., and Amatruda, C. S.: Developmental diagnosis: normal and abnormal child development; clinical methods and pediatric applications, New York, 1947, Harper & Row, Publishers.
19. Gesell, A., and others: The first five years of life, New York, 1940, Harper & Row, Publishers.
20. Gesell, A., and others: Infant and child in the culture of today; the guidance of behavior, New York, 1943, Harper & Bros.
21. Gesell, A., and others: The child from five to ten, New York, 1946, Harper & Bros.
22. Gesell, A., Ilg, F. L., and Ames, L. B.: Youth, the years from ten to sixteen, New York, 1956, Harper & Row, Publishers.
23. Grubbs, J.: The Johnson behavioral system model. In Riehl, J. P., and Roy, Sr. C., Conceptual models for nursing practice, New York, 1974, Appleton-Century-Crofts.
24. Guyton, A. C.: Textbook of medical physiology, ed. 5, Philadelphia, 1976, W. B. Saunders Co.

25. Hurlock, E. B.: Child development, ed. 5, New York, 1972, McGraw-Hill Book Co.

26. LeMasters, E. E.: Parents in modern America; a sociological analysis, ed. 3., Homewood, Ill, 1977, Dorsey Press.

27. Lewin, K.: Field theory in social science; selected theoretical papers, New York, 1951, Harper & Row.

28. Lourie, R. S.: The concern of one generation for the next, Children, Nov.-Dec. 1970, pp. 234-235.

29. Maslow, A. H., The farther reaches of human nature, New York, 1971, The Viking Press, Inc.

30. Mead, M.: Culture and commitment; a study of the generation gap, New York, 1970, Natural History Press, Doubleday & Co., Inc.

31. Menyuk, R.: The development of speech, New York, 1972, Bobbs-Merrill.

32. Mussen, P. H., Conger, J. J., and Kagan, J.: Child development and personality, ed. 4, New York, 1974, Harper & Row, Publishers.

33. Nursing Development Conference Group: Concept formalization in nursing; process and product, Boston, 1973, Little, Brown and Company.

34. Orem, D. E.: Nursing; concepts of practice, New York, 1971, McGraw-Hill Book Co.

35. Philips, I.: Youth, permissiveness and child development, Pediatrics 40:1-4, Jan., 1972.

36. Piaget, J.: The moral judgment of the child, New York, 1965, The Free Press.

37. Piaget, J., and Inhelder, B.: The psychology of the child, New York, 1969, Basic Books, Inc., Publishers.

38. Rogers, C.: On becoming a person, Boston, 1961, Houghton-Mifflin Co.

39. Rogers, M.: An introduction to the theoretical basis of nursing, Philadelphia, 1970, F. A. Davis Co.

40. Rudolf, A. M., editor: Pediatrics, ed. 16, New York, 1977, Appleton-Century-Crofts.

41. Sullivan, H. S.: The interpersonal theory of psychiatry, New York, 1953, W. W. Norton & Co., Inc.

42. Sutterly, D. C., and Donnelly, G. A.: Meeting nursing needs throughout the life cycle. In Kintzel, K. C., editor: Advanced concepts in clinical nursing, Philadelphia, 1971, J. B. Lippincott Co., pp. 49-67.

43. Timiras, P. S.: Developmental physiology and aging, New York, 1972, Macmillan Publishing Co., Inc.

44. Toffler, A.: Future shock, New York, 1970, Random House.

45. Vetter, H. J., and Smith, B. D., editors: Personality theory; a source book, New York, 1971, Appleton-Century-Crofts.

46. White, R. W.: Competence and the psychosexual stages of development. In Rosenblith, J. F., and Allinsmith, W., editors: The causes of behavior, ed. 2, Boston, 1966, Allyn & Bacon, Inc.

47. Williams, C. D., and Jelliffe, D. C.: Mother and child health; delivering the services, New York, 1972, Oxford University Press.

48. Yarrow, L. J., and others: Infancy experiences and cognitive and personality development at ten years. In Stone, L. J., Smith, A. J., and Murphy, L. B., editors: The competent infant; research and commentary, New York, 1973, Basic Books, Inc., Publishers, p. 1274.

49. Ziai, M., editor: Pediatrics, ed. 2, Boston, 1975, Little, Brown and Company.

# CHAPTER 2

# Child nursing today . . . and tomorrow

Child health maintenance has become an increasing concern as relationships between health during early life and later development have become more clearly understood. The history of nursing in relation to children specifically demonstrate a responsiveness to this concern growing over the years. Because for many people a major portion of life covers their own childhood years combined with the years of rearing their children, nursing care of the child is an integral part of comprehensive health care for families of all stages of development.

## HISTORY OF NURSING CARE OF CHILDREN
### Past history

As recently as one century ago the recognized health needs of children were primarily only those that occurred during periods of acute illness. Children were reared in extended families and were needed to assume many responsibilities for the survival of the family. Major life-threatening illness may have resulted in hospitalization, or the child may have been cared for in the home by family members or women in the community who volunteered their services. Many of the diseases of the time, such as severe diarrhea and tuberculosis, were the result of unsanitary dairies and diseased cattle. Only at the beginning of the twentieth century was it realized that sterilization of milk was related to problems of health. Milk stations were established to help mothers learn the proper preparation of milk for children and to provide a place to receive medical care. It was from these stations that child welfare clinics and their visiting nursing programs evolved.

Hospital care of children at the turn of the century often involved strict isolation because of the infectious nature of most of the illnesses. When, after World War I, the problems of asepsis and isolation received more emphasis, children became the victims of increasing isolation from all that was familiar and secure to them for prolonged periods of time. It was not until after World War II, when the effects of maternal deprivation were discovered and studied, that nurses and physicians began to question the practices of prolonged isolation of children from mothers and the sterility of the deprived environments of hospitals. Educational programs for nurses began to include courses in growth and development and psychology, and a deeper understanding of children's needs and behavior began to emerge.

The growing need for day-care facilities became evident just before 1900 as thousands of rural families and a large number of immigrant families were lured to the urban area by rapid industrialization. Early day-care facilities were usually converted houses, overcrowded with children ranging in age from two weeks to six years. Food was of poor quality, and personnel were often unskilled and untrained. In decades since the day-care services of the United States have remained sparse and are largely initiated and maintained by private businesses or by charitable organizations. Standards of quality in care are sometimes regulated by local, state, and more recently federal governments, but existing services are of predominantly poor quality. Of significance is the fact that the United States is the only industrialized nation in the world that does not provide basic child-care services for its citizens. The lack of adequate day-care services coupled with the absence of adequate standards by which to evaluate and regulate existing facilities attests to the critical nature of the present national dilemma in relation to care for preschool age children.[45,46,61]

Table 2-1 summarizes the development of day-care services in this country. It should be noted that the focus of day-care legislation has been on selected target groups of children or selected, limited services, rather than on comprehensive child care. By 1970, over 60 different programs for child care and child development had been established, with over \$1.3 billion in federal funds spent annually. These programs were not organized into a comprehensive plan for total services to all children but rather provided isolated services to selected groups of children for a specified period of time and for specific purposes. This trend is not in accord with the statements of intent, such as the Declaration of Interdependence cited in Chapter 1.

In 1909 the White House Conference on Care of Dependent Children was held in response to concern over the deplorable conditions for children who were working in factories for long hours. This conference resulted in the formation of the Children's Bureau, which was first under the Department of Labor and later under the Department of Health, Education, and Welfare. Since this Bureau was established, the federal government in the United States has conducted regular White House Conferences on Children to consider the health and welfare of children in this country.

Antibiotics and vaccines, whose use became widespread during the 1940s, have dramatically changed the health status of children. Commu-

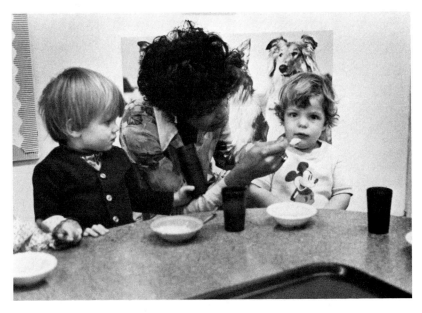

**Fig. 2-1.** Adequate day-care services provide optimal nutrition, well-prepared workers, and an environment of nurturance for the development of physical, learning and thought, social and inner competencies.

**Table 2-1.** Landmarks of day-care development in the United States*

| Date | Event | Services | Funding |
|------|-------|----------|---------|
| 1870-1914 | Industrial Revolution<br>World War I | Day care—all ages | Private |
| 1914 | Social worker involvement | Nursery school<br>   3 years and over | Tax supported |
| 1933 | Works Project Administration | Child care<br>   Infant—school age | Federal |
| 1941 | World War II | Day care<br>   Preschool | Danham Act Federal |
| 1945-1950 | Maternal deprivation studies<br>   by Spitz and Bowlby | Decreased—seen as "abnormal" | Federal Aid to Dependent Children |
| 1962 | Social Security Act amended | Day care | Federal |
| 1965 | Economic Opportunity Act | Head Start programs | Federal |
| 1967 | Title IV funds<br>Social Security Act | Day care | Federal |
| 1967 | Work Incentive Program | Day care | Federal |
| 1968 | School Lunch Act | Food and kitchen equipment | Federal |
| 1968 | Handicapped Children's Early<br>   Education Assistance Act | Day care for handicapped preschoolers | Federal |

*Data obtained from Parker, K., and Knitzer, J.: Day care and preschool services; Trends and issues, Atlanta, Georgia, 1972, Avatar Press.

nicable diseases have become a relatively minor health problem with the combined effects of antibiotics for treatment and immunizations for prevention. Because many of the health problems of children, such as accidents, infectious illness, and nutritional disorders, are often preventable or most effectively treated during early stages, the practice of pediatric nursing and medicine has become a specialty emphasizing the preventive aspects of care.

In 1948 the World Health Organization was formed as a special agent of the United Nations. Because a primary objective of this organization has been maternal and child health, it has remained a major force influencing the health and welfare of children around the world.[26,68,73]

## Trends of today

Highly specialized areas of nursing within the scope of pediatrics have emerged in recent years to meet special demands for specific groups of children. Adolescent and child psychiatric nursing, care of high risk newborn infants, care of the mentally retarded or birth defect child, and nursing care for the child with metabolic problems such as cystic fibrosis have developed.[26,72,73]

Today nursing has emerged with generally accepted philosophical commitments.[13] These may be stated in relation to child nursing as follows:

1. Every child, regardless of color, creed, or economic status, has the right to health, happiness, and an optimal environment for growth.
2. The basic responsibility for providing basic needs and protecting the child's health and happiness rests with the family. Society shares this responsibility but also protects the child and family's right to independence, autonomy, and primary responsibility for their own destiny.
3. The basic goal of child nursing, as part of society, is to promote the ability of children and families to attain, retain, or regain health.
4. Child health care is meaningful to the extent that it is provided within the family's life style and health state, and to the extent wished by them.

There are many complex problems in the world that interfere with the realization of these utopian commitments. The economic structure of most societies in the modern world does not allow for equal health care to all people. Nevertheless, the commitment to this ideal is strong enough that many significant efforts are continually supported in an attempt to provide better health care for mothers and children. The World Health Organization promotes many programs that enhance the health status of mothers, infants, and children throughout the world. Individual countries have attempted to find ways of providing more equalized health care for all citizens, and many are continuing to search for and implement programs that improve the effectiveness of care. The United States government and private agencies have been in the process of developing economic programs to provide health care for the most needy segments of society, notably the poor, the elderly, and mothers and dependent children.[4,16,30,43,66]

Another great barrier to the provision of adequate health care for all children is the cultural and societal gap between the segment of society offering health care and other segments of society who need the services offered. In Western cultures this is often conceptualized as a middle class versus minority group problem. Offering health care in a culturally acceptable manner is a challenge that has received more attention by the health care professions in recent years.

Within the profession of nursing there is beginning to emerge a renewed sense of direction and identity that provides for unity. A visibly autonomous, responsible practice of nursing is developing on a sound and scientific basis. It focuses on the individual and his or her family, is initiated through the nursing assessment, and then proceeds into need identification, plan formulation, and objective evaluation of the process. A setting or a situation does not define and delegate nursing responsibilities, but rather the characteristics of nursing itself direct nursing care.

### The future

Changes in current health care systems point clearly toward certain features of health care delivery of the future. First, there is wide acknowledgment of the concept of comprehensive health care. It has been firmly demonstrated that most effective programs for optimal health incorporate all aspects of health care and educa-

tion. This approach necessitates the implementation of a team of health care workers.*

The National Commission for the Study of Nursing and Nursing Education has directed, implemented, and facilitated national efforts toward innovation and team development between the major professions of nursing and medicine.[38,39] The American Nurses' Association and the American Academy of Pediatrics have particularly encouraged development of team relationships between medical and nursing groups specializing in child care through conferences held jointly for mutual deliberation of professional problems in the team approach to child health care.[12] Joint basic education for all health care professionals is recognized as a most important step toward comprehensive health care team development. Many educational centers are creating opportunities for students in medicine, nursing, pharmacy, dentistry, social work, health education, nutrition, and administration to learn, share, and discover together.[69]

Consumers are becoming recognized as an important part of the team in delivering health care services. They are able to define what care is most acutely needed, to establish priorities, and to define what is culturally acceptable to the group receiving care.[35,58,70,75]

## IMPLEMENTING HEALTH CARE FOR CHILDREN

In the effort to provide health services for a group of people, goals must be determined that are appropriate to the needs of the consumer. This requires careful consideration for each setting and situation, but a few general guidelines, which are drawn from the philosophic commitments of child health care, may be offered. Goals that need further definition by a team may be (1) what changes in community health care are desired, (2) what areas of health care are to receive priority, (3) in what manner the consumer can realistically use the services offered, (4) how many people are to be served, and (5) how the services can be designed to be comprehensive and family-centered in scope. In

---

*References 10, 23, 28, 33, 55, 69, 77.

addition the specific goals for medical care, nursing care, dentistry, nutrition, social work, counseling, education, and every other specialty must be incorporated into the overall plan.

## Definition of goals
### General goals of comprehensive health care

The general goal of health care is to promote the individual's motivation to seek health and use personal resources to attain, maintain, or regain optimal health and function.[57] To understand this goal more thoroughly, it is necessary to consider a definition of the concept of health. Imogene King, in *Toward a Theory for Nursing*, presents the following definition of the concept of health:

Health is a dynamic state in the life cycle of an organism which implies continuous adaptation to stresses in the internal and external environment through optimum use of one's resources to achieve maximum potential for daily living. Health relates to the way an individual deals with the stresses of growth and development while functioning within the cultural pattern in which he was born and to which he attempts to conform.*

This concept of health is further enhanced when we consider the idea that health for any individual is most meaningful when defined by that individual.[19] The concept of health in many parts of the world incorporates a significant amount of disease or illness. Some individuals fail to cope with a very occasional illness. For some, maximum potential for daily living is severely limited by physical or mental handicaps, and yet the person may consider himself or herself healthy. The King definition provides a general guide for the nurse in identifying the goals of health care as defined jointly with the individual receiving care.

The identification of health care as "comprehensive" further defines the way in which the ideal of "health" is most effectively attained. The health care system incorporates many groups that contribute, through knowledge and services, to the attainment of health for individuals and communities. These groups in turn are concerned with all aspects of society that affect the group's health, such as political decisions, financial concerns, legal protection of individuals, community support for programs that render health and care services to all members of the community, and the provision of a healthy environment. The goal for the system of health care, then, is that the individual be considered as a total being, with each health care need having some provision within the total system of care.

The team effort requires that professional, technical, and consumer groups join together in some organized effort to work cooperatively toward attainment of specific and general goals. The problems and risks in attempting such a cooperative effort are significant but not insurmountable. One concern is the loss of individualized, continuous, personalized care and relationship development between the individual and the health care agent. Nurses, physicians, social workers, and counselors have long shared a desire to protect the relationship of trust that is formed between the professional helper and the individual served. In defining each of their roles, the members of a health care team must consider how this aspect of health care is to be provided when it is deemed important.

Another related problem is how the individuals offering health care services are going to utilize overlapping skills and talents without duplicating services and yet maintain the responsibility for functioning within the full scope of personal ability. Within a health care team each worker is prepared with unique skills and abilities, such as the diagnostic and treatment capabilities of the physician. There are also multiple overlapping skills, such as the ability of the nurse, physician, social worker, and dietitian to obtain a nutritional history. It is the obligation of each worker to come to the health care team equipped to demonstrate personal and professional capabilities and then to determine collaboratively how these talents can best be used to meet the goals of the group.[3,7,13,57]

## Process of child nursing

The nurse is specifically equipped to help a family seek health and use their own resources

---

*King, I. M.: Toward a theory for nursing: General concepts of human behavior, New York, 1971, John Wiley & Sons, Inc., p. 24.

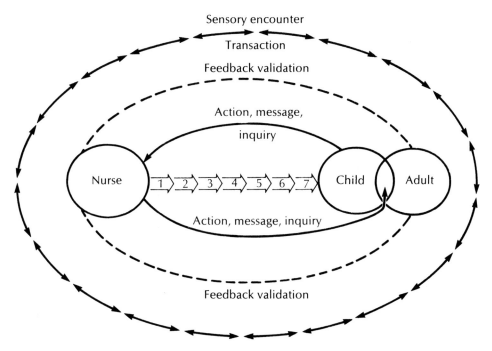

**Fig. 2-2.** Process of child nursing care. The seven components of nursing action are (1) identify values and goals to be attained, (2) identify structure, process, and outcome standards and criteria for goal attainment, (3) measure degree of attainment of selected standards and criteria, (4) interpret available data, (5) identify alternative nursing actions, (6) select the course of action, and (7) implement the course of action. Evaluation of the nursing process is accomplished by review and audit of each component in comparison with professional standards of practice.

to attain, maintain, or regain health. In a unique way the nurse is equipped with knowledge of the multiple factors affecting total health, which enables the nurse to serve the child and family in defining and attaining individual health goals. A nurse is broadly prepared in psychosocial, family, and multidisciplinary approaches to health care and shares with the medical profession an understanding of the biologic and psychologic aspects of health and disease.

Nursing care of the child involves specific, purposive processes in the acts of nursing assessment and management of health care.[11,21,22,34,40] It is stressed that the process of nursing care remains the same regardless of the nurse's employment or setting. The tasks performed and the information gathered in rendering nursing care become meaningful and relevant by the process that occurs between the nurse and the child and the family. These processes are depicted in Fig. 2-2. In this diagram

the child and the significant adult are represented as overlapping, separate units, for each shares overlapping concerns, and communication from each significant person involved in a particular child health problem is essential in formulating reliable and relevant nursing judgment and management.[25] The nurse and the child/adult units are seen as being separate human entities within an encompassing transaction sensory encounter circle. Each sends the other some kind of communicative message through action, verbal message, or inquiry. This is represented as a solid arrow in the direction of the message sent. The person receiving the message then gives some form of feedback or validation indicating receipt of the message. This is represented as a broken arrow in the direction of the feedback sent, signifying the fact that this feedback is not always sent or perceived in a totally accurate manner. Sometimes the communication sent is inadequate; at other times there is an inadequacy in the perception of the message by the receiver or in perception of the feedback.

The nucleus of the model represents the nursing actions that are indicated. These actions incorporate all components of the nursing process and the steps indicated to achieve quality assurance, as will be described in later sections of this chapter. Use of these actions also provides for testing standards of nursing practice. The seven components* of action occur continuously throughout the nurse-client interaction and are described as follows:

1. *Identify values and goals to be attained.* The nurse and the child/adult client mutually determine the personal, cultural and professional values that influence goal attainment, and select the goal to be reached. Mutual participation is essential for effective achievement of goals. When mutual participation is not possible, the nurse assumes a role of advocate for the child/adult client and uses professional standards of care to determine the best course of action given the nature of the situation.

2. *Identify structure, process, and outcome standards and criteria for goal attainment.* The nurse identifies the structure of the health care system, particularly those factors within it that exist to facilitate or hinder goal attainment, such as physical facilities, staffing patterns on the health care team, monetary resources, and characteristics of the care givers. The process needed to attain the goals is also identified, including the actions of the various members of the health care team that are needed. The outcome is finally identified, including the criteria by which the nurse and the child/adult client will determine that adequate goal achievement has occurred.

3. *Measure degree of attainment of selected standards and criteria.* The nurse uses measurements and assessment tools to measure and document the child/adult state of well-being or movement toward attainment of the health care goal. If complete goal attainment is not projected, the differences in actual attainment and goal are described.

4. *Interpret available data.* The data are interpreted in light of the initial goals, assessment of the adequacy of the state of well-being, and in terms of developmental norms and cultural expectations. The interpretation is summarized in a statement of a nursing problem, nursing diagnosis, or health need. These statements are needs or problems of the child/adult that are subject to nursing intervention. A diagnosis represents a problem statement supported by evidence of the etiology of the problem, whereas a problem is any health problem for which the etiology is uncertain or unknown, and intervention is directed primarily to resolution of the problem rather than direct alteration of the etiology. A health need represents the client's need for specific health maintenance, promotion, and prevention of illness whether or not a health deficit exists. The Minnesota Nursing Problem Classification for Children and Youth, presented in the Appendix (p. 884) is referred to throughout this text as a means of labeling and classifying each of these forms of nursing problem.

5. *Identify alternative nursing actions.* The nurse, in consultation with the child/adult client and the health care team, determines the alternative actions that may be selected to meet the desired goal.

6. *Select the course of action.* In accord with the values of the health care team and the child/adult client, the preferred action is selected. This step involves a critical stage of client advocacy and may present the most difficult challenge of the nursing process. Determining the course of action that is in the best interest of the child and the adult, as well as professionally sound, may lead to conflict. Because of this potential, the first stage of values clarification cannot be overemphasized, for that early determination of relevant values will enable the nurse to serve as an effective advocate for the child.

7. *Implement course of action.* All actions indicated in the plan for the selected approach are implemented, with full accounting of the structure, process and outcome criteria in relation to each action.

---

*Adapted from ANA model for Quality Assurance, Committee for Implementation of Standards for Nursing Practice, 1975.

Upon completion of the action, the process of nursing care is reviewed in entirety, with reevaluation and reassessment of the values and goals, structure, process and outcome criteria, measurement tools, interpretation, and courses of action. This repetitive cycle provides for ongoing evaluation and monitoring of the quality of care, as well as identification of the areas that need alteration or improvement.

When the nurse uses this process skillfully, a valuable transaction process of validation, reevaluation, and reciprocal relationship is formulated, which enables the nurse and the child/adult to each continually participate in the formulation of goals to be achieved. Within the framework of sensory encounter and transaction, the nurse specifically is executing the acts of skilled nursing judgment based on the assessment (described in following sections) followed by nursing intervention and management. The child and adult remain an integral part of the nursing acts through the transaction and communication processes that are ongoing and continuous.

## Incorporating the conceptual model into nursing practice

The totality of the nursing experience is so complex that we can only conceptualize small parts of it at a time. In Chapter 1 and in the present chapter several concepts in relation to nursing care of the child have been presented. The interrelationships between these ideas and the practice of nursing needs to be fully explored and understood in order for the nurse to attempt sound, unified, purposeful nursing care of children.

*The basic goal* governing all of nursing care is to promote individual motivation to seek health and use personal resources to attain, maintain, or regain optimal health and function. This goal offers the nurse a general guiding focus for all nursing care of children.

*The processes of nursing care* (see Fig. 2-1) provide the conceptualization of nursing behavior and acts. These processes describe how the nurse approaches nursing acts and interactions; they are features of all that the nurse does. The process of quality assurance, which is inherent in the process of nursing care and provides for implementation of the standards of nursing care, encompasses the seven basic components of nursing action.

*The conceptual framework for nursing care of the child,* as presented in Chapter 1; provides for the nurse who works with children, either as a general nurse practitioner or as a specialist in child care, the added dimension that is unique and essential in child health care. Although all people of all ages are involved in one of life's developmental stages, children are unique in the developmental requirement of gradually gaining the adultlike competency to assume total responsibility for their own behavior and maintenance of life and health. The framework, which incorporates multiple factors influencing children's attainment of their own unique competency in physical, learning and thought, and social and inner development, gives the nurse a broad basis for orderly consideration of the child as a total human being and exercising nursing judgment and intervention that is relevant to the particular child at a particular point in life.

## Communicating nursing care to the health team

As the nurse serves the consumer within a team of health care workers, one of the most crucial aspects of nursing care is communicating effectively the nursing care given to the child and family to other team members who are serving the same child and family. Nurses have traditionally used nurses' notes, charts, referral forms, and nursing care plans in an effort to provide continuous, timely communication regarding ongoing nursing care. Because of growing implementation of the comprehensive team, a unified approach to communication among all health care professionals emerged. No longer is it useful to have separate records for each person involved in rendering health services.

Weed's approach to record-keeping has been demonstrated to provide a valuable approach to health care practice in hospitals and communities.[6,56,63,71] Further development of the problem-oriented record for nursing practice has led to a systematic approach to record keeping and communication that provides for:

1. Memory and recall of facts relating to pa-

tient care regardless of who enters the facts or the time or setting in which the event occurred

2. A tool whereby the practitioner can learn and analyze his or her own data and that of other health care workers in an orderly, organized manner

3. A tool for evaluation of the effectiveness of total health care

Each component will be described and is illustrated at the conclusion of each unit.

The *data base* is the initial evaluation of the child. The information to be included in the data base is defined in advance for all children seen by a given practitioner in a given situation. The data base is comprised of the initial statement of the client concerning the reason for seeking health care, a profile of the child/adult unit, the past history of the child, parents and family, review of physiologic systems, data obtained from the physical assessment, data obtained from psychosocial assessment, and any testing or laboratory data obtained. The data base concludes with a summary of the child's physical, learning and thought, social, and inner competencies. The conceptual framework for nursing care of the child gives one general definition for content of the data base, but further definition depends upon the circumstances of the health team and the immediate needs of the child and family. The health history and nursing assessment provide the major source for gathering the initial data base, but other sources for social, environmental, and cultural information may be used. The more comprehensive the data base, the more accurate and relevant will be the identification of problems.

The *problem list* is extracted from the information obtained in the data base. For the purposes of this text, the problem list will be titled the *health status* list. This terminology indicates inclusion of health maintenance, promotion and prevention of illness needs that are usually not conceptualized as "problems" but that are real health care needs requiring planned nursing intervention. This list is entered at the front of the client's record and is permanent. Each health need or problem is dated, titled, and numbered consecutively as it is entered, and the list becomes an index to the entire record, for prog-

ress notes are made relative to each problem by number. All known problems are listed—physiologic, psychologic, and socioeconomic. A problem title is not listed as a diagnosis unless it can be unquestionably confirmed by the data. Titles begin as subjective symptoms (e.g., blurred vision) and are changed as more information becomes available (acute myopia). Each health care worker contributes to the same central problem list and to the other components of the record.

*The initial plan* is designed for each health need or problem identified separately. This may be part of the initial assessment, or this description and evaluation process may be employed as new problems arise. Within the body of the record, the problem is referred to by number and title, and the following information is then recorded:

1. *Subjective data* (S). The problem from the adult's or child's point of view. Often a direct quote from the informant is given to convey more completely the person's own perception of the problem.

2. *Objective data* (O). The direct physical observations, laboratory findings, or behavioral observations made by the nurse which are pertinent to the present problem.

3. *Assessment* (A). The criteria that can be identified in delineating the problem are listed in detail. It may not be possible to make a diagnosis, but a summary statement of the subjective and objective findings can be made that reflects possible diagnostic criteria. Often the nurse will encounter indications of problems that are beyond the scope of nursing diagnosis and treatment. In such a case the nurse articulates nursing observations and refers the child to another health care team member for further delineation of the problem. A diagnosis is never assigned until sound criteria are demonstrated. Advance delineation of adequate diagnostic criteria by the members of a health care team is helpful for consistent implementation of team health care.

4. *Plan* (P). The plan is stated in terms of the client care goals and the expected outcomes of selected nursing actions. These goals are refined to indicate what the child/adult client is expected to accomplish. A statement of behav-

ior and of the expected behavior traits is included in the objectives of the plan. Behavior statements can include such expectations as the client identifying, demonstrating, explaining, or describing the expected outcomes. A statement of specific traits includes such things as understanding, achieving an improved physiologic state, or a specific alteration in behavior. Subsequent implementation of the plan may then be conducted in an organized, purposeful, and efficient manner, or changed in specific response to the unfolding needs of the child.

5. *Nursing orders* are defined as a process of implementing the client care objectives as stated in the initial plan. The nursing orders identify the specific nursing interventions necessary in meeting the client care objectives. Nursing intervention indicates actions that are directed toward the prevention, alleviation, or elimination of the problem or toward maintenance of the present state of well-being. Nursing orders are specific written directions for specific nursing actions. The components of nursing orders include the person responsible for carrying out the nursing action, the specific action to be taken, when the action is to be carried out, and how the action is to be accomplished.[67] Nursing orders are to be identified for each client objective. When the nursing actions are entered in the record, the corresponding problem number is recorded with it to provide access to other components of the record related to the same problem.[67]

6. *Progress notes* serve as a tool in the evaluation process of the client's achievement of goals. Each progress note entry should be identified by date, problem number, and problem title. Each problem should be discussed in the progress notes as to the assessment of change in status, their relationship to the progress of other problems, and the relationship to previous progress. Narrative notes, presented in the SOAP format, flow sheets, and summaries, may be included in the progress notes. This presentation allows for monitoring of progress, systematic modification of plans of care, and accurate identification of level of resolution of each problem. Progress notes and related data are entered by all members of the health care team in continuing sequence. They are made according to the format of the problem assessment and plan formulation in relation to each existing or new problem that is identified. A flow sheet may be developed for recording frequently obtained data for a specific problem. For example, if a child is seen at frequent intervals because of a nephrotic syndrome, all of the data to be obtained at each visit, such as urinalysis results, blood pressure, observations of physical features, and so on, might be entered on a flow sheet to facilitate comparison from one visit to another. However, the numbering systems for each problem allows one to identify and quickly compare all data obtained in relation to a single problem over a period of time. In addition, health care over an extended period of time can be critically evaluated, and learning from past experience is maximized for the practitioner.

7. *The discharge summary* is a statement presenting salient information about the child/adult client, including the nursing and medical diagnoses and other significant demographic and descriptive events. A summary statement is then included about the progress of each of the identified problems and presented in the SOAP format. This allows for evaluation of the total activities of care as initially planned and provides direction for future care.[67]

## Responsibility for action

Each member of the health care team is vitally concerned with individual as well as group responsibility for the acts they perform in seeking to attain their goals. Professional workers need to know through performance demonstration what skills and abilities their fellow workers possess. They need assurance that a given level of responsibility, accountability, and competence will be assumed in order for natural trust to develop. The consumer, as a member of the team as well as the recipient of the services offered, is particularly aware and actively interested in the competency of the workers and the quality of services.

Ethical and legal aspects of nursing practice and health care, which have developed as changes have occurred, have generated much debate. Because the nursing process involves making skilled nursing judgment and executing nursing intervention and management, the nurse is professionally obligated to assume direct and individual responsibility for demonstrating and maintaining competency to perform the highest quality of skill possible. In so doing, legal and ethical protection is also maintained. Employers provide supervision and expectations for officially sanctioned behavior in the form of a job description. Professional employees should carefully participate and determine the appropriateness of these expectations for their own level of competency. There are several steps that are indicated in demonstrating this competency.

First, the professional nurse in the United States is obligated to obtain licensure in the state in which practice is conducted. This mandatory licensing is the minimal demonstration of competence as a professional nurse who has completed a given level of basic preparation for the practice of nursing and who is capable of meeting the basic requirements of the Nurse Practice Act of that state.

Second, the nurse has the opportunity to join professional organizations that encompass the entire profession of nursing or are restricted to an area of specialized interest. These organizations provide timely exposure to the issues and problems encountered by the profession as a whole. They give the nurse an opportunity to relate to members of allied professions through joint conferences and interprofessional tasks centered on areas of mutual interest. They also provide the nurse a channel through which to exert legislative, political, and legal influence in relation to community and administrative decisions affecting health care and professional practice.

Third, the nurse has available several resources for continuing education. Particularly when a nurse wishes to become specialized in an area of nursing practice that offers a great personal challenge, programs for developing specialized knowledge and skill in the area of choice are widely available. Short-term continuing education through schools of nursing are frequently offered, and most education programs, either of the specialized or continuing education type, offer some manner of certification indicating the type of educational experience gained by the nurse and the particular performance competencies that should be expected. In addition to the more formal education programs the nurse has readily available professional journals and publications that assist in the personal pursuit of knowledge. Colleagues in a professional setting can often assist one another in finding relevant application of knowledge and ideas discovered through literature exploration.

Fourth, job recognition and legal/ethical protection rise from performance demonstration of the actual competency of the individual. Demonstration involves the performance of those acts of which the individual is capable, as well as visible judgment of not attempting those things that are beyond the individual's capability. The mutual trust that develops when professional colleagues experience the professional ability of one another develops into a colleagueship that gives support for and confidence in one another. Legally, an individual employee is held personally responsible for all acts performed in the line of duty. The employer may defend the actions of an employee if that action is deemed to be within the realm of officially sanctioned behavior by the employer. This is a very fine distinction and often the decision, when questions arise, depends heavily upon the level of trust developed among the persons involved. With the establishment of the Professional Standards Review Organizations in 1973, the concept of quality health care was incorporated as a professional obligation to provide this fundamental human right. All professions involved in health care delivery have begun to examine their own practices and to develop methods and procedures to evaluate the quality of practice of the individual as well as of the professional group. The nursing profession has begun this examination through the joint efforts of the American Nurses' Association Divisions of Practice and the Congress on Nursing Practice. Generic standards and specialized standards of care have been developed whereby the quality of nursing care may be ascertained.[1] The standards for maternal-child health are presented at the conclusion of this chapter.

Fifth, just as recognition and protection arise from the trust and relationship of confidence among professional colleagues, trust and a re-

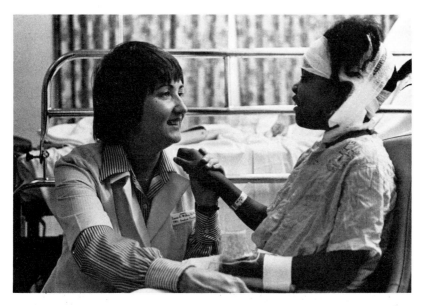

**Fig. 2-3.** Skill in careful listening must be consciously developed. Here the nurse positions herself in such a manner that she can "hear" the child's nonverbal as well as verbal communication.

lationship of confidence between the nurse and the consumer give rise to another source of recognition and protection for the nurse. Mutual trust indicates that the consumer (1) understands the nature of the services that may be expected from the nurse and (2) is satisfied with the manner in which these services are rendered and (3) senses the advocacy role provided by the nurse in protecting his or her own health and in participating in the achievement of the individual's own health care goals.

Finally, the nurse may provide some degree of personal protection from legal action by subscribing to a plan of professional liability insurance. As nurses have assumed a more independent and autonomous function in health care systems in recent years, the need to provide their own insurance protection for professional practice has increased.[26,53,59]

## NURSING ASSESSMENT OF THE CHILD

The ability of the nurse to utilize all observational skills to reassess the continuing health status of a child is crucial for meaningful nursing care. Every sensory modality is used. The information received is integrated with knowledge and understanding of the phenomena of life, health, and illness to formulate skilled nursing judgment.

### Modalities of assessment
*Listening*

The nurse listens for every significant sound and message that is conveyed by the child or adult. The child's heart, lungs, and abdominal sounds are auscultated through use of the stethoscope. Diagnostic decisions based on auscultation usually require physician evaluation, but recognition and description of sounds ordinarily encountered, as well as unusual sounds, are the responsibility of the nurse.[36,37,64]

Listening as the child or parent speaks is one of the most valuable tools available to the nurse. This talent seems deceptively simple, but accurate, complete listening ability requires concentration and practice.[14] Attentive receiving of what the child or adult is seeking to convey demands that the nurse lay aside personal needs to talk, to say things, to get the job done, and concentrate on the needs of the child or parent to convey his or her own message. This listening ability also conveys to the child and adult that they are indeed quite important to the nurse and that their messages are important and necessary.

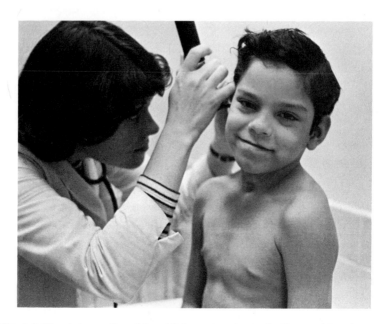

**Fig. 2-4.** Visual observation of the child's ear is enhanced with use of the otoscope.

Skill in careful listening must be consciously developed by the person who desires to use it. Most conversation is barely listened to in everyday life. A serious attempt at trying to understand and help another person, while appearing very much like everyday conversation, has the characteristic of at least one of the communicators giving active, serious attention and response to the messages sent. The less obvious, nonverbal messages sent through action, gestures, facial expression, tone of voice, and by things deliberately not said are also attended and integrated with verbal messages.[52,74] These are often the real, important messages regardless of what the words may transmit. The concept of active listening as a therapeutic tool will be discussed later in this chapter.

Specific concerns in gathering verbally conveyed material through the health history and interview are reviewed most appropriately for each of the developmental stages during childhood and will appear within the discussion of assessment for each of the age groups in the following units.

### Visual observation

Visual observation has been discussed in the preceding section as a part of the listening pro-

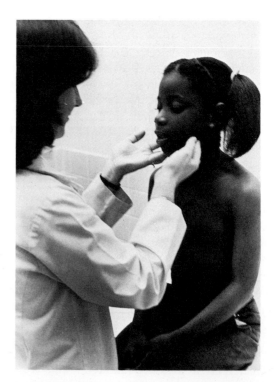

**Fig. 2-5.** The sense of touch conveys information not available through other senses, such as characteristics of temperature, texture, and size and shape of subcutaneous structures.

cess. In addition to the communicative messages that the child or adult may be sending, the nurse is alert to signs of physical impairment or difficulty. For example, children who are having trouble seeing objects at a distance will squint their eyes and strain their heads and necks in an effort to see more clearly. Children who have difficulty with fine motor coordination will exhibit this difficulty when asked to perform some fine motor task.

The nurse observes the color and character of the child's skin, mucous membranes, hair, and nails.[54] These surfaces reflect many important physiologic processes of the body, as well as signs of health care and hygiene practice.

To enhance the ability to observe orifices of the child's body and to see their characteristics more clearly, a light source such as a small flashlight is essential. An otoscope is necessary for visualization of the eardrum, and an ophthalmoscope is needed for visualization of the eye grounds.

The multitude of possible visual observations are too numerous to list. Specific important observations that are indicated by the child's age and developmental stage are discussed in detail in later chapters. As with the skill of listening, the skill of attending to each visual observation available during an encounter with a child is one that requires discipline.

### Touch

The power of the nurse's touch in the comforting and healing process has long been acclaimed. The information available to the nurse through the sense of touch has also been recognized. Characteristics of high fever (warmth), dehydration (dryness), and circulatory inadequacies (cold) can be observed through the sense of touch. Characteristics of the child's ability to move and respond physically, such as symmetry of strength in the shoulders or arms, are observed through feel. The child also is asked to respond to touch sensations such as weight, cold, or heat, in order to assess the integrity of the neurologic system. Palpation of various areas of the body, such as the infant's fontanel or the child's abdomen, conveys valuable information. Percussion of the surface of the body can give clues as to size of various or-gans or composition of spaces (e.g., air or fluid in the lungs).

### Integration of information

Information gathered and simply listed serves no useful end. Gathering information becomes relevant and is meaningful only as it is integrated in some useful fashion with knowledge of human growth and development, health principles, illness signs and symptoms, and a personal knowledge of the uniqueness of the individual child. The conceptual framework for nursing care of the child as presented in Chapter 1 is designed to assist in this task.

## Evaluating childhood competencies
### Physical competency

The level of physical competency to be expected of any child is defined by averages and norms established for several traits for each age and stage of life and by the uniqueness of the individual child. Averages are obtained by measuring the growth or performance of many children on a given trait and determining the mathematical average. When children who represent many different social and cultural groups are measured, the average is considered more truly representative of all children. If, however, a particular group of children tend to be quite different from all other children for a given trait, it is more useful to obtain an average that represents just that group of children. For example, average expected height and weight charts have been established that were determined using a comprehensive, representative group of children of all ages.[27] If, however, the nurse is working with a particular group of children who tend not to follow the growth pattern norms of the larger group, averages for the particular group would be more useful in making an interpretation of height and weight patterns for an individual child within the group.[18,50]

Physical competency expectations have been described more completely than any of the other competencies. When a child tends to deviate from the expected pattern or average, however, it is often very difficult to determine the meaning of the deviation for this particular child. The uniqueness of the individual is often lost in seeking to understand the academic questions

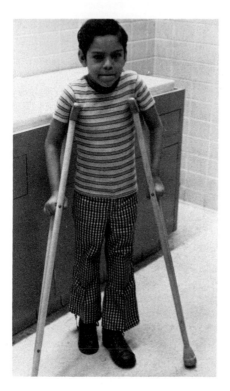

**Fig. 2-6.** Each child at each stage of development has an optimal level of physical competency. Here a 10-year-old boy achieves mobility with the use of crutches after paralysis caused by Guillain-Barré disease.

of what is causing or what has influenced the deviation. Society often is cruel to children who exhibit physical traits that are not considered abnormal but are uncommon. A boy who is extremely short, though normal, is placed in an extremely difficult social situation. The girl who is hefty and strong is likewise normal, although unusual in a way that is not socially acceptable. Thus the interaction of all variables influencing development becomes an important factor in determining health needs. Averages or norms are simply a map giving general direction and expectation.

Growth charts for height and weight, chest measurements, and head circumference are available for large, representative groups as well as for a few sociocultural groups of children (see Appendix). The use of growth grids can be extremely helpful if a pattern is obtained over extended periods of time and proportions of each growth parameter are compared.[44] For in-

stance, a child who over a period of three years, remains in the fiftieth percentile for height and the twenty-fifth percentile for weight, with a head circumference around the mean, might be recognized to be constitutionally average in height, slender, but not necessarily underweight. Investigation of the build characteristics of relatives and the nutritional adequacy of the diet would aid in making such a judgment. On the other hand, a child who throughout early childhood is just above the average for both height and weight and whose weight percentile slowly begins to rise during the preadolescent years would be recognized as beginning to be overweight.

Expectations for dental development, as well as norms for temperature, pulse rate, respiration rate, and blood pressure are also available (see Appendix).

Estimating the adequacy of development of traits for which norms are not measurable is enhanced by the use of various screening tools and by physical observation. The Denver Developmental Screening tool is useful for estimating development of preschoolers in the areas of gross motor, fine motor, language, and personal-social skills. Developmental expectations in neurologic functioning, visual acuity, and hearing responses are described for each developmental stage in subsequent chapters (see Chapters 9, 10, 12, 14, and Appendix).

Laboratory determinations that are important in routine health supervision are urinalysis and hematocrit or hemoglobin. Normal values for various ages are found in the Appendix. Other laboratory determinations may be used by the nurse during periods of illness or in particular situations. For example, a child who is being observed during a periods of rheumatic heart disease might be monitored for erythrocyte sedimentation rate, C-reactive protein, white blood cell morphology, and electrocardiogram traits.

Estimating the adequacy of nutrition is an important aspect in judging physical competency at each developmental stage. Typical patterns of eating occur for each age group, and nutritional needs of children and adolescents are specific and well documented, affecting all areas of growth and development. These are discussed in detail in later chapters.

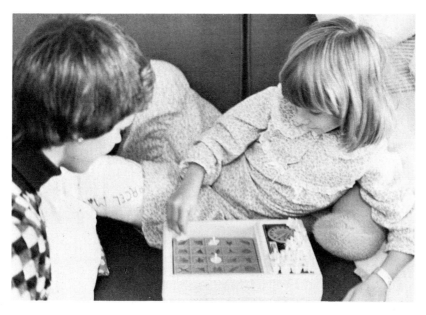

**Fig. 2-7.** Development of learning and thought competency is stimulated for this hospitalized child with the use of a learning game that requires matching of geometric shapes.

Physical activity patterns in relation to exercise, sleep and rest, and elimination processes are to be documented as accurately as possible. Often families develop patterns of activity that are not in the best interest of healthy development for the children and yet do not necessarily inhibit adequate growth and development. Again, skilled nursing judgment must be developed to determine the desirability for nursing intervention. For example, a young couple may be accustomed to being up very late at night, and they enjoy the company of their young child during the late hours. If this style if not interfering with the child's total rest needs or behavior traits and the time is a valuable social occasion for the family, the pattern should not be questioned. If, however, the child does not sleep during day hours to compensate for total needs and becomes unusually irritable, the family needs to consider some alternative pattern for socialization.

### Learning and thought competency

Developmental guidelines for learning and thought ability are less well defined than those for physical competency. Piaget[47,51] has provided important evidence in recent years re-garding cognitive, language, and thought abilities of children. Psychologists during the past 50 years have developed useful tools for the estimation of intelligence and reasoning abilities of children.[15] The actual measurement of these abilities is beyond the scope of nursing assessment, but several screening tools are available for detecting lags in development. The child who has not yet entered school is particularly vulnerable to a number of factors that may produce a lag in learning and thought competency. Lack of environmental stimulation has been demonstrated to produce significant difficulty in learning during the school years, and it may be reversible if detected and intervention is begun early. Because the nurse or the health care team is often the only professional group who has access to the child and is able to screen for problems in this area during the preschool years, attention to this area of functioning is crucial. Learning and thought competency interacts increasingly with competencies in other areas of ability as the child grows older and as the need to assume more personal responsibility for health and living grows.

Speech and language development may be indicated by the child's ability to recall past

**39**

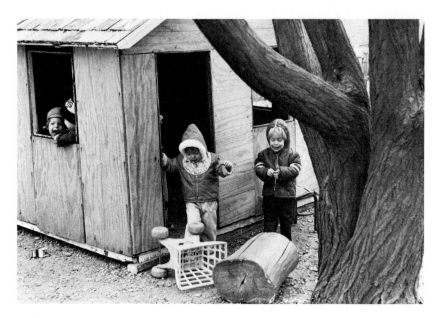

**Fig. 2-8.** During early childhood the development of social competency includes role-playing adult tasks and behaviors in a peer group.

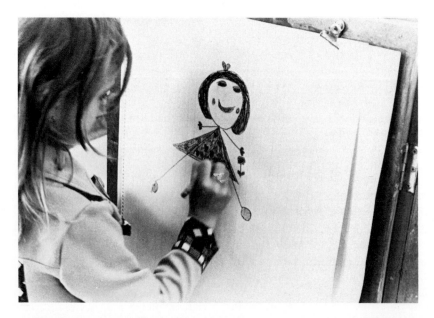

**Fig. 2-9.** The child's self-portrait reveals inner perceptions of her body and self.

events, discuss forthcoming events, and describe abstract concepts, such as "cold," "funny," "near," and "love." Adequacy of neurologic functioning gives an indication of learning and thought competency. Tools that can be used in assessing learning and thought competency include the "Draw-a-Person" test, the Peabody Picture Vocabulary test,[20] and school readiness and achievement tests.

The perceptions of the child and the parent regarding the child's learning and thinking ability should also be taken into account. The accuracy of these perceptions needs to be considered, and any factors that are recognized by the child or the parent are regarded as important evidence related to the child's ability. The accuracy of this ability contributes to the nursing assessment of inner competency as well.

### Social competency

Social competency during the early years of life is primarily defined by the age and stage of development of the child, but as age progresses it is more predominantly defined by the society of which the child is a member and the point in historical time that the particular society exists. For example, the family in Western societies has traditionally been the acceptable social unit in which children are to be reared. This unit is now changing in form and style. The nurse is able to describe the social abilities of the child as they are observed or reported and can draw some inferences regarding the acceptability of these behaviors based on the standards that apply to the child. The greatest asset in making an adequate judgment regarding social competency is the nurse's ability to know, understand, and conceptualize standards for social behavior that apply to the child when those standards are not those that apply to the nurse.[9]

Assessment tools that can be used for social competency include the Vineland Social Maturity Scale.[17] The nurse can use a standard interview plan to obtain data regarding the child's family structure and function and the nature of interactions with the peer group. If possible, these interactions should be observed directly and considered along with data regarding the child's perceptions of these interactions. A child

may appear to interact in a desired, healthy manner but harbor feelings of inferiority in relation to the peer group.

### Inner competency

Evidence available to the nurse in regard to inner competency is the most indirect of all observations made. Yet this is the realm of functioning of the individual that is the most pervasive, and even minor or transient disorders cause extreme concern on the part of adults in the child's life. Judgments in this area in actual practice often require making large inferences based on relatively minute pieces of evidence. Signs of inner suffering or pain are often overlooked unless there is some socially unacceptable or troublesome behavior on the part of the child. Because competency in each of the other three areas significantly conditions and influences a child's self-concept, any unusual developmental trait signals concern for the child's inner self.

Inner competency, or the self-concept, may be conceptualized as including three major components: structure, function, and quality. Each of these components encompasses a wide range of ideas, which may be useful in conceptualizing the many phenomena that comprise inner competency.

*Structure* may be represented by four major continuums that describe the nature of inner competency. These are:

1. Rigid—flexible
2. Accurate—inaccurate
3. Simple—complex
4. Broad—narrow

It should be remembered that we are not speaking of an object but are speaking of structure in the sense that one speaks of the structure of logic or of an argument. It has form in a conceptual sense that may be described by the above traits.

*Function* of inner competency is represented by those aspects that describe what this structure does for the person or how it works. It includes such things as:

1. Self-evaluation
2. Prediction of success or failure
3. Obtaining personal survival, acceptance,

comfort, enhancement, competence, and actualization or realization

4. Instigation of behavior mediated by one's own desires and values or by the society's desires and values

Finally, the *quality* of inner competence may be conceptualized in terms of one major continuum ranging from self-approval, high self-esteem, and self-acceptance to self-disapproval, low self-esteem, and self-rejection.[41]

The nurse's personal concept of inner competency greatly influences the clues in the child's behavior and environment on which the nurse bases inferences about the adequacy of development. The philosophic, religious, and psychologic ideas that have been adopted during the years of development and education shape the notions that define, for a particular nurse, adequacy of the child's inner competence. Care must be cultivated in allowing the standards and values of the child's own culture and family to predominate in formulating this definition of adequacy.

Significantly deviated functioning in self-esteem and personality development is detected with relative ease. However, the child who is suffering with a relatively low level of self-esteem or guilt feelings or feelings of inadequacy may not be able to freely or convincingly reveal this suffering until a level of trust and rapport is developed with an admired adult. The nurse who is able to identify and describe traits, behavior, or verbal messages that suggest concern for a child's inner feelings and development may not be the appropriate person to fully explore and diagnose such a disorder. Again, frequent contact with the child and his or her total environment often create a special advantage in the initial detection of inadequate development, but referral for diagnosis or treatment may be indicated.[29]

## NURSING MANAGEMENT OF CHILD HEALTH NEEDS

Once the identification of specific health care needs is accomplished, the nurse proceeds with the formulation of a plan for management and implements this plan through specific nursing acts. This entire process of need identification and plan formulation and implementation is governed by several crucial factors:

1. The nurse's level of competence
2. The context of this particular nurse-child or family relationship

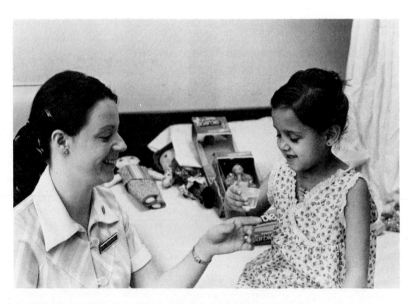

**Fig. 2-10.** Administering drugs to children requires an understanding of the hazards and factors concerning drug effects in children.

3. The child and family's own desires, aspirations, and goals

Health needs that are clearly identified but are not subject to management by the nurse because of one of the above factors are attended by another member of the health care team who can adequately fulfill the necessary criteria. Conflict between the nurse's personal aspirations and goals and those of the child or family may occur, and on occasion the child may be in conflict with the family's goals. For example, the parents of a child with mild myopia may prefer not to purchase glasses, and the nurse may react indignantly or angrily to this decision. The adolescent girl may desire family planning counsel against the wishes of her family. Resolution of such conflict is difficult, and each professional health worker will encounter occasion to work through such a conflict situation, resolving it in his or her own manner.

## Identification of needs based on the data base

The process and the data of the nursing assessment provide the evidence upon which needs are identified and defined. When a problem or a need cannot be clearly identified, the nurse makes a judgment regarding the weight of existing evidence and either leaves the existing evidence with no further investigation or makes plans to obtain further evidence. When a need has been clearly identified from the nurse's point of view, validation may be necessary with the child or family. For example, when a child clearly has a severe injury, validation is immediate and only the exact nature of the injury may need further exploration. If, on the other hand, the nurse feels that subjective and objective evidence suggests that a child is suffering from a nutritional deficiency, the validation may come from other members of the health care team as complex evidence of the child's status is obtained, and the deficiency may become a realization for the child's mother or caretaker only gradually.

## Formulating a plan

When nursing intervention is deliberately planned and articulated, the possibility for success is greatly increased, and the evaluation process, which is essential for the development of clinical expertise, is possible.[40] Success is also enhanced with the involvement, on a meaningful and sincere level, of the child and the family. Plans that are unrealistic and not attainable for the child will surely go unfulfilled.[5] The plan that evolves may not be ideal from the nurse's point of view, but it may assist the child toward an improved health status.

## Implementing the plan

The nurse is prepared with several modalities for implementation that characterize nursing practice.

### *Physical care related to specific needs or problems*

Physical care by the nurse is most commonly associated with periods of dependency, as during infancy or debilitation. During these periods physical care is an essential part of therapeutic and restorative care. Although not as acutely essential when the child is more independent and well, there are frequent instances when physical care is needed that the nurse is particularly prepared to respond to. For example, the nurse may give first aid care following an accident, give care to a child suffering from a minor illness while visiting the home to teach the mother fundamental principles of basic nursing care, or assist a young mother in early attempts to breast-feed her infant. Acquisition of the physical, technical skills for nursing care is often the first encounter with nursing that a student experiences, and these skills remain essential throughout nursing. Many skills depend upon the setting in which the nurse works. A nurse caring for high risk infants acquires abilities that are certainly foreign to the nurse working in homes. The process through which physical skills are employed, however, remains the same for all nurses. Full description of technical and physical skills is beyond the scope of this text, but a few skills are discussed and illustrated as they are particularly important for specific age groups.

Drugs are frequently administered to children for health problems and in the prevention of illness. Immunizations, discussed in detail in later chapters, are frequently administered independently by nurses with standard guidelines, standing orders, or protocol for management determined in advance by the health team. These drugs, as with all others employed by the nurse in any setting, are subject to each of the hazards and factors concerning drug effects in children. It is imperative that the nurse understand completely the following special hazards and considerations when administering drugs to children:

**Age.** Children are often more sensitive to the effects of specific drugs than are adults, or they exhibit effects that are not seen in adults. For some drugs, such as most antibiotics, age does not significantly affect the desired dosage. Infants and children are not simply small adults, and dosage should not be calculated from adult doses by formula. Rather, the dosage for each drug used and the specific effects on infants and children should be learned as such, or a resource on the specific drug should be consulted before administration.

**Weight, blood volume, and body surface area.** Body weight is not a satisfactory index for determining dosage for most drugs, because it does not provide an accurate index of blood volume, which is the critical factor in determining concentration of an administered drug. Body surface area is more nearly accurate in estimating drug dosage, since it more closely correlates with blood volume. However, dosage recommendations for specific drugs should be carefully considered in making an estimate (see nomogram for estimating body surface area, Appendix.

**Route of administration.** Drugs intended by the manufacturer to be administered by a given route can *never* be administered by a different route. The drug is formulated for effective utilization and safety by the route indicated only.

**Rate of metabolism and excretion: time of administration.** The young infant metabolizes and excretes most drugs at a slower rate than do older children or adults. When the function of the organs associated with excretion of a specific drug is impaired, the rate of excretion is greatly altered. Therefore, timing of repeated dosages or amounts of dosages should be altered accordingly.

**Tolerance.** Progressive reduction in response to certain drugs sometimes occurs after repeated administration. When prolonged use of a drug is necessary, physician supervision is desired to judge the potential hazard or risk of tolerance.

**Pathologic state.** The effects of some drugs are changed or determined by the pathologic condition of the individual. Aspirin, for example, reduces body temperature only when the temperature is elevated.

**Form in which the drug is administered.** Whether the drug is administered in liquid, tablet, capsule, or injectable form influences the action of the drug. Because there is a wide choice of forms available for most drugs used with children, the specific action of each form must be understood.[31,48,49,60,76]

### Teaching and counseling

Teaching and counseling within nursing require a level of expertise and skill that goes beyond the mere giving of information or "support." There is often the opportunity and need for skillful employment of basic principles of learning in the one-to-one or small group nursing encounter. A few of the principles that are particularly important in relation to child nursing will be reviewed here, and the reader is referred to more complete resources on teaching and learning for further study.

1. Readiness and motivation are essential for learning to occur. This places a very real limitation on the learning capability of young children, but as soon as they develop the readiness or the ability to learn and experience a need to learn a particular thing, they will be able to learn. Fatigue, illness, hunger, pain, or other discomfort interferes with readiness and ability to learn. Often motivation must be aroused by the person who desires to teach. If a mother needs to learn and understand certain essential principles of nutrition, the nurse may need first to arouse her desire to acquire this information and then motivate her to use it.

2. Rewarded behavior is perceived as desirable and is learned. Children are *inadvertently* taught some behaviors by receiving some kind of reward for the behavior. For example, a child who acts obnoxious and silly in the presence of company may irritate the guests eventually, but

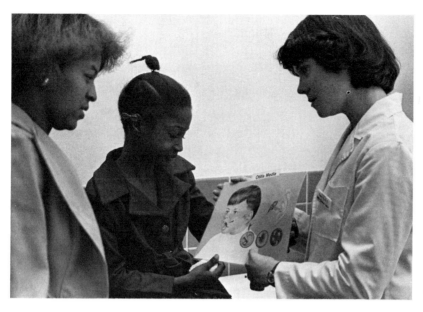

**Fig. 2-11.** The nurse has determined the readiness and motivation of the child and mother to learn specific details of the child's health problem and includes both in teaching.

their initial response of laughter and humor perpetuate repetition of the behavior. In nursing, concern for a sign of illness may inadvertently teach the child or the family to repeat the illness behavior.

3. Repetition and practice result in learning. When the nurse wishes to teach a child a health care skill, such as the use of dental floss, her success is greatly enhanced when this skill is demonstrated, slowly explained, reviewed again, and then performed by the child for the nurse. Success is further enhanced if, after a period of a day to two, the child is asked to repeat the performance for the nurse and to report on success at home. The longer a behavior is practiced, the more lasting the learning is likely to be.

4. The simpler the lesson, the more likely will be the learning. Regardless of intellectual capacity, a point that is made in a few dynamic words facilitates comprehension and learning.

5. Ideas are communicated more completely and effectively when they are experienced through more than one sensory channel. If a child or adult sees a picture of what the nurse is discussing, learning is enhanced.[8,42]

Counseling differs from the teaching-learning situation in that information acquisition is not necessarily involved in the interaction. The person who is being helped usually has a need or a problem with which he or she needs assistance. The nurse may not be prepared to function as a fully qualified, professional counselor, yet certain counseling situations occur in the nursing process that require some skill and understanding in the basic helping relationship. The child or family may ask the nurse for advice on a certain problem that, in reality, is their decision to make. Giving advice, even when the advice is sought by the person needing help, is seldom helpful in solving a problem. Instead, skilled counseling involves helping the person to recognize all alternatives available, to consider the probable outcomes for each available alternative, and to make his or her own choice in the matter. When the problem is difficult to identify, advanced skills in counseling are required and a nursing referral is desirable.

One important counseling skill that can be used effectively by the nurse is *active listening*. This approach involves the skill of listening as described earlier in this chapter, with the added dimension of reflecting back to the child or adult the listener's perception of what has been said or implied, always responding to the affect messages as well as the content.[24] For example:

**45**

MOTHER: (In a distressed tone of voice) I honestly don't know what to do about these temper tantrums. I think I get it figured out, then he has a tantrum and all my plans go to pot. I end up screaming and spanking him. My husband is even worse.

NURSE: I know this is terribly frustrating. You seem to be thinking and planning what you are going to do about the next tantrum, and then you find it doesn't work (mother nods). Apparently this is just as frustrating for your husband.

MOTHER: Yes, only he gets even more upset and blames me for not being able to handle the child.

NURSE: The two of you have a difference of opinion over how to manage?

MOTHER: (calmer now) Oh no, not really. We have really tried to plan what we're going to do together. But I'm with Billy all day and he can't understand why our plans fall apart.

NURSE: Being with a child all day is hard, and I can tell that you resent being blamed for the problem continuing. (Mother nods.) Tell me about your plans that haven't seemed to work.

Here the nurse is eliciting real information. The mother has an opportunity to clear up a misunderstanding the nurse seems to have about husband-wife conflict. Her anxiety and distress are acknowledged and begin to dissipate. Arbitrary advice-giving is avoided by the nurse. Once the mother's approaches are understood, the two can work together toward a meaningful, helpful resolution.

### Referral, additional data-gathering, and team mobilization

Throughout the discussion thus far the idea of referral and team mobilization has occurred repeatedly. This very important management tool is one of the contributions that the nurse can make toward successful team operation. Ideal, optimal health care for all people cannot be realized within most health care systems of today or of the future. But because the goal is there for the nurse and the health care team, progress toward better health care for more people can be realized. Each team member assumes responsibility for mobilizing the team when it is appropriate, either for additional data gathering or for assumption of some aspect of health care. Once a referral is made, there are two reasonable types of outcome for the nurse. One is that additional follow-through care is

needed and provided in relation to the problem or in relation to other nursing care needs. The other outcome may be that nursing care by the nurse giving the referral is no longer desirable.

The act of terminating a relationship with a child or adult may be more difficult in some instances than continuing. For example, a nurse who had maintained a long and satisfying relationship in a clinic with a child and her parents referred the child to the physician because of several signs of illness. The child's problem was medically diagnosed as acute lymphocytic leukemia. A nurse on the health team who specialized in working with families and children with similar circumstances in the hospital, in the clinic, and at home was asked to assume primary nursing care for the child and family. A satisfying relationship between the child, family, and specialist nurse was developed. Since there were no other children in the family, the nurse making the referral terminated the formal, professional relationship with the family. Personal expressions of concern as they were appropriate were continued, but the professional services of this particular team member were adequately assumed by another person who was able to offer additional help required because of the illness.

Another crucial aspect of team mobilization and follow through is teaching the family and child to independently know when and how to obtain needed health services and follow-through care. As the central member of the health care team, the consumer should become proficient in expressing the need for care and resources of the health team. When the consumer can and does assume this part of the responsibility, professional talents are more efficiently distributed in areas of need.

## Evaluation of the quality of care

Arbitrary maxims that presently govern many nursing acts are increasingly subject to systematic, objective review and evaluation. As more complete and thorough documentation is utilized, demonstration of sound nursing practice can more completely be evaluated. Outcomes that are considered successful and adequate should be examined for critical features that tend to recur in all similar successful situations.

When the outcome is less than desirable, the instance should be objectively and thoroughly evaluated by all with the goal of determining how nursing care can be improved in all similar situations. This process, rather than presenting a threat to the nurse, should be eagerly pursued in self-evaluation and peer evaluation, because nursing care is improved and understood in all respects. Because the ultimate services rendered to the child and family are of central concern for the nurse, and not the aggrandizement of that which is admirable in the nurse, total evaluation should be desired, sought, and pursued by each practitioner.[32,62,65]

The means of evaluating the effectiveness of care is accomplished using three major steps: (1) implementation of the process of nursing care as presented in Fig. 2-1, (2) recording of each component of nursing action using the problem-oriented record, and (3) audit of the nursing record using a professionally accepted standard. Implementation of the nursing process and the problem-oriented record have been discussed in earlier sections of this chapter.

The Maternal-Child Health Standards of nursing practice developed by the American Nurses' Association[1] provide a professionally accepted standard by which the audit of the nursing record may be accomplished. These standards are based on the premise of individual responsibility and accountability of the nurse in providing the right of all people to receive the benefit of the delivery of optimal health services.[1] The standards of maternal-child health nursing practice contain 13 major standards with an accompanying rationale and factors that specify those dimensions to be evaluated in review of the quality of nursing care. The standards, rationale, and assessment factors are as follows:

## STANDARD 1*

Maternal and child health nursing practice is characterized by the continual questioning of the assumptions upon which practice is based, retaining those

---

*American Nurses' Association: Standards of maternal-child health nursing practice, Kansas City, Mo., 1973. Reprinted by permission.

which are valid and searching for and using new knowledge.

**Rationale:** Since knowledge is not static, all assumptions are subject to change. Assumptions are derived from knowledge or findings of research which are subject to additional testing and revision. They are carefully selected and tested and reflect utilization of present and new knowledge. Effective utilization of these knowledges stimulates more astute observations and provides new insights into the effects of nursing upon the individual and family. To question assumptions implies that nursing practice is not based on stereotyped or ritualistic procedures or methods of intervention; rather, practice exemplifies an objective, systematic and logical investigation of a phenomenon or problem.

### Assessment factors

Therefore in practice, the Maternal and Child Health Nurse:
1. Critically examines and questions accepted modes of practice rather than relying on ritualistic or routinized modes of practice.
2. Utilizes current and new knowledge in identifying and questioning the validity of the assumptions which form the bases of nursing practice.
3. Continuously expands and improves nursing practice by utilizing theories and research findings in search of alternative solutions.
4. Actively shares new knowledge and approaches with colleagues and others in the community.

## STANDARD II

Maternal and child health nursing practice is based upon knowledge of the biophysical and psychosocial development of individuals from conception through the childrearing phase of development and upon knowledge of the basic needs for optimum development.

**Rationale:** A knowledge and understanding of the principles and normal ranges in human growth, development and behavior are essential to Maternal and Child Health Nursing Practice. Concomitant with this knowledge is the recognition and consideration of the psychosocial, environmental, nutritional, spiritual and cognitive factors that enhance or deter the biophysical and psychological maturation of the individual and his family.

### Assessment factors

Therefore in practice, the Maternal and Child Health Nurse:
1. Observes, assesses and describes the develop-

**47**

mental level and/or needs of the individual within the family before performing any actions.

2. Involves the individual and family in the assessment and planning of care.

3. Works with individuals and groups utilizing knowledge of the psychosocial, environmental, nutritional, spiritual and cognitive factors inherent in the family or group environment.

## STANDARD III

The collection of data about the health status of the client/patient is systematic and continuous. The data are accessible, communicated and recorded.

**Rationale:** Comprehensive care requires complete and ongoing collection of data about the client/patient to determine the nursing care needs and other health care needs of the client/patient. All health status data about the client/patient must be available for all members of the health care team.

### Assessment factors

1. Health status data include:
   - Growth and development
   - Biophysical status
   - Emotional status
   - Cultural, religious, socioeconomic background
   - Performance of activities of daily living
   - Patterns of coping
   - Interaction patterns
   - Client's/patient's perception and satisfaction with his health status
   - Client/patient health goals
   - Environment (physical, social, emotional, ecological)
   - Available and accessible human and material resources
2. Data are collected from:
   - Client/patient, family, significant others
   - Health care personnel
   - Individuals within the immediate environment and/or the community
3. Data are obtained by:
   - Interview
   - Examination
   - Observation
   - Reading records, reports, etc.
4. Format for the collection of data:
   - Provides for a systematic collection of data
   - Facilitates the completeness of data collection
5. Continuous collection of data is evident by:
   - Frequent updating
   - Recording of changes in health status

6. The data are:
   - Accessible on the client/patient records
   - Retrievable from record-keeping systems
   - Confidential when appropriate

## STANDARD IV

Nursing diagnoses are derived from data about the health status of the client/patient.

**Rationale:** The health status of the client/patient is the basis for determining the nursing care needs. The data are analyzed and compared to norms.

### Assessment factors

1. The client's/patient's health status is compared to the norm to determine if there is a deviation, the degree and direction of deviation.
2. The client's/patient's capabilities and limitations are identified.
3. The nursing diagnoses are related to and comparable to the totality of the client's/patient's health care.

## STANDARD V

Maternal and child health nursing practice recognizes deviations from expected patterns of physiologic activity and anatomic and psychosocial development.

**Rationale:** Early detection of deviations and therapeutic intervention are essential to the prevention of illness, to facilitating growth and developmental potential, and to the promotion of optimal health for the individual and the family.

Early detection requires that minute deviations be recognized, often before the individual or his family is aware that such deviations exist. The nurse has a unique opportunity to observe and assess the patient and his family, particularly in the community setting.

### Assessment factors

Therefore in practice, the Maternal and Child Health Nurse:

1. Demonstrates a thorough understanding of the range of normal body structure and function by detecting signs and symptoms which are not within normal limits.
2. Identifies the variety of coping mechanisms which may serve an adaptive function or represent maladaptive patterns of response.
3. Searches for improved means of detecting impairment of physical and emotional function.
4. Searches for improved means of detecting physical, psychological or environmental situations which may lead to impaired functioning.
5. Informs the individual and family in recognizing and understanding deviations.

## STANDARD VI

The plan of nursing care includes goals derived from the nursing diagnoses.

**Rationale:** The determination of the desired results from nursing actions is an essential part of planning care.

### Assessment factors

1. Goals are mutually set with the client/patient and significant others:
   - They are congruent with other planned therapies.
   - They are stated in realistic and measurable terms.
   - They are assigned a time schedule for achievement.
2. Goals are established to maximize functional capabilities and are congruent with:
   - Growth and development
   - Biophysical status
   - Behavioral patterns
   - Human and material resources

## STANDARD VII

The plan of nursing care includes priorities and the prescribed nursing approaches or measures to achieve the goals derived from the nursing diagnoses.

**Rationale:** Nursing actions are planned to promote, maintain and restore the client's/patient's well-being.

### Assessment factors

1. Physical measures are planned to manage /prevent or control specific client/patient problems and clearly relate to the nursing diagnoses and goals of care, e.g. ADL, use of self-help devices, etc.
2. Psychosocial measures are specific to the client's/patient's nursing care needs and to the nursing care goals, e.g. techniques to control aggression.
3. Teaching-learning principles are incorporated into the plan of care and the objectives for learning stated in behavioral terms, e.g. specification of content for learner's level, reinforcement, readiness, etc.
4. Approaches are planned to provide for a therapeutic environment:
   - Physical environmental factors are used to influence the therapeutic environment, e.g. control of noise, control of temperature, etc.
   - Psychosocial measures are used to structure the environment for therapeutic ends, e.g. paternal participation in all phases of the maternity experience.
   - Group behaviors are used to structure interaction and influence the therepeutic environment, e.g. conformity, territorial rights, locomotion, etc.
5. Approaches are specified for orientation of the client/patient to:
   - New roles and relationships
   - Relevant heatlh (human and material) resources
   - Modifications in the plan of nursing care
   - Relationship of the modifications in the nursing care plan to the total care plan
6. The plan includes the utilization of available and appropriate resources:
   - Human resources—other health professionals
   - Material resources
   - Community
7. The plan is an ordered sequence of proposed nursing actions.
8. Nursing approaches are planned on the basis of current knowledge.

## STANDARD VIII

Nursing actions provide for client/patient participation in health promotion, maintenance and restoration.

**Rationale:** The client/patient and family are provided the opportunity to participate in the nursing care. Such provision is made based upon theoretical and experiential evidence that participation of client/patient and family may foster growth.

### Assessment factors

1. The client/patient and family are kept informed about:
   - Current health status
   - Changes in health status
   - Total health care plan
   - Nursing care plan
   - Roles of health care personnel
   - Health care resources
2. The client/patient and family are provided with the information needed to make decisions and choices about:
   - Promoting, maintaining and restoring health
   - Seeking and utilizing appropriate health care personnel
   - Maintaining and using health care resources

## STANDARD IX

Maternal and child health nursing practice provides for the use and coordination of all services that assist individuals to prepare for responsible sexual roles.

**Rationale:** People are prepared for sexual roles through a process of socialization that takes place from birth to adulthood. This process of socialization, to a large extent, is carried out within the family structure. Social control over child care increases in importance as humans become increasingly dependent on the culture rather than upon the family unit.

The culture of any society is maintained by the transmission of its specific values, attitudes and behaviors from generation to generation. Attitudes and values concerning male and female roles develop as part of the socialization process. Attitudes toward self, the opposite sex and parents will influence the roles each individual assumes in adulthood and the responsibilities accepted.

### Assessment factors

Therefore in practice, the Maternal and Child Health Nurse:

1. Utilizes resources available in the social and behavioral sciences to help her understand the attitudes and values of individuals and families with whom she is working.
2. Utilizes opportunities available to her to promote those attitudes and values conducive to emotional and physical health and family solidarity, without imposing her own value system.
3. Encourages society to provide the resources needed to help people prepare for responsible sexual roles.
4. Interprets to other health personnel the needs of individuals and families as she sees them and attempts to understand the needs as seen by other health personnel.
5. Works with other health personnel to develop services which promote optimal health and family solidarity.

### STANDARD X

Nursing actions assist the client/patient to maximize his health capabilities.

**Rationale:** Nursing actions are designed to promote, maintain and restore health. A knowledge and understanding of the principles and normal ranges in human growth, development and behavior are essential to Maternal and Child Health Nursing Practice.

### Assessment factors

1. Nursing actions:
   • Are consistent with the plan of care.
   • Are based on scientific principles.
   • Are individualized to the specific situation.

• Are used to provide a safe and therapeutic environment.
   • Employ teaching-learning opportunities for the client/patient.
   • Include utilization of appropriate resources.
2. Nursing actions are directed to the physical, psychological and social behavior associated with:
   • Ingestion of food, fluid and nutrients
   • Elimination of body wastes
   • Locomotion, exercise
   • Temperature and other regulatory mechanisms
   • Self-fulfillment
   • Relating to others

### STANDARD XI

The client's/patient's progress or lack of progress toward goal achievement is determined by the client/patient and the nurse.

**Rationale:** The quality of nursing care depends upon comprehensive and intelligent determination of the impact of nursing upon the health status of the client/patient. The client/patient is an essential part of this determination.

### Assessment factors

1. Current data about the client/patient are used to measure his progress toward goal achievement.
2. Nursing actions are analyzed for their effectiveness in goal achievement of the client/patient.
3. The client/patient evaluates nursing actions and goal achievement.
4. Provision is made for nursing follow-up of particular clients/patients to determine the long-term effects of nursing care.

### STANDARD XII

The client's/patient's progress or lack of progress toward goal achievement directs reassessment, reordering of priorities, new goal setting and revision of the plan of nursing care.

**Rationale:** The nursing process remains the same, but the input of new information may dictate new or revised approaches.

### Assessment factors

1. Reassessment is directed by goal achievement or lack of goal achievement.
2. New priorities and goals are determined and additional nursing approaches are prescribed appropriately.

3. New nursing actions are accurately and appropriately initiated.

## STANDARD XIII

Maternal and child health nursing practice evidences active participation with others in evaluating the availability, accessibility and acceptability of services for parents and children and cooperating and/or taking leadership in extending and developing needed services in the community.

**Rationale:** Knowledge of services presently offered parents and children is the first step in determining the effectiveness of health care to all in the community. When it is recognized that needed services are not available, accessible or acceptable, the nurse takes leadership in working with consumers, other health disciplines, the community and governmental agencies in extending and/or developing these services. Services must be continually evaluated, expanded and changed if they are to improve the health and well-being of all parents and children within our society.

## Assessment factors

Therefore in practice, the Maternal and Child Health Nurse:

1. Applies and shares the cultural and socioeconomic concepts which help her understand the differences in the unique needs of individuals and families.
2. Recognizes the need for available health services for all parents and children in the community.
3. Utilizes the services and resources presently available.
4. Works with consumers, nurse colleagues, other health disciplines, the community and governmental agencies in evaluating the availability, accessibility and acceptability of services to all parents and children in the community.
5. Participates actively with significant others in initiating changes in the delivery of health services and/or developing new services to enable each individual in the family to function at his optimum capacity and to enhance family unity.

In order to assist the reader in making application of the model for the nursing process, the framework of child competencies, the problem-oriented record, and audit of the nursing record, case studies are presented in each unit of this text. The reader is provided guidelines for evaluation of each case according to the following factors (see Case Audit Guide, p. 896 of the Appendix):

1. The application of the framework of child competencies.
2. Achievement of the components of the nursing process, or those actions represented in the nursing process model.
3. Adequacy of the use of the problem oriented record.
4. The nursing care standards which are appropriate to determine the quality of care.

## STUDY QUESTIONS

1. What are the major laws affecting your local community that specifically protect the health and welfare of children?
2. Describe the features of at least one major agency or program in your community that offers comprehensive health care for children and families. Compare these features with the ideas presented in this chapter.
3. Prepare a statement of your personal definition of health. If necessary, give specific examples of instances that for you would constitute a major health problem, illness, minor illness, reasonable health, and optimal health. Discuss and compare ideas with classmates. Identify, if possible, social and cultural norms that influence your definition of health.
4. List the steps the nurse may take to demonstrate professional competency. Give the means by which you as a professional nurse may take these steps in your own state (e.g., what professional organizations are available to you, how can you go about joining them, what is the cost, the benefit?).
5. Describe in your own words the following concepts:
   a. The basic goal governing nursing care
   b. The processes of nursing care
   c. The nursing assessment
   d. Nursing intervention and management
   e. The conceptual framework for nursing care of the child.
6. Discuss the use of the problem-oriented record in the example presented at the conclusion of this unit. Does it present a comprehensive understanding of the family? What factors have been overlooked? Is the plan adequate? Is adequate follow-through indicated for the plan? Is there evidence that planning includes the family?
7. Practice your own listening skills by engaging in an interview or serious conversation with a friend or classmate. Carefully write down all the messages that you hear, and present the written ideas to the sender for validation. Discuss your misperceptions with him or her, and attempt to discover the source of misunderstanding.
8. Practice your visual observation skills by watching, with another student or friend, a specified event or oc-

casion (such as children on a playground or a group of people in a restaurant). As you watch, carefully record all that you see happening. Compare and discuss your observations.

9. Discuss the resolution of a conflict between a family's desires and health care goals and those of the nurse.

10. Using a case from your own clinical experience, evaluate your record according to the standards of nursing practice. Present a summary of the accomplishment of each standard and the factors you might need to improve as you continue to relate to the child and family.

## REFERENCES

1. American Nurses Association: Standards of maternal-child health nursing practice, Kansas City, Mo., 1973, The Association.

2. Ansley, B.: Patient-oriented recording; a better system for ambulatory settings, Nurs. '75, **5:**52, Aug. 1975.

3. Bates, B.: Nurse-physician dyad; collegial or competitive? In Three challenges to the nursing profession, selected papers from the 1972 American Nurses' Association Convention, 1972.

4. Bates, B.: Nursing in a health maintenance organization, Am. J. Public Health **62:**992, July, 1972.

5. Becker, M. H., Drachman, R. H., and Kirsch, J. P.: Predicting mothers' compliance with pediatric medical regimens, J. Pediatr. **81:**843, Oct., 1972.

6. Bonkowsky, M. L.: Adapting the POMR to community child health care, Nurs. Outlook **20:**515, Aug., 1972.

7. Brunetto, E., and Birk, P.: The primary care nurse; the generalist in a structured health care team, Am. J. Public Health **62:**785, June, 1972.

8. Bugelski, B. R.: The psychology of learning applied to teaching, ed. 2, New York, 1971, Bobbs-Merrill.

9. Caldwell, M.: The social biology of human beings. In Cooke, R. E., editor: The biological basis of pediatric practice, New York, 1968, McGraw-Hill Book Co.

10. Chabot, A.: Improved infant mortality rate in a population served by a comprehensive neighborhood health program, Pediatrics **47:**989, June, 1971.

11. Chappell, J. A., and Drogos, P. A.: Evaluation of infant health care by a nurse practitioner, Pediatrics **49:**871, June, 1972.

12. Child health care in the '70's. Proceedings of the Eastern Regional Workshop for Registered Nurses, Physicians, Educators on Pediatric Nurse Association Programs, June 14-15, 1971, New York, 1972, American Nurse Association.

13. Chioni, R. M., and Panicucci, C.: Tomorrow's nurse practitioners, Nurs. Outlook **18:**32-35, Feb., 1970.

14. Combs, A. W., Avila, D. L., and Purkey, W. W.: Helping relationships; basic concepts for the helping professions, Boston, 1971, Allyn & Bacon, Inc.

15. Cronbach, L. J.: Essentials of psychological testing, ed. 3, New York, 1970, Harper & Row, Publishers.

16. Crook, W. G.: Utilization of allied health workers; does it solve the basic problem? Letter to the editor, Pediatrics **49:**477, March, 1972.

17. Deloughery, G. L.: History and trends of professional nursing, ed. 8, St. Louis, 1977, The C. V. Mosby Co.

18. Doll, E. A.: Vineland Social Maturity Scales, Circle Pines, Minn. 1965, American Guidance Service, Inc.

19. Dugdale, A. E.: For best results, make and use your own growth charts, Clin. Pediatr. **11:**191, April, 1972.

20. Dunn, H.: High level wellness for man and society, Am. J. Public Health **49:**786, June, 1959.

21. Dunn, L. M.: Peabody Picture Vocabulary Test, Minneapolis, 1965, American Guidance Service, Inc.

22. Ford, B., and Berlinger, M.: Caring—a priority in pediatric nursing. In Duffey, M., and others, editors: Current concepts in clinical nursing, vol. 3, St. Louis, 1971, The C. V. Mosby Co., p. 128.

23. Ford, L. C.: The changing role of the nurse in well child care. In Duffey, M., and others, editors: Current concepts in clinical nursing, vol. 3, St. Louis, 1971, The C. V. Mosby Co., p. 128.

24. Gazda, G. M., Walters, R. P., and Childers, W. C.: Human relations development; a manual for health services, Boston, 1975, Allyn and Bacon.

25. Gordon, T.: Parent effectiveness training, New York, 1970, P. H. Wyden, Inc.

26. Grant, W. W.: The child plus the parent equal one patient; an important lesson, Clin. Pediatr. **11:**433, Aug., 1972.

27. Growth Charts: Medical World News. Dept. M., 1221 Avenue of the Americas, New York, N.Y. 10020.

28. Haggerty, R. J.: Do we really need more pediatricians? Pediatrics **50:**681, Nov., 1972.

29. Hughes, J. G.: Synopsis of pediatrics, ed. 4, St. Louis, 1975, The C. V. Mosby Co.

30. Hunt, J. H.: Prospects of national health insurance, Nurs. Admin. **1:**20-25, March-April, 1971.

31. Hussar, D. A.: Drug interactions—good and bad, Nurs. '76 **6:**61, Sept., 1976.

32. Jelinek, R. C., and others: A methodology for monitoring quality of nursing care, DHEW Publication No. (HRA) 76-25, U.S. Dept. of Health, Education and Welfare, Bethesda, Md., Jan. 1974, DHEW.

33. Kaplan, R. S., Lave, L. B., and Leinhardt, S.: The efficacy of a comprehensive health care project; an empirical analysis, Am. J. Public Health **62:**931, July, 1972.

34. King, I. M.: Toward a theory for nursing; general concepts of human behavior, New York, 1971, John Wiley & Sons, Inc.

35. Kramer, M.: The consumer's influence on health care, Nurs. Outlook **20:**574-578, Sept., 1972.

36. Lehmann, J.: Auscultation of heart sounds, Am. J. Nurs. **72:**1242, July, 1972.

37. Littman, D.: Stethoscopes and auscultation, Am. J. Nurs. **72:**1239, July, 1972.

38. Lysaught, J. P.: An abstract for action, New York, 1971, McGraw-Hall Book Co.

39. Lysaught, J. P.: From abstract into action; progress report from the National Commission on Nursing and Nursing Education, Nurs. Outlook **20:**173-179, March, 1972.

40. Mauksch, I. G., and David, M. L.: Prescription for survival, Am. J. Nurs. **72:**2189, Dec., 1972.

41. McCandless, B. R.: Adolescents; behavior and development, Hinsdale, Ill., 1970, The Dryden Press, Inc.

42. Murray, R., and Zentner, J.: Guidelines for more effective health teaching, Nurs. '76, **6:**44, Feb., 1976.

43. Nader, P. R., Emmel, A., and Charney, E.: School health service; a new model, Pediatrics **49:**805, June, 1972.

44. Owen, G. M.: The assessment and recording of measurements of growth of children; report of a small conference, Pediatrics **51:**461, March, 1973.

45. Parker, K., and Knitzer, J.: Day care and preschool services; trends and issues, Atlanta, Ga., 1972, Avater Press.

46. Payne, P. A.: Day care and its impact on parenting, Nurs. Clin. North Am. **12:**525, Sept., 1977.

47. Piaget, J.: The language and the thought of the child, New York, 1965, The World Publishing Co.

48. Plein, J. B.: Drug dosing for pediatric patients, Nurse Practitioner **2:**35, Sept.-Oct., 1977.

49. Pochedly, C., and Ente, G.: Adverse hematologic effects of drugs, Pediatr. Clin. North Am. **19:**1065, Nov., 1972.

50. Pryor, H. B., and Thelander, H. E.: Growth comparisons of urban and rural children in southern Mexico with randomly selected California children, Clin. Pediatr. **11:**411, July, 1972.

51. Pulaski, M. A.: Understanding Piaget—an introduction to children's cognitive development, New York, 1971, Harper & Row, Publishers.

52. Reik, T.: Listening with the third ear, New York, 1948, Grove Press.

53. Ridge, J. L.: Legal implications of rendering health care to the community, Clin. Proc. Child. Hosp. **27:**52, Jan., 1971.

54. Roach, L. B.: Color changes in dark skins, Nurs. '72 **2:**19, Nov., 1972.

55. Roemer, M. I.: Rural health care, St. Louis, 1976, The C. V. Mosby Co.

56. Schell, P. L., and Campbell, A. T.: POMR—not just another way to chart, Nurs. Outlook **20:**510-514, Aug., 1972.

57. Schlotfeldt, R. M.: Nursing is health care, Nurs. Outlook **20:**245-246, April, 1972.

58. Schumaker, C. J.: Change in health sponsorship. II. Cohesiveness, compactness and family constellation of medical care patterns, Am. J. Public Health **62:**931, July, 1972.

59. Scott, W. F.: Some aspects of the pediatric nurse associate having legal implications. In Child health care in the '70's. Proceedings of the Eastern Regional Workshop for Registered Nurses, Physicians and Educators on Pediatric Nurse Associate Programs, June 14-15, 1971, Boston, New York, 1972, American Nurses' Association.

60. Shirkey, H. C.: Dosage (posology). In Shirkey, H. C., editor: Pediatric therapy, ed. 5, St. Louis, 1975, The C. V. Mosby Co. p. 19.

61. Siegel, E.: Child care and child development in Thailand, Sweden, and Israel—their relevance for the United States, Am. J. Public Health **63:**396, May, 1973.

62. Starfield, B., and Scheff, D.: Effectiveness of pediatric care; the relationship between processes and outcome, Pediatrics **49:**547-552, April, 1972.

63. Thoma, D., and Pittman, K.: Evaluation of problem-oriented nursing notes, Nurs. Admin. **2:**50, May-June, 1972.

64. Traver, G. A.: Assessment of thorax and lungs, Am. J. Nurs. **73:**466, March, 1973.

65. Tucker, S. M. and others: Patient care standards, St. Louis, 1975, The C. V. Mosby Co.

66. Turner, I. R.: Free health centers; a new concept? Am. J. Public Health **62:**1348, Oct., 1972.

67. Vaughan-Wrobel, B., and Henderson, B.: The problem-oriented system in nursing; a workbook, St. Louis, 1976, The C. V. Mosby Co.

68. Wallace, H. M., and Goldstein, H.: Child health care in the United States, Pediatrics **55:**176, Feb., 1975.

69. Walsh, M. E.: On nursing's role in health care delivery, Nurs. Outlook **20:**592-593, Sept., 1972.

70. Weaver, J. L.: National health policy and the underserved; ethnic minorities, women, and the elderly, St. Louis, 1976, The C. V. Mosby Co.

71. Weed, L. L.: Medical records, medical education, and patient care, Cleveland, 1970, Press of Case Western Reserve University.

72. Williams, C. D., and Jelliffe, D. B.: Mother and child health; delivering the services, New York, 1972, Oxford University Press.

73. Williams, J. K.: The pediatric nurse in the past hundred years, Clin. Proc. Child. Hosp. Jan. 1971.

74. Wilson, L. M.: "Listening" in behavior concepts and nursing intervention, coordinated by C. E. Carlson, Philadelphia, 1970, J. B. Lippincott Co.

75. Wing, K. R.: The Law and the public's health, St. Louis, 1976, The C. V. Mosby Co.

76. Yaffe, S. J.: Drug interactions, I. Pediatrics **49:**452, March, 1972.

77. Zahourek, R., Leone, D. M., and Lang, F.: Creative health services; a model for group nursing practice, St. Louis, 1976, The C. V. Mosby Co.

# CHAPTER **3**

# Understanding family and society

The basic social unit of most societies, the family, has provided focus for inquiry and study for individuals and disciplines over several decades. Most people grow up and develop within a family, and they remain in contact with this unit of society more consistently throughout life than with any other segment of society. Because the family provides the setting for development during the early years of life, it provides a most important influence on personality, behavior, and subsequently upon group characteristics.

Because family and society have undergone many intense, dramatic, and rapid changes in recent decades, much speculation has arisen regarding the role of the family in the future. Some have predicted its total demise; others have stated that the functions of the family will change from those of socialization, placement or status, and reproduction to providing security, affection, and guidance. The premise upon which this text is based, however, is that the family unit is growing in significance and function. Changes that have been documented in recent years represent neither the demise of the family unit nor a change in essence, but rather the flexibility and adaptation of the family to the demands of an increasingly complex society. The family unit is one that maintains the stability of a society in a way that no other established social unit can. Stability does not demand inflexibility or rigidity. Although these may be features of an individual family, the family demonstrates far more flexibility than most other social units and yet provides the most predominant source of security available to its members.

The family exists within the framework of society, culture, and environment. As such it generates the multiple factors that influence development of the child, and it becomes a significant concern for the nurse who works with children.

## CULTURE AND ENVIRONMENT

Human environment shapes human culture, and in turn the culture influences the environment. Each element of a child's experience is important to the child in gaining an understanding of who he or she is as a human being.

### The meaning of culture

Culture may be conceptualized as the generalized patterns of behavior that a group of people evolve in carrying out the essential tasks of daily living. Although these generalizations may be described and are useful in understanding a social group, they often assume an aura of artificiality. When any generalization is applied to an individual within a culture, we find that many of the traits either do not apply or to some degree misrepresent the reality of the situation. The descriptions do, however, provide an understanding of influencing traits, and they form a basis for understanding the way in which people behave in society. For example, many cultures do not sanction pregnancy out of wedlock but provide for some resolution of the problem when it does occur. The fact that such a pregnancy occurs may not be typical of the cultural pattern, but cultural patterns influence the individual and group reaction to the unusual event. In other instances, the woman may choose to bear a child as a single woman without regard for the prevailing cultural norm.*

Anthropology, which provides for formal study of cultures, has generated comparisons among many of the world's cultures that provide valuable insight into human nature. Developmental and behavioral traits of children that appear universally are said to be basic, fundamental human features. On the other hand, when behavioral responses to certain similar events are noted to vary among cultures, it is believed that these traits are shaped and determined by the culture. Margaret Mead,[57] in her significant studies, noted that adolescence in many societies generates upheaval and disequilibrium, but for some groups there are very different or virtually no behavioral responses to the physical changes of puberty. It is believed, then, that the physical changes of puberty are not actually the cause of the behavioral response seen in Western cultures, but rather in some way the culture shapes and causes the response.

### Effect of culture on growth and development

The growing child is subject to the influences of culture from the moment of conception. The culture of the parents affects the child's nutritional heritage, and it continues to dictate the kinds and quality of food that is eaten. The practices of childbirth that each culture adopts influence the stress or lack of stress that is experienced at birth. From the moment of birth the child experiences the pattern of child-rearing that is sanctioned by the culture and is not exposed to patterns that are foreign to that of the family's culture. The child learns the language of the family, which provides the means by which to think consciously and form the concepts that are common to others in the society. Children learn the abstractions that are possible through the use of language. They assume traits that are encouraged for survival and success in the social milieu. Behaviors are assumed that are appropriate for each stage of development as defined within the culture. Clothing is defined by the culture, and health habits defined by the culture are adopted by the child throughout the process of growth and development.

On the other hand, it is recognized that there is an important interaction between the child and the culture. Although people are shaped by the culture, it is also people who create it. The child inherits the possibility for the entire range of human behavior. Behaviors that are most commonly adopted are those that are sanctioned by the culture.

However, through the growing years all children exhibit behaviors that are either ignored or are disapproved, and they tend not to be repeated. When such behaviors persist, the child is either thought of as possessing a "disorder" or is considered highly gifted and unusually talented. Some relatively minor deviations, such as those that are ignored as unimportant, often give rise to changes that are seen to develop through the years. Changes in behavioral patterns often occur from necessity and demands of the environment or circumstances in the world. At such a time persons who have maintained the ability to behave in slightly different ways and in ways that particularly suit the demands of the moment become shapers of a new cultural trait.

An individual's "native responses," or the particular inborn preferences to behave in a certain manner, may be congruent with the culture or in conflict with it. Different cultures seem to tolerate varying degrees of deviancy from the typical pattern, and the greater complexity of modern, technologic cultures has fostered the growth of widely varying individual behavior.[18]

Within a nation as large as the United States, with individuals from many different ethnic and social backgrounds, there is significant variation. Subgroups or subcultures exist that can be clearly identified and described. In reaction to the growing necessity to live and work harmoniously together in an increasingly crowded

---

*References 3, 12, 32, 33, 45, 59, 62.

world, there has been a tendency for people to lose their cultural identity. People are encouraged to use the standard English language to foster the ability to speak with all persons and to communicate more effectively in the American academic and business worlds. However, the loss of ethnic identity that is suffered by individuals in this process is keenly felt, and many groups seek actively to resist or to resolve the conflict of living "between" two different cultures in a way that allows them to be successful in one and not lose the identity of the other. The American Indian family in particular is caught in this difficult struggle. The demands of living and surviving in Anglo societies require that American Indians adopt ways of behaving and acting that are in significant disharmony with the culture of their people, but the Indian culture often does not provide a means of sustenance.[9,53]

### Helping different cultural groups

Nurses at some point come in contact with people and families who are in some manner culturally different from themselves. Some work exclusively with culturally different groups. Poverty, which touches all ethnic groups, entails cultural elements that are particularly strange and foreign to most nurses. People of different cultural groups are much more likely to be misunderstood than understood. We all bring expectations to a relationship that color the interpretations and assumptions that we make of other people. Even when working with people of our own cultural groups, we tend to view them as possessing all the value traits typical of our culture. Middle-class children are expected to be goal-oriented and striving, but in reality they may have no desire to strive toward a particular goal.[20,27,61]

The two most predominant problems that arise between people of different cultures are those of communication and value differences. These two factors are intimately intertwined and interdependent, but they will be considered separately for purposes of discussion.

**Spoken communication.** Spoken language, which is a primary tool of communication, is often taken for granted. The language most easily used by people is that with which they have grown up and integrated into their thought and feeling patterns. The individual who attempts to help another person usually assumes that the words spoken are understood, that the listener

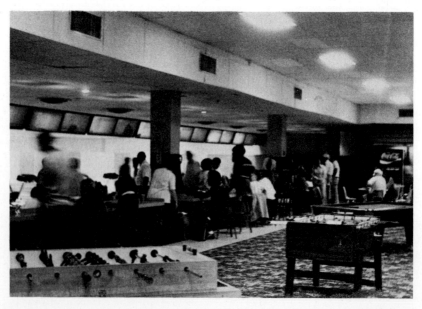

**Fig. 3-1.** Clothing, behavior, and social activities are defined by the culture of the family.

perceives the situation in the same manner as the helper does, that the person wants to solve the problem or receive the help being offered, and that the person has the resources to mobilize himself or herself and seek the goals outlined. These assumptions may be false in the best situation, but when two persons of different cultural backgrounds are trying to work together, there are frequent misunderstandings that may not be recognized.

The language used by persons of lower socioeconomic groups, regardless of ethnic background, is particularly puzzling to the middle-class professional person. The English of ghetto or rural America often appears limited, strange, or underdeveloped because of apparent grammatical errors and misuse of words. Rather than being incorrect, such forms of language have been described as full, but nonstandard, English. The meanings that are conveyed by the very consistent well-ordered but different grammatical rules are often not possible to duplicate through standard English. For example, speakers of the nonstandard American black dialect can make a distinction between a momentary action and one that is continuous or habitual. "She busy" or "He workin" conveys the fact that a person, at this point in time, is busy or is working. "She be busy" or "He be workin" conveys the fact that the person is habitually busy or working.[83] Even though the same basic language is being used, transformation or translation of exact meanings from one form of the language to another is most often impossible or too difficult to accomplish in ordinary conversation. The nurse who is highly sensitive to the messages of a child or family can overcome the differences between language forms and will find that it is possible to adopt the language form of the family with little difficulty once the meanings of the dialect are understood. The rewards for this effort in the form of mutual respect and successful communication are well worth the effort.

**Nonverbal communication.** Another primary means of communication is that of nonverbal communication, or the transmission of signals and meanings between people without the use of verbal language. Nonverbal communication includes such behaviors as vocal sounds that do not carry speech meanings, such as grunts, laughs, or cries; body movements and gestures; signals conveyed in distancing established between people; and touch. Behaviors associated with each of these means of communications acquire meanings that are specific to the culture or subculture and that members of a culture use to convey signals one to another. Without awareness, people within a culture acquire understanding of these signals and rely upon these signals to round out, or complete, the verbal language messages that are used.

Verbal sounds that do not carry speech meanings, or paralanguage, include the vocal sounds of grunts, laughs, and cries, as well as the tonal quality of the sounds and inflections. The use of such sounds is determined by the culture, and their specific meaning needs to be understood by the nurse. In some subcultures, cries of alarm may be appropriately used by adults and children alike and by both sexes; in other subcultures, such expressions are restricted to

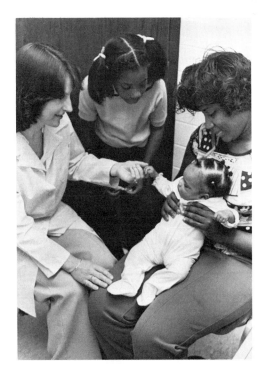

**Fig. 3-2.** The individuals in this interaction are conveying nonverbal messages by their body positions, eye contact, facial expressions, and touch.

specified situations or their use is restricted to persons of a certain age or sex. Tonal inflections and qualities convey affective messages such as the certainty with which a person speaks or messages of hostility or affection. In most cultures a high-pitched tone of voice carries an affectionate message, regardless of the word message that is spoken.[10,13,78,80]

Body motions include hand gestures, facial expression, eye movement, and posture. Body movements tend to increase in frequency and intensity when the emotion that is felt increases in intensity. The culture develops certain specific gestures to convey specific meanings, as well as body postures that are appropriate for specific situations. Generally, when people are attentive to one another, there is an increase in eye-to-eye contact and body posture tends to be open and leaning in the direction of each person involved.[6,24]

Signals conveyed in distancing between people, or proxemics, involve the culturally defined and socially acceptable distance that is automatically established when two or more people interact. The concept of proxemics is based upon the assumption that all people have a nonphysical boundary or territory that is not supposed to be invaded except when there is an emotional feeling of intimacy between the two or more people interacting. The amount of space tolerated by people before intrusion is felt is defined by the culture; some cultural groups expect spatial closeness in interactions with health care providers; others expect spatial distance. In any event the client will interpret the spatial behavior according to their own cultural definitions, the this behavior makes a significant contribution to the communication process.[29,30]

Touch is one of the most powerful tools of communication and as such is of primary importance in the interaction between people who are emotionally intimate with one another. Montague[60] has described the effect of tactile experience upon human development. The quality and quantity of touch experiences is universally important for the healthy growth and development of the child; however the specific messages that the child learns to convey through certain types of touch are highly specific to the culture. In some cultures, touch of any sort is relatively forbidden between people of any age, except in specific situations and between people of certain defined relationships. In other cultures, touch is a relatively frequent occurrence and is observed between all people who interact, but the kinds of touch used is still governed by the touch behaviors that convey the messages acceptable to the cultural group. For example, if a handshake is used for greeting another person, its use may be restricted to persons of a specific sex or age group. Further, the nature of the handshake conveys feelings of relative warmth or friendliness or other feelings such as passivity or power. The length of time for which the parties continue to grasp their hands in a handshake may convey intense feelings of warm emotion or a power struggle. The difference in meaning is known to each of the parties involved because of the nature of their relationship, and the cultural significance of the touch experience.[25,44]

Touching another person involves tactile experiences and perceptions that are rooted in early intimate life experiences and that are prone to carry intense emotional meanings, often associated with dependency. A willingness or desire for dependency or passivity can be expressed through touch, as by the person who shakes hands in a passive manner or who allows another person to lead him or her to another room in spite of verbal protest. The specific meanings of all touch interactions are highly dependent upon the culture and the nature of the relationship between the people who are interacting. Through an understanding of the subculture definition of such specific meanings, the nurse can use touch as a powerful means of communicating in a manner acceptable to the client group served.

### Values

When we communicate, we send both the content message of the words being spoken and the message of who we are and what we believe. Thus values are pervasive in all that we do as human beings. Values are important for the survival of a culture or a group of people as an intact group. They give a focus, or an orientation, for human beings and their relationships to the world and other people, to health and illness, to what is desirable and undesirable. Sanchez[74] describes the differences between middle-class American value systems and those of Spanish-surnamed people, which tend to be representative of those groups who are disadvantaged economically. These will be discussed briefly to illustrate possible conflicts that can occur when opposing values are encountered, but it should be remembered that judgments about individuals within either culture cannot be drawn from these general statements.

In terms of interpersonal relationships, the middle-class American orientation tends to be toward individualism. The purposes of the individual take precedence over those of the group. Some subcultures of America tend to stress the group, either vertically, where group hierarchy and authority are stressed, or horizontally, where each member of the group by definition supports purposes of the entire group. The situation defines which type of group loyalty or group identity emerges.

Time orientation for middle-class America emphasizes what is new and future-bound over what is old or present-bound. Other groups stress the present, with little regard for the past or for the future. Thus there is little need to plan for the future or to take steps to ensure what tomorrow will bring.

In relation to nature the middle-class American tends to believe that people are able to control nature and that they can control their own fate if they so desire. By contrast, some groups tend to feel helpless and weak in the face of nature, and no amount of struggle or desire will change what nature wills.

The contrast in orientation toward activity is related to the ideas about nature. The middle-class tendency is toward striving, achievement, and success as measured by outside standards. Other cultural groups tend to react to what the inner nature dictates at the moment and to respond spontaneously to present moods, feelings, desires, and impulses.

Finally, middle-class American groups tend to view people as human but perfectible. If they try hard enough, people can become the perfect individuals that were intended. In contrast, other groups view people as both innately good and evil, that they will always remain a mixture of two dichotomous traits; the thought of changing this state of affairs is not conceptualized.

In reflecting over these differences, we can understand a few reasons for the mutual frustration that is experienced when health care workers seek to effect changes in behavior among poverty-stricken groups. Health care requires advanced planning, individual and group effort to change the way things are, a consistent effort toward an often ill-defined, far-removed goal which, when it finally arrives, may not be easily recognized. The goal of good health is not something you feel, taste, see, or touch. For many people it is merely the absence of disease. The fact that a long list of health practices will simply aid in avoiding disease in the long run is a difficult, if not impossible, notion to conceptualize. It is easy to recognize a bad toothache when it is hurting, but the idea of brushing your teeth every night just to avoid another bad toothache at some unknown point in the future may be impossible to incorporate from another orientation. An even more difficult concept for some groups of people is that of mental health, because this concept is often defined in an entirely different frame of reference. The conflict between a smaller culture, such as that of Mexican-Americans, and the dominant culture within which they exist subjects the members of the smaller group to a great amount of stress and vulnerability to mental anguish. Yet to take steps to alleviate this suffering in the future is often, for some people, incomprehensible.

The nurse does communicate values to the child and the family. The family, likewise, communicates indicators of their own values. Recognizing these messages and interpreting them accurately and finally accepting them and incorporating them into nursing care can be a significant step toward working successfully with people of different cultural groups. This understanding needs to be more than a superficial recognition of facts that can be gleaned from a group of people. There needs to be a certain degree of experiencing the life of the people with whom the nurse works and development of an appreciation for the way in which they live. When poverty or its consequences cannot be overcome, this becomes the framework of life.

Health care workers can allow and encourage parents and children to use the forms of language that are most comfortable for them. There may be a point when the use of standard English is desirable for success in the world of school and work, but in a health care relationship the use of nonstandard English is more appropriate in expressing the intimate needs and dilemmas of everyday life and health problems.

The expectations that the family holds for the health care relationship need to be understood. If the family expects health care workers to be authority figures and tell them what to do, some degree of authoritarian telling and directing is highly desirable. When this is accomplished in a manner that is kindly and in accordance with the desires of the family, the relationship is enhanced.

When a family has in some manner demonstrated that they wish to move toward integration with the dominant culture rather than the subculture, support and help toward this goal are appropriate. If there has not been such an expression, this lack of mobility should be recognized and accepted. Often a family wishes to improve their standard of health and living without movement away from the subculture. This distinction is extremely important, because false expectation for movement away from the culture can destroy desired efforts toward better health and living. Understanding why a family is not motivated toward a life that is better (by middle America's standards) may be difficult. When children suffer from malnutrition and disease, that suffering obviously needs relief, and the health care system exists to provide relief and care. But plans and goals for health care must remain appropriate to the resources and desires of the family.*

### The environment

For several centuries people have exerted some effort to improve health through environmental control. The germ theory of disease led to the recognition that isolation and confinement contribute to prevention of spread of disease. Impure water and food were identified as sources of illness, and means of controlling the quality of water and food products were devised. Guarantee of a minimal level of quality in composition of prepared foods, both in relation to actual content and control for contamination, has become a governmental concern in many countries.

Within recent decades environmental control has widened and become a major concern, since problems of pollution have reached life-threatening proportions. The monumental problems of waste disposal, which once only related to pest control and spread of disease, have now become problems of conservation of human life, because by-products that create air, water, and land pollution have threatened our very existence. Animal and vegetable food sources have been threatened, as well as the health of human beings. The problem is no longer confined to the large cities of the world, and the problems of one country affect many others around the world. While the primary source of control comes through group and social action, the health professions are intimately concerned with interpretation and documentation of the effects of environmental problems upon health. Characteristics of each community must be thoroughly known and understood by the nurse working within the community, and they should be documented particularly when an environmental trait becomes a factor in the life of children and families. Individual responsibility for control of environmental problems can have a significant effect when unified recognition and attack are implemented.

In addition to the effects of waste pollution of the earth, problems such as noise, overcrowding, and transportation hazards affect people in all parts of the world. Physical harm, as well as psychologic stress, grows with the increasing complexities of maintaining life in a technologically dependent society and preserving health within that environment.*

### THE FAMILY

To understand the total environment of the child, the family in which the child lives must be described and understood as accurately as possible. The behaviors that are visible to the

*References 17, 19, 35, 41, 42, 51, 68, 74, 77, 83.

*References 15, 16, 52, 56, 69, 75, 84.

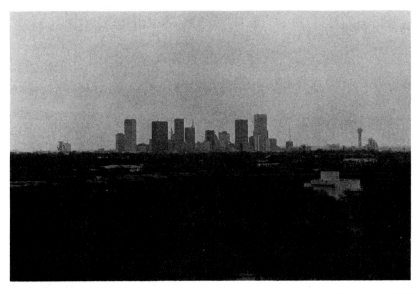

**Fig. 3-3.** Air pollution problems in large cities are related to respiratory illness and debilitation. Steps necessary to eliminate harmful deposits in the air are gradually being identified.

nurse may not be representative of what the child experiences in everyday life, but they should be carefully described and continually revised as more complete understanding evolves. Evaluative assumptions about traits must be carefully avoided. The goal is objective observations that represent as completely as possible the total.

The disciplines of anthropology, sociology, and psychology have sought in recent years to study the modern family in industrialized nations and extract an understanding of what is happening. The widely divergent points of view that have developed are beyond the scope of this text, but it is possible to predict that the patterns, structures, and functions of family life that will be observed by health care workers are increasingly complex and divergent. Experimentations in alternatives to the family for the purposes of child-rearing, such as the kibbutz in Israel, have demonstrated that successful child-rearing is not totally dependent upon the family as we have known it in the past. Indeed, many of the patterns of family living in America today may be startling and strange to the beginning health care worker.[37,38,43,63]

## Definition of family unit

The family has been defined at different times in history in different ways. In recent years, most traditional definitions of the family have become inadequate as people in society have become more flexible in the establishment of roles and relationships with one another, and as the traits and needs of society have changed. People in recent years have formed ties and affectional bonds without establishing legal relationships such as marriage or adoption, and the development of significance in one another's lives increasingly does not depend on such legal ties or genetic relationship. For the purposes of this text, the family is defined as any child or children and their consistent caretaker or caretakers and other persons who the child or caretaker identifies as significant to them. Usually this group of people resides together in the same household, although there are often people identified as significant who do not reside with the family. Also, not all persons residing in the same household are necessarily members of the family. People of genetic relationship are usually considered to be part of the family, but membership in the family does not depend

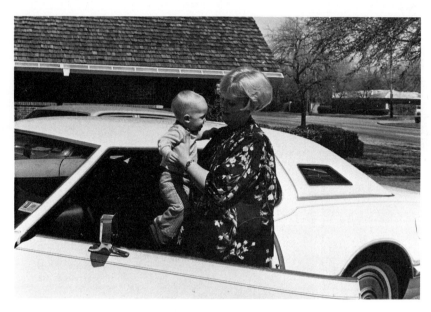

**Fig. 3-4.** This mother is utilizing the resources of a day-care center for child care in order to strengthen the family's economic resources and pursue individual career development.

upon genetic or legal ties. The major focus for the nurse who is working with a child is the identification of the primary caretakers, and all persons who provide a source of support for this primary relationship.

## Change in the idealized American family

The stereotypical American family is less predominant now than it once was in American society, but the stereotype continues to exert a significant influence on the expectations that people hold for normal family life. The stereotype consists of a white, middle-class married mother and father living together in a neat house in the suburbs with two or three children. The father earns sufficient income to provide the needs of the family as well as luxury purchases, trips, and vacations. The mother provides care for the home, emotional support for all members, and is active in community activities on a volunteer basis. The family is harmonious, spends work and playtime together sharing their mutual interests and goals, and together they work out the few problems that they encounter.[76]

In reality, less than half of the population in the United States live within such family units.[76] For example, by the mid-1970s there were an estimated 26 million children of wage-earning mothers, with eight million in female-headed households in the United States.[70] The many changes in society in recent years have created a significant impact on people, particularly women and children. The idealized emphasis on love, affection, and sexual intimacy between men and women who are married has produced a climate for unrealistic expectations for happiness and satisfaction, unmanageable sex-role expectations, and limited resources for coping with the stress of child-rearing.[47,70]

The impact on society of the mid-twentieth century wave of feminism and the general re-evaluation in society of what it means to be "human" have yielded unprecedented changes in the structure and function of the family. This movement has brought forth significant societal shifts of value, relation, and identity affecting people of all ages and economic levels. The role expectations that have been engrained as a part of the idealized family myth have been found to be inadequate for the small nuclear family,

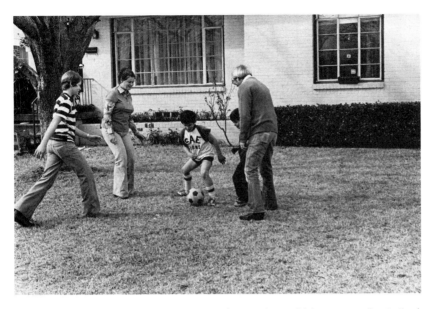

**Fig. 3-5.** Family group activities today center around recreation and leisure according to the family's economic resources. Such group activity predominates when children are young.

given the social and economic stress of existing independent of extended family support. There is increased awareness among women and men of the stifling effect of the traditional nuclear family unit on the mental health and personal development of the woman. The growing dissatisfaction of both women and men with the constraints of sex-role behaviors has led to a major trend toward androgenous parenting roles in which either the woman or the man can assume both provider and nurturing roles, with an emphasis on the personhood of the individual. In addition, parents are relying increasingly on individuals or groups outside the family, such as schools, day-care centers, and babysitters, to share the many dimensions of child-rearing. Increasingly, adults are selecting alternate life styles to the idealized American family and are either living alone, living within adult groups, or living with children in family forms that do not conform to the ideal myth. Probably the most prevalent style of living where children are involved is that of the single parent either living alone with biologic or adopted children either by choice or because of a marital separation or divorce. Many single parents share house-

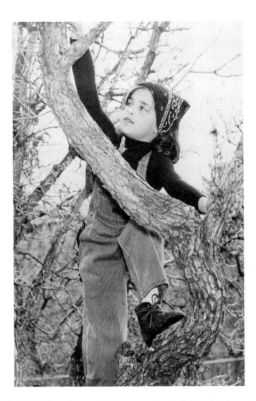

**Fig. 3-6.** The older child expresses individuality through independent choices of clothing and activities.

**63**

holds or in other ways share resources for child care.*

The American family has made a definitive shift away from the development of close family ties and the pursuit of group goals toward the pursuit of individual goals and purposes. Because the mother no longer must devote long hours and great energy on tasks of housekeeping and custodial care, she has become increasingly oriented toward personal fulfillment of her individual goals. Thus new ways of developing the family as a group have emerged and center more around recreation and leisure than around the acts of sustaining life and living. Individuation of all family members becomes increasingly apparent as financial resources and emotional maturity increase. While this trait has generated pessimistic predictions for the future of family life in America, it has been a necessary response to the demands of increasing technology and industrialization, and it may be an important factor in individuals developing the ability to survive in societies of the future.

Along with the goals of individuation, the nuclear family in America has become more isolated from in-laws and other relatives. Thus the extended family is relatively uncommon. Resources from members of the family who are older and more mature are often lacking in the young American family. This leads to an absence of the stresses and strains experienced when several generations try to coexist under one roof, but an increasing dependence upon social institutions other than the family during times of need or stress has also emerged. This factor in American life has been very significant for the health care of children. Young mothers increasingly depend upon physicians, nurses, social workers, and mass media for advice and direction in the rearing of children, a function that previously was filled by a grandmother or other older woman in the family. However, the existence of extended families continues in some form for most people, particularly during times of stress. Grandmother is often present when a new baby is born or when illness occurs.

One of the primary functions of the family

*References 1, 8, 11, 14, 22, 23, 34, 46, 47, 48, 55, 65, 66, 70, 73.

universally is the transfer of culture and socialization. In recent decades this function has occurred in a manner that is different and more conducive to cultural change than at any point in history, because the child and the parent tend to influence one another mutually. In the past the parent was the sole authority influencing, directing, teaching, and indoctrinating children in the family. Increasingly today, as young people have become better educated than their parents, the child and adolescent have assumed the roles of teacher and trend setter for the parents, and the resulting "gap" between generations has emerged. The structure and shaping of personality, behavior, and values, which formerly occurred for children within a family, have become less dictated and possibly ignored. The resulting upheaval, lack of identity, and alienation that occur during adolescence have been disturbing to society. As the educational achievement of the forthcoming generation of parents evolves to resemble more closely that of their offspring, the outcome for family life is yet to be observed.[58]

Ideally, roles of family members have been described and proclaimed through the culture. The biologic functions of bearing children remain constant, but little else has continued to be a consistent trait of role function for mother, father, or children. While confusion, conflict, and stress have arisen out of role uncertainties and changes, individuals and families have increasingly learned to live with and accept a wider range of possibilities for life style than was previously possible. The outcomes for children, when analyzed under existing cultural orientations and theories, may be significant. Masculinity and femininity have begun to represent highly individualistic traits, with the dichotomies that were formerly perpetuated merging into a more singular notion of individual humanness.[5,70] The man of the family is no longer the exclusive breadwinner, and as a result the ability to provide for his family can no longer be considered a sign of masculinity. Finding an identity and appropriate role function within the emerging system is increasingly complex and difficult.

The changes and challenges in the modern family emphasize growing demands and stresses placed upon the family unit. Many apparent signals of destruction and demise of the family may in fact be useful responses facilitating survival in the world of the future. The basic human needs of children may be successfully met through other societal sources, and it appears that a combination of family and society is emerging to fill functions formerly exclusively that of families. But the family, which remains the most constant element offering security, continues to be a most important influence upon the child.[2,4,7,66]

## Family assessment

To make accurate judgments regarding a child's health and to provide adequate health care, the nurse must obtain an accurate assessment and understanding of the child's family within the context of the cultural group. The family assessment may be obtained in any setting, but the accuracy and detail of the assessment is greatly enhanced if all or a portion of the assessment is conducted in the home environment, and if all members of the identified family participate. Portions of the interview are conducted with the adult member or members only present or with only the child or children present.

A comprehensive family assessment includes the actual responses to the interview as well as behavioral observations and affective messages. If there is an observed incongruence between verbal responses and family behavior, the behaviors are described in detail. If the behaviors

**Table 3-1.** Stage-critical family developmental tasks through the family life cycle*

| Stage of the family life cycle | Positions in the family | Stage-critical family developmental tasks |
| --- | --- | --- |
| 1. Married couple | Wife<br>Husband | Establishing a mutually satisfying marriage<br>Adjusting to pregnancy and the promise of parenthood<br>Fitting into the kin network |
| 2. Childbearing | Wife-mother<br>Husband-father<br>Infant daughter or son or both | Having, adjusting to, and encouraging the development of infants<br>Establishing a satisfying home for both parents and infant(s) |
| 3. Preschool-age | Wife-mother<br>Husband-father<br>Daughter-sister<br>Son-brother | Adapting to the critical needs and interests of preschool children in stimulating, growth-promoting ways<br>Coping with energy depletion and lack of privacy as parents |
| 4. School-age | Wife-mother<br>Husband-father<br>Daughter-sister<br>Son-brother | Fitting into the community of school-age families in constructive ways<br>Encouraging children's educational achievement |
| 5. Teenage | Wife-mother<br>Husband-father<br>Daughter-sister<br>Son-brother | Balancing freedom with responsibility as teenagers mature and emancipate themselves<br>Establishing postparental interests and careers as growing parents |
| 6. Launching center | Wife-mother-grandmother<br>Husband-father-grandfather<br>Daughter-sister-aunt<br>Son-brother-uncle | Releasing young adults into work, military service, college, marriage, etc., with appropriate rituals and assistance<br>Maintaining a supportive home base |
| 7. Middle-aged parents | Wife-mother-grandmother<br>Husband-father-grandfather | Rebuilding the marriage relationship<br>Maintaining kin ties with older and younger generations |
| 8. Aging family members | Widow/widower<br>Wife-mother-grandmother<br>Husband-father-grandfather | Coping with bereavement and living alone<br>Closing the family home or adapting it to aging<br>Adjusting to retirement |

*From Duvall, E. M.: Marriage and family development, ed. 5, Philadelphia, 1977, J. B. Lippincott Co., p. 179. Reprinted with permission.

and verbal messages are congruent, this observation is described as supportive evidence of the nursing diagnosis. It is imperative that the nurse record and acknowledge the family's own perceptions and their own cultural frame of reference. Verbal statements or behaviors that are different from the nurse's own may tend to be overlooked or interpreted incorrectly from the nurse's frame of reference. All dimensions of the family's life and culture need to be recorded objectively, with the assessment reflecting the values of the family rather than those of the nurse.[39]

### Family development stages and tasks

From the comprehensive data of the family assessment, the nurse determines the family's stage of development and the ways in which the family is achieving fulfillment of the functions or tasks relative to their stage of development. Duvall[21] has presented a useful conceptualization of stages of family development and the related developmental tasks for the family. These are summarized in Table 3-1. These stages of development best suit a cohesive family unit; if the family lacks cohesiveness or has experienced major changes in membership, the assessment of the stage of development must be qualified in accord with the circumstances of the particular family. For example, if an identified family unit consists of two adults sharing a household, joining children from two formerly different families of different age groups, the new family comprises a complex family unit with at least two stages of development coexisting. Duvall's stages of development and a description of the assessment of the critical developmental tasks are as follows:

*Stage 1*. Married couple with children. In today's society legal marriage may not be the basis for the relationship, but the adults may still define themselves as a family unit. The critical family development tasks include establishment of a mutually satisfying adult relationship and fitting into a kinship network. When the adults make a decision to adopt or give birth to a child, the anticipation and adjustment to the promise of parenthood becomes a focus of family development and a primary health maintenance need.

*Stage 2*. Child-bearing family. For purposes of categorization, this stage is identified as a family with the oldest child under 30 months of age. A family may bear children after the oldest child reaches this age, but it is anticipated that previous experience in accomplishing the developmental tasks of this period will facilitate further development as each new child arrives. In a complex family unit, this may not be the case, and the family may need to accomplish these tasks with a new child's arrival, regardless of the age of the oldest child. The stage-critical tasks during the child-bearing phase include establishing a home milieu that is satisfying for the adults and the new child and adjusting to and encouraging the development of the child. This involves the establishment of the parental roles of providing for the child's physical health and the economic support for this provision, as well as assuming the nurturing interactions vital to the child's learning and thought, social, and inner development. In a family consisting of a single adult, external support systems for the provision of these needs must be identified and their adequacy assessed.

*Stage 3*. Family with preschool child. This stage is defined as a family with the oldest child between the ages of 2½ to 6 years of age. The primary tasks for the family in this stage of development include adaptation of the home environment and adult life styles to the critical needs and interests of preschool children and coping with the energy depletion and lack of privacy for the adult family members. The particular physical, learning and thought, social and inner development needs of the preschool child require specific home environment traits that promote stimulation and means of experience and exploration by the child. When the child spends portions of time in a day-care facility or in another home for partial care, the adequacy of that environment in relation to developmental needs must also be assessed.

*Stage 4*. Family with school children. This stage is defined as a family with the oldest child between the ages of 6 and 13 years. The primary tasks of family development are encouraging the children's educational achievement within the framework of their capacity and becoming involved in the community of school-age families in ways that augment the child's social development. Of particular importance in assessing the family's success during this stage of development is viewing social and educational goals in terms of the family's culture and their own defined goals. When the family belongs to a subculture and their primary orientation is to that subculture and yet the child must perform and fit into a larger predominant society, the conflicts experienced by the family between the two cultures must be assessed and taken into account in planning for health maintenance and intervention.

*Stage 5.* Family with teenager. This stage is defined as a family with the oldest child between the ages of 13 and 20 years. During this stage the family tasks center on balancing freedom with responsibility as the teenager matures and gains independence and separation from the family unit and the establishment of adult interests and careers less centered on the family unit. The degree of individuation established previously in family interactions will greatly influence the success of the family in accomplishment of these tasks, as will the family power structure and the use of shared power. Family communication patterns often change during this period of development as the adult members begin to communicate with the teenagers as adults rather than children.

*Stage 6.* Family as a launching center. This stage is defined from the time that the first child leaves the home environment to the time the last child leaves home. The primary tasks involve maintaining a supportive home base for the young adult member and releasing the young adult into his or her new living pattern with appropriate rituals and assistance.

*Stage 7.* Middle-aged parents. This stage is defined as the period of time between the departure of the last child until retirement. The primary tasks of this stage are the rebuilding of the adult relationships within the family and establishment of a means of maintaining kinship ties with older and younger generations of the family.

*Stage 8.* Aging family. This stage is defined as the period from retirement to the death of the adult members. The major tasks include adjustment to retirement, closing the family home or adapting to the needs of aging, and coping with bereavement and living alone without significant family ties.

In assessing the family, overlap between each of these stages will be evident. Further, the overlap between generations presents a complex situation for many families. The health care provider in child care is usually concerned primarily with assessment of the family of procreation or the identified family of the child and the primary adult caretakers. The adult member's family of orientation, or the family in which they were reared and the family system that consists of the child's grandparents, uncles, aunts and cousins, may be a significant component of the family system that needs to be assessed for a complete understanding of the child's family milieu. The interrelated family tasks originating from the family of procreation and the family of orientation need to be identified and the impact on the growth and development of the child and family assessed.

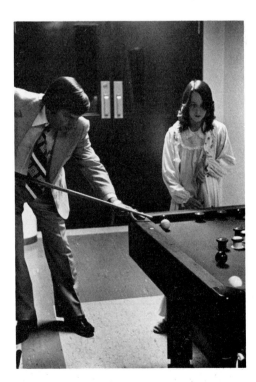

**Fig. 3-7.** Parent and child mutually participate in cultural and social pursuits. The father centers upon the child's hobby, and the child's personality, behavior, and values are gradually influenced.

### Members and interrelationships

The individuals comprising a family unit are important to the child. As discussed earlier, the individuals who comprise the family unit consist of the child or children residing in this household, the primary caretaker or caretakers, and all other persons who are identified as significant to the family unit.

Usually it is sufficient to identify those members of the family living within the same household, but another member, such as a grandparent or aunt, may be equally important if the child spends a significant amount of time with that relative or friend. Friends who are not related biologically or by marriage ties may, in reality, comprise part of a family unit. Young women may share households for the purposes of child-rearing when fathers and husbands are absent.[71]

The manner in which the individuals of a household relate to one another may be difficult to observe accurately, because the presence of a nonfamily member usually motivates a person's "best" behavior. While more accurate behavior begins to become visible as a relationship of trust develops between a health care worker and family, the child is often an indicator of the adequacy of interrelationships within the family life. Often, to the chagrin of adults, children reveal through words or actions the interpersonal traits of those around them. The behavior that is learned primarily by imitating and modeling the significant people in the child's life tells accurately the nature of interpersonal experience.

Traits that are particularly important to identify include the degree of dependency between the family members, the predominance of strife or harmony among members of the family, and characteristics of family life that produce cohesiveness among the group and that perpetuate its existence in the present form. Again, outside standards that are imposed upon visible observations create evaluative judgments. Although these need to be carefully avoided, characteristics of the family are crucial to understanding the child and must be explored.

Assessment data that reflects the interrelationships among family members includes a description of the identified family members and their own description of the nature of their relationship. A family pedigree, such as that presented on p. 80, gives a picture of the family members and the basic identifying information, as well as summary information regarding the nature of the interrelationships among members. The family's description of their household use of space, provisions for privacy, identification of sleep and living spaces for various members of the family gives an indication of the family's definitions of respect for individual time and space as well as an indication of sharing of space and intimacy within the family. A description of the tasks and roles that various family members fulfill in relation to other family members is indicative of dependency relationships, the degree of autonomy of family members, and the nature of the activities that are shared or not shared among members. A de-

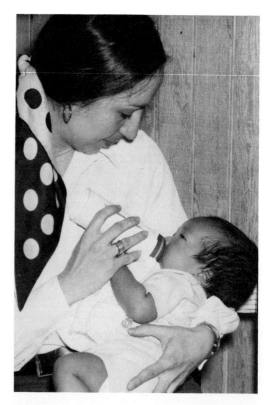

**Fig. 3-8.** A family may be composed of mother and child, or there may be several other members in addition. The relationship of the infant and mother is a primary one that is influenced by the total family constellation.

scription by each person within the family of what he or she feels is expected of him or her and a description of his or her expectations of others in the family is another indicator of the degree of dependency or autonomy existing among family members. The way in which decisions are made in the family and the family's means of solving problems is one of the most important sources of information related to power relationships and the use of power within the family.

Healthy family relationships consist of respect for individual members, adequate provision of the dependency and nurturing needs of the children, and shared use of power within the family, with the children participating in decision making but the adults in the family maintaining guidance and setting limits. There is a respect for the individuality of each family member, and adult members are actively involved in pursuit of their own interests and development. All family members are free and active in pursuit of individual goals.[54]

### Resources of the family

As families experience daily living, internal and external resources are essential for maintenance of the group as a unit. There must be some means of financial support and sustenance. Further, the family must have a sufficient degree of common sense about the management of money to exist within the limits of resources available to them. It is recognized that the amount of money that a family has to live on is not nearly as indicative of their success in "making ends meet" as is their ability to manage their money. Some families with very little income manage more adequately than families with a generous, regular income. How a family manages can be determined to some extent by the presence of loans and debts accrued in the course of meeting minimal living expenses. Stress on family living created by economic strife, growing out of either lack of adequate income or inadequate money management skill, is greatly underestimated. Families who could otherwise succeed satisfactorily for a long period of time often find the stresses of economic problems too great to sustain any number of other strengths that they may have.

Resources for assistance during times of stress or crisis are also important to a family. In addition to financial reserves or emergency loan sources, the family needs to have available resources for emotional support, help with household chores, and relief from child care when unusual circumstances occur. If such resources are known to be present, they are easily identifiable.

### Adult social history

The adult member or members of the family are vital influences on the physical, learning and thought, social and inner development of the child members of the family. Adults who themselves experienced a satisfying childhood and who had healthy attachments with adults during their own childhood are better able to provide for the nurturing needs of children. Further, adults must have satisfying dimensions of their own adult lives in order to provide for the needs of children. The memories and perception of adult members of their own child experiences, specifically the nature of discipline and punishment during childhood, and the nature of gratification and rewards given are important in determining the way in which they will behave with their children. Adults who experienced a loss before about the age of 15 years are at greater risk for developing personal and family interrelationship problems. If they indicate some means of dealing openly with their feelings and sense of loss throughout their years of development into adulthood, they may have developed a means of attaining and maintaining good mental health, which will positively affect this family unit. The adult relationships that exist within and outside of the family unit are important to the family. Healthy adults have mature reasons for forming adult attachments, such as mutually shared interests and goals in life, shared opinions and feelings toward life, and the dimensions of living that provide a sense of meaning for existence. There are active involvements with other adults outside of the family unit that provide for diversion, relate to professional or career goals, or give a sense of relationship and validation in the form of friendship. The adults are able to discuss openly their concerns for themselves and their children and can identify their own and one another's strong and weak points.

### Means of child-rearing

Although methods and prescriptions for child-rearing abound in Western society today, families seldom succeed in total adherence to a particular method. They may be able to relate details of the manner in which they would like to rear their children and to some degree succeed. But the task of everyday living with children is great, and the intellectual knowledge of a way to deal with a child is not sufficient to cope with the emotional reactions and interactions of everyday living. Children do not always respond as a particular "method" would have them, and in their own humanness react to the approaches of the parent just as the parents did during their childhood. Nevertheless, modes of mothering and fathering entail traits of discipline, affection, guidance, physical contact, modeling of behavior, teaching, verbal interaction, and provision of needs that can be described, independent of a specific child-rearing approach or developmental theory. These traits are believed to be particularly significant in the development of physical, learning and thought, social, and inner competencies.

Physical contact has been demonstrated to be a basic, essential component of successful child-rearing.[7,31,60] As children grow older, cultural inhibitions against tactile contact with other people often prohibit physical contact, but during infancy and early childhood it should be apparent that some significant person is providing a generous amount of physical contact.

Traits of discipline need to be identified in regard to at least three components that are independent of method. No two adults agree consistently on the way discipline is to be employed, and throughout life children experience differences of approach within the home and between home and other institutions of society. However, the child should be exposed consistently to some form of positive reinforcement. Discipline is often perceived as punishment, but self-control and discipline are accomplished through knowledge of what is acceptable and pleasing as well as through knowledge of what is not acceptable. The child's behavior patterns should reflect a sufficient proportion of acceptable behavior that is self-directed and indicative of some understanding of what is acceptable for the stage of development.

Punishment should be dealt as fairly as possible at the time of the undesired behavior, and it should be appropriate to the child's age and without physical harm. Total consistency in discipline, including punishment, is humanly impossible, but the child should have an adequate notion of which behaviors will incite adult members of the family to punishment and under what conditions the behavior is displeasing. These conditions for punishment provide the child with a sense of controlling impulses for unacceptable behavior.

Appropriate discipline for the stage of development of the child is necessary. There should be gradual lessening of parental restraint and control and guidance and a concomitant assumption of control by the child for his own behavior. Physical punishment, if used at all, should lessen as a child enters school. Positive reinforcement should remain an important part of interactions between adults and children throughout the development of the child.

### Life-style

As discussed in Chapter 1, life-styles greatly affect the development of the child. These involve many of the factors of interrelationships, resources of the family, and dominant means of child-rearing. Interests, hobbies, leisure activities, and things that the family share are important in healthy living. The way in which a family accomplishes daily living reflects highly individual styles of living, none of which are necessarily superior to another. The degree to which a family relies on other institutions for socialization is a life style trait that can be identified.

Young adults bring to a new relationship the styles of living from their own childhood, and no two are alike. A great deal of compromise and restructuring of daily living habits is required. Thus each child experiences home life that is different from all others. In-laws often express surprise or displeasure with the traits that a young couple evolve, which leads to uncertainty, stress, or some degree of alienation from the parents. But whether a family eats meals at an appointed hour or at varying times or whether they bathe in the morning or the evening has little to do with the success and health of the family. The family's life-style should reflect some component that satisfies the needs for affiliation of each individual member and that serves to promote the cohesiveness of the group as long as that cohesiveness is possible or desired. Basic health care needs and nutrition should be met, but the way in which they are executed fits into a total constellation of unique activities.[72]

## The family in crisis

A crisis for a family may be defined as any event that causes stress within the family group. Individual stress may or may not be present. For some families a normal developmental change, such as the oldest child leaving home for the first time, may precipitate a crisis for the group. Parenthood itself is seen as a crisis during the initial stage and at other crucial points during the parenting experience. Whether an event becomes a crisis for a family depends upon three conditions.

First, the nature of the event or situation itself may be so severe that similar conditions would constitute a crisis for any family. Poverty, with its accompanying constant stresses, is overwhelming for families with the best of resources. Death of a family member constitutes a major stress for families, as does disorganization through divorce or long absence of a parent who must earn a livelihood away from the family.

Second, resources of the family, including role structure, emotional maturity of adult members, and their previous experiences with stress, greatly influence how a given event affects the family. The arrival of the first or second child may constitute a crisis for a family, but after the arrival of several children and a greater maturity in coping with changes within the family, the arrival of a child may no longer be stressful.

Third, the definition that the family makes of the event and whether they perceive it as a threat to their status, goals, and objectives determine how stressful it will be. Some families define frequently occurring ordinary events as crises, while others seldom react with stress to

relatively common events. Minor illness may cause great stress for some families, while another family that experiences great physical hardship through major disability continues to function without stress.

Crisis events particularly affect the lives of children, because they are often innocent victims not equipped with the maturity and experiential resources to know how to cope adequately. During times of crisis, adults tend to concentrate attention on their children with extraordinary intensity, as if they can somehow find relief in their misery if their children are cared for and their future ensured. In the emotionally charged situation of stress parents often need but seldom receive help in adequately resolving the effects of unusual stress with minimal effect on the lives of their children.[50,54,64,79]

### Divorce and dissension

Divorce and marital dissension are stressors in the lives of many children in today's society. Among the Western nations the United States has the highest divorce rate. Furthermore, almost 70 percent of the divorcing couples have children under the age of 18 years, and almost one in seven children in the United States are children of divorce. This does not include the number of permanent separations or desertions, which are estimated to equal the number of legal divorces. About 85 percent of divorced persons eventually remarry, and of these 40 percent divorce again. An estimated 80 percent of third marriages end in divorce, yielding a significant number of children who have endured this trauma more than once.[1]

How severe this event becomes for the child and how lasting are the effects depend to a great extent on the three factors discussed in the previous section. The culmination of discord within the family in the actual divorce begins a long process of reorientation and restructuring of life for the children involved. Success depends on the resources, mental health of the parent with whom they reside, the age and developmental stage of each child, and other factors influencing the situation. Divorce itself cannot be condemned, because often this is the best alternative available to parents. The event may, in fact, bring relief after many months of conflict. The child's inner suffering, possible feelings of guilt over the situation, wishes and hopes for a happier family life, and the way in which the child works out these inner problems will significantly affect the course of his or her entire life. Seeking counsel and help for children during a time of family discord is virtually impossible for most parents, because their own suffering and humiliation over the inadequacies of the family immobilize action toward available help. Stress that produces intense reactions often precipitates illness and symptoms of illness that bring the family to health care workers when they might not seek help for mental anguish.[1,81]

### Poverty and economic stress

The dilemma of poverty has been with mankind throughout recorded history. In modern times the industrialization of society and the social reforms that made movement out of poverty possible have altered ways of socially dealing with problems created by poverty. Frequently overlooked, however, is the problem of the middle-class family with an adequate income that suffers unexpected financial burden or the family that is totally unequipped to manage financial resources available to them. Although these problems differ from those of the family suffering from poverty, the trap is just as ominous and overwhelming. Children in either instance suffer emotional stress created by the economic dilemma. They may suffer physical harm because of poor nutrition, inadequate clothing or heating, or inadequate health care during times of illness. To expect families to maintain themselves indefinitely under the stress of economic crises may be expecting too much.

### Illness and disability

When an illness or disability occurs for any member of the family, the children are significantly affected. The loss of ability to earn a living by an adult member throws the family into the additional stress of economic failure. Mental illness particularly affects the lives of children. It alters affectional ties, which they need from the adult member who becomes ill, and the children may suffer the social stigma that continues to plague the family suffering from mental illness. When a child within the family is stricken by mental or physical illness, the family experiences stress in a slightly different way, since children who are cared for adequately simply are not expected to be ill. An accident in which a child is seriously injured, the birth of a disabled child, or the onset of life-threatening illness produces a potentially severe crisis for parents who feel guilty and responsible for the suffering of their child.[26,49,53]

Helping families during times of stress often becomes a great challenge for the nurse. Having entered nursing to help people, the nurse responds with the desire to be helpful and to relieve suffering. Success is therefore defined by relief of the stressful situation. In reality this is often not possible. The nurse can provide one source of help and can open the way to community and health care resources, but the burden of relieving the plight of many families is impossible to bear. In many cases, as when helping a poverty-stricken family or when working with a family whose child is dying, the nurse must define goals in increments that are attainable and realistic and seek in some manner to offer what is within reasonable reach.

## Health maintenance problems and nursing intervention

Once the complete family assessment has been obtained, the nurse and the family determine the priorities of health maintenance needs and the extent to which the family is meeting or can meet these needs independently or which problems require nursing intervention. In the following section, examples of family health maintenance problems are discussed, including possible deviations from health that may exist. In addition, nursing approaches that can be used in relation to health maintenance and health deviation are discussed.

### Provision of safe home environment

Regardless of the developmental stage of the child, the family must provide for the child's physical safety. Safety includes arrangements of furnishings that allow for physical activity within the home without undue hazards, special protection from accidental injury such as falls from stairs or ingestion of nonfood substances, and provision of adequate supervision of activity. Deviations from a safe home environment range from the absence of such provisions to the presence of unusual hazards that endanger the child's safety. Health maintenance begins with adult attentiveness to the existence of possible hazards as well as knowledge of the child's developmental stage and the special hazards that exist for the child in relation to developmental stage. The nurse uses the assessment of the home environment and the adult perception of the child's developmental stage to determine the need for health maintenance and nursing intervention.

Nursing intervention primarily is focused on family teaching in regard to home environment safety, as well as teaching in regard to developmental safety needs of the child, with emphasis on anticipation of the coming year. Home environment safety teaching may involve home visits and assessment of changes in the home environment that the adult members have made to enhance home safety. The effectiveness of developmental teaching may be assessed in progressive interviews to determine changes toward increasing accuracy in the adult percep-

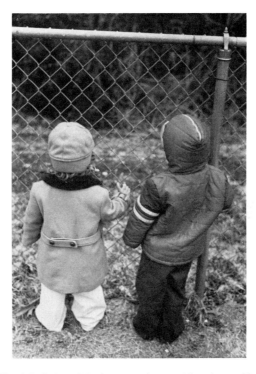

**Fig. 3-9.** Safety of the home environment is enhanced by devices that limit the child's range of mobility.

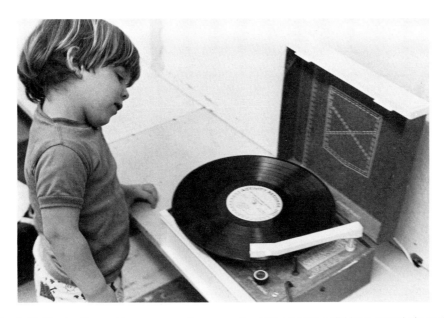

**Fig. 3-10.** The family provides a means of sensory stimulation for this child by a record player that the young child can operate independently.

tion of the child's developmental needs. Subsequent chapters of this text provide descriptions of each developmental stage and the implications of each stage for the safety of the child.

### Provision of home environment stimulation

The family provides stimulation for the child by its very existence; however the quality of stimulation that exists must be assessed in accord with developmental needs of the child. Appropriate sensory input in visual, auditory, kinesthetic, and tactile modes is necessary for the child's healthy development. Sufficient social interaction and freedom for imitation and play are the primary means of providing home environment stimulation. The type of social interaction and play experiences provided should be in accord with the developmental needs of the child.[66] For example, the preschool child needs ample opportunity to initiate social interaction and to engage in such play as make-believe and imitation with space and toy objects provided for such play. The assessment of space provisions for play within the home and of the toy and play objects provided is an important aspect of determining the adequacy of stimulation that the child experiences. The space and toy objects need not be elaborate or expensive in quality or quantity but should reflect adult understanding of the child's actual developmental needs and competencies. Deviations from health include absence of social interactions or insufficient social interactions observed between the child and adult, inappropriate social interactions for the child's developmental stage, absence of sufficient space or toy objects for play, and inappropriate space or toy objects for the child's stage of development.

Nursing intervention for this health maintenance problem is often focused on teaching of developmentally appropriate stimulation for each child in the family. Many adults do not realize the function that social interaction and play serve in promoting the child's development and do not know how to provide for these needs within the home. Selection of age-appropriate toys and play objects may be a particular problem for middle-class or affluent families who are eager for their children to achieve social and in-

tellectual success early in life. By contrast, families experiencing social or economic stress often do not provide sufficient adult social interaction for the children in the family. The specific needs of the family are planned and evaluated in accord with their particular needs.

### Development of parenting competency

Closely related to the provision of home environment stimulation is the problem of parenting competency. Parenting competency requires that the family's economic needs are met for food, shelter, and clothing, and that the nurturing needs are met in accord with the developmental stage of the children. Guidance and discipline, including positive reinforcement and a reward system, as well as the predominant style of communication and use of power within the family, are important dimensions of assessment in determining the need for development of

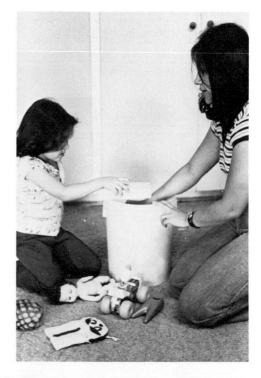

**Fig. 3-11.** Parenting competency includes the ability to provide guidance for the child in developing a sense of responsibility. Here mother participates with the child in picking up toys, thus providing social interaction as well as guidance.

parenting competency. Health deviations include inappropriate means of guidance and discipline, imbalance in the use of punishment and positive reward, and inadequate communications or use of power.

Nursing intervention includes teaching and counseling. If the adults in the family have an adequate knowledge of what is required for effective parenting but do not manage to put their knowledge into practice in the home, counseling is required to assist them in development of the needed abilities. The nurse and adult members of the family mutually define the nature of the parenting needs for development and set goals for attainment of specific parenting behaviors. Role playing of parenting situations that are evolving or that present difficulty for the adults can be effective in giving the parent experiences of the desired behavior, as well as provide the nurse the opportunity to reinforce achievement of the desired behavior. Such an approach also helps the nurse and the adults to explore alternate parent behaviors and project the possible effectiveness of each. Guidance in the use of shared power within the family while maintaining parental authority can also be accomplished through the use of role playing. Parent groups often provide an effective means of achieveing these counseling goals, since the benefit of sharing problems and alternate solutions can be of benefit.[28,40,48,54] Another important dimension of counseling in regard to parenting competency is exploring with the adult the memory and perception of their own experience in being parented as a child. Most adults tend to parent as they themselves were parented, in spite of the fact that they may cognitively desire to use a different approach. Working through the anxieties related to personal change and achievement of new behaviors is an important dimension in the achievement of behavioral change.[36]

### Developmental transition

A developmental transition within the family can be stimulated by a number of events, including developmental changes for any member of the family or changes in social or economic status. Such changes stimulate various responses on the part of the family and may be conceptualized as a normal crisis. The family response usually includes a period of relative disorganization and decreased function followed by a period of coping and integrating new behaviors, expectations, and interrelationships among members. When a developmental transition is anticipated because of a developmental change that is predicted for a family member or because of an anticipated social or economic change, assessment of the usual patterns of coping within the family, including the use of power and the style of communication, are vital to planning nursing intervention and establishment of priorities with the family.

Nursing intervention includes provision of support systems from the community and health care delivery system as appropriate to the nature of the developmental transition. For example, if the birth of a new child is anticipated, health care for the pregnant woman and the new infant is one priority. In addition, there may be teaching, guidance and counseling needs associated with the nature of the event itself or the family may need specific guidance in developing adequate coping mechanisms such as improved communication patterns within the family. The event may provide a needed stimulus for change within the family that results in achievement of increased family health and function, in spite of the turmoil experienced during transition. Active nursing care during this developmental transition is important.[67,82]

### STUDY QUESTIONS

1. Identify aspects of your own cultural inheritance which you tend to perpetuate and those which you actively have sought to change. Compare these orientations with colleagues and discuss implications for the future.
2. Discuss current efforts within your community that attempt to control the environment for healthier living. Are the efforts sufficient to meet the real problems? Which problems need further attack? How can individuals participate in environmental changes?
3. Describe your own experience with either the family of your childhood or the family in which you are a parent. What roles can be identified, and how have the purposes of the family group been facilitated? Identify the nature of the traits discussed in this chapter.
4. Recall a recent crisis situation that affected your life or someone close to you. What internal resources were available for coping, and what external resources were utilized? What features of the event led to the development of a crisis situation?

**REFERENCES**

1. Anthony, E. J.: Children at risk from divorce; a review. In Anthony, E. J., and Koupernik, C., editors: The child in his family; children at psychiatric risk, vol. 3, New York, 1974, John Wiley & Sons, Inc., p. 461.
2. Bane, M. J.: Here to stay; American families in the twentieth century, New York, 1976, Basic Books, Inc., Publishers.
3. Becker, M. H., Drachman, R. H., and Kirscht, J. P.: A new approach to explaining sick-role behavior in low-income populations, Am. J. Public Health 64:205, March, 1974.
4. Benedek, T.: The family as a psychological field. In Anthony, E. J., and Benedek, T., editors: Parenthood; its psychology and psychopathology, Boston, 1970, Little, Brown and Co.
5. Bennett, M., and Walker, L.: The double bind of motherhood. In Duffey, M., and others, editors: Current concepts in clinical nursing, vol. 3, St. Louis, 1971, The C. V. Mosby Co., p. 220.
6. Birdwhistell, R. L.: Introduction to kinesics, Louisville, Ky., 1952, University of Louisville Press.
7. Brandes, N. S.: Family togetherness and other fairy tales; a psychiatrist looks at family closeness, Clin. Pediatr. 11:516, Sept., 1972.
8. Brandwein, R. A., Brown, C. A., and Fox, E. M.: Women and children last; divorced mothers and their families, J. Marriage Family 37:498, Aug., 1975.
9. Brodt, E. W.: Urbanization and health planning; challenge and opportunity for the American Indian community, Am. J. Public Health 63:694, Aug., 1973.
10. Byers, P.: Rhythms, information processing and human relations; toward a typology of communication. In Klopfer, P., and Bateson, P., editors: Perspectives in ethology, vol. 2, New York, 1975, Plenum Publishing Corp.
11. Carey, W. B.: Adopting children; the medical aspects, Children Today 3:10, Jan.-Feb., 1974.
12. Cassel, J.: Epidmiological perspective of psychosocial factors in disease etiology, Am. J. Public Health 64:1040, Nov., 1974.
13. Chomsky, N.: Reflections on language, New York, 1975, Random House.
14. Clavan, and Vatter, E.: The affiliated family; a device for integrating old and young, J. Gerontol. Soc., pp. 407-411, Winter 1972.
15. Committee on Environmental Hazards, Massachusetts Chapter, American Academy of Pediatrics: What are the environmental hazards to the health of children? Clin. Pediatr. 13:322, April, 1974.
16. Cropp, G. J.: Effects of air pollution on health, J. Environ. Health 35:22, May-June 1973.
17. Crow, M. M., Bradshaw, B. R., and Guest, F.: True to life; a relevant approach to patient education, Am. J. Public Health 62:1328, Oct., 1972.
18. Damon, W.: The social world of the child, San Francisco, 1977, Jossey-Bass Publishers.
19. Dennison, D.: Social class variables related to health instruction, Am. J. Public Health 62:814, June, 1972.
20. Downs, F. S.: Technological advances and the nurse-family relationship, J. New York State Nurses' Assoc. 5:30-34, Aug. 1974.
21. Duvall, E. M.: Family development, ed. 4, Philadelphia, 1971, J. B. Lippincott.
22. Eiduson, B. T.: Looking at children in emergent family styles, Children Today 3:2, July-Aug. 1974.
23. Eisenberg, L.: Caring for children and working, Pediatrics 56:24, July 1975.
24. Ekman, P., and Friesen, W. V.: Head and body cues in the judgment of emotion; a reformulation. I. Perceptual and motor skills XXIL:711-724, June, 1967.
25. Frank, L. K.: Tactile communication, Genetic Psychol. Monograph 56:211-251, Nov. 1957.
26. Glasser, P. H., and Glasser, L. N., editors: Families in crisis, New York, 1970, Harper & Row, Publishers.
27. Glittenberg, J.: Adapting health care to a cultural setting, Am. J. Nurs. 74:2218, Dec., 1974.
28. Gordon, T.: Parent effectiveness training, New York, 1970, Peter H. Wyden, Inc.
29. Hall, E. T.: The silent language, Garden City, N.Y., 1959, Doubleday and Co.
30. Hall, E. T.: The hidden dimension, Garden City, N.Y., 1966, Doubleday and Co.
31. Harlow, H. F.: The nature of love, Am. Psychol. 13:673, 1958.
32. Heger, D. T.: A supportive service to single mothers and their children, Children Today 6:2, Sept.-Oct. 1977.
33. Heisel, J. S., and others: The significance of life events as contributing factors in the diseases of children, J. Pediatr. 83:119, July 1973.
34. Helson, R.: The changing image of the career woman, J. Social Issues 28:33, Jan., 1972.
35. Henderson, L. M.: Nutritional problems growing out of new patterns of food consumption, Am. J. Public Health 62:1194, Sept., 1972.
36. Horowitz, J. A., and Perdue, B. J.: Single-parent families, Nurs. Clin. North Am. 12:503, Sept., 1977.
37. Howell, M. C.: Employed mothers and their families. I. Pediatrics 52:252, Aug., 1973.
38. Howell, M. C.: Effects of maternal employment on the child. II. Pediatrics 52:327, Sept., 1973.
39. Hrobsky, D. M.: Transition to parenthood; a balancing of needs, Nurs. Clin. North Am. 12:457, Sept., 1977.
40. Hughes, C. B.: An eclectic approach to parent group educations, Nurs. Clin. North Am. 12:469, Sept., 1977.
41. Irelan, L. M.: Low-income life styles, Washington, D.C., 1967, U.S. Dept. of Health, Education and Welfare, Social and Rehabilitation Service.
42. Jeffers, C.: Unstereotyping black families in America. In Where we are; a hard look at family and society, New York, 1970, Child Study Association of America, p. 64.
43. Johnston, C. M., and Deisher, R. W.: Contemporary communal child rearing; a first analysis, Pediatrics 52:319, Sept., 1973.
44. Jourard, S.: The transparent self, Princeton, N.J., 1964, D. Van Nostrand Co.

45. Katz, S. H., and Wallace, A. F. C.: An anthropological perspective on behavior and disease, Am. J. Public Health **64**:1050, Nov., 1974.

46. Keller, S.: The future role of women, Ann. Am. Acad. Polit. Social Science **408**:1, July, 1973.

47. Keniston, K.: All our children; The American family under pressure, New York, 1977, Harcourt, Brace, Jovanovich.

48. Kiernan, B., and Scoloveno, M. A.: Fathering, Nurs. Clin. North Am. **12**:481, Sept., 1977.

49. Koch, C., Minuchin, S., and Donovan, W. M.: A case of somatic expression of family and environmental stress, Clin. Pediatr. **13**:815, Oct., 1974.

50. Krim, A. S.: Families in crisis, Children Today **3**:2, Jan.-Feb. 1974.

51. Langelloto, E.: Involving parents in a children's clinic, Children **18**:202, Nov.-Dec. 1971.

52. Lave, L. B., and Seskin, E. P.: Air pollution, climate, and home heating; their effects on U.S. mortality rates, Am. J. Public Health **62**:909, July, 1972.

53. LeMasters, E. E.: Parents in modern America; a sociological analysis, ed. 3, Homewood, Ill., 1977, The Dorsey Press.

54. Lewis, J. M., and others: No single thread, New York, 1976, Brunner/Mazel.

55. McBride, A. B.: Can family life survive? Am. J. Nurs. **75**:1648, Oct., 1975.

56. McNamara, J. J.: Hyperactivity in the apartment bound child, Clin. Pediatr. **11**:371, July, 1972.

57. Mead, M.: Sex and temperament in three primitive societies, New York, 1935, The New American Library.

58. Mead, M.: Culture and commitment; a study of the generation gap, New York, 1970, The Natural History Press.

59. Messer, J. W., and others: A comparative survey of five common market foods in low and high income economic areas, Am. J. Public Health **63**:1074, Dec., 1973.

60. Montagu, A.: Touching; the human significance of the skin, New York, 1971, Columbia University Press.

61. Morsell, J. A.: Ethnic relations of the future, Ann. Am. Acad. Polit. Social Science **408**:83, July, 1973.

62. Muhich, D. F., and Johnson, B. J.: Youth and society; changing values and roles, Pediatr. Clin. North. Am. **20**:771, Nov., 1973.

63. Myers, J. K., and others: Life events and mental status, J. Health Social Behavior **13**:398, Dec., 1972.

64. Newman, L. R.: Family stresses in the 1970's; what does the pediatrician have to learn and transmit? Clin. Pediatr. **13**:987, Nov., 1974.

65. Norton, A. J., and Glick, P. C.: Changes in American family life, Children Today **5**:2, May-June, 1976.

66. Perdue, B. J., and others: "Mothering." In Smoyak, S., editor: Nurs. Clin. North Am. Symposium on Parenting, **12**:491, Sept., 1977.

67. Peters, L.: The family and family therapy. In Hall, J. E., and Weaver, B. R., editors: Nursing of families in crisis, Philadelphia, 1974, J. B. Lippincott Co.

68. Redmann, R. E.: Black child—white nurse; a nursing challenge and privilege. In Duffey, M., and others, editors: Current concepts in clinical nursing, Vol. 3, St. Louis, 1971, The C. V. Mosby Co., p. 106.

69. Reverby, S.: A perspective on the root causes of illness, Am. J. Public Health **62**:1140, Aug., 1972.

70. Rich, A.: Of woman born, New York, 1976, W. W. Norton and Co., Inc.

71. Rubin, L. B.: Worlds of pain; life in the working-class family, New York, 1976, Basic Books, Inc., Publishers.

72. Sagar, M.: A mother's ability to love her child. In Duffey, M., and others, editors: Current concepts in clinical nursing, vol. 3, St. Louis, 1971, The C. V. Mosby Co., p. 141.

73. Samson, J. M.: The emerging significance of sexuality, Main Currents Mod. Thought **29**:186, May-June 1973.

74. Sanchez, V.: Relevance of cultural values for occupational therapy programs, Am. J. Occup. Ther. **28**:1, Jan.-Feb., 1964.

75. Sargent, F.: Man—environment—problems for public health, Am. J. Public Health **62**:628, May, 1972.

76. Smoyak, S.: Symposium on parenting; introduction, Nurs. Clin. North Am. **12**:447, Sept., 1977.

77. Spaulding, M. R.: Adapting postpartum teaching to mother's low-income life-styles. In Bergersen, B. S., and others, editors: Current concepts in clinical nursing, vol. 2, St. Louis, 1969, The C. V. Mosby Co., p. 280.

78. Stern, D. N., and others: Vocalizing in unison and in alternation; two modes of communication within the mother-infant dyad, Ann. N.Y. Acad. Sciences **263**:89, Sept. 19, 1975.

79. Straus, M. A.: Leveling, civility and violence in the family, J. Marriage Family **36**:13-29, Feb., 1974.

80. Trager, G. L.: Paralanguage; a first approximation, Studies in Linguistics **13**:112, 1958.

81. Weiss, R. S.: Marital separation, New York, 1975, Basic Books, Inc., Publishers.

82. Williams, F. S.: Intervention in maturational crises. In Hall, J. E., and Weaver, B. R., editors: Nursing of families in crisis, Philadelphia, 1974, J. B. Lippincott.

83. Wilson, M. E.: The significance of communication in counseling the culturally disadvantaged. In Wilcox, R., editor: The psychological consequences of being a black American, New York, 1971, John Wiley & Sons, Inc.

84. Zepp, E. A., Thomas, J. A., and Knotts, G. R.: The toxic effects of mercury; a survey of the newer clinical insights, Clin. Pediatr. **13**:783, Sept., 1974.

# Patrick—FAMILY ASSESSMENT*

Cheryl Boyd Hundley

## HEALTH STATUS LIST

| Onset | Date | No. | Active | Date | Inactive/resolved |
|-------|------|-----|--------|------|-------------------|
| 1/15/78 | 1/15/78 | 1 | Incomplete data base | | |
| 9/72 | 1/15/78 | 2 | Developmental tasks of young adulthood | | |
| 9/72 | 1/15/78 | 2A | Establishing an intimate bond | | |
| 6/77 | 1/15/78 | 2B | Change in career goal | | |
| | 1/15/78 | 2C | Change in anticipated life style | | |
| 1/15/78 | 1/15/78 | 3 | Need for knowledge and anticipatory guidance for child-rearing | | |
| | 1/15/78 | 3A | Safe home environment | | |
| | 1/15/78 | 3B | Developmentally stimulating home environment for child | | |
| 12/17/74 | 1/15/78 | 3C | Parenting | | |
| 12/17/74 | 1/15/78 | 3D | Child health maintenance | | |

## FAMILY ASSESSMENT

### I. General data

**Number of members in the family:** Three—father, Robert (28); mother, Marjorie (28); child, Patrick (3).

**State of development of the family:** Intimacy vs. self-isolation

**Members not living in the household:** None

**Household space and privacy arrangements:** Apartment dwelling. 2 bedroom, den, 2 baths, living-dining and kitchen. Parents have own bedroom and bath.

**Description of the home environment:** Uncrowded with furniture; placement for clear traffic ways. Neat, clean and uncluttered. Door opens into enclosed courtyard. In kitchen there is a child's table and chair. There are safety devices in outlets and a device on doorknob to outside, preventing Patrick from getting outside. They have a small dog. There is no play equipment in the courtyard.

**Income:** How do you manage to make ends meet:
Robert—custodian job $460/monthly; new business $450/monthly (expects this to increase)
Marjorie—manages apartment complex. Rent and utilities as salary.

*Tool adapted from Family Assessment Tool by Patsy Kaiser and Donna Kem, Texas Woman's University, Denton, Texas.

Child health
maintenance

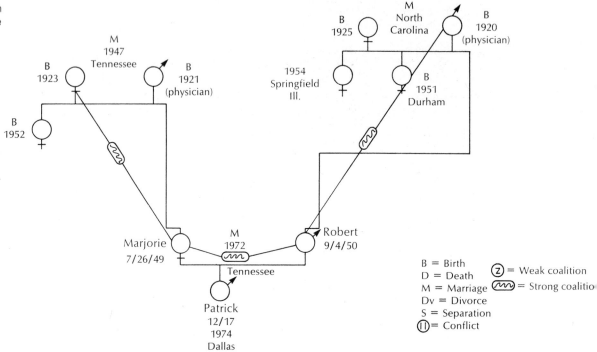

B = Birth
D = Death    ⓩ = Weak coalition
M = Marriage   ∿ = Strong coalitio
Dv = Divorce
S = Separation
Ⓘ = Conflict

**Transportation available:** One car. Robert uses most of the time. Wife has friends she relies on for transportation or husband rearranges schedule so she can have car.

**Child care arrangements:** Mother at home and cares for child. Child to mother's-day-out at local church, 6 hours, 2 times weekly.

**Emergency resources:** Stocks, $6500 (half is mortgaged for new business); savings, $1000; insurance, group health, term life on husband, $100,000.

**Eating patterns:** All eat breakfast together and supper. Mother and child have lunch. Sit at table for meals.

**Leisure activities:** Have lunch together on mother's-day-out. Occasionally to dinner and a movie. Read a lot at home in evenings. Take child fishing or to park weekly.

**Adult friends and relationships outside of family:** Good friends with two couples. No family nearby. Extended families live out of state.

**Time spent with friends:** Visit weekly with friends. Children are included in this. Mother frequently has coffee with nearby friends.

**Community activities and organizations:** Active in church. Robert is part-time (3 hours) seminary student and they sometimes are involved with school-related activities.

## II. Adult social history

**Adult relationships as defined within the family:** Robert sees himself as provider, she sees herself as homemaker and caretaker. Both expressed mutual responsibility for decision-making.

**How adult relationships were formed:** Met in college. Worked in a church organization as friends for a year before dating. Dated one year. Engaged six months.

**What they consider best about their relationship:** Their "commitment to one an- other" for a viable healthy relationship.

**What they consider to be worst about their relationship:** Ineffective communication, i.e., verbalizing feelings. Through marriage counseling this past year they are dealing with this.

**What was life like for you as a child growing up?**
Marjorie—Remembers a pleasant childhood, a sense of security. Believes parents cared about each other and children.
Robert—Also expressed positive reflections. Felt secure and loved. Perceives parents as having loving relationships, committed to one another.

**Any losses before the age of 15?** None for either parent.

**As a child, what practice did your parents use in discipline?**
Marjorie—Parents raised voices. Was infrequently spanked.
Robert—Only remembers two instances when spanked, otherwise verbally disciplined. Remembers that he was raised to think that "being angry was not nice."

**What things did you enjoy as a child?**
Robert—Yearly family vacations each time to a different place. Enjoyed sports, scouts, and piano activities.
Marjorie—Family had houseboat so she enjoyed water sports. Family also camped out together.

III. **Family interactions** (Complete for each family member.)

**ROBERT**

**General health status:** Stable. No acute or chronic illness or disability.

**Role in family:** Sees himself as provider and leader. Wants to be an effective role model for son and helpmate to wife.

**Family tasks:** Assists wife in managing apartment complex. Assists her with grocery shopping. Bathes son and puts to bed after reading to him.

**Life events in previous year:** 1/77 quit full-time graduate work after three years. Changed from career goal of ministry to being self-employed businessman. Anticipates buying a home. Seemed excited about new directions of his career and about the decision to have a different life style with a higher standard of living.

**Previous coping mechanisms:** To stress or conflict, until last year, reacted passively. Since counseling, is learning to verbalize appropriately his feelings, especially when he does not "like" or is "angry with" wife.

**Developmental state:** Intimacy versus self-absorption.

**Expectations of self:** Provide for family comfortably—imbue son with emotional health and Christian concepts and have sound marriage.

**Expectations of family:** To be a loving, emotionally healthy viable unit.

**Description of child-adult relationships:** Loves Patrick and "feels good" about their relationship but often "gets frustrated" with him.

**Perception of how decisions are made:** Thinks wife and he talk and select a decision acceptable to both; not a "Do what I say" situation.

**Perception of how problems and conflicts are solved:** In past, before counseling, interpersonal problems and conflicts were not openly acknowledged. Since counseling, they can verbalize about conflicts within the relationship as the first step to problem solving.

81

## MARJORIE

**General health status:** Stable. Several years ago had fever of unknown origin for a year. No diagnosis was made. No recurrences. Occasional gastritis (ulcer ruled out medically).

**Role in family:** Wife, full-time mother, homemaker, helpmate to husband.

**Family tasks:** Provide a clean comfortable relaxing home for husband and child. Believes children have advantages with a full-time mother.

**Life events in previous year:** 1/77 husband quit school. 6/77 new business started. 1/78 anticipate buying a new home. Robert quit full-time graduate work in the seminary 1/77. Having difficulty deciding exactly what he wanted to do about finishing school. They saw a marriage counselor who has helped them surface and verbalize the more basic question of how they desired to live. Prior to this time, they visualized their life as one not oriented toward materialism but serving a church. Since then, he has worked through a desire to change his life chosen career from the ministry to that of a businessman. She feels positive about the change. They both expressed a desire to have a higher standard of living and to express their Christian commitment in other ways than through the ministry.

**Previous coping mechanisms:** In stressful situations becomes dominant and assertive "telling everyone what to do." Trying not to do this as much.

**Development state:** Intimacy vs. self-absorption.

**Expectations of self:** Wants emotional health and desires to raise emotionally healthy and Christian children.

**Expectations of family:** Wants a viable happy family and to live with some of the comforts of life.

**Description of child-adult relationships:** Believes she and Patrick have a good relationship and perceives that he feels secure. Thinks behavior is "attention getting" at times.

**Perception of how decisions are made:** Monthly they sit down and discuss outcome of decisions as to discipline, etc. about son. Thinks decisions are derived from mutual discussion.

**Perception of how problems and conflicts are solved:** Trying to interact differently with husband so they can use conflict creatively and learn to solve problems based on true feelings and perceptions. The counselor has assisted them in deriving this process which she thinks is mutually satisfying.

## IV. Child-rearing

**How do you correct the child when he/she misbehaves?** Initially they give one warning. Unsociable behavior—child gets put to bed with an explanation. Tantrums or open violation of established rules, he gets spanked. After both measures they reiterate reason for action and that they love him. They will hold him after that if he desires. Talk to him about it being "OK to be mad" but that there are acceptable ways of showing anger.

**How do you reward the child for good behavior?** Praise; hugs; say how "big" he is.

**What do you agree that the child should learn in life?** "That he should know Christ," "be able to love," "be able to have inner control," "be assertive," and "be sensitive to others."

**On what do adult members disagree regarding child-rearing?** Claimed no disagreement or couldn't think of anything at this time.

**How do you think the child responds to your disciplining/guidance/control?** When they are consistent, behavior of child changes toward desired outcome. Expressed the difficulty of always being consistent.

**When do you feel closest to the child?** When reading to him while holding, when they play with Patrick.

**When do you feel the most distant/strange to your child?** When he's loud and obnoxious.

**Adult description of each child, including developmental stage and anticipation of events of the coming year.** See child as needing to learn to control "obnoxious" behavior which erupts. Plan to have another child and planning for how sibling rivalry will affect Patrick. Plan to move and buy a home this year. Think this will allow them more privacy as there are many people in and out of apartment as they manage the complex. After three years of this, they find this stressful to their private life. Think a home with yard and another neighborhood is a better climate for Patrick. No specific developmental tasks given for child.

## V. Summary of family's communication

**Clarity of speech:** Speech is distinct, appropriate volume and loudness.

**Topic changes/consistency:** Topic completed consistently before change in subject.

**Ratio of agreement/disagreement between members:** No disagreement in this encounter with family.

**Intensity of feelings conveyed:** Feeling tones appropriate to words expressed.

**Speaking order:** Altered in response to inquiries and to subject changes.

**Commitment to family goals:** Equally committed to similar goals.

**Patterns of communication:** Exchange ideas individually and then compared expressed thoughts.

## VI. Summary of family assessment

**Level of family functioning**
  **Stage of maturity:** Moving through developmental tasks appropriately.
  **Open/closed:** Family is an open system.
  **Degree of individuation:** Concerned with their own goals for child and marriage. Would like comfortable way of life as dictated by middle-class standards.
  **Degree of dependency:** Mostly a self-sufficient unit.

**Family strengths**
  • Similarly stated life goals.
  • Commitment to long-term relationship.
  • Ability to seek guidance professionally when necessary.

**Active or potential problems**
  • No extended family in the area.
  • No regular babysitter for activities they desire not including child.
  • Possibility of new business venture not succeeding.
  • Not being able financially to buy a home at this time.
  • Adapting to a new neighborhood and people should they move into a home.
  • Social isolation of Patrick; not many opportunities for interactive play with peers.

**INITIAL PLAN**

1/15/78 **No. 1 Incomplete data base**

**S** Expressed need for information to intelligently prepare child for a sibling. Are thinking of having child within a year. Seemed to desire further interventions and contacts.

**O** In first encounter with client's information about relationships, communication patterns may not be altogether accurate. Other interactions and observations of the family unit may be necessary to correctly identify manifest as well as latent needs of the family.

**A** Family appears to be working through developmental tasks of the young adult and as parents of a preschooler.

**P** Obj. 1 The family should demonstrate desire for future interactions to provide information for further need identification

1/15/78 **No. 2 Developmental tasks of young adulthood**

2,A Establishing an intimate bond

**S** Both expressed commitment to one another and have cooperated in an effort through marital counseling to establish a more effective communication.

**O** Communication between the couple was accompanied by congruent feeling tones. Perceived was an openness and honesty about the problems and outcomes in their efforts to enrich their relationship. There was mutual interchange, clarity of speech and affect, and completion of topic discussion.

**A** An intimate viable relationship is in part accomplished by creating an intimate system of communication that allows for exchange of confidences, feelings, and for predictability of each other's responses. Also necessary for an intimate bond is planning ahead for a stable relationship, concurring on how life should be lived, and establishing themselves as a pair in their eyes and in the eyes of families and friends. The inability to be intimate leads to isolation. They appear to be accomplishing intimacy thus moving through a major task of the stage of intimacy versus isolation (self-absorption), which is appropriate to their age and station in the life span.

**P** Obj. 1 The couple should continue to create an effective communication system that allows for intimacy.

2,B Change in career goal—Robert

**S** Changed goal from the ministry to business. Expresses relief and excitement about the change. Is eager about building his own business. Will take only a 3-hour course at school as he is almost finished with degree. Wife is pleased with changes. Both expressed anticipation at planning for higher standard of living they feel was not possible with prior career plans. Mortgaged half of investments to buy equipment for business.

**O** Business equipment in house. Both seemed to realize the risks of self-employment but talked more about how this would affect their life-style. Feeling tones again congruent with communication. Role change for Robert from a student to a full-time employed person.

**A** Becoming established in a profession or vocation that gives personal satisfaction, economic independence, and· a feeling of contributing to society is a task of young adulthood. A person's work can be viewed as a tool function, or a way to earn a living, a means of helping others, or as central to the self. A person with a sense of self-confidence and a positive self-image is more flexible, able to change, and admits new attributes to himself. Through self-knowledge and insights he or she has found the energy and strength to change. Job satisfaction increases in occupations of entrepreneurial, professional, and management natures. People selecting these occupations often have high achievement needs.

**P** Obj. 1 The couple should demonstrate the ability to cope with events related to career goal change.

2,C Change in anticipated life-style

**S** Plan to buy a home in the suburbs in a few months after living in and managing an apartment complex. Used to having rent and utilities supplied in exchange for management of apartments. Said that disruptions of phone calls and apartment dwellers as managers decreased privacy they desire. Want now a materially higher standard of living. Have one car, which Robert uses for business.

**O** No mention of wife being more isolated from present nearby friends and further independence restricted with no car readily available in a suburban home. They now live in city with public transportation and close-by shopping, laundry, parks, health care facilities.

**A** May not be aware of adjustments and expense of moving into and maintaining a home. Robert being self-employed may not have initially a predictable income. Marjorie may be more isolated with a new neighborhood, no friends nearby, and not having a car should they move. They will not have closeness of facilities in suburbs as they presently do. Will have more privacy without interruptions from managing apartments. Establishing and managing a home is a developmental task of the young adult. Maintaining privacy and supplying adequate housing, space, equipment, and materials for life, comfort, health and recreation are also developmental tasks of this era.

**P** Obj. 1 The couple should be able to cope with events produced by chosen life-style.

1/15/78 **No. 3 Need for knowledge and anticipatory guidance for child-rearing**

3,A Safe home environment

**S** Expressed that it would be nice if son had a yard to play in. Don't "like" son when he is "obnoxious." Relates son has "attention-getting" behavior.

**O** Safety devices used on doorknob and in outlets. Courtyard is enclosed. Pathways in house are clear. No specific knowledge of child's developmental stage and inherent hazards in relation to the stage.

**A** The most common cause of death at this age is accidents. Injury control and safety of a child is a major responsibility for parents. The environment should be kept as safe as possible while teaching safety precautions to the child. Preschoolers need clear-cut, simply explained rules, explained on a consistent basis. As child learns to protect himself, recognition and praise should be given. Health maintenance for a family begins with parental knowledge of the child's developmental stage and the hazards for the child developmentally.

**INITIAL PLAN—cont'd**

1/15/78 **No. 3  Need for knowledge and anticipatory guidance for childrearing—cont'd**

Patrick is entering the stage of initiative vs. guilt affectively and cognitively is entering the phase of preconceptual thought. Physically he is mastering large and small muscle coordination and movement, and his growth is slowing. He can undress and help dress self and can toilet alone with simple clothes. Intervention should be directed toward family teaching of home safety, developmental safety needs with anticipation of developmental events for the coming year.

**P**  Obj. 1  The family should provide a physically safe home environment for Patrick.

Obj. 2  The family should plan for forthcoming developmental safety needs for Patrick.

3,B  Developmentally stimulating home environment

**S**  Parents feel a home would be a better environment for Patrick. They visit each week with friends who also have children. Patrick goes to mother's-day-out twice a week. They hold son and rock him at intervals throughout the day. They read to him.

**O**  No mention as to types of toys or play environment appropriate for Patrick. No mention of nearby playmates or need for peer play for child.

**A**  Sensory input in the visual, auditory, kinesthetic, and tactile modes is necessary for healthy development. Social interaction and freedom for imitation and play are the main channels for providing home environment stimulation. Space and play objects need to be geared to allow imitative and make-believe play. Play for a preschooler has elements of reality, and there is a sincerity about it. The preschooler is intrusive in play and may attack playmates accidentally or purposefully. Needs space for rigorous gross motor activities. Has consuming curiosity and is always exploring. The child progresses from solitary and parallel play to cooperating a longer time in a larger group. The time of separation from parents increases in length and frequency and eventually he should orient from family to a peer group. Purposes of play for the preschooler include establishing concerns and friendships for others, learning cooperation and sharing, expressing creativity, imagination, imitating and learning about adult roles and social activity, building self-esteem, and having fun and expressing joy. Play needs to give the preschooler a sense of power and provide experiences for assimilation, which is necessary for cognitive foundations of intellectual thought.

**P**  Obj. 1  The parents should demonstrate knowledge of developmental stimulation and purposes of play for the preschooler.

Obj. 2  The parents should provide experiences for appropriate developmental stimulation for Patrick.

3,C  Parenting

**S**  Expressed difficulty with being consistent with guidance and discipline of child. Goals for child include being able to love, to be Christian, to have inner control, to be assertive, and to be sensitive to others. They agree and follow through with a discipline regimen. Both parents discipline child. Both expressed no negative perceptions of how they were parented. Monthly evaluation of how they are parenting child.

3,C   Parenting—cont'd

**O**   No conflicts or contradictions between verbal accounts of how they discipline. Feeling tones of being frustrated with disciplining child was consistently perceived. No opportunities were manifest to see the practice of cognitively stated regimen of discipline. They provide for child's economic and nurturing needs.

**A**   Parenting competency requires that family's economic needs and nurturing needs are met and that they are appropriate to the developmental level of the child. A positive reward and reinforcement system. Style of communication and use of power within the family are components to be assessed to determine parenting ability.

Sometimes methods of guidance and discipline are stated cognitively but are not followed through in actual practice. Most adults tend to parent as they were parented as a child. The child learns how to behave through opportunities to develop self-control and by imitating parents. The child needs consistent, fair, kind limits to be secure. Limits preserve the child's and parent's self-respect. He must be able to predict the behavior of others in order to inhibit or change some of his behavior. Parents must communicate to the child (in his effort to control his own inner impulses) that he should not be afraid of his impulses but learn to control them.

**P**   Obj. 1   The parents should demonstrate adequate knowledge of requirements for effective parenting.

3,D   Child health maintenance

**S**   Patrick is 3 years old. Born 12/17/74 in Dallas.

**O**   None.

**A**   To provide sound and appropriate intervention the competencies of the child must be assessed. Identify physiologic, psychologic, sociologic, and environmental stressors of the child are the basis for providing primary care of health maintenance.

**P**   Obj. 1   The child should demonstrate normal development in all parameters.

## NURSING ORDERS

1/15/78 **No. 1 Incomplete data base**

Obj. 1 The family should demonstrate desire for future in-
teractions to provide for further need identification.
  A. Make one appointment for another interview at    C.S.*
     family's convenience for two weeks, 1/30/78
  B. Inquire as to how they perceive these interac-    C.S.
     tions for meeting their needs at this time (1/30)

**No. 2 Developmental tasks of young adulthood**

2,A Establishing an intimate bond.

Obj. 1 The couple should continue to create an effective
communication system that allows for intimacy.
  A. In subsequent interviews continue to assess    C.S.
     the adequacy of communications. (1/30)
  B. Assist them to utilize their skills as they plan    C.S.
     ahead for normative crisis, i.e., planning for
     new home, moving to another neighborhood,
     planning another child, and preparing for
     sibling rivalry. (1/30)
  C. Educate them as to the developmental tasks    C.S.
     necessary for the young adult and the tasks for
     a viable marriage (1/30).

2,B Change in career goal—Robert

Obj. 1 The couple should demonstrate the ability to cope
with events related to career goal change.
  A. Obtain more concrete data about how they    C.S.
     plan to cope should business not proceed as
     planned. (1/30)
  B. Explore the depth of their commitment to new    C.S.
     goals and fears they may have. (1/30)
  C. Encourage wife to positively recognize his    C.S.
     achievements. (1/30)
  D. Explore the existence and source of motivation    C.S.
     of achievement needs individually. (1/30)

2,C Change in anticipated life-style

Obj. 1 The couple should be able to cope with events
produced by chosen life-style.
  A. Have each relate their perception of how life    C.S.
     they think will be when they move into a home
     and changes they foresee. (1/30)
  B. Explore their ability to plan financially to support    C.S.
     a home. Provide budgeting and financial infor-
     mation by referral if necessary. (1/30)
  C. Explore how they will be able to cope with un-    C.S.
     expected costs of family life after financial com-
     mitment to a home. (1/30)
  D. Determine if Marjorie is prepared to supple-    C.S.
     ment income should necessity require. (1/30)

*Clinical specialist.

1/15/78 **No. 2 Developmental tasks of young adulthood—cont'd** **PERSONNEL**

E. Determine if they have investigated community facilities for health care, recreation, public transportation, and community organizations, schools, and churches where they are planning to buy a home. Refer to Chamber of Commerce for this type of information.　　C.S.

1/15/78 **No. 3 Need for knowledge and anticipatory guidance for childrearing**

3,A　Safe home environment

Obj. 1　The family should provide a physically safe home environment for Patrick.

A. Investigate safety for prevention of burns, ingestion, and car safety in next home visit. Share information about accidents as cause of death.　　C.S.

B. Teach parents to give recognition and praise to compliance with safe behavior. (1/30)　　C.S.

C. Have parents teach Patrick his full name and address and phone number and how to utilize police or adults in service roles for help.　　C.S.
Parents

D. Phrase safety rules positively; impress that he must obey simple commands.　　Parents

E. Teach him to look for and get away from cars.　　Parents

Obj. 2　The family should plan for forthcoming developmental safety needs for Patrick.

A. Teach parents events to anticipate in his physical, cognitive, and emotional development within the year, i.e., gender identity, egocentric thought, imaginative thought.　　C.S.

B. Provide literature pertinent to Patrick's developmental level. (1/30)　　C.S.

C. Teach them that "obnoxious" and intrusive behavior is a hallmark of his developmental age. (1/30)　　C.S.

D. Teach them that he will be sexually curious about his own body. (1/30)　　C.S.

3,B　Developmentally stimulating home environment for child.

Obj. 1　The parents should demonstrate knowledge of developmental stimulation and purposes of play for the preschooler.

A. Teach parents the modes for sensory input for developmental stimulation. (1/30)　　C.S.

B. Assess adequacy of space, play objects. (1/30)　　C.S.

C. Inquire as to types of TV programs Patrick watches. Encourage "Sesame Street," "Electric Company," "Mr. Rodger's Neighborhood" with input from mother reinforcing content. (1/30)　　C.S.

## NURSING ORDERS—cont'd

1/15/78   **No. 3  Need for knowledge and anticipatory guidance for childrearing—cont'd**     **PERSONNEL**

      D. Give literature to parents about purposes of play and how to promote development. (1/30)

      E. Outline a sample stimulation program appropriate for Patrick with parents' input.     Parents C.S.

Obj. 2  The parents should provide experiences for appropriate developmental stimulation for Patrick.

      A. Educate parents as to function of social interactions in preschool period.     C.S.

      B. Assess the quality and quantity of peer contact for Patrick (church, mother's-day-out experiences, ages of friends' children).     C.S.

      C. Explore how they will provide peer interactions for Patrick in the event of another sibling.     C.S.

3,C  Parenting

Obj. 1  The parents should demonstrate adequate knowledge of requirements for effective parenting.

      A. Arrange a home visit to observe further interactions of parents and child in discipline situation. (1/30)     C.S.

      B. Offer parenting literature (later discuss reactions) and helpful techniques. (1/30)     C.S.

      C. Teach parents to convey authority without anger or threat.     Parents C.S.

      D. Help the child express resentment when restrictions are imposed—"I realize you don't like the rules but . . ."     Parents

      E. Use positive suggestions, rather than commands.     Parents

      F. Control of the situation by parents should child lose control—removing from stimulating event, distraction, encouraging him to think through the problem.     Parents

      G. Offer parents an option of going to local parenting group.     C.S.

      H. Assess further the use of power within the family.     C.S.

3,D  Child health maintenance

Obj. 1  The child should demonstrate normal development in all parameters.

      A. With permission perform a physical examination and D.D.S.T. on Patrick. (1/30)     C.S.

      B. Talk with Patrick about his activities and friends. (1/30)     C.S.

      C. Observe child in a spontaneous play situation in the home if possible. (1/30)     C.S.

      D. Obtain a health history from the parents (illnesses, immunizations, accidents, etc.) (1/30)     C.S.

**REFERENCES**

Eshleman, R. J.: The family, Boston, 1974, Allyn & Bacon, Inc.

Murray, R., and Zentner, J.: Nursing assessment and health promotion through the life span, Englewood Cliffs, N.J., 1975, Prentice-Hall, Inc.

Satir, V., Stachowaick, J., and Taschman, H.: Helping families to change, New York, 1976, Jason Aronson, Inc.

# Prenatal development and care

The period of life from conception to birth is the most mysterious of all developmental stages. The importance of this stage of life is increasingly recognized as indications of lasting and significant effects of events during gestation become known. There remain many unanswered questions surrounding the nature of the fetal experience and the nature of this experience on the child's future personality and physical health. In this unit we will consider briefly some of the areas of knowledge regarding prenatal existence and indicate issues that are important to health care for the fetus and mother.

In Chapter 4, "The Unborn Child," we will consider (1) a review of the physiology of the reproductive systems and of conception, (2) a summary of the developmental features of fetal life, and (3) a summary of the principles of heredity.

The purposes of Chapter 5, "Providing a Healthy Prenatal Environment," are to (1) consider the ways in which healthy maternal physiology during pregnancy may be promoted and (2) present features of nursing assessment and care of the mother and fetus before labor and delivery.

# The unborn child

The mystery of life before birth has fascinated scientists, philosophers, and theologians for centuries. When a child is conceived, many events take place that greatly affect the entire life of the individual. Some of these events are presently beyond human control. Others have only recently been discovered and described for the first time, and this new knowledge has led to speculation and experimentation with ways to protect and ensure a better life for mankind. Many established beliefs about optimal care for the expectant mother and her child have been reconfirmed as sound; others have been changed or discarded with new understanding of the phenomena of fetal life. The nurse whose attention is centered upon children and families needs to understand the presently available concepts and ideas in order to implement the nursing process. Particularly in working with older children, adolescents, and young mothers, interpretation and teaching of reproductive phenomena are essential. Understanding the nature of heredity and fetal development aids in obtaining relevant and complete prenatal information.

## THE BEGINNING OF LIFE

The ability to bear children is a complex interaction of many factors for men and women. It is recognized that psychologic and higher men- tal processes are important in reproductive functions, but these interactions are not at this point accurately described or understood. The elaborate social tasks that accompany sexual maturation, pairing, mating, and child-bearing in human cultures are also known to influence the physical reproduction, but the nature of this influence is as yet speculative.

### Physiology of reproduction
#### *Maternal reproductive cycle*

Female reproductive function involves cyclic activity, a series of interactive processes that oc- cur among the various structures and hormones of the body. The primary structure and hor- mones involved in this rhythmic activity are de- picted in Fig. 4-1. The cerebral cortex, which is presumed to mediate emotional and psychic re- sponses and stimuli, influences the action of the sexual cycle. Beginning at puberty and ending gradually during menopause at age 40 to 50, this cycle involves primarily the anterior pituitary, ovaries, and uterine lining. When pregnancy occurs, the cycle is interrupted temporarily and hormonal functions change for the duration of the pregnancy.

The major hormones secreted by the pituitary during the cycle are the gonadotropic hor- mones, primarily the follicle stimulating hor- mone (FSH), the luteinizing hormone (LH), and

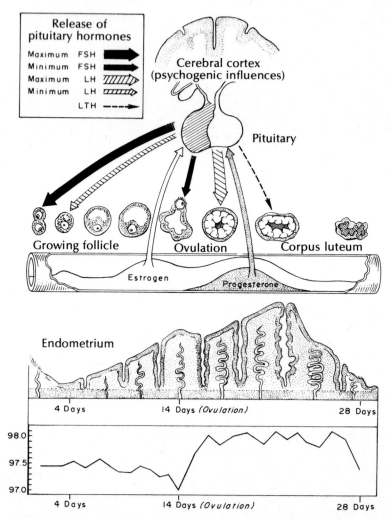

**Fig. 4-1.** Diagram illustrating the interrelationships among the cerebral, hypothalamic, pituitary, ovarian, and uterine functions throughout a usual 28-day menstrual cycle. The variations in basal body temperature are also illustrated, although this may not be demonstrated universally in women.

the luteotropic hormone (LTH). There is evidence that suggests that the luteotropic hormone is not functional during human reproductive cycles except during production of milk by the breasts. For this reason, LTH is often referred to as a prolactin or lactogenic hormone when human cycles are described. The ovaries supply estrogens and progesterone.

The function of these hormones is usually studied in animals, most commonly rats and rabbits. Studies of human hormonal function are relatively limited, and thus understanding of the human cycle is far from complete. The human cycle differs in several important ways from

that of animals, but the similarities that can be observed lead to the assumption that when it is not possible to describe human function directly, animal function provides models that are close enough for most practical inferences. As newer methods of study are developed, human function has been more accurately ascertained, but much work still needs to be completed.

FSH, LH, and LTH are secreted by the anterior pituitary and regulate ovarian function. During childhood, gonadotropic hormones are not produced, and the ovaries remain essentially dormant. FSH stimulates growth of the ovaries and follicles. The ovum grows, followed by proliferation of tissues around the ovum that comprise the follicle. At the time that FSH production is at its height, several follicles have increased in size and one has reached maturity—the point at which release of the ovum is possible. During the period of accelerated growth of the follicle, LH production begins and continues to act synergistically with FSH until the final stages of follicular fluid production and growth are accomplished. LH seems to be particularly necessary for the follicle finally to rupture and release the ovum. LH also serves as the stimulus for the secretion of estrogens by the follicle and from the corpus luteum, which forms from the follicular cells after ovulation occurs. The lutein cells continue to secrete estrogens actively and begin progesterone production. This continues until gradual involution of the corpus luteum about 12 days following ovulation. LTH contributes to this process of luteinization in some species. When LH is no longer produced in quantities, menstruation begins and another cycle is initiated.

The estrogens are a group of related hormones, which all seem to have similar effects known as estrogenic effects. The three major estrogens known are β-estradiol, estrone, and estriol. The primary function of these compounds is to stimulate proliferation of tissues of the sexual organs and other tissues related to reproduction. During the menstrual cycle, growth of uterine endometrium and development of glands that nourish and aid in the implantation of the ovum are stimulated. In addition, estrogens affect the mucosal lining of the fallopian tubes by causing proliferation of glandular tissues and increased activity of the cilial lining of the tubes. This aids in transport of the ovum through the fallopian tubes and into the uterus. At puberty the estrogens play a significant role in development of sexual characteristics (see Chapter 14).

Progesterone acts to promote the secretory functions of the proliferated endometrium and prepare it for the implantation of the fertilized ovum. It also decreases motility of the uterine muscle, thus facilitating retention of the newly developing embryo. This also stimulates secretory development of alveoli and lobules of the breasts, but actual secretion of milk does not occur in response to progesterone. Estrogens and progesterone act synergistically to cause the production of LH and FSH to subside, thus providing a negative feedback mechanism to the anterior pituitary, which allows recycling to occur. This mechanism seems to be mediated by the hypothalamus, but the exact manner in which this happens has not been ascertained.

Awakening basal body temperature varies in response to the endocrine cycle that has just been described. As seen in Fig. 4-1, basal body temperature is low during the phase of dominant estrogen production. A slight drop occurs at about the time of ovulation; during the period of progesterone secretion the temperature rises over that observed during the first half of the cycle. This phenomenon is useful in the timing of fertilization when pregnancy is desired.[5,9,11]

### Paternal reproductive system

The anterior pituitary functions in much the same manner for the regulation of the male reproductive system as for the female. FSH and LH (also known as interstitial cell–stimulating hormone, or ICSH) are secreted by the pituitary in response to the hypothalamus, and they work synergistically to control the production of testosterone and other male sex hormones produced throughout the body. Testosterone is the primary hormone for male sexual characteristics and reproductive function. This hormone is produced by the interstitial cells of Leydig, which lie between the seminiferous tubules in the testes. These cells are numerous in the fetus and newborn male infant and after puberty. At these stages relatively large amounts of testosterone are secreted. LH primarily stimulates the production of testosterone, and small amounts of FSH greatly potentiate the function of LH. When the total amount of testosterone becomes excessive, a negative feedback mechanism occurs to stop the production of LH and FSH, thus cutting the stimulation for further testosterone production.

The function of testosterone in stimulating the development of secondary male sexual characteristics is described in Chapter 14. In relation to reproduction, FSH is necessary for primary spermatogenesis to occur, and testosterone controls secondary spermatogenesis, or full maturation of the sperm. When spermatozoa form in the seminiferous tubules, they pass through the vasa recta into the epididymis. After 18 hours to 10 days in this area the spermatozoa develop the power of motility and the ability to fertilize an ovum. The capability of the sperm to travel in a normal, straight fashion is essential for fertilization to occur. This ability is enhanced by a neutral or slightly alkaline environment and by exposure to basal body temperature that is slightly higher than that of the testes. The increase in temperature encountered within the female body, while facilitating motility of the sperm, also shortens the life of the sperm, so that survival beyond 24 to 72 hours is not possible.

When appropriate neural and psychic stimuli lead to erection of the penis and ejaculation, reflex centers of the spinal cord begin to emit rhythmic sympathetic impulses that initiate emission of the spermatozoa. Peristaltic contractions of the ducts of the testes, epididymis, and vas deferens cause expulsion of the sperm into the internal urethra. Contractions involving the seminal vesicles and prostate gland cause the expulsion of seminal and prostatic fluids along with the sperm. These fluids, along with that formed by the bulbourethral glands, form the semen. Ejaculation is accomplished by further impulses from the spinal cord to the skeletal muscle at the base of the erectile tissue. Similar neural impulses from the spinal cord occur during coitus for the female, but the role that these impulses play in successful fertilization is not known, although they are believed to facilitate fertilization.[5,9,11]

### Factors leading to effective fertilization

Culmination of union between male and female sex cells and the beginning of life require several crucial factors, not all of which are fully understood. When the ovum lies within the fallopian tube and is penetrated successfully by a sperm cell, a zygote is formed and mitotic division of cells begins. Both of the sex cells have to be in a proper state of maturity before union can occur. A period of about five hours within the fallopian tube is required for both the sperm and the ovum in order for penetration to occur. The sperm must possess high motility and must be able to secrete an enzyme or enzymes that aid in the dissolution of the membrane surrounding the ovum at the point of entry. Although only one sperm penetrates the ovum successfully, it appears that a minimal sperm count of about 35,000,000/ml of semen is required for fertilization to occur. Although the process of spermatogenesis requires the slightly lower temperature maintained in the male testes, fertilization requires the basal temperature of the abdomen. The sperm must be uniform in size and shape, and they must be normally formed. The fallopian tube must be free from adhesions or obstructions, so that transport of the ovum and zygote may occur. The period of fertility for the female is believed to be within 24 hours of ovulation, since this places the ovum in the fallopian tube, where fertilization most commonly occurs within the lifespan of the sperm.[5,11]

### Factors leading to successful implantation

Transport of the ovum into the uterine cavity usually requires about three days. This period of time appears to be required for the developing zygote because secretions from the glands lining the tube seem to be important for the developing organism. When the uterine cavity is entered, the ovum remains unattached for an additional four or five days, and it receives nutrition from endometrial secretions. The cells that have formed around the developing zygote secrete enzymes that begin to digest and liquefy the endometrial lining and initiate conditions for attachment of the zygote and the beginning of the development of the placenta.

The event of fertilization triggers the production of greater amounts of progesterone. This hormone has already stimulated the formation of endometrial cells rich in glycogen, proteins, lipids, and minerals, and the extra supply of progesterone stimulates further development of these nourishing cells, known as decidua. The decidua provides nutrition for the embryo for 8 to 12 weeks, but the placenta begins to function within a week after implantation and also contributes to the nourishment of the developing organism. Excessive motility of the uterine muscle during this period interferes with effective implantation, and the pregnancy is not maintained. This is the principle of some drugs that are employed for the purpose of birth control, as well as of the intrauterine device for this purpose.[5]

## PRINCIPLES OF HEREDITY

Several concepts have been introduced in preceding sections that refer to genetic factors in the beginning of life. These are briefly described here and related to development.

### Chromosomes and genes

Chromosomes are contained within the nucleus of the cell and are composed of a double strand of deoxyribonucleic acid (DNA), which carries the genetic codes. The arrangement of amino acids comprising DNA varies to form different genes, which are attached to one another. The genes dictate by way of ribonucleic acid (RNA) the synthesis of enzymes that in turn control body metabolism. This ongoing process requires (1) essential proteins from which to build new cells and cell components, (2) energy,

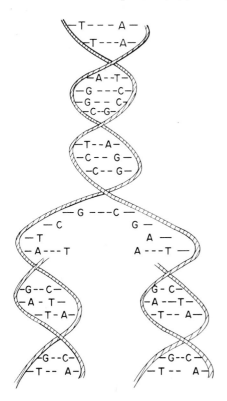

**Fig. 4-2.** Schematic representation of the duplication of a strand of DNA.

which derives primarily from the energizing molecule of adenosine triphosphate (ATP), and (3) molecules to form the linking structures, primarily hydrogen, oxygen, and phosphorus.

It is hypothesized that there are some genes for the specific functions of structure and building of body proteins and other genes for regulation and control of the structural genes. Alterations in the system, as when certain mutations occur, interfere with the normal regulation of cell production, and some aspect of normal body function is altered. A mutation is a change that occurs in the gene itself or in the configuration of the chromosome. Such changes are permanent and may be passed on to subsequent offspring. Factors causing mutations of genetic material are usually unknown, but it has been demonstrated that environmental hazards such as radiation, ingestion of drugs and other toxic substances, stress, and aging may be associated with mutations.

The ability of chromosomes to duplicate themselves is the significant property that allows for continuation of the species. Watson and Crick[7,9] in the early 1950s suggested a model for the replication of DNA, which has been confirmed through later studies. The chromosome, which is arranged in a double helical strand, contains nucleotides that are bound together in pairs by a phosphate group of the sugar of each nucleotide. The four nucleotides of DNA are adenine (A), which always pairs with thymine (T), and guanine (G), which pairs with cytosine (C) (Fig. 4-2). When replication occurs, the helical strands unwind, and each single strand of DNA serves as a template for the formation of a new double structure.[5,6,10,11]

### Cell division
#### Mitosis

The process by which autosomal, or the non-reproductive, cells of the body duplicate and increase in number is known as mitosis. This is illustrated diagrammatically in Fig. 4-3, which shows the major stages in cell duplication. The action of various components of the cytoplasm is not illustrated, and continuing investigation is needed to fully understand many facets of cell division that are not mentioned here. A few phenomena are known or hypothesized, which

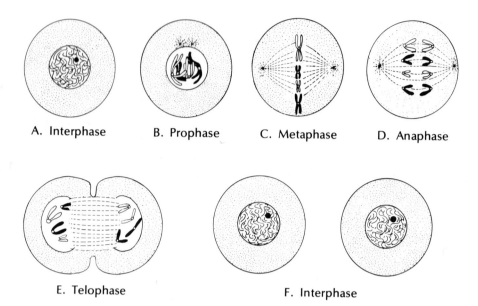

A. Interphase    B. Prophase    C. Metaphase    D. Anaphase

E. Telophase        F. Interphase

**Fig. 4-3.** The major stages of mitosis. The white chromosomes represent those inherited from one parent; the black from the other parent.

are important in understanding certain problems that occur during intrauterine and later life and in understanding the phenomena of human variation. Each new offspring is a unique individual unlike any before; the inheritance that is received from the mother and father combines in such a way that the infant carries their traits in his or her own unique way, and passes some of these on to future generations.

Mutation, described above, is one way in which variation occurs in human beings. The rate and incidence of mutation are not known, but mutation is presumed to occur with increasing frequency as age increases. Mutations do not always give rise to abnormalities or disease, and they may not be recognizable if the effect for the individual is within normal limits and does not interfere with life and health. Therefore, at the present time the study of mutations is pursued in relation to undesirable effects.

As chromosomal duplication progresses, small pieces of chromosomal material dissociate from the original configuration, and several phenomena may then happen. The material may become lost within the body of the cell and cease to participate in the reproductive process. This condition most often leads to death of the cell or the individual organism. The material may cross over, or exchange, with material from

a paired chromosome. This contributes to the variable inheritance that is possible, since the major portion of the genetic material contained on the chromosome may be inherited from one parent, with only a small portion now deriving from the other.

Material that becomes detached may attach itself to a chromosome of another pair. This phenomenon, known as translocation, is thought always to result in some abnormality.

Another type of unusual event may occur in the process of separation of the chromosomal pairs to the opposite poles, when one or more pairs do not separate. This event, known as nondisjunction, leads to one of the daughter cells containing none of the genetic material for that pair and the other daughter cell containing twice the chromosomal material. This extra chromosome leads to a condition known as trisomy when it occurs very early in cell duplication of the ovum. When it occurs later, it gives rise to a condition known as mosaicism. The term mosaicism refers to the fact that cells may be found in the body that reflect both overendowment and underendowment of genetic material.*

---

*References 1, 5, 6, 7, 10, 11.

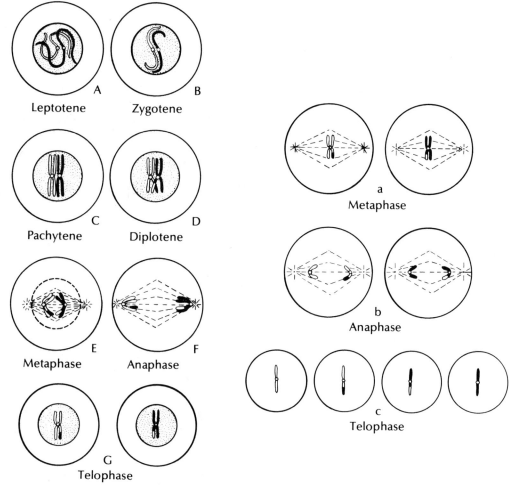

**Fig. 4-4.** The major stages of meiosis. *A* through *G* indicate the first meiotic division; *a* through *c* indicate the second meiotic division, culminating in four daughter cells, each containing one half of the original number of chromosomes.

*Meiosis*

The phenomenon of meiosis occurs only in the sexually reproductive cells, and it results in daughter cells that contain only half of the original number of chromosomes. Fig. 4-4 illustrates diagrammatically the process of meiosis and the mechanisms by which variation and resection occur in chromosomal material passed to the individual offspring. The human cell contains 23 pairs of chromosomes, or a total of 46. Each parent contributes 22 autosomes and 1 sex chromosome. The sex chromosomes are known as the X and Y pair (see Fig. 4-5). The Y chromosome carries genetic information that leads to

male characteristics, and the normal chromosomal pattern for men contains one each of the X and Y chromosomes. Females, on the other hand, possess two X chromosomes. The father is capable of passing to an offspring either sex chromosome, whereas the mother can only contribute the X chromosome. The fertilizing sperm cell contains either an X or a Y chromosome, and the sex of the offspring is determined as soon as the chromosomes from each parent pair to form the first nucleus of the ovum. If the sperm contains a Y, the child will be a boy; if it contains an X, the child will be a girl.

**101**

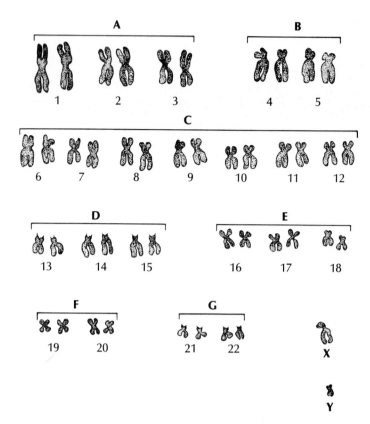

**Fig. 4-5.** Reproduction of human chromosomes during metaphase. The chromosomes are arranged according to a standard system known as a karyotype. This is often provided as a tool in genetic counseling.

### Oogenesis

During fetal development of the female, primary oocytes, precursors to the mature ovum, are formed from the germinal epithelial cells of the fetal ovaries. These total approximately 500,000 by birth. A few more primary oocytes and the surrounding granulosa cells may develop during infancy and childhood, but the majority of the oocytes develop to prophase of the first meiotic division before birth. These cells remain dormant at this stage until the time of ovulation of each particular oocyte, when maturation of the follicle occurs. Shortly before ovulation, the first meiotic division resumes and is completed. The second meiotic division begins with ovulation and is completed to the time of fertilization. This accomplishes the final maturation of the ovum containing 23 unpaired chromosomes. Thus the process of oogenesis involves a long period of development spanning anywhere from 12 to 50 years, and the age of the maternal gamete is believed to be an important factor in fetal outcome.

During the divisions that occur in meiosis, the cytoplasm of the oocyte divides unevenly, so that instead of producing two daughter cells that are equal in size and function, one cell becomes the large ovum and the others small, rudimentary cells incapable of reproduction.[1,10,11]

### Spermatogenesis

The entire process of spermatogenesis occurs in the seminiferous tubules of the testes after sexual maturation is reached. The spermatogonia, which lie at the periphery of the tubules, undergo the first and second meiotic divisions and within 75 days produce four mature sperm cells, each containing 23 chromosomes and having the capability of motility.[10,11]

## Factors affecting inheritance

Classic genetics, which began as a science with the publication of Mendel's paper in 1866, offered several hypotheses regarding the nature of inheritance, which are still accepted today. Many of these concepts are oversimplified for human genetics; multiple factors in the processes of metabolism and reproduction yield results that are not totally and accurately explained by the propositions. While the propositions may be demonstrated in lower forms of life, such as plants, bacteria, and flies, they are demonstrable in humans only in rare instances and through indirect evidence. Traits that cause illness, disability, or shortening of life are most easily studied in relation to inheritance. Although there seem to be unexplained factors in the ineritance of most human traits, the basic tenets of classic genetics are useful in studying family histories and in offering counseling for afflicted families.[7,8,12]

### Autosomal dominance and recessive inheritance

Each chromosome of a pair contains homologous genes that carry codes for the same traits. Since each gene pair is inherited from each of the individual's parents, the information carried is often for different effects. Each gene of a pair is known as an allele, and although they code the same type of information, they often give detectably different effects. For example, a trait such as skin color may require a specific gene for a particular aspect of shading. One allele may produce a very light skin shade, while the other may produce a darker skin shade. The trait that will be manifest for the individual depends upon the dominance of one allele over the other. This concept of dominance and recessiveness is a relative matter, because an allele that is dominant in combination with one gene may not be dominant in combination with another. In fact, it is supposed that genes influence the expression of one another in such a way as to cause a "mixing" effect in expression. In other cases both alleles may be fully expressed, as occurs when a person carries both A and B blood types. When a person carries the same gene rendering the same trait expression from each parent, he or she is *homozygous* for that condition. When the person carries two different alleles, he or she is *heterozygous*. When a genetic trait (genotype) is typically not expressed in the physical traits of individuals (phenotype) unless the individual is genetically homozygous for the trait, the condition is thought to be recessive in nature. That is, if the dominant trait were present genetically, the dominant trait, not the recessive trait, would be expressed physically.

### Variable expressivity

Genetic traits in humans seem to have variable expressivity, or penetrance. Several members of a family may develop a disease or condition that is known to be inherited, and yet one person is severely affected while another is only mildly affected. The same condition may tend to be more severe within one family than in another. Factors leading to variable expressivity are not well defined at this point.

### Pleiotropy

Genes set a series of events into action, which are often secondary and very different from the primary effect of the specific gene. Again, this phenomenon has been studied and understood in relation to undesirable traits. A gene that leads to absence of an essential enzyme is said to exert the primary effect of enzyme deficiency. As a result of this condition, many severe secondary effects may occur, which range from physical differences and abnormalities to metabolic, life-threatening consequences. For example, an infant who is born with phenylketonuria lacks the enzyme phenylalanine hydrolase as a primary effect of the gene. Among many secondary effects the child will develop very light blond hair regardless of the genetic characteristics for shades of hair that were inherited from the parents.

### Genetic heterogeneity

It is becoming clear that many disorders that appear superficially to be the same condition are in reality different genetic conditions, resulting from different genes and inheritance patterns. The muscular dystrophies, once thought to be one disorder, are now described as several distinguishable conditions. Until it is possible to study genetic factors governing inheritance in humans more directly, many problems of this sort will remain.

### Sex-linked inheritance

The specific pattern of inheritance that occurs on the X chromosome is more clearly subject to scrutiny by the indirect methods used in human genetics than are autosomal traits. The Y chromosome is not known presently to contain information other than that rendering maleness, and only a few rare conditions of abnormality have been associated with the Y chromosome. Conditions that demonstrate sex-linked recessive inheritance, such as classic hemophilia, are known to be coded from the X chromosome. For this reason the condition is almost always expressed physically by the male offspring of the mother who is the carrier. Females can only exhibit a recessive X chromosome gene when they are homozygous for the condition. Females in the family almost always inherit one X chromosome containing the dominant and desirable trait, thus preventing expression of the undesirable condition.[4,5,7] Fig. 4-6 illustrates a typical pattern of inheritance of a sex-linked recessive trait. Male to male transmission of the trait does not occur; it is not possible to detect female carriers until a male descendent has been affected.

## EMBRYONIC STAGES OF DEVELOPMENT

The stages of physical development that occur throughout embryonic life are well delineated and described for each of the structural systems of the body. Metabolic functions, particularly endocrine and neurologic functions, are less completely understood. There have been efforts to demonstrate the effect of various prenatal factors on subsequent behavior and personality of the child, but the isolation of a cause-and-effect relationship between specific influences, such as maternal stress or maternal nutrition, on long-term characteristics of the child has not been possible. The following description of embryonic development is that which is expected under normal conditions. The development of the embryo depends upon these events occurring at a specified critical period and in a specific order. When cells do not develop adequately at the necessary point in time and sequence, abnormality in structure or function occurs, since it becomes impossible for development to proceed normally. Various effects of influencing factors on gestational development will be explored in Chapter 5.

### First trimester

The first three months of pregnancy are critical for the development of the child. These

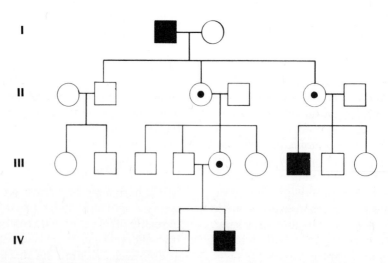

**Fig. 4-6.** Pedigree showing typical sex-linked recessive inheritance. The females who are carriers are indicated by a dot within the circle; males who are affected are indicated by blackened squares.

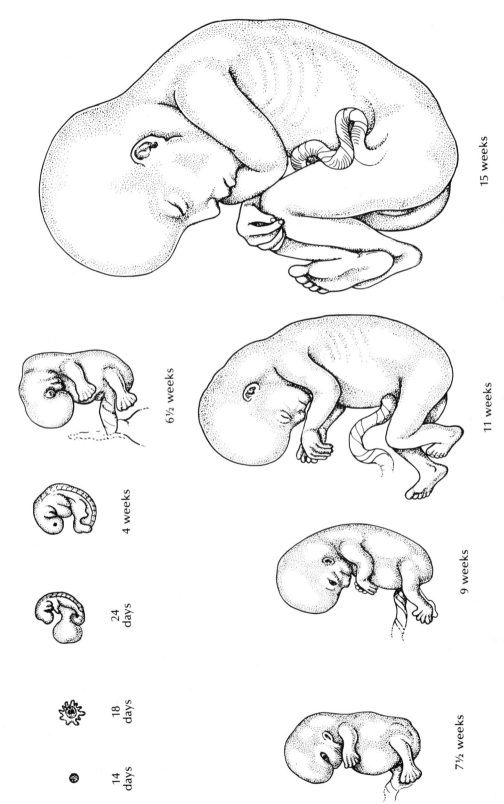

**Fig. 4-7.** The actual size of human embryos at early stages of development. Comparison of the relative stages of external development is also indicated.

14 days

18 days

24 days

4 weeks

6½ weeks

7½ weeks

9 weeks

11 weeks

15 weeks

weeks are characterized by extremely rapid cellular growth and differentiation of tissues into essential organs. By the time implantation occurs during the second week of gestation, tissues have begun to develop into distinct layers, differentiating according to types. These become the precursors of different body tissues. The rudiments of the central nervous system have begun to develop, and within a few days of implantation blood cells that are clearly those of the developing organism have formed. By the end of the fourth week of gestation, the blood cells and rudimentary circulatory system have become fairly well formed in the trunk. The heart has assumed major anatomic characteristics and has begun to pulsate. The respiratory and gastrointestinal systems have developed in rudimentary stages, as have the skeletal and muscular systems of the trunk. The nervous system is in a critical stage of development; the groove that forms the spinal cord is accomplishing closure, and rudimentary structures for the major sensory organs of the eye and ear are developing. Limb buds are distinguishable by this point in gestation.

At the fifth week of gestation, the embryo has a marked C-shaped body, accentuated by the presence of a rudimentary tail and large head folded over a large, protuberant trunk. Fig. 4-7 illustrates the relative shape and size of the human embryo at about this stage of development in contrast to earlier and later stages. The relatively large nervous system, heart, liver, and precursor to the genitourinary tract account for the external appearance of the embryo at this stage of development. Each of the systems has now been established in at least primordial form, and the umbilical cord organizes as a distinct unit. Blood vessels have extended into the head and limbs. The skin has developed a second layer of epidermis. Five brain vesicles can be distinguished, and the nerve and ganglial tissues are more fully developed.

At the sixth week of development the heart reaches definitive form characteristics of the human organ, with all septa intact, and the circulatory pathway that characterizes fetal life is established. Limbs are now recognizable as arms and legs, although ossification of skeletal tissue has not yet occurred. The embryonic head and face are approaching a critical stage of development, because the ridges of the jaws, the tissues that form the tongue and palate, are widely separated. The eyes are set at 160 degrees, and the external ear is in a very low-set position close to what seems to be the shoulder. The intestine begins to elongate and form loops, and the stomach begins to differentiate and assume the rotated position. The lungs now have formed the lobes with the bronchi beginning to branch. The liver begins to produce blood cells. Although a gonad, which is the precursor to both male and female gonads, is distinguishable, it is impossible to determine the sex of the embryo, because differentiation has not yet occurred.

Significant events occur in the gastrointestinal and genitourinary tract during the seventh week of gestation; until approximately this point the rectum and the bladder-urethra are part of the same structure with no external opening. During this period the rectum separates from the bladder-urethra, and each forms into a separate tube. Shortly thereafter, the urethral and anal openings form. Fetal circulation is further established with final formation of the inferior vena cava and the differentiation of the cardiac valves. Eyelids begin to form over the lens of the eyes, and nerve fibers to the sensory areas of the head are more completely developed.

At the end of the eighth week, and before the end of the second month of gestation, the embryo reaches the fetal stage of development. It has not yet begun to assume a "human" appearance, but several external features are surprisingly advanced. The fingers and toes are well formed at this point, and it begins to assume a more nearly erect posture. Glands of the body, such as the thyroid, adrenals, and those lining the intestine, are nearing more mature development. The liver is very large, and the diaphragm is formed. The main blood vessel system has completed development, and the lymphatic system has begun formation. Testes and ovaries are distinguishable as such, but external differentiation of sex is still impossible. Definitive muscles have formed for all parts of the body, and the fetus is capable of movement. The eyes have begun to converge rapidly, and the cerebral cortex has formed. Olfactory lobes are visible, but the nose is still flat and the nostrils are not yet open.

The tenth through twelfth weeks of development are particularly crucial for the development of the face and mouth, since during this period the palate fuses completely, lips separate from the jaw, the cheeks become distinguishable as facial features, and the nasal septum forms the nasal passages. The kidney becomes functional in that it acquires the ability to secrete urine, and the bladder expands into a sac. External genitalia become distinguishable as male or female, and internal sex organs begin definitive development for the appropriate sex. The lungs acquire definitive shape. Enucleated red blood cells are predominant in the circulation, and the bone marrow begins to produce blood cells. Ossification of the skeletal system begins, hair follicles begin to appear on the face, and the nail beds of the fingers and toes are apparent. The spinal cord reaches definitive internal structure, and the brain reaches the general structural characteristic of the human organ. Essential structures of the eye are formed and arranged in characteristic organization; the eyelids are fused.

By the end of the first trimester of pregnancy, the fetus is not yet capable of extrauterine life, but essential formation of the body structures is complete. Growth and maturation proceed throughout the remainder of gestational life, with many essential developmental events occurring that lead to the ability to sustain life. The most hazardous point of prenatal existence has passed, for the primary, crucial period of genetic endowment has been determined, and the delicate miracle of formation of human structure and rudimentary function from a single cell has been accomplished.

## Second trimester

Early in the second trimester, at about the sixteenth week of gestation, the fetus assumes a "human" appearance. The face has formed with the eyes close to the nasal bridge, the trunk and limbs have grown larger in proportion to the head, and hair begins to appear on the head. Metabolic function begins to develop with the acquisition of more mature glands; the pituitary, gonads, tonsils, and lymphatics acquire defini-

tive structure and begin to function. Meconium begins to accumulate in the intestine, indicating some activity of smooth as well as skeletal muscle. The lungs remain functionally immature throughout the second trimester, but their structure is primarily completed by the end of the sixteenth week. Blood formation becomes a function of the spleen. The bones of the entire skeletal system are indicated, and joint cavities begin to form. Muscular movements of the fetus are detectable by the mother early during the second trimester.

By the twentieth week of gestation, lanugo has developed over the entire body, and vernix caseosa begins to appear. Myelinization of the spinal cord begins and continues through infancy and toddlerhood. The function of blood formation lessens in the liver and increases in the bone marrow. Enamel and dentin begin to form in the primary tooth buds. The nostrils open. Growth and maturation of functional development proceed throughout the second trimester until, at about the twenty-eighth to thirty-second week of gestation, the fetus is theoretically capable of sustaining extrauterine life.

## Third trimester

The lungs, which are essential for viability, do not achieve adequate maturity until late in the third trimester. Pulmonary branching, formation of the alveoli, and the ability of the lungs to secrete surfactant remain grossly immature so that at any point prior to the thirty-sixth week of gestation the infant is in jeopardy of not being able to adequately exchange gases in the lungs and support extrauterine life. Recent advances in the study of amniotic fluid for the ratio of lecithin and sphingomyelin offer promising avenues for assessing the ability of the lung to produce surfactant and for estimating the gestational age of the infant.

During the third trimester, which is a period of rapid growth and weight gain, the fetus collects fat in subcutaneous tissue, which changes his appearance from that of a wrinkled, lean fetus to a rounded, smooth infant. The maturation of the skin, with further development of epidermal layers, contributes to a pinkish coloring rather than the red appearance typical of the younger fetus. The gonads achieve final structural form, and in the male the testes begin to descend into the scrotal sac late in the third trimester.

Cerebral fissures appear rapidly during the third trimester, and myelinization of the brain begins. All of the sensory organs become functional, although at birth the sensory abilities of the infant remain immature and primitive. Reflexes begin to appear by the beginning of the third trimester, but only the Moro reflex is typically present during the early weeks of this period of gestation. The ability to suck begins to appear at about the thirtieth week, but as reflexes appear they are immature and rapidly exhaustible. As the fortieth week, or term, approaches, the reflexes and neuromuscular capacity of the infant increase greatly, thus enhancing the infant's chance for surviving extrauterine life.

### The placenta and fetal membranes

Throughout embryonic and fetal life the primary source of nourishment is from the placenta. This essential organ begins to develop at the time of implantation, when integration of the embryonic cells and the cells of the decidua begins. The chorionic and amniotic membranes, which surround the fetus throughout gestation, also begin to form in connection with the placenta, as does the amniotic fluid, which provides a support medium for the developing infant and protection from injury.

The basic structure of the mature placenta (Fig. 4-8) provides for the interchanges that occur between the mother and the fetus in the processes of providing nourishment for the fetus and excreting fetal waste materials. Maternal blood flows through the intervillous spaces; the chorionic villi contain the fetal vessels. The unique structure of the tissues between the two circulatory systems allows for exchange of certain molecules but prevents mixing of the two blood supplies. Previously it was supposed that the placenta offered a barrier to most toxic influences from the maternal system, but the existence of this barrier has not been substantiated. Large molecules cannot pass, and there are fac-

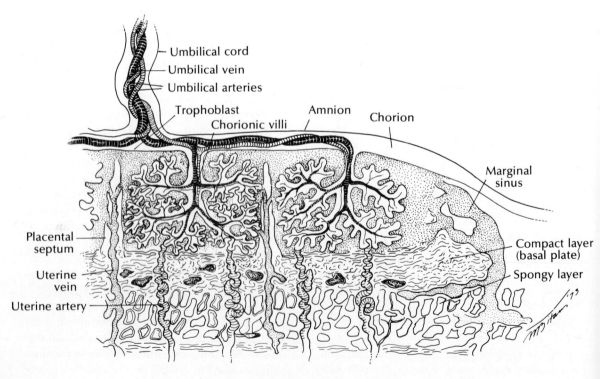

Umbilical cord
Umbilical vein
Umbilical arteries
Trophoblast
Chorionic villi
Amnion
Chorion
Marginal sinus
Placental septum
Compact layer (basal plate)
Uterine vein
Spongy layer
Uterine artery

**Fig. 4-8.** Structure of the mature placenta.

tors that inhibit certain exchanges, but the exact function of the placenta in the exchange of substances is not clearly understood.

Inspection of the placenta after birth reveals important clues of the adequacy of gestational life. The placenta contains distinctive lobules, known as cotyledons, which number from 14 to 30 and are incompletely separated from one another by thin septal partitions. The tissue of the placenta appears dark red, with the spongy maternal side darker than the shiny fetal side, which has a gray, glassy appearance. The umbilical cord normally rises from near the center of the placenta, and the membranes rise smoothly from the rim. Abnormal insertion of the cord, necrotic areas of the placenta, abnormal insertion of the membranes, or two umbilical vessels rather than three, are signals of possible problems initiated during gestation but which may not be immediately apparent in the infant.

The fetus, who has continued to gain strength and maturity during the later weeks of gestation, assumes a position with the head resting in the lower maternal pelvis. Fig. 4-9 illustrates the relationship of the fully developed fetus to the placental and membrane structures. The membranes provide protection from infection for the fetus as well as a container for the amniotic fluid. As birth begins, the membranes rupture, causing the loss of amniotic fluid. When labor is imminent, this often stimulates strengthening of uterine contractions, but when rupture of the membranes is premature, risk to the infant from infection is great.

At the time that gestation nears completion, the placenta decreases gradually in function. This decrease is thought to be one possible stimulus for the onset of labor. When gestation proceeds beyond the point of fetal development, there is considerable risk to the infant's well-being because its source of nourishment and waste disposal is continually declining.[2,3,4]

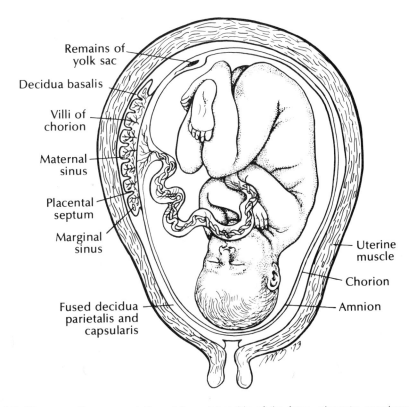

Remains of yolk sac

Decidua basalis

Villi of chorion

Maternal sinus

Placental septum

Marginal sinus

Fused decidua parietalis and capsularis

Uterine muscle

Chorion

Amnion

**Fig. 4-9.** Diagrammatic representation of the relationship of the fetus, placenta, membranes, and uterus near the end of gestation.

## STUDY QUESTIONS

1. Interview a young mother or expectant mother to ascertain important clues to possible hereditary and developmental prenatal factors. Relate the information from the mother to the information reviewed in this chapter.
2. Describe the point during gestation when abnormalities are most likely to occur for the following structures:
   a. Heart and great vessels
   b. Mouth
   c. Gastrointestinal tract
   d. Skeletal system
   Why are they particularly vulnerable at this point in development?
3. Relate your knowledge of possible means of family planning to the processes of reproduction. How does each approach interfere with reproduction, and what steps are taken to reestablish reproduction when this is desired?
4. Describe traits that you can identify as inherited among the members of your family. Is there evidence of dominance or recessiveness? Variability of expression? Pleiotrophy? Sex-linked inheritance?

## REFERENCES

1. Alfi, O. S.: Genetic disorders in adolescents and young adults, Pediatr. Clin. North Am. **20**:865, Nov., 1973.
2. Arey, L. B.: Developmental anatomy; a textbook and laboratory manual of embryology, ed. 7, Philadelphia, 1965, W. B. Saunders Co.
3. Charnock, E. L., and Doershuk, C. F.: Developmental aspects of the human lung, Pediatr. Clin. North Am. **20**:275, May, 1973.
4. Dobbing, J.: The later growth of the brain and its vulnerability, Pediatrics **53**:2, Jan., 1974.
5. Guyton, A. C.: Textbook of medical physiology, ed. 5, Philadelphia, 1976, W. B. Saunders Co.
6. Hsia, D. Y.: Human developmental genetics, Chicago, 1968, Year Book Medical Publishers, Inc.
7. Moore, J. A.: Heredity and development, ed. 2, New York, 1972, Oxford University Press.
8. Reisman, L. E., and Matheny, A. P.: Genetics and counseling in medical practice, St. Louis, 1969, The C. V. Mosby Co.
9. Selkurt, E. E., editor: Physiology, ed. 4, Boston, 1976, Little, Brown and Co.
10. Thompson, J. S., and Thompson, M. W.: Genetics in medicine, Philadelphia, 1966, W. B. Saunders Co.
11. Timiras, P. S.: Developmental physiology and aging, New York, 1972, Macmillan Publishing Co., Inc.
12. Valentine, G. H.: The reproductive counseling process, Clin. Pediatr. **16**:233, March, 1977.

# Providing a healthy prenatal environment

Philosophers, theologians, and lawyers continue to debate the moment at which a human fetus assumes a spirit and the inalienable rights of all humans. But for health and protection, the moment of conception begins the important period of prenatal life when sustenance and nurturance are totally dependent upon the mother's body, her health, and well-being.[34] The developing fetus is to some extent protected from many potential hazards which threaten its well-being, because within the uterus the fetus lives in a constant thermal environment, where only those substances that cross the placenta can enter from the external environment. The mysteries of the hazards of prenatal life have puzzled humankind for centuries, and most cultures are rich with folklore surrounding the gestational period. Scientific investigations have provided some evidence that more accurately guides health care workers in helping a mother reach a satisfactory conclusion of her pregnancy. Because of the bothersome infant mortality rate in the United States and several other medically advanced countries, care of the expectant mother has received intensive scrutiny, with the demonstrated result that, indeed, the infant's chances for survival are enhanced when the mother receives optimal health care during pregnancy.

## SUPPORTING MATERNAL PHYSIOLOGY
### The folklore of prenatal influences

In every known human culture there are strong beliefs about factors and influences that either enhance or endanger the outcome of pregnancy.[25] These attitudes are superstitious, and they tend to be most prevalent when the culture has been relatively unexposed to advances of modern science. In spite of the availability of advanced knowledge in a society, however, the attitudes and beliefs of the culture persist to an amazing degree and become expressed in unexpected forms, depending upon the strength of cultural influences and idiosyncrasies of the individual mother and her family. These attitudes commonly involve strict limitations, or taboos, on certain kinds of behavior or exposure to certain specified influences. These may be either external influences, such as ingestion of certain foods, exposure to some form of "evil eye," or participating in some specific activity, or internal influences (from within the mother herself), such as a sudden fright, anger, frustrations, or peace and tranquility.

Some of the food taboos, as well as other beliefs to be discussed, may not seem logical or conceivable to a person of another culture or belief, yet these ideas persist tenaciously. Often the person who is practicing them is not fully convinced of their worth but is afraid to break the taboos just in case they should turn out to be correct. In many cases, where no harm is done, the belief or practice is important to the mental health or social well-being of the pregnant woman and her family.

Particularly prevalent are the many superstitions regarding the appropriateness of foods during pregnancy. The animism typical of the life and cultures of primitive societies is evident in common beliefs and food taboos. A particular trait of an animal or animal product that is forbidden for consumption during pregnancy is often said to become a trait of the child. Some aboriginal tribes of Australia forbid the eating of porcupine; consumption of this usual dietary meat may lead to a child who is humpbacked. An African tribe of the Bantu in eastern Portuguese Africa forbids the eating of eggs lest the child be bald forever. Characteristics of the animal or food product are often said to affect the child in utero in other ways, such as the snake being able to scare the child or the frog or eel causing the child to be born too suddenly or too soon. In Madagascar pregnant women are not to eat the snout of an animal for fear of causing cleft lip or palate in the unborn child. In some cultures food taboos apply to the father of the unborn child also; he and his wife may each affect the unborn child by eating specified foods.

Beliefs surrounding external influences also reflect animism and belief in spirits typical of primitive cultures. In some modern cultures the spiritual reasons for attitudes and beliefs toward external influences have been lost, but the practices persist with the members of the culture, who do not fully understand why this should be so. A pregnant woman must not, in some tribes, walk across a stream for fear that her unborn child will be carried away by the spirits of the water. In many tribes elaborate precautions are taken to protect the mother and unborn child from a variety of evil spirits, which may visit them and bring harm to the mother or the child. Effects of the moon and its cycles are particularly troublesome for many cultures, and an eclipse of the moon is often believed to possess magical powers that harm the unborn child.

Certain things that a woman usually does during the course of her everyday work become forbidden during pregnancy in the fear that the act will cause certain characteristics in the unborn child or will harm the child in some way. The use of a knife to cut fish or meat is said to bring the risk of stabbing the unborn child or cutting off the limbs. Tying knots or twisting yarn and/or walking around in circles have all been associated with causing some problem with the cord of the unborn child, such as knotting of the cord or strangling the infant with the cord around the neck. In some cultures these same hazards are said to result from the father's tying an animal with a rope.

Another type of influence derives from things with which a mother comes in close contact or looks upon during pregnancy. Looking upon something dead is said to cause the infant to be born dead. Looking upon a deformed or unsightly person, animal, or statue is said to result in a child who is similarly affected. Likewise, a mother is said to be able to produce a handsome or beautiful child by looking at beautiful things or people or by being close to them during pregnancy.

In some cultures the infant is said to be affected by the ways in which a mother dresses or behaves, by changes in her external appearance, or by the food she craves. Distorting her facial expression may cause the infant to be permanently disfigured in the same manner. Holding her breath at any time during pregnancy may cause her infant to be unable to breathe when he is born. Among the most persistent beliefs surrounding pregnancy in most modern societies are those concerning the emotions that the mother feels during pregnancy. Birthmarks are commonly said to be the result of fright or food cravings during pregnancy, and the shape of the mark reveals the object or animal that frightened the mother or the food craved. Other cultures have associated birthmarks with eating certain foods, such as strawberries. Objects of clothing or adornment worn by the mother during pregnancy are often associated with birthmarks; if there is no taboo concerning the wearing of such articles, many cultures seek a post hoc explanation of the mark by pointing to some article, such as a necklace or particular piece of clothing frequently worn by the mother during pregnancy.

Superstitions regarding when and to whom the pregnancy is announced also involve the potential endangering of the well-being of the child. If the impending birth is announced too early or too widely, the child is more likely to be endangered. Purchasing needed infant clothing before birth is often identified as an undesirable action that will result in disaster for the child. Going into high places, being confined in small enclosures, viewing a frightening movie, thinking bad thoughts, and feeling envious of another person are all associated with undesirable outcomes for the infant. On the other hand, a mother is said to be able to influence the development of desirable traits in her infant by doing certain things during pregnancy. She will have a child with a sweet disposition if she thinks good, kind, gentle thoughts during pregnancy; she will produce a muscially talented child if she associates often with music.[8,35]

Mothers in modern societies are often reluctant to reveal their underlying motivation for behaving in a certain way or for avoiding certain foods, behaviors, or experiences. The commonly experienced fear of giving birth to an infant who is abnormal in some respect often leads to practices that the expectant mother may reject or oppose under other circumstances. When these practices are in opposition to recommendations of the health care of modern science, the conflict that results may be inordinately disturbing for the mother and family unless in some tactful manner the matters can be explored and understood. The result sought must in some satisfactory manner facilitate the physical and emotional health of the mother and avoid pitfalls endangering the health of mother or infant. In many instances there is no sound reason for a conflict to exist between practices arising from folklore and those of adequate health care, for many folklore practices do not violate basic principles of health.

## Interactions among general factors influencing the mother and fetus

Several important factors are thought to be so pervasive that they invariably interact with all other influences that affect the health and well-

being of the mother and fetus. Several circumstances, such as geographical location and time of the year or lunar cycle at which conception occurs, have been demonstrated to bear a statistical relationship with fetal outcome, but the relationships remain obscure and not fully tested. Furthermore, many of the supposed influences on the health of the fetus are such that intervention is virtually impossible, even if the nature of the relationship were fully understood. The factors mentioned in this chapter, while not completely understood in terms of the nature of the effect, are considered to be amenable to social and individual intervention, with a potentially beneficial outcome.

### Socioeconomic resources

Probably the single most pervasive factor affecting the health of mothers and unborn children around the world is that of the socioeconomic resources available to them. In countries where all people receive equivalent health care during pregnancy regardless of family income, this effect is virtually eliminated, because care has a greater effect on health than larger personal income. Infant death rates, the commonly used indicator of adequacy of maternal and infant health care, have been effectively and significantly reduced when groups of mothers who are known to be at risk for high rates of infant death are given adequate prenatal care.[2,8,32] Other indices of desirable fetal outcomes, such as birth weight, gestational age at birth, subsequent development of the child, and condition of the placenta at birth, have likewise indicated the striking disadvantage that occurs in the face of inadequate socioeconomic resources.[1,12,14,18,39]

These associations offer us no explanations. The fact that the parents are poverty-stricken or financially burdened is not the direct cause of the unborn child's disadvantage; direct causes arise from accompanying factors, such as inadequate nutrition, illness (which occurs more frequently and without adequate medical care), ignorance, and social stress. Regrettably, the exact importance of each factor is unknown, and in fact conflicting evidence regarding each of the suspected influences leads to a great deal of confusion and disagreement concerning necessary intervention. Thus it becomes practical to speak of the general matrix of socioeconomic disadvantage as important, for under these conditions the important specific influences combine to create the disadvantage for the unborn child and lead to risk for the well-being of mother and child.

### Genetic inheritance

The genotype of the fetus has been suspected to render particular susceptibility to certain kinds of hazards, but the relationship is still unclear. It appears that some individual infants are more apt to develop congenital anomalies in response to environmental hazards than others. A family trait of sensitivity to drugs, pollutants, or infections that seems to occur in older children and adults appears somehow accentuated for the fetus.[2,40]

### Maternal age and parity

The risk of undesirable outcome of pregnancy for the infant is significantly related to the mother's age at the time of delivery and to the number of previous pregnancies she has had. Generally speaking, the younger mother with multiple pregnancies (three or more under age 20) is particularly handicapped in producing a healthy infant. Mothers who are first pregnant during the middle teenage years are also more likely to have an infant who is not well at birth. The rate of infant prematurity and illness in the first month of life is sharply higher for this mother than for the older mother. The mother's optimum age for bearing the first child, in terms of her own well-being, seems to be at about the age of 18, but the risk for the infant continues to be higher than for the mother who is in her 20s. After the age of 30, the risk for both the mother and infant begins to rise significantly. A greater number of inherited conditions appear in infants born to mothers after age 30 to 35 years, with the risk after age 40 rising sharply. Infant deaths from all causes begin to rise after the maternal age of 30. The exact reasons for these relationships are largely speculative, except for the case of the older mother who gives birth to a child with an inherited condition, where evidence suggests that a breakdown of chromosomal material occurs with increasing age.

Statistics describing the general association between maternal age, parity, and fetal outcome are not to be confused with an explanation for infant risks. Mothers of lower socioeconomic groups and minority cultures are overrepresented in the younger and older age groups with increased parity in all age classifications, suggesting once again that multiple factors comprising the social condition of these mothers in reality represent multiple interacting causes for increased risk to infants. Biologically it is presumed that maternal physiology cannot support many pregnancies in rapid succession, and as age increases the ability to cope with stresses of pregnancy decreases. These presuppositions seem to be demonstrated for all sociocultural groups. However, the fact remains that for some reason disadvantaged mothers of all ages and stages of parity suffer an increased risk of producing an infant who is not well, as illustrated by Fig. 5-1 in relation to prematurity. Data that are potentially available for such evaluations are not often compiled in a manner that can be examined and probed for clues to underlying problems, and often the effort is futile. Associations, once again, are discovered, but causes remain elusive.*

### Pervasive environmental factors

Factors in the maternal environment, such as level of irradiation, pollution of the air, water, and food, that increase the psychologic and physiologic stresses of daily living are becoming increasingly important for all humans, and particularly for the unborn. The effects of certain sources of pollution on the ability to reproduce and rear offspring are well documented in current animal populations of the world. Although it is impossible to make direct inferences from animals to humans, there is evidence that specific substances, such as trace metals and radiation, produce certain kinds of teratogenic, or harmful, effects on human infants. These effects are similar to those of drugs and diseases discussed in the next section, but the important feature of environmental sources of harm lies in the fact that these substances are usually undetectable by the individual or family, and thus in-

*References 2, 8, 12, 16, 18, 27, 39.

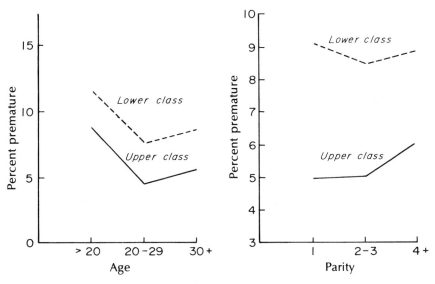

**Fig. 5-1.** Prematurity rates by maternal age and social status *(left)* and by parity and social status *(right).* (Based on data from Donnelly, J. F., and others: Maternal, fetal and environmental factors in prematurity, Am. J. Obstet. Gynecol. **88:**918, 1964. Graphs from Birch, H. G., and Gussow, J. D.: Disadvantaged children: Health, nutrition, and school failure, New York, Grune & Stratton, Inc. Used by permission.)

dividual protection and safeguard are virtually impossible. Social action and societal control of environmental pollutants are required for the protection of unsuspecting individuals.[8,37,40]

### The role of the placenta

It has long been known that the placenta supplies the fetus with essential nutrients, provides for the excretion of wastes, and protects the fetus from harmful substances. These functions have each been confirmed but are not sufficiently understood to allow prediction of which substances will cross the placenta and which will not. This was formerly believed to be controlled by molecular size, with the heavier molecules not passing the placenta. This, in fact, may be a factor, but it is not the mechanism by which placental transfer occurs. Diffusion, facilitated diffusion, and active transport are all demonstrated to participate in the transfer mechanisms of the placenta. Pinocytosis, a form of active transport, has been demonstrated to transport larger lipid and protein molecules through the membranes.[43] Currently, a substance is presumed to be transferable to the infant unless substantial evidence indicates otherwise. This leads to increased concern with regard to drug use during

pregnancy and provides the safest guideline for maternal ingestion of materials.

### Specific influences and their effects

The study of specific, potentially hazardous influences and of the optimal levels of potentially beneficial influences on the developing human fetus is severely limited by the ethical requirements of human research. Animal studies give some direction and aid in contrasting less well-controlled findings of human studies, but generally the results on animals have limited value in understanding human reproductive phenomena. The discussions of each of the factors considered here will be limited, therefore, to findings of human studies.

### Maternal nutrition

The large volume of evidence regarding the general effects of adequate nutrition on the viability, growth, and development of the unborn child conclusively indicates that, in humans, this is one of the most important variables for satisfactory health and well-being of the fetus. Maternal malnutrition during pregnancy, which is usually a life-long state of inadequacy, has been implicated as exerting a possible terato-

**115**

genic effect on the fetus. The principal fetal system that is usually damaged is the central nervous system, leading to impaired intelligence performance later in life; malnutrition may also be associated with neuropsychiatric disorders.[18,49]

Poor maternal nutrition during pregnancy is less well understood. It is presumed that there is a possible direct effect of depriving the fetus of essential nutrients for growth and development and an indirect effect of contributing to development of maternal disease states that interfere with pregnancy. However, there is evidence that the effects of poor nutrition are most severe for the young adolescent, who herself still has growth requirements, and for the mother with accumulated effects of several pregnancies, at which time prolonged poor nutrition more directly affects the fetus. Nutritional deficiencies of the mother during her own fetal, infancy, and childhood years contribute to the development of structural and physiologic disadvantages for supporting a growing fetus. Maternal stature and pelvic development, which evolve from prior nutritional state as well as genetic endowment, may influence the difficulty of labor.[18] There is suggestive evidence that improvement of the diet of pregnant women who have been poorly nourished throughout life does not always appreciably improve their ability to produce healthy offspring. Poor nutrition throughout the life of the mother may be more significant than the inadequacy of the diet during pregnancy. This evidence superficially appears to conflict with the evidence supporting the proposition that the fetus derives most of the raw materials for development from the maternal diet and not, as formerly believed, from the mother's body structure and reserves. Maturity and development of all functional systems, such as essential enzyme systems, appear to depend heavily upon a lifetime of adequate nurturance. Thus utilizing dietary elements effectively may be impaired in the mother who has been poorly nourished. Further study is required to fully understand these aspects of nutrition.[49]

A major portion of families who eat poorly also suffer from socioeconomic limitations and they are often strongly influenced by dietary practices of a subculture. These factors compound efforts to fully understand the influence of poor nutrition on fetal well-being. Although differences in food habits and beliefs that are culturally based are important, the factor that keeps the diet inadequate in basic nutrients continues to be poverty. It seems apparent that cultural differences in type of diet lose nutritional significance as adequate economic resources become available. Families of all cultural groups who are relatively affluent tend to choose and eat foods from each of the four basic food groups, although the manner of preparation and seasoning continues to vary according to cultural practices.[2]

Evaluation of specific features of the diet and determination of essential levels of nutritive components that are optimal during pregnancy are complicated by the current inability to examine, under normal physiologic conditions, nutritive requirements of the fetus and the functional capacity of the human placenta.[13,48] The additional dietary demands of the mother, which exceed those of the nonpregnant woman of comparable age, have been estimated, and investigations leading to this knowledge have added greatly to understanding of normal physiologic adjustments made during pregnancy. Ideas regarding the demands of pregnancy have changed substantially as it has become understood that the woman herself requires more metabolic energy and structural resources to adequately support pregnancy.[38]

Calorie requirements during pregnancy exceed those of the nonpregnant woman by about 200 kilocalories each day, resulting in a weight gain of about 25 pounds. If, at the end of 20 weeks' gestation the woman has not gained at least 10 pounds, she should be considered a high risk mother in jeopardy of delivering an ill infant. The former belief that limitation of weight gain by limiting caloric intake during pregnancy was desirable was founded on the unsound notion that any weight gain, whether in the form of fat or liquid, was related to the development of toxemia. Although there is considerable variation among women in the rate of gain and in the total gain during pregnancy, it is now recognized that to limit weight gain by limitation of caloric intake is seriously hazardous to the well-being of the fetus. Low maternal weight gain, as well as being underweight at the onset of pregnancy, is associated with infants who are underweight for gestational age and risk the hazards of impaired neonatal adjustment that accompany low birth weight. The woman who is overweight at the time of conception also risks endangering the fetus if an attempt is made during pregnancy to lose her own body weight. The effects of ketoacidosis, which occurs as a result of caloric limitations, have been associated with neuropsychologic defects in infants.[31] Thus with the exception of the presence of specific disease states in the mother, it is advisable to eat a well-balanced diet according to appetite.[20,30,31]

The well-balanced diet of the pregnant woman is similar to the diet needed by all humans, with specific increases of certain components as recommended by the Food and Nutrition Board of the National Research Council.[4,38] These recommendations are based on research findings available to the date of publication, and they are constantly subject to revision as new findings emerge. It is well to approach the diet of a pregnant woman in terms of the food that is offered to the entire family. Asking a mother to feed herself differently from other family members is usually an unrealistic and unacceptable idea. It may be tempting to recommend that limited resources be directed to upgrading nutrition for the mother and fetus, but such recommendations are futile if family needs are not considered.

Protein requirements during pregnancy are estimated to be about 1.2 gs/kg/day, as opposed to the nonpregnant woman's requirement of about 1.0 g/kg/day. It is usually advisable that animal protein constitute the major source of protein during pregnancy, since these contain the most complete supply of essential amino acids, but achieving this goal may be virtually impossible when resources are limited. Because the protein requirement of the family diet is the most costly, money management problems must first consider this essential component, and a larger proportion of nonanimal protein sources may be necessary.

The most important increase of intake during pregnancy aside from the calorie and protein re-

quirements is minerals. Increase in protein foods usually provides the essential minerals needed in increased amounts, particularly phosphorus and calcium. Calcium is mainly deposited in the fetus during the last month of gestation. The rapid deposition at this time requires a good supply stored from the early months of pregnancy to meet this demand and to minimize depletion of maternal calcium supplies. One quart of cow's milk each day supplies about 1 g of calcium; the requirement of the pregnant woman is estimated to be about 1.2 g per day. Other protein foods consumed in adequate amounts supply the extra amounts needed.

Vitamin supplementation, a common practice among American physicians, is of unsubstantiated value. If the woman's diet is well balanced and adequate in amount, the food sources of vitamins and minerals should be adequate to meet the needs of pregnancy with the exception of the needs for iron. It has been convincingly demonstrated that supplementation with 30 to 60 mg of ferrous iron during the last three to four months of pregnancy can be beneficial in building and protecting maternal iron stores.[30,38] Some evidence exists regarding the desirability of folic acid supplementation, particularly in the face of potential or real anemia or multiple pregnancy.

Fats and carbohydrates are needed in an amount that will supply the caloric requirements during pregnancy. Although a portion of the caloric increase is supplied by protein increase, protein components are needed for the body-building requirements of pregnancy and fetal growth. Fats and carbohydrates remain the most important sources of energy, and they also supply essential vitamins and minerals. Supplementation of additional vitamins and minerals, while not known to cause harm to the mother or fetus if conducted within reasonable limits, is usually a costly way to achieve nutritional improvement when compared with the cost of improving the dietary intake of the mother and family. The related benefits of increasing consumption of needed components that exist in the form of food may be of more importance than is currently recognized.

The practice of pica, or the eating of nonfood substances, by pregnant women occurs with significant frequency among economically deprived black Americans to warrant special consideration. This phenomenon is known to exist among small children, particularly when hunger and poor nutrition are a common state of affairs. The practice is not limited to pregnant women of black or economically deprived groups. The hunger and poor nutrition of the economically deprived pregnant woman, combined with normal cravings for food or nonfood substances, lead to a culturally acceptable practice of eating such materials as starch, mud, clay, soap, or plaster. While this practice has been known to exist for centuries among many groups of people, it is not understood in relation to possible harm that can develop or the causes for the practice occurring more commonly during pregnancy than at other times during adult life. The effect that has been most reliably associated with pica is the presence of iron deficiency anemia, but whether this condition would be present in the absence of pica is not known.[7]

### Drugs during pregnancy

Until 1961 only a few cases of malformation in humans had been attributed to drugs. Among these, quinine, which causes abortion, malformations, and possibly deafness, had been identified. The teratogenic effects of most drugs that are studied in animals are difficult or impossible to implicate in humans, as no well-controlled study is possible that examines the interaction of all complex variables that operate in humans. As a result of a tragic inadvertent human experiment with the tranquilizing drug thalidomide in the early 1960s, this drug has been confirmed as a teratogenic drug for the human fetus. The experience with this drug has led to an extremely conservative approach in the administration of any drug for pregnant women. However, the fact remains that during the most critical early weeks of development, a woman usually is not aware of the fact that she is pregnant.

At the time that thalidomide was first introduced in 1956 it was thought to be effective against influenza. When it was later found to have a sedative effect on humans, it quickly gained popularity and increased in use. The experimental data available on the drug at the time was scanty and of questionable value, but the features of being highly effective as a sedative with an amazingly low degree of acute toxicity even in high doses appealed greatly to manufacturers and to practitioners. The incidence of certain types of malformations of the limbs and ears, which had been exceedingly rare prior to this date, followed the sales figures by three-quarters of a year and abruptly declined by the end of July 1962, about six months after the drug was removed from the market. The period of human sensitivity to the drug has been demonstrated to be between the twenty-eighth and forty-second day after conception. The severity and type of malformation that follows depend upon the exact point within this period that the drug is ingested by the mother.[8,21,47]

Table 5-1 summarizes data regarding other drugs that are currently ingested by women in the general population either through prescription or from over-the-counter sources, with an indication of the suspected effects on the fetus and the strength of evidence relating the drug to the particular effect.*

The fetal response to drugs, as illustrated by the thalidomide incident, is a serious interference with normal growth and development of any of the systems of the body that happen to be developing during the first trimester at the time of drug ingestion. The mechanism for this occurrence is largely speculative. As the fetus matures during the later half of pregnancy, its response to drugs that cross the placental barrier seems to more closely resemble that of the neonate. The mechanisms of absorption, distribution, metabolism, and excretion of drug substances occur according to the ability of the fetal organs to adequately perform these functions. Differences in drug action at different fetal stages may be dependent upon the level of maturity of a series of interdependent mechanisms that are developing at differential rates during fetal life.[6,29,33,43] There is also the possibility that drugs alter the placenta itself or that the placenta reacts differentially to this influence at different stages of pregnancy.[19,43]

*References 6, 19, 24, 26, 29, 33, 44, 46, 50.

*Maternal metabolic factors*

Fetal sustenance, growth, and development are vitally dependent upon the many endocrine and metabolic adjustments that occur during pregnancy. The placenta participates in providing necessary estrogens, progesterone, and gonadotropin to sustain pregnancy and to trig-ger the other endocrine adjustments of the maternal system. These adjustments involve primarily the pituitary, adrenal cortex, and thyroid. Fetal endocrine function appears to be regulated independently from that of the mother, but evidence elucidating the interrelationships of the functions of the two systems is con-

**Table 5-1.** Adverse effects of drugs during fetal life*

| Drug | Effect on fetus | Dependability of evidence |
|---|---|---|
| **Analgesics and antipyretics** | | |
| Acetylsalicylic acid | Hemorrhage, anatomic sequelae | Suggestive |
| **Anticoagulants** | | |
| Dicumarol | Hemorrhage, fetal death | Conclusive |
| **Antihistamines** | | |
| Meclizine | Congenital malformations | Doubtful |
| **Antihypertensives and/or diuretics** | | |
| Ganglionic blocking agents | Impaired neonatal adjustment | Suggestive |
| Nitrites | Methemoglobinemia | Suggestive |
| Reserpine | Impaired neonatal adjustment | Suggestive |
| Thiazides | Thrombocytopenia | Conclusive |
| Acetazolamide | Anatomic malformations | Suggestive |
| **Antimalarials** | | |
| Quinine | Fetal death, deafness | Suggestive |
| **Antimicrobials** | | |
| Chloramphenicol | Impaired neonatal adjustment | Suggestive |
| Gantrisin | Hemolysis, kernicterus, jaundice, methemoglobinemia | Suggestive |
| Novobiocin | Hyperbilirubinemia | Suggestive |
| Penicillin | Growth retardation | Doubtful |
| Streptomycin | Deafness, vestibular disturbances | Suggestive |
| Tetracycline | Retarded skeletal growth | Suggestive |
| | Pigmentation of teeth, hypoplasia of enamel | Conclusive |
| | Cataract, limb malformations | Doubtful |
| **Endocrines** | | |
| Methyltestosterone | Masculinization of female fetus | Conclusive |
| Progesterone | Masculinization of female fetus | Suggestive |
| Methimazole | Goiter | Conclusive |
| Stilbestrol | Deafness | Suggestive |
| Corticosteroids | Anatomic malformation | Conclusive |
| **Narcotics and other addicting drugs** | | |
| Barbiturates | Impaired neonatal adjustment which may be accom- | Conclusive |
| Heroin | panied by permanent neurologic sequelae; these | |
| Meperidine | effects most severe when addiction is confirmed | |
| Morphine | Anatomic malformations | Suggestive |
| Nicotine | Low birth weight for gestational age | Suggestive |
| **Tranquilizers** | | |
| Thalidomide | Limb deformities, ear and facial nerve deformities | Conclusive |

*Abstracted from references 6, 19, 24, 26, 29, 33, 44, 46, 50.

fusing and insubstantial. It is apparent that therapeutic doses of some of the endocrine products administered as drugs produce undesirable effects on the fetus (see Table 5-1).

The prevalence of anemia during pregnancy even in the face of relatively rich social and economic resources is a major threat to the well-being of the fetus. The source of anemia cannot always be detected. In fact the anemia may occur in spite of a totally well-balanced, adequate diet, because even this diet may not meet the increased demands for iron during pregnancy. Fetal and placental growth, development, nourishment, excretion of wastes, and total function are dependent upon the adequacy of the mother's blood system. Inadequate hemoglobin levels or low concentration of red blood cells is destined to interfere with adequate functioning of the fetal processes that sustain life.

The diabetic mother is in a particularly hazardous reproductive position. The mother's hyperglycemia is thought to stimulate the fetal pancreas to overproduce insulin during fetal life. This hyperinsulinism is in turn responsible for the increased body fat and typical overgrown appearance of the infant. The increased incidence of anomalies in infants of diabetic mothers and the impaired ability to adjust to extrauterine life are less clearly understood, but they seem to also be related to the metabolic stress of hyperinsulinism stimulated by the maternal system.[8,43]

### Infectious illness

Maternal infections occurring during the first trimester of pregnancy often result in severe consequences for the fetus. Fetal death and malformations are conclusively related to certain infections, particularly viral illness. Pregnancy appears to render many women more susceptible to viral illness. Most viruses are subject to placental transfer, and the rapidly developing tissue of the embryo seems to be more vulnerable to viral attack than at later periods of fetal life. Rubella, which produces mild symptoms in childhood and adulthood, results in severe defects of the eyes, ears, heart, and central nervous system of the fetus. This virus can also induce chronic infection, which leads to serious postnatal disability. The prevention of

rubella through vaccination has made it possible to avoid the possibility of teratogenic effects of rubella, but this protection must be achieved before child-bearing ensues, for the vaccination can lead to effects similar to the disease.[8,43]

Cytomegalic inclusion disease and toxoplasmosis cause serious central nervous system defects in the fetus. Other infections have been implicated in the development of various fetal complications but are less well understood and documented.

Infections during the later months of pregnancy can also affect the fetus. Measles, scarlet fever, and smallpox have been known to affect the fetus during the last months of gestation, resulting in severe infections that endanger the life and well-being of the infant but that do not result in the teratogenic effects that accompany early infections. Syphilis is well known as an infection of later pregnancy, for although the disease is preventable and treatable, it is still initiated during pregnancy and can remain undetected in the mother throughout the perinatal period. About 30% of all affected fetuses die, and the symptoms of those who survive vary widely. The infant may be born with localized mucocutaneous lesions, coryza, anemia, and generalized septicemia. Often, however, the infant appears healthy at birth, and symptoms appear during the second to sixth week of life. Occasionally a child survives without symptoms for two or more years, when wide variation in manifestations of the disease occur. Relating the illness with congenital infection is difficult (see Chapter 18).

### Immunologic factors

Immunologic phenomena of pregnancy continue to elude the scrutiny of modern science. The ability of the mother to nurture an organism that is immunologically foreign to herself defies all currently understood mechanisms of immunology. Further, selected maternal immunologic protection is transferred to the fetus. If the mother has developed antibodies for infectious diseases such as measles, chickenpox, hepatitis, poliomyelitis, whooping cough, and diphtheria, the antibodies pass readily across the placenta and confer immunity to these diseases, which lasts for several months after birth. Some antibodies seem to be excluded from the fetal circulation, such as antibodies to dust, pollen, or other common allergens.[8]

The most commonly encountered interference with fetal development that results from antibody transfer is in relation to incompatibility of maternal and fetal blood factors, resulting in varying levels of hyperbilirubinemia and erythroblastosis fetalis. Maternal antibodies that are developed against Rh positive blood cells or the major blood types cross the placental membranes and destroy the circulating fetal cells, with devastating effects on the fetus. The severity of the effects is dependent upon the level of isoimmunity developed in the mother and on a complexity of inadequately understood factors, which seem to be best described as maternal idiosyncrasies.[3,8,31]

### Emotional factors

Folklore surrounding pregnancy is rich in most cultures with implications regarding the influence of maternal emotions upon the pregnancy. Tendencies among scientific investigators to reject such ideas as unsound have interfered with the pursuit of inquiry into this mysterious phenomenon. It is now generally accepted that the emotional state of the mother does in some manner affect the fetus and the outcome of pregnancy, but exactly what these effects are and how they occur remain totally elusive. It is difficult to separate the effects of traits during pregnancy from the effect of the same trait during early infancy and childhood, since the maternal disposition tends to persist and continues to exert influence on the growth and developing child.

Maternal "stress" and "anxiety" have been related to the degree of undesirable physiologic responses to pregnancy that the mother experiences, such as nausea and vomiting, backaches, or headaches. Habitual abortions and infertility problems have been related to psychogenic disturbances. Psychotherapy has been conclusively demonstrated to effectively interrupt an abortion pattern or infertility syndrome and to enable a woman to successfully complete pregnancy. The woman who begins pregnancy with inadequate psychic reserves and strengths is particularly vulnerable to the stresses that become manifest and the emotional conflicts and moods that ordinarily accompany the pregnant state. The stresses, anxieties, and being unable to cope lead to behavior that otherwise would not be typical for the mother, such as taking drugs, bizarre eating patterns, or susceptibility to accidents. Each of these behavioral sequelae results in physiologic disturbances for the fetus.

Emotions are mediated in the physiologic systems through neuroendocrine responses. It has been speculated that the effects of emotions on the fetus are physiologic responses to endocrine stimulation. However, demonstration of a direct connection and endocrine effect on the fetus has not yet been possible.[3,5,18,43]

## ASSESSMENT AND CARE OF THE MOTHER AND FETUS

Adequate prenatal care requires the efforts of an appropriate team of health workers who cooperatively assist the mother and family to achieve a desirable outcome of pregnancy. Monitoring of maternal and fetal responses throughout pregnancy reveals deleterious conditions and makes intervention possible. Equally important to the well-being of the unborn child is prevention of exposure to many known hazards of pregnancy. Maintenance of health for the family can significantly enhance the chances of producing a healthy infant.[51]

Unfortunately, this health care goal may cause a great deal of conflict for the mother and family; not all pregnancies occur intentionally, nor is every birth anticipated with joy and happiness. Cultures provide ways of resolving or coping with this problem, but the individual family may find their personal conflict even greater when cast against the values and attitudes of society. Societal changes in many countries in recent decades have increased alternatives available to couples in planning and controlling the size and rate of growth of families, but conflicting situations continue to occur. During times of stress, such as that imposed by an unexpected pregnancy, the health care system may be avoided as part of the total reaction to avoid the reality of the unwanted birth. The mother and fetus are then subject to problems of fear, guilt, anxiety, distress, and the accompanying physiologic hazards that tend to occur.

**121**

When pregnancy is a welcome event, the ability and motivation of the mother and family to participate in their own health care are extremely significant. Socioeconomic, educational, or psychologic limitations may severely handicap a family in carrying out the health practices that are desired during gestation. When these factors are understood by the health care worker, strengths of the individual family can be called upon to achieve as much as possible, thereby accomplishing some improvement that may prove beneficial for the unborn child.[15,22,23,28]

## Ongoing assessment of the mother and fetus

Factors known to influence the growth and development of the fetus have been discussed to provide guidelines for assessment of the mother and fetus. Detailed family, social, and medical histories are desirable in alerting the health care team to potential problems for the mother or for the fetus. When an inheritable trait such as diabetes is found in the mother's history, particular attention to the possible development of diabetes is stressed. If the mother is found to have ingested drugs in the past, a detailed accounting of all drugs taken, particularly since the onset of pregnancy, is helpful in determining the mother's risk of having an affected infant.

Palpation and auscultation of the uterus and its contents, with ongoing estimation of growth in size, provide one of the most important indices of fetal well-being. Visualization and palpation of the cervix and vagina give information of the adequacy of these structures for labor and delivery, plus possible clues of maternal infections. The mother's bony pelvis is measured early during pregnancy to determine the adequacy of size and shape. This information provides an important determinant for the course of labor and delivery. Pelvic-infant disproportion cannot be predicted with complete accuracy, but a number of severe problems may be detected with accurate measurements. As the fetus grows in size, it becomes possible to palpate and determine its position, a matter of increasing importance as delivery approaches. The mother's breasts are inspected and monitored in regard to the physiologic development accompanying pregnancy. Circulatory adequacy of the lower extremities is monitored.

The health and integrity of all maternal systems are determined at an early point in pregnancy and are monitored throughout the course of pregnancy. Particular attention is given to those systems most intimately involved in the reproductive process and to those that have been identified as sources of potential problems for this particular mother. The use of the problem-oriented medical record facilitates studious attention to the idiosyncratic details of each mother's pregnancy; although many features of pregnancy tend to be universal for all mothers, seldom is a pregnancy encountered in which there is not some particular detail that is of special importance for the individual mother.

Regular monitoring of weight gains and blood pressure and routine laboratory data are needed to provide evidence of the health of all maternal systems. Repeated hemoglobin or hematocrit measures estimate the adequacy of the blood system and are particularly significant because of the prevalence of anemias during pregnancy. Routine examinations of the urine provide important indices of general maternal well-being, as well as specific evidence of the adequacy of function of the renal system. Serologic tests for syphilis, as well as vaginal smears for the detection of a variety of other infections, are particularly important in detecting the presence of potentially harmful diseases that may be treated effectively. Determination of the mother's blood type characteristics (and sometimes those of the father) are essential. Although maternal chest roentgenograms may be desired in areas where the incidence of tuberculosis is high, the risk of maternal or fetal damage from exposure to radiation justifies postponement of this procedure until the postpartum period. When a roentgenogram is indicated for specific reasons, a reasonable level of safety can be accomplished by shielding the mother's abdomen with a lead apron and using a 6-foot filtered x-ray beam with the defining cone limiting the beam to the thorax as much as possible.[31]

The adequacy of the mother's psychologic resources for coping with pregnancy may be estimated through her past history of mental health and her physiologic, social, and psychologic responses to the pregnancy. Other family members may also provide information regarding the mental health of the mother. Although some mood and personality changes during pregnancy are expected, an alarming change in the mother arouses an expression of concern or frustration in family members.

Pregnancy is a developmental event for the mother, regardless of her age or past experience with bearing children. Tanner[41] has attempted to describe and demonstrate the specific developmental and psychologic events that are expected to occur during pregnancy. Each of the features described interacts with and overlaps others, so that a mother may be involved in more than one task at any given point in pregnancy. Normal regressions or reexperiencing of a task that was previously encountered is not uncommon, but the description of each feature may facilitate accurate and comprehensive estimates of the psychologic health of the mother throughout pregnancy.

Usually at the onset of pregnancy the mother exerts a considerable amount of energy, time, and thought in working through the idea of being pregnant. During this time there is usually a predominance of mood changes and of ambivalent feelings about the pregnancy, even if it was planned and wanted. There is a preoccupation with bodily changes that take place during the early weeks.

As this task is resolving, the mother begins to ready herself psychologically to end pregnancy, a shift that occurs at about the time that fetal movement is first felt. A neutral, reserved, or negative feeling toward body changes and size increments emerges, and the mother begins to try to imagine what the infant's physical appearance is like. The task of perceiving the fetus as a separate object is characterized by assigning a sex to the child. Acute awareness of the responses of the fetus, with an effort to assess their adequacy, and recognition of the fact that death or abnormality of the fetus is a real possibility indicate processes in identifying the fetus as separate.

Finally, the mother exhibits behaviors that indicate preparation and readiness to assume a care-taking relationship with the infant. In some cultures this does not occur until just before or after the delivery of the infant, but when integration of the pregnancy and perceiving the fetus as a separate being have been satisfactorily completed, it is believed that completion of the care-taking relationship follows easily and naturally. The mother who is involved in this particular task expresses definite plans about feeding the infant, and she makes plans for household and infant care when the baby comes home. When the prospects of the infant's crying and interruption of sleep during the night are mentioned, the mother responds with a mood of acceptance and some idea as to how these situations will be handled. Finally, plans for labor and delivery are completed, with general conveyance of satisfaction in understanding what is to happen and what is expected of her.[19,36]

### Nursing care

Probably the most important aspect of nursing care during the prenatal period is appropriate teaching. The assumption that a mother who is experienced or well educated understands and knows all that she needs to know about her own care during pregnancy is fallacious and dangerous to the well-being of the infant. It is essential that the nurse knows that the mother understands adequate health practices during pregnancy, including needs and guidelines for exercise, sleep, rest, nutrition, clothing, bathing, dental care, and regular health supervision. Teaching aids in the form of audiovisual media or reading material that is appropriate for the mother's level of understanding and interest may enhance her ability to participate in the recommended practices. In addition, help and instruction or demonstration in the mother's own home may be beneficial in guiding her to an understanding of how she can realistically incorporate adequate health care into her existing daily life style.

Without unduly alarming the mother the nurse must determine that the mother is aware of danger signs that merit immediate attention during pregnancy. These are:
1. Any vaginal bleeding
2. Swelling of the face or fingers
3. Severe or continuous headache
4. Dimness or blurring of vision

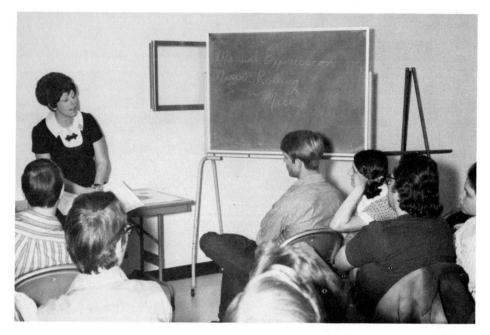

**Fig. 5-2.** Group classes may be helpful for expectant mothers and fathers in understanding pregnancy, labor, delivery, and infant care.

5. Abdominal pain
6. Persistent vomiting
7. Chills or fever
8. Dysuria
9. Escape of fluid from the vagina

Finally, nursing care may incorporate actual preparation for labor and delivery. Under optimal conditions the mother and father both understand each alternative available in regard to the conduct of labor and delivery, and they select the approach that most adequately suits their needs. Community- or agency-sponsored group classes that concentrate on preparation for specified approaches to the labor and delivery experience are often available, as are classes that prepare the mother for breast-feeding. Some approaches involve the father initimately and are beneficial for those couples desiring this type of approach.[42] If the mother is not in a position to include the father in her parturition experience, such an approach would be an inappropriate choice. When a specific approach is not designated and preparation for labor and delivery is largely a matter for the mother and the health care worker who will be most intimately involved in her labor and delivery, individual teaching and preparation may accompany regular health supervision during the later months of pregnancy. It is necessary for the mother to understand exactly what to expect of each detail for this particular labor and delivery. Visiting the area where labor and delivery will occur and "walking through" the process of getting into the system often facilitate a prior familiarity; this promotes psychologic and physical comfort when the actual event arrives.

The decision regarding breast- or bottle-feeding should be a major focus in prenatal teaching. The circumstances of the family before delivery need to be assessed in order to provide realistic counseling regarding the decision to breast or bottle feed. Their economic status, ability to provide sound nutrition for the mother and infant, and emotional climate of the family are important factors in advising a mother as to the preferred feeding approach. The mother needs to understand the facts of each approach to feeding, and develop her own motivation and reasons for choosing one method or another. The relative economy, convenience, and benefit to the infant of breast-feeding in the first few weeks of life are important factors for the moth-

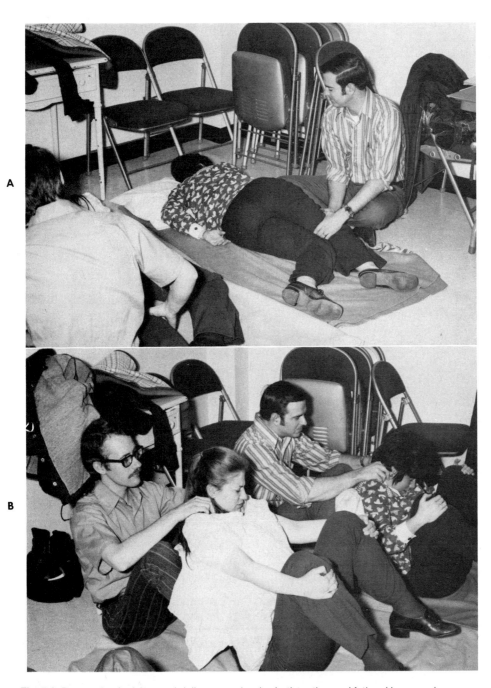

**Fig. 5-3.** Preparation for labor and delivery may involve both mother and father. Here couples prepare for **A,** early stages of labor and **B,** later stages of labor, using natural childbirth approaches.

**Table 5-2.** Composition of mature human milk and cow milk*

| Component | Human milk | Cow milk |
|---|---|---|
| Water (100 ml) | 87.1 | 87.3 |
| Energy (kcal/100 ml) | 75 | 69 |
| Total solids (g/100 ml) | 12.9 | 12.7 |
| Protein | 1.1 | 3.3 |
| Fat | 4.5 | 3.7 |
| Lactose | 6.8 | 4.8 |
| Ash | 0.21 | 0.72 |
| Proteins (% of total protein) | | |
| Casein | 40 | 82 |
| Whey proteins | 60 | 18 |
| Vitamins per liter | | |
| Vitamin A (IU) | 1,898 | 1,425 |
| Thiamine ($\mu$g) | 160 | 440 |
| Riboflavin ($\mu$g) | 360 | 1,750 |
| Niacin ($\mu$g) | 1,470 | 940 |
| Pyridoxine ($\mu$g) | 100 | 640 |
| Pantothenate ($\mu$g) | 1,840 | 3,450 |
| Folic acid ($\mu$g) | 20 | 30 |
| $B_{12}$ ($\mu$g) | 0.3 | 4 |
| Vitamin C (mg) | 43 | 1 |
| Vitamin D (IU) | 21 | 13 |
| Vitamin E (mg) | 6.6 | 1.0 |
| Vitamin K ($\mu$g) | 15 | 60 |

*From Macey, I. G., and Kelly, H. J.: Human milk and cow's milk in infant nutrition. In Kon, S. K., and Cowie, A. T., editors: Milk: the mammary gland and its secretion, vol. 2, New York, 1961, Academic Press, Inc., p. 265; and Committee on nutrition, American Academy of Pediatrics: Composition of milks, Pediatrics **26:**1039, 1960.

er to understand, but if family and individual circumstances indicate that breast-feeding would be undesirable or stressful, these factors should not become sources of the development of guilt feelings.[10,11,17,45]

Table 5-2 presents a comparison of the nutritional components of human and cow's milk. It should be remembered that variation among individual mothers and individual cows occurs. This variation is significant for the infant who is breast-fed, but is not significant for the bottle-fed infant because the composition of cow's milk formulas is carefully regulated by the manufacturers by combining the milk of many cattle in preparing the specific commercial formula. Composition of each commercial preparation may be obtained from the manufacturer.[9]

If the mother decides to breast-feed her infant, preparation of the breasts and nipples should begin about three months before expected delivery. The mother should begin to learn manual expression of milk and may be able to express colostrum as the delivery date approaches. She needs to rub the nipples and areola with a coarse cloth several times a day to toughen the skin in readiness for the effects of the infant sucking. Her emotional readiness for breast-feeding needs to be developed by providing counseling and guidance as to what she might expect regarding her ability to provide adequate nutrition for the infant, the infant's behavior during breast-feeding, and how to recognize signs of adequate nutrition and feeding in the infant (see Chapter 7).

**STUDY QUESTIONS**

1. In a culture with which you are familiar, identify folklore beliefs that seem to actually enhance the health and well-being of the fetus. What physiologic or psychologic phenomena are related to the belief, and what scientific rationale for the observed benefit can be described?
2. Identify environmental and community health hazards for people living in an area of your community that is economically deprived. Discuss the possible relationships of these factors to the unborn child and maternal health and steps that would be needed to correct them. What resources or action is available for an individual mother and her family to protect themselves against these hazards?
3. Give detailed, specific recommendations for prenatal care that you would give to a pregnant mother, and describe the rationale for each recommendation in terms of the health of the fetus. Compare your recommendations with those of a health care worker (nurse, midwife, physician) who has participated in prenatal care for a number of years. Discern which features of maternal care can vary in the detail of "how to do it," and which are defined closely by the requirements of the fetus.
4. Interview a woman in the child-bearing age group in regard to her past health care practices and features of present health care which potentially affect the fetus. Identify the strengths and inadequacies of various health habits with plans for nursing care during pregnancy that would incorporate these features of already established health care.
5. Identify resources in your community that currently exist for preparation of parents for birth and delivery. Identify the specific approach used, if any, and features of the programs that are important in making a choice. How do organized programs differ from preparation offered to pregnant mothers in various private office, clinics, or community health care agencies offering prenatal care? Is a resource available for preparation for breast-feeding? What is the cost or enrollment requirement? Examine the specific recommendations for maternal self-care that

are offered through these resources and judge their adequacy in relation to care of the fetus.

6. Examine a copy of the pamphlet, *Prenatal Care,* Children's Bureau Publication Number 4-1962 or some similar publication intended to guide the mother in prenatal care. Assess the adequacy of the information contained and various features of the material, such as reading ability required or cultural features that are incorporated. How can the material be incorporated into a teaching program for mothers who would not appropriately use this particular piece of literature?

## REFERENCES

1. Birch, H. G.: Malnutrition, learning and intelligence, Am. J. Public Health **62:**773, June, 1972.
2. Birch, H. G., and Gussow, J. D.: Disadvantaged children; health, nutrition and school failure, New York, 1970, Harcourt, Brace, and World, Inc.
3. Chinn, P. C., and Mueller, J.: Advances in the treatment of Rh negative blood incompatibility of mothers and infants, Mental Retard. **9:**12, Feb. 1971.
4. Christakis, G., editor: Nutritional assessment in health programs, Am. J. Public Health (suppl.) vol. 63, part 2, Nov. 1973.
5. Colman, A. D., and Colman, L. L.: Pregnancy; the psychological experience, New York, 1971, Herder and Herder, Inc.
6. Done, A. K.: Perinatal pharmacology, Ann. Rev. Pharmacol. **6:**189, 1966.
7. Dunston, B. N.: Pica during pregnancy. In Bergersen, B. S., and others, editors: Current concepts in clinical nursing, vol. 2, St. Louis, 1969, The C. V. Mosby Co., p. 268.
8. Ferreira, A. J.: Prenatal environment, Springfield, Ill., 1969, Charles C Thomas, Publisher.
9. Fomon, S. J.: Infant nutrition, ed. 2, Philadelphia, 1974, W. B. Saunders Co.
10. Galant, S. P.: Biological and clinical significance of the gut as a barrier to penetration of macromolecules; Practical implications with respect to breast feeding, Clin. Pediatr. **15:**731, Aug., 1976.
11. Gerrard, J. W.: Breast-feeding; second thoughts, Pediatrics **54:**757, Dec. 1974.
12. Gilien, N. R.: Determinants of birth weight. In Duffey, M., and others, editors: Current concepts in clinical nursing, vol. 3, St. Louis, 1971, The C. V. Mosby Co., p. 169.
13. Gluck, L.: Appraisal of the fetus and neonate; growth, development, nutrition. In Abramson, H., editor: Symposium on the functional development of the fetus and neonate, St. Louis, 1971, The C. V. Mosby Co., p. 68.
14. Grant, J. A., and Heald, F. P.: Complications of adolescent pregnancy; survey of the literature on fetal outcome in adolescence, Clin. Pediatr. **11:**567, Oct., 1972.
15. Hott, J. R.: The crisis of expectant fatherhood, Am. J. Nurs. **76:**1436, Sept., 1976.
16. Jekel, J. F., and others: A comparison of the health of index and subsequent babies born to school-age mothers, Am. J. Public Health **65:**370, April, 1975.
17. Jelliffe, D. B., and Jelliffe, P.: Alleged inadequacies of human milk; common misapprehensions and errors, Clin. Pediatr. **16:**1140, Dec., 1977.
18. Joffe, J. M.: Prenatal determinants of behavior, New York, 1969, Pergamon Press.
19. Juchau, M. R., and Dyer, D. C.: Pharmacology of the placenta, Pediatr. Clin. North Am. **19:**65, Feb. 1972.
20. Lechtig, A., and others: Effect of food supplementation during pregnancy on birthweight, Pediatrics **56:**508, Oct., 1975.
21. Lenz, W.: Malformations caused by drugs during pregnancy, Am. J. Dis. Child. **112:**99, Aug., 1966.
22. Marquart, R. K.: Expectant fathers; What are their needs? Matern. Child Nurs. **1:**32, Jan.-Feb. 1976.
23. May, K. A.: Psychologic involvement in pregnancy by expectant fathers, J. Obstet. Gynecol. Neonatal Nurs. **4:**40, July-Aug. 1975.
24. McNiel, J. R.: The possible teratogenic effect of salicylates on the developing fetus; brief summaries of eight suggestive cases, Clin. Pediatr. **12:**347, June, 1973.
25. Mead, M., and Newton, N.: Conception, pregnancy, labor the puerperium in cultural perspective, Rev. Med. Psychol. **4:**22, 1962.
26. Modell, W., editor: Drugs of choice 1978-1979, St. Louis, 1978, The C. V. Mosby Co.
27. Morris, N. M., Udry, R., and Chase, C. L.: Shifting age-parity distribution of births and the decrease in infant mortality, Am. J. Public Health **65:**359, April, 1975.
28. Obrzut, L. A. J.: Expectant fathers' perceptions of fathering, Am. J. Nurs. **76:**1440, Sept., 1976.
29. Palmisano, P. A., and Polhill, R. B.: Fetal pharmacology, Pediatr. Clin. North Am. **19:**3, Feb., 1972.
30. Pomerance, J.: Weight gain in pregnancy; How much is enough? Clin. Pediatr. **11:**554, Oct., 1972.
31. Pritchard, J. A., and MacDonald, P. C.: William's obstetrics, ed. 15, New York, 1976, Appleton-Century-Crofts.
32. Promoting the health of mothers and children fiscal year 1971: Report of the Maternal and Child Health Service, Health Services and Mental Health Administration, U.S. Dept. of Health, Education and Welfare, Stock No. 1730-0017, Washington, D.C., 1971, U.S. Government Printing Office.
33. Rane, A., and Sjoqvist, F.: Drug metabolism in the human fetus and newborn infant, Pediatr. Clin. North Am. **19:**37, Feb., 1972.
34. Ratner, H.: Commonwealth vs. Brunelle. II. Humanity of the fetus, Child Family **9:**159, 1970.
35. Rich, A.: Of woman born; motherhood as experience and institution, New York, 1976, W. W. Norton Co.
36. Rubin, R.: Maternal tasks in pregnancy, Maternal-Child Nurs. J. **4:**143, Fall 1975.
37. Scanlon, J.: Human fetal hazards from environmental pollution with certain non-essential trace elements, Clin. Pediatr. **11:**135, March, 1972.
38. Shank, R. E.: A chink in our armor, Nutrition Today **5:**2, Summer 1970.
39. Smiley, J., Eyres, S., and Roberts, D. E.: Maternal and

infant health and their associated factors in an inner city population, Am. J. Public Health **62:**475, April, 1972.

40. Susceptibility of the fetus and child to chemical pollutants, Pediatrics Supplement, vol. 53, no. 5, part 2, May 1974.

41. Tanner, L. M.: Developmental tasks of pregnancy. In Bergerson, B. S., and others, editors: Current concepts in clinical nursing, vol. 2, St. Louis, 1969, The C. V. Mosby Co., p. 292.

42. Tanzer, D., and Block, J.: Why natural childbirth? A psychologist's report on the benefits to mothers, fathers, and babies, New York, 1972, Doubleday and Co.

43. Timiras, P. S.: Developmental physiology and aging, New York, 1972, The Macmillan Publishing Co., Inc.

44. Vaughn, V. C., III, and McKay, R. J., editors: Nelson's Textbook of pediatrics, ed. 10, Philadelphia, 1975, W. B. Saunders Co.

45. Weichert, C.: Breast-feeding; first thoughts, Pediatrics **56:**987, Dec., 1975.

46. When a mother smokes during pregnancy, will it affect her baby? Clin. Pediatr. **13:**485, June, 1974.

47. Whipple, D. V.: Dynamics of development; Euthenic pediatrics, New York, 1966, McGraw-Hill Book Co.

48. Wilson, J. G.: Physiology of development. In Cooke, R. F., editor: The biologic basis of pediatrics, New York, 1968, McGraw-Hill Book Co., p. 1394.

49. Winick, M., editor: Nutrition and fetal development, New York, 1974, John Wiley & Sons.

50. Zellweger, H.: Anticonvulsants during pregnancy; a danger to the developing fetus? Clin. Pediatr. **13:**338, April, 1974.

51. Zimmerman, H. S., and others: The mothers' center; women work for social change, Children Today **6:**11, March-April 1977.

# Sallie L.—ANTEPARTAL MOTHER*

Cheryl Boyd Hundley

## HEALTH STATUS LIST

| Onset | Date | No. | Active | Date | Inactive/resolved |
|-------|------|-----|--------|------|-------------------|
| 2/1/78 | 2/1/78 | 1 | Incomplete data base | | |
| | 2/1/78 | 2 | Need for knowledge and anticipatory guidance during the antepartal period | | |
| 1/30/78 | 2/1/78 | 2,A | Nutrition | | |
| 6/77 | 2/1/78 | 2,B | Preparation for baby | | |
| ? | 2/1/78 | 3 | Lack of financial resources | | |
| | 2/1/78 | 4 | Child-rearing tasks of parent with pre-schooler | | |
| 5/74 | 2/1/78 | 4,A | Parenting | | |
| ? | 2/1/78 | 4,B | Safety of home environment | | |
| ? | 2/1/78 | 4,C | Child health maintenance | | |
| | 2/1/78 | | | 5/15/74 | Labor and delivery of Darla |
| | 2/1/78 | | | 11/77 | Impetigo—Darla |

Client ___**Sallie L.**___ Sex __F__ Age __20__ B.D. __6/30/57__

Date __2/1/78__ Race __Black__

**Information sources:** Sallie L.—reliable
Clinic records

### PRENATAL PROFILE
#### Present health status

Now eight months pregnant (gravida ii, para i). Prenatal course has been uncomplicated until last clinic visit where CBC revealed "iron-deficiency anemia." Since diagnosed as pregnant 8/30/77 has had a weight gain of 18 pounds. Date of LMP (first day) June 1, 1977. EDC is estimated March 8, 1978. First "felt life" sometime in late November.

### Vital signs

2/1/78   B/P 126/80   AP = 82/regular   R = 20/min   T = 98.4° F

Ranges:   B/P since 8/30   130/70-120/80   AP = 72-82 min   R = 18-22/min
T = 98.0-98.6

2/1/78   FHT 145/min   FHT is heard by obstetrician 11/15

Range:   FHTs   140-150/min

---

*Tool adapted from Family Assessment Tool by Patsy Kaiser and Donna Kem, Texas Woman's University, Denton, Texas.

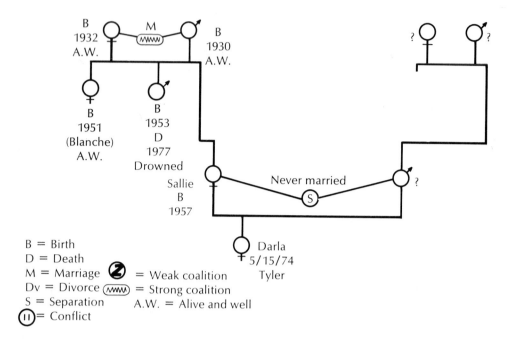

B = Birth
D = Death
M = Marriage  = Weak coalition
Dv = Divorce (MWW) = Strong coalition
S = Separation    A.W. = Alive and well
(II) = Conflict

## Laboratory

Urinalysis reports trace of sugar and no albumin (specimen taken at 1 PM 1/30)

1/30    Hgb 10 g       Hct 33
        Ranges:    Hgb 11-10.5 g       Hct 37-33

1/30    Negative sickle cell

8/30    Class I pap smear

## Medications

Ordered 1/30 Multivitamins with iron (100 mg) daily.

## History

Cannot recall any major illnesses or surgeries. Had "something done" during a postpartal check after delivery of first child but doesn't know what it was or reason. Denies discomforts of heartburn, nausea, constipation, hemorrhoids, backache, or leg cramps. States her ankles are starting "to swell" some. She denies smoking. Has a "drink sometimes." Has not been taking vitamins.

## Nutrition

Skips breakfast sometimes. Usually has lunch and dinner. Presently not on a supplemental food program (food stamps, WIC). Upon inquiry, evaded questions about types and quantity of food intake at each meal. Presently she is not employed and has recently moved from her parents' home with her 3½-year-old daughter. Her parents live 80 miles away in a small town where she previously was working as a waitress and her mother cared for her little girl. She now lives in the inner city. Uses local city clinic for health care. Will go to county hospital for labor and delivery. States "things are much different here" than at home.

## Prenatal fantasies

Dreams that the child will be a boy. Tries not to get upset or in arguments as she believes this is "not good" for the baby.

## FAMILY ASSESSMENT

### I. General data

**Reason for interview:** Client seen in the home for antepartal care after having recently been diagnosed in clinic with iron-deficiency anemia. Client presents several concerns: financial needs, health needs, adjustments to new community, and preparation for new baby. Sister and children not at home this visit.

**Number of members in the family:** Five—Sallie L. (20); Darla L. (3½); Sallie L.'s sister, Blanche (26); Blanche's daughter, Michelle (8); Blanche's son, Terry (11)

**Members not living in household:** There are no fathers or husbands in the household.

**Household space and privacy arrangements:** Sallie and Darla have one room in the five-room house. The room has a door on it. There are twin beds (Sallie sleeps in one and Darla sleeps in the other). There is a chest-of-drawers with a TV on top. The living room contains two couches, and much of the furniture is crowded up against the wall. Everyone shares the same bath.

**Description of the home environment:** The home was clean but cluttered. There are small gas heaters in the rooms. Pathways generally are clear. The house is a small frame located in the inner city neighborhood. They are located across the street from a park. Sallie is living with her sister after moving from a nearby small town where she was living with her parents. Not visible were any toys, books, and indoor space for play for the children. There is no evidence of preparations for the baby in regard to space, a crib, clothing, diapers.

**Income:** No child support. No income from employment. No public assistance. Sister's income and sources not known at this time.

**How do you manage to make ends meet?** "My sister's been real good to me and helps me out." Plans to get a job after having baby. Does "not want to go through the trouble of getting welfare" right now.

**Transportation available:** Lives near busline. Car outside house is not working. Uses bus to get to clinic.

**Child care arrangements:** Takes care of Darla. Takes her wherever they go. An aunt who lives nearby will care for Darla and baby when she returns to work.

**Emergency resources:** None.

**Eating patterns:** Skips breakfast sometimes. She and Darla eat together in their room for lunch and supper.

**Leisure activities:** Go to park when it's not too cold as it's right across the street. Watch TV.

**Adult friends and relationships outside of family:** Doesn't know anyone here except sister and aunt.

**Time spent with friends:** None.

**Community activities and organizations:** Occasionally will go to the church down the street.

### II. Adult social history

**Adult relationships as defined within the family:** There is no traditional husband-wife bond. She has never been married.

**How adult relationships were formed:** Pregnant by a man she knew "awhile." Does not know where he is now.

**What do they consider best about their relationship?** Not applicable.

**131**

**What was life like for you as a child growing up?** Grew up in a small town with her brother and her sister. Stated her parents have always "been together."

**Any losses before the age of 15:** None.

**As a child, what practice did your parents use in discipline?** "Got after me" with words. Sometimes got spanked.

**What things did you enjoy as a child?** Playing with siblings.

III. **Family interactions** (Complete for each family member.)

**SALLIE L.**

**Identity within family:** Mother to Darla. Sister to Blanche.

**General health status:** See prenatal profile.

**Role in family:** Is a mother and caretaker of Darla, while Sallie seems like a dependent or child to her sister.

**Family tasks:** Helps with housework. Cares for Darla.

**Life events in previous year:** 5/77 her brother was drowned in a pond accidentally. 7/77 moved to the city.

**Previous coping mechanisms:** Tries "to make the most" of something that happens. States she doesn't get "real mad" but tries to be calm when something upsets her.

**Developmental state:** Intimacy vs. isolation (self-absorption).

**Expectations of self:** Wants Darla to be loved and happy. Desires to be a good mother. Wants to get a job.

**Expectations of family:** To love and to help her and her children.

**Description of child-adult relationships:** Sallie loves Darla and believes she feels "wanted." She and Darla enjoy drawing together.

**Perceptions of how decisions are made:** She "does what she thinks is best" for herself and Darla.

**Perception of how problems and conflicts are solved:** Most of time tries to wait and see how things are going to turn out. Stated she and her sister got along real well. No mention of how she and parents related as to problems or conflicts.

**DARLA L.**

**Identity within family:** Daughter. Niece.

**General health status:** Healthy except for recent case of impetigo of legs in 11/77. Had an ear infection last year, mother cannot remember exactly when. Was a "healthy baby." Was on formula for six months. Appears well developed and well nourished. Very active and inquisitive. Points out that "mommy's tummy sticks out." Was toilet trained by 2½. Sleeps soundly all night. Has not had frequent colds. Mother believes "shots" are up to date.

**Role in family:** "I'm mommy's girl."

**Family tasks:** Helps mommy.

**Life events in previous year:** Death of uncle 5/77. Moved to city 7/77.

**Previous coping mechanisms:** Mother states Darla sometimes has toileting accidents when she's real upset, like when they moved.

**Developmental state:** Initiative vs. guilt—affective. Preconceptual stage of cognitive development.

**Expectations of self:** Wants to be a "good girl."

**Expectations of family:** Wants a brother to play with.

**Description of child-adult relationships:** Child not able to respond to this.

**Perceptions of how decisions are made:** Believes her mother decides everything.

**Perceptions of how problems and conflicts are solved:** No response.

## IV. Child-rearing

**How do you correct the child when he/she misbehaves?** "I scold her most of the time." She sometimes spanks her.

**How do you reward child for good behavior?** I say "that's a good girl."

**What do you agree that the child should learn in life?** Wants Darla to get an education and to be happy.

**On what do adult members disagree regarding child-rearing?** Not applicable.

**How do you think the child responds to your *discipline/guidance/control?*** Most of the time she does what I want her to. If not, she gets a little spanking.

**When do you feel closest to the child?** When she holds Darla.

**When do you feel distant/strange to your child?** When she "acts up."

**Adult description of each child, including developmental stage and anticipation of events of the coming year.** She sees Darla as a real alive little girl who likes to play and who is "always asking questions." In the next year wants Darla to come to love the new baby but knows she will probably be "jealous."

## V. Preparation for new baby

**What concerns do you have for this new child?** Wants the baby to be "healthy and normal."

**What changes in your life style do you anticipate when the baby arrives?** Believes she'll be busy with the frequent feedings and will be tired trying to care for both children. Will have to work to support her children. Believes Darla will be jealous for a while but hasn't said much to her except she may get a new brother soon.

**Preparations for the arrival of the baby:** Has some diapers and some clothes. There was no mention of getting a crib, and there is not space for one in Sallie's room. She does not have a washer and dryer for washing child's things.

**How are they prepared for sibling rivalry?** Not sure how Darla will adjust and there was no stated plan to deal with "jealousy" of the baby.

## VI. Summary of family's communication

**Clarity of speech:** Speaks slowly, softly. Sometimes difficult to understand. Darla's speech is rapid and sometimes difficult to understand.

**Topic changes/consistency:** Completes a topic with interviewer before changing subject.

**Ratio of agreement/disagreement between members:** Mother verbally scolded Darla, who protests but minds her.

**Intensity of feelings conveyed:** Emotional feelings congruent with subject matter most of time. Seems passive at times in conversation.

**Speaking order:** She usually spoke to Darla. She allowed interviewer to initiate topics of conversation.

**Commitment to family goals:** Seems sincerely concerned about happiness and welfare of the family.

**Patterns of communication:** Mother-child communication. Unable to assess interactions between Sallie and sister.

## VII. Summary of family assessment

### Level of family functioning

**Stage of maturity:** Sallie not moving through all tasks for young adult as expectant parent with preschooler.

**Open/closed:** Mostly closed.

**Degree of individuation:** Seems to be a developing matrilocal family.

**Degree of dependency:** Totally dependent upon extended family supports.

**Family strengths:** Genuine love and affection.

### Active or potential problems

- Lack of finances for essentials of living and on-going health care.
- Inadequate preparation physically and psychologically for forthcoming baby.
- Sibling rivalry.
- Iron deficiency anemia—in-depth nutritional assessment 2/8/77
- Incompletion of life tasks appropriate to developmental level of Sallie.
- Social isolation of Darla from peers.

## INITIAL PLAN

2/1/78  **No. 1 Incomplete data base**

**S**  None

**O**  Time not sufficient this visit for a nutritional assessment or for in-depth assessment of Darla. No interaction yet with other people living in the household.

**A**  Additional data is necessary for accurate identification of health needs requiring intervention.

**P**  Obj. 1  The family should demonstrate motivation for further interactions with clinical specialist.

2/1/78  **No. 2 Need for knowledge and anticipatory guidance during antepartal period**

2,A  Nutrition

**S**  Occasionally "skips" breakfast but eats with daughter for lunch and supper. Not employed and not receiving assistance from public programs or funds. Takes a vitamin now.

**O**  Avoided direct questions about foods she eats. 2/1 Hemoglobin 10 g with range of 11-10.5 g since 8/77. No obvious means of financial support. No easy transportation for grocery shopping. In third trimester of pregnancy. Gained 18 lbs. A multivitamin with iron is now prescribed.

**A**  In the third trimester of pregnancy a hemoglobin of 10 or below is indicative of iron deficiency anemia. This indicates depletion of mother's iron stores in the liver. Iron deficiency results eventually into anemia of hypochromic, microcytic type. Behaviors resulting are manifested as fatigue, irritability, decreased attentiveness and decreased ability to concentrate. Deficiency of iron occurs when there is a chronic deficiency in dietary iron. Pregnancy is a common condition in which iron deficiency anemia occurs, brought on by a combination of iron utilization by the fetus and borderline dietary intake. Late anemia of this type is characterized by marked hypochromia and microcytosis. Reticulocyte count is normal in uncomplicated iron deficiency anemia. Prematurely born and congenitally defective infants are more often born to mothers who have inadequate nutrition antepartally. Iron is essential for hemoglobin formation, fetal development, and fetal storage of an iron reserve.

**P**  Sallie should be able to:
Obj. 1  Correct iron-deficient condition with assistance of health workers.
Obj. 2  Identify food groups and nutrients basic to adequate nutrition.
Obj. 3  Provide nutritionally sound diet for her family and herself.

2,B  Preparation for the baby

**S**  Concerned that the baby be "healthy and normal." Anticipates she'll be much busier with two children. States she has a few clothes and diapers for the baby. Expects daughter to be jealous.

**O**  No space for a crib or no crib for the child. No mention of obtaining or creating these. No obvious source of funds to provide necessities for baby. No consistent preparation of Darla as to what to expect when new baby gets here. Not taking advantage of public funds during this time period to help prepare materially. Has made tentative plans for child care so she can work

## INITIAL PLAN—cont'd

2/1/78 **No. 2 Need for knowledge and anticipatory guidance during antepartal period—cont'd**

after child is born. Left a familiar support unit and is getting adjusted to a new environment. No husband to help share care of children.

**A**   Unable to financially provide equipment and space at a most basic level for the infant. May not perceive this as necessary. Does not conceptualize a new baby as a crisis. The entrance of a new baby into a family structure is considered a maturational crisis. The infant's addition causes each person's role to change as the family's structure is altered. Successful coping with reorganization will be manifest in satisfaction with role modifications. When families do not perceive or plan for entry of a new infant, disintegration and chaos can result in frustration and standstill. Intervention is then necessary to facilitate adaptation. The critical tasks of the child-bearing phase include establishing a home environment that is satisfactory for the adults and the child and for the adjustment of the family.

**P**   The family should:
Obj. 1   Perceive and plan for change created by a new infant.
Obj. 2   Receive intervention should a chaotic situation develop.

2/1/78   **No. 3 Lack of financial resources**

**S**   Not working. Does not want to go through trouble of getting assistance at this time. No child support. No emergency funds. Plans to work after baby's birth. Has experience as waitress.

**O**   Dependent on sister for shelter, food, and necessities. Having baby at county hospital. No visible means of income. Has always been financially dependent on extended family.

**A**   Mother, in stage of intimacy vs. self-isolation, is not meeting expenses and not managing a residence. Since she has been financially dependent, she may not have realistic knowledge about the cost of living. Black matriarchal families are "multiproblem" families in which mothers usually live alone with one or two children or with parents. The majority of these families are under $2,000 a year income level with low income threshold being $3,936 (1970). This type of family faces the greatest difficulty in meeting daily demands of existence. Usually recipients of public funds also utilize services that educate persons for financial and home management, for employment, and services to secure housing.*

**P**   Obj. 1   The mother should be aware of all available resources and employment opportunities.

2/1/78   **No. 4 Child-rearing tasks of parent with a preschooler**

4,A   Parenting

**S**   Believes Darla will be "jealous" of new baby. Child seems to respond to mother's verbal admonitions. Has just explained to Darla that she is going to get a new brother. Darla is aware of mother's "tummy sticking out." Mother states Darla has toilet accidents when stressed.

**O**   Mother is not giving Darla enough explanation to prepare child and to decrease sibling rivalry in the future.

---

**136**   *Eshleman, J. R., The family, Boston, 1974, Allyn and Bacon, Inc. pp. 221, 234.

**A** The arrival of a new baby changes life for the preschooler as she is no longer the center of attention, she must accept affection being given to the newborn and the newborn gets more attention than she. As a result a preschooler may regress. She may show hostility toward the mother or try to harm the baby. Parents can benefit from anticipatory counseling to foster readiness in parenting in a sibling-rivalry situation. Parents can plan to move the child to another room well before the arrival of a new infant. Any changes affecting the older child should be made well in advance if possible. The older child may behave in a way to get parental attention. This may involve misbehaving or acting disruptively. There may be increased whining, increased requests for help, clinging behaviors, and increased use of "no."

**P** Obj. 1 The mother should demonstrate knowledge of parenting in a sibling rivalry situation.

4,B Safety of home environment

**S** Takes Darla to park. Anticipates she will have to adjust to new baby in forthcoming year.

**O** Mother does not have knowledge of developmental hazards ahead for Darla. Physical safety features in home are not obvious. There are gas heaters near doorways. Pathways are partially occluded with crowded furniture. No safety devices in outlets.

**A** Knowledge of existence of possible hazards includes physical hazards and special hazards associated with the child's developmental stage. Health maintenance as a function of the family begins with attention to these factors. The home environment and adult's perception of the child's developmental stage give clues to the safety of the home environment.

**P** The mother should:
Obj. 1 Demonstrate techniques for making home safe for preschooler.
Obj. 2 Identify developmental milestones for Darla over the next year.

4,C Child health maintenance

**S** Darla is 3½, born 5/15/74. Mother believes "shots" are up-to-date. Had impetigo in November.

**O** None

**A** An interview and physical exam and DDST will give information about the basic structure of the child in all parameters. This data can be used for more accurate problem identification as a basis for more pertinent intervention.

**P** Obj. 1 Darla should demonstrate optimum growth and development appropriate to her age.

Case

Prenatal
development
and care

## NURSING ORDERS

2/1/78   **No. 1 Incomplete data base**                       **PERSONNEL**

Obj. 1   The family should demonstrate motivation for further interactions with clinical specialist.

    A. Plan a visit 2/8/78 at Sallie's convenience.         C.S.*

    B. Give family phone number where nurse can be reached.         C.S.

2/1/78   **No. 2 Need for knowledge and anticipatory guidance during antepartal period**

2,A   Nutrition

Obj. 1   Correct iron-deficient condition with assistance of health workers.

    A. Teach Sallie the reasons for taking the vitamin and iron capsule as prescribed. Interpret directions so she understands them.         C.S.

    B. At next clinic visit collaborate with physician to obtain serum iron level and total iron binding capacity as well as CBC and peripheral smear. (2/14)         C.S.

    C. Assess Sallie for symptoms and signs of anemia in assessment and physical exam. (2/8)         C.S.

    D. Teach Sallie the behaviors associated with iron-deficiency anemia. (2/8)         C.S.

Obj. 2   Identify food groups and nutrients basic to adequate nutrition.

    A. During nutritional assessment ascertain her knowledge of the basic four and essential vitamins and minerals. (2/8)         C.S.

    B. Provide pamphlet explaining this information. (2/8)         C.S.

    C. Using this information have her make a sample grocery list reflecting this knowledge. (2/15)         C.S.

    D. See if she qualifies for the WIC program, which includes nutritional teaching of the recipient. (2/3)         C.S.

Obj. 3   Provide nutritionally sound diet for her family and herself.

    A. Ascertain the exact amount of money available to family. (2/8)         C.S.

    B. Determine grocery shopping habits, types of food purchased, and who grocery shops. (2/8)         C.S.

    C. Determine if family qualifies for food supplement program (i.e., food stamps, WIC) and refer. (2/3)         C.S.

    D. Determine who prepares and how foods are prepared. (2/8)         C.S.

    E. Schedule a visit during a meal time if possible. (2/15)         C.S.

---

*Clinical specialist.

2/1/78  **No. 2  Need for knowledge and anticipatory guidance during**    PERSONNEL
**antepartal period—cont'd**

2,B  Preparation for the baby

Obj. 1  The family should perceive and plan for change created by a new infant.

A.  Have mother pretend baby is here. Ask her how    C.S.
she will handle getting rest, coping with Darla's
demands. Ask her to describe how she coped
after Darla was born. (2/8)

B.  Explain the changes that family members under-    C.S.
go when there is a change in family structure.
(2/8)

C.  2/8 Ask her how she plans to create a bed and a    C.S.
space for the baby. Assist her if necessary in doing this. Have her describe preparations she
made for Darla. (2/8)

D.  Ascertain if she would be able to go to local    C.S.
childbirth preparation classes. (2/8)

Obj. 2  Intervention services should be available if a chaotic
family situation develops

A.  Assess further the family interactions specifically    C.S.
those of Sallie and sister to determine help and
support available to Sallie. (2/8)

B.  Talk with sister as to how this is affecting her life    C.S.
and family. (2/15)

C.  Ascertain the adjustments the sister foresees for    C.S.
herself and her children. (2/15)

D.  Intervene to facilitate adjustments after baby's    C.S.
birth if necessary. (3/78)

2/1/78  **No. 3 Lack of financial resources**

Obj. 1  The mother should be aware of all available financial
resources and employment opportunities.

A.  Call county and city departments for services    C.S.
and funds available to Sallie at this time. (2/8)

B.  Share this information with Sallie. (2/8)    C.S.

C.  Ask Sallie if she would be willing to work with the    Sallie
employment agency now to see if they could be    C.S.
making plans to assist her with future employment. (2/8)

D.  Ascertain dollar figures as to income and ex-    C.S.
penses and the specific sources of income (if
any). (2/8)

E.  Investigate the cost for care at the county hospi-    C.S.
tal and advise client. (2/15)

F.  Encourage Sallie to use any funds available to    C.S.
her at this time.

G.  Investigate local child care facilities available to
Sallie when she returns to work.

## NURSING ORDERS—cont'd

2/1/78   **No. 4 Child-rearing tasks of a parent with a preschooler**      **PERSONNEL**

4,A    Parenting

Obj. 1    The mother should demonstrate knowledge of parenting in a sibling rivalry situation.

     A. Teach mother the behaviors to expect from Darla when the new baby arrives and that these are normal. (2/15)    C. S.

     B. Ask her to talk with Darla more about the baby and that she still loves her as much as ever.    C. S.

     C. Encourage Sallie to give Darla the status of "big sister" and have her help with preparations for the baby.    C. S.

     D. Talk with Sallie about new sleeping arrangements soon for Darla so she can make room for the baby and so Darla will be used to a new sleeping room.    C. S.

     E. Talk with Darla to ascertain her perception of the situation.    C.S.

     F. Encourage mother to have Darla play with a doll that is "Darla's baby" to be used later in imitative behavior after baby comes.    C.S.

4,B    Safety of home environment

Obj. 1    The mother should demonstrate techniques for making home safe for preschooler.

     A. Teach mother that accidents are a major killer and maimer of small children.    C.S.

     B. Teach mother not to allow running in the house to avoid falls on the gas heater.    C.S. / Sallie

     C. Encourage her to purchase safety devices for electric outlets.    C.S. / Sallie

     D. Teach her to turn handles in on cooking pans on the stove.    C.S. / Sallie

     E. Teach mother to have clear-cut simple safety rules for Darla.    C.S. / Sallie

     F. Teach the child her full name, address, and phone number and how to use the services of the fireman and the police.    Sallie

     G. Attend the child closely while she is playing.    Sallie

Obj. 2    The mother should identify developmental milestones for Darla over the next year.

     A. Teach mother the major developmental needs of Darla over the next year.    C.S. / Sallie
- Need to identify with parent of same sex
- Need for increased peer association
- Need for imitative play
- Purposes of play

     B. Inventory Darla's toys and books and play areas. Work with mother to maximize and improvise space and materials for play.    C.S. / Sallie

2/1/78   **No. 4   Child-rearing tasks of a parent with a preschooler —cont'd**                    **PERSONNEL**    Case

4,C   Child health maintenance

Obj. 1   Darla should demonstrate optimum growth and development appropriate to her age
A. Interview Darla and perform a physical exam and D.D.S.T.                                          C.S.
B. Observe Darla in a play situation if possible                                                    C.S.

## PROGRESS NOTES

2/8/78 **No. 2  Need for knowledge and anticipatory guidance during the antepartal period**

2,A  Nutrition

**S**  Sallie is taking iron capsules and vitamins. Takes them "like I'm supposed to." Had "some blood tests" at last clinic visit. She drinks a glass of milk every day and is having cereal for breakfast. Has a sandwich and Coke for lunch most of the time—either cold cuts or peanut butter. May have hamburger or bacon and eggs for supper. Occasionally has a piece of fruit.

**O**  Client qualifies for WIC program. Diet is not adequate in all four food groups. Doesn't have basic knowledge of food groups. Reviewed the basic four and the requirements for the pregnant woman. Is willing to participate in the WIC program. Eats what sister provides. Has no money for food. Serum iron and total iron-binding capacity results not known. Client seems tired, pallor of nail beds upon blanching. Pale mucosa of eyes. Visit was not during a meal time.

**A**  Client data reflects on-going iron deficiency anemia. Will benefit from the WIC program nutritionally, and this should assist in learning better dietary habits. Child needs to have CBC to also assess for anemia. Arranged next visit over the lunch hour.

**P**  Continue with present plan. Add E to Obj. 1 of nursing orders.
E. Sallie will go to local WIC headquarters for evaluation, nutritional assistance, and teaching. (2/10/78)

2,B  Preparation for the baby

**S**  Mother assisted Sallie with Darla when she was born, allowing Sallie to rest when necessary. Aware that she does not have this resource now. Plans to rest when new baby will be napping. Did not have a baby bed with Darla. Plans to sleep with the new baby when it arrives. Has made no plans for a baby bed.

**O**  Explained to Sallie next visit we can make a bed with a box and a pillow and cover with contact paper. She agreed to do this. Seemed relieved for help. Instructed her to talk with her sister about how sister could assist her with Darla and letting her get some rest after baby gets here and make a plan to cope. We'll discuss this next week. Doesn't want to hassle with local childbirth classes because of no place to leave Darla and lack of transportation. Will start preparing her in the next home visits.

**A**  Mother needs assistance to plan forthcoming coping strategies. Is not oriented to future planning as is typical of persons who are having difficulties in meeting the demands of daily living. Needs preparation for childbirth.

**P**  Continue with present plan. D.C. action D under Obj. 1 of nursing orders. Next visit have mother provide a box and pillow for making a bed. Nurse will bring contact paper.

### No. 3  Lack of financial resources

**S**  Is still unsure about receiving any public assistance but will consider again as she recognizes her financial need. Doesn't know sister's income, and she doesn't have any.

**O** Informed Sallie of monies available to her. Encouraged her to have an appointment with local employment office soon so they can be looking for her in the interim. Unable to locate a child-care agency to care for Darla. Will continue to search for a child-care arrangement for her.

**A** Mother needs assistance at this time in all areas with no income. At this time seems motivated for employment after child gets here. Is having much difficulty in meeting everyday needs of herself and family.

**P** Continue with present plan.

### No. 4   Child-rearing tasks of a parent with a preschooler

4,A   Parenting

**S** Mother expressed appreciation for information about behaviors to expect from Darla and how she can manage her behavior. States she will talk with child more about the new baby and reinforce her love to the child. Will talk to her sister about Darla maybe sleeping in another room with the other children.

**O** Darla has a doll. Suggested to the mother she reinforce doll as Darla's baby so she can imitate Sallie. Mother appears genuinely concerned about effect of new baby on Darla. Darla knows "mommy's tummy is big and we're getting a brother."

**A** Sibling rivalry can create coping problems for a new parent and affect the older child's self-esteem if the situation is not handled in a positive way. Education about sibling rivalry should facilitate adjustment of all to the new baby.

**P** Continue with the present plan. Add G to Obj. 1 of nursing orders.
G. Review with Sallie how the doll play and further preparation of Darla has increased her readiness for a new brother or sister.

4,B   Safety of home environment

**S** None.

**O** Outlined the major developmental needs for Darla within the next year and methods for facilitating the development. Unable to assess the safety of the home environment at this time or to give physical safety guidelines.

**A** "Home Inventory for Ages 3-6" will give data about child's environment as to the adequacy for stimulating cognitive, affective, and physical development. Need to assess this environment for a plan to stimulate the child. Will do safety teaching and assessment next visit.

**P** Continue with the present plan. Add C to Obj. 2 of nursing orders.
C. Do "Home Inventory" next visit. (2/16)

## NURSING ORDERS

2/8/78 **No. 2   Need for knowledge and anticipatory guidance during antepartal period**

2,A   Nutrition                                                    **PERSONNEL**

Obj. 1   Correct iron-deficient condition with assistance of health workers.
Add E to Obj. 1.
E. Sallie will go to local WIC headquarters for evaluation, nutritional assistance, and teaching. (2/10/78)                                C.S.
Sallie

2,B   Preparation for the baby

D.C. D. Add E to Obj. 1.
E. Next visit have mother provide a box and a pillow for making a bed. Nurse will bring contact paper.      Sallie
C.S.

### No. 3   Lack of financial resources

Continue with same orders.                                          C.S.

### No. 4   Child-rearing tasks of parent with a preschooler

4,A   Parenting

Continue with same orders. Add G to Obj. 1 of nursing or-     C.S.
ders.

G. Review with Sallie how the doll play and further preparation of Darla has increased her readiness for a new brother or sister.

4,B   Safety of home environment

Obj. 2   The mother should identify developmental milestones for Darla over the next year.
Continue with same orders. Add C to Obj. 2. of              C.S.
nursing orders.
C. Do "Home Inventory" next visit. (2/16).

4,C   Child health maintenance

Obj. 1   Darla should demonstrate optimum growth and development appropriate to her age.
Continue with present orders.                              C.S.

**S**      None.

**O**      None.

**A**      Home visit time was limited. Will plan to do physical exam and DDST next visit as previously planned.

**P**      Continue with present plan.

A. Teach mother that accidents are a major killer and maimer of small children.    C.S.    Case

B. Teach mother not to allow running in the house to avoid falls on the gas heater.    C.S.
Sallie

C. Encourage her to purchase safety devices for electric outlets.    C.S.
Sallie

D. Teach her to turn handles in on cooking pans on the stove.    C.S.
Sallie

E. Teach mother to have clear-cut simple safety rules for Darla.    C.S.
Sallie

F. Teach the child her full name, address, and phone number and how to use the services of the fireman and the police.    Sallie

G. Attend the child closely while she is playing.    Sallie

Obj. 2 The mother should identify developmental milestones for Darla over the next year.

A. Teach mother the major developmental needs of Darla over the next year.    C.S.
Sallie

- Need to identify with parent of same sex
- Need for increased peer association
- Need for imitative play
- Purposes of play

B. Inventory Darla's toys and books and play areas. Work with mother to maximize and improvise space and materials for play.    C.S.
Sallie

4,C   Child health maintenance

Obj. 1   Darla should demonstrate optimum growth and development appropriate to her age

A. Interview Darla and perform a physical exam and D.D.S.T.    C.S.

B. Observe Darla in a play situation if possible    C.S.

## REFERENCES

Brunner, L. S., and Suddarth, D. S., editors: The Lippincott manual of nursing practice, Philadelphia, 1974, J. B. Lippincott Co.

Erickson, M. L.: Assessment and management of developmental changes in children, St. Louis, 1976, The C. V. Mosby Co.

Eshleman, J. R.: The family, Boston, 1974, Allyn & Bacon, Inc.

Murray, R., and Zentner, J.: Nursing assessment and health promotion through the life span, Englewood Cliffs, N.J., 1975, Prentice-Hall, Inc.

Murray, R., and Zentner, J.: Nursing concepts for health promotion, Englewood Cliffs, N.J., 1975, Prentice-Hall, Inc.

Ravel, R.: Clinical laboratory medicine, ed. 2, Chicago, 1973, Year Book Medical Publishers, Inc.

Standeven, M. V.: Social sensitivity in health care, Nurs. Outlook **25:**640-643, 1977.

# The newborn

The first day, week, and month have been identified as the periods of greatest risk during childhood. In the previous chapter we considered the developmental period that takes place before birth, and now we turn to the period that begins as labor and delivery begin and progresses through the first month of life.

In Chapter 6, "Labor, Delivery, and Initial Adaptation," we consider (1) the effects of events during labor and delivery on the fetus and (2) nursing care measures that are directed specifically toward the welfare of the fetus and the newborn through the first few hours, when the major adaptation takes place.

The purposes of Chapter 7, "Nursing Assessment and Care of the Newborn Infant," are to (1) present the principles of care of the newborn infant during the first month of life, (2) describe the complete assessment of the newborn infant, (3) describe estimation of gestational age, and (4) describe features of the early parent-child relationship and ways to promote adequate parenting.

Chapter 8, "Newborns at Risk," deals with the problems that can be encountered during the crucial first few weeks of life. Consideration of these hazards is intended to help the nurse who is beginning to work with newborns who have problems such as those discussed here and to assist in early detection of problems and identification of neonatal factors of importance in the history of the older child. The purpose of this chapter is to (1) consider the social and economic problems of care of the ill infant, (2) discuss selected neonatal problems, and (3) consider the implications of these kinds of health problems for the infant's family.

# CHAPTER 6

# Labor, delivery, and initial adaptation

The dramatic process of birth is probably the most significant single event in life. In many cultures it is celebrated yearly. In all cases the effects and possible scars of the birth process become a part of the individual's anatomy and physiology for the rest of his or her life. Successful completion of the transition from intrauterine to extrauterine life is highly dependent upon prenatal factors, which were discussed in Unit II. Onset of labor and delivery marks the end of one phase of life and the beginning of another, with multiple implications for the future safety and health of the newborn. The primary purpose of the health care team during this important event is to achieve safe and optimal progression through the various stages of labor and delivery for both mother and infant.

In the past, obstetric care concentrated on the mother, with very little attention directed to the fetus. The newborn who was abnormal or ill commanded some attention from pediatricians and other medical specialists. However, minimal effort was directed systematically toward understanding the birth process in terms of effect on the fetus and defining optimal care of the normal newborn. Recent research and application of new understanding have greatly increased the concept of care of the fetus and newborn during labor and delivery.

## LABOR AND DELIVERY: FETAL NURSING
### Processes of labor
*Events through the third stage*

The precise cause of labor is not known. Several theories have been considered as explanations of why labor begins. There probably exists an interaction among several factors, including distension of the uterus, mechanical irritation, progesterone deprivation, posterior pituitary action, and localized progesterone activity.[34] The early onset of labor, as in the case with twins or in the presence of an excessive amount of amniotic fluid, may be explained by hyperextension of the uterine muscle. Labor usually begins at the end of 40 weeks, or the equivalent of ten normal menstrual cycles. This fact suggests that some hormonal control, which participates in controlling menstrual cycles, also contributes to the onset of labor. When pregnancy has reached term, emotional or physical factors such as a fall, diarrhea, or a mental shock can begin labor.

The placenta may also play an important factor in beginning labor. Special hormones may be produced when the placenta has reached term and may be responsible for inducing labor. Placental aging, resulting in dropping of blood levels of estrogen and progesterone, is also believed to be an influential factor. This has a parallel in the menstrual cycles. With deterioration of the corpus luteum, blood levels of estrogen and progesterone drop, with menstruation beginning a few days later.

Labor may be conveniently divided into three distinct stages. The first stage is that of cervical dilatation. It begins with the first true labor pain and ends with complete dilatation of the cervix. The presenting part of the fetus begins to press on the cervix and lower uterine segment as well as on the nerve endings around the cervix and vagina. The upper uterine segment is the active contractile portion, which becomes thicker as labor advances and accomplishes retraction of the lower uterine segment and cervix, pushing the fetus downward. The lower uterine segment is the thin-walled, passive portion through which the baby descends. Many mothers, particularly those delivering their first child, need help and guidance in determining whether labor has in fact begun. The concepts of true labor and false labor are further contrasted in Table 6-1. Signs of true labor may be summarized as follows: (1) the escape of the plug of mucus that has corked the cervical canal mixed with a minimal amount of blood, known as bloody show; (2) regular uterine contractions; (3) painful contractions; (4) palpable hardening of the uterus during contractions; and (5) pain felt both in the back and the front of the abdomen. Examination of the mother's cervix and vaginal canal reveals that the cervix has begun to dilate and that the presenting part of the fetus has begun descent into the birth canal but remains in a fixed posi-

tion between contractions. Bulging or rupture of fetal membranes is a frequent result.[34]

The mechanisms of the first stage of labor accomplish two important changes in the cervix, namely effacement and dilatation. Effacement refers to shortening of the cervical canal from a structure of 1 to 2 cm in length to one in which the canal is replaced by a mere circular orifice with almost paper-thin edges. Dilatation refers to the enlargement of the cervix from an orifice a few millimeters in size to an aperture large enough to permit passage of the baby. The primary forces that accomplish these changes are uterine contractions retracting the cervix and bringing about pressure of the membranes or the pressure of the presenting fetal part against the cervix and lower uterine segment. Effacement usually begins before the onset of the actual labor through the mechanism of Braxton-Hicks contractions, which are painless, irregular contractions of the uterus that occur throughout pregnancy.

During the second stage, descent of the baby through the birth canal is accomplished. The upper uterine segment increases greatly in thickness. Abdominal muscles are auxiliary forces, which assist in accomplishing descent and expulsion during the second stage.

At some point during the first or early second stage of labor, the amniotic membranes rupture spontaneously, or they may be ruptured artificially. Once this occurs and the amniotic fluid escapes, the progression of labor tends to be an irreversible process. As descent of the fetus begins, the mother cannot resist contracting her

**Table 6-1.** Contrasting features of false labor and true labor

| True labor | False labor |
| --- | --- |
| Pains at regular intervals | Irregular pains |
| Intervals gradually shorten in length | No change |
| Duration and severity of contraction increase | No change |
| Pains start at the base of the spine and move upward into the abdominal region | Pain remains in the front |
| Walking increases intensity of contractions | No change |
| Association between the degree of uterine hardening and intensity of pain | No relationship |
| Bloody show is often present | No show |
| Cervix becomes effaced and dilated | No change |
| Descent of the presenting part begins | No descent |
| Head of fetus in a fixed position between contractions | Head remains free |
| Sedation will not stop true labor | Efficient sedative will stop labor |

abdominal walls and diaphragm and pushing downward during uterine contractions. This process is repeated at varying intervals and with ever increasing force and strain. When the head is presenting, this force is applied directly to the fetal spinal column. The curve of the fetal spine tends to straighten, adding power to the push of the head downward. The fetal spine is usually parallel to the midline axis of the mother's abdomen or is slightly to one side. The head accommodates to the mother's pelvis as it passes through the vaginal canal by turning first to one side and then the other. Finally the head crowns, with the diameter of the occiput being visible at the level of the perineum. When the head is born, the neck straightens, turning the head to one side in alignment with the position of the shoulders. When the shoulders pass through the pelvis and accommodate to the shape of the birth canal, the body continues to rotate. The posterior shoulder is usually born over the perineum first, and the anterior soon follows under the symphysis pubis. The body quickly follows and the infant is born.[34,41]

The third stage begins after the infant is completely born and lasts until expulsion of the placenta is complete. Placental separation usually takes place within 5 to 30 minutes after completion of the second stage. Signs that indicate that placental detachment has occurred include a rush of blood from the vagina, lengthening of the umbilical cord outside the vulva, rise of the uterine fundus and the abdomen as the placenta passes from the uterus into the vagina, and the uterus becoming very firm and globular. It is essential to examine the placenta to determine whether or not any parts are missing and remain in the uterus and to detect any abnormalities that may aid in determining the infant's condition and expectations for the transition to extrauterine life.

Areas of necrosis on the placenta, an excessively small placenta, or abnormal anatomy of the lobes, membranes, and vessels of the placenta give clues suggesting abnormal or inadequate functioning of the placenta during intrauterine life. The normal placenta weighs from 500 to 600 g, and a normal cord is approximately 18 inches in length. At the time of delivery the maternal side (the spongy, dull side) of the placenta should appear dark red, with irregularly shaped lobes. The fetal surface (the shiny side) of the placenta should appear reddish purple, with the vessels attached firmly and deeply into the placental mass and veins visibly extending over the entire surface. The cord should contain three vessels, two arteries, and one vein. The most common vascular anomaly is the absence of one umbilical artery, a condition that is sometimes associated with other fetal anomalies.[31]

Placental transfer of molecules may change in the last week of pregnancy as the efficiency of the placenta decreases. In addition, compression, decreased uterine pressure, and placental blood flow during contractions influence the transfer of molecules. The biochemical status of the fetus is altered noticeably during even a normal uncomplicated delivery. Alteration of normal oxygen and carbon dioxide exchange between mother and fetus is reflected in acid-base analyses of blood from the umbilical cord and the infant following birth. Oxygen levels fall, carbon dioxide tension rises, and pH falls. The infant must accomplish recovery and readjustment from this normal biochemical birth asphyxia in adapting to extrauterine life.[4,30] The occurrence of this kind of event is considered a medical and anesthesiologic problem at any other time in life. While most infants seem to recover adequately, observation and evaluation of the infant's progress are essential to protect him or her from developing difficulty.

### The use of drugs during labor

The factors that influence the effect of drugs in the fetus that were discussed in Chapter 5 apply to drugs administered during labor, but the effects and processes may be altered during labor and delivery. These factors may be summarized as follows:[10]

1. Potency of the drug agent
2. Placental transfer of drugs
3. Maternal and fetal blood flow
4. Molecular size of the drug agent
5. Concentration gradient across the placental membrane
6. Distribution, absorption, and excretion of the drug by the fetus
7. Biochemical status of the fetus
8. Maternal disease

**Table 6-2.** Summary of factors related to drugs commonly used during labor*

| Class | Effect on mother | Effect on fetus | Agents and factors related to use | Miscellaneous |
|---|---|---|---|---|
| Inhalation agents | Analgesia, anesthesia | Usually no significant depression with analgesic dosage. Asphyxiation and slow onset of respiration with anesthetic dosage. | Nitrous oxide mixture containing 40%-60% for brief periods produces moderate analgesia. Mixtures containing 75% for several minutes produce anesthesia. Cyclopropane 3%-5%, mixture for brief periods produces analgesia. Anesthetic dosage depends on depth and duration of administration. Crosses placenta within 1.5 minutes; is used safely within 6-10 minutes of delivery. Methoxyflurane, diethylether, halothane used in some centers with good effect in carefully selected cases; may lead to maternal toxicity during conditions such as induction of labor or maternal disease. | Used during second stage. Action potentiated by barbiturates, phenothiazides, and potent analgesics. |
| Barbiturates | Sedation, amnesia, anesthesia | Controversial; depression usually occurs correlated with the administered dosage. Deleterious effects of mild-to-moderate barbiturate depression have not been defined. These drugs may offer some protection to CNS following asphyxia. | Secobarbital: short-acting; seems to have no adverse effect on 1 or 5 minute Apgar score if given before last 25 minutes before delivery. Thiopental: ultra shortacting; used IV to induce or maintain general anesthesia; considerable risk of neonatal depression when used immediately before delivery, as placental transfer is almost immediate. | All cross placenta rapidly; infants born within several hours of administration have significant blood barbiturate levels as long as the fourth day of life. |
| Regional anesthetics | Localized anesthesia | Variable from no effect to profound depression. Greatest hazard occurs with improper technique in administering paracervical block or caudal anesthesia. | Procaine (ester group): fairly long latent period between administration and action; short duration of action, poor ability to penetrate tissues. Lidocaine, prilocaine, mepivacaine (amide group) acts more rapidly than ester group, longer duration and better penetration of the tissues. | Amides are more poorly metabolized by the fetus than are esters. When either group is used for spinal anesthesia, hazard of maternal hypotension with decreased blood flow to the uterus is present. Use of these agents with cesarean sections less hazardous for the fetus than general anesthesia. |
| Phenothiazines (tranquilizers) | Generally unsubstantiated; believed to produce sedation, relieve anxiety, | Generally unsubstantiated. Cross placenta rapidly; apparently no adverse effects. | Chlorpromazine: substantial alpha-adrenergic blockage resulting in epinephrine reversal and norepinephrine unresponsiveness, leading to possible maternal hypotension. This effect may impair neonates temperature-regulating capability. | |

*See references 1, 10, 34, 41.

**Table 6-2.** Summary of factors related to drugs commonly used during labor—cont'd

| Class | Effect on mother | Effect on fetus | Agents and factors related to use | Miscellaneous |
|-------|------------------|-----------------|-----------------------------------|---------------|
| Phenothi-azines—cont'd | potentiate analgesic action, and prevent nausea and vomiting | | Promethazine: uncertain benefits in obstetric use; mainly noted for antihistiminic and mild sedative effect. | |
| Narcotics | Analgesia | Varying levels of depression, depending on dosage and time of administration. Peak effect is during second and third hour following IM or subcutaneous injection. Infants born within an hour of administration or after the third hour exhibit minimal effect. | Morphine: seldom used because of reports of severe neonatal depression. Careful usage, however, is probably as safe as the other narcotics. Meperidine: thought to be the safest narcotic, but this is unsubstantiated. | Narcotic antagonists (nalorphine, levallorphan) should be available when these agents are in use. However, they may not always reverse respiratory depression in infants, possibly because of action of metabolites of narcotics rather than action of narcotics themselves. |

Drugs administered to the mother during labor affect the fetus primarily by exaggerating the degree of fetal asphyxia and/or influencing the rate and quality of the infant's recovery, adaptation, and neurologic behavior. Studies of visual attentiveness, sucking behavior, and neurologic and electroencephalogram features of infants born after maternal sedation suggest that depressant effects of drugs may last as long as four days after birth.[11,20,33]

Understanding of specific actions of drugs remains limited. For this reason, only a limited number of drugs are used during labor and with varying degrees of confidence. The nurse is obligated to be entirely familiar with drugs administered to the mother and to apply whatever information is available regarding fetal effect to the care of the infant after delivery, as any therapeutic agent given to the mother has a potential for adversely affecting the fetus and newborn. In addition, carefully documented observations of infants who were exposed to maternal drugs during labor contribute significantly to the advancement of knowledge and evaluation of long-term effects of drugs. Table 6-2 summarizes current known factors related to drugs commonly used during labor. Rapid growth and change in the fields of pharmacology and anesthesiology require constant study and attention by health care team members who participate in perinatal care of mothers and infants.

*Fetal assessment*

In the past there has been a dearth of knowledge regarding a relationship between the condition of the fetus and future development of the child. Recent advances in perinatal medicine and research, even though in an early stage of development, have resulted in a growing understanding, which carries great implications for nursing care. The collaborative study* on cerebral palsy, mental retardation, and other neurologic and sensory disorders of infancy and childhood from 1957 to 1970 indicated that children with a five-minute Apgar score of 0 to 3 exhibit three times as many neurologic abnormalities at 1 year of age than do children of comparable birth weights with a five-minute Apgar score of 7 to 10. (For a discussion of Apgar scoring, see p. 159.) Since other similar evidence has developed, concerted efforts have been directed toward reducing the frequency of newborns with

---

*The National Institute of Neurological Diseases and Stroke, the National Institutes of Health, Bethesda, Maryland.

low Apgar scores and, in turn, toward reducing neonatal morbidity and mortality.[20]

Nursing care for the mother and fetus has been greatly enhanced by fetal monitoring techniques. Even when continuous mechanical monitoring of the fetal heart rate patterns is not used, nursing care is facilitated by a thorough understanding of principles of fetal assessment. When a mother and fetus are in a known or suspected high risk category, mechanical and nonmechanical monitoring is particularly helpful in attempting to deliver the infant with as little compromise as possible.

The range of normal fetal heart rate is generally accepted to be between 120 and 160 beats per minute. However, knowledge of the rate alone, particularly when sampled between uterine contractions, is of little value in assessing fetal condition.[21]

Three patterns of fetal heart rates have been described by researchers, denoting the time re-

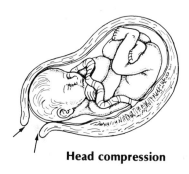

**Head compression**

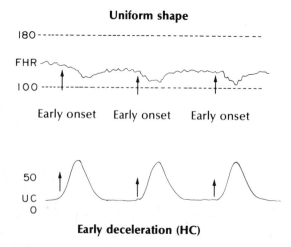

**Early deceleration (HC)**

**Fig. 6-1.** Early deceleration, usually associated with head compression.

lationship between the onset of uterine contractions and onset of change in fetal heart rate. Because of some confusion arising from the use of different terminology for similar events, an agreement was reached to use terminology based on Hon's work.[27,28] Formerly used synonyms for the various patterns are indicated to facilitate the reader's understanding.

Early deceleration (type I dip, early bradycardia, or V-shaped bradycardia) is a pattern in which uterine contractions are relatively uniform and the fetal heart rate deceleration pattern is also uniform, reflecting uterine amplitude (Fig. 6-1). Onset of rate deceleration coincides with the onset of the uterine contraction and is thought to be the result of compression of the fetal head and fetal vagal stimulation. This pattern is thought to be innocuous to the fetus.

Late deceleration (type II dip, late bradycardia, or U-shaped bradycardia) begins late during the phase of uterine contraction and is believed to be caused by asphyxial depression of cardiovascular centers of the central nervous system and of the heart itself (Fig. 6-2). This ominous pattern is often associated with maternal diabetes, hypertension, toxemia, or placental insufficiency. The appearance of late deceleration is usually associated with abnormal acid-base and blood gas status in the fetus, and monitoring of these values is desirable. Often immediate obstetric intervention is indicated, but immediate administration of oxygen to the mother may modify the pattern.

Variable deceleration (Fig. 6-3) occurs in 80% to 85% of cases of clinical fetal distress. The fetal heart rate does not reflect uterine amplitude or timing. The variability is thought to be caused by acute hypoxia and strong vagal stimulation; it is often associated with cord compression. For this reason the usual intervention of choice is repositioning the mother and monitoring for any change in the fetal heart rate pattern. A maternal supine position is particularly adverse for the fetus, because pressure is exerted on the inferior vena cava of the mother, decreasing uterine blood flow. Improvement in the fetal heart rate pattern will be noted within 10 to 20 minutes if positioning was contributing to the problem.

Interpretation of patterns not clearly defined

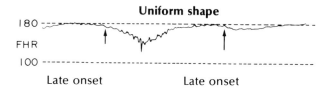

**Uteroplacental insufficiency**

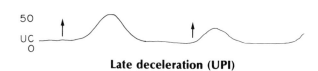

**Late deceleration (UPI)**

**Fig. 6-2.** Late deceleration, usually associated with uteroplacental insufficiency.

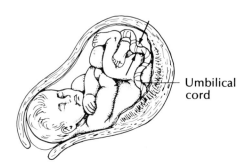

**Umbilical cord compression**

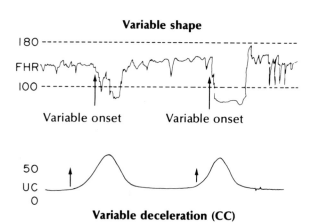

**Variable deceleration (CC)**

**Fig. 6-3.** Variable deceleration, usually associated with cord compression.

by the major categories requires skilled obstetric judgment. Such patterns are usually assumed to be the most ominous sign of fetal welfare, and obstetric intervention is mandatory.

The limitations of using only stethoscopic auscultation of fetal heart rate are serious when the fetus is known to be at risk or is subjected to some undesirable influence during labor and delivery. However, for most instances of normal labor and delivery, stethoscopic auscultation is valuable and can be understood more completely by application of knowledge derived from fetal heart rate patterns monitored mechanically. The normal range of fetal heart rate is between 120 and 160 beats per minute as determined between uterine contractions. Auscultation of the fetal heart rate throughout the course of uterine contractions to determine the adequacy of the pattern is difficult but most important in adequately determining the well-being of the fetus. [19,38]

Equipment used to monitor these patterns incorporates either ultrasonic or electronic techniques. Familiarity with the manufacturer's recommendations for use and interpretation of readings is necessary to obtain optimal benefit for the mother and fetus. Ultrasonic monitoring is based on the use of a Doppler signal of high-frequency sound waves that transmit well through water and soft body tissues. The signals of uterine contractions and fetal heart rate are both monitored transabdominally, which enables monitoring before and after the membranes have been ruptured. [9]

Electronic monitoring is used only after the membranes have ruptured and is obtained by applying the fetal electrode to the presenting part and inserting a catheter electrode into the uterus for uterine contractions. [25] With either method the mother may move and turn, and nursing care measures can be continued without interruption.

Although it is profitable to study patterns of the fetal heart rate and uterine contractions, the majority of mothers deliver without this procedure. Auscultatory monitoring of the fetal heartbeat is imperative and is, in fact, enhanced by an understanding of its limitations. Counting fetal heartbeats throughout and just after a contraction, rather than waiting for relaxation, is

required. Any arrhythmia, persistent tachycardia, or bradycardia is noted, and intervals between auscultation are shortened to determine more exactly the extent of the trait. [5]

Fetal electrocardiography is a more difficult monitoring procedure than fetal heart rate pattern monitoring, but it will probably yield proportionately greater understanding as equipment and data interpretation become more accessible to a greater number of practitioners.

Monitoring of fetal blood pH and blood gases is an important adjunct to effective use of fetal heart rate pattern monitoring. Ranges of acceptable blood gas levels depend on the method used, and the nurse should be aware of the limits determined for a given setting. Fetal pH is well standardized, with the lower limit of acceptability being 7.25. When a fetal heart rate pattern is questionable or when a decision is required regarding obstetric intervention, data obtained from frequent sampling of fetal blood clarify the extent of fetal asphyxia.

Diligent nursing observations are essential for effective and optimal care by each member of the health care team. Ominous signs of fetal distress, which have long been recognized, include passage of meconium by a fetus in a vertex presentation at any point during labor and delivery, sudden thrashing or tumultous movements of the fetus, and maternal bleeding. [5,26,42]

### Nursing care of the mother and fetus

Many aspects of care are required from professional members of the health team, but a woman's family or significant friends may be an important part of her care during labor and delivery. The observation of many practitioners suggests that the way labor and delivery are experienced by the mother has a great deal to do with the way in which the mother is able to fill the mothering role for the infant. When significant people are available and willing to help her by support, encouragement, and physical care, nursing assistance is often needed to encourage their participation and sharing that is satisfying for the mother and her family. The mother may be functioning at a disadvantaged level of ability during labor and delivery, with her dependence on others heightened considerably. When people are present who have established a sharing, trusting relationship, the mother is more able to give to her infant in the mothering process. This is particularly true when the mother has planned and prepared for a particular method of childbirth using minimal medication and requiring a great deal of her own participation.[43]

As long as the mother is healthy, presentation of the fetus is normal, and the fetus is in good condition, the mother may walk about or lie down as she wishes. Her condition, progress, and the condition of the fetus are monitored periodically by one of the methods described above. In addition, the progress of labor may be followed by rectal or vaginal examinations to note the station of the presenting part and degree of dilatation of the cervix. These examinations should be conducted often enough to ensure safe conduct of labor.

It is desirable that the first stage of labor be conducted over a period of time ranging from 4 hours for a multipara to approximately 12 hours for a primipara. During normal labor it is desirable that the mother refrain from eating solid foods because of the danger of vomiting and aspiration during the latter parts of labor and delivery. She does, however, need fluids and some source of energy such as clear soup or fluids containing sugar.

During the first stage of labor the mother must be encouraged to continually relax with contractions. Bearing down is to be avoided because it does not improve the progress of labor. During the second stage, however, when the cervix is fully dilated, bearing down becomes helpful in pushing the baby through the birth canal. Probably one of the most important aspects of care during the second stage is the support that the mother receives from those with her. Even when she has had past experiences with delivery or when she is coping adequately with the demands of labor utilizing the principles and techniques learned during preparation for labor and delivery, she needs continual reinforcement and reassurance regarding the progress of labor and the safety of her infant.[17,34]

Assistance and reassurance for the mother when progress is not satisfactory require a great deal of professional skill and care. When fetal monitoring is used, the nurse may give reassurance by explaining the purpose of the various leads and keeping the mother informed regarding the information that the monitoring approach is yielding. False optimism can be more difficult to cope with eventually, because most mothers have a heightened sensitivity to any clues that might be interpreted as ominous signs. A period of silence or a whispered conference outside her door may create images of the worst disaster in the mother's mind.[9,25,36]

Physical care that promotes the mother's comfort and rest during labor is very important. Back rubs, frequent positional changes, assistance with elimination, provision of clean and dry linen, and assistance in keeping the skin dry and mucous membranes moist become progressively more significant to the mother as labor progresses. Such care given to the mother affects the well-being of the fetus in many instances. Positional changes lessen the chances for severe cord compression and/or decreased uterine blood flow. Brief periods of oxygen administration to the mother may be important in aiding the fetus through a brief period of stress, which may be detected indirectly by the mother or nurse.

Matousek[26] has recommended several features essential to adequate fetal nursing. Complete observation is essential, including:

1. Any unusual fetal activity, described as precisely as possible
2. Presence of meconium when the membranes rupture or at any point thereafter
3. Fetal heart rate auscultation
4. Duration of any tachycardia or bradycardia continuing after a contraction

When an unusual sign is observed, there must be prompt reporting with complete description of the unusual signs to the physician. Current fetal signs, as well as the former fetal patterns, are related to the following conditions of the fetal environment:

1. Maternal vital signs
2. Medications administered; amount and time given
3. Frequency, type, and duration of uterine contractions
4. Intactness of the membranes and the presence or absence of meconium
5. Bleeding, with an estimate of the amount lost externally

6. Other significant changes in the mother's condition that occur at or near the time of altered fetal signs

## Physiology of the fetus and newborn

There is a relatively orderly continuum of adaptation from fetal to extrauterine life. The events pass unnoticed and with relative ease in many cases. When difficulty occurs, however, care of the infant depends upon understanding the normal events of adaptation during this period. Since normal transition is dependent upon a rather fine balance of chemical, physiologic, and anatomic changes, stress is ultimately hazardous. Infants have demonstrated a relative resistance to the stress of anoxia; they can survive longer in an oxygen-free environment than can an adult. The search for a metabolic or biochemical basis for this relative tolerance has yielded no complete answer, and the long-term effects of mild oxygen deprivation are not known. Skillful detection of impending danger to the neonate from any stress can be a life-saving and health-protecting measure.

### Respiratory system

The most important and life-dependent change at the moment of birth is the establishment of respiration. The first inspiratory effort is mammoth. A negative pressure of up to 70 cm $H_2O$ is required to move between 12 and 70 mm of air in to the lungs. The normal negative pressure of about 20 cm $H_2O$ is sufficient to move air into the lungs once initial expansion is established. Obligatory respiratory effort greater than the normal pressure required continues to decline until a relatively stable, easy rhythm is established. Lung expansion greatly increases the capillary bed absorptive surface areas for gas exchange. The presence of surfactant, a lipoprotein secretion, facilitates expansion and prevents collapse of the alveoli with expiration (see Chapter 8).

### Circulatory system

Dramatic anatomic changes occur in the heart and circulatory systems. Placental circulation ceases with the cutting of the cord or the complete detachment of the placenta. There is a relative rise in left atrial pressure and drop in inferior vena cava pressure, resulting in effective functional closure of the foramen ovale during the first 24 hours of life. There is still controversy over the exact mechanism of closure of the foramen ovale and the ductus arteriosus. Murmurs resulting from incomplete closure of these structures are not unusual in the neonatal period. The ductus arteriosus is probably not closed for several days, and it either becomes functionally ineffective or a normal reversal in flow continues before true closure occurs.

The sudden decrease in vascular pressure, which occurs with the expansion of the lungs at the moment of inspiration, causes the rush of blood flow through the capillary beds of the lungs for the first time. This vascularization of the lungs contributes to the dramatic changes in the blood flow through the greater vessels surrounding the heart and lungs.

There is a rise in plasma protein and hemoglobin concentration occurring from a few minutes to three hours after birth. This is thought to be a result of a shift of plasma fluid from the vascular compartment, plus a loss of cellular water from the erythrocyte. This shift in turn may be the result of the redistribution of blood flow and capillary leakage. The altered pH, $PCO_2$ and $O_2$ saturations at birth and their return to normal may account for the water lost from the erythrocyte. These factors may also be related to the edema of the neonatal period. In term infants this is usually confined to the presenting parts, but in the premature infant it is more generalized.[12,23,29]

### Gastrointestinal system

At birth the digestive and absorptive mechanisms necessary to handle the complex sugars present in human milk, as well as protein and fat, are present. The neonate's source of energy for the first few hours is carbohydrate, with fat becoming important by the second day of life. Protein metabolism begins by the third day. Brain tissue continues throughout life to be dependent upon carbohydrates as the source of energy.

The liver is limited in its function, especially in the ability to conjugate bilirubin and corticosteroid. Glycolysis occurs more rapidly in the first 12 hours of life than it does after three days.

Lowered surrounding temperatures cause an increase in the metabolic rate, which in turn continues to contribute to metabolic acidosis or at least keeps the balance just on the acidotic side so that respiratory efforts to correct the imbalance remain relatively neutral. Increased metabolism is further mediated by adrenal medulla compounds (epinephrine, norepinephrine), which delay or disturb the adaptation of pulmonary circulation.

### Renal system

Renal capacity is generally considered adequate in the normal term infant. However, stress of dehydration, excess solutes in oral fluids, tissue catabolism, or illness brings out the limited adaptive capacity of the neonatal kidney.[1]

### Nervous system

The nervous system of the neonate is incompletely integrated at birth but is fully functional in a life-sustaining sense. Clinical signs of adaptation described by Desmond and colleagues[15] are basically related to the functioning of the autonomic nervous system, which is believed to be the most crucial system during transition. This is the overall integrator and stimulator for maintenance of respiration, acid-base control, compensation of imbalance, and temperature control.

During the first oscillation, the infant is responding to the massive stimuli of birth. Responses of the autonomic nervous system to the stimulation of the delivery process are demonstrated by the infant's behavior. This is reflected in a massive wave of sympathetic system activity. Normal, healthy newborns will cry, look around with a wide-eyed expression, and move vigorously. Their heart and respiratory rates are slightly elevated, and they are likely to discharge urine, stool, and mucus from the mouth. After this first reactive period, infants exhibit a reversal of these signs, and enter a period of sleep and relative calm. The respiratory and heart rates decrease, they exhibit very little spontaneous motion and are not likely to discharge mucus, urine, or stool. If an effort is made to stimulate them or to elicit neurologic responses, only minimal response will be ob-

tained, and they will easily resume the appearance of deep sleep.

After a period of time, ordinarily ranging from two to six hours, infants spontaneously experience the second reactive period, which resembles closely the active, alert behavior exhibited during the period immediately after birth. The intensity of the behavior is not as pronounced, but the same characteristics are again present. They then go through slowly declining periods oscillating between rest and stimulation. At any point during the periods of stimulation the newborn is at risk from the common hazards present during the period immediately after birth including respiratory, circulatory, and neurologic complications.

The implications of this adaptation process are great. First, the newborn probably benefits from being allowed to pass through the normal physiologic stabilizing process with a minimal amount of disturbance and a maximal degree of observation. Bathing and feeding, for instance, should be delayed until behavior and physiologic mechanisms are stabilized. This point usually occurs between 4 and 8 hours of age. The nurse's most reliable guideline, however, is individual behavior, not clock hours of life.

Mucus, which newborns tend to regurgitate during this period, is a normal product of intrauterine life and probably originates in the lungs and gastrointestinal tissues. The amount of mucus produced varies greatly. Some controversy remains regarding the efficacy of gastric suctioning for alleviation or prevention of mucus being regurgitated into the upper esophageal tract where it remains as a danger for aspiration. Certainly, when the production of mucus reaches a level at which aspiration becomes an obvious hazard, suctioning should be employed. Suctioning of mucus from the mouth with a simple bulb syringe may be of some benefit, but the more effective approach is to remove material from the esophagus, then the stomach.[37]

## NURSING CARE OF THE NEONATE
### Apgar scoring and assessment at delivery

Assessment of the newborn begins as soon as the infant is born. The times of the first inhalation, the first cry, and the onset of sustained

**Table 6-3.** Apgar scoring

| Sign | Score | | |
|---|---|---|---|
| | **0** | **1** | **2** |
| Heart rate | Absent | Slow (below 100) | Over 100 |
| Respiratory effort | Absent | Weak cry, hypoventilation | Good; strong cry |
| Muscle tone | Limp | Some flexion of extremities | Active motion, extremities well flexed |
| Reflex irritability | No response | Grimace | Cry |
| Color | Blue, pale | Body pink, extremities blue | Completely pink |

respiration are noted. Apgar scoring provides a simple and easily applied clinical measure for evaluation of the infant's general condition.[2,40] The score has been validated by a wide variety of studies, and its usefulness in determining the condition of the infant, as well as predicting future adaptation and neurologic development, is well established.[1] The scoring is made at 1 minute and 5 minutes of age and may be repeated until the infant's condition has stabilized. The total score is obtained by adding the values allotted to observations of heart rate, respiratory effort, muscle tone and reflex irritability, and color as indicated in Table 6-3.

The heart rate is best followed when the observer listens with a stethoscope. This is the most important of the five signs, and response of the heart rate after resuscitative measures is a good prognostic sign. Failure of the heart to respond after artificial expansion of the lungs indicates the need for closed chest cardiac massage. For the purposes of Apgar scoring, a rate over 100 beats per minutes is assigned a value of 2, a rate under 100 is assigned a value of 1, and a score of zero is assigned if the heart beat is absent. However, tachycardia, or a heart rate over 160, is indicative of moderate, recent asphyxia and is considered an ominous sign. Such an infant should be carefully observed during the adaptation period. Bradycardia is indicative of serious distress of longer duration and some form of resuscitation is probably indicated.

Respiratory effort is the second most important sign. A score of 2 is given for vigorous, effective respirations; a score of 1 is given if respirations are present but are ineffective and irregular, and zero is assigned if apnea is present at the time of the scoring.

Active, vigorous flexion and extension of arms and legs are given a score of 2. A score of 1 is assigned when the infant moves the extremities, but they do not resist passive extension. A score of zero is assigned when the infant is completely limp or flaccid.

Reflex irritability refers to the response of the infant to any form of stimulation. In some cases where nasopharyngeal suctioning is conducted, the response of the infant to the passage of the catheter may be noted. A brisk slap with the palm of hand to the sole of the feet is recommended for an infant who is not otherwise stimulated by such procedures as suctioning. Flicking the soles with the fingers or spanking the buttocks are not recommended because of the danger of inadvertently injuring the infant. If the infant cries, a score of 2 is assigned. A grimace is assigned a score of 1, and no response is assigned a score of zero.

Color is the least important of the five observations but is the most easily obtained. If the infant is pink over the entire body, including hands and feet, a score of 2 is given. One point is given when the hands and feet remain blue. A score of zero is assigned if the whole body is blue or colorless.

Further nursing assessment may be conducted soon after the infant is born, depending upon the condition and needs of the infant.

### Care during the adaptation period

There are four major needs toward which nursing care and observation of the neonate are directed during the first day of life:

1. Provision of adequate respiration
2. Provision of warmth
3. Provision of safety
4. Provision of nutrition

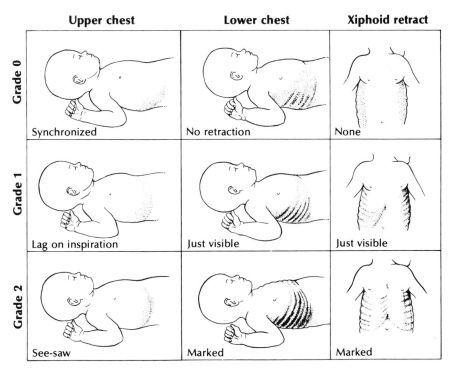

**Fig. 6-4.** Silverman-Andersen score of respiratory difficulty. (From Silverman, W., and Andersen, D. H.: A controlled trial of the effect of water mist on obstructive respiratory signs, death rate, necropsy findings among premature infants, Pediatrics **17**:1, 1956.)

## Provision of adequate respiration

The first requirement is presence of an open airway. Most infants need minimal suctioning of the mouth and nasopharynx to achieve this. In some cases deep suctioning or intubation of the trachea is required. These procedures should be skillfully performed by any member of the health care team who is present at the time of need.[37] Nurses who work with neonates are required, therefore, to develop skill in the choice and manipulation of resuscitation equipment and in administering a wide range of resuscitative techniques. Once the airway is clear, the infant may be administered oxygen or air by mouth-to-mouth or mask and bagging techniques. If the infant's respirations are further inhibited by poor exchange of gases at the alveoli and circulatory levels, oxygen administration is imperative. A variety of suctioning equipment that is easily portable should be available in the delivery room area. The nurse in any setting can apply the technique of postural drainage to help an infant discharge mucus or other material that may be obstructing a full exchange of gases.

Continuous observation and evaluation of the quality of respiration are imperative, because this is the basis upon which the decision is made to assist the infant in some way. An infant with an Apgar score of 6 or below should receive a thorough continuing clinical description of respirations as to severity, presence, and location of retractions, nasal flaring, chin lag, paradoxical action of the chest and abdomen (see-saw action), and grunting that is audible with or without a stethoscope (Fig. 6-4). Infants experiencing difficulty should receive constant surveillance and care, being allowed to rest and conserve energy as much as possible. Nursing care measures and techniques administered to enhance respiratory effort, such as suctioning or positive pressure insufflation of the lungs, should be administered with skill and dexterity so as not to prolong handling or cause excessive stimulation or tiring.

## Provision of warmth

From an ambient intrauterine temperature of approximately 100° F, the infant is suddenly thrust into a room as cool as 70° F. In addition, the infant is wet with amniotic fluid, which in-

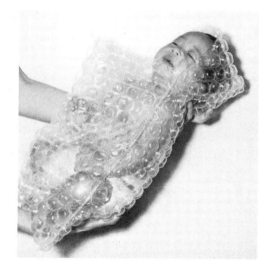

**Fig. 6-5.** An infant may be wrapped in a plastic swaddler to provide protection from heat loss from conduction, evaporation, and convection. Protection from radiant heat loss must be provided from an additional source, but this kind of protection alone is effective in minimizing the stress of heat loss during the first one to four hours after delivery.

creases the cooling effect by means of evaporation. In a hospital setting, equipment that provides warmth by radiation or conduction may be provided. Again, thorough familiarity with such equipment is mandatory for maximum benefit to the infant and protection from misuse resulting in burning. Thorough drying of the infant is beneficial in reducing the period of time exposed to evaporation. In many cases improvised sources of heat can be used, including lamps, blankets heated in an oven, or warmth from the mother's body. The smaller or younger the infant is at birth, the greater the need for supportive measures for heat control, as thermoregulating ability is immature or unreliable for a small or low gestational age infant. The ideal ambient temperature and humidity for infants of a given gestational age or condition at birth are unknown; however, most infants do not tolerate overheating (above a skin temperature of 96° F). Humidity levels in the air affect the temperature-regulating ability of the body, as well as loss of body water through the skin. High levels of humidity (about 50%) have been demonstrated to be of some benefit to premature infants.[1,14,32]

## Provision of nutrition

Benefits of feeding within the first eight hours of life are well demonstrated for infants of diabetic mothers, and implications for normal newborns have been drawn. The occurrence of hypoglycemia and hyperbilirubinemia in all infants has been demonstrated to be reduced for infants fed during the first eight hours.[4,5] An initial feeding of 10% glucose in water may be given to the infant between 4 and 12 hours of age or when the infant is observed to have completed the oscillation periods of the adaptation process. A breast-fed infant may feed as soon as the mother desires after delivery and as often as the infant is hungry. The most important nutrient for the neonate during the first 24 hours is carbohydrate to sustain needed sources of energy and maintain biochemical homeostasis. Maternal colostrum is rich in carbohydrates. Formula may be started at any point. A solution of glucose and water is usually chosen during the first 12 hours because of the tendency toward mucus production, increasing chances of aspiration.[22]

## Provision of a safe and clean environment

Some term infants can roll completely over, thus it should never be assumed that the infant will not roll off a bed or table. The infant is also particularly vulnerable to infection during the neonatal period. Immature blood and metabolic defenses against microorganisms render him or her more susceptible to infections. Infection affects the infant's blood and nervous system more readily than is usual for the child or adult. Silver nitrate or some other acceptable drug is instilled in the infant's eyes as prophylaxis against gonorrheal infection.

## Care of the family at the time of birth

When the mother and father or other significant people are actively participating in the delivery experience, consideration and care offered to them in relation to the condition of the infant at birth are of prime importance. Their primary expressed concern is for the health and well-being of the infant. For each member of the family the birth of an infant represents a personal event in their own development. Producing a healthy, well-formed infant is often a meaningful step in the development of the self-concept of the parents. Becoming a grandparent also represents certain inner self and social developmental accomplishments. Coping adequately with the realization of these anticipated events depends upon a number of complex factors that precede and accompany the birth. Assistance with the usual developmental tasks is discussed in more complete detail in Chapter 7.[6,8,13,43]

Unless the infant encounters unforeseen difficulty adapting to immediate extrauterine life, the mother and father should be able to see their infant, to examine, and to hold him or her. The physiologic and emotional experience for the parents offers an optimal climate in which to begin the parenting relationship with this infant, and they should be allowed their innate right to experience it as fully as they desire.

It is impossible to fully conceal an unforeseen problem such as a congenital malformation. Such an event is the realization of the worst fears, of shattered hopes and dreams. Many mothers who were partially anesthetized at the time of delivery recall immediate realization that something was wrong. A simple, brief explanation to the family at the time of delivery that the infant has a deformity or is experiencing difficulty is more easily grasped and resolved than is suspicion, which creates uncertainty and anxiety. Questions about the infant's prognosis can be answered honestly and briefly.

The health care team should carefully consider the responsibility of each member in the event of an emergency or unusual circumstance at the time of delivery, so that efficient and effective action can be instituted to handle every aspect of the situation. This should always include emotional care and support for the mother and family, and ideally this requires the full attention of one of the profession team members.[39,44]

## HOME DELIVERY
JEAN TILLMAN
### Background and trends in home delivery

Since the early 1970s, a small percentage of the total natural births have occurred at home, and this number is increasing across the United States.[16,18] This trend appears to be occurring primarily among the young, educated population. General reasons given for the increase include the trend toward the natural life style, a desire for greater mother-child contact, and greater participation by the father in the birth process. Many couples wish to have family and friend support during birth and to avoid a mechanized, cold, illness-oriented, dehumanizing hospital. Others feel that gaining personal control and taking an active as opposed to a passive role during the experience of birth is a reason to avoid the hospital. While finances may play a part in the decision to deliver at home, the knowledge that 90% to 96% of all births are spontaneous and without complications is also a factor. A general defiant, rebellious attitude toward the establishment may also be present.

The public's interest in childbirth at home seems to have coincided with two larger social trends. The desire fostered by the women's movement to gain control over one's life and body has extended to this uniquely feminine area, along with a resentment against the male-dominated practice of obstetrics. At the same time, there has been a general movement toward distrust of technology, authority, and esoteric expertise in every phase of life, from home repairs to food production.[7,24,35] These trends have caused traditional hospital birth to be re-evaluated by many young couples, creating a new consciousness of its faults and advantages.

The general public is asking for acceptance of childbirth as a normal phenomenon. They do not care to be treated as if they were ill or as if they will become ill if they do not take all the precautions deemed necessary by the traditional medical establishment. Informed mothers have cited objections to the utilization of oxytocin (Pitocin), artificial rupturing of membranes, and monitoring labor with mechanical devices—practices that have become common in many hospitals in the United States. The use of enemas, drugs, forceps, fundal pressure, and intravenous fluids are routine procedures that many feel decrease the naturalness and control of the delivery process while increasing the risks to mother and infant. A lack of choice in the position for labor and delivery, along with routine use of episiotomies, are further reasons couples object to hospital birth.[38]

To be able to give birth in a familiar environ-

ment that is cheerful and pleasant as opposed to one that is sterile and illness oriented and in a place where cross-contamination by staff members and other patients does not exist decreases tension, fear, and anxiety, making the birth experience more enjoyable. This experience can then be celebrated with family and friends who have provided assistance, strength, encouragement, and companionship. This chance to rejoice with family and friends rather than alone or with strangers is a major incentive for childbirth at home. As a part of the total family experience, the couples choosing childbirth at home are eager to be able to breast-feed the infant at the time of delivery, to have the infant with them as a family group for the period following delivery, and to be able to watch the infant's adaptation to extrauterine life as a part of the family. The choice is often based on the assumption that control over all of these advantages is lost if delivery is conducted in the hospital.

When a couple considers home delivery and chooses instead to have birth in the hospital, the major reason given is for the security of the hospital. Equipment and personnel are perceived as being available for both the mother and infant in the event that anything goes wrong. Further, insurance coverage only applies for a hospital delivery, which constitutes a financial consideration for many couples. In other instances the woman may choose hospital birth because she wants to assume a passive role and to be assured of being taken care of. She may have no help at home and may desire the period of time after the delivery to rest and be free from the responsibility of caring for the infant and other children. Some women do not view birth as a natural process and willingly assume the "sick" role. Others find the psychologic and emotional aspects of birth unimportant and do not value mate involvement and therefore do not view home delivery as advantageous. For many women, there is simply no choice, or they do not have an awareness of delivery alternatives that might be available to them.

## Criteria for safety in home delivery

In deciding to deliver at home, a woman needs to recognize that labor and delivery are unpredictable, with potential complications for the mother and the infant. If complications arise, the home may not have the equipment to deal with the problem nor qualified personnel to intervene immediately and decrease the risks involved in the complication. Friends and family may not be able to remain calm and rational during a stressful situation. The psychologic risk of delivery at home must be considered, for if anything does go wrong, causing permanent damage or death, the mother and father may subject themselves to unfounded guilt or will not be able to accept what has happened without fixing blame.

Rather than leave young couples to proceed unprepared with a home delivery, several organizations have been formed that recognize the risks of home delivery and that provide a needed resource to help the couple minimize the risks and prepare for the delivery. These organizations include HOMEBIRTH, The Association for Childbirth at Home, the National Association of Parents and Professionals for Safe Alternatives in Childbirth, and Home Oriented Maternity Experience (H.O.M.E.).

HOMEBIRTH* is a nonprofit organization of parents interested in reclaiming control over the birth experience. They provide guidelines and information for birth at home, thereby decreasing the risks involved. The organization has a resource center to help prospective parents locate home birth resources in their specific geographic area. They provide an educational series of six classes aimed at preparing parents specifically for childbirth at home. The classes are taught by trained leaders and are supplemented by a lending library, selected reprints, films and slides, private counseling, and referrals to medical specialists in the area.

The purposes of HOMEBIRTH are as follows: (1) to establish an educational and informational group that will provide instruction and promote childbirth at home, (2) to conduct research and compile statistics on childbirth at home and make this research available to all members of the community, (3) to provide educational and informational instruction to parents desiring childbirth at home, (4) to train and instruct individuals in the birth experience, and (5) to provide this information to the broadest spectrum of people with varied experiential,

economic, and cultural backgrounds. It is the official policy of HOMEBIRTH that deliveries be professionally attended in the home. Members do not assume primary responsibility for assistance at a birth in place of legally qualified professional workers, and they are expected by the organization to comply with the legal requirements of the jurisdiction in which the birth takes place.

HOMEBIRTH has established prerequisites for home delivery. An absolute requirement is comprehensive prenatal care with a physician who is aware of the couple's plan to deliver at home. Adequate pelvic measurements and above average nutrition are required, along with a good obstetric history. Contraindications for delivery at home include serious hereditary and familial abnormalities, sickle cell disease, metabolic disease, anemia, heavy smoking, excessive multiparity, placental separation, maternal infection or drug addiction, and cardiovascular or renal disease.

The couple is required to acquire an understanding of what can be predicted and what cannot be predicted during the course of labor and delivery. A woman can know the general condition of her pelvis, the fetal position and presentation, her obstetric history and general health, but the type of uterine contractions, degree of joint mobility, and the ultimate fetal presentation are not predictable until the process of labor and delivery proceeds.

At the time of delivery, the mother and attendants should shower, wear clean clothes, and scrub their hands. Clean linen should be used and a sterile field maintained around the perineum. It is recommended that a car or ambulance be available, with ample gasoline, and that the home delivery be conducted at a location within a 15-minute drive of the local hospital and not further than a 30-minute drive. Added precautions that may be available at the home include oxygen, suction, and blood pressure equipment and a fetascope. If the membranes have been ruptured over 24 hours or if there is an abnormal presentation or premature labor, hospitalization is recommended.

Alternatives to hospital or home birth are presently not available in most communities in the United States. However, in response to the public concern and demand for more humanis-

*89 Franklin Street, Suite 200, Boston, Mass. 02110

tic care, many hospitals are revising their approach to the care of mothers and children to provide a more humanistic, family-centered experience. Mobile delivery units and short-term maternity clinics/motels are being designed to provide a setting for delivery that combines the advantages of the services of the hospital with the advantages of home delivery.[44]

## STUDY QUESTIONS

1. Observe an infant during the first few hours of life and describe all signs of physiologic adaptation that you can detect. What nursing care is given to the infant during this period of time? Explain the rationale for each aspect of care given, and determine the soundness of the practice that you observe. If an alternative plan of care is indicated, describe this and give your rationale.
2. Give an Apgar score to an infant at one and five minutes after delivery simultaneously with a more experienced scorer. Compare your scores, and discuss the rationale for each score given.
3. Describe ways in which you would provide for each of the essential needs for care during the immediate postpartum period if the infant were delivered at home or in some other place away from a hospital. Particularly include the situation where the delivery is not expected. What provisions would you include if you were planning for such a delivery?
4. Describe signs of the infant's behavior and physical features that you might observe to confirm the adequacy of functioning of each of the major systems involved in the adaptation process.
5. Describe how the event of giving birth to an infant contributes to the mother's and/or father's further development of each of the four major competencies: (1) physical, (2) learning and thought, (3) psychosocial, and (4) inner self.

## REFERENCES

1. Abramson, H., editor: Resuscitation of the newborn infant and related emergency procedures in the perinatal center special care nursery, ed. 3, St. Louis, 1973, The C. V. Mosby Co.
2. Apgar, V.: Proposal for a new method of evaluation of the newborn infant, Cur. Res. Anesthesiol. Analg. 38: 260, 1953.
3. Arms, S.: Immaculate deception, Boston, 1975, Houghton-Mifflin Co.
4. Babson, S. G.: Feeding the low-birth-weight infant, J. Pediatr. 79:694, Oct., 1971.
5. Babson, S. G., Benson, R. C., Pernoll, M. L., and Benda, G. I.: Management of high-risk pregnancy and intensive care of the neonate, ed. 3, St. Louis, 1975, The C. V. Mosby Co.
6. Bean, M.: Birth is a family affair, Am. J. Nurs. 75:1689, Oct., 1975.
7. Boston Women's Health Book Collective: Our bodies, ourselves, New York, 1971, Simon & Schuster, Inc.
8. Brown, M. S., and Hurlock, J.: Mothering the mother, Am. J. Nurs. 77:438, March, 1977.
9. Case, L. L.: Ultrasound monitoring of mother and fetus, Am. J. Nurs. 72:725-727, April, 1972.
10. Cavanagh, D., and Talisman, M. R.: Prematurity and the obstetrician, New York, 1969, Appleton-Century-Crofts, pp. 328-344.
11. Cohen, S. N., and Olson, W. A.: Drugs that depress the newborn infant, Pediatr. Clin. North Am. 17:835-850, Nov., 1970.
12. Cooke, R. E., editor: The biological basis of pediatric practice, New York, 1968, McGraw-Hill Book Co.
13. Crummett, B. D.: Transitions in motherhood, Matern. Child Nurs. J. 4:65, Summer, 1975.
14. Dahm, L. S., and James, L. S.: Newborn temperature and calculated heat loss in the delivery room, Pediatrics 49:504, April, 1972.
15. Desmond, M. M., and others: The clinical behavior of the newly born, J. Pediatr. 62:307-325, Nov., 1963.
16. Edwards, M.: Unattended home birth, Am. J. Nurs. 73:1332, Aug., 1973.
17. Goodwin, B.: Psychoprophylaxis in childbirth. In Duffey, M., Anderson, E. H., Bergerson, B. S., and others, editors: Current concepts in clinical nursing, ed. 3, St. Louis, 1971, The C. V. Mosby Co., pp. 194-203.
18. Haber, C.: Grass roots movement toward home delivery, Valley Advocate, 2:7, May 28, 1975.
19. Hasselmeyer, E. G.: Indices of fetal welfare. In Bergerson, B. S., Anderson, E. H., Duffey, M., and others, editors: Current concepts in clinical nursing, vol. 2, St. Louis, 1969, The C. V. Mosby Co., pp. 298-318.
20. Hellmuth, J., editor: Exceptional infant, vol. 1, The normal infant, New York, 1967, Brunner/Mazel, Inc.
21. Hon, H. E.: An atlas of fetal heart rate patterns, New Haven, Conn., 1968, Harty Press, Inc.
22. Johnson, N. W.: Breast-feeding at one hour of age, Matern. Child Nurs. 1:12, Jan.-Feb. 1976.
23. Karlburg, P.: Respiratory physiology during infancy and childhood, Acta Anaesthesiol. Scand. (Suppl.) 37:10-17, 1970.
24. Kraft, S.: Birth at home, Valley Advocate 2:1, May 28, 1975.
25. Lasater, C.: Electronic monitoring of mother and fetus, Am. J. Nurs. 72:728-730, April, 1972.
26. Matousek, I.: Fetal nursing during labor, Nurs. Clin. North Am. 3:307, 1968.
27. Measurement techniques and interpretation of fetal heart frequency patterns: Application Note 700, Palo Alto, Calif., 1969, Hewlett-Packard Co.
28. Mueller-Heuback, E., and Adamsons, K.: Approaches to the fetus-intrapartum and intrauterine. In Abramson, H., editor: Symposium on the functional physiopathology of the fetus and the neonate; clinical correlations, St. Louis, 1971, The C. V. Mosby Co., pp. 43-60.
29. Oliver, T. K., editor: Neonatal respiratory adaptation, Washington, D.C., 1963, U.S. Department of Health, Education and Welfare, Publication No. 1432.

30. Papageorgiades, G.: Transplacental passage of fetal red cells into the maternal circulation in normal, abnormal and instrumental deliveries, Clin. Pediatr. 15:42, Jan. 1976.

31. Peltonen, R., and Peltonen, T.: Immediate information expected by the neonatologist from the placenta, Clin. Pediatr. 15:743, Aug., 1976.

32. Phillips, C. R. N.: Neonatal heat loss in heated cribs vs. mothers' arms, J. Obstet. Gynecol. Neonatal Nurs. 3:11, Nov.-Dec. 1974.

33. Pilon, R. N.: Anesthesia for uncomplicated obstetric delivery, Am. Fam. Physician 9:113, Jan., 1974.

34. Pritchard, G. A., and MacDonald, P. C.: Williams' obstetrics, ed. 15, New York, 1976, Appleton-Century-Crofts.

35. Rich, A.: Of woman born; motherhood as experience and institution, New York, 1976, W. W. Norton and Co.

36. Rich, O. J.: How does the patient use the nurse during labor? In Duffey, M., Anderson, E. H., Bergerson, B. S., and others, editors: Current concepts in clinical nursing, vol. 3, St. Louis, 1971, The C. V. Mosby Co.

37. Roberts, J.: Suctioning the newborn, Am. J. Nurs. 73:63, Jan., 1973.

38. Russin, A. W., O'Gureck, J. E., and Roux, J. F.: Electronic monitoring of the fetus, Am. J. Nurs. 74:1294, July, 1974.

39. Sasmor, J. L., Castor, C. R., and Hassid, P.: The childbirth team during labor, Am. J. Nurs. 73:444, March, 1973.

40. Scanlon, J. W.: How is the baby? The Apgar score revisited, Clin. Pediatr. 12:61, Feb. 1973.

41. Smith, B. A., Priore, R. M., and Stern, M. K.: The transition phase of labor, Am. J. Nurs. 73:448, Feb., 1973.

42. Strickland, M. D.: Fetal assessment techniques; challenge to the nurse practitioner. In Duffey, M., Anderson, E. H., Bergerson, B. S., and others, editors: Current concepts in clinical nursing, vol. 3, St. Louis, 1971, The C. V. Mosby Co., pp. 179-188.

43. Swartz, R.: A father's view, Children Today 6:14, March-April 1977.

44. Timberlake, B.: The new life center, Am. J. Nurs. 75:1456, Sept., 1975.

# CHAPTER 7

# Nursing assessment and care of the newborn infant

The newborn period is indeed a critical time in life. The predominant concern of new mothers is expressed in the often heard question, "Is my baby all right?" Equipped with skills and knowledge, the nurse is able to help the parents resolve this question. Adequate nursing care for parents and neonate during the first few crucial days of life can be an important influence in establishing a healthy, satisfying start for the family into which the baby has been born.

The basis upon which care is provided is a complete nursing assessment. Contrary to the impression that all newborn infants are alike, each provides a slightly different challenge because of complexities of individual responses to life, individual needs, and unique personal anatomy and physiology. In addition, the mother and father respond to their infant in ways that differ from those of other parents, and each begins very early to contribute to the ongoing development of their young child.

Assessment during the newborn period includes parental health histories and pertinent aspects of pregnancy, labor, and delivery. The nurse performs a thorough physical evaluation of the infant to obtain information regarding anatomic features and functional responses to extrauterine life. Many ongoing observations comprise a constantly revised nursing evaluation. The infant's evolving patterns of eating, responses to handling, adequacy of sleep, waking behavior, changes in weight, and continuing evaluation of adaptation to extrauterine life are obtained and utilized.

## PRIMARY PRINCIPLES OF CARE OF THE NEWBORN

Because human infants are almost totally helpless and dependent upon others for their needs, their well-being and health are directly related to the quality of care given. A few basic factors characterize an adequate quality of care given to newborn infants. These principles guide nursing care, but they also should characterize care given by parents and should be observed in hospital or home.

### Conservation of energy

During the first few weeks of life, the infant's energy reserves and ability to generate energy are limited. Excessive crying, handling, or stimulation tolerated by an older infant is exhausting to the newborn. Young infants do not sleep for long periods of time, and their sleep and waking periods are erratic. Depending on dispositional traits, the needs for holding and cuddling vary greatly. This type of handling is soothing and comforting and provides for energy conservation.

## Provision of warmth

All term infants do not possess a totally reliable ability to maintain body temperature or to compensate for heat loss. Body heat is lost by the four basic mechanisms of convection, conduction, radiation, and evaporation. Controlling for one source of heat loss does not ensure protection from loss of heat from another. For example, infants may be placed under a radiant heater to control heat loss by radiation. If, however, they are placed on a cold metal surface without clothing, or if a draft is passing continuously through the room, they will still lose heat by means of conduction, convection, or evaporation.

## Protection from infection or injury

The most important protective procedure that can be employed by nurses and mothers in the hospital or home is frequent and thorough hand-washing before handling. The importance of hand-washing before handling a young infant cannot be overemphasized. In addition, ongoing surveillance for infection in a hospital nursery aids in identifying other sources of infection.

Constant care to prevent injury is also mandatory. The infant is never placed on an unguarded surface or close to objects that may cause injury, such as safety pins, scissors, or tools.

Measures that contribute to keeping the infant clean are employed for his or her comfort and protection. The use of plain water or a mild cleansing agent is adequate, unless an infection or known contaminant is present in the environment. Bactericidal soaps that are known to be safe for newborns may be used in this case. Daily bathing may be drying to the skin but may be preferred by mothers as a socialization experience with the child. Thorough cleansing between diaper changes is mandatory for maintaining a rash-free diaper area.[18]

## Provision of contentedness and comfort

A period of crying, exposure, and handling is tiring and distressing. The natural response to cuddling and comforting restores stable behav-

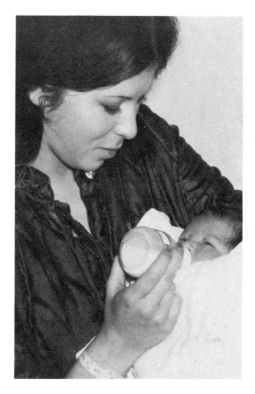

**Fig. 7-1.** The mother is encouraged and assisted with her chosen method of feeding and in establishing close contact with her infant while feeding.

ior and contributes to a sense of security. The need of the newborn infant for tactile sensation has been impressively documented. Adequate care during this time of life is closely associated with frequent physical cuddling, and the infant's behavioral response is significant.

## Provision of nutrition

Mothers who have chosen to breast-feed should be encouraged to nurse the infant immediately after delivery, as this stimulates contraction of the uterus for the mother and allows the infant to have an early experience of nutritive sucking during the period of intense autonomic stimulation. This early experience in sucking is believed to facilitate successful breast-feeding for the mother and the infant; it also provides early intake of colostrum, which may allay hypoglycemia for the infant.

A bottle-fed infant is fed either glucose and water or formula during the first period of autonomic nervous system stimulation. There needs to be suction equipment readily available to keep the infant's airway clear during and after feeding, as during each period of autonomic system stimulation to prevent aspiration of milk or water.

The preferred approach to feeding the infant in the hospital is on the basis of infant demand. Using this approach, the infant receives optimal amounts of feeding, and the frequency of feeding provides some protection against periods of hypoglycemia (see Chapter 8). Intervals between feeding should be recorded and monitored to assure adequacy of fluid and calorie intake for either bottle- or breast-fed infants.[11]

## NURSING ASSESSMENT OF THE NEWBORN

Assessment of the health and well-being of the infant can yield valuable evidence indicating the adequacy of genetic inheritance, fetal development, and adaptation to extrauterine life. Because many of the responses observed for the newborn differ from those of the older infant, a detailed discussion of each aspect will be presented.

### Maternal history

Knowledge of the health status of the mother during pregnancy aids greatly in predicting the course of the newborn. The history of labor and delivery, particularly the timing and identification of drugs administered during labor, is important in anticipating the infant's condition at birth.

The maternal health history should include traits of prenatal care, including the time when prenatal care was begun, frequency of prenatal visits, results of blood and urinary testing throughout pregnancy, and trends in blood pressure changes that occurred during pregnancy. The extent of maternal weight gain should be recorded and evaluated in light of the mother's nutritional pattern during pregnancy. The mother's ability to assume responsibility for her own health care during pregnancy is an important indication of her future ability to care for the health needs of the infant. Her patterns of social interaction and the emotional and social support resources available to her are essential components of the maternal health history.

Maternal metabolic disorders present a special problem in relation to newborns; in every case there is some level of interaction between the pregnancy and the disease. For example, with the availability of insulin the combination of pregnancy and diabetes mellitus has become a common occurrence, and perinatal infant mortality and morbidity as the result of this condition have become major problems. The more severe the diabetic condition and the earlier the age of maternal onset, the more critical the influence on the pregnancy and likewise the greater the influence of the pregnancy on the diabetic condition. Abortion, premature labors, and intrauterine or neonatal deaths occur in about 25% of all diabetic pregnancies. Infants who are large for gestational age are common and produce mechanical difficulties in labor that sometimes necessitate a cesarean section. Hydramnios, congenital malformations, hypoglycemia, and anoxia are common. All infants born of mothers with a known diabetic condition should be placed under extremely close nursing surveillance in an isolette because of their extreme susceptibility to complications during the first 24 to 48 hours. Conversely, mothers of all infants considered to be large for gestational age should be tested thoroughly for the presence of early stages of a diabetic condition.[31]

### Infant history

Even at 1 hour of age, the newborn's brief personal history provides useful information in predicting the course of adaptation and defining relevant nursing care. The Apgar score, which was discussed in detail in Chapter 6, correlates closely to the ability of the infant to continue the adaptation process beyond the first few moments of life and throughout the newborn period.

Careful documentation of the neonate's behavior and reactions to extrauterine life during the first few hours provides useful predictive information as well as a baseline from which to evaluate future behavior. An accurate birth weight is essential if body weight obtained on subsequent days of life is to have meaning. The percentage of weight change since birth reflects adequacy of fluids and nutrition during the first week. Daily calculation of this change can lead to early detection of a variety of problems. One approach to this calculation is indicated in the following:

1. Determine 1% of birthweight:

$$
\begin{array}{r}
3060 \text{ g birthweight} \\
\times .01 \\
\hline
30.60
\end{array}
$$

2. Determine difference between birthweight and today's weight:

$$
\begin{array}{r}
3060 \text{ g birthweight} \\
-2980 \text{ g today} \\
\hline
80 \text{ g change}
\end{array}
$$

3. Divide the change by 1% of birthweight, yielding the percentage of change:

$$
\begin{array}{r}
2.61\% \\
30.6 \overline{)80.000} \\
\underline{612} \\
1880 \\
\underline{1836} \\
440 \\
\underline{306} \\
134
\end{array}
$$

Further evidence of the adequacy of total fluid and calorie intake may be estimated by recording the amount taken with each feeding. Approximate requirements are 150 ml of fluid and 100 calories per kilogram of body weight over each 24-hour period. Protein requirements are estimated as 2 to 4 mg per kilogram of body weight.[11]

In addition to the initial body weight, other body measurements are obtained to provide a baseline for future measurements. The head circumference and measurements of the anterior fontanel are important measurements for future determination of adequate growth in head size, which is known to be an important indicator of brain growth.[12] The head circumference measurement must be accurate to be useful. The circumference is measured with a plastic tape, paper tape, or other type of tape that can be pulled taut around the occipital to frontal circumference of the head. The tape is placed and pulled taut three times to assure accuracy of measurement. The average of the three measurements is used as the "true" circumference, which is entered on a standardized head growth grid to begin sequential plotting of this measurement. Measurement of the frontal fontanel and body length are obtained and recorded in the infant's initial data base.

Detailed observation of the infant's initial adaptation following delivery has been described in Chapter 6. As the infant continues adaptation during the first few days of life, physiologic responses of the neurologic, respiratory, and cardiovascular systems are particularly observed for increasing stabilization and maturity. The time of temperature stabilization and stabilization of the autonomic system responses to delivery are described and recorded. The time and response of the infant to initial feedings become important information for assessing adequacy of nutrition and changes in body weight.

In addition to the physical dimensions of the infant's history, the infant's behavior and responses to mother and other family members are observed. The infant's ability to focus on mother's face when first held should be noted. The infant should respond to being held and cuddled by becoming calm and relaxed during the first few hours of life.[21]

## Physical competency
### General observations

While the infant is resting, the posture naturally assumed and general appearance should be observed. The degree of extension of extremities, coloring, ease or difficulty in respiration, and nature of spontaneous movement provide knowledge of developmental maturity as well as general state of health. An infant who exhibits any abnormal behavior, such as grunting or other difficulty in breathing, an appearance of exhaustion, or frequent jittery movement, should be placed in an incubator where maximal observation can be conducted continuously.

The infant's color and general skin condition are evaluated repeatedly. The skin should be free of abrasions, rashes, or cracking. The presence of such conditions should be noted and documented thoroughly, even though they may be within the limits of normal variation (such as birthmarks, milia, mild drying and peeling of the skin around the ankles, wrists, and trunk, peripheral cyanosis of the hands and feet, forceps marks, and rashes in the absence of papules). Elasticity of skin turgor is further indication of adequacy of hydration.

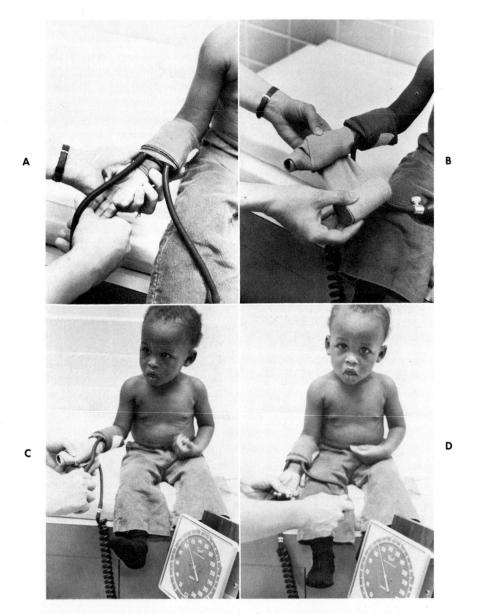

**Fig. 7-2.** The flush method may be used to obtain an estimate of blood pressure for an infant or toddler. **A,** A blood pressure cuff of about 2-inch width is placed above the wrist. **B,** A compression bandage is wrapped around the extremity distal to the cuff. **C,** The cuff is inflated, then the compression bandage removed. **D,** As the cuff is gradually deflated, the mean blood pressure is read when the first appearance of flushing of the hand (or foot in the lower extremity) occurs.

Cyanosis that persists and includes the entire face or body or occurs regularly with feeding or crying or increases in severity is indicative of neonatal distress and requires further nursing evaluation and medical attention.

Yellow coloring of neonatal jaundice is an-

other concern. Blanching the tip of the nose or the gumline by applying pressure facilitates estimating presence and degree of jaundice. Time of onset and ongoing estimation of changes in degree of jaundice are documented. Mild jaundice requires blanching to detect. This fine determination may require a second observer for confirmation, since the ability to visualize a slight yellow cast varies. Moderate jaundice is a yellow cast to the skin that does not require blanching to detect. Severe jaundice appears brownish yellow and involves the sclera of the eye.

Accurate observation of the infant's vital signs is essential for responsible nursing judgments of the health status of the infant. The temperature should be taken in the axilla rather than the rectum of the infant because of the very real danger of perforation of the rectum or colon, as these structures are relatively small and fragile. Insertion of a rectal thermometer also causes vagal stimulation, which effects cardiac and gastrointestinal function. When a mercury thermometer is used, the temperature is measured for five minutes holding the infant's arm firmly against the thorax, providing a measurement that has been determined to be as accurate as that obtained rectally.[9] When using an electronic thermometer, the time required for accurate measurement should be used following the manufacturer's recommendation.

The heart rate and respiratory rate should both be obtained by auscultation of the chest with a stethoscope. A full minute of auscultation is required for accurate rate determination, due to the irregularity of rhythm of the heart and respirations of the newborn. A full minute's count of each of these rates is recorded on the infant's record numerically and on a graph for sequential comparison over the newborn period.

During the newborn period the blood pressure is obtained using a flush method, as auscultation of the diastolic and systolic pressures is usually not possible. A blood pressure cuff about 2 inches in width is placed above the wrist or ankle, and a compression bandage is wrapped around the extremity distal to the cuff. The cuff is then inflated to about 200 mm Hg, the compression bandage is removed, and the cuff is gradually deflated at a rate of about 5 mm Hg/sec. The pressure is read when the first appearance of flushing occurs distal to the cuff. This represents the mean blood pressure. If the infant cries during the procedure, the value cannot be considered as accurate.[23,32]

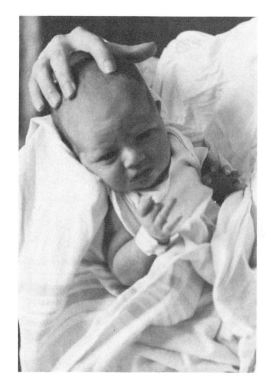

**Fig. 7-3.** The infant's anterior fontanel is palpated. Here the lateral boundaries are indicated.

### Head and sensory organs

The most important measurement to be obtained, next to body weight, is head circumference measured at the greatest diameter of the head, occiput to frontal areas. Without an initial baseline circumference, changes in head size during the first few months of life are impossible to document as to severity or extent. It is imperative that this initial measurement be obtained on all infants. Head circumference may be plotted on a chart such as that shown in the Appendix to determine adequacy of head size. Measurement of anterior and posterior fontanels may also be helpful in evaluating a problem in head growth at a later date.[30] Chest circumference, which is measured at the level of the nipples, is useful as a comparison against the head measurement. The neonate's chest is normally slightly smaller than the head.

Symmetry of facial features and degree of molding of the skull are noted in detail. Placement of the features of the face and head are noted and documented. The ear is normally in

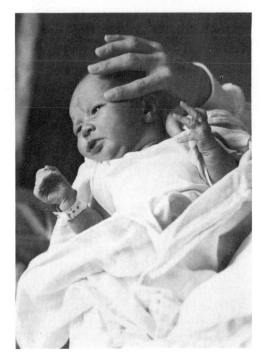

**Fig. 7-4.** Normal placement of the ear in relation to the eye is indicated in a horizontal plane.

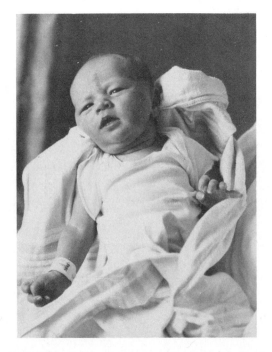

**Fig. 7-5.** Symmetry of facial expression and movement is noted. The infant is stimulated to open his eyes, and reactions of the pupils, ability to fixate, and coordination of eye movements are observed.

alignment with the outer canthus of the eye. Should facial features appear to be irregular or have an unusual appearance, they should be described as accurately and objectively as possible. Drawings or diagrams may be useful in communicating the exact appearance at the time of observation. Trauma to neurologic pathways of the face and head may result in temporary paralysis of the musculature of this area, a matter of grave concern for parents.

The pattern of hair growth over the scalp should be noted. A normal pattern of hair growth consists of a single parietal whorl over the posterior scalp, with most of the hair growing toward the hairline around the scalp. There is often an upsweeping pattern of the anterior scalp hair, commonly known as a cowlick.[37] Major differences in hair growth patterns should be described and recorded. Infants with curly hair may not have an easily discernible hair growth pattern.

Thorough palpation and inspection of the skull reveal the degree of molding, the presence of and differentiation between caput succedaneum and cephalhematoma, separation or overlapping of sutures, or abrasions of the skull, which may be the result of trauma during delivery. Caput succedaneum is swelling occurring under the scalp and is not limited to suture lines of the skull. The swelling appears very shortly after delivery and begins to dissipate within three or four days. Cephalhematoma, on the other hand, is swelling resulting from an accumulation of fluid under the skull and is limited to suture line boundaries. Swelling begins to occur after the first day of life and continues to increase, becoming large enough to cause obvious disconfiguration of the head. Regression is very slow and may not fully disappear until the infant is 3 months of age.[42]

The newborn's eyes are observed for any drainage or irritation. Instillation of silver nitrate or other opthalmic prophylactic in the delivery room may cause some irritation of the eyelid. Upright positioning, dimming of the light source, and shading of the eyes from direct light may stimulate the infant to open his or her eyes. Each pupil is observed for reaction to light and equality of reaction. Eye movements are observed for symmetry and coordination.

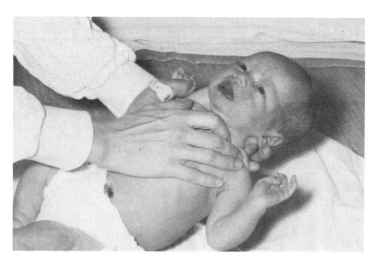

**Fig. 7-6.** The neck and shoulders are palpated for detection of masses, asymmetry, or injury.

Some ocular incoordination during the first month is within normal limits but should be fully described. The neonate is able to focus on a human face and follow movement to the midline.[14]

The mouth is inspected visually. The entire hard and soft palate should be visualized clearly. The patency of each nostril may be evaluated by briefly obstructing the airflow through the opposite nostril and mouth and observing for respiratory effort through the nostril that remains free.

The tympanic membranes are not usually available for visualization because of an accumulation of vernix in the small ear canal. The infant may be screened for the ability to hear by using a loud sound stimulus and observing for a Moro-like reflex. Ringing a bell or whistling may cause movement.

The neck and shoulders are palpated for detection of masses, asymmetry, and injury. The patency of the clavicles is determined, as these bones are susceptible to trauma during delivery. The head is fully extended in all directions to determine adequacy of range of motion and neck muscle function.

### Chest and abdomen

The rate and nature of heart and respiration sounds should be carefully evaluated while the infant is at rest by auscultation in each of the four quadrants of the chest from the front and from the back. Only the normal sound of air moving in the lungs should be present in any of the four quadrants. Sounds of grunting or the crackling noise of moisture in the lungs is a signal of immediate or impending danger for the neonate. Functional heart murmurs of the newborn period are common and usually reflect incomplete closure of fetal structures of the circulatory system. These benign sounds should be differentiated by the physician from more serious murmurs indicating congenital malformations. Any persistent increase in the heart rate above 160 or a respiratory rate above 50 per minute during periods of rest should lead the nurse to form a more detailed evaluation of the infant's well-being and to alert medical staff of the possibility of impending danger.

The abdomen is also auscultated to determine the presence of intestinal activity. Bowel sounds should be heard at any point after birth and should occur with sufficient frequency so that there is no difficulty in determining their presence. The abdomen is palpated gently to detect abnormal masses and to locate the spleen and liver. The area of the spleen is approached on the infant's left side by applying gentle pressure with the fingers placed close together. The spleen should be palpable just under the left costal margin. During the neonatal period the liver is palpated at the level of the costal margin, or no more than 1 cm below. The cord and the surrounding abdominal surface are inspected carefully. Any redness or discharge from this area should alert the nurse to apply increased measures to protect the infant from infection until the cord is completely healed.

Femoral pulses are palpated at the inner aspect of the vertical tendons in the groin. Excessive pressure may obstruct the pulse. It is important to determine the quality and presence of the pulse on each side, indicating intact circulatory patterns to the extremities.

The genitalia are inspected thoroughly. Edema of the labia or scrotal sac occurs in response to maternal hormones during pregnancy. The male scrotum is inspected for symmetry. The presence of descended testes is observed by gently palpating downward from the groin to the scrotal sac. It is neither necessary nor desirable to retract the foreskin. Female infants usually have a white discharge, with bloody spotting occurring in some infants. Adequacy of urinary stream may be observed in either male or female for strength and direction of flow. The anus is also inspected for patency.

The entire spinal column is inspected and palpated to detect any irregularities or deviations. A small dimple at the base of the spinal column is indicative of late embryologic closure of the spine and may indicate the possibility of spina bifida occulta or other irregularities of the spinal column, particularly if there is a history of minor deviations in the infant's family.

### Extremities

The hands normally assume a clenched fist position. Variations, such as overlapping of fingers or outward positioning of the thumb, are sometimes characteristic of infants with chromosomal disorders. The palmar surface is inspected for a normal crease pattern and coloring. A persistent paleness of the palm is suggestive of inadequate hemoglobin level. The simian crease, a single crease across the infant's palm, may accompany chromosomal disorders and commonly occurs with Down's syndrome.[19]

Range of motion of all joints is evaluated. Particular attention is given to the infant's hips. The hands are placed over the thighs with the fingers extended from the knee to the tip of the

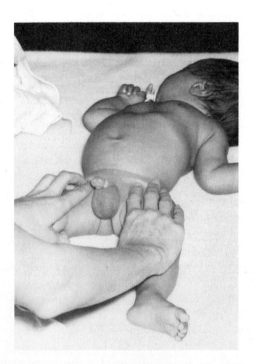

**Fig. 7-7.** Femoral pulses are palpated at the inner aspect of the vertical tendons in the groin.

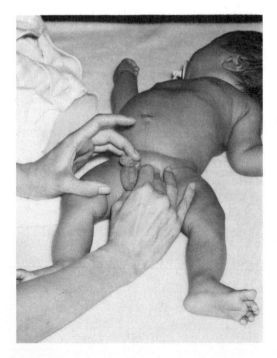

**Fig. 7-8.** The presence of descended testes is observed by gently palpating downward from the groin to the scrotal sac.

femur. When the hips are abducted 90 degrees, the index finger will palpate movement of the joint, detecting any click that may be present. This is known as Ortalani's sign. Other signs of possible hip joint abnormality include painful crying with abduction, resistance to full 90-degree abduction, and asymmetry of thigh and buttock areas. These conditions may also occur with normal hip joints, but should they be noted in connection with a click or inequality of length of the legs, a physician should evaluate the possibility of hip defects.[20]

A very common orthopedic trait in infancy is mild incurvation of the ankles. The feet are cradled in the examiner's hands and observed for resting position and spontaneous movement. If incurvation is present, the degree of incurvation can be estimated. It should also be noted whether spontaneous motion corrects the incurvation or tends to accentuate it, since this information may be helpful in differentiating between incurvation caused by fetal positioning and that caused by structural imbalance of the legs and ankles. If motion accentuates the con-

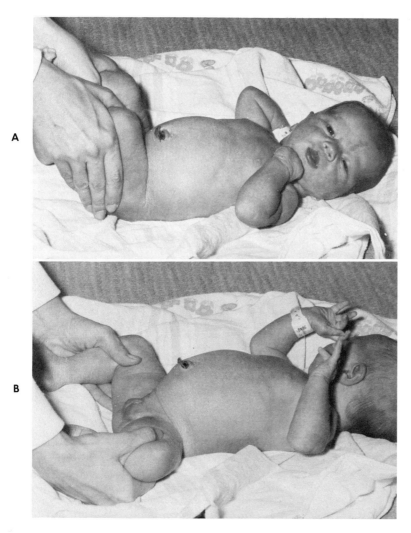

**Fig. 7-9.** Observation of the motion of the hip joints is conducted by full abduction with palpation. **A,** The examiner's index finger is placed along the thigh with the finger palpating hip motion as, **B,** the hips are brought to a full 90-degree angle.

dition or alignment cannot be achieved passively, there is a possibility that orthopedic correction will be needed.

### Neuromuscular development

Neuromuscular responses are most reliably present after the second day of life and when the infant is rested. An infant who is tired, sleepy, hungry, or excessively stimulated may not respond adequately to neurologic testing.

Responses of the eyes, as described on p. 174, should be noted in relation to the examination of sensory organs. The infant's strength of suck is best observed during feeding. A rooting response, which consists of the infant turning toward a stroke on the cheek, is also well developed in the term infant. The hands will spontaneously grasp a finger placed on the palm. This palmar grasp should be strong, equal on both sides, and should increase in strength as the examiner exerts a tug away from the grasp.

The Moro reflex may be elicited by numerous methods. This is probably the most important of all newborn neurologic responses, because it correlates with gestational age as well as with the degree of neurologic impairment that may be present at birth. The most reliable and specific method of eliciting the Moro reflex is sudden movement. The child is supported under the back and head, and the head and trunk are allowed to drop backward through approximately 30 degrees. Arm and leg responses are noted. The necessary component of the reaction is outward extension of the arms and fingers. The legs may also exhibit an extension movement, and there may be a subsequent brief, jittery movement in the position of extension followed by slower, smoother, encircling movement of the arms and hands.

The Babinski reflex consists of the flaring of the toes when the sole of the foot is stroked gently. This is a normal neonatal response as opposed to indicating neurologic insult in the older child or adult. Placing a thumb or finger on the sole elicits plantar grasp. The toes flex in a grasping motion. The cry elicited by a pain stimulus to the foot indicates intact neuropain pathways to lower extremities. A pinch on the sole is the stimulus of preference. Flicking the

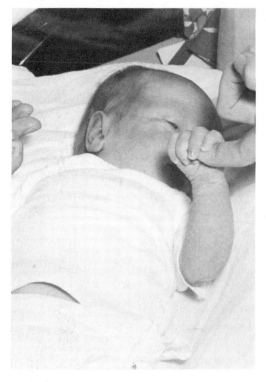

**Fig. 7-10.** The palmar grasp is strong, equal on both sides, and increases in strength as the examiner exerts a tug away from the grasp.

fingers against the sole or pin pricks are more prone to result in injury.

Evidence of neuromuscular development of the neck and shoulder muscles is demonstrated by pulling the infant by the arms from a supine to a sitting position. Head lag will vary among infants but should not be demonstrated to the extent shown in Fig. 7-14 for a normal term infant.

The term infant who is placed in a prone position should respond simultaneously by making crawling motions with the legs, lifting the head away from the surface, and turning the head to one side. A gentle stroke to one side of the spinal column elicits incurvation of the trunk. Several attempts should be made at various time intervals, since this response is often not reliably present until the third or fourth day of life. A stepping reflex is elicted by touching the infant's soles to the table surface when he or she is held in a standing or upright position. Each leg should be observed to lift as if the infant were stepping across the surface of the table.

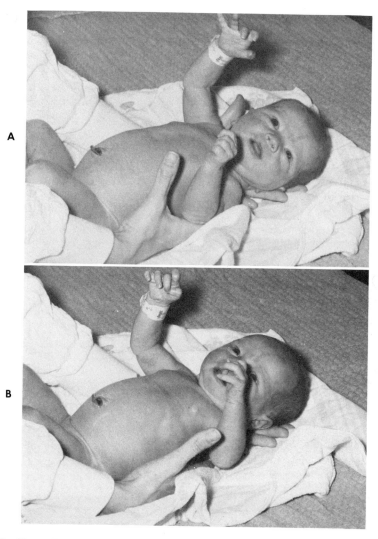

**Fig. 7-11.** The Moro reflex is one of the most important of all neonatal reflexes. **A,** The response is not symmetrical, since one hand is not seen to form the tense normal reaction of the **C** shape. **B,** When the reaction is elicited the second time, symmetry is observed in each arm and hand.

Transillumination is an extremely desirable routine screening procedure for early detection of certain central nervous system defects, which otherwise might not be detected in the first week of life. A totally blackened room must be used. A flexible rubber cone is attached to a standard flashlight. When the light is placed on the frontal region, the area of transillumination should be noted. Generally this should not exceed 1 to 2 cm beyond the cone of the flashlight. Gently and slowly sliding the flashlight to the parietal and temporal areas should reveal a gradually decreasing area of transillumination around the cone. As the light is moved to the occipital area, the zone of transillumination should be minimal or absent. Limits of normalcy are yet to be established, but findings exceeding these rough guidelines indicate that further neurologic evaluation or careful follow-through monitoring of neurologic development is warranted.

### Estimation of gestational age

Estimation of gestational age is dependent upon a number of observations that, as a total impression, suggest the stage of development.

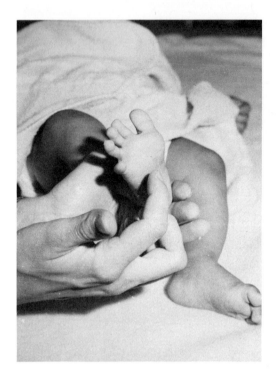

**Fig. 7-12.** The Babinski reflex consists of flaring of the toes when the sole of the foot is gently stroked from the heel toward the toes.

This judgment is recognized as extremely important for adequate nursing care. The mother's expected date of confinement, though consistent with the actual birthdate of the infant, may be misleading in relation to the developmental maturity of the infant.

Infants who are developmentally immature, yet whose birth weights fall within the acceptable range of normal limits for term infants, are at particular risk. They may be given nursing care appropriate for infants who have reached a mature state of development, but because of their immaturity are extraordinarily vulnerable to stress. The obviously small premature infant may also exhibit inconsistencies in relation to estimated degree of prematurity as compared to the actual degree of developmental maturity exhibited.

Infants who have been undernourished during intrauterine life, although they may indeed be several weeks premature, may exhibit a more advanced level of developmental maturity than would be expected for their size and weight. The ability to adapt to and sustain ex-trauterine life is more closely related to the degree of developmental maturity than birth weight.

**Tissue development.** Features of tissue development include characteristics of skin and hair, subcutaneous tissue, muscle tone, and cartilage formation (Fig. 7-16). The skin of a premature infant is fragile and translucent. Veins are visible over the head and face, and tissue is soft and delicate to the touch. Fine, downy hair is distributed over most of the body, especially over the forehead, back, and shoulders. The postmature infant, by contrast, lacks body hair. The skin appears shiny, cracked, and feels like thin crinkly paper. This is known as "parchment skin" and is indicative of prolonged uterine life.

Fingernails and nailbeds also give gestational age clues. Nails normally do not extend beyond the fingertip and often have a mildly cyanotic coloring. Excessively long nails or nailbeds having a yellow or brown meconium staining suggest postmaturity accompanied by fetal distress.

Subcutaneous tissue is noted to be lacking in the premature infant. When drawn together, the skin creases closely, and bony parts are readily palpated. Infants of any gestational age may exhibit this characteristic if they have suffered fetal malnutrition during a portion of the pregnancy. Such an infant may also be termed dysmature. Sole creases in the term infant are well developed over the entire plantar surface, while the sole of a premature infant is smooth and shiny over the portion toward the heel (Fig. 7-17).

Muscle tone and development may be estimated with the scarf sign (Fig. 7-18). An arm is drawn across the chest and the head turned toward the shoulder. No resistance is felt in the premature infant. The term infant resists the pull of the arm, and the chin will not easily move beyond alignment with the elbow. The degree of head lag suggests the extent of muscle development of the head and trunk.

Ear cartilage in the premature infant is soft and pliable, feeling more like skin than cartilage. The auricle may be easily folded forward; should the infant lie upon the folded ear, it will remain folded when he assumes another position. The head is minimally molded. The skull bones and suture lines are soft, pliable, and

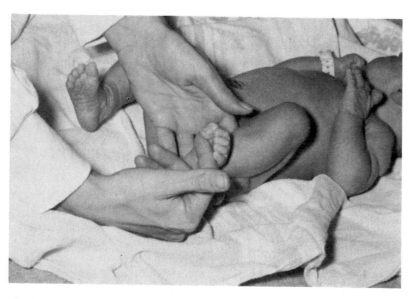

**Fig. 7-13.** A plantar grasp is elicited by placing a finger across the ball of the infant's sole.

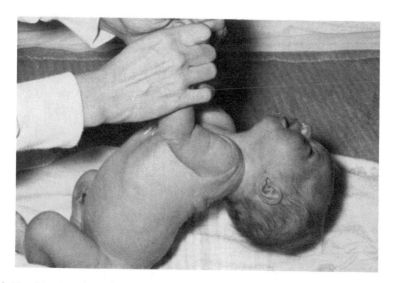

**Fig. 7-14.** Head lag is observed by pulling the infant from a supine to a sitting position. Strength of neck and shoulder muscles is felt as the infant makes an effort to pull himself up. The degree of head lag shown here is excessive (more than 45 degrees) for a normal term infant.

delicate. The term infant's ear cartilage, on the other hand, is soft, but well developed and firm. The auricle will not fold forward with ease and springs back to the original position.[8,22]

**Neurologic development.** Most of the reflexes are not present before 28 weeks' gestation, but as early as 26 weeks, the infant may have a weak cry, barely apparent Moro reflex, and a feeble grasp. As neurologic integration progresses, a weak exhaustible rooting reflex and suck begin to appear. Further details of the appearance of various reflexes at roughly equivalent gestational ages are shown in Table 7-1.

**Appearance and behavior.** Behavior of the infant is evaluated for signs of gestational age. The degree of flexion of the extremities, quality of movement, and alert behavior are described

**181**

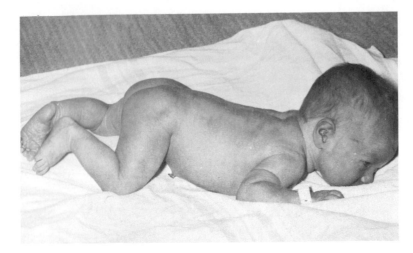

**Fig. 7-15.** The term infant who is placed in a prone position should respond spontaneously by making crawling motions with his legs, lifting his head away from the surface, and turning his head to one side.

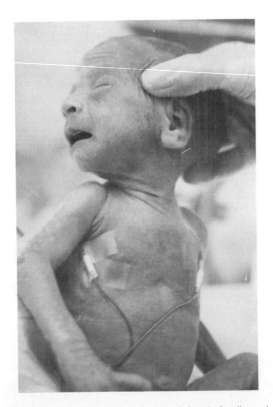

**Fig. 7-16.** The skin of the premature infant is fragile and translucent; fine, downy hair is distributed over most of the body, especially over the forehead, back, and shoulders. Subcutaneous tissue is lacking.

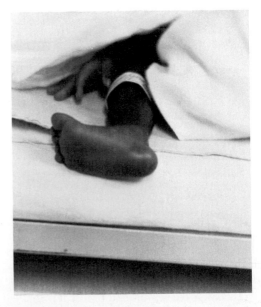

**Fig. 7-17.** Sole creases that are less developed toward the heel indicate lower gestational age.

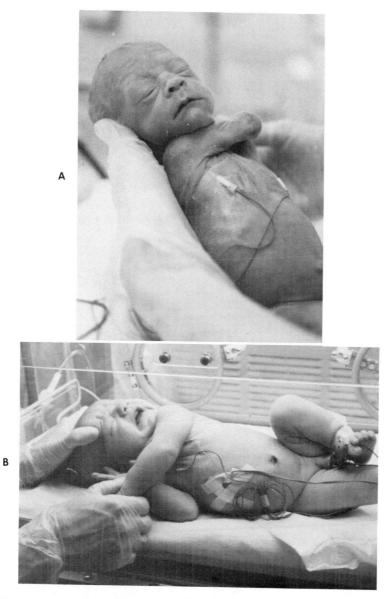

**Fig. 7-18.** The scarf sign estimates muscle tone and development. **A,** The premature infant's arm is drawn across his chest and the head turned toward the shoulder. No resistance is felt. **B,** The infant who is near term resists the pull of the arm, and the chin will not easily move beyond alignment with the elbow.

**Table 7-1.** Appearance of neurologic signs

| Reflexes | 24 Weeks+ | 28 Weeks+ | 32 Weeks+ | 34 Weeks+ | 37 Weeks+ | 41 Weeks+ |
|---|---|---|---|---|---|---|
| Moro | Barely apparent (exhaustible) | Complete (exhaustible) | Good | Complete | Complete | Complete |
| Grasp | Feeble | Fair | Solid (involves arm) | Solid | May pick infant up | As before |
| Rooting | Minimal | Good | Good | Good | Good | Good |
| Suck | Absent | Present | Improving | Strong (synchronized with swallow) | As before | As before |
| Pupillary response | Absent | Absent | Present | Present | Present | Present |
| Trunk incurvation | Present | Present | Present | Present | Present | Present |
| Automatic walk | Absent | Absent | Absent | Minimal | Fair on toes | Good on heels |
| Cry | Feeble (exhaustible) | Brief, high pitch | Good | Good | Good | Good |

in detail. The normal term infant draws the arms and legs close to the trunk and exhibits almost continuous movement (in some cases being able to roll independently from a prone to supine position). Lying prone, the normal term infant flexes and moves the extremities and head. The premature, on the other hand, lies with the extremities extended. The facial expression is one of complete exhaustion or worry (Fig. 7-19). The arms, legs, and facial muscles make occasional, brief, twitching movements, which are largely uncoordinated. A stable premature may also make effective crawling motions, but the position of extension is assumed for periods of rest. If the legs are drawn toward the trunk, they frog outward rather than tuck under.[8,22]

### Learning and thought competency

Assessment of learning and thought competency during the newborn period is often overlooked but provides an important basis for future assessment. The evaluation of infant reflexes provides the core of learning and thought competency assessment during the newborn period. Reflexive behavior is the theoretical basis for all future learning, according to Hebb, Piaget, and other learning theorists.[29] During the first month of life the inborn reflexes make it possible for the infant to make orienting responses to light or sound, to grasp an object placed in the palm of the hand, to suck when the lips are touched, and to raise the head from the surface when in a prone position. The infant is able to focus attention briefly on an object, showing preference for a human face. These early responses, which are observed as a part of the nursing assessment, provide the basis for future learning in that complex neural associations are formed as these responses are repeated over and over during the first month of life.[29,36]

These reflexive abilities form the behavioral basis for the processes of conditioned and reinforcement learning, which predominates throughout infancy. The predominant reinforcers of early infancy include food, visual patterns with a preference for human faces, light presentation, the human voice, maternal heartbeat, movement of a mobile and movement of the infant's body.[36] These experiences have been demonstrated to reinforce the infant's behavior; the newborn can and does respond to these stimuli in preference to other environmental stimuli. Observation of the infant's ability to turn the head and to visually attend or cry in response to stimuli in the environment is an important indicator of learning and thought competency in the newborn period.

### Social and inner competency

The development of social and inner competency is dependent upon the nature of the attachment formed between the infant and mother and other significant persons. Therefore, assessment of reciprocal attachment behavior of both the mother and the newborn during their interaction is an essential component of the newborn assessment. It has been documented

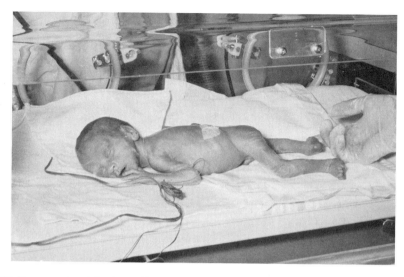

**Fig. 7-19.** The premature infant's position at rest is one of extension of extremities. His head is minimally molded, and his facial expression is one of exhaustion.

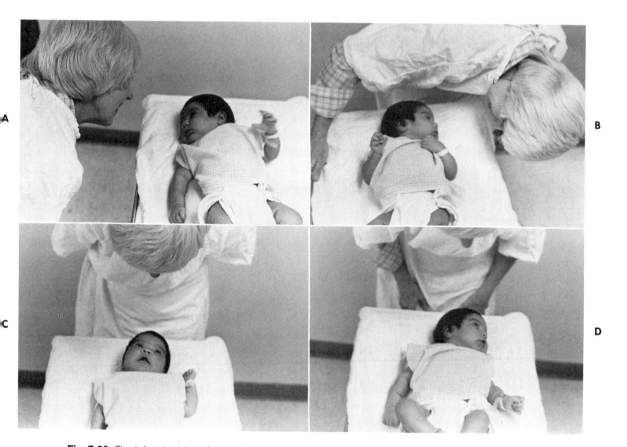

**Fig. 7-20.** The infant is able to focus attention on the human face and follow movement to the midline. **A,** The infant demonstrates ability to focus on the nurse's face. **B,** The nurse engages the infant's attention and, **C,** moves her face slowly to the midline, observing the infant's ability to follow her movement. **D,** She regains focus on her face at the midline.

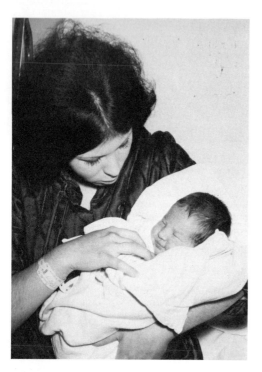

**Fig. 7-21.** Initially the mother begins to get acquainted with her infant through visual inspection and small areas of physical contact.

that early events during the newborn period have a significant and long-lasting effect on the mother and the infant and that there is a sensitive period in the first few minutes and hours of life during which it is necessary for the mother and father to have close contact with their infant in order for later development to be optimal.[21] If there is a separation during this period, or if circumstances that create stress for the parents exist, the behaviors of early attachment will occur, but more time may be required and there may be more effort required of the parent.[21]

Of the interactions originating in the mother that affect the infant, the following may be observed and described as a component of the nursing assessment:

1. *Touch.* The usual initial response of the mother to the infant, whether the infant is dressed or undressed, is to gently stroke the infant's face with her fingertips. Subsequently, she strokes other areas of the body, often the hands, arms, and other parts of the head. As the initial acquaintance progresses, she begins to use her palms in stroking the infant. When the initial contact is during the first few minutes after delivery, this occurs within the first three minutes of contact. When there is a delay in the initial contact, progressing to use of the palms may be delayed for several days.[21]

2. *Eye-to-eye contact.* During the initial contact and for the first several days, the mother will express a strong desire for the infant to open his or her eyes. She holds the infant in the en face position in order to obtain parallel eye-to-eye contact and often talks to the infant in an effort to stimulate and seek eye contact.[21]

3. *High-pitched voice.* Mothers speak to their infants in a noticeably higher pitched voice than that used in everyday conversation. It has been documented that infant's have a preference for the female voice and respond with greater sensitivity to speech in the high-frequency range.[21]

4. *Entrainment.* When the mother speaks to the infant, the infant responds with body movements that are rhythmically coordinated with the rhythm of the speech. Regardless of the mother's language, the infant can be observed to move in coordination with the speech of the mother. Although this movement may be difficult to perceive, when the mother pauses for a breath or accents a syllable, the infant may be observed to move some part of the body, such as lift an eyebrow, move a hand, or lower a foot.[21]

5. *Time-giver.* During the first few days of life, the mother helps the infant establish biorhythmicity; she responds to alert states by giving the infant her time and attention. She seeks time with the infant and is pleased to have the infant in an alert state in order to interact. In a rooming-in setting or a setting where she chooses when and how often she has the infant with her, she will seek time with the infant when the infant is alert and will choose to have the infant cared for by the nurses or family members when the infant is likely to be asleep.[21]

Of those interactions originating with the infant that affect the mother, the following should be observed as a part of the nursing assessment:

1. *Eye-to-eye contact.* When the mother holds the infant in the en face position and his or her eyes open, there is an observable period of mutual gazing, with the infant showing a prefer-

ence for the mother's face, particularly her eyes. The infant will follow the movement of the mother's face, maintaining a gaze into her eyes as she moves. This interaction is considered to be the most powerful stimuli for the maternal care-taking response. It often stimulates the mother to talk to the infant and to express pleasure with the infant's traits and behavior.

2. *Cry.* The cry of the infant stimulates a significant increase of blood flow to the mother's breasts, a phenomena that cannot be directly observed but that will be reported by the mother either spontaneously or in response to inquiry. The mother will be observed to respond to the infant's cry by attending to the infant, either to check the diaper, pick up the infant, or feed the infant.

3. *Licking and sucking.* When the infant is placed in a breast-feeding position immediately after delivery, the first response is to lick the mother's nipple. This causes erection of the nipple, and also initiates the secretion of oxytocin, which promotes uterine contraction, facilitating delivery of the placenta and reducing maternal bleeding.

4. *Entrainment.* The process of entrainment has been described above from the maternal perspective. When the mother speaks and the infant moves, she is likely to continue talking to the infant. If the infant does not respond, the mother is not likely to continue talking to the infant. Klaus and Kennell have called this principle "You cannot fall in love with a dishrag."[21]

The importance of providing an environment where these behaviors can emerge and continue cannot be overemphasized. If the setting provides for these interactions to occur and they do not, the nurse needs to assess physical or psychosocial circumstances of the family that might be interfering with the initial attachment between the infant and the family. The actual behaviors of the mother and the infant should be documented in detail as to the nature of the behavior, the time of occurrence, and the frequency of occurrence. This assessment provides a basis for planning nursing intervention during infancy to facilitate optimal family relationships and attachment for the infant.[5,21,24,35,39]

Another dimension of social and inner competency concerns the temperament of the infant. To the extent that the infant's temperament is in harmony with that of the family, their adjustment together will be adverse or relatively easy. Behavioral individuality of the newborn can be observed, and Farrar[10] has developed a tool specifically for this purpose. The infant is observed in states of sleep, hunger, satiety, and after stimulation. The intensity of the infant's behavior during each of these states is recorded, and an assessment of the infant's behavioral style is made. This assessment is used as a basis for counseling and guidance with the family and for teaching them the types of behavioral clues that their infant is likely to use during the early months of life.[10]

Nursing care during the newborn period is planned and implemented to provide for the needs of the newborn and mother during the first days of adjustment and adaptation and also to provide for a foundation of health maintenance during the weeks ahead. Once the family leaves the health care setting after delivery of the infant, health care resources can be limited and relatively inaccessible, particularly for matters of daily routine health care. If the family is inexperienced in caring for an infant or if the family is experiencing another physical, emotional, or social stress, optimal adjustment during the newborn period may be difficult to achieve.

The following section presents a discussion of the common health problems faced by a family with a newborn infant. Nursing management related to each of these problems takes into account not only the period of time in the health care setting immediately after delivery, but also the first few weeks of the new family's adjustment.

## Nutrition and feeding

Many hospitals provide some planned program of group or individual teaching for new mothers in relation to breast- or bottle-feeding.[1] Many such programs provide a useful learning experience for mothers, as well as provide an opportunity for social interaction among mothers. However, this approach alone serves a limited function in relation to nutrition and feeding. One concern that is often neglected is the new father's role in feeding and nutrition and that of other members of the household. In addition, many mothers are still debating whether to breast- or bottle-feed, reevaluating their earlier decision in this regard, and have many questions regarding the effect of either method on their family life-style. Knowledge of infant and family nutrition is often lacking. Each of these factors needs to be taken into account in planning nursing care for the family during the newborn period.[4,6]

The mother who has decided to breast-feed her infant may be troubled by doubts and false beliefs in the first few weeks of her infant's life because breast-feeding has been surrounded by superstitions and false tales for centuries. For instance, it is often believed that there is no nourishment from the breasts for the infant until the milk comes in, which for many mothers is believed to be on the third or fourth day, when breast engorgement occurs. In reality, colostrum is present several weeks before delivery, and it is present in sufficient amounts at delivery to nourish the infant for several days. Colostrum, a yellowish substance, has a lower mean energy value than does mature breast milk, but it is higher in ash content, particularly sodium, potassium, and chloride. The major changes from colostrum to mature milk are accomplished by the tenth day after delivery.

A primary concern for many mothers who are considering or have decided to breast-feed is their probability of success. Concerns may center on the sufficiency of the amount of milk the mother can provide, the size or shape of the mother's nipples, or the problems in meeting the demands for feeding the infant in light of the other demands on her time and energy. If the mother is going to return to work at some point after the birth of the infant, she may have questions regarding the effect of such a change in her schedule on the feeding of her infant. Success in breast-feeding is dependent upon her mental attitude and that of her family toward each of these factors. She needs to feel confident in her ability to provide adequate amounts of milk and to have the infant respond to her offering the breast with strong nutritive sucking. Care and protection of her breasts and nipples must be accomplished with relative ease and comfort. Her family must be supportive of breast-feeding to the extent that they assist with household chores and provide understanding and support for the feeding demands of the infant. If the other adults in the family are accustomed to receiving much physical and emotional care and support from the mother, their needs must be acknowledged and provision made for setting these aside as the new infant is integrated into the family. The entire family must be involved in planning for the mother's return to work and the feeding transitions that are probably necessary. The problem of the mother's fatigue level during breast-feeding needs to be discussed with the adult family members so that they can anticipate the mother's need for rest and alleviation of demands and responsibilities without developing feelings of guilt. The family needs to be able to communicate openly regarding their needs and desires and work out satisfactory compromises and agreements in conducting the usual affairs of the family. The nurse can use and teach the mother to use relaxation exercises to help combat the feelings of fatigue that will inevitably occur.[34]

The concern is often expressed as to whether the mother will be able to produce sufficient amounts of milk to fully nourish the infant. A real problem with insufficient milk supply seldom occurs, and thus it is reasonable to assure a healthy mother desiring to breast-feed that she will be able to fully nourish her infant with breast milk for several weeks. An adequate supply of milk depends upon the infant adequately emptying both breasts at fairly regular intervals around the clock. The production of prolactin by the anterior pituitary of the mother is stimulated by the sucking of the infant, which in turn stimulates further milk production. Oxytocin, produced simultaneously by the posterior pituitary, causes the smooth muscle cells surrounding the milk-producing glands to contract, forcing mature milk into the ducts that lead to the nipple openings. This process causes a let-down sensation in the breasts, which becomes a familiar sensation for the mother in response to the infant's sucking and may be stimulated by the crying of her infant when feeding is imminent. Discussion of these sensations with the mother can reassure her that she is producing milk normally.

## Initiation of breast-feeding

Optimal initiation of breast-feeding occurs just after delivery when the infant is stimulated, sucking spontaneously, and the mother experiences the eager ecstasy of first holding the infant and providing the closeness and warmth of first offering her breast to the infant. When the infant first breast-feeds, several hours after delivery, stimulation and readiness to suck is not as strong, and the mother will need assistance and encouragement in initiation of feeding. The infant should be first presented in a hungry state, and the mother and infant should be positioned comfortably. The mother's comfort may be difficult to achieve at first; she may feel awkward and ill at ease in any position. Help her in finding the position of greatest comfort, lying down or sitting. Position the infant in such a manner that the mother and infant can comfortably assume an en face position in relation to one another, as the infant usually opens his or her eyes to gaze at the mother while feeding, a response that is rewarding and encouraging for the mother. Stroke the infant's cheek and mouth to stimulate rooting toward the nipple. Assist the mother in stimulating her nipple so that it becomes erect and ready for the infant to grasp. The infant should achieve a firm grasp of the areola, with the gums approximating the edge of the areola. Assuming an adequate grasp during early feeding will prevent nipple soreness that otherwise occurs when the infant's gums grasp at the base of the nipple. The mother may support her breast with her hand, massaging gently the area around the areola to stimulate the flow of milk. If there are firm, engorged areas in the breast, teach the mother to gently massage these areas while the infant is feeding to stimulate the flow of milk in this area. This kind of massage is important in the prevention of mastitis, which sometimes occurs when milk does not flow from areas of the breast. The mother needs to be aware of her infant's temperament in relation to feeding and know that the infant's responses to breast-feeding will mature as they both become accustomed to feeding. By observing the infant's responses to the first few feedings, the nurse can explain the general nature of the infant's temperament so that the mother may understand and respond appropriately. For example, some infants eagerly grasp the nipple and attempt to suck but lose the nipple in their excitement to feed. These infants need comforting and calming by the mother to help them relax and get a firm hold on the nipple. Other infants will initially grasp

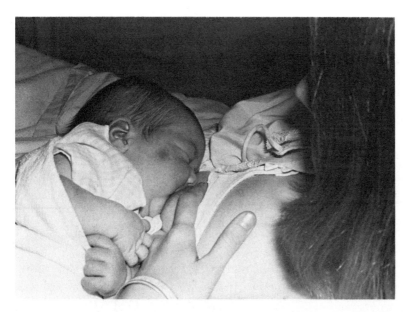

**Fig. 7-22.** The infant should achieve a firm grasp of the areola, with the gums approximating the edge of the areola.

the nipple effectively but only gradually begin to suck effectively. The mother needs to anticipate that the infant will begin to suck, given a few minutes.[34]

### Establishing a breast-feeding routine

It is recommended that the mother nurse from both breasts at each feeding, alternating the side on which she begins feeding. The length of time that the infant nurses from the first breast may vary with the mother, but it is usually from about five to ten minutes. The nurse needs to discuss the infant's feeding behavior with the mother and help her become sensitive to the cues that she can use in determining the time to change feeding from one breast to the other. The first breast should become relatively unengorged and soft to touch before moving to the second breast. Usually the infant will show signs of wanting to rest or needing burping within the first few minutes of feeding. Depending upon how eagerly and effectively the infant has fed, the mother may continue on the same breast or change at this time.

The mother needs to understand the infant's cues, which she will use to determine the frequency of feeding the infant. The signs of satiety that the infant will be expected to demonstrate include sleeping and relaxation toward the end of a sufficient feeding. The infant will remain relatively sleepy and inactive for about two hours if the feeding has been sufficient in amount. In addition, the infant will demonstrate a satisfactory weight gain through the first months of life. During the first few weeks of life, the mother needs to understand that her infant's individual temperament will cause variations in the amount of time he or she will remain satiated between feedings and that the period between feedings is likely to vary throughout the day and night. As their routine at home becomes established, the infant will probably establish periods of the day when the desire to feed is more frequent—often in the afternoon and early evening. Most infants begin to sleep for longer periods during the night within the first month and may not awaken to be fed for four to six hours. This natural tendency is an advantage in providing rest for the family during the night; however they need to anticipate more difficult periods of coping with fussiness, which are bound to occur.

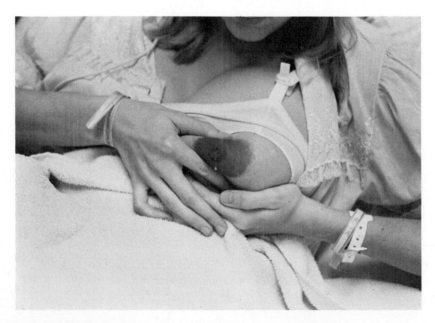

**Fig. 7-23.** This mother is learning to manually express milk from her breast to relieve excessive engorgement. She has applied pressure to the breast with her left hand, and as she releases the left hand pressure, she gently applies pressure around the areola. This action is repeated, rotating each hand around the breast and the areola.

### Care of the breasts and nipples

For both breast-feeding and bottle-feeding mothers, care of the breasts is of great importance. As engorgement occurs, the bottle-feeding mother will need assistance in coping with the discomfort until milk production subsides. Ice packs are recommended as soon as the mother's breasts become firm and tender. A firm-fitting bra provides support for the breasts.

The mother who is breast-feeding will also experience the discomfort of engorgement. Frequent feeding of the infant will provide some relief and is beneficial in establishing the flow of milk. The mother may need to manually express small amounts of milk between feedings or just before feeding if the engorgement interferes with the infant's ability to grasp the nipple. To express milk from the breast, the mother supports the breast with her hand on the same side as the breast being expressed. With the thumb and fingers of the other hand, she grasps the areola. Gentle pressure is first applied to the breast, then the thumb and finger around the areola are gently squeezed. The thumb and finger are rotated around the areola each time it is compressed so that all ampulae are emptied. Any areas of the breast that are particularly firm should be gently massaged to assure adequate emptying.

The nipples are particularly important in breast care. Initial soreness and tenderness are inevitable for a mother who is first breast-feeding. She needs to learn to clean her nipples with mild soap and water before each feeding and observe for any cracking of the skin. After feeding the mother should air-dry the nipples. She may need to use dry heat in the form of light. A goose-neck lamp with a 20-watt bulb may be positioned about 18 inches from the breasts for five to ten minutes several times a day. To facilitate the let-down reflex before nursing and decrease the infant's need for hard sucking while the nipples are tender, the mother may use warm wet compresses on the breasts before feeding.[34]

### Excretion of drugs in human milk

The factor of maternal drugs being excreted in milk is a seldom considered and very important factor for the breast-feeding mother. If drugs are prescribed, this factor should be considered and discussed by the health care team. The mother needs to know of this factor when she uses any nonprescription drug. The exact mechanism for excretion of drugs in human milk is not known, but it has been demonstrated that drugs taken by the mother do appear in human milk.[27] The newborn infant changes rapidly in the ability to tolerate and metabolize drugs, and this ability can vary within a brief period of time. The infant's ability to combine potentially harmful materials with glucuronic acids, one of the principle detoxifying mechanisms, is generally not fully functioning in the infant under 1 month of age. Other enzyme systems important in the metabolism of drugs, such as acetylation and oxidation, are also deficient. Oxidation, for example, is an important factor in the metabolism of drugs such as sulfisoxazole, which is found in significant quantities in breast milk of mothers given this drug for postpartum urinary tract infections.[27] The immature enzyme system, combined with the infant's incompletely developed renal function, render the infant susceptible to the accumulation of toxic levels of drugs, with a resulting range of symptoms such as jaundice, irritability, vomiting and diarrhea.[27] Table 7-2 summarizes the excretion of commonly used drugs and the significance of this for the breast-feeding infant.

### Bottle-feeding

Many of the concerns and problems of breast-feeding mothers are similar for bottle-feeding mothers. Establishment of a feeding routine is very similar, with the difference that other members of the family may be involved in meeting the infant's feeding demands at different times of the day or night. This may offer some advantages to the mother and also provides the infant close interaction with other family members. However, it also may be a factor creating disagreements as to when the infant should be fed, how much, and for how long. If these areas of concern can be discussed with all adults in the family during the newborn period and each member of the family demonstrates a congruent understanding of the feeding needs of the infant, their adjustments in balancing their responses to the infant for feeding will be mini-

*Text continued on p. 200.*

**Table 7-2.** Drugs excreted in human milk and the possible significance for nursing infants*

| Drug | Excreted | Quantity excreted | Significance |
|------|----------|-------------------|--------------|
| **ANTIHISTAMINE DRUGS** | | | |
| Diphenhydramine (Benadryl) | Yes | | Not significant in therapeutic doses to affect child. |
| Trimeprazine tartrate (Temaril) | Yes | | Not significant in therapeutic doses to affect child. |
| Tripelennamine (Pyribenzamine) | Yes | | Only bovine studies reported to date; apparently not enough is excreted to be significant in therapeutic doses. |
| **ANTIINFECTIVE AGENTS** | | | |
| Amantadine (Symmetrel) | Possible | | Not to be administered; personal correspondence with the manufacturer suggests it will be found in maternal milk; may cause vomiting, urinary retention, skin rash. |
| Ampicillin (Polycillin, Amcill, Omnipen, Penbritin, Principen, others) | Yes | 0.07 $\mu$g/ml | Not significant in therapeutic doses to affect child. |
| Carbenicillin disodium (Pyopen, Geopen) | Yes | 0.265 $\mu$g/ml one hour after administration of 1 g | Not significant in therapeutic doses to affect child. |
| Cephalexin (Keflex) | No | | |
| Cephalothin (Keflin) | No | | |
| Chloramphenicol (Chloromycetin) | Yes | Half blood level 2.5 mg/100 ml | Infants have underdeveloped enzyme system, immature liver and renal function, may not have glycuronide system adequately developed to conjugate chloramphenicol; caution advised. |
| Chloroquine (Aralen) | No | After daily dose of 0.6 g no traces could be found in milk of 105 subjects | Not significant in therapeutic doses to affect child. |
| Demethylchlortetracycline (Declomycin) | Yes | 0.2-0.3 mg/500 ml | Not significant in therapeutic doses to affect child. |
| Erythromycin (Ilosone, E-mycin, Erythrocin) | Yes | 0.05-0.1 mg/100 ml 3.6-6.2 $\mu$g/ml | Higher concentrations have been reported in milk than in plasma. |
| Isoniazid (Nydrazid) | Yes | 0.6-1.2 mg/100 ml same concentration in milk as in maternal serum | Infant should be monitored for possible signs of isoniazid toxicity. |
| Kanamycin (Kantrex) | Yes | 1 g given intramuscularly gave a concentration of 18.4 $\mu$g/ml | Infant should be monitored for possible signs of kanamycin toxicity. |
| Lincomycin (Lincocin) | Yes | 0.5-2.4 $\mu$g/ml | Not significant in therapeutic doses to affect child. |
| Mandelic acid | Yes | 0.3 g/24 hr following maternal dose of 12 g/day | Not significant in therapeutic doses to affect child. |
| Methacycline (Rondomycin) | Yes | | Same precautions as with tetracyclines. |
| Methenamine (Hexamine) | Yes | | Not significant in therapeutic doses to affect child. |
| Metronidazole (Flagyl) | Yes | Level comparable to serum | Apparently not significant in therapeutic doses; caution should be exercised due to its high milk concentrations. |

*From O'Brien, T. E.: Excretion of drugs in human milk, Am. J. Hosp. Pharm. **31:**844-854, Sept., 1974.

**Table 7-2.** Drugs excreted in human milk and the possible significance for nursing infants—cont'd

| Drug | Excreted | Quantity excreted | Significance |
|------|----------|-------------------|--------------|
| **ANTIINFECTIVE AGENTS—cont'd** | | | |
| Nitrofurantoin (Furadantin) | Yes | | Not significant in therapeutic doses to affect child. |
| Nalidixic acid (NegGram) | Yes | 3.9 μg/liter | Not significant in therapeutic doses, however one case of hemolytic anemia in an infant was attributed to nalidixic acid. |
| Novobiocin (Albamycin, Cardelmycin) | Yes | 0.36-0.54 mg/100 ml | This antibiotic has been used to treat infections among infants with no untoward effects reported. |
| Oxacillin (Prostaphlin) | No | | |
| Paraamino salicylic acid | No | | |
| Penethamate (Leocillin) | No | 24-74 μg/100 ml | Animal study suggests it be avoided. |
| Penicillin G potassium | Yes | Up to 6 units/100 ml | Controversy exists among authors; some feel that the risk of sensitivity symptoms must be looked for, others feel the small amount is insignificant; parent should be told to inform physician that infant has been exposed to penicillin. |
| Penicillin, benzathine (Bicillin) | Yes | 10-12 units/100 ml | Clinical need should supersede possible allergic responses. |
| Pyrimethamine (Daraprim) | Yes | | Detected in human milk but no conclusions drawn; apparently not significant in therapeutic doses. |
| Quinine sulfate | Yes | 0-0.1 mg/100 ml after maternal dose of 300-600 mg | Not significant in therapeutic doses to affect child. |
| Sodium fusidate | Yes | 0.02 μg/ml | Not significant in therapeutic doses to affect child. |
| Streptomycin | Yes | Present for long periods in slight amounts given as dihydrostreptomycin | Risk should outweigh benefit of nursing; to be avoided. |
| Sulfanilamide | Yes | After maternal dose of 2-4 g daily 9 mg/100 ml in milk | Not significant in therapeutic doses; may cause a rash. |
| Sulfapyridine | Yes | 3-13 mg/100 ml after maternal dose of 3 g daily | To be avoided; has caused skin rash. |
| Sulfathiazole | Yes | 0.5 mg/100 ml after dose of 3 g/day | Not significant in therapeutic doses to affect child. |
| Sulfisoxazole (Gantrisin) | Yes | Concentration similar to plasma level | To be avoided during first two postpartum weeks; may cause kernicterus. |
| Tetracycline HCl (Achromycin, Steclin, Sumycin, others) | Yes | 0.5-2.6 μg/ml after maternal dose of 500 mg q.i.d. | Not enough to treat an infection in an infant; however, it has been hypothesized that there may be a sufficient amount to cause discoloration of the teeth in the infant; the antibiotic, however, may be largely bound to the milk calcium. |
| **ANTINEOPLASTICS** | | | |
| Cyclophosphamide (Cytoxan) | Yes | | To be avoided, as are other antineoplastic drugs; nursing should be discontinued. |

**193**

*Continued.*

**Table 7-2.** Drugs excreted in human milk and the possible significance for nursing infants—cont'd

| Drug | Excreted | Quantity excreted | Significance |
|---|---|---|---|
| **AUTONOMIC DRUGS** | | | |
| Atropine sulfate (ingredient in many products, both prescription and nonprescription) | Yes | Less than 0.1 mg/100 ml | Should not be administered for two main reasons: (1) it inhibits lactation, and (2) it may cause atropine intoxication in the infant. |
| Carisoprodol (Soma, Rela) | Yes | May be present in breast milk at concentrations 2-4 times maternal plasma | Not to be administered, based upon manufacturer's recommendation; infant may be exposed to a series of adverse reactions ranging from CNS depression to gastrointestinal upset. |
| Ergot (Cafergot) | Yes | | Avoid where possible; may cause symptoms in infants ranging from vomiting and diarrhea to weak pulse and unstable blood pressure. |
| Hyoscine | Yes | Trace amounts | Not significant in therapeutic doses to affect child. |
| Mepenzolate bromide (Cantil) | No | | |
| Methocarbamol (Robaxin) | Yes | Small amounts | Not significant in therapeutic doses to affect child. |
| Propantheline bromide (Pro-Banthine) | No | | |
| Scopolamine | Yes | | Not significant in therapeutic doses to affect child. |
| **BLOOD FORMATION AND COAGULATION** | | | |
| Bishydroxycoumarin (Dicumarol) | Yes | | Therapeutic doses can be administered without deleterious effect on infant; infant should be monitored with mother. |
| Ethyl biscoumacetate (Tromexan) | Yes | 0-0.17 mg/100 ml; no correlation with dosage | Not significant in therapeutic doses; infant should be monitored with mother. |
| Iron Ferrous sulfate Iron-dextran (Feosol, Imferon) | Yes | | Not significant in therapeutic doses to affect child. |
| Phenindione (Hedulin, Dindevan) | Yes | | To be avoided; may produce a prothrombin deficiency in infant; one case of massive hematoma reported in an infant receiving drug in maternal milk. |
| Warfarin sodium (Coumadin) | Yes | | Infant should be monitored with mother; benefit should outweigh possible risk. |
| **CARDIOVASCULAR DRUGS** | | | |
| Dextrothyroxine (Choloxin) | Yes | | Not significant in therapeutic doses to affect child. |
| Guanethidine (Ismelin) | Yes | | Not significant in therapeutic doses to affect child. |
| Methyclothiazide and deserpidine (Enduronyl) | Yes | | Same precautions as with reserpine and thiazide diuretics. |
| Methyldopa (Aldomet) | Yes | | Studies performed on bovines; nothing reported in humans. |

194

**Table 7-2.** Drugs excreted in human milk and the possible significance for nursing infants*—cont'd

| Drug | Excreted | Quantity excreted | Significance |
|------|----------|-------------------|--------------|
| **CARDIOVASCULAR DRUGS—cont'd** | | | |
| Propranolol (Inderal) | No | | |
| Reserpine (Serpasil, others) | Yes | | May produce galactorrhea. |
| **CENTRAL NERVOUS SYSTEM DRUGS** | | | |
| Alcohol | Yes | Small amounts | It appears that moderate amounts of alcohol have little, if any effect on the nursing infant. |
| Amitriptyline (Elavil) | No | | |
| Aspirin | Yes | Moderate amounts | It could cause a bleeding tendency by interfering with the function of the infant's platelets or by decreasing the amount of prothrombin in the blood. Risk is minimal if mother takes aspirin just after nursing and if the infant has an adequate store of vitamin K. |
| Barbiturates | Yes | | It appears that in therapeutic doses the barbiturates have little or no effect on the infant; one case was reported where high doses had a hypnotic effect on one infant; it is best to avoid administering, since barbiturates serve as inducing agents for hepatic drug metabolizing enzymes. |
| Barbital (Veronal) | Yes | 4-5 mg of diethylbarbituric acid/ 500 ml of milk detected after a single dose of 500 ml | Significant quantities, avoid administration; produced marked sedation in infant. |
| Bromides (Bromo-Seltzer; many nonprescription sleeping aids) | Yes | 0-6.6 mg/100 ml | Not to be administered; reactions range from rash to drowsiness. |
| Caffeine | Yes | 1% of that ingested | Not significant in therapeutic doses to affect child. |
| Chloroform | Yes | | One study performed in 1908 reported that a nursing infant slept for eight hours; not significant in therapeutic doses. |
| Chloral hydrate (Noctec, Somnos) | Yes | 0-1.5 mg/100 ml | Not significant in therapeutic doses. |
| Chlorazepate (Tranxene) | Yes | | Not to be administered based upon manufacturer's recommendation; may cause drowsiness. |
| Chlordiazepoxide (Librium) | Yes | | Not significant in therapeutic doses to affect child. |
| Chlorpromazine (Thorazine) | Yes | 4.15 mg/ml after daily dose of 200 mg in dogs | Not significant; may cause galactorrhea. |
| Codeine | Yes | | Not significant in therapeutic doses to affect child. |
| Cycloheptenyl ethyl barbituric acid (Medomin) | Yes | | Not significant in therapeutic doses to affect child. |

*Continued.*

**Table 7-2.** Drugs excreted in human milk and the possible significance for nursing infants—cont'd

| Drug | Excreted | Quantity excreted | Significance |
|---|---|---|---|
| | | **CENTRAL NERVOUS SYSTEM DRUGS—cont'd** | |
| Desipramine (Norpramin) | No | | |
| Dextroamphetamine (Dexedrine) | No | | |
| Diacetylmorphine (Heroin) | Yes | | Not enough to prevent withdrawal in addicted infants. |
| Diazepam (Valium) | Yes | 51 ng/ml after 4 days of diazepam; 28 ng/ml of N-demethyl-diazepam | Recent studies recommend that this drug be avoided during nursing; infant reported as lethargic and experienced weight loss; may cause hyperbilirubinemia. |
| Diphenhydramine (Benadryl) | Yes | | Not significant in therapeutic doses to affect child. |
| Flufenamic acid (Arlef) | Yes | | Excreted in small amounts; no recommendations |
| Hydroxyphenbutazone (Tandearil) | Yes | 0 in 53 of 55 mothers | Conflicting reports; both conclude that it would have no significant effect in therapeutic doses. |
| Imipramine (Tofranil) | No | | |
| Indomethacin (Indocin) | Yes | | Not significant in therapeutic doses to affect child. |
| Lithium carbonate (Eskalith, Lithane, Lithonate) | Yes | Same in child's serum as in mother's milk, 0.3 mEq/liter | Infant should be monitored for possible signs of lithium toxicity. |
| Mefenamic acid (Ponstel) | Yes | | Not significant in therapeutic doses to affect child. |
| Meperidine (Demerol) | Yes | | Not significant in therapeutic doses to affect child. |
| Meprobamate (Miltown, Equanil) | Yes | Present in milk at 2-4 times maternal plasma level | Infant should be monitored for possible signs of meprobamate toxication if therapy is to be continued. |
| Mesoridazine besylate (Serentil) | Yes | | Not significant in therapeutic doses to affect child. |
| Morphine | Yes | Small amounts | Not significant in therapeutic doses to affect child. |
| Pentazocine (Talwin) | No | | |
| Phenobarbital (Luminal, others) | Yes | | To be avoided where possible; serves as an inducing agent for hepatic drug metabolizing enzymes. |
| Phenylbutazone (Butazolidin) | No | 0.63 mg/100 ml 1.5 hrs after mother injected (i.m.) with 750 mg | No side effects noted among group studied, but because of possible lethal reactions infant should be closely monitored. |
| Phenytoin (Dilantin) | Yes | | Not significant in therapeutic doses although one case of methemoglobinemia was associated with phenytoin. |
| Piperacetazine (Quide) | Yes | | Manufacturer suggests it may have a great potential for excretion in milk. |
| Primidone (Mysoline) | Yes | | To be avoided, may cause undue somnolence and drowsiness. |

**Table 7-2.** Drugs excreted in human milk and the possible significance for nursing infants—cont'd

| Drug | Excreted | Quantity excreted | Significance |
|------|----------|-------------------|--------------|
| **CENTRAL NERVOUS SYSTEM DRUGS—cont'd** | | | |
| Prochlorperazine (Compazine) | Yes | 0.4-1.5 mg/100 ml in dogs after daily dose of 200 mg | Not significant in therapeutic doses to affect child. |
| Propoxyphene HCl (Darvon) | Yes | 0.4% of dose to mother found in stomach of nursing rat | Not significant in therapeutic doses to affect child. |
| Salicylates | Yes | 1.0-3.0 mg/100 ml of sodium salicylate detected 4 hours after maternal dose of 4 g | Not significant in therapeutic doses; high doses (5 g/day) have been reported to cause a rash in infant. |
| Thiopental sodium (Pentothal) | Yes | | Not significant in therapeutic doses to affect child. |
| Thioridazine (Mellaril) | Yes | | Not significant in therapeutic doses to affect child. |
| Tranylcypromine (Parnate) | Yes | | Not significant in therapeutic doses to affect child. |
| Trifluoperazine (Stelazine) | Yes | 0.4-1.5 mg/100 ml in dogs after daily dose of 200 mg | Not significant in therapeutic doses to affect child. |
| **DIAGNOSTIC AGENTS** | | | |
| Carotene (natural product found in carrots) | Yes | | One incident reported where infant turned yellow; mother ate 2-3 lbs of carrots per week; not significant in average quantities. |
| Iopanoic acid (Telepaque) | Yes | | Not significant in therapeutic doses to affect child. |
| **ELECTROLYTIC, CALORIC, AND WATER BALANCE** | | | |
| Cyclopenthiazide (Navidrex) | No | | |
| Cyclamate (Sucaryl) | Yes | | Not significant in therapeutic doses to affect child. |
| Furosemide (Lasix) | No | | |
| Hydrochlorothiazide (Hydrodiuril, Esidrix, others) | Yes | | To be avoided, based on manufacturer's recommendation; no specific adverse effects reported in infants to date. |
| Spironolactone (Aldactone) | No | | |
| Thiazides | Yes | | To be avoided based on manufacturer's recommendation; no specific adverse reactions reported in infants to date. |
| **EXPECTORANTS AND COUGH PREPARATIONS** | | | |
| Potassium iodide | Yes | 3 mg/100 ml | To be avoided, may affect infant's thyroid. |
| **GASTROINTESTINAL DRUGS** | | | |
| Aloe | Yes | | Controversial, one author claims it may give rise to catharsis in some infants, others feel its presence is insignificant. |

*Continued.*  **197**

**Table 7-2.** Drugs excreted in human milk and the possible significance for nursing infants—cont'd

| Drug | Excreted | Quantity excreted | Significance |
|------|----------|-------------------|--------------|
| **GASTROINTESTINAL DRUGS—cont'd** | | | |
| Anthraquinone (Dorbane, Dorbantyl, Danthron, Peri-Colace, Doxidan, Dialose-Plus) | Yes | | One animal study found it present in milk and in "significant" amounts; another human study did not detect it; a third human study detected it and felt it best not to administer it to nursing mothers, as it may cause catharsis in the infant. |
| Cascara | Yes | | Avoid where possible; reported to have increased gastric motility in infant. |
| Emodin (found in cascara sagrada) | Yes | | Avoid where possible; reported to have increased gastric motility in infant. |
| Phenolphthalein (found in many nonprescription laxative products) | Yes | | Not significant in therapeutic doses to affect child. |
| Rhubarb | Yes | | Not significant in therapeutic doses to affect child. |
| Senna | Yes | | Not significant in therapeutic doses; high doses may cause diarrhea in nursing infant. |
| **HORMONES AND SYNTHETIC SUBSTITUTES** | | | |
| Carbimazole (Neo-Mercazole) | Yes | | Not to be administered; antithyroid may cause goiter in nursing infant. |
| Chlormadinone- (Estalor-21) | Yes | | Possible effects must be weighed against risk of pregnancy; see contraceptives (oral). |
| Chlorotrianisene (Tace) | Yes | | Avoid where possible estrogenic substances may be in breast secretions. |
| Contraceptives (oral) | Yes | | Possible effects must be weighed against risk of pregnancy; may inhibit lactation if administered during first prenatal weeks; possible gynecomastia in male infant. |
| Corticotropin | Yes | | Destroyed during passage through gastrointestinal tract; its presence in milk is unimportant. |
| Cortisone | Yes | | No human study; among animals a 50% lower weight than control; retarded sexual development; exophthalmus. |
| Dihydrotachysterol (Hytakerol) | Yes | | May cause hypercalcemia. |
| Estrogen (oral contraceptives) | Yes | 0.17 $\mu$g/100 mg | Possible effects must be weighed against risk of pregnancy; see contraceptives (oral). |
| Ethisterone (Pranone) | Yes | | To be avoided; may cause significant skeletal advancement. |
| Fluoxymesterone (Halotestin, Ora-testryl, Ultandren) | | | Used to suppress lactation. |
| Iodides (nonradioactive) | Yes | After a dose of 0.6 g (as potassium salt) 68 mg was recovered | To be avoided, chronic use may affect infant's thyroid gland. |

**Table 7-2.** Drugs excreted in human milk and the possible significance for
nursing infants—cont'd

| Drug | Excreted | Quantity excreted | Significance |
|---|---|---|---|
| **HORMONES AND SYNTHETIC SUBSTITUTES—cont'd** | | | |
| Liothyronine sodium (Cytomel) | No | | |
| Lyndiol | Yes | | To be avoided; caused a diminution in milk protein and milk fat. |
| Lynestrenol (oral contraceptive under investigation) | Yes | | Possible effects must be weighed against risk of pregnancy; see contraceptives (oral). |
| Medroxyprogesterone acetate (Provera) | No | | |
| Mestranol (estrogenic compound found in several oral contraceptives) | Yes | | Possible effects must be weighed against risk of pregnancy; see contraceptives (oral). |
| Norethisterone ethanate (progesterone contraceptives) | Yes | | Possible effects must be weighed against risk of pregnancy; see contraceptives (oral). |
| Norethynodrel (Enovid) | Yes | 1.1% of dose | Possible effects must be weighed against risk of pregnancy; see contraceptives (oral). |
| Norethindrone (Norlutin) | Yes | | Possible effects must be weighed against risk of pregnancy; see contraceptives (oral). |
| Phenformin HCl (DBI) | Yes | | Not significant; does not exert hypoglycemic effect on normal subject. |
| Pregnane-3 ($\alpha$), 20 ($\beta$)-diol | Yes | | Although it may cause unconjugated hyperbilirubinemia in breast fed infants it was regarded as not being significant enough to stop nursing. |
| Thiouracil | Yes | Higher in milk than in blood 9-12 mg/100 ml | To be avoided; may cause goiter in nursing infant or agranulocytosis. |
| Thyroid | Yes | | Not significant in therapeutic doses to affect child. |
| Tolbutamide (Orinase) | Yes | | Not significant in therapeutic doses to affect child. |
| **RADIOACTIVE AGENTS** | | | |
| Gallium-67 (gallium citrate) | Yes | | Avoid where possible, radionuclides are generally contraindicated during nursing, or nursing should be temporarily stopped. |
| Iodine radioactive (131I) | Yes | Total in 48 hours of milk: 1.3 microcuries after maternal dose of 29.5 microcuries | To be avoided; affects infant's thyroid gland. |
| Sodium, radioactive as sodium chloride | Yes | 0.5-1.3% of dose per liter of milk | Not significant in therapeutic dose, although it seems best to avoid the radionuclides if possible. |
| **SERUMS, TOXOIDS, AND VACCINES** | | | |
| Diphtheria antibodies | Yes | Less than 0.30% of dose administered | Of no value in conferring passive immunity to infant. |

*Continued.*

**Table 7-2.** Drugs excreted in human milk and the possible significance for nursing infants—cont'd

| Drug | Excreted | Quantity excreted | Significance |
|---|---|---|---|
| **SKIN AND MUCOUS MEMBRANE PREPARATIONS** | | | |
| DDT | Yes | 5 mg/100 ml | The concentration is higher in human milk than in bovine milk; DDT poisoning. |
| **VITAMINS** | | | |
| Calciferol (vitamin D) | Yes | | Caution advised; may cause hypercalcemia. |
| Cyanocobalamin (vitamin $B_{12}$) | Yes | 0.1-0.4 $\mu$g/liter | Not significant in therapeutic doses to affect child. |
| Folic acid | Yes | 0.7 $\mu$g/liter | Not significant in therapeutic doses to affect child. |
| Phytonadione (vitamin $K_1$, Aquamephyton) | Yes | | Not significant in therapeutic doses to affect child. |
| Thiamine (vitamin $B_1$) deficiency | Yes | 10-13 $\mu$g/liter | A lack of this B vitamin in the nursing mother (beriberi) causes the excretion of a toxic substance, methylglyoxal, which has caused infant death. |
| **MISCELLANEOUS AGENTS** | | | |
| Allergens (eggs, wheat flax seed, peanuts, cottonseed, etc.) | Yes | | May cause allergic response in sensitive child. |
| Colchicine | Yes | | A 1929 study indicated that this drug may pass into milk; no adverse effect reported. |
| Fluorides (found in many toothpastes) | Yes | | Not significant in quantities ingested; excess could affect tooth enamel. |
| Hexachlorobenzene[1,23] | No | | Avoid use as an insecticide; has caused infant mortality. |
| Mercury | Yes | | Environmental contaminant; signs of mercury intoxication and CNS effects. |
| Nicotine | Yes | 0.4-0.5 mg/liter; 11 to 20 cigarettes/day | In moderation, no effect; not more than 20 cigarettes/day. |
| Ribonucleic acid (RNA) | Yes | | Particles from human milk contain a reverse transcriptase and high molecular weight RNA that serves as a template; these particles have two features diagnostic of known RNA tumor viruses. |

mized. Selection of formula and method of preparation needs to be discussed. If possible, it is desired that the mother demonstrate her ability to prepare the formula properly, particularly if she will be mixing her own formula. She needs to demonstrate understanding of the proper proportions and of the hazards that exist in using overconcentrated or underconcentrated proportions. Discuss with her the possibility of other family members or baby sitters preparing the formula so that their understanding can be determined as well.

### Supplemental feedings and addition of solid foods

A breast-feeding mother needs to discuss the use of supplemental feedings. She needs to understand the effect of such feedings on her milk supply and be ready to use manual expression to relieve discomfort or to maintain the milk supply, particularly if supplemental feedings will be used regularly when she is not available to breast-feed the infant. The need to supplement breast milk with cow's milk because of an inadequate supply of mother's milk is rare. The mother should be encouraged to use frequent feedings during the first one or two weeks to stimulate the production of milk. She may need to consult her community health nurse or physician during this period for reassurance concerning the adequacy of the amounts of milk and growth of the infant. Once her milk supply is well established, the mother may want to plan for times away from the infant for work or relaxation or plan for other members of the family to feed the infant in order to have this kind of family experience for other family members and the infant.

Addition of solid foods will be of more concern later in infancy, but many mothers are tempted to add cereals during the first month of life, particularly when they believe that periods of fussiness are due to hunger. The mother needs to be prepared to cope with periods of fussiness and understand that as long as the infant is gaining weight appropriately and getting sufficient amounts of milk to produce satiety behavior after eating, an infant's fussiness is probably not due to hunger. Means of comforting an infant during a period of fussiness may be difficult for the family, but if they anticipate such times and plan together to assist in caring for the infant, their adjustment will be eased.

### Prevention of hypoglycemia

Of the several fluid and electrolyte imbalances that can occur during the normal course of the newborn's first week, the most important and frequent is hypoglycemia. It is believed that even mild, temporary occurrences of low blood sugar during the newborn period can lead to some forms of neurologic impairment, although such direct relationships have not been fully demonstrated. The infant with mild hypoglycemia will have a variety of symptoms that are almost imperceptible, such as jitteriness of movement, mild cyanosis, or listlessness (see Chapter 8). Periodic screening with a simple Dextrostix (Ames) testing on all infants is desirable to detect infants who may be reaching a particularly dangerous blood sugar level. It is recommended that any infant whose blood sugar is estimated to be less than 45 mg/100 ml Dextrostix be given a feeding of 10% glucose water immediately. The occurrence of mild hypoglycemia can be effectively prevented by early feedings and feeding the infant subsequently by demand as recommended earlier in this section. The nurse should monitor the time intervals of feedings on demand to assure that the infant is feeding frequently enough to maintain an adequate blood sugar level.[41]

### Maintenance of body temperature

Because of the newborn infant's limited ability to regulate body temperature in response to exposure to environmental conditions, attention must be given to maintenance of conditions that protect the infant from undue cold or heat stress. Optimal methods of warming infants after the initial cold exposure of delivery and of maintaining optimal body temperature remains controversial. It is known that cold exposure of delivery is a stimulus for respiration and that episodes of exposure to cooling stimulate the infant's development of cold adaptation responses.[28] However, infants who experience cooling or who are not adequately protected from heat loss are prone to development of acidosis and hypoglycemia, whereas infants who are warmed rapidly are prone to the development of apnea.[26,28] Further investigation is needed to determine more precisely the nature of the infant's responses to cooling and warming, as well as methods for optimal care in this regard. Presently, it is generally accepted that the infant's body temperature should not fall below 36° C, and that the infant should demonstrate maintenance of a body temperature of 37° C as an indicator of body temperature stabilization. Warming of infants in a servocontrolled incubator or radiant heat crib using a skin probe placed 2 cm above the umbilicus in the midline is the recommended approach for warming infants who have a low body temperature or who do not maintain an adequate body temperature under usual environmental conditions. During procedures such as physical assessment, laboratory studies, bathing, weighing, and diaper changing, care should be taken to protect the infant from unnecessary heat loss by means of evaporation, conduction, convection, or radiation. Periodic monitoring of the ambient air temperature and humidity is necessary to assure optimal environmental conditions in the health care setting.

The mother may need guidance regarding provision of optimal levels of warmth for the infant at home. Concerns such as clothing the infant, optimal home temperature settings, and dressing the infant for going outside may need to be discussed. The newborn infant should be dressed in clothing similar to that of the other family members for comfort in the home but needs extra protection when exposed to cold outdoor temperatures.

### Hygiene

Bathing and care of the infant's body is a primary concern for health care workers. The importance of healthy, intact skin is vital for adequate function of the skin as a defense against infection and in regulating fluids and electrolytes as well as body temperature. The skin of the newborn is particularly prone to breakdown, particularly in the diaper area, skin folds, and pressure points. The skin is prone to drying, particularly for infants who are born past the date of maturity. Each infant should be provided individual packages of clothing and crib linens, as well as individual equipment for bathing and routine skin care, such as bath basin, mild soap, and skin lotion if desired. Strict attention to hand-washing by all persons who handle each infant in a health care setting has been determined to be the most effective means of controlling the occurrence of *Staphylococcus aureus* and other microorganisms on the skin of infants.[3]

The infant's first bath after delivery is usually given within a few hours after birth. Policies of each health care setting vary regarding the time of the first bath, the extent to which vernix is removed, agents for cleansing the skin, and for cord care. These policies should be periodically reviewed and revised in accord with recent research findings. For example, the use of hexachlorophene is unjustified based on research

evidence of its toxicity and limited effectiveness in combating virulent strains of staphylococcus.[3]

The mother needs to have the opportunity to care for her infant during their stay in the health care setting so that her ability and ease may be observed and established. She may need assistance and teaching and reassurance, particularly if this is her first experience in handling an infant. Even for an experienced mother, the nurse needs to make sure that she understands the need for special care of the cord and thorough cleansing of the cord stump and for care of the circumcision if this procedure has been done for her male infant. She needs to be aware of signs of infection of these areas in particular and prepared to intervene if such signs occur. Her plans for diapering and laundering of diapers need to be discussed in order to assist her selection of methods that are optimal in prevention of skin reactions due to inadequate laundering or allergic reactions to laundry agents used.

### Sleep

That the infant's pattern of sleeping is innately different from that of adults is well recognized, but most families expect their newborn infant to sleep much more than in fact they do. The newborn spends about one third of every day in a state of wakefulness. The pattern of sleeping is characterized primarily by active, rapid-eye movement (REM) sleep, which occurs for brief intervals frequently throughout the day and night. Initially, there is little or no difference in the pattern of sleep during the day or night, but by the end of the first week of life, most infants begin to exhibit longer periods of sleep during the night.[35] The mother needs to be aware of her infant's states of sleeping and waking, for optimal interaction between the mother and the infant are dependent upon her ability to respond to the infant appropriately in accord with the state of consciousness. She will find it helpful for her own well-being to plan rest periods for herself during her infant's periods of sleep.

### Stimulation and play

Assessment of maternal behaviors that form the basis for attachment between the infant and mother provide a basis for teaching the mother approaches for stimulation of her infant. If the mother exhibits an active involvement in maternal attachment behaviors, she will likely stimulate the infant spontaneously. If she is not involved with the infant, she may be assisted in this process through teaching infant care and stimulation. Her reluctance may involve lack of experience or hesitancy to handle and become acquainted with the newborn. Her ability to recognize her infant's state of consciousness is important in her ability to provide appropriate interactions for the infant. Her mothering role during infancy involves providing appropriate stimulation when the infant is receptive to such stimulation and mediating for the infant during periods of excessive stimulation. Thus when the infant is distressed and crying, she responds by picking up the infant, which usually calms him or her and helps the infant to achieve and perhaps maintain an active alert state. If this does not work, she may feed the infant or change the diaper. This action serves an important function for the infant's learning ability, for perception of environmental stimuli is optimal during states of active alertness. The mother's spontaneity in maintaining interaction with the infant during active alertness, as opposed to leaving the infant alone, is important in providing needed stimulation for learning. All family members participate in this important function for the infant. Nursing teaching may be directed to their learning how to play simple games with the infant, to engage the young infant's attention, and to plan for appropriate play objects for the infant. Parents need to have realistic expectations for the infant's responses during the newborn period. For example, a mobile over the infant's crib provides important visual stimulation during the newborn period, but active kicking and movement to cause movement of the mobile will not occur until later in infancy.

## Promoting initial mother-infant interaction

Each of the nursing care measures described above serves to assist the mother in establishing interactions with her infant. The importance of providing a health care setting that facilitates rather than interferes with the spontaneous opportunities for interaction cannot be overemphasized. The mother must have the opportunity to spend uninterrupted time with her infant to learn the infant's temperament and changes in states of alertness and to experience the infant's responses to her presence, while at the same time receiving support and assistance from competent nurses.[33] In addition to facilitating spontaneous interaction between the mother and infant, the nurse must be alert to obstacles that interfere with the unfolding of this capacity and intervene to lessen these obstacles.

To establish a relationship with the infant, the mother needs to obtain information about the infant either by direct experience with the infant or from others in the health care setting. She must think through and develop her attitudes about herself in the new role of mother of this infant, and she needs to validate her impressions of the infant and herself by interacting with others in the environment. She must also develop new skills in mothering this infant. If she is a new mother, all skills of taking care of the infant and nurturing the infant are new and probably different from anything that she has previously experienced. If she has other children, many of the skills will be familiar, but the individuality of the new infant will present different challenges in forming a relationship as well as alter to some extent her relationships with others in the family.[5]

In discovering the real infant now in her presence, the mother is testing and altering her preconceived notions of what she expected this child to be. During the prenatal period the mother imagined what the child would be like, and this "dream child" will affect her perception of the infant. The infant's behavior in response to the mother also influences her perception of him or her and contributes to her concept of herself as a mother. If the infant responds in a manner that she perceives as positive, she develops an early positive concept of herself and the infant.[5]

One other component in identifying the infant as an individual is the process of ascertaining his or her completeness and wholeness. This takes much more "work" for the mother than the first examination of the baby's body. Indeed, some mothers are not able to really see and comprehend their newborn during the first

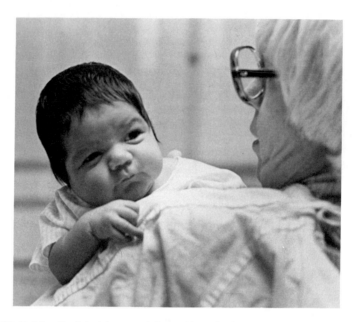

**Fig. 7-24.** Holding the infant in an upright position stimulates a state of active alertness.

few contacts. They may require several inspections and be extremely hesitant to look beyond the edge of the blankets, even though they have been assured of the infant's physical perfection. There is also a concern for the infant's ability to perform bodily functions adequately. The first wet diaper, the first cry, and the first time the baby opens his or her eyes are all important events in helping the mother to come to the realization that her infant is intact physically.

The nurse can facilitate positive interactions between the mother and infant by assisting the mother to recognize the infant's spontaneous states of active alertness and teaching her to interact with the infant in such a manner as to elicit positive responses. Further, the mother can be assisted in calming the infant when distressed in order to restore active alert states and enhance opportunities for positive interaction. False beliefs about spoiling the infant during the newborn period by picking him or her up should be discussed, and the mother reassured that for this developmental stage, prompt response to the infant's state of distress is necessary for learning and for emotional development. The mother needs to understand that prompt response to the infant's crying during this period of life when it is the only means of communicating needs gives the child a basis for trusting that mother will respond to needs expressed in a more mature fashion later.[5]

The mother often needs assistance in thinking through her role as a mother. She needs to perceive realistic expectations for herself but be confident in her ability. She needs to have a sense of support and resource people within and outside of the family to whom she can turn when she needs help without feeling as if she has somehow failed as a mother. For example, she needs to be aware that instances occur when she is not capable or willing to meet the demands of the infant. If she knows of others who can assume the responsibility for periods of time, giving her time to rest or pursue some positive activity to restore her psychologic equilibrium, she will be able to resume the care of her infant. The other members of the family may need to be involved in counseling in this regard and a foundation laid for future adult interactions that promote optimal care for the mother and infant.

### Promoting initial father-infant interaction

Just as important as the initial basis for attachment between mother and infant is the at-

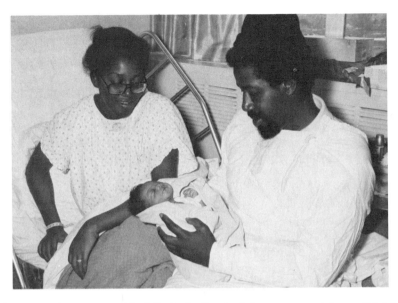

**Fig. 7-25.** Increased awareness of the father's significant role in pregnancy, delivery of his infant, and development of the early family relationships has led to encouraging his participation in the events of childbirth.

tachment between the father and the infant. Research evidence has begun to appear in the literature that substantiates the fact that early contact with the infant is important in releasing the father's innate potential for the development of his bond with the infant, a process that has been termed "engrossment."[15] Fathers who witness the delivery of the infant have consistently reported the witnessing of the birth as an experience of extreme elation, a peak experience, or a "high." Fathers who either have the opportunity to witness the birth or who see and hold the infant shortly after birth feel a strong sense of attraction to the infant and focus attention on the infant and characteristics of the infant. They are able to respond to the infant's normal reflex activity and behavior with great interest and feel increasingly a sense of belongingness toward the infant. As much as possible, the father needs to be involved in the nursing teaching and counseling that is provided in the health care setting. When the father is given the opportunity to develop engrossment with the infant, his involvement in all dimensions of infant care and responsibility is increased, and there develops a sense of sharing of the nurturing role that was traditionally relegated to the mother alone.[13,15] This trend is consistent with

the developing life-style of many families and needs to be promoted during this early family experience with the new infant (see Chapter 3).

Of particular importance for fathers are visual and tactile experiences with the infant. Fathers often recall in great detail physical characteristics of the newborn and describe their own infant as being beautiful and perfect. Experiences with the newborn consistently result in father's reporting a sense of increased self-esteem, self-importance, and worth.[13,15] Contrary to traditional beliefs, the intimate involvement of the father with the infant and mother in the health care setting does not increase rates of infection nor does it result in disturbance to other families in the setting. Including the father in formal and informal group teaching experiences and in the care of the infant in the health care setting is a valuable opportunity for the development of healthy family relationships.[13,15]

## Planning for health maintenance during infancy

Before the family leaves the health care setting after delivery, the nurse and family should review their plans for health maintenance during infancy. The first screening procedure conducted after the initial period of adaptation is screening the infant for phenylketonuria (PKU). This screening procedure is now required by law in most states. It should not be done before the fourth day of life and only after the infant has been on milk for at least 24 hours. If the infant leaves the health care setting before obtaining this screening test, provision needs to be made for obtaining the test at a community health care center.[16,17]

The parent's needs for family planning should be discussed. If the couple has not previously made a decision regarding provision for family planning after the birth of the infant or if they have not reevaluated their previous method in light of their changing needs as parents of a new infant, the couple will need continued health guidance with respect to this important dimension of family health. The couple may have questions regarding sexual intimacy during the coming weeks. The nurse needs to discuss their concerns openly and offer suggestions as to approaches that may be used for sexual intimacy until the new mother is comfortable with vaginal sexual intimacy, and her safety has been determined with complete healing of vaginal tissues.

## NURSING CARE OF THE NEWBORN

The first few days of life are significant for both mother and child. We have explored the dimensions of the infant's competency. The mother is also undergoing a time of great physical adjustment in returning to a nonpregnant state. Furthermore, psychologic tasks and events typically occur that have great importance for the family. These events are not important in the sense that they alone hold a great influence on the child's eventual personality development, but rather they often begin a pattern for future behavior and attitudes that becomes a part of the parent-child relationship.

In planning and implementing nursing care for the new family unit, the most important single principle that can universally apply is *relevance to the unique family.* The nature of the family, including cultural, religious, economic, personality, and emotional factors, needs to be considered. Each of the important variables will not be known to the health care team, but all families will give clues that will guide and direct nursing responses. Many clues during this period are subtle. Awareness and knowledge of common needs of families facilitate efficient identification of needs for a particular family. For example, new parents often feel uncertain of their own ability to handle and care for their infant. This message is seldom stated this way. They may feel uncertain but resolve the uncertainty and gain confidence as the infant responds to their first few attempts in a manner that is satisfying. A cue for nursing assistance may come as a rather indirect question, such as "Is he getting enough to eat?" While it is entirely appropriate to give parents information that answers their questions, this may not be enough to satisfy their desire to become more certain of their ability to care for the child. This may be a slow and arduous process. Successful completion can be made only by the mother and father individually. Each has strengths he or she brings to the relationship; each has weaknesses. The primary goal is to begin laying the foundation during the first few days after birth to facilitate movement through this task as the parents are ready to respond.

One way in which parents may be aided in these tasks is to conduct the nursing assessment with the mother and father present, encouraging them to participate and ask questions. It may be discouraging to watch an experienced nurse handle their baby with complete confidence and ability, but encouraging the parent to simply feel the baby's grasp or elicit a rooting response may help them to gain confidence in interacting with the baby. This can be an excellent opportunity for teaching. Many immediate questions may arise about physical features the mother has noticed. "Is his soft spot too big?" "Why is her skin so dry?" "Will the marks on his face go away?" The questions may seem simple and of little consequence to the nurse. They may not seem appropriate, or it may appear that the mother would know the answers. Regardless, the concerns of the parents are real to them at the moment. The content of the question as well as the answer may be of very little importance; the essential fact is that they are beginning to know this infant.

Anticipatory guidance is also important during the first few weeks of life. While some of the information conveyed to parents may be lost during the days to come, they can be introduced to health resources available when questions or problems arise. There may be a specific person to contact, or a book or pamphlet may be available. The parents need to know signs of common illness in infancy and how to respond when these signs appear. They should also be aware of resources available for well-child care, and definite plans should be made for the first well-child health visit. Problems of health maintenance during the first few weeks will vary with the experience and resources of the family. Some mothers need very detailed teaching with repeated demonstrations of infant care tasks such as bathing, feeding, and routine diaper changing. There may be a need to teach the family basic health maintenance, exploring in detail how they might improve the health environment of their home through better hygiene or nutrition. Fads and fancies in infant and health care may be the center of concern for parent-nurse dialogue.

Teaching and demonstration of each of the principles of care of the newborn that were discussed earlier in this chapter are important for the parents. Their understanding of the special physical requirements of the young infant will significantly enhance their ability to give adequate care to the infant during the first few weeks at home and will provide guidelines for their own judgments in regard to specific instances that require a decision. For example, they may be undecided about taking the infant to a social event during the early weeks following the infant's birth. If they understand the infant's needs for conservation of energy, provision of warmth, protection from infection and injury, provision of contentedness and comfort, and provision of nutrition, they will be able to make a sound judgment regarding taking the infant away from home. They will be able to determine whether they can reasonably assure that each of these needs will be met under these circumstances or any other, and they will make their own judgment.

When the family's resources appear to be limited in providing for the basic needs of the infant, the most crucial need must be ascertained, and this area of need becomes the area of teaching and concentration for this particular family at this particular time. For example, a mother may be observed to need help primarily with nutritional concerns, and the other areas of need are, for the time being, of secondary concern. She is able to respond to only one area of concern at this particular time. She seems to be able to give the infant reasonable comfort and warmth, and does not expend his or her energy reserves unreasonably. She is not able to protect the infant from injury or infection reasonably, and her provision of warmth and comfort is sporadic and unpredictable. If she can reasonably understand and provide for nutrition in a way that protects him or her from infection and provides adequate cuddling and personal contact, some progress is made in these areas as well as in the area of provision of nutrition, but the major concern of nutrition is the one that is emphasized for the mother's understanding.

Each family and infant is individual. Infants express definite preferences for positions of sleep, eating behavior, positions of comfort, and amount of physical contact and cuddling. Activity levels vary greatly, and there is considerable variation in the amount of sleep infants require.[1,2,38,40] Parents vary in their degree of flexibility and ability to accept infants of different types. Although probably no single trait of either parents or infant can be designated as an adverse sign for future development, a combination resulting in an unsatisfactory experience in relating during the early days may be the primary step in the development of a pathologic relationship. The challenge for the nurse is to (1) facilitate movement toward a mutually satisfying early experience, (2) evaluate the experience according to the physical and emotional behavior of the parents and child, and (3) provide for further assistance when difficulty arises and when such assistance is acceptable to the family.

**STUDY QUESTIONS**

1. Based on the primary principles of care of the newborn, give detailed recommendations for the mother's early care of her infant, including day-to-day concerns of cleansing the infant, feeding, including the infant in family activities, and shopping excursions. Give your rationale for each specific recommendation.
2. Explore the literature and other resources suggested in

the chapter for help with breast-feeding, and describe in detail specific recommendations and ways of helping a breast-feeding mother that you might employ. If you have the opportunity, try your plan with a mother who is beginning to breast-feed. Describe the areas of concern expressed by the mother in which you feel you were able to provide some help and those areas in which you needed more preparation.

3. Observe an infant under 1 month of age and describe in detail all relevant visual observations that you can make. Determine the areas in which you need to feel, auscultate, or handle the infant in order to obtain accurate and complete information regarding the well-being of the infant. If possible, complete the nursing assessment and describe in detail your findings.

4. Conduct a complete assessment of a newborn infant and validate your findings with those of an experienced nurse. Formulate a health status list based on your assessment, including health problems and health maintenance needs of the infant and family. Formulate the nursing plan and nursing orders related to each health status problem. Defend your nursing plan with evidence from literature that indicates the rationale for the plan.

5. Observe a parent-infant interaction, perhaps during a feeding. Describe as objectively as possible the behavior of the infant and of the parent. Does the behavior appear to be conducive to the development of a sound parent-infant relationship? Give specific examples of behavior that support the judgments you make.

## REFERENCES

1. Bird, I. S.: Breast-feeding classes on the post-partum unit, Am. J. Nurs. 75:456, March, 1975.
2. Bowlby, J.: Attachment and loss, vol. 1, Attachment, New York, 1969, Basic Books Publishing Co., Inc., pp. 235-298.
3. Bressler, R., Walson, P. D., and Fulginitte, V. A.: Hexachlorophene in the newborn nursery, Clin. Pediatr. 16:342, April, 1977.
4. Brown, R. E.: Breast-feeding in modern times, Am. J. Clin. Nutr. 26:556, May, 1973.
5. Clark, A. L., and Affonso, D. D.: Infant behavior and maternal attachment; two sides of the coin, Am. J. Matern. Child Nurs. 2:94, March/April, 1976.
6. Cole, J. P.: Breast-feeding in the Boston suburbs in relation to personal-social factors, Clin. Pediatr. 16:352, April, 1977.
7. Craig, M. E.: Normal neonatal behavior patterns; the first week of extrauterine life, Bull. Nurse-Midwives vol. 15, Nov., 1970.
8. Dubowitz, L. N. S., Dubowitz, V., and Goldberg, C. L.: Clinical assessment of gestational age in the newborn infant, J. Pediatr. 77:1, 1970.
9. Eoff, M. J. F., Meier, R. S., and Miller, C.: Temperature measurement in infants, Nurs. Res. 23:457, Nov.-Dec., 1974.
10. Farrar, C. A.: Assessing individuality in the newborn, J. Obstet. Gynecol. Neonatal Nurs. 3:15, May/June, 1974.
11. Foman, S. J.: Infant nutrition, ed. 2, Philadelphia, 1974, W. B. Saunders Co.
12. Germany, L. D., Mason, P. A., and Rosman, P.: Reliability of head circumference measurements in the newborn, Clin. Pediatr. 15:891, Oct., 1976.
13. Gollober, M.: A comment on the need for father-infant postpartal interaction, J. Obstet. Gynecol. Neonatal Nurs. 5:17, Sept.-Oct., 1976.
14. Goren, C. C., Sarty, M., and Wu, P. Y. K.: Visual following and pattern discrimination by newborn infant, Pediatrics 56:544, Oct., 1975.
15. Greenberg, M., and Morris, N.: Engrossment; the newborn's impact upon the father, Am. J. Orthopsychiatry 44:520, July, 1974.
16. Holtzman, N. A., Meek, A. G., and Mellits, E. D.: Neonatal screening for phenylketonuria. IV. Factors influencing the occurrence of false positives, Am. J. Public Health 64:775, Aug., 1974.
17. Holtzman, N. A., Mellits, E. D., and Kallman, C. H.: Neonatal screening for phenylketonuria. II. Age dependence of initial phenylalanine in infants with PKU, Pediatrics 53:353, March, 1974.
18. James, L. S.: Hexachlorophene, Pediatrics 49:492, April, 1972.
19. Johnson, C. F., and Opitz, E.: Unusual palm creases and unusual children, Clin. Pediatr. 12:101, Feb., 1973.
20. Kadkhoda, M., and others: Congenital dislocation of the hip—diagnostic screening and treatment, Clin. Pediatr. 15:239, March, 1976.
21. Klaus, M. H., and Kennell, J. H.: Maternal-infant bonding; the impact of early separation or loss on family development, St. Louis, 1976, The C. V. Mosby Co.
22. Korones, S. B.: High-risk newborn infants; the basis for intensive nursing care, ed. 2, St. Louis, 1976, The C. V. Mosby Co.
23. Long, M., Dunlop, J. R., and Holland, W. W.: Blood pressure recording in children, Arch. Dis. Childhood 46:636, Aug., 1971.
24. Ludington-Hoe, S. M.: Development of maternicity, Am. J. Nurs. 77:1170, July, 1977.
25. Montagu, A.: Touching; the human significance of the skin, New York, 1971, Columbia University Press, pp. 81-160.
26. Motil, K. J., Blackburn, M. G., and Pleasure, J. R.: The effects of four different radiant warmer temperature setpoints used for rewarming neonates, J. Pediatr. 85:546, Oct., 1974.
27. O'Brien, T. E.: Excretion of drugs in human milk, Am. J. Hosp. Pharm. 31:844, Sept., 1974.
28. Perlstein, P. H., Hersch, C., Glueck, C. J., and Sutherland, J. M.: Adaptation to cold in the first three days of life, Pediatrics 54:411, Oct., 1974.
29. Phillips, J. L., Jr.: The origins of intellect; Piaget's theory, San Francisco, 1969, W. H. Freeman and Co.
30. Popich, G. A., and Smith, D. W.: Fontanels; range of normal size, J. Pediatr. 80:749, May, 1972.
31. Pritchard, J. A., and MacDonald, P. C.: Williams' Obstetrics, ed. 15, New York, 1976, Appleton-Century-Crofts.

32. Rance, C. P., Arbus, G. S., Balfe, J. W., and Kooh, S. W.: Persistent systemic hypertension in infants and children, Pediatr. Clin. North Am. **21:**801, Nov., 1974.

33. Ratsoy, M. C.: Maternity patients make decisions, Can. Nurse **70:**42-44, April, 1974.

34. Roberts, F. B.: Perinatal nursing; care of newborns and their families, New York, 1977, McGraw-Hill Book Co.

35. Schaffer, R.: Mothering, Cambridge, Mass., 1977, Harvard University Press.

36. Sheppard, W. C., and Willoughby, R. H.: Child behavior; learning and development, Chicago, 1975, Rand McNally College Publishing Co.

37. Smith, D. W., and Gong, B. T.: Scalp hair patterning as a clue to early fetal brain development, J. Pediatr. **83:**374, Sept., 1973.

38. Spaulding, M. R.: Adapting postpartum teaching to mothers' low-income life-styles. In Bergersen, B. S., Anderson, E. H., Duffey, M., and others, editors: Current concepts in clinical nursing, vol. 2, St. Louis, 1969, The C. V. Mosby Co., pp. 280-291.

39. Stern, D.: The first relationship; mother and infant, Cambridge, Mass. 1977, Harvard University Press.

40. Tanner, L. M.: Assessing the needs of new mothers in a postpartum unit. In Duffey, M., Anderson, E. H., Bergerson, B. S., and others, editors: Current concepts in clinical nursing, vol. 3, St. Louis, 1971, The C. V. Mosby Co., pp. 204-209.

41. Van Leeuwen, G.: The nurse in prevention and intervention in the neonatal period, Nurs. Clin. North Am. **8:**509, Sept., 1973.

42. Yasunaga, S., and Rivera, R.: Cephalhematoma in the newborn, Clin. Pediatr. **13:**256, Mar., 1974.

# CHAPTER 8

# Newborns at risk

There is no time in childhood when health and well-being hold such meaning and impact as during the newborn period. Parents and family are usually anticipating and hoping for an infant who is normal and healthy. In all families and cultures the experience of giving birth to a child who is not well holds some special significance, often in relation to spiritual attitudes and beliefs. The mystery of a life begun with tragedy and disaster for a small, helpless, innocent child has been too great for humankind to cope with alone. When the infant survives, the impact of this experience follows the child and family throughout life.

The primary purpose of this chapter is to present sufficient information regarding the problems of the newborn to permit any nurse working with newborns, particularly in the first few days of life, to recognize signs of illness and make provisions for adequate care for the newborn. Early detection of neonatal problems, sound early intervention, and coordination between all health care facilities and specialized high risk care centers is imperative for improving the health and decreasing death rates among infants. For more detailed information related to these and other problems of the newborn, the reader is referred to the references at the end of the chapter.

## PROVISION OF SPECIALIZED CARE
### Society and the newborn at risk

Societies respond to the problems of illness during the newborn period in different ways according to the predominant beliefs of the culture and their level of scientific advancement. Where there are too many children, providing for another is too great a burden. The child who is not healthy may be left to die. Death during infancy may bring sorrow, but the overwhelming press of living is the greater sorrow. Where children are highly valued, either for their own existence or as a means of gaining security, status, or solidarity for the family, illness or death during infancy is a source of grave distress.

Health science advances have greatly enhanced the prognosis and survival of infants in the modern world. It is societal values, however, which generally dictate the extent to which the resources of science will be used to help the newborn infant who is at risk. The extent to which society is willing to invest in the life just begun, with no guarantee of the outcome, is an issue that health care professions continually face. The nature of many health and life-threatening problems in infancy requires intensive, elaborate medical and nursing care. The expense of a prolonged hospitalization is more than the young family alone can bear.

**Table 8-1.** Classification of newborns by gestational age groupings in neonatal mortality and morbidity*

| | Gestation (weeks) | Deliveries (%) | Mortality rate (%) | Neonatal deaths (%) | Special problems |
|---|---|---|---|---|---|
| Immature | 20 to 27 | 0.4 | 95+ | 26 | Generally incapable of extrauterine existence |
| Premature | 28 to 33 | .8 | 70 to 14 (mean 32) | 23 | Capillary hemorrhage; periodic breathing (apnea and cyanosis); hyperbilirubinemia; susceptibility to infection; respiratory distress syndrome |
| Preterm | 34 to 37 | 7.5 | 9.6 to 1.7 (mean 3.6) | 22 | Respiratory distress syndrome; hyperbilirubinemia; hypoglycemia |
| Term | 38 to 42 | 88.3 | 0.8 to 0.2 (mean 0.3) | 28 | Minimal problems unless complicated |
| Postterm | 43+ | 2.9 | >0.5 | 1 | Dysmaturity; intrauterine asphyxia; hypoglycemia, dystocia; meconium aspiration; polycythemia |

*Adapted from Babson, S. G., and Benson, R. C.: Management of high-risk pregnancy and intensive care of the neonate, ed. 2, St. Louis, 1971, The C. V. Mosby Co.

## Occurrence of neonatal mortality and morbidity

About 50,000 infants in the United States die each year before they reach 1 month of age. This figure, which represents about half of all deaths during childhood, is particularly disturbing since prevention or correction of many of the problems is possible, as noted in previous chapters. Another 40,000 infants born in the United States yearly suffer from severe congenital malformations, which may or may not be correctable. At least 90,000 infants born yearly will be mentally retarded (IQ score below 70). Retardation can often be traced to illness or injury during the neonatal period. Another 150,000 children born each year in the United States will have difficulty in school because of learning disabilities. It is estimated that the wastage of human potential from the death and disorders occurring in the neonatal period exceeds that from all other major health problems, including cardiovascular disease, cancer, and accidents.[3,87]

The single most pervasive problem continues to be prematurity. These infants are especially prone to illness, and this disadvantage, added to the delicate ability to sustain extrauterine life, contributes significantly to the mortality rate during the neonatal period. Table 8-1 summarizes the rate of death and illness that occurs in all gestational age groups, showing the particular risks of infants born before term.

## Special care facilities

The patterns of occurrence of death and illness in infancy have led to special efforts in recent years by health care professions to direct attention to efforts that extend fetal life and improve the quality of care given to any infant who is not healthy at birth. Throughout the United States and Canada, regional care facilities have been established that offer intensive services to ill pregnant women and newborn infants in the entire region. Increasingly, regional high risk perinatal centers have been established that provide a unified approach to the high risk pregnant mother and the fetus, with a primary goal to improve the health of both individuals and extend intrauterine life as long as possible. These facilities also offer educational services to the health professions of the area to improve care for pregnant women and newborn infants. The great expense involved in offering care and the elaborate medical and nursing resources that are needed have made regional planning and organization of regional services necessary in order for optimal care to be available for all mothers and infants who need it. In most areas the major resource intensive care unit provides the maximal level of care needed by the most severely affected mothers and infants, with transportation available to all areas of the region where infants are born. The medical and nursing personnel of the surrounding areas utilize the major resource unit's information and consultation services to improve the care of those mothers and infants who do not need to be transported to the intensive care unit. These centers are also actively involved in generating evidence regarding the effects of special care on infant death rate and on the future life and development of infants who survive. The initial evidence available suggests that recently developed measures that prevent neonatal death also prevent damage to the quality of life, and that most infants who survive will progress to adult life as useful citizens.[20,87,103]

The advanced knowledge and skill required of nurses who administer care to infants in intensive care settings exceed the scope of this discussion. Usually six months to a year of supervised experience in a regional intensive care facility is required to develop a desired level of nursing ability. However, a beginning level of knowledge of the approaches developed in these neonatal centers has had a great impact on the quality of care possible for all infants. The majority of infants who suffer illness or complications during the neonatal period do not require the full expert services available in the intensive care center, but they have profited by the improved methods of care that are possible in any infant care facility. In addition, understanding of the roles, functions, and methods of the neonatal or perinatal intensive care center enhances coordination of care between the center and other health care facilities in the region. Adequate judgment and early determination of the infant's level of need are dependent upon awareness of the full scope of care available to newborn infants.

An integral component of a regional network for care of the high risk mother and infant is a well planned and equipped transport system. It is estimated that 3% to 6% of infants born in the smaller community hospital need to be transferred to a larger regional center.[3] Most regional centers have developed criteria for transfer of infants and a communication network that can be used by all health care facilities in the area. In addition the center provides the transport equipment and highly specialized, experienced nurses and physicians to conduct the transfer of infants.[3] Many regional centers also have devel-

oped provisions for retransfer of convalescent infants to the community center, which provides for improved family contact with the infant and local supervision of teaching the family to care for the infant.[71]

## Developmental prognosis of high risk infants

Before 1960, studies in the United States and other countries documented a high prevalence of severe handicaps among low birth weight infants and infants who were ill during the neonatal period.[3,42,107,121] Since the development of mother and infant high risk care facilities, research evidence consistently documents the marked improvement in not only the survival rate of these infants but also in their developmental prognosis.* For example, in a five-year follow up study of 176 premature infants conducted by Teberg and others, 67% of the children were found to be developmentally and neurologically normal for their age, with no difference in outcome for those children weighing less than 1,000 and 1,500 g at birth.[121] Studies by Harrod[48] and Johnson[57] revealed few, if any, residual cardiopulmonary symptoms in infants who survived mechanical ventilation and severe respiratory distress during the newborn period. The improved outcome for survivors of early birth and illness has been consistently attributed to improved fetal monitoring during labor and delivery accompanied by improvement in Apgar scores at birth and to aggressive neonatal care, particularly monitoring of biophysical, biochemical, and metabolic factors.[3,42,107,121]

Another factor in the improvement of care has been increased attention and effort directed to continuing education of health care workers in the community hospital, as well as in the regional center, which results in rapid clinical application of recent research findings that define improvements in nursing and medical management.[42] The incidence of retrolental fibroplasia, for example, was formerly presumed to arise from the state of prematurity. With the discovery in 1951 of the destructive effects on the retina of high oxygen tension in the blood, it was recognized that the low gestational age in-

*References 4, 35, 42, 107, 117, 121.

fant is extremely vulnerable to the damaging results, but the cause is not prematurity. As progress has been made in understanding the dynamics of oxygen's effects, greater reliability in controlling and preventing the occurrence of this tragic effect has evolved.[67,82,53]

Another prognostic concern for infants who receive intensive care as newborns is related to the quality of parenting that develops after the period of hospitalization. The low birth weight infant is three times more likely to experience physical and emotional abuse and neglect than the average infant.[3,65] Approaches to the prevention of this major problem are increasing in all intensive care centers and are described in detail later in this chapter.

### Legal and ethical issues

The multitude of activities and decisions involved in the care of the high risk newborn raises serious and agonizing ethical and legal problems for all health care workers and for the parents of the infant. The range of legal and ethical concerns is great and includes such issues as the right to life, the definition of the quality of life, sources of responsibility and duty, distribution of limited resources for care, population control, and genetic control. Each nurse involved in the care of a newborn infant who is not well will encounter the difficult choices that confront the health care team in caring for the infant and family. The basic principles outlined in Chapter 2 are pertinent to the development of legal and ethical responsibility in newborn care.

When confronted by such difficult legal and ethical problems as exist in newborn care, it is the responsibility of the health care team to formulate their own guidelines for sound action. The guidelines should include a definition of negligence, criteria for withholding, maintaining or discontinuing resuscitation, approaches to be used in gaining consent of parents or other legally responsible individual, criteria for making decisions in the face of limited resources, and accepted standards of quality for care.[58,68] A set of ethical propositions that may be used as a basis for such guidelines was formulated in 1974 by a group of specialists in neonatal care.[58] These propositions recognize the parents as responsible for the well-being of their infant, a principle that is widely accepted in society today. The nurse who maintains a very special relationship to the infant and the family is intimately involved in assisting the parents in fulfilling their responsibilities for making very difficult decisions and understanding the alternatives available to them.[47,58,68]

## HEALTH MAINTENANCE FOR THE INFANT AND FAMILY

Care of the newborn infant who is ill requires careful attention to maintenance and promotion of optimal health, including provision of environmental conditions that promote attainment of health. Special provisions and approaches are needed to accomplish these health care goals. These provisions are discussed in the following section and are needed by all infants experiencing stress in the newborn period. Specific techniques are not discussed here in detail; constant improvements are made in equipment and techniques requiring highly specialized skill and experience. The purpose of this discussion is to present the primary problems encountered by the high risk newborn and the principles that govern their management.

### Environmental control

Control of the incidence and spread of infection in newborn nurseries is a major concern, particularly in the intensive care nursery where adequate care requires the involvement of a multitude of health care personnel and elaborate equipment. Details of infection surveillance techniques, essential hygienic techniques to be used by all persons entering a nursery, and management of nursery epidemics of infection are fully presented in *Standards and Recommendations for Hospital Care of Newborn Infants* published by the American Academy of Pediatrics (1976). This publication should be readily available for all nursery personnel, and periodic evaluation of the practices of each newborn care facility should be conducted. The most important principle involved in control of infection has been well documented to be adequate handwashing. An iodinated detergent is recommended for an initial three-minute scrub for all persons entering the nursery, including parents and visitors. Before each contact with any infant, a 15-second handwashing is recommended. Other approaches for the prevention of propagation of infection by personnel have been used and may be used in a particular nursery; however recent trends have been to simplify techniques used and maintain strict surveillance of the techniques that are used, as well as monitor the rate of appearance of microorganisms in the nursery area.[67]

Meticulous aseptic technique is essential in the use of material and equipment where an invasive procedure is used. When a catheter, needle, or tube is used for a diagnostic or therapeutic purpose, the equipment must be adequately sterilized and the technique followed must include rigid rules of asepsis. All equipment used in caring for the infant must be frequently cultured to determine the presence of microorganisms. Of particular concern is any equipment with which water or moisture is in frequent contact, because of the tendency for these areas to harbor gram-negative organisms known as "water bugs." All such equipment should be regularly sterilized, usually on a daily basis.[67]

Environmental control of temperature and humidity is an important nursing consideration for any newborn infant but particularly for the infant who is experiencing problems. Thermoregulation is a problem of maintaining a balance between the losses that occur and the heat production that is generated by the body.

The premature infant has limited resources for producing body heat, particularly in the face of stress. In fact, he or she may be able to generate body heat only when not exposed to heat losses. Therefore, the use of incubators and radiant heat cribs has developed as an important aspect of care of the infant with problems. Incubators provide the advantage of maximal observation of the infant while allowing for a certain degree of control of the temperature, humidity, and oxygen concentration of the environment.[77] Radiant heat cribs provide a special advantage in accessibility to the infant, and control of other aspects of the environment is provided with other specialized equipment. Most incubators and heat cribs used in care of the high risk newborn are equipped with a Servo-control

mechanism. A probe is attached to the infants skin about 2 cm above the umbilicus at the midline, which serves to regulate the amount of heat produced by the crib. Optimal skin temperature has been estimated to be approximately 36.7 degrees C. The recommendations of the manufacturer should be carefully observed and the equipment monitored frequently for accuracy of performance.[134]

The equipment that is employed in the care of infants cannot provide adequate control unless the mechanisms of heat production and loss are understood thoroughly by the nurse. The premature infant is particularly subject to losses because of a large exposed surface area, which is further increased by a relaxed, extended posture and by the lack of insulating body fat. The infant does possess a layer of brown adipose tissue peculiar to the newborn, which participates in the production of body heat. This fat is located around the scapulas, neck, and thoracic inlet, sternum, kidneys, and adrenals. It generates heat, which warms the blood flowing through it, thus contributing to the production of body heat. The newborn is not able to shiver in the face of cold stress, a response that is extremely important in the thermoregulating mechanisms of older children and adults. The major source of heat production is the increase of metabolic rate, a defense that can be maintained only very briefly in the face of cold stress.[67,83,118]

The mechanisms of heat loss become extremely important when a large number of mechanical devices are used in the care of the infant. When oxygen is forced into an incubator or hood, heat loss by convection is a danger because of the velocity of flow of air and the lowered temperature of the gas being administered. To combat this effect, oxygen is warmed and the flow is directed away from the infant's body if possible.

Humidity in the oxygen is desirable to combat the drying effect of oxygen, and the moisture contributes to control of heat loss by evaporation. A minimum of body surface moisture can vaporize into surrounding air in which the moisture content is high. When the infant's body is covered with amniotic fluid or bath water, losses from evaporation are greatly exaggerated and represent a real threat to the premature infant.[83,118] The ambient air of the nursery should be maintained at between 40% and 60% relative humidity. The relative humidity of incubators, which can be more precisely controlled, should be maintained at around 50%.[134]

Radiation of body heat to cooler solid objects in the environment most commonly occurs in relation to incubator walls that are at a temperature that is excessively low. The internal air temperature of the incubator may be at an acceptable level, but an adjacent cold wall will still provide a source of radiant heat loss. Wall temperature is most effectively controlled by the environment of the room outside of the incubator; exposure of the incubator to a cold draft from a doorway or window will cool the solid parts and render the infant prone to heat loss.[83,118]

Conduction of body heat to solid objects in direct contact with the infant's body is a serious hazard whenever the infant is laid on a new surface. The mother's bed, a table top, a counter surface, or a crib surface that has not been previously occupied will all be about the temperature of the room air and thus provide a significant heat gradient against which the infant may lose heat.[83]

Other environmental factors that may affect the infant at risk have been inadequately investigated. The level of noise in the environment, the intensity and duration of light, and the kinesthetic motion to which the infant is exposed are beginning to be investigated by nurse scientists.[62] There is evidence for older people that the physiologic rhythms of the body may depend upon regular exposure to periods of lightness and darkness. Whether or not the newborn infant is affected by constant exposure to bright light or constant noise as exists in intensive care nurseries remains to be investigated.[8]

## Feeding and nutrition

Recent improvements in the developmental prognosis of premature and ill infants can be attributed to a large extent to substantial improvements in providing adequate nutrition for these infants. Low birth weight infants are born at a time when brain development is progressing at a rapid rate. A significant brain growth spurt

begins in the human fetus during the third trimester of gestation and lasts through the first year and a half following the fortieth week of gestation. There is increase in the size of neurons and glial cells as well as development of myelination. Enzymatic activities of the brain are also increasing and developing. During fetal life the infant is provided all essential proteins by transport through the placenta from maternal circulation. After birth, these nutrients must be supplied to the infant, but the premature infant's immature ability to synthesize these nutrients creates a significant nutritional barrier. Research is underway to discover the nature of metabolic deficiencies of preterm infants and effective means of providing nutritional requirements to meet the growth needs of the infant in light of metabolic immaturity.[24,41,97]

There are two methods currently available by which the ill infant can receive nutrition. He or she may be given formula through a nipple or a tube leading to the stomach or may be given intravenous solutions, which supply either par-

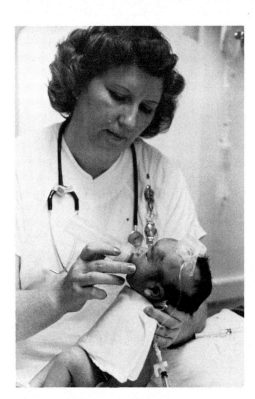

**Fig. 8-1.** The infant who is just beginning to suck is held and encouraged in developing this ability.

tial or complete nutritional requirements. Decisions regarding either approach must be shared by medical and nursing personnel who are caring for the infant.* Nursing personnel may be involved in the preparation of parenteral solutions, the ongoing supervision and administration of the fluids, and monitoring of the infant's response to the feeding. Since total nutrition may be maintained via this route for prolonged periods of time in high risk infants, nurses must become intimately familiar with the procedures involved and the risks for the infant. Both long-term and short-term intravenous feeding requires thorough understanding of fluid and electrolyte components of the solution being administered and the possible effects on the infant. The extremely delicate balance in the rate of flow required for the newborn necessitates the use of mechanical devices that automatically regulate the rate of flow. The device must be continually checked for accuracy, but adequate, safe manual regulation of intravenous fluid for a newborn infant is virtually impossible.[111]

Formula feeding of infants requires consideration of several major nutritional problems that exist for the newborn, particularly for premature infants. There is currently no known substitute for the intrauterine form of nutrition that the premature infant receives under normal circumstances. An ill term infant often is not in the same position physiologically as the well infant to metabolize and receive feedings. Differences in the effects of feedings on premature or ill infants are known to exist, but they are only partially understood. The enzyme systems of the premature infant are probably important clues to understanding his absorption, utilization, and excretion processes. These infants develop abdominal distention and regurgitate or vomit when oral feedings are given too rapidly, but the exact reason for these occurrences is not understood and has not been adequately investigated.[97]

There is confusion concerning the composition of feedings for the premature infant because of disagreement concerning the clinical effects of the various basic nutrients in different proportions. The basic nutrients needed by all

**Table 8-2.** Range in daily feeding requirements of low birth weight infants per kilogram of body weight*

| Nutrient requirements | First week of life | Active growth period |
|---|---|---|
| Water (ml) | 80-200 | 130-200 |
| Calories | 50-100 | 110-150† |
| Protein (g) | 1-2 | 3-4 |
| Glucose (g) | 7-12 | 12-15 |
| Fat (g) | 3-4 | 5-8 |
| Sodium (mEq) | 1-2 | 2-3 |
| Potassium (mEq) | 1-2 | 2-4 |
| Chloride (mEq) | 1-2 | 2-3 |
| Calcium (mEq) | 1-2 | 3-5 |
| Phosphorus (mEq) | 1-2 | 2-4 |
| Magnesium (mEq) | — | 0.5-1.0 |
| Iron (mg) | | 1.5-2.0 |

*From Babson, S. G., Benson, R. C., Pernoll, M. L., and Benda, G. I.: Management of high-risk pregnancy and intensive care of the neonate, ed. 3, St. Louis, 1975, The C. V. Mosby Co., p. 109.
†Calorie requirements of over 120/kg apply to infants with perinatal undergrowth.

humans are known to be essential for the premature infant, but there is wide difference of opinion as to the appropriate proportions of each component.[3,41]

Table 8-2 summarizes recommended daily feeding requirements of low birth weight infants.

Water must never be overlooked as an essential nutrient for the newborn. One of the high risk infant's most immediate and continuing risks is that of water depletion, and replacement of the normal large physiologic insensible loss of water is essential. The usual recommended intake for infants is 110 to 150 ml/kg/24 hours, but the low birth weight infant needs a finer evaluation and estimation as the days and hours progress. Babson[2] recommends progressing to 100 to 120 ml/kg/24 hours by the first week of age for the stable premature, then to 130 to 150 ml/kg/24 hours by the second week of age. The infant's responses to feedings individually determine the progression rate that can be attained.

The ability of the immature infant to metabolize and synthesize human or cow's milk protein is not fully known.[97] Further, controversy remains regarding the relative values of human protein versus cow protein, even when the cow's milk protein is denatured and adjusted to

*References 12, 17, 51, 70, 110, 130.

a more humanlike concentration. There is a preference in the United States for a highly concentrated protein formula for the undergrown or premature infant in order to obtain intrauterine growth rate levels quickly.[2,3,25,64,125] Such a formula would deliver 3 to 4 g of protein per kilogram every 24 hours. The potentially dangerous renal solute load of highly concentrated formulas (exceeding 30 Kcal/ounce) must be considered. The exact ability of high risk infants to handle solutes is still debated, and some evidence exists that central nervous system damage can occur as a result of a high solute load.[25]

Animal fat is less effectively absorbed by the low birth weight infant than by the term infant. Formula manufacturers have resolved this problem either by skimming cow's milk partially or by replacing it with vegetable oils. Either type of formula promotes growth if the essential requirement of calories (from 120 to 130 Kcal/kg/day) is met through some source.[25]

Carbohydrate utilization has been very reliably demonstrated in the small infant. This dietary element is identified as the single most important nutrient during the early hours of life for all infants but particularly for the low birth weight infant who is unusually susceptible to hypoglycemia and hyperbilirubinemia.[25,32,67,96]

The issue of allowances for vitamins and minerals is generally less well defined than for the basic dietary components. Most prepared formulas are enriched with the various vitamins, minerals, and trace elements at a level considered acceptable or necessary for the term infant. The low birth weight infant does not consume, until later, sufficient amounts of formula to provide the supposed needs defined either in terms of the standards for older infants or in terms of symptomatic responses to inadequate intake of a specific element. Therefore, it is recommended that supplementation of vitamins, minerals, and particularly iron begin within the first week of life. The amount of supplementation is balanced with the intake from other sources as these increase.[24,25,36]

The choice of whether to feed the formula by nipple or tube depends upon the infant's ability to suck with enough vigor to consume an adequate amount. When this ability is just beginning to develop it is important to allow the infant to nipple feed for at least one or two feedings a day, or the infant may lose the desire or ability to suck if this practice is delayed. The practice of gavage feeding is an extremely important aspect of care of the premature infant, since nutrition may be supplied before sucking is present without the use of intravenous techniques. The procedure exerts a physiologic effect, however, and must be understood for sound, safe administration. Passage of the tube causes vagal stimulation, which in turn can cause bradycardia. The newborn infant is an obligatory nose breather, and thus intubation through the nose is not recommended because it obstructs adequate exchange of gases. The rate of flow of formula should be similar to that expected if the infant were nipple feeding, usually about 1 ml/min, until the amount of formula exceeds 20 ml, at which point the time should be limited to 20 to 25 minutes.[19]

Measurement and plotting of body weight loss and gain is important in estimating the adequacy of nutritional intake for the premature infant. The pattern of initial weight loss for low birth weight infants is different from that of the term infant, in that there is a greater percentage of birth weight loss due to the greater percentage of body fluid in the immature infant. The lower the initial birth weight, the greater the percentage of loss and the longer the period of time for the infant to begin to regain body weight. The premature weight chart in the Appendix reflects the expected weight curves for infants at various birth weights and should be used to plot sequential measurements of body weight.[56]

## Monitoring of vital signs and support of gas exchange

One of the most important advances in the care of the premature or ill infant is the development of electronic monitoring of the infant's heart and respiratory rates. The monitors present electrical hazards in the nursery and must be continually evaluated for safety. Their reliable function can never be totally taken for granted; however, the extremely delicate balance with which an infant at risk maintains heart and respiratory function makes the continuing monitoring of these parameters important in adequate nursing care.

The repeated and frequent occurrence of apneic episodes in premature infants is more adequately managed by monitoring devices, since attention is immediately drawn to the infant when the alarm sounds alerting the onset of apnea and the resulting anoxia. The infant is stimulated to breath again, and the period of anoxia is prevented or shortened. This in turn prevents further depression and acidosis.

Heart and respiration rates are monitored using equipment that measures impedance across the chest by means of electrodes placed over the anterior chest. The manufacturer's recommendations for placement of the electrodes is important for accurate function of the monitor. The monitor provides an alarm that is sounded when the heart or respiratory rate falls below a minimum level determined by the operator. The recommended lower limit for the heart rate is 80 beats per minute; for the respiratory rate the monitor is set at either 20 breaths per minute or by duration of apnea, usually 10 to 15 seconds.[3,114]

When the infant experiences apneic episodes, the nurse observes the infant's condition and provides gentle stimulation if apnea is in an early stage. Suction of the nasopharynx is often indicated, as well as resuscitation with a bag and mask using an air-oxygen mixture.[3]

When support of gas exchange requires the use of oxygen, either intermittently or continuously, the infant's blood gases should be monitored regularly. This may be accomplished by periodic blood sampling from a heel prick or venipuncture or the use of an indwelling umbilical vessel catheter. The indwelling catheter poses several risks to the infant, such as infection, perforation and hemorrhage, thrombosis, and cardiac arrythmias. However, the benefits of arterial blood samples for monitoring outweigh the risks involved, particularly when catheterization techniques are used with vigilant precaution.[27]

Monitoring oxygen concentrations and oxygen consumption is important as a means of regulating the amount of oxygen intake. Weekly assessment of retinal changes by an experienced opthalmologist is essential to protect the infant against development of retrolental fibroplasia if oxygen is used over a period of time at any level of concentration.[3,73,82]

Temperature monitoring can be associated

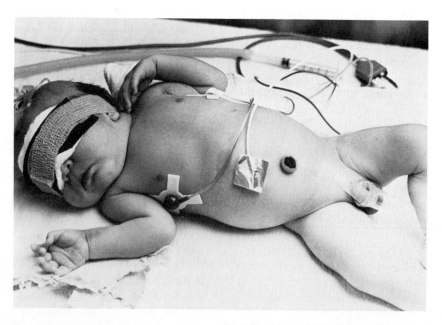

**Fig. 8-2.** Needle electrode leads to the monitoring equipment provide safe monitoring with a minimum of damage to the infant's skin. The infant's heart rate and respiratory rate are being monitored.

with the control mechanism of the incubator or heated crib, and the infant's own demands for increases in ambient temperature regulate the temperature of the surrounding air, much as a thermostat in a room.[7,54] Regular manual monitoring of temperature remains essential to assure adequate function of servo-control mechanisms.

Blood pressure determinations in premature infants have been more easily and accurately obtainable since the development of Doppler ultrasound blood pressure measurement equipment. As measurements of systolic and diastolic values are more adequately studied, the use of this vital sign in premature infants will increase in aiding clinical management. The flush method of obtaining a blood pressure estimate described in Chapter 7 is recommended as a reliable estimate when a more exact monitoring technique is not available or not deemed necessary.[128]

## Stimulation and support of optimal development

The infant who is born prematurely and placed in a special care nursery experiences sensory stimulation that is very different from either the fetus of the same gestational age or the mature infant born at term. The effects of the type of sensory stimuli that occur in most intensive care nurseries is not known, but these stimuli can be recognized as extremely different from those that are known to promote healthy learning and social and inner competency. Further, the relative absence of day-night cycles and constant exposure to light and noise are not conducive to the establishment of diurnal biologic rhythms.

Some research attention has been focused on the provision of planned stimulation programs for critically ill newborns.[8,14,105] Initial results indicate that such infants benefit physically and psychologically from such a program. The parents are usually involved in the stimulation program, which provides an important source of contact and involvement with the infant and is a means of developing continuity between hospital and home care. The stimulation programs that have been developed approximate the experiences of good home care for any infant, including visual, tactile, and kinesthetic stimulation. In addition, provisions are made for cyclic periods of relative quiet and darkness, especially during night hours. The stimulation

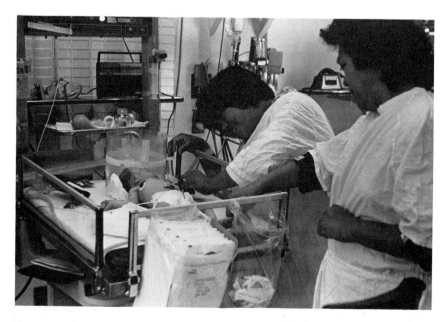

**Fig. 8-3.** This newborn's mother and grandmother are participating in a stimulation program for the infant; their contact with the infant also promotes the development of attachment with the infant.

programs used include stroking the infant, holding his or her hands, talking to the infant in a high-pitched voice, holding and rocking the infant, presenting various visual stimuli known to induce infant response, eliciting a following and gazing response to a human face (preferably that of the parents), providing color stimuli in the form of mobiles, colored blankets, and clothing, and providing music. The infant is assessed for physiologic stability and strength, as well as developmental level using the Brazelton Neonatal Assessment Scale.[13] The family is interviewed to involve them in planning for a stimulation program that will suit their family style, promote their learning about their infant, and encourage their interaction. The nurse plans and revises the stimulation program in accord with the needs and responses of the infant and the family.[14,105]

### Support of family interactions

The birth of a preterm or ill infant initiates an agonizing crisis of fear, guilt, disappointment, and grief for the family. The reaction of each family is individual and is influenced by the multitude of factors that exist in their psychologic field, including their style of living, family interactions, whether or not they planned and wanted this child, their religious beliefs, and their hopes and fantasies for the unborn child. The practices and routines of modern hospitals caring for preterm and ill infants has contributed to, rather than alleviated, the distress that is experienced by the family.[65] When such an infant is born, attention is focused on the survival needs of the infant and the infant is separated from the mother with little or no explanation given the mother or the family. Further, hospital rules and regulations inhibit family interaction with the infant rather than promote them. It is often assumed that the family might as well begin to face the possibility of the death of their infant and that they will be glad and able to assume grateful parenting responsibilities if their infant lives. Substantial research evidence has emerged that renders these practices and assumptions unjustified and is based largely on the recognition of the increased chance that such infants will experience child abuse and neglect.[3,65] It was only in the mid-1960s that the

practice of strict isolation of the infant from the mother began to be investigated, primarily from the point of view of the impact of her presence on the infection rate in nurseries. The data of these studies indicated that mothers' presence in nurseries did not increase the risk of infection.[65] Separation of the mother from the infant during the critical first few days of life has recently been studied extensively, with consistent results indicating the negative effect of this separation on the psychologic development of the child, the development of mothering capacity, and on the development of healthy parent-child interactions. When the infant is visibly deformed or life is seriously threatened, separation compounds, rather than eases, the trauma experienced by the family.[5,15,30,65] Where newborn care settings have begun planned programs to facilitate family interactions during this critical period, the results consistently document their effectiveness in alleviating the initial stress of the family, improving the quality of development of the child, and improving

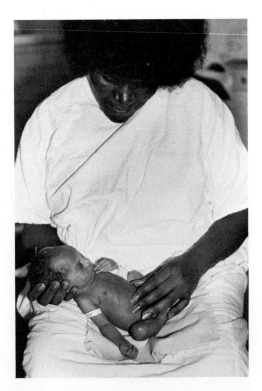

**Fig. 8-4.** The mother's first contact with her preterm infant often involves a guarded exploration of the infant's body.

the long-range quality of family interactions.[5,14,63,65,67]

In working with parents, there are at least seven goals that must be accomplished to promote healthy adjustment to the birth of a high-risk infant. These include:

1. Helping the mother and father adapt their previous conceptualized image of the ideal normal infant to the infant who has been born
2. Assisting the parents in resolving the guilt felt in producing a high-risk infant
3. Facilitating the parents' building of a close affectional tie with the infant by providing for mutual interaction from the earliest possible moment
4. Encouraging and teaching the parents to care for the infant while the child is hospitalized in order to develop confidence and competence in their ability to care for the child at home
5. Facilitating the family's mutual resolution of the crisis they are experiencing
6. Recognizing and helping the parents with individual needs, particularly those stresses they might be experiencing that detract from their ability to cope with the birth of this infant. Common problems include preexisting conflict in the family, the fact that the infant was unplanned and unwanted, financial stress compounded by the expense of this infant, interruption of other family goals, and low self-esteem on the part of the parents.
7. Providing for continuity of care when the infant leaves the hospital[65]

### Initial encounter for the family

Regardless of the condition of the infant, the mother needs to see her infant at the time of birth and be given simple, direct information regarding her infant's condition. Studies have repeatedly confirmed the negative effects of withholding information from the mother and of delaying her seeing the infant. Knowing the reality of her infant's condition alleviates fears and fantasies of the unknown and provides the mother with real information that she can begin to incorporate from the beginning.[15,28,30] If the infant's condition permits, the mother should be

encouraged to touch the infant. Other family members also need early experience in seeing and touching the infant, along with simple and direct information as to the infant's condition. When the mother is not capable of having this early experience, provision should be made for such contact as soon as possible.

At the time of the initial encounter, the mother needs to know what to anticipate in the first few hours, where the infant will be, what uncertainties exist, when to expect to have more information, when to expect to see the infant again and where, and who will be involved in the care of the infant. As soon as possible, the family needs to be brought together or a supportive friend needs to join the mother and this small group should be assisted in establishing mutual support for one another. Their questions need to be answered, and common concerns experienced by parents under these circumstances should be acknowledged in a brief and direct fashion.

### Facilitating parent-infant interaction

From the beginning, the parents should be viewed as the infant's primary care-givers and assured of their important role in caring for the infant. They should always have access to information regarding the infant and opportunities to contact the infant. The means of achieving this access needs to be explained to them. Concurrently, their own needs with regard to acceptance of the infant, dealing with their emotional crisis, and resolving the many problems that arise need to be met outside of the nursery setting. Group sessions with other parents of infants in the nursery are helpful and provide a network of mutual support among the parents.[65] Individual counseling and guidance sessions may be needed in meeting the family's particular needs.

From the early days of life and during periods when the infant is critically ill, the role of the parents as care-givers may be limited to psychosocial interaction with the infant. During these periods they can be involved in planning for the infant stimulation program and begin to acquire a few technical abilities that they can use in caring for the infant. As their readiness develops, they can assume responsibilities for daily care activities such as bathing and clothing, skin care, and feeding. Parents often develop skill in many technical procedures involved in the care of their infant, particularly when such procedures may be needed after the infant is discharged. They learn how to respond to periods of apnea, percussion of the chest, suction of the nasopharynx, and special feeding techniques. Initially, the parents are likely to experience great emotional conflicts in approaching the infant as care-giver. They are likely to feel afraid, incompetent, or angry, while at the same time wanting to approach the infant and provide care. When the nurse senses hesitancy, a direct acknowledgment of the parent's feelings serves to open communication between the nurse and parent and reassures them that such feelings are not abnormal or bad. Encouraging the family to go ahead and interact directly in the care of the child removes some of the fear and feelings of incompetence and begins to build a bridge of interaction that helps sustain the parent through the difficult transition. They may find it easier to avoid becoming closer to the infant, even though they want very much to do so. They cannot be encouraged to take an approach for which they are not ready, but they often need encouragement to take a difficult step for which they are prepared. Carefully planned nursing intervention is based upon the nurse's astute assessment of the mother and other significant family members, knowledge of the developing parent-infant relationship, and knowledge of the effects of illness or prematurity upon the development of the relationship.[5,15,30,65,82]

## SPECIAL NEONATAL PROBLEMS
### Birth weight and gestational age problems

The importance of accurately classifying infants according to both parameters of gestational age and weight cannot be overemphasized. Previous sections have included discussions of the impaired ability of premature infants to adjust to extrauterine life. While birth weight in most instances is consistent with that expected for gestational age, there are infants who are either small or large for gestational age. A graph for classification of newborns by birth weight and gestational age appears in the Appendix; it gives the mortality risk for infants classified on both factors simultaneously.

### Causes

One prevalent cause of low birth weight is multiple pregnancy. For reasons that are unknown, racial groups other than Caucasians produce more twins and triplets than do Caucasians. The occurrence of twin pregnancies is about 1 in 90 pregnancies, triplets occur in 1 in $90^2$ instances, quadruplets 1 in $90^3$ instances, and so forth. Identical twinning, resulting from the abnormal division of a single fertilized ovum, is usually an inherited trait and accounts for about one third of all instances of twinning. Most often there is a single chorionic membrane and single placenta, but occasionally there are two separate or fused placentas and separate chorionic membranes. Identical twins are particularly prone to abnormal development resulting from crowding, circulatory and nutritional competition, and cord entanglement and compression. Fraternal, or dizygotic, twinning is a chance occurrence resulting from the fertilization of two ova. There are always two chorions and two placentas, although the two placentas may have fused during growth and development.[3]

Abnormalities of placental structure or function are related to many instances of prematurity and low birth weight. Implantation of the placenta near or covering the internal os of the cervix (placenta praevia) results in poor placental functioning, delivery of the placenta before delivery of the infant, and some loss of maternal or infant blood. Premature separation of the placenta occurs in varying degrees and can lead to premature delivery. In some cases bed rest and restriction of activity can prolong the gestational period, but thorough medical evaluation and supervision are necessary to make a decision that leads to safe care for both the mother and the fetus.

Incompetency of the cervix, which occurs with about 2% of all premature or immature deliveries, is a disorder of the cervix resulting from injury or congenital weakness. The cervix is unable to contain the fetus. The weaker the cervical structure, the earlier will be the premature delivery. Cervical cerclage has been performed surgically to prolong the gestational period with some success.[3]

Maternal metabolic disorders invariably interact with pregnancy, and premature delivery is often inevitable. The mother who has hyperthyroidism or hypothyroidism requires close medical supervision throughout pregnancy; with adequate medical control, the outlook for the newborn is favorable. Maternal diabetes mellitus complicates at least one out of every 325 pregnancies, and many women tend to exhibit signs and symptoms of diabetes during pregnancy only. The incidence of congenital anomalies in infants of diabetic parents is about five times that of nondiabetic parents. Prematurity is masked by the infant's large size for gestational age. The risk is actually increased, because superficially the infant appears at birth to be healthy and large. On closer examination, the infant is recognized to be only as mature as gestational age would indicate and exhibits all of the external and neurologic characteristics appropriate for that age. Such an infant is prone to develop hyaline membrane disease, hypoglycemia, acidosis, hypocalcemia, and hyperbilirubinemia. Degenerative changes in the placenta are common.[3]

Maternal toxemia, or preeclampsia-eclampsia, is a complex of symptoms that occurs in pregnant women only after the twenty-fourth week of pregnancy. The symptoms include hypertension, generalized edema, and proteinuria. The eclamptic stage of the disorder is characterized by convulsions, and the outlook for the fetus is grave. Close medical management of preeclampsia can prolong gestation with minimal risk to the mother and the infant, but judicious early termination of pregnancy may be indicated.

Urinary tract infections during pregnancy contribute significantly to premature delivery, fetal death, and maternal morbidity. If a woman has a history of bladder or kidney infections, she is more likely to develop a urinary tract infection during pregnancy. About 15% of all pregnant women experience symptomatic urinary tract infections, and another 5% to 10% develop asymptomatic bacteriuria.[3] If the infection is treated effectively during pregnancy, the outlook is good for the fetus. However, if the infection persists, the likelihood of fetal death or premature delivery is increased threefold.[3]

Despite the availability of human Rh immunoglobulin (RhoGAM) for the prevention of maternal isoimmunization to the fetal blood group antigen, instances of Rh factor incompatibility still occur, with the resulting hemolytic disease of the fetus and the necessity to terminate pregnancy early in order to save the life of the infant.[3]

Premature rupture of the membranes occurs in about 15% of all pregnancies. The degree of prematurity may not be severe, and labor and delivery occurring within a few hours or days present few problems to the infant who is near full gestational age. When the infant is younger, the time between the rupture of the membranes and spontaneous labor and delivery tends to be prolonged, and the infant suffers the disadvantages of immaturity and exposure to infections before delivery.[3]

### Factors that predispose to illness

Review of the embryologic stages of development in Chapter 4 and the gestational age assessment in Chapter 7 will provide a general understanding of the disadvantages suffered by the infant who is born before term. Essentially, the preterm infant enters extrauterine existence inadequately prepared to sustain life, growth, and development independently. The skin and mucous tissues are thin and delicate, rendering the infant particularly susceptible to injury, invasion by infectious organisms, and insensible water loss. The small anatomic size of structures places body parts in proximity to one another, promoting rapid communication of infection from one area of the body to another. The infant's fragile capillary structures easily succumb to injury, and blood loss in small quantities amounts to great percentages for the premature infant. The smaller and less mature the infant, the greater percentage of body weight is fluid content. Fluid losses occur in greater percentages than for older infants and with increased hazards. The premature infant's susceptibility to cerebral hemorrhage is at least partially related to capillary fragility, but other factors, such as anoxia, probably contribute to this problem, which remains one of the major causes of death among premature infants, even though they receive optimal medical and nursing care.

Metabolic enzyme systems of the premature infant remain a challenge to researchers who are seeking to understand the phenomena that account for the inability to cope successfully with extrauterine life. The lack of surfactant production in the lungs and the immature ability of the liver to conjugate bilirubin have been the most thoroughly investigated disorders, but major gaps in understanding continue to exist. Speculation regarding the underlying physiology of the fetus and premature infant continues to guide many areas of medical and nursing management of the premature infant in his struggle to sustain life. The premature infant is like the fetus of a certain age in many developmental respects, but the event of birth induces the circulatory, gastrointestinal, renal, metabolic, and respiratory changes that occur in the full-term infant. These changes require the onset of functions for which the infant is not fully equipped. The premature infant is, in summary, at risk of developing each of the special neonatal problems that are discussed in the following sections, and thus these conditions are often equated with prematurity.

## Disturbances in fluid and electrolyte metabolism and acid-base balance
### Pathophysiology

Low birth weight and low gestational age infants, as well as those suffering from other neonatal problems, are particularly jeopardized by an impaired ability to maintain the delicate balance between fluids and electrolytes and acids and bases. The total percentage of body water in infancy is an important contributing factor. Table 8-3 indicates a comparison between the approximate percentage of body weight that is accounted for by water contained in the body fluid compartments of premature infants as opposed to term infants and adults. This comparison illustrates the importance of the relatively small percentage volume of the plasma, because this crucial portion of body water is the portion by which the volume and biochemistry of the interstitial (and subsequently the intracellular) spaces are mediated. The infant will exchange about one half of the total extracellular fluid volume every 24 hours, whereas the adult exchanges only about one seventh of this volume in 24 hours. This rapid rate of exchange, coupled with the inability of the immature renal system to conserve water, contributes significantly to the immediate crisis

**Table 8-3.** Body fluid compartments

| | Estimated percentage of total body weight | | |
|---|---|---|---|
| | Intracellular water | Plasma | Extracellular interstitial water |
| Premature infant | 23% | 5% | 60% |
| Full-term infant | 30% | 5% | 45% |
| Adult | 50% | 5% | 15% |

occurring in premature infants when even very slight volume losses are not replaced.[34]

The basic principles of electroneutrality and tonicity of body fluids operate for the premature as for the systems of all individuals. The premature infant's particular disadvantage in regulating the pH of the body's fluids results from an impaired ability to buffer the concentration of hydrogen ions under stress. When the accumulation of $CO_2$ occurs, as when respiratory function is impaired, the infant cannot maintain the appropriate balance of bicarbonate ion and carbonic acid buffering system without assistance. Further, the buffering power of hemoglobin is reduced, since this important molecule may be in short supply in the prematurely born infant and may be further depleted with blood loss. The immaturity of the kidney in both the premature and the full-term infant requires the loss of a large volume of water in order for small amounts of nitrogenous wastes to be excreted. The regulatory function of the mature kidney in conserving or excreting hydrogen ions in response to an imbalance is simply not reliably present in the newborn infant; the adrenocortical, parathyroid, and ADH factors, which ordinarily control these renal functions, may be undeveloped.

The higher metabolic rate of all infants is a further significant factor in the development of water and electrolyte imbalances. Stresses imposed by prematurity or illness further increase the metabolic rate, tissue production of $CO_2$ increases, and the demand for oxygen increases. To the extent that the respiratory system is impaired in its ability to take in oxygen and eliminate $CO_2$, the infant's dependence on anaerobic metabolism increases and the resulting production of lactic and pyruvic acids further compounds the rapidly developing acidosis.

A significant stress factor leading to increased metabolic rate during infancy is the loss of body heat. The premature infant is particularly vulnerable to this stress, because of the limited ability to regulate body temperature. As body temperature falls, the development of uncompensated acidosis progresses, and the infant's condition is seriously jeopardized.*

### Causes of disturbances

Labor and delivery, under totally adequate circumstances, result in mild acidosis in the neonate. Complications of this process greatly contribute to the development of a serious acidotic condition, which is further complicated by the infant's impaired ability to physiologically compensate under stress. Blood losses and prolonged periods without adequate oxygenation are particularly hazardous to the infant's fluid and electrolyte balance. Acid-base imbalance can occur as a component of all of the problems encountered by high risk newborn infants, and the signs and symptoms are often subtle and less remarkable than those of the primary disorder. Imbalances occur as a result of cold stress, during respiratory compromise, with gastrointestinal disorders, with infections, with disorders of the central nervous system, and after surgery. Many of the therapeutic procedures produce hazards related to acid-base and fluid and electrolyte imbalances, such as the insensible water loss that occurs with the use of radiant heaters and phototherapy.[32,67]

### Nursing problems

Skilled nursing intervention specifically directed toward the correction of fluid and electrolyte imbalances in the newborn requires advanced knowledge and skill. Nursing care in relation to respiratory difficulty that affects acid-base disturbance is discussed in the following section. The beginning practitioner may primarily be involved in appropriate prevention and early detection of imbalances by maintaining the infant's body temperature, providing for adequate exchange of oxygen and carbon dioxide, and astutely observing symptoms suggesting the development of an imbalance. The subtlety of signals that neonates exhibit makes this type of observation critical. They may appear only restless or irritable before they experience a major crisis and medical intervention is imperative immediately. Therefore, laboratory measurements hold increased importance in monitoring infants vulnerable to or suffering from fluid and electrolyte problems. Accurate, repeated laboratory determinations of blood pH, $Pco_2$, and $Po_2$ are required, and in many instances plasma bicarbonate and calculation of base excess or deficit are also necessary. Knowledge of the standard normal values established by the laboratory is essential in interpreting the acid-base status of the infant at any time and in guiding nursing and medical management of imbalances.[52] Table 8-4 indicates the changes that occur in the blood pH, $Pco_2$, and blood bicarbonate in conditions of compensated and uncompensated acid-base disturbances.

The pH is a measure of hydrogen ion concentration. It is normally within the range of 7.35 to 7.44. The pH is the end result of buffer activity and it does not provide information as to whether the disturbance is a respiratory or a metabolic problem. It is used to monitor the effectiveness of the infant's ability to compensate for a disturbance and buffer the hydrogen ion and as a general indicator of the effectiveness of therapeutic management.[67]

$Pco_2$ is the partial pressure of the portion of carbon dioxide dissolved in plasma. This reflects the degree of efficiency of ventilation and therefore deviations from normal reflect disorders of the respiratory system. It may be obtained from an arterial source or from a capillary stick. The range of normal values for a newborn infant is from 30 to 37 mm Hg.[67]

$Po_2$ is the partial pressure of oxygen carried in the blood. The $Po_2$ measurement of arterial blood reflects the effectiveness of movement of oxygen from the lungs to the blood. Because of the variation that exists in the partial pressure of oxygen in various blood compartments, the arterial source is essential to obtain an accurate assessment of the effectiveness of oxygen therapy. Estimates of the $Po_2$ from capillary samples are usually not sufficiently accurate to be useful.

*References 50, 64, 67, 79, 106, 115, 129.

**Table 8-4.** Attributes of acid-base disturbances according to type and degree of compensation*

| Disturbance | Blood pH | Blood Pco² (mm Hg) | Blood HCO₃⁻ (mEq/L) |
|---|---|---|---|
| Normal | 7.35 to 7.44 | 30 to 35 | 20 to 24 |
| Metabolic acidosis | | | |
|    Uncompensated | Lowest | Normal | Low |
|    Partially compensated | Low | Low | Low |
|    Fully compensated | Normal | Lowest | Low |
| Metabolic alkalosis | | | |
|    Uncompensated | Highest | Normal | High |
|    Partially compensated | High | High | High |
|    Fully compensated | Normal | Highest | High |
| Respiratory acidosis | | | |
|    Uncompensated | Lowest | High | Normal |
|    Partially compensated | Low | High | High |
|    Fully compensated | Normal | High | Highest |
| Respiratory alkalosis | | | |
|    Uncompensated | Highest | Low | Normal |
|    Partially compensated | High | Low | Low |
|    Fully compensated | Normal | Low | Lowest |

*From Korones, S. B.: High risk newborn infants; the basis for intensive nursing care, ed. 2, St. Louis, 1976, The C. V. Mosby Co., p. 125.

The neonatal range of normal is from 48 to 58 mg Hg.[67]

Plasma bicarbonate is a measure of total bicarbonate concentration, and it reflects this aspect of the buffering capacity of the system. Normal values range from 20 to 24 mEq/liter.

Base excess or deficit indicates the quantity of blood buffer base remaining after hydrogen ion is buffered. This reflects the combined blood buffering capacity of both the components of plasma bicarbonate and hemoglobin. This value is calculated rather than measured directly by the laboratory using an acid-base nomogram. To calculate the base excess or deficit, the hemoglobin concentration and any two of the following measurements must be known: blood pH, $Pco_2$, plasma bicarbonate, or total carbon dioxide content of the plasma. The normal range is from +4 to −4 mEq/liter, with a normal value of zero.[67,79]

Control of the environment and provision of feeding and nutrition (described earlier) are important means by which the nurse facilitates the infant's fluid and electrolyte and acid-base balance. In addition the nurse must give careful attention to the management of intravenous fluids. A wide range of fluids is used in care of the newborn, and many are discussed in the following sections, which concern specific disorders. The most commonly used substance for the direct regulation of acid-base balance is sodium bicarbonate. The dose of sodium bicarbonate is calculated as follows:

$$\text{mEq of NaHCO}_3 \text{ to be given} = \text{base deficit} \times 0.3 \times \text{body weight in kilograms}$$

The factor 0.3 represents the approximate percentage of body weight composed of extracellular fluid. The dose of sodium bicarbonate must be diluted because the alkaline pH is likely to damage the tissues near the site of infusion.[67]

Fluid therapy is usually begun with 10% dextrose in water at a dose of 65 to 70 ml/kg of body weight per 24 hours. A hypotonic electrolyte solution is usually added by the second day, and if the infant is not able to take gastrointestinal feedings by the third day, an amino acid-glucose-electrolyte solution is used.[67]

Constant attention must be given to the prevention of insensible water loss. The smaller the infant, the more precarious is the achievement of water balance, due to the large total body surface area, thin skin, and immaturity of the renal system. Accurate measurement of body weight is the fundamental means by which

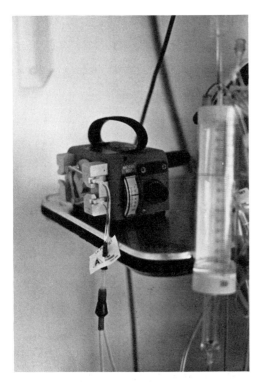

**Fig. 8-5.** An infusion pump such as that shown here is required to maintain consistency of the minute flow rate for small infants. Monitoring of the amount of fluid that passes through the volutrol assures adequate functioning of the mechanical pump.

monitoring of insensible water loss is accomplished. If the infant loses more than 10% of birth weight in the first three days or 5% in any single day, water losses are excessive and there is danger to the infant's fluid and electrolyte balance.[67] The function of the renal system may be estimated in part by frequent Clinitest determinations, which reflect the metabolism of sugar. If the results are consistently 3+ or 4+, the concentration of intravenous dextrose solution must be decreased.[67]

Careful monitoring and adjustment of the rate of infusion of IV fluids is critical for the newborn. An infusion pump is essential to maintain the constancy of the minute flow rate required by small infants. The equipment and the site of administration must be checked frequently to monitor the adequacy of performance of all components of the infusion system.[67]

## Disturbances interfering with effective gas exchange

### Pathophysiology of neonatal cardiopulmonary disorders

The establishment of respiratory and circulatory functions necessary to maintain extrauterine life occurs with apparent ease and efficiency for the healthy term infant. The most dramatic changes occur within a few minutes of birth, and the adaptation of all systems to extrauterine function is essentially complete within a few days. By contrast, the premature infant is faced with a difficult and prolonged period of adaptation in respiratory and circulatory function, and the impairment creates a vicious cycle of events that further inhibits the adequate development of extrauterine functioning.[100] Similar phenomena may occur for a term infant who is born with congenital malformations or who suffers from an infection.

Initial insufflation of the lungs requires pressures of about 70 cm $H_2O$ negative intrathoracic pressure, rapidly decreasing within a few breaths to 15 to 20 cm $H_2O$ pressure to move air in and out of the lungs.[21] If collapse of the alveoli occurs after the onset of respiration, pressures required to reopen the alveoli begin to increase and may approach the level needed with the first breath. When the infant is required to exert this much negative pressure with each breath on his or her own, over and over again, the amount of energy required is too great to sustain life indefinitely.

The first inspiratory effort is probably stimulated by multiple physical, chemical, and neuroendocrine responses at the moment of birth. The great inspiratory pressure required to initially expand the lungs is thought to be increased for the low gestational age infant, and sensitivity to the stimuli that ordinarily initiate breathing is diminished. Thus the first inspiratory effort may be a weak gasp or it may not occur. In other instances the infant may begin to breathe without observable difficulty but after a period of time may develop grunting, which initially may be audible only with a stethoscope. This may be the first sign of respiratory deficiency. Retractions begin to appear and increase in severity as the effort requires to expand the lungs increases.

**227**

With the establishment of respiration during the first few breaths, the normal effort required to move air into and out of the lungs decreases as the functional residual capacity of the lungs is established. This involves the retention of a certain volume of air in the alveoli at the end of expiration. This capacity represents the ability of the alveoli to remain partially expanded, a phenomenon necessary for continued lung function. Maintaining partial expansion depends upon the presence of surfactant, a lipoprotein material that minimizes the surface tension of the alveolar surface.[39] As air moves in and out of the lungs, the alveoli must be able to respond to changes in volume with minimal resistance, or the effort to breath becomes great and collapse of the alveolar sacs is imminent. If residual capacity is not maintained, atelectasis of the lungs occurs. When an infant exhibits an expiratory grunt, he or she is making a physiologic effort to maintain a residual capacity in the lungs against forces that may be causing collapse of the alveoli. These forces are most commonly associated with an absence or a shortage of surfactant, or hyaline membrane disease. The grunting sound arises from the partial closure of the glottis against the expiratory flow of air, retaining a portion of air that would otherwise escape. Through this mechanism the infant can raise the arterial $P_{O_2}$ by 10 to 20 mm Hg.

Problems with pulmonary circulation occur concurrently with the development of respiratory difficulty. Under ordinary circumstances the capillary surface of the lungs increases greatly as a result of decreased pulmonary vascular resistance at the time that respiration is established. When for some reason oxygen uptake does not occur sufficiently to maintain a physiologically homeostatic level of $P_{O_2}$, chemoreceptors sense the deprivation and the capillary bed of the lungs constricts, causing increased resistance, or a tendency to return to fetal patterns of blood flow. Adequate gas exchange in extrauterine life is further hampered, carbon dioxide levels increase, acidosis develops, and the cycle worsens.[55,67,131] Fig. 8-6 diagrammatically illustrates these interrelationships.

The nature of the fetal circulatory system (see Chapter 6) makes it possible for the fetus to survive severe congenital abnormalities of the

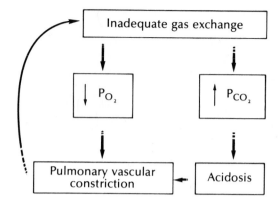

**Fig. 8-6.** The interrelationships between inadequate gas exchange and the development of acidosis and hypoxemia. Once the cycle begins, assistance is needed to intercept worsening of the condition.

heart as long as one side of the heart can deliver blood from the great veins to the aorta. Blood can bypass nonfunctioning chambers that are both proximal and distal to the heart. This accounts for the ability of the fetus with cardiac abnormalities to survive and to grow normally during fetal life. When the infant shifts from oxygen dependence from the placenta to the lungs, there is a sudden increase in arterial blood oxygen tension, which is one of the factors that initiates constriction of the patent ductus arteriosus. Inflation of the lungs produces a marked reduction in pulmonary vascular resistance. The pulmonary vessels, which were supported by a fluid medium, become suspended in air, reducing extravascular pressure. Pulmonary arterial pressure falls and pulmonary blood flow increases greatly. Systemic vascular resistance rises with clamping of the umbilical cord. Along with these changes the return of blood flow to the left atrium is increased and raises left atrial pressure, which in turn closes the patent foramen ovale. The changes result in a division of the formerly single circulatory pathway to a pathway compatible with gas exchange originating in the lungs.[102]

Because of the intrinsic relationship between cardiac function and pulmonary function during the newborn period, differentiating symptoms of underlying cardiac or pulmonary disorders is often difficult. Adequate function of both systems is essential for survival.[102] The following section presents a summary of the common disorders that occur in these systems at birth.

## Common cardiopulmonary medical diagnoses

**Apnea of prematurity.** Approximately 30% of preterm infants of less than 32 weeks' gestation and almost all of those of less than 30 weeks' gestation have apneic periods severe enough to cause bradycardia, cyanosis, and possible asphyxia. Apnea is also likely to be caused by temperature variations above and below that of thermoneutrality (skin temperature of 36 degrees C), airway obstruction, vasovagal response to feeding, hypoglycemia, hypocalcemia, infection, or intracranial hemorrhage. When apneic episodes persist, the underlying pathophysiology must be determined for adequate management of the infant. Symptomatic management of apnea must be instituted in any event. The monitoring techniques described previously in this chapter are most important for early detection and intervention in cases of apnea and are essential to prevent asphyxia. Careful monitoring and management of insensible water loss and temperature of the ambient air and the infant's body are important preventive measures. Suction equipment must be readily available and must be used before artificial aeration of the lungs. Often, suctioning the nasopharynx is sufficient to stimulate the infant to breathe alone. When the infant suffers repeated or severe apneic attacks, periodic treatment with a bag and mask is used. The nurse must acquire skill in using the bag and mask to assure that the air pressure exerted is sufficient to expand the lungs but does not produce excessive pressure, which might damage the lungs. When apnea episodes are severe or frequent, the infant may be intubated to provide continuous transpulmonary distending pressure, which serves to maintain a functional residual capacity and alveolar stability for the infant.[3,10,29,67] Orally administered theophylline (2 to 3 mg/kg every six hours) may be used to combat severe apnea and may be used as an alternate to mechanical ventilation.[109,124]

**Hyaline membrane disease (respiratory distress syndrome).** Approximately 25% to 35% of all preterm infants suffer from hyaline membrane disease. The lower the birth weight of the infant, the more likely the possibility of developing this respiratory disease. From 20% to 30% of all infants who develop the disease die, with twice the number of male infants suffering lethal effects as female infants. The underlying pathophysiology arises from diminished production of surfactant in the lung parenchyma, which is essential for maintaining alveolar expansion and stability.[67] Factors associated with hyaline membrane disease include asphyxiation during labor and delivery, which further reduces surfactant production, and the presence of acidosis, hypoxemia, hypovolemia, and hypothermia.[3]

Hyaline membrane disease is essentially a developmental problem in that it arises from the infant's immature ability to synthesize surface-active pulmonary lecithin, a process that increases sharply at about 35 weeks' gestation. To predict the maturity of the unborn fetus, the ratio of lecithin and sphingomyelin (L/S ratio) may be obtained from the amniotic fluid. When the densitometric ratio of these compounds reaches 2 to 1 or more, sufficient maturity has been reached that the infant will not develop hyaline membrane disease. Earlier periods of development reflect a relatively lower concentration of lecithin and higher for sphingomyelin.[3,40,67]

The infant with hyaline membrane disease is inactive and assumes a froglike position. There is an expiratory grunt, sternal and costal retractions, and flaring of the nares. Fine rales are heard at the end of inspiration, with reduced movement of air in the lungs. The respiratory rate is increased, and the infant experiences frequent periods of apnea. Blood gas and pH changes are not specific for hyaline membrane disease but are important in monitoring the severity and progress of the illness. The blood pH falls (under 7.25), the $P_{CO_2}$ rises (above 55 mm Hg) and the arterial $P_{O_2}$ falls (under 45 mm Hg). The medical diagnosis is based on clinical signs and symptoms and interpretation of the chest roentgenogram.[3]

Management is focused on the support of respiration and maintenance of adequate fluid and electrolyte and acid-base balance. Continuous positive airway pressure is a valuable measure in the treatment of infants with hyaline membrane disease and may prevent the necessity of using a respirator. Oral feeding is delayed, which may necessitate the use of parenteral alimentation.[3,38,67] Detailed descriptions of these measures are found in previous and following sections of this chapter.

**Meconium aspiration syndrome.** Aspiration of meconium-contaminated amniotic fluid occurs as a result of hypoxia in utero, which causes increased fetal respiratory activity. Meconium is passed into the amniotic fluid in about 10% of all pregnancies, and aspiration may occur gradually, as in the case of placental insufficiency with chronic fetal distress, or suddenly, as when there is premature separation of the placenta or prolapse of the cord. The presence of meconium-stained fluid in the lungs prevents complete expansion of the lungs on delivery, interferes with adequate resuscitation, and impairs the exchange of gases. The infant who is not treated immediately after delivery has an increased chance of developing pneumothorax and pneumonia. The presence of meconium-stained amniotic fluid before delivery is the first signal that meconium aspiration may have occurred. The infant will exhibit an increase in inspiratory effort and tachypnea, and rales may be heart in the chest. Immediate suctioning of the trachea is imperative to clear the airway and prevent complications of respiratory distress. Without the benefit of early suctioning of the trachea, the death rate of infants with meconium aspiration syndrome is 28%. Tracheal lavage with normal saline solution may be needed if there is aspiration of tenacious meconium. Positive pressure should not be applied to the airway until the airway is known to be cleared. The stomach of the infant should also be suctioned to prevent further aspiration of regurgitated fluid. Many infants who have suffered from meconium aspiration need the benefit of full intensive care for support of respiration and management of fluids and electrolytes and acid-base balance until full recovery occurs.[3,43,67,127]

**Obstructive emphysema of the newborn (transient tachypnea, respiratory distress syndrome type II).** Obstructive emphysema of the newborn results from the delayed absorption of fetal lung fluid trapped in the interstitial spaces and engorged periarterial lymphatics. This is a relatively mild disorder, and the infant usually recovers within a few days with adequate care. Differentiation of obstructive emphysema from hyaline membrane disease may be difficult at first, for the infant may exhibit similar signs and symptoms. The infant has an expiratory grunt, which represents an attempt to get rid of trapped alveolar air. The respiratory rate is elevated, but there is seldom the appearance of significant retractions or rales. Cyanosis may appear, and the blood gas determinations are similar to that for mild hyaline membrane disease. With sound management to support respiration and the balance of fluids and electrolytes and the blood pH, these infants are quickly able to establish their own ability to exchange gases effectively.[3,67]

**Pneumothorax and pneumomediastinum.** Pneumothorax and pneumomediastinum are the most common forms of extraneous air leaks of the chest. These disorders occur spontane-

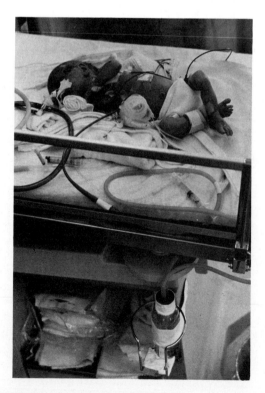

**Fig. 8-7.** A chest tube and gravity suction is provided to relieve tension of accumulated air in the chest.

ously in newborns who appear to be normal, as well as those with respiratory abnormalities. They also occur in conjunction with positive pressure ventilation and continuous distending pressure techniques, although the extent to which these procedures contribute to air leaks is not known.[46] Overdistension of distal air sacs precedes the rupture of these sacs and escape of air into the interstitial spaces. Medical diagnosis depends upon interpretation of the chest roentgenogram. The infant exhibits increasing tachypnea, rapid development of cyanosis, falling blood pressure, increased anteroposterior diameter of the chest, a shift of apical cardiac impulse, and increased resonance of percussion of the chest. In some instances the infant will recover with conservative treatment, but for many infants the condition is life-threatening and the accumulated air must be aspirated and a chest catheter inserted with continuous or intermittent suction to relieve tension. The infant may need oxygen therapy. Transillumination of the chest has been found to be effective in detecting air leaks of the lung.[3,67,133]

**Congenital anomalies of the respiratory tract.** Anomalies of the respiratory tract are infrequent, but the malformations that have been observed are numerous. Whenever an infant exhibits respiratory difficulty immediately after delivery, the possibility of respiratory tract anomalies should be considered. Choanal atresia results from stenosis of the posterior nares that open into the nasopharynx. This malformation produces dramatic symptoms due to the fact that newborn infants are nose breathers, and this passage is blocked, leaving the infant essentially without an airway. Cyanosis and severe retractions are apparent immediately. An oral airway must be inserted and maintained until surgical correction can be completed.

The most common malformation observed is tracheoesophageal fistula. The most frequent form is atresia of a segment of the esophagus, which divides it into an upper blind pouch and a lower portion that is connected to the stomach, and a fistula joining this lower esophageal segment with the trachea. The infant exhibits distinctive symptoms of accumulation of secretions in the mouth and pharynx requiring urgent and frequent suctioning, continuous or sporadic res-

piratory distress, and repeated regurgitation of feedings. Observation of the accumulation of secretions and respiratory distress should alert the nurse to consider the possibility of a tracheoesophageal fistula, withhold feedings, and attempt to pass a catheter into the esophagus. Astute observation for the placement of the tube in the stomach can provide evidence as to whether an anomaly exists, but medical diagnosis depends upon interpretation of the roentgenogram. Surgical intervention is imperative; the earlier the surgical correction, the greater the infant's chances for survival. Postsurgical pneumonia and septicemia are the major causes of death after successful surgical correction, provided other congenital anomalies are not present.[3,67]

**Congenital heart disease.** Respiratory difficulty is an inevitable problem for infants with congenital heart disease. It is usually preceded by congestive heart failure, and the infant will exhibit tachypnea, fatigue or difficulty in feeding, and an enlarged liver. A gallop rhythm of the heart may be observed. A patent ductus arteriosus is the most common congenital problem resulting in heart failure and pulmonary edema. There is a high mortality rate among infants with cardiac anomalies, and complications of surgery are difficult to combat. The anomalies that account for the greatest percentage of deaths among infants with cardiac anomalies include hypoplastic left heart syndrome, coarctation of the aorta, transposition of the great vessels, hypoplastic right heart syndrome with pulmonary atresia or stenosis, tetralogy of Fallot, truncus arteriosus, endocardial cushion defect, and ventricular septal defect[3,67] (see Chapter 18).

**Shock.** Shock is a state of severe circulatory failure in which cardiac output does not meet tissue requirements. It can occur as a result of severe blood loss, septic shock in the face of severe infections, severe heart failure due to congenital heart disease, excessive or inappropriate use of positive pressure to the airway, and as a result of metabolic disturbances such as hypoglycemia or adrenal insufficiency. The infant exhibits tachycardia, tachypnea, pallor, poor filling of blanched skin, decreasing urinary output, and lowered blood pressure. Supportive care of the infant's temperature, respirations, acid-base balance and fluids and electrolytes is basic. Diagnosis and correction of the underlying cause of shock may require some time, but every effort should be made to determine the cause and correct it quickly. Expansion of blood volume is accomplished by giving blood or Plasmanate, 5 to 10 ml/kg of body weight, over a two- to five-minute period.[3,67]

### Nursing problems

The primary nursing problem associated with cardiopulmonary disorders in the newborn is the provision of the exchange of gases. This problem requires four major areas of intervention. These are (1) clearing the airway, (2) administration of oxygen, (3) provision of a functional residual capacity in the lungs, and (4) assisted ventilation. These measures also contribute significantly to the management of acid-base imbalances, because they interrupt the cycle of inadequate gas exchange and acidosis.

Clearing the airway with adequate precautions to avoid trauma and infection is vitally important before positive pressure air is introduced during resuscitation or assisted ventilation, because obstruction interferes with efforts to provide for flow of gases. Suctioning alone

may suffice, but occasionally endotracheal intubation with visualization is necessary to clear the passages of tenacious material (Fig. 8-8). The constant accumulation of mucus, secretions, and orally administered feedings, if not effectively swallowed and cleared by the infant who is ill, makes it necessary to suction the infant regularly to lessen the hazard of aspiration of these materials into the lungs.

The administration of oxygen to an ill or low gestational age and low birth weight infant is a continuing major concern; it is vitally necessary to the survival and well-being of many of these infants, but the hazards are great. The use of oxygen during the neonatal period became conservative after the discovery of the relationship between retrolental fibroplasia and the partial pressure of oxygen in the retinal arteries. However, many infants simply could not survive or escape central nervous system depression or damage with the oxygen levels of 40% or lower thought to be safe in preventing eye damage. The discovery was then made that the ability of these infants to absorb oxygen at the level of lung-blood exchange in the alveoli is limited, and that the level of partial pressure of oxygen in the blood is severely jeopardized. When this occurs, administration of higher concentrations

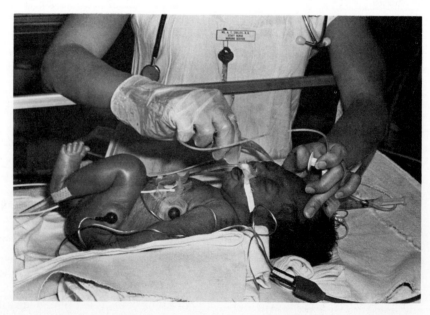

**Fig. 8-8.** Suctioning of the airway is the first step in providing artificial support for exchange of gases.

of oxygen, exceeding the 40% level, is required to attain a partial pressure of oxygen that is compatible with metabolic demands, or a $PaO_2$ of approximately 50 mm Hg. As the use of oxygen has once again increased, a resurgence in the incidence of retrolental fibroplasia has occurred, because the $PaO_2$ levels in infants are again exceeding a safe range. Careful monitoring of the blood gas levels of oxygen is mandatory in adequate oxygen administration. In addition, regular assessment of the retina by an experienced ophthalmologist is required to determine the possibility of early retinal changes in an infant receiving any concentration of oxygen over a period of time. When detected early, such changes may be reversible, thus preventing the occurrence of retrolental fibroplasia.[82] Methods of administration have been improved with the use of head boxes, bag and mask therapy, continuous positive airway pressure, continuous negative chest wall pressure therapy, intubation practices, and oxygen-air mixing, so that the measured concentration of ambient oxygen more reliably represents the real concentration that is reaching the alveolar space.

It has also been recognized during recent years that high levels of inspired oxygen are toxic to the neonatal lung, causing a thickening of the alveolar tissue and a permanent impairment of the gas exchange ability of the lungs. An inspired concentration of over 60% seems to result in this damage, but the duration of therapy is also significant. The point of damage in relation to duration is not known.

The best guide in the administration of oxygen seems to be to use the lowest inspiratory concentration $(F_1O_2)$ possible over the shortest possible period of time. When ambient concentrations of over 30% to 40% are required to maintain life and well-being for any period of time exceeding two to three days, the infant should be transported to a neonatal center where there are resources for frequent monitoring of blood gases, and expert administration and nursing care can be provided. Predicting this circumstance before it actually occurs is of great benefit to the infant, since the earlier the institution of expert care, the more satisfactory will be the outcome for the infant.[3,67]

Artificial provision of a functional residual capacity in the lungs (continuous distending pressure breathing) has developed as an important adjunct in the care of infants with respiratory distress who can breathe spontaneously. The

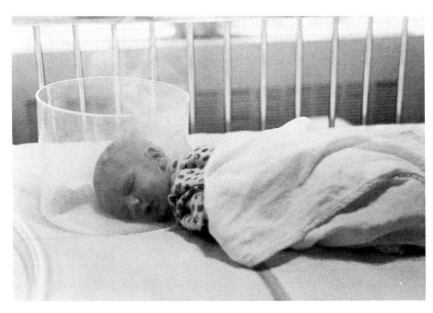

**Fig. 8-9.** The head box provides a reliable means of administering oxygen and with it a reasonable control of the percentage of ambient oxygen can be achieved. The oxygen is mixed with air for the desired concentration level, warmed, and humidified.

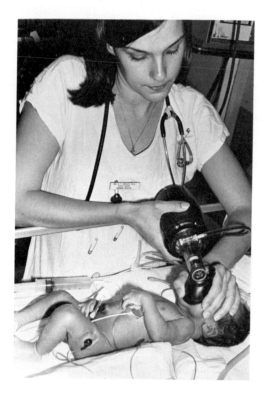

**Fig. 8-10.** A bag and mask is used for intermittent ventilatory assistance or for emergency resuscitation. The mask must fit snugly around the infant's face, and the bag must be capable of delivering greater than 40% concentration of oxygen.

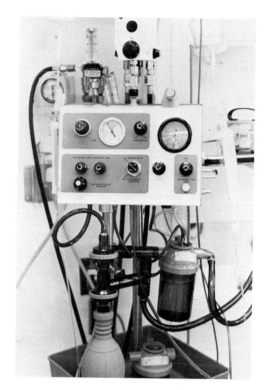

**Fig. 8-11.** A mechanical respirator designed for infants is used to provide continuous assisted ventilation. Fig. 8-7 shows placement of the endotracheal tube through the infant's nose from this mechanical device.

effect is similar to that accomplished when the infant grunts, and the need for artificial ventilation and for prolonged administration of high levels of inspired oxygen has been significantly decreased. A nasal or endotracheal tube is usually used, but a face mask that maintains a solid seal can also be used. The difficulty of maintaining a seal and the resulting damage to facial tissues make some form of intubation preferable. Expired air is directed through a system that is partially occluded with an adjustable clamp to maintain an end-expiratory pressure above zero, usually 5 to 15 mm Hg. Measured concentrations of oxygen, which is warmed, humidified, and mixed with air, are provided for inspired air. Because alveolar collapse is prevented, the functional capacity of the lungs is maintained and supported throughout the period when surfactant is not being produced in hyaline membrane disease or when other pathologic changes leading to collapse would other-

wise occur in other forms of respiratory disease. The lungs are able to exchange gases effectively, and the need for high levels of inspired oxygen is decreased. The damaging, permanent results of both high concentrations of inspired oxygen and alveolar collapse are avoided, and the improved outcome for the infant is remarkable.*

Continuous negative pressure to the chest has also been developed as a means of providing positive end-expiratory pressure in the lungs. The infant is placed in a device that provides a lower than atmospheric pressure to the entire body below the neck. The infant's head is in an oxygen hood at an atmospheric pressure in which the $F_1O_2$ is regulated. The negative pressure to the chest expands the thorax and prevents collapse of the alveoli at end-expiration. This method eliminates the need for nasal tubes, endotracheal tubes, or face masks.[18,67]

*References 1, 23, 61, 67, 88, 99.

Ventilatory assistance may be accomplished manually or mechanically. Manual methods include the emergency use of mouth-to-mouth resuscitation, which can be life-saving to an infant when sudden or unexpected respiratory distress occurs. External cardiac massage is usually necessary at the same time, and if the infant survives, expert continuing care is needed.

The bag and mask form of manually assisted ventilation avoids the necessity for mouth-to-mouth resuscitation. The mask must be of a size and shape that will seal around the infant's face, and the bag should be capable of delivering high concentrations of oxygen. Bag and mask insufflation of the lungs is frequently employed on a regular basis for infants who are experiencing some interference with totally adequate respiration. Although they may be able to adequately maintain respiration for indefinite periods of time, weakness of the accessory muscles that accomplish expansion of the chest prevents ventilation of the entire lung field. The occurrence of the periodic deep breath, or sigh, which is an important feature of totally adequate ventilation, may be missing. Periodic, regular application of bag and mask ventilation assures full expansion of the entire lung field, and boosts the infant's borderline capacity to maintain adequate oxygen levels in the blood.

Mechanical ventilation in the form of either positive or negative pressure is a complex procedure requiring the most expert nursing and medical care. Because the machine is not able to respond homeostatically to the constantly changing function and requirements of the infant, nursing and medical personnel must utilize a vast array of resources to determine the physiologic function of the infant's systems. They then manipulate the machine in such a manner that it adequately provides the kind of ventilation that is optimal for the infant at any given moment.

The greatest hazard in providing ventilatory assistance of any kind is imposing excessive pressure in the lungs. Particularly when emergency positive pressure assistance is applied, the zeal with which assistance is offered too often results in excessive pressure gradients and the development ultimately of pneumothorax. Further, adequate gas exchange is inhibited, because air is trapped in the pleural cavity without adequate escape; the lungs are compressed and the entry of inspired air is blocked. Mouth-to-mouth resuscitation and bag and mask insufflation require careful attention to provision of escape of air introduced to the lungs. Most bag and mask apparatuses do not provide for adequate monitoring of the amount of pressure being delivered with each puff of air, and the practitioner's skill in estimating the adequacy of this pressure is crucial, requiring practice and supervised learning. It is impossible to measure the exact amount of pressure needed by the infant at any time, but the rise and fall of the chest and auscultation for air movement in and out of the lungs provide guidelines for maintaining a balance between delivering pressures that are too great and delivering pressures that are not sufficient to accomplish gas exchange.[46]

## Neonatal infections
### Pathophysiology related to infection

For reasons not completely understood, infection during the neonatal period is distinctly different from infection during later infancy and childhood. Organisms that do not result in illness later in life are often pathogenic for the newborn, and, conversely, some organisms that cause serious disease later in life do not seem to cause disease during the neonatal period. The pattern of disease, regardless of the offending organism, is entirely different from that observed during later life. As mentioned earlier, gestational age, delicacy of the tissues, proximity of parts, and impaired ability to compensate for imbalances in the system are all related to the newborn's particular vulnerability to infections. Once an organism invades the system, devastating and rapid progression occurs, very often resulting in serious illnesses such as pneumonia, septicemia, or meningitis. The newborn infant displays only nonspecific and subtle signs of illness during infection, and these become perceptible only after the disease has progressed to an advanced stage. The infant with seriously advanced septicemia may exhibit only malaise and disinterest in feeding.[3,67]

Neonatal infections are associated with hemolytic anemia, which for the premature infant is a particular hazard. Hyperbilirubinemia may be a sign that infection is present, but it does not occur early enough in most instances to be of value in detecting the presence of infection. Hepatic damage resulting from the infectious agent, as well as direct hemolysis during infection, accounts for the presence of hyperbilirubinemia.

The defenses of the newborn against the invasion of infectious agents are sufficiently different from those of older individuals to bear special consideration. The thin, delicate tissues of the mucous membranes and skin are often the site of invasion. They provide little defense against invasions because of their delicacy and the lack of immunosuppressive agents. The inflammatory response of newborn tissues is often very different, if it is exhibited at all.

The immunologic defense system best understood is the immunoglobulin system of the lymph and plasma cells. Some maternal immunoglobulins are transferred across the placenta and render a degree of protection for the newborn. However, a significant portion of this transfer occurs during the last trimester of gestational life, and the premature infant lacks this advantage of the older, term infant.

Maternal IgG, which contains antibodies specific to the majority of bacterial and viral organisms, first appears in fetal tissues at about the third month of gestation and continues to accumulate throughout fetal life until a level equivalent to that of the mother's own IgG level is attained at term. The infant's resistance is equivalent to the mother's own ability to resist infection—an ability built up in response to exposure to specific organisms throughout her lifetime. At birth the maternal IgG molecules begin to disappear as normal catabolism takes place, and the infant begins to produce IgG antibodies. At about 3 months of age the maternal supply is depleted, and the infant's own supply is about half of the maternal quantity he had at birth. For most newborns IgG antibodies supply protection against most of the common bacterial and viral agents that attack older children and adults, except the enteric gram-negative rods. IgM, which supplies maternal protection against these organisms, is not transported across the placenta, and the infant's supply is not built against these specific organisms until they are encountered in extrauterine life. The gram-negative rods account for a significant proportion of infection during the newborn period, and the lack of defense against them is probably a significant factor.

IgM levels in the newborn are greatly increased if he or she was exposed to certain infections during fetal life, such as syphilis, rubella, cytomegalovirus, or herpes virus. The ability to produce IgM antibodies begins early in gestational life and continues throughout fetal life, but the response of specific IgM production is greatly stimulated during early neonatal life to the extent that the infant is exposed to infectious agents.

IgA does not cross the placenta and is not produced by the newborn infant in significant quantities. This level continues to be very low until several weeks of age, at which time a gradual increase begins as production is stimulated.[67]

### Infectious agents and factors in their spread

The most frequently involved agents in neonatal infections are the bacterial organisms that comprise the normal flora of the mother's intestinal and genital tracts. These organisms enter the uterus through the cervix and infect the chorion, amniotic membrane, and possibly the amniotic fluid. Such infections may not infect the fetus, but detection of such exposure is important in early detection and treatment of newborn infection. Prolonged rupture of membranes and prolonged labor are associated with an increased risk of infection.[67]

Gram-positive cocci, generally group B streptococci and staphylococci, account for 15% to 25% of the incidence of pneumonia, septicemia, and meningitis in the neonatal period. The worldwide epidemic of staphylococcal infections in nurseries during the 1950s and 1960s led to important discoveries of the mechanisms of infection transmission in hospital nurseries and to ways of keeping transmission at a minimum. Nursery personnel, equipment, linens, airborne particles, and other infants have all been identified as sources of infection. Stringent hygienic measures and isolation techniques were developed as a result of the tragic experiences with staph infections in nurseries, but many of the measures were never identified clearly as being related to infection control. The epidemiologic features of this experience have been impossible to fully understand, and for some obscure reason the incidence of staph infections in nurseries subsided, either as a result of the natural life cycle of the organism, a mutation of the species, or as a result of the control efforts undertaken in nurseries.[37,66]

The gram-negative rod organisms, known as "water bugs" because of their tendency to grow and thrive in water, produce 75% to 85% of all cases of neonatal pneumonia, septicemia, and meningitis. *Escherichia coli, Pseudomonas aeruginosa, Klebsiella, Aerobacter, Proteus,* and *Flavobacterium* are among the common organisms that are identified. The increased use of equipment in which water is either stored or can accumulate is probably related to the great increase in incidence of these infections in recent years. Careful attention to regular cleaning and care of all equipment, particularly incubators, is an important factor in the control of these infections in nurseries.[31,45]

Viruses can cause postnatally acquired infection, but more commonly they are involved in prenatal infection acquired through the placenta or from the vaginal tract. When these organisms invade the fetus early during gestation, congenital malformations and severe lasting effects are produced. When the infection occurs later in pregnancy, the infant may escape permanent effects, but serious illness during the neonatal period is often present, and the viable virus is harbored by the infant for several months after birth.[92]

Thrush, a fungal infection caused by *Candida albicans,* is acquired through the maternal vaginal tract at the time of delivery. It is a commonly occurring infection seen in all nurseries. The infant may demonstrate a disinterest in feeding, but the typical white membranous plaque that forms on the tongue and mucous membranes of the mouth and throat is the most characteristic sign. Within a week of appearance of the mouth lesions the infant will exhibit a typical cherry-red, raw-skin rash of the buttocks if the infection is not treated. Transmission from one infant to another can occur via the hands of personnel. Gentian violet or nystatin is used in specific treatment.[106]

### Medical diagnoses related to infection

**Pneumonia.** Congenital pneumonia is evident at birth or within 48 hours. It is acquired before delivery, often in association with premature rupture of membranes, prolonged labor, maternal infections, or premature delivery. The outlook for the infant is grave. At birth, the infant is flaccid, pale, and cyanotic. Respirations are rapid and shallow, often with retractions of the chest, and rales are sometimes evident. If the infant is born at term, there may be an elevation in temperature; if the birth is premature, there may be a subnormal body temperature. The organisms most frequently involved are *Escherichia coli* and other enteric organisms and group B streptococci.[3,67]

Pneumonia acquired after delivery is most often caused by *Pseudomonas aeruginosa,* penicillin-resistant staphylococci, and enteric organisms. The infant usually becomes ill after the first 48 hours of life, and exhibits increase in respiratory rate, poor feeding, and aspiration during feeding. The outlook for the infant is better than that for the infant with congenitally acquired pneumonia, but effective antibiotic therapy instituted early during the course of the illness is essential.[3,67]

**Septicemia.** This generalized infection characterized by proliferation of bacteria in the blood can occur in the newborn infant rapidly without any signs that the infant is developing a problem. The early symptoms are vague and not specific to the infection, with the only signs being lethargy, loss of weight, and poor feeding. Some infants develop vomiting and diarrhea, abnormal respirations, jaundice, or hypoglycemia. A variety of skin lesions occurs after the onset of the illness, such as pustules, furuncles, and subcutaneous abscesses associated with streptococcal and staphylococcal organisms and occasionally with *P. aeruginosa* and *E. coli. P. aeruginosa* produces a typical localized purplish cellulitis that breaks down to a black, gangrenous ulcer. Meningitis develops in about one third of all infants with septicemia, although symptoms of this secondary infection may not be present.

Medical diagnosis is made by blood culture, which takes at least 24 hours for growth. The spinal fluid and urine must also be cultured in order to accurately identify the organism involved in the infection. Other laboratory data are useful in making decisions regarding treatment before the results of cultures are obtained. Leukocytes in peripheral blood less than 4000/mm³ are commonly associated with septicemia. White blood cell counts of over 30,000 may be present. A platelet count of less than 150,000 mm³ (thrombocytopenia) commonly occurs. Determination of the infant's IgM is often elevated (over 20 mg/100 ml in the first week of life), but this elevation is usually not evident for several days after the onset of the infection.[3,33,67]

**Meningitis.** Meningitis occurs more frequently in premature than in term infants and is usually associated with the same maternal problems and causative organisms as those for septicemia. The outlook for the infant is grave, with a fatality rate of 35% to 60%, and approximately half of those infants surviving suffer severe central nervous system handicaps. General symptoms are similar to those of septicemia. Often the only specific sign is tension of the anterior fontanel. The infant may exhibit opisthotonos, coma, or convulsions; stiffness of the neck (Kernig's sign) rarely occurs.

Medical diagnosis is confirmed from spinal fluid abnormalities and culture of spinal fluid. Spinal fluid sugar content is low, protein elevated, polymorphonuclear leukocytes are predominant, and the white cell content of the fluid may vary from 20 to several thousand per cubic millimeter.[3,67]

**Diarrhea.** The enteropathogen, *E. coli,* is the most frequent and important of the organisms causing primary diarrhea in infants. It can cause rapidly spreading epidemics in a nursery even though careful precautions are taken to prevent its spread. Because of this, when this organism is identified in an infant, the infant must be placed in strict isolation and all infants in the nursery cultured and treated for the infection. Early signs of the infection are a refusal to feed and weight loss and lethargy, often preceding the appearance of diarrhea stools by one or two days. As the illness progresses, the infant becomes toxic, dehydrated, and acidotic.

An ashen gray color is indicative of vasomotor collapse and impending death associated with severe metabolic acidosis and dehydration.[3,67]

**Urinary tract infection.** Urinary tract infections in the newborn are more common than is generally recognized. It occurs more often in male infants than in female infants, which is the reverse of the sex distribution in older children. In addition, it is not usually associated with an underlying anomaly as it is in older children. The most frequent early sign is a body weight loss of more than 10% during the first five days for an infant who otherwise appears to be doing well. If the symptoms occur after the first week of life, fever, jaundice, or cyanosis may be exhibited. The organisms involved in urinary tract infection are usually gram-negative enteric rods. Medical diagnosis is made by obtaining two consecutive urine cultures by suprapubic aspiration.[3,67]

**Conjunctivitis.** Conjunctivitis may be acquired from the nursery environment or from the mother during delivery. The infant develops swelling and redness of the conjunctiva, with varying amounts of purulent exudate. The causative organisms include staphylococcus, *P. aeruginosa,* and enteric organisms. Gonorrheal infection causes a serious infection, and although the source of infection occurs during delivery, symptoms may not emerge for several days or weeks. Early diagnosis and treatment are essential to prevent destruction of tissues of the eye and other complications, such as arthritis.[3,67]

### Nursing problems

Nursery infection control programs are well outlined in the 1976 revision of *Standards and Recommendations for Hospital Care of Newborn Infants* published by the American Academy of Pediatrics. The elaborate rituals that grew out of the staphylococci epidemics are no longer practiced, but sound control measures based on scientific evidence have become vitally important in the day-to-day conduct of safe nursery care. The single most important practice in infection protection is *thorough handwashing* by every individual who comes in contact with any infant. Nurses who handle and care for several infants frequently are identified as the source of infection transmission from equipment to infant to another infant in rapid succession. Physicians, technicians, and parents can enter and safely handle infants within a nursery as long as the principle of careful hand-washing with an effective antiseptic agent is observed. Regular culturing of organisms from equipment and selective culturing of organisms taken from personnel are important features of adequate infection control programs. The information obtained gives the best basis for sterilization procedures, cleaning, and storage of equipment and other items used in the care of infants. Special isolation of infected infants is not usually indicated if the nursery area is not unduly crowded and an adequate program to prevent the spread of infection is in effect.

Umbilical catheters and other equipment used in intravenous fluid administration provide a dangerous potential source of direct infection and must be continually evaluated for the safety of methods in sterilization, storage, and use.[119]

Administration of drugs used in the treatment of neonatal infection is an important aspect of nursing care of the infected neonate. There are only a limited number of antibiotics available for safe administration during the neonatal period, and the fact that the causative organisms are not known at the time that therapy must begin greatly complicates the therapeutic decisions that must be made. Cultures are obtained before therapy is instituted, and a decision regarding the choice of drug must be made based on known infection patterns. The fact that bacterial organisms develop drug-resistant strains further frustrates efforts to effectively treat neonatal infections.[60,78,85,106]

Drug interactions are an important factor in their administration, particularly when they are being administered intravenously. Thorough familiarity with the manufacturer's recommendations regarding the use of the drug should be obtained before it is administered.

Table 8-5 indicates antibiotics used in treatment of newborn infections, the dose, route of administration, indications for use, and known hazards to the infant.

The safe intramuscular administration of drugs to a newborn infant is of utmost impor-tance. The small premature infant particularly has very poorly developed muscular and subcutaneous tissue, and the only acceptable site for injection is the anterior lateral thigh. Blood vessels and major nerve pathways are close to other available sites in older infants. The problem is complicated when the infant must receive frequent injections over a prolonged period of time, because the tissue available for administration is subject to becoming necrotic and painful. Meticulous attention to the location of a suitable, safe site, with sound technique of administration, is imperative.[3,11]

## Hematologic disturbances
### Pathophysiologic considerations

Blood volume of the newborn infant is approximately 90 mg/kg of body weight, but this volume may be significantly altered by the time that the cord is clamped at delivery. As much as one third of the total fetal blood volume is contained in the placenta at the time of birth, and approximately half of this volume is transferred to the infant within a minute after delivery if the cord is not clamped. In prematurely born infants the practice of late clamping of the cord is believed to result in some benefit by raising the blood volume and the hemoglobin level.

Capillary fragility and permeability, which are characteristic of the premature infant, result in extravascular leakage of plasma constituents. This is thought to be a primary mechanism producing both the edema commonly noted in the premature infant and the slight rise in hemoglobin level that occurs during the first week of life. The premature infant, however, is in serious jeopardy of anemia for several months after birth, because the ability to produce red blood cells is not sufficient to meet the demands of rapid body growth. In addition the life span of red blood cells is shortened, and hemolysis is not compensated by erythropoietic processes for several weeks.[69,80]

Most premature infants have high concentrations of fetal hemoglobin, which is the primary form of hemoglobin formed during fetal life. Fetal hemoglobin possesses, for reasons not totally understood, a greater affinity for oxygen than does adult hemoglobin. This is one factor that may account for the neonate's ability to

**Table 8-5.** Antibiotic therapy*

| Drug | Dose | Indication | Hazards |
|---|---|---|---|
| Kanamycin sulfate<br>Limit to 7-12 days<br>Supplied as Kantrex<br>(75 mg/2 ml) | 15 mg/kd/day, divided into two doses (IM) | Gram-negative pathogens, coliform bacteria, *Proteus, Neisseria,* and *Mycobacterium* | Ototoxic if dose excessive or prolonged; renal damage, particularly if fluid intake low |
| Gentamicin | Less than 7 days: 5 mg/kg/24 hr (IM) divided into 2 doses; more than 7 days: 7.5 mg/kg/24 hr in 3 doses | *Klebsiella-Aerobacter, Pseudomonas, Proteus,* staphylococci, *Escherichia coli, Salmonella* | Toxic to vestibular system; nephrotoxic |
| Potassium penicillin G (aqueous) | 50,000-100,000 units/kg/24 hr, divided into 2 doses (IM or IV) for infants less than 7 days; for older infant, divide into 3 doses | Hemolytic streptococci, pneumococci, and some strains of staphylococci | Procaine products avoided when muscle mass reduced |
| Ampicillin | 50 mg/kg/24 hr (IM or IV); divided in 2 doses for infants less than 7 days; preterm infants over 7 days, 100 mg/kg/24 hr in 3 doses; term infants over 7 days of age, 150 mg/kg/24 hr in 3 doses | Most gram-positive organisms, most gram-negative organisms, *Salmonella, Haemophilus influenzae, Streptococcus faecalis, Proteus mirabilis,* and *Escherichia coli* | Dangers not delineated for newborn infant |
| Nafcillin, sodium methicillin (Staphcillin) | 100 mg/kg/24 hr, divided into 2 doses (IM or IV) for infant under 7 days; 200-300 mg/kg/24 hr in 4 doses for infants over 7 days | Penicillinase-resistant staphylococci | Low order of toxicity |
| Carbenicillin | 200-400 mg/kg/24 hr (IV), divided in 3 doses for infants under 7 days; 4 doses for older infants | *Pseudomonas, Proteus* | SGOT elevation |
| Colistimethate sodium (Colistin), 5-7 days | 5-8 mg/kg/24 hr, divided into 2 doses (deep IM) | *Pseudomonas* | Nephrotoxicity; overgrowth of *Candida* |
| Polymyxin B sulfate, 5-7 days | 3.5 to 5 mg/kg/24 hr, divided into 2 doses (IM) | *Pseudomonas* | May have cumulative nephrotoxicity with kanamycin |
| Neomycin | 50-100 mg/kg/24 hr, in 4 doses (by mouth only) | Pathogenic *Escherichia coli* and gram-negative organisms producing diarrhea | No significant intolerance |
| Nystatin (Mycostatin) | 200,000 units, divided into 4 doses daily (by mouth only) | Local candidal infections | No significant intolerance |
| Amphotericin B | 0.25-1 mg/kg/24 hr (by slow IV infusion) | Systemic yeast and fungous infections | Gastroenteritis; nephrotoxicity; dangers not specified for immature infant |

*From Babson, S. G., Benson, R. C., Pernoll, M. L., and Benda, G. I.: Management of high risk and intensive care of the newborn, ed. 3, St. Louis, 1975, The C. V. Mosby Co., pp. 122-123.

withstand longer periods of oxygen deprivation and for his tolerance of a $Po_2$ level that is lower than that tolerated by the adult.[90]

The breakdown of erythrocytes occurs as a natural physiologic process as the life span of these cells ends and the components of the cells are catabolized. The life span of the neonatal red cell is shorter than the adult cell (from 80 to 100 days as compared to 120 days for the adult). The hemoglobin molecule of the cell is broken into the heme and globin fragments. Globin is a protein and is utilized by the body as such. The heme fragment is formed into unconjugated (indirect reacting) bilirubin in the reticuloendothelial cells, which are located primarily in the spleen and liver. This form of bilirubin is bound to albumin in the plasma through a special affinity between the two molecules. In this bound form it cannot leave the vascular space and penetrate the cells. The bound unconjugated bilirubin is transported to the liver; to the extent that it is freed from the albumin molecule it enters the liver cells, where conjugation with the glucuronide radical occurs. This process involves a complex series of reactions that depends upon many factors, including a supply of oxygen, glucose, and the enzyme glucuronyl transferase. The conjugated form of bilirubin (direct reacting) is water-soluble as compared to the fat-soluble unconjugated (indirect reacting) form, and the water-soluble form can be excreted through the gastrointestinal and renal systems effectively. In the normal newborn the activity of glucuronyl transferase is greatly diminished, resulting in a significantly decreased ability to conjugate bilirubin. This results in an elevated level of bilirubin until the enzymatic activity of glucuronyl transferase becomes functional.

In about half of all term neonates the level of bilirubin exceeds 4 to 6 mg/100 ml of serum and becomes visible as a yellow pigment in the skin on the third day of life, and not before. The unconjugated, unbound form of bilirubin is available to invade skin and unmyelinated nerve tissues. When this quantity is excessive and the invasion of these tissues is great, damage to central nervous system tissue occurs, and the infant is subjected to permanent effects of kernicterus.[22,76] The exact level at which damage occurs is not known, but therapy is usually considered when the unconjugated form in the serum exceeds 12 mg/100 ml.[67]

The elevation of bilirubin and the resulting jaundice that occurs during the normal course of neonatal life are usually resolved spontaneously by the end of the first week, and the infant suffers no undesirable effects. For the premature infant, this phenomenon occurs as in the term infant, but the bilirubin level rises more rapidly and the jaundice will be apparent by 48 hours of life, resolving more gradually through the ninth or tenth day. A number of abnormal conditions may cause hyperbilirubinemia and jaundice, which are entirely unrelated to this usual physiologic process. In addition the physiologic process may be exaggerated by an abnormal condition, such as polycythemia, or by an increased number of red blood cells, as might occur with an excessive placental transfusion at the time of birth.[3,67]

Infants who are breast-fed occasionally experience a period of hyperbilirubinemia and jaundice appearing during the second week after breast-feeding is initiated and persisting for as long as three to ten weeks. Temporary discontinuation of breast-feeding may be necessary if the levels of unconjugated bilirubin rise to potentially dangerous levels, but permanent interference with breast-feeding is not indicated. A form of pregnanediol, which is excreted in breast milk, is thought to temporarily interfere with the infant's glucuronyl transferase activity. Undesirable effects of the elevated bilirubin level may be inhibited by the advanced myelinization of nervous tissue that has occurred by the age that breast milk hyperbilirubinemia appears.

### Common hematologic medical diagnoses

**Anemia.** The premature infant's natural propensity for anemia has been described in a previous section. In addition, anemia can be caused by blood loss and by a number of primary disorders. An initial measurement of the infant's hematocrit at birth can serve as a useful baseline from which to determine serious conditions leading to the development of anemia. Blood loss in the infant can occur as a result of fetal-maternal transfusion in utero, bleeding from tearing of the cord or placenta, fetal rupture of the spleen or liver, loss of blood to the placenta resulting from holding the infant above the level of the placenta before clamping of the cord, birth trauma, inadequate cord clamping, coagulation defects, and hemolytic disorders such as erythroblastosis fetalis, red blood cell enzyme defects, or drug-induced disorders of the blood. Infection, insufficient iron intake, and vitamin E deficiency may also be associated with anemia. Frequent and continuous sampling of the blood of the small premature infant can become a source of chronic blood loss, substantial enough in amount to require replacement of blood volume. Transfusions are often required to maintain an adequate hemoglobin level for the premature infant, particularly if the blood loss is serious and sudden, if the infant has an underlying hematologic disorder, or suffers from the shock syndrome.[3,67]

**Polycythemia.** Polycythemia is present when the venous hematocrit is over 65% or the hemoglobin is over 22 g/100 ml. It occurs when the fetus receives a transfusion of blood from the placenta before or after birth or from a twin in utero. It also occurs as a result of increased erythropoiesis in small-for-date infants, dysmature infants, and infants who experienced chronic fetal distress. The infant usually has a flushed appearance and may not exhibit any other symptoms. Symptoms such as lethargy, poor feeding, cyanosis, seizures, grunting respirations, hyperbilirubinemia, and heart failure are usually indicative of hyperviscosity of the blood. Partial exchange transfusion with plasma is used to lower the venous hematocrit to approximately 55%.[3,67]

**Thrombocytopenia.** Thrombocytopenia is a severe deficiency of platelets in the blood, which are essential for effective coagulation. Platelets are below 50,000/mm$^3$ and often fall below 10,000/mm$^3$. Petechial hemorrhages are visible over the entire body and head of the infant. This condition occurs in association with severe infections, severe erythroblastosis fetalis, congenital leukemia, autoimmune responses from the mother, and as a result of maternal drugs, particularly thiazides. Treatment of the underlying condition is essential, and platelet transfusions may be used to reduce the bleeding tendency.[3,67]

**Hyperbilirubinemia.** The expected physiologic course of the newborn infant was described above with regard to destruction of red blood cells. Hyperbilirubinemia can occur as a result of this process, in conjunction with infections, congenital enzyme deficiency, congenital red blood cell abnormality, an enclosed hemorrhage, such as cephalhematoma, or can be induced by drug toxicity.

Maternal-fetal blood group incompatibility, usually a difference in Rh or ABO factors, is the most commonly occurring cause of abnormal red blood cell destruction in the newborn. The mother's blood contains antibodies against the blood factor of the fetus, and these are transmitted across the placenta, attacking the fetal red blood cells—a condition known as erythroblastosis fetalis. When the disorder is severe, hydrops and fatal damage to the fetus can occur before birth. When damage has not progressed to this point, the infant is subject to a prolonged period of hyperbilirubinemia and anemia due to the continuing destruction of red blood cells by the maternal antibodies that continue to circulate in the infant's system. Exchange transfusion with blood that will not be destroyed by the maternal antibodies is the treatment employed, and this procedure, though beset with many hazards of its own, can enable an infant to survive without damage until his own blood cells are produced in sufficient amounts to sustain life without the hazard of destruction from maternal antibodies.[3]

The development of maternal antibodies in Rh-negative mothers may now be prevented with the use of anti-D gamma globulin to unsensitized mothers. Total prevention of this newborn disease is thus possible, but it is imperative that the drug be administered at every occasion when sensitization is possible, that is, with every delivery or abortion.[59,84]

### Nursing problems

Procedures that must be undertaken for an infant who suffers hematologic disorders are often complicated and hazardous. Blood transfusions to replace blood loss or to exchange the infant's blood volume require intensive, expert medical and nursing supervision. The infant's fluid and electrolyte balance is severely jeopardized during these replacements, and heart failure may occur as an effect of the procedure. Undesirable reactions to donor blood occur in newborns as in older persons. Infection is a routine hazard of blood administration, and the nurse must be alert to this complication in the hours following the procedure.[16,84]

The administration of albumin increases significantly the capacity of the blood to carry bilirubin and to attract it from extravascular tissue into the circulation, where it is available for transfer through the hepatic excretion system. This enhances the excretion of bilirubin and is often employed in conjunction with exchange transfusions. Certain drugs, notably the sulfa

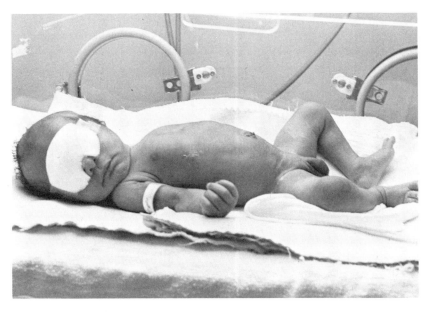

**Fig. 8-12.** High-intensity fluorescent lights provide phototherapy for the infant.

drugs, compete for the albumin binding sites available to bilirubin and significantly decrease the excretion of bilirubin from the body.[116]

Phototherapy for hyperbilirubinemia (Fig. 8-12) demands careful nursing attention to the adequacy of function of the equipment. The high-intensity light used in therapy may be damaging to the retina of the eye, and for protection a shield must be maintained over the eyes.[67,75,89,112] During this treatment the nurse must be aware of the infant's needs for periodic visual stimulation and physical cuddling and of the mother's needs to establish eye-to-eye contact with the infant. These aspects of care are discussed in earlier sections, but they bear special mention here. Many infants who undergo this procedure are essentially healthy with no condition that justifies disruption of the provision of adequate family-centered care. However, the isolation that occurs when the infant is placed under intense lighting too frequently leads to disruption of such care.[3,67,81,94,120]

## Neuromuscular and structural tissue disorders

### Pathophysiologic considerations

The basic structure of the skin, bone, muscle, and nervous systems is completed before the time of viability, and development of these tissues is thought to continue for the preterm infant as it would in the intrauterine environment, unless adversely affected by events after delivery. Abnormal neurologic signs for gestational age are therefore considered to most often be the result of adverse effects after delivery and constitute the major concern with regard to long-term prognosis for the infant.

Abnormal neurologic signs frequently occur and may be either transient or persistent. Because of the immaturity of central nervous system myelination, the infant's response to specific stimuli is generalized, and signs such as hyperirritability, exaggerated response to stimuli, localized twitching, rhythmic repetitive jerks of one or more muscle groups (myoclonus), cannot be correlated with a specific central nervous system lesion. Such signs occur in association with a wide range of problems, as described below.

Cerebrospinal fluid volume appears to be proportionately increased over that of a fetus of the same age or the term infant. This may account for a widened area of transillumination that persists even after 40 weeks of gestational age is reached.

Behavior of the premature infant is recog-    **243**

nized to be different from either that of the fetus at a comparable gestational age or the term infant. The origin of typical premature behavior is not known but is thought to arise from the fact of neurologic stimuli that occur at birth, hypoxia, or any number of other chemical stimuli that occur as a sequela to premature birth. The infant's behavior includes jerky movements of the extremities occurring frequently, even during sleep, a muted cry, and frequent facial grimaces, even though the infant's muscle tone is generally flaccid.

Asymmetry of movement or muscle tone is abnormal at any gestational age and may be associated with injury to the nervous system, paralysis, or bone fracture. Hypotonia is related to a wide range of disorders, including low gestational age, genetic disorders such as Down's syndrome, and hypoxia.

Abnormalities of bony structures are congenital anomalies arising from hereditary influences or intrauterine exposure to teratogenic substances such as drugs or viruses. Surgical intervention is often required for partial or complete correction of the abnormality or to provide for the survival of the infant. Such abnormalities often give rise to other problems during the neonatal period, such as feeding problems or fluid and electrolyte and acid-base balance problems.[3,67]

### Common neuromuscular and structural tissue disorders diagnoses

**Seizures and hyperactivity.** Seizures and hyperactivity must be differentiated from the typical jerky movements exhibited by the preterm infant. A severe tremor of an extremity, sometimes of prolonged duration, or generalized body convulsions, are usually indicative of serious underlying pathology and a poor prognosis for the infant. Approximately 30% of infants exhibiting convulsions die. Less than half of those infants who survive achieve intact neurologic function later in life. The earlier the convulsion appears, the more serious is the infant's prognosis. Seizures and hyperactivity occur as a result of fetal or neonatal asphyxia, intracranial hemorrhage, meningitis, hypoglycemia, hypocalcemia and other metabolic imbalances, and in association with various congenital malforma-

tions. When a convulsion is observed, the infant is placed in an incubator with oxygen supplementation, intravenous solutions are instituted for symptomatic relief, and diagnostic laboratory measures are obtained. The recommended intravenous solutions are 25% glucose, 2 to 4 ml, 10% calcium gluconate solution, 1 to 2 ml/kg of body weight, and 50% solution of magnesium sulfate, 0.1 to 0.2 ml/kg of body weight. Phenobarbital sodium may be used to control convulsions if they persist.[3,6,67,123]

**Lethargy and hypotonia.** A premature infant whose obligatory reflexes are absent or depressed for the age of maturity may have suffered asphyxia during birth or some other form of injury. Any change from an active to a relatively inactive state is a sign for alarm during the newborn period, as such a change is often the first and only sign of impending serious illness. The most commonly associated conditions in which lethargy emerges early are intracranial hemorrhage, infection (primarily meningitis), hypoglycemia, and fluid and electrolyte imbalance. Measures must be taken to determine the underlying cause and treat the infant appropriately.[3,67]

**Hydrocephalus and microcephalus.** Detecting abnormal changes in head size after birth requires an accurate head measurement at birth recorded and charted on a growth graph. Head size above 2 standard deviations from the mean for the infant's gestational age is suspect for hemorrhage, inflammation, or congenital hydrocephalus. An infant whose head size increases more than 1.2 cm/week for a three-week period should also be regarded as having a possible disorder in head size and brain growth. As the infant matures, an increase in the size of the head suggests obstruction of spinal fluid circulation or the effects of fluid accumulation from sodium retention or hypoproteinemia. The infant may exhibit bulging of the frontal fontanel, separation of the cranial sutures, excessive head growth, and asymmetric or extensive transillumination of the head (see Chapter 18).

A head size below 2 SD from the mean for gestational age may indicate an injured or maldeveloped brain, and the infant should be observed for continued overlapping of sutures, inadequate growth in head circumference (under 0.7 cm/week), and developmental delay.[3,67]

**Infants of drug-addicted mothers.** The teratogenic effects of drugs taken during pregnancy has been discussed in Chapter 5. Drugs that cause maternal addiction may lead to congenital malformations but also lead to addiction in the fetus and the resulting necessity for withdrawal after delivery. Barbiturates, alcohol, amphetamines, and narcotics have all been observed to cause withdrawal symptoms in the newborn. Heroine addiction has produced particularly serious effects in the newborn infant. Symptoms of withdrawal vary but usually occur within 24 hours of birth. If the mother was on methadone, withdrawal can begin as late as two to three weeks after birth. Common symptoms include hypertonicity, irritability, tremors, vomiting, and diarrhea. Occasional symptoms include tachypnea, elevation of temperature, convulsions, and a high-pitched cry. Drugs may be used to control central nervous system symptoms, and close attention must be given to nutritional intake and fluid and electrolyte balance. The blood glucose level must be carefully monitored, with early intervention for hypoglycemia.*

### Nursing problems

The major nursing challenge related to problems of the neuromuscular system is prevention of events that might cause harmful effects to the premature infant's neuromuscular system. Monitoring to prevent and detect early periods of apnea, support of respirations, and careful behavioral observation of the infant are fundamental to preserving the infant's intact neurologic capacity. Skill and expertise in early intervention when a problem is detected is also essential.

Nursing planning and implementation of the infant stimulation program described earlier in this chapter is another important nursing measure related to development of the neuromuscular system. Planned stimulation should be carefully balanced with measures to provide rest, particularly when the infant is critically ill. During such periods the amount of handling and unnecessary stimulation should be minimal

---

*References 3, 72, 95, 98, 101, 126.

to conserve the infant's limited energy resources.

Postsurgical care for the newborn incorporates all measures of health maintenance, with particular attention to maintaining adequate gas exchange, provision of nutrition, acid-base and fluid and electrolyte balance, and prevention of infection. Involvement of the parents as the primary care-givers should be maintained, with particular nursing care directed to meeting their needs for understanding the surgical procedure and the infant's progress.

## Metabolic problems

Many of the limitations of the preterm infant's ability to maintain homeostasis have been discussed in detail. Of particular concern are limitations in pulmonary and renal function, as well as immaturity of enzyme systems. Metabolic problems during the newborn period are related primarily to renal function and function of the enzyme systems. The most common metabolic problems are hypoglycemia and hypocalcemia. Either of these problems can occur in conjunction with many of the neonatal problems discussed in previous chapters, or they can occur as a single problem.

### Medical diagnoses related to metabolism

**Hypoglycemia.** Normal blood sugar concentrations fluctuate widely in the newborn as in the older individual. However, concentrations that persist below 30 mg/100 ml in term infants or below 20 mg/100 ml in low birth weight infants are considered to be the lower limits of tolerance. Blood sugar levels become abnormally low if gluconeogenesis in the liver is diminished. if insulin production is excessive, or if the carbohydrate-regulating hormones, such as cortisol, epinephrine, and glucagon, are deficient. Table 8-6 indicates the most common forms of hypoglycemia during infancy and the underlying pathologic mechanism for each.

During fetal life, the heart, skeletal muscle, and the liver of the fetus store glycogen, reaching levels above those found in adults. However, in the face of fetal distress, these stores are rapidly depleted. At birth the normal energy cost of respiration, thermoregulation, and muscle activity quickly depletes even the nor-

**Table 8-6.** Causes of neonatal hypoglycemia*

| Clinical entity | Mechanism | Duration |
|---|---|---|
| Intrauterine malnutrition | Low liver glycogen store | Transient |
| Fetal asphyxia | Glycogen depletion | Transient |
| Cold stress | Glycogen depletion | Transient |
| CNS hemorrhage | Unknown | Transient |
| CNS malformation | Unknown | Transient |
| Adrenal hemorrhage, insufficiency | Ineffective catecholamine response | Transient |
| Infants of diabetic mothers | Increased plasma insulin activity | Transient |
| Erythroblastotic infants | Increased plasma insulin activity | Transient |
| Maternal tolbutamide, chlorpropamide | Hyperinsulinism | Transient |
| Abrupt stop of intravenous glucose, ≥10% | Hyperinsulinism | Transient |
| Glycogen storage disease (types I and II) | Defective glycogen breakdown | Protracted |
| Galactose intolerance (galactosemia) | Defective conversion of galactose to glucose | Protracted |
| Islet cell tumor | Hyperinsulinism | Protracted |
| Cyanotic congenital heart disease with congestive failure | Unknown | Transient |
| Hypopituitarism | Adrenal insufficiency | Protracted |
| Septicemia | Unknown | Transient |

*From Korones, S. B.: High risk newborn infants; the basis for intensive nursing care, ed. 2, St. Louis, 1976, The C. V. Mosby Co., p. 205.

mal term infant's glycogen stores, and several days may be required to restore sufficient glycogen stores to a level at which the infant can withstand stress. A serious danger exists for the infant whose glycogen stores are depleted, in that blood glucose is the sole source of energy that can be used for metabolism in the brain.

The symptoms of hypoglycemia are subtle and not specific to the disorder. Table 8-7 indicates the most frequently observed symptoms associated with hypoglycemia, and the approximate percentage of incidence of these symptoms among symptomatic infants. The determination of hypoglycemia rests solely with blood sugar determinations, as defined above.[67,91,93,113,122]

Infants of diabetic mothers deserve particular mention, for the incidence of pregnancy for diabetic women has increased considerably as effective means of management of diabetes has been developed. The incidence of congenital defects, illness, and death is high for these infants, even though at birth they may appear to be normal infants. During fetal life, the fetal pancreatic islet cells are overstimulated to produce insulin, probably in an effort to supply insulin for the mother and to combat the high blood glucose level in the fetal circulation. After birth, the infant's islet cells continue to produce excessive amounts of insulin, which produces hypoglycemia within two to four hours.

**Table 8-7.** Nonspecific symptoms occurring with neonatal hypoglycemia

| Symptom | Approximate percentage of incidence among all symptomatic infants |
|---|---|
| Tremors | 75% |
| Cyanosis | 75% |
| Convulsions | 50% |
| Apnea, irregular respirations | 50% |
| Listlessness | 25% |

This fetal pathophysiology is associated with excessive growth and development of fatty tissue, so that these infants are large for gestational age. Because of the rising prevalence of gestational diabetes, which may go undetected during pregnancy, all infants born large for gestational age must be observed for signs of neonatal complications, and the mother evaluated for this condition.[3,44,67]

**Hypocalcemia.** Deficiencies in calcium are common among preterm infants, with reduced parathyroid activity and renal immaturity. Approximately 30% of preterm infants weighing less than 2,000 g birth weight develop hypocalcemia (less than 7 mg/100 ml) before 48 hours of age. Various forms of stress during the neonatal period lead to hypocalcemia, such as asphyxia, which tends to cause increased corticosteroid and thyrocalcitonin release, which in turn can result in lowered serum calcium. Treatment of acidosis with bicarbonate tends to decrease the ionized portion of serum calcium. Symptoms of hypocalcemia, like those of hypoglycemia, are difficult to detect. They include twitching of the extremities, jitteriness, a high-pitched cry, and seizures.[3,67]

### Nursing problems

The major focus of nursing care is prevention and early detection and intervention. Screening all infants for hypoglycemia during the first three days of life is an important measure in detecting infants who are not suspected of being in danger from hypoglycemia. A dextrostix indication of blood sugar below 50 mg/100 ml indicates the need for oral intake of glucose to prevent further development of hypoglycemia. Early feeding of infants as a preventive measure has been discussed earlier in this chapter.

## Gastrointestinal problems
### Pathophysiology

The premature infant has several traits of immaturity and deficient function of the gastrointestinal tract that give rise to a variety of problems, several of which have been discussed previously in this chapter. The sucking reflex is often weak, and the infant has limited or no ability to take oral feedings. The cardiac sphincter of the immature infant is lax and intestinal mobility is depressed, causing easy regurgitation and delay in evacuation of the intestinal tract. Intestinal enzyme mechanisms are immature and may not be able to provide for complete digestion and absorption. The capacity of the stomach may not be sufficient to accommodate the calorie and fluid requirements of the small infant. Many gastrointestinal problems of the newborn are congenital abnormalities, requiring surgical intervention for the infant to sustain life.[3,67]

### Common gastrointestinal medical diagnoses

**Necrotizing enterocolitis.** Necrotizing enterocolitis has been recently recognized and described as a significant problem among high risk infants, occurring in approximately 5% of all infants admitted to intensive care setting. It is often fatal for the infant, and the etiology is un-

known. It appears to be associated with stress such as hypoxia or infection. The illness is characterized by ischemic necrosis of the gastrointestinal tract leading to perforation. Surgical intervention is often indicated to remove seriously damaged portions of the tract in order to prevent perforation. The infant begins to retain gastric contents, vomit bile-stained fluid, has abdominal distension, apneic episodes, poor skin color, and palpable loops of the bowel. Gastrointestinal feedings must be discontinued promptly and parenteral alimentation used until the gastrointestinal tract heals sufficiently to tolerate resumption of intake.*

## Death of an infant

Death is a relatively frequent experience in high risk newborn care centers and occasionally occurs in all newborn care settings. Death is a very difficult experience for all concerned, including the family and the health care professionals who have cared for the infant and the mother. The discussion of facilitating family interactions in this chapter laid the foundation for working with the family of the infant who is dying or who has died. The health care professional group must give some time and attention to dealing with their own feelings and establish mutual understanding of how they as a group will work with the family of the infant who is in danger of dying or who dies. The usual inclination of health care workers has been to protect the family from involvement with the seriously ill or dying newborn in an effort to ease the suffering they experience. As was discussed earlier, even though the family may have great difficulty in dealing with this crisis, their involvement and contact with the actual events experienced by the infant facilitates eventual resolution of the grief that they experience.

During periods when the infant's prognosis is grave, families often begin expecting the infant to die and begin to grieve for the infant. Their unwillingness to maintain contact with the infant must be acknowledged and honored, but every effort made to help them maintain a guarded optimism and understand the accurate conditions that exist for the infant. Close early

---

*References 3, 9, 49, 67, 86, 104.

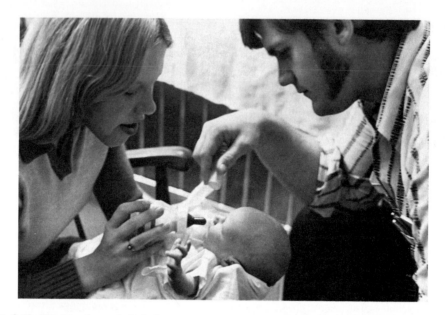

**Fig. 8-13.** "We have to say hello before we can say goodbye." Shawn Griffin Cox has an inoperable congenital heart defect and a life expectancy of only a few days or weeks. Close early contact with their infant is valued by the parents in "making the most" of the time they have with their son. (Name used at the request of the parents.)

contact with the infant who eventually dies or suffers long-lasting handicaps is of crucial benefit in the family's adjustment to the actual outcome and shattered hopes.

After the death of the infant the family should be given the opportunity to come to the nursery and to see and hold their infant in privacy, with some one of the health care team present if they so desire. They may need time to ask questions and to talk about their feelings. Often there are overwhelming feelings of guilt and failure; offering reassurance of the infant's condition leading to death may help the family begin to construct a realistic understanding of the facts of the death. In working through the death over the weeks to come, the family may need to return to the nursery and talk with the nurses and physicians who cared for the infant. Continued counseling should be available to assist them in this grief work.[67,108,135]

## STUDY QUESTIONS

1. Determine the location of the neonatal intensive care unit that serves your geographic area. If possible, visit this facility and describe the particular services that it offers to newborns, their families, medical and nursing personnel in surrounding institutions, and the research that is being conducted in relation to medical and nursing care.

2. Describe in your own words the interrelationships that exist between the control of fluid and electrolyte balance in the newborn infant and the respiratory, circulatory, hematologic, and renal systems.

3. Investigate the specific features of a congenital malformation and describe the nursing care considerations that particularly relate to the maintenance of fluid and electrolyte metabolism and exchange of gases. Also, describe the specialized nursing considerations that are imposed by the malformation.

4. Study the medical and nursing record of an infant who has undergone surgery during the neonatal period. Indicate the nursing care problems that were identified in relation to the infant's needs. Discuss these in relation to the ideas presented in this chapter.

5. Compare the composition of breast and cow's milk. Indicate the special advantages of each in the light of the nutritional needs of premature infants. How can the deficiencies of each be compensated?

6. Interview a member of the nursery health care team in a nursery, either intensive care or one that offers care to all newborn infants. Describe the ways in which this nursery promotes the parent-child relationship during the newborn period, with particular attention to the care for the family when an infant is premature or ill. In what ways does this individual see that changes could be made to enhance parent-child interaction during hospitalization?

## REFERENCES

1. Affonso, D., and Harris, T.: Continuous positive airway pressure, Am. J. Nurs. **76:**570, April, 1976.
2. Babson, S. G.: Feeding the low-birth-weight infant, J. Pediatr. **79:**694, Oct., 1971.
3. Babson, S. G., Benson, R. C., Pernoll, M. L., and Benda, G. I.: Management of high-risk pregnancy and intensive care of the newborn, ed. 3, St. Louis, 1975, The C. V. Mosby Co.
4. Babson, S. G., and Henderson, N. B.: Fetal undergrowth, relation of head growth to later intellectual performance, Pediatrics **53:**890, June, 1974.
5. Barnard, M. U.: Supportive nursing care for the mother and newborn who are separated from each other, Mat. Child Nurs. **1:**107, March-April 1976.
6. Berger, A., Sharf, B., and Witer, S. T.: Pronounced tremors in newborn infants; their meaning and prognostic significance, Clin. Pediatr. **14:**834, Sept., 1975.
7. Black, I. F. S., Kotrapu, N., and Massie, H.: Application of Doppler ultrasound to blood pressure measurement in small infants, J. Pediatr. **81:**932, Nov., 1972.
8. Blennow, G., Svenningsen, M. W., and Almquist, B.: Noise levels in infant incubators (adverse effects?), Pediatrics **53:**29, Jan., 1973.
9. Bliss, V. J.: Nursing care for infants with neonatal necrotizing enterocolitis, Mat. Child Nurs. **1:**37, Jan.-Feb., 1976.
10. Boros, S. J., and Reynolds, J. W.: Prolonged apnea of prematurity; treatment with continuous airway distending pressure delivered by nasopharyngeal tube, Clin. Pediatr. **15:**123, Feb., 1976.
11. Brandt, P. S., Smith, M. E., Ashburn, S. S., and Graves, J.: Intramuscular injections in children, Am. J. Nurs. **72:**1402, Aug., 1972.
12. Brans, Y. W., and others: Feeding the low birth weight infant; orally or parenterally? Preliminary results of a comparative study, Pediatrics **54:**15, July, 1974.
13. Brazelton, T. B.: Neonatal behavior assessment scale (Clinics in developmental medicine, No. 50), Philadelphia, 1973, J. B. Lippincott.
14. Brown, J., and Hepler, R.: Stimulation—a corollary to physical care, Am. J. Nurs. **76:**578, April, 1976.
15. Butani, P.: Reactions of mothers to the birth of an anomalous infant; a review of the literature, Mat. Child Nurs. J. **3:**59, Spring 1974.
16. Canale, V. C.: The acute anemias of the perinatal period. In Abramson, H., editor: Resuscitation of the newborn infant and related emergency procedures; principles and practice, ed. 3, St. Louis, 1973, The C. V. Mosby Co., p. 249.
17. Cashore, W. J., Sedaghatian, M. R., and Usher, R. H.: Nutritional supplements in small premature infants, Pediatrics **56:**8, July 1975.
18. Chernick, V.: Continuous negative chest wall pressure therapy for hyaline membrane disease, PCNA **20:**407, May 1973.
19. Chinn, P. L.: Infant gavage feeding, Am. J. Nurs. **71:**1964, Oct., 1971.
20. Cranley, M. S.: When a high risk infant is born, Am. J. Nurs. **75:**1696, 1975.
21. Creasy, R. K., and Parker, J. T.: Prenatal care and diagnosis. In Rudolf, A. N., editor: Pediatrics, ed. 16, New York, 1977, Appleton-Century-Crofts, p. 121.
22. Crichton, J. U., and others: Long-term effects of neonatal jaundice on brain function in children of low birth weight, Pediatrics **49:**656-670, May, 1972.
23. Cumarasamy, N., and others: Artificial ventilation in hyaline membrane disease; the use of positive end-expiratory pressure and continuous positive airway pressure, Pediatrics **51:**629, April, 1973.
24. Dallman, P. R.: Iron, vitamin E, and folate in the preterm infant, J. Pediatr. **85:**742, Dec., 1974.
25. Davidson, M.: Formula feeding of normal term and low birth weight infants, Pediatr. Clin. North Am. **17:**913, Nov., 1970.
26. Deaton, D. W., and others: Oxygen administration for neonatal intensive care, J. Pediatr. **80:**1039-1041, June, 1972.
27. Dorand, R. D., Cook, L. N., and Andrews, B. F.: Umbilical vessel catheterization; the low incidence of complications in a series of 200 newborn infants, Clin. Pediatr. **16:**569, June, 1977.
28. Drotar, D., and others: The adaptation of parents to the birth of an infant with a congenital malformation, Pediatrics **56:**710, Nov., 1975.
29. DuBrow, I. W., Chen, J. W., and Wong, P. W. K.: Bradycardia preceding apneic attacks in low-birth-weight infants; the relationship of recognition and management, Clin. Pediatr. **15:**119, Feb., 1976.
30. DuHamel, T. R., Lin, S., Skelton, A., and Hantke, C.: Early parental perceptions and the high risk neonate, Clin. Pediatr. **13:**1052, Dec., 1974.
31. Eichenwald, H. F.: Bacterial infections of the newborn. In Abramson, H., editor: Resuscitation of the newborn infant, ed. 3, St. Louis, 1973, The C. V. Mosby Co., p. 326.
32. Eisengart, M. A., Gluck, L., and Kessen, M.: Early feeding of premature infants; effect on blood sugar and gross motor activity, Biol. Neonate **17:**151, 1971.
33. Escobedo, M. B., Barton, L. L., Marshall, R. E., and Zarkowsky, H.: The frequency of jaundice in neonatal bacterial infections, Clin. Pediatr. **13:**656, Aug., 1974.
34. Fanaroff, A. A., and others: Insensible water loss in low birth weight infants, Pediatrics **50:**236, 1972.
35. Fitzhardinge, P. M.: Growth and development in low-birth-weight infants, Pediatrics **56:**162, Aug., 1975.
36. Fomon, S. J.: Infant nutrition, ed. 2, Philadelphia, 1974, W. B. Saunders Co.
37. Franciosi, R. A., Knostman, J. D., and Zimmerman, R. A.: Group B streptococcal neonatal and infant infections, J. Pediatr. **82:**707, April, 1973.
38. Garvey, J.: Infant respiratory distress syndrome, Am. J. Nurs. **75:**614, April, 1975.
39. Gluck, L.: Surfactant: 1972, Pediatr. Clin. North Am. **19:**325, May, 1972.
40. Gluck, L., and Kulovich, M. V.: Fetal lung development; current concepts, Pediatr. Clin. North Am. **20:**367, May, 1973.

41. Goldman, H. I., and others: Late effects of early dietary protein intake on low-birth-weight infants, J. Pediatr. 85:764, Dec., 1974.

42. Grassy, R. G., and others: The growth and development of low birth weight infants receiving intensive neonatal care, Clin. Pediatr. 15:549, June, 1976.

43. Gregory, G. A., and others: Meconium aspiration, J. Pediatr. 85:848, Dec., 1974.

44. Guthrie, D. W., and Guthrie, R. A.: The infant of the diabetic mother, Am. J. Nurs. 74:2008, Dec., 1974.

45. Hable, K. A., and others: Klebsiella type 33 septicemia in an infant intensive care unit, J. Pediatr. 80: 920-924, June, 1972.

46. Hall, R. T., and Rhodes, P. G.: Pneumothorax and pneumomediastimum in infants with idiopathic respiratory syndrome receiving CPAP, Pediatrics 55:493, April, 1975.

47. Harris, C. H.: Some ethical and legal considerations in neonatal intensive care, Nurs. Clin. North Am. 8: 521, Sept., 1973.

48. Harrod, J. R., and others: Long-term follow-up of severe respiratory distress syndrome treated with IPPB, J. Pediatr. 84:277, Feb., 1974.

49. Hartline, J. V.: Continuous intragastric infusion of elemental diet, Clin. Pediatr. 16:1105, Dec., 1977.

50. Heird, W. C., Grebin, B., and Winters, R. W.: The stabilization of disorders of water, electrolyte and acid-base metabolism in newborn infants under intensive care. In Abramson, H., editor: Resuscitation of the newborn infant, ed. 3, St. Louis, 1973, The C. V. Mosby Co., p. 240.

51. Heird, W. C., and Winters, R. W.: Total parenteral nutrition, J. Pediatr. 86:2, Jan., 1975.

52. Hunt, C. E.: Capillary blood sampling in the infant; usefulness and limitations of two methods of sampling, compared with arterial blood, Pediatrics 51:501, March, 1973.

53. Hunt, J. V.: Long-term outlook for high-risk infants. In Rudolf, A. M., editor: Pediatrics, ed. 16, New York, 1977, Appleton-Century-Crofts, p. 183.

54. Indyk, L.: Monitoring in children. II. Temperature and blood pressure, Clin. Pediatr. 11:157, March, 1972.

55. James, L. S.: Physiology and biochemistry. In Abramson, H., editor: Resuscitation of the newborn infant and related emergency procedures; principles and practice, ed. 3, St. Louis, 1973, The C. V. Mosby Co.

56. Jaworski, A. A.: New premature weight chart for hospital use, Clin. Pediatr. 13:513, June, 1974.

57. Johnson, J. D., and others: Prognosis of children surviving with the aid of mechanical ventilation in the newborn period, J. Pediatr. 84:272, Feb., 1974.

58. Jonsen, A. R., Phibbs, R. H., Tooley, W. H., and Garland, M. J.: Critical issues in newborn intensive care; a conference report and policy proposal, Pediatrics 55:756, June, 1975.

59. Judelsohn, R. G.: Erythroblastosis; the potential for eradication, Am. J. Public Health 64:997, Oct., 1974.

60. Kaplan, J. M., and others: Pharmacologic studies in neonates given large dosages of ampicillin, J. Pediatr. 84:571, April, 1974.

61. Kattwinkel, J., and others: A device for administration of continuous positive airway pressure by the nasal route, Pediatrics 52:131, July, 1973.

62. Katz, V.: Auditory stimulation and development behavior of the premature infant, Nurs. Res. 20:196, May-June 1971.

63. Kennedy, J. C.: The high-risk maternal-infant acquaintance process, Nurs. Clin. North Am. 8:549, Sept., 1973.

64. Kilderberg, P., and Winters, R.: Infant feeding and blood acid-base status, Pediatrics 49:801-802, June, 1972.

65. Klaus, M. H., and Kennell, J. H.: Maternal-infant bonding; the impact of early separation or loss on family development, St. Louis, 1976, The C. V. Mosby Co.

66. Korones, S. B.: The immune response to perinatal infection. In Abramson, H., editor: Resuscitation of the newborn infant, ed. 3, St. Louis, 1973, The C. V. Mosby Co., p. 346.

67. Korones, S. B.: High risk newborn infants; the basis for intensive nursing care, ed. 2, St. Louis, 1976, The C. V. Mosby Co.

68. Ladimer, I.: Resuscitation of the newborn infant; legal and ethical aspects. In Abramson, H., editor: Resuscitation of the newborn infant; principles and practice, ed. 3, St. Louis, 1973, The C. V. Mosby Co., p. 366.

69. Lahey, M. E.: The erythrocyte; physiologic considerations. In Cooke, R. E., editor: The biologic basis of pediatric practice, New York, 1968, McGraw-Hill Book Co., p. 421.

70. Landwirth, J.: Continuous nasogastric infusion feedings of infants of low birth weight, Clin. Pediatr. 13: 603, July, 1974.

71. Leake, R. D., Loew, A. D., and Oh, W.: Retransfer of convalescent infants from newborn intensive care to community intermediate care nurseries, Clin. Pediatr. 15:293, March, 1976.

72. Lipsitz, P. J.: A proposed narcotic withdrawal score for use with newborn infants, Clin. Pediatr. 14:592, June, 1975.

73. Lister, G., Hoffman, J. I. E., and Rudolph, A. M.: Oxygen uptake in infants and children; a simple method for measurement, Pediatrics 53:656, May, 1974.

74. Lubchenco, L. O., Searls, D. T., and Brazie, J. V.: Neonatal mortality rate; relationship to birth weight and gestational age, J. Pediatr. 81:814-822, Oct., 1972.

75. Lucey, J. F.: Neonatal jaundice and phototherapy, Pediatr. Clin. North Am. 19:827, Nov., 1972.

76. Maisels, M. J.: Bilirubin; on understanding and influencing its metabolism in the newborn infant, Pediatr. Clin. North Am. 19:447, May, 1972.

77. Marks, F. H.: Infant incubators, Nurs. '72, 2:26, Nov. 1972.

78. McCracken, G. H., and others: Clinical pharmacology of penicillin in newborn infants, J. Pediatr. 82:692, April, 1973.

79. Mikal, S.: Homeostasis in man, Boston, 1967, Little, Brown and Co.

80. Miller, H. C.: Prematurity. In Cooke, R. E., editor: The biologic basis of pediatric practice, New York, 1968, McGraw-Hill Book Co., p. 1514.

81. Mims, L. C., and others: Phototherapy for neonatal hyperbilirubinemia—a dose-response relationship, J. Pediatr. 83:659, Oct., 1973.

82. Miyazaki, Y., Van Leeuwen, L., and Van Leeuwen, G.: Retrolental fibroplasia; a continuing dilemma for the pediatrician, Clin. Pediatr. 16:1091, Dec., 1977.

83. Moth, K. J., and Blackburn, M. G.: Temperature regulation in the neonate; a survey of the pathophysiology of thermal dynamics and of the principles of environmental control, Clin. Pediatr. 12:634, Nov., 1973.

84. Naiman, J. L.: Current management of hemolytic disease of the newborn infant, J. Pediatr. 80:1049-1059, June, 1972.

85. Nelson, J. D., and McCracken, G. H., Jr.: Clinical pharmacology of carbenicillin and gentamycin in the neonate and comparative efficacy with ampicillin and gentamycin, Pediatrics 52:801, Dec., 1973.

86. Nutting, P. A.: Reduction of gastroenteritis morbidity in high risk infants, Pediatrics 55:354, March, 1975.

87. Oberman, J. W.: The high risk infant; changing concepts, Clin. Proc. Child. Hosp. Natl. Med. Center 28:114, May 1972.

88. O'Boyle, M. P., Fletcher, A. B., and Avery, G. B.: Objective early criteria for ventilatory assistance in hyaline membrane disease, Pediatrics 51:748, April, 1973.

89. Odell, G. B.: The photodynamic action of bilirubin on erythrocytes, J. Pediatr. 81:473-483, Sept., 1972.

90. Oski, F. A.: The unique fetal red cell and its functions, Pediatrics 51:494, March, 1973.

91. Pagliara, A. S., and others: Hypoglycemia in infancy and childhood. I. J. Pediatr. 82:365, March, 1973.

92. Philip, A. G. S., and Larson, E. J.: Overwhelming neonatal infection with ECHO 19 virus, J. Pediatr. 82:391, March, 1973.

93. Pildes, R., and others: A prospective controlled study of neonatal hypoglycemia, Pediatrics 54:5, July 1974.

94. Preliminary report of the committee on phototherapy in the newborn infant, J. Pediatr. 84:135, Jan., 1974.

95. Rahbar, F.: Observations on methadone withdrawal in 16 neonates, Clin. Pediatr. 14:369, April, 1975.

96. Rabor, I. F., and others: The effects of early and late feeding of intra-uterine fetally malnourished (IUM) infants, Pediatrics 42:261, 1968.

97. Raiha, N. C. R.: Biochemical basis for nutritional management of preterm infants, Pediatrics 53:147, Feb., 1974.

98. Reveri, M., Pyati, S. P., and Pildes, R. S.: Neonatal withdrawal symptoms associated with glutethimide addiction in the mother during pregnancy, Clin. Pediatr. 16:424, May, 1977.

99. Rhodes, P. G., and Hall, R. T.: Continuous positive airway pressure delivered by face mask in infants with the idiopathic respiratory distress syndrome; a controlled study, Pediatrics 52:1, July, 1973.

100. Rigatto, H., and Brady, J. P.: Periodic breathing and apnea in preterm infants. I. Evidence for hypoventilation possibly due to central respiratory depression, Pediatrics 50:202-218, Aug., 1972.

101. Rothstein, P., and Gould, J. B.: Born with a habit; infants of drug-addicted mothers, Pediatr. Clin. North Am. 21:307, May, 1974.

102. Sahn, D. J., and Friedman, W. F.: Difficulties in distinguishing cardiac from pulmonary disease in the neonate, Pediatr. Clin. North Am. 20:293, May, 1973.

103. Samansky, H., and Strobel, K.: Care of the critically ill newborn; in an infant care center, Am. J. Nurs. 76: April 1976.

104. Santulli, T. V., and others: Acute necrotizing enterocolitis in infancy, Pediatrics 55:376, March, 1975.

105. Scarr-Salapatek, S., and Williams, M. L.: A stimulation program for low birth weight infants, Am. J. Public Health 62:662, May, 1972.

106. Schaffer, A. J., and Avery, M. E.: Diseases of the newborn, ed. 4, Philadelphia, 1977, W. B. Saunders Co.

107. Schlesinger, E. R.: Neonatal intensive care; planning for services and outcomes following care, J. Pediatr. 82:916, June, 1973.

108. Seitz, P. M., and Warrick, L. H.: Perinatal death; the grieving mother, Am. J. Nurs. 74:2028, Nov., 1974.

109. Shannon, D. C., and others: Prevention of apnea and bradycardia in low birthweight infants, Pediatrics 55:589, May, 1975.

110. Shaw, J. C. L.: Parenteral nutrition in the management of sick low birthweight infants, Pediatr. Clin. North Am. 20:333, May, 1973.

111. Sinclair, J. C., Driscoll, J. M., Heird, W. C., and Winters, R. W.: Supportive management of the sick neonate, Pediatr. Clin. North Am. 17:863, Nov., 1970.

112. Sisson, T. R. C., and others: Phototherapy of jaundice in the newborn infant. II. Effect of various light intensities, J. Pediatr. 81:35-38, July, 1972.

113. Snyder, C. H.: Conditions that stimulate epilepsy in children, Clin. Pediatr. 11:487, Aug., 1972.

114. Stein, I. M., and Shannon, D. C.: The pediatric pneumogram, Pediatrics 55:599, May, 1975.

115. Stern, L.: The newborn and his thermal environment, Cur. Prob. Pediatr. 1:3, Nov. 1970.

116. Stern, L.: Drugs, the newborn infant, and the bindings of bilirubin to albumin, Pediatrics 49:916-917, June, 1972.

117. Stewart, A. L., and Reynolds, E. O. R.: Improved prognosis for infants of very low birthweight, Pediatrics 54:724, Dec., 1974.

118. Sulyok, E., Jequier, E., and Prod'hom, L. S.: Respiratory contribution to the thermal balance of the newborn infant under various ambient conditions, Pediatrics 51:641, April, 1973.

119. Symansky, M. R., and Fox, H. A.: Umbilical vessel catheterization; indications, management and evaluation of the technique, J. Pediatr. 80:820-826, May, 1972.

120. Tan, K. L.: Comparison of the effectiveness of single-direction and double-direction phototherapy for neonatal jaundice, Pediatrics 56:550, Oct., 1975.

The newborn

121. Teberg, A., and others: Recent improvement in outcome for the small premature infant, Clin. Pediatr. **16:**307, April, 1977.
122. Tsang, R. C., and others: Neonatal hypocalsemia in infants with birth asphyxia, J. Pediatr. **84:**428, March, 1974.
123. Tsiantos, A., and others: Intracranial hemorrhage in the prematurely born infant, J. Pediatr. **85:**854, Dec., 1974.
124. Uauy, R., and others: Treatment of severe apnea in prematures with orally administered theophylline, Pediatrics **55:**595, May, 1975.
125. Valman, H. B., and others: Protein intake and plasma amino-acids of infants of low birth weight, Br. Med. J. **5790:**789-791, Dec. 25, 1971.
126. Vargas, G. C., and others: Effect of maternal heroin addiction on 67 liveborn neonates, Clin. Pediatr. **14:**751, Aug., 1975.
127. Vidyasagar, D., and others: Assisted ventilation in infants with meconium aspiration syndrome, Pediatrics **56:**208, Aug., 1975.
128. Virnig, N. L., and Reynolds, J. W.: Reliability of flush blood pressure measurements in the sick newborn infant, J. Pediatr. **84:**594, April, 1974.
129. Voda, A. M.: Body water dynamics, a clinical application, Am. J. Nurs. **70:**2594, Dec., 1970.
130. Winters, R. W.: Total parenteral nutrition in pediatrics, Pediatrics **56:**17, July, 1975.
131. Woodrum, D. E., and others: The effect of prematurity and hyaline membrane disease on oxygen exchange in the lung, Pediatrics **50:**380-386, Sept., 1972.
132. Wu, P. Y. K., and Hodgman, J. E.: Insensible water loss in preterm infants; changes with postnatal development and non-ionizing radiant energy, Pediatrics **54:**704, Dec., 1974.
133. Wyman, M. L., and Kuhns, L. R.: Accuracy of transillumination in the recognition of pneumothorax and pneumomediastimum in the neonate, Clin. Pediatr. **16:**323, April, 1977.
134. Yashiro, K., and others: Preliminary studies on the thermal environment of low-birth-weight infants, J. Pediatr. **82:**991, June, 1973.
135. Zahourek, R., and Jensen, J. S.: Grieving and the loss of the newborn, Am. J. Nurs. **73:**836, May, 1973.

# Jason—PROBLEM-ORIENTED RECORD

## HEALTH STATUS LIST

| Onset | Date | No. | Active | Date | Inactive/resolved |
|-------|------|-----|--------|------|-------------------|
|  | 10/28/77 | 1 | Incomplete data base |  |  |
| 10/17 | 10/28/77 | 2 | Low birth weight, preterm baby |  |  |
|  |  | 2,A | Gestational maturity |  |  |
|  |  | 2,B | Nutrition |  |  |
| 10/17 | 10/28/77 | 3 | Complications following pro-longed rupture of membranes |  |  |
| 10/17 | 10/28/77 | 3,A | Neonatal sepsis ——————→ | 10/28/77 | Neonatal sepsis |
| 10/17 | 10/28/77 | 3,B | Jaundice ——————————→ | 10/28/77 | Jaundice |
| 10/17 | 10/28/77 | 3,C | Anemia ——————————→ | 10/28/77 | Anemia |
| 10/17 | 10/28/77 | 4 | Systolic murmur —————→ | 10/28/77 | Systolic murmur |
| 10/17 | 10/28/77 | 5 | Maternal-infant bonding |  |  |

Infant **Jason B.** Sex Male Age 11 days Gestational age 38 weeks
Date 10/28/77 Race Black
Mother Mary Lou B. 502 Hudson St. Father Solomon B. 502 Hudson St. Phone 607-5332

### Religious preference
Baptist

### Employment status
Mother—housewife
Father—machinist

### Insurance
Group plan from employer—covers infant care

### Reason for seeing infant
10/28 Infant, now stable, is dismissed and ready to be taken home. According to staff and records the parents have not interacted with the infant and have not come to take him home since notified of his dismissal. 10/26. Public health nurse has visited home and approved as acceptable for baby. Infant and family may need assistance with the attachment process.

**MOTHER PROFILE**

Mary B. (Mrs. Solomon) 502 Hudson St. (Mother not available for an interview at this time.)

## PRESENT HEALTH STATUS

Age 22, gravida ii, para ii. Record reveals involution progressing without puerperal infection; membranes ruptured 10/14. Admitted 10/17 for delivery of infant. Dismissed 10/20 without infant.

## PRIOR MEDICAL-SURGICAL EVENTS

Record reveals none.

## PRENATAL HISTORY WITH THIS CHILD

**Medical supervision**

Monthly visits to area city clinic—diagnosed with iron-deficiency anemia 9/30/77. Hemoglobin 12 g at time of dismissal.

**Prenatal classes**

None documented.

**Nutrition and diet**

Record reveals weight gain of 25 pounds at time of admittance. Unable to obtain this information from the record. Multipurpose vitamins with iron prescribed during pregnancy.

**Illnesses, infections, complications**

None.

**Treatments and procedures**

None.

**Describe your reaction when you first felt the baby move**

Obtain this data 10/31 at home visit if possible.

**Planned or unplanned pregnancy?**

Record reveals unplanned.

**Describe home preparations made for the new baby**

Record does not reflect this information. Obtain during home visit. P.H.N. has not yet submitted this information to staff from her visit.

**Describe how bringing home a new baby will change the life of each member of the family**

Record does not reflect this data. Obtain in a home visit.

**Helping persons available**

Record does not reflect this information.

**Named the baby?**

Jason Michael

LIFE CHANGE EVENTS (DATES)

Death (family, close friend)_____ New baby __10/17/77__

Divorce _____ Marital separation _____ Return to school _____

Injury, illness __10/17/77—hospital stay for infant__

Retirement _____ Change of residence _____

**Pedigree (include chronic, inherited conditions, allergies, causes of death, illness in siblings)**

○ = Female
□ = Male
? = Unknown
A.W. = Alive and well
B.D. = Birthday

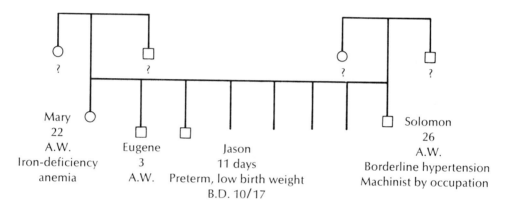

COURSE OF LABOR AND DELIVERY
**Duration**

4 hours. Birth time 0407 10/17/77

**Type of delivery**

Low forceps, spontaneous vaginal delivery

**Medications and anesthesia (types, durations, reactions, satisfaction with)**

Demerol 50 mg 0305 (10/17)
Pudendal block—delivery room

**Episiotomy**

Midline

**Fluids–blood–blood loss**

300 ml E.B.L.
1000 ml $D_5$/LR to keep open
No blood. Blood type A positive.

**Attended by significant other**

Record does not reflect this information.

**Held and/or nursed baby on delivery table**

Record does not reflect this information.

FATHER/MOTHER–INFANT INTERACTION

No opportunity in hospital to observe any parent-infant interaction. Obtain data on the home visit.
Touches infant _____
Touching pattern, what parts of hands used, where she touches infant
Eye-to-eye contact between them
High pitched voice _____
Entrainment _____
Holding and feeding positions
 Personnel does not always hold infant to feed. Infant is propped in bassinet with one hand behind head and bottle held in mouth with the other.
State of alertness of infant
 Infant does not follow with eyes movements of nurse's head from side to side. Alerts slowly when held en face. Most alert when talked to by nursery personnel.

**INFANT PROFILE**
**Present health status**

Stable physiologically since delivery. Sent to low-birth-weight nursery to rule out sepsis following prolonged rupture of membranes. Coombs, serology were negative. After losing 45 g from 10/17 to 10/20, weight increments progressed at 15 to 30 g daily.

Jaundice appeared 10/21 (bilirubin = 6.8 mg/100 ml total) and was resolved as of 10/25. Cultures of umbilicus, urine negative. Blood type B+ (mother A+)

No meconium staining. No respiratory distress or resuscitation in immediate neonatal period and none subsequently. No fever since birth (T = 97.8 to 98.8 Ax).

Taking nourishment from bottle since birth (see nutrition).

Initial P.E. on 10/17 reflects an "active baby" and "normal," except for right-sided maxillary swelling of soft tissue, without erythema of edematous tissues, "notched upper gum," and grade I systolic murmur heard at third left I.C.S.

10/17   Gestational age estimated at 36 to 38 weeks. (Gestational age not calculated with "Clinical Estimation of Gestation Age" chart for baseline data.) Mother's E.D.C. 11/17/77.

Heart rate range (10/17-10/27) = 150 to 160 per minute apically. Respiratory rate range 50 to 60 per minute.

**Laboratory**

| 10/17 | Hgb = 12.9 | Hct = 38.7 | Reticulocytes = 4.1% | MCV = 105³ | WBC = 20.8 |
|-------|------------|------------|----------------------|------------|------------|
| 10/20 | Hgb = 15.1 | Hct = 40.6 | WBC = 13.8 | | |

Infant discharged on 10/26/77.

NEONATAL STATUS

Risk  Preterm/low birth weight—secondary care nursery

Apgar  9/9

Abnormalities: Cleft in upper gum at midline of mouth.
10/17   Wt 1985 g   Length 43.5 cm
10/17   Head circumference 31 cm   Chest circumference Not done 10/17

**Nutrition**

Has progressed from taking Similac with iron (20 calories per ounce) 35 ml every three hours to 75 ml every four hours with a weight gain of 215 g since 10/20 (weighed 1945 g). Present weight 2160 g. Meconium stool 10/18. Transitional stools. No diarrhea. Burping. Little or no regurgitation of formula.

**Medications**

10/17   Aquamephyton   IM

10/17   Tetracycline ophthalmic ointment to eyes.

PSYCHOLOGIC PROFILE                                                                    Case

### 10/28   Sensory motor                              **Comments**

___No___ Turns head toward sound outside of vision

___Yes___ Searches for sound with eyes               Only after repeated at-
                                                      tempts

___No___ Infant watches hand in front of eyes

___Yes___ Follows a slowly moving object or face with eyes    Only after repeated at-
                                                      tempts

___No___ Stops ongoing activity in response to vocalizations

___Yes___ Infant gets hand into mouth; can reinsert if examiner removes

___No___ Follows disappearing object to point of disappearance    Needs auditory and visual
                                                      following stimulation

___Yes___ Crying                                     Vigorous

___Yes___ Sucking                                    Vigorous, coordinated

___Yes___ Variations of breathing pattern and change of activity

### 10/28   Trust vs. mistrust                         **Comments**

___Yes___ Enjoys eating, sucking activity

___No___ Follows voices and eyes                     Not readily

___No___ Relaxed mother-infant interaction           There is no mother-infant
                                                      interaction. No records
                                                      or reports of visits and
                                                      of mother holding baby
                                                      since birth. Personnel
                                                      unable to contact par-
                                                      ents so baby can be
                                                      taken home.

___No___ Able to sleep after feeding and handling by mother.

___No___ Infant quiets in mother's presence during feeding, changing, holding, comforting.

SOCIAL PROFILE

*See* father/mother–infant interaction.

### Position of child in family

Second born. Both children are boys.

### Life-style of family

No information available from record. Obtain on home visit.

### Pattern of family visits to mother and nursery

There is no record of calls or visits on the logs or records. Baby dismissed for two days, and home is approved for arrival of baby. Parents cannot be located to *again* inquire as to why they have not come to take baby home.

### Other caretakers for the baby

No information.

ENVIRONMENTAL PROFILE

10/28   Plan to obtain this profile in home visit.
Space for infant
Number of people in the home
Population denstiy
Infestations
Fire hazards

The newborn

Medications/poisons
Crime
Availability of transportation

PHYSICAL PROFILE
**Measurements (taken 10/28/77)**
Head 32.5 cm    Chest 27.5 cm    Wt. 2160 g    Length 46 cm
Gestational age Estimated 36-38 weeks
Vital signs AP = 140/min    Resp = 50/min    T = 98.8 Ax

**Neuromuscular system**

Posture, muscle tone (recoil, strength)
 Quick recoil of extremities. Can raise infant to sitting position and he can hold head up momentarily.
Activity level; states of alertness
 Physically active but is not reacting optimally to visual and auditory stimulation.
Cry/vocalizations
 Strong cry. Infant made no vocalizations during examination.
Reflexes
 See chart for neurologic exam on "Clinical Estimation of Gestational Age"

| | | |
|---|---|---|
| Babinski Present | Sucking Present | Plantar Present |
| Rooting Present | Stepping Immature | Moro Present |
| Crawling Present | Tonic neck Present | |
| Hand grasp Present | Fencing Not tested | |
| Landau Not applicable | Incurvation of trunk Present | |

**Skin**

Color (cyanosis, jaundice, pale, pink)
 Sclerae pink. Blanching at nose, gums, and trunk negative for jaundice.
Texture (dryness, turgor)
 Turgor reflects hydration.
Presence of:
 Milia None
 Vernix (color) None
 Lanugo None
 Erythema toxicum None
 Mongolian spots One spot extending from midline of sacrum to midline of left buttock
 Ecchymosis, petechiae, edema
  Edema over R maxillae near TMJ the size of a quarter.
  No redness. No crepitus of the joint.
  No ecchymosis or petechiae.

**Head**

Fontanels (size, pressure)
 Anterior-4 × 5 cm    Sponginess 1-2 cm surrounding anterior. Center firm. No bulging.
 Posterior-finger tip
Suture lines/molding
 No signs of molding remaining. Sutures without wide separation.
Shape of head (caput, cephalhematoma)
 Normocephalic in size and shape. No cephalhematoma.
 Transillumination negative.
Face (symmetry)
 Bilateral movement and symmetry of the face except for R sided edema (see edema above)
Eye (scleral hemorrhage, discharge, red reflex)
 Red reflex present. Pupils equal, round, and react to light. Test for convergence not definitive.
 Negative for ptosis, discharge, or scleral hemorrhage.
Ear (shape, set, amount of cartilage)

Well-defined auricle incurving to lobe. Springs to original position. Ears in line with outer canthus of eyes. Gross hearing intact.

Nose (patency, flaring, discharge)

Patent. Negative for discharge. No flaring with quiet respiration.

Mouth (gums, precocious teeth, Epstein's pearls, palate)

Upper gum notched in midline. Lower jaw slightly receded from upper jaw. Smooth coordinated sucking with arched palate. Tongue in midline. Negative for precocious teeth or Epstein's pearls.

### Neck (mobility, edema, openings)

Full ROM of neck. Negative for edema, openings, opisthotonos, or nodes and masses. Can turn head from side to side.

### Chest (clavicles, engorgement, excursions, symmetry, nipples)

Bilaterally equal symmetry and movement of the chest. Breast tissue is 3-5 mm under well-defined nipples. Palpation negative for nodes, masses. Acromion process elevates in response to pressure on sternal aspects of clavicles.

Lungs (movement, auscultatory sounds)

Rate, 50 per minute. Paradoxical breathing. No flaring of nares at rest, no retractions. Conjunctivae pink, extremities warm. Chest clear to auscultation. P.E. negative for systemic cyanosis.

Heart (PMI, murmurs, size, pulses)

A.P., 140 per minute rate varying slightly with respiration. $S_1$ loudest at apex; $S_2$ loudest in pulmonic area—splits on inspiration. No murmurs heard. Not able to palpate PMI. Pulses bilaterally equal in carotids and femorals. Extremities perfused.

### Abdomen (contour, bowel sounds, liver, spleen, umbilicus, femorals)

Protuberant. Bowel sounds present. Umbilicus clean and dry and stained with triple dye. Musculature tenses when crying. Palpation for liver, spleen, and kidneys negative.

### Urinary (location of meatus, characteristics of urine and voiding)

Normal placement of meatus; no spadias. Urine clear, yellow. No other openings visualized.

### Genitalia (labial swelling, descended testes, spadias, hernias)

Testes descended. Uncircumcised normal male anatomy. Palpation negative for inguinal hernias.

### Rectum/anus (patency, stools)

Patent. Transitional stooling.

### Back and spine

Vertebral column in midline with no palpable defects. No openings or pilonidal dimple at sacrum.

### Extremities (palmar creases, ROMs, hip abduction)

Negative Ortalani's sign. Full passive ROM without crepitus. Nails well developed. Feet negative for clubbing. No extra digits.

## INITIAL PLAN

10/28/77 **No. 1  Incomplete data base**

**S** Mother dismissed from hospital on 10/20. Unable to talk with her or any family member at this time.

**O** Unsuccessfully tried to phone family at home, 10/28, after working with baby, 10/28.

**A** Need mother's and family's input for data for accurate identification of health problems needing professional intervention. Lack of parental calls and visits need aggressive followup.

**P** The family should be available for interview with clinical specialist.

10/28/77 **No. 2  Low birth weight, preterm infant**

2,A  Gestational maturity

**S** EDC, 11/17/77. Gestational age estimated between 36 and 38 weeks by physician.

**O** Birth weight 1985 g (4 lb, 6 oz), head circumference 31 cm, length 43.5 cm. No resuscitation or respiratory distress at any time. No chart of base-line assessment for estimation of gestational age in record. 10/28 gestational chart reflects development of 38-39 week infant, except for unchanging preterm sign of immature stepping reflex (beginning tiptoeing). Weight gain up to 2160 g, head circumference, 32.5 cm, and length 46 cm on 10/28.

**A** A preterm baby is one 37 weeks old (including thirty-seventh week). A term infant is one 38-42 weeks old. Babies are classified by weight and gestational age as immaturity is a considerable risk factor in neonatal adjustment. Immature infants have the highest mortality rate. Body length and head circumference are better guides to maturity than body weight as term infant circumferences are greater. Jason's head circumference of 31 cm falls on the mean for a preterm infant of 36-37 weeks at birth. Objective data indicate increase in growth and progressive neurologic development. The neurologic assessment provides useful information as to adequacy of physiologic development of the neuromuscular system. Developmental assessment may reveal clues in the environmental and interpersonal world of the child. Monitoring physical growth patterns and vital signs provides a sound basis for determining adequacy of function of all systems involved in growth.

**P** Jason should demonstrate continued growth and development.

2,B  Nutrition

**S** Nursery personnel state infant has always been able to take nourishment from a bottle. Records indicate progressive increase in amount of formula taken at feedings. (35-75 ml per feeding). Similac with iron (75 ml) is ordered six times daily.

**O** Infant took 70 ml of Similac with iron after examination by nurse. Suck is vigorous and coordinated. Burps well after 20-30 ml without regurgitation. Nursery personnel do not always hold infant in their arms to feed. Mother has not held baby to feed him. He has had no diarrhea. Taking 450 ml formula per day (20 calories per ounce.)

**A** Although Jason did not receive a formula with higher protein content as suggested for low birth weight infants, he has steadily grown. Low birth weight infants need 3-5 g of protein daily. Prepared formulas contain only 1.5% protein. The usual recommended intake is 110-150 ml of formula per kilogram every 24 hours. Infant needs to be held while eating as a sense of satisfaction and enjoyment associated with body contact heightens an infant's sense of well-being and may, in fact, stimulate development.

**P** The infant should demonstrate adequate nutrition for growth and development.

10/28/77 **No. 3 Complications following prolonged rupture of membranes**

3,A Neonatal sepsis

**S** Mother stated membranes ruptured 10/14. Recorded observations of mother do not reflect puerperal infection.

**O** Order by physician to admit to nursery to rule out neonatal sepsis on 10/17. Cultures revealed normal flora. Axillary temp range from 98.4 to 99. Negative serology. No immediate jaundice. Umbilical cord clean and dry. No diarrhea or vomiting. No pneumonitis or respiratory inflammatory process signs and symptoms. No antimicrobials given (except to eyes). WBC range from 13.8-20.8. Hemoglobin initially low but elevated to normal limits (10/17 = 12.9, 10/20 = 15.1). Data does not reflect sepsis.

**A** Criteria for admission to secondary nursery can include infants born after prolonged rupture of membranes with signs of contamination and low birth weight. The purpose is to observe and to monitor the infant suspected of developing an infection for 24-48 hours.

Neonatal sepsis, a generalized bacterial disease, is one of the most common problems in the neonatal period and is a major contributor to nursery mortality. Because of the seriousness of its consequences physicians tend to overdiagnose neonatal sepsis. Generalized sepsis may lead to meningitis and hyperbilirubinemia leading to kernicterus. Occurrence of sepsis in the preterm infant is most frequent. After rupture of membranes inflammatory changes occur in the umbilical cord in six hours and after 24 hours the incidence of infection greatly increases. While data does not reflect sepsis following premature rupture of membranes (PROM), infant should be observed and protected as his defenses are immature.

**P** Obj. 1 The infant should not demonstrate signs and symptoms of neonatal sepsis.

Obj. 2 The infant should not acquire an infection post hospitalization.

3,B Jaundice

**S** None.

**O** On 10/21 total bilirubin elevated to 6.8T. By 10/23 jaundice was resolved as confirmed by lab. P.E. revealed negative signs for jaundice. Neonatal sepsis was never manifest. Negative Coombs. Infant B+, mother A+ blood type. No cephalhematoma. By 10/21 Hgb and WBC within normal limits.

**INITIAL PLAN—cont'd**

10/28/77    **No. 3    Complications following prolonged rupture of membranes—cont'd**

**A**    Bilirubin is the end product of heme released from hemoglobin when the RBC undergoes hemolysis. In a preterm infant total bilirubin reaches a peak level by four or five days and declines to normal levels in three to four weeks and is "physiologic." The age of onset, the maturity and clinical status of the infant and the rate of increase in bilirubin levels are parameters in determining course of therapy. Data does not reflect hyperbilirubremic due to sepsis or immaturity.

**P**    Obj. 1    The infant should not demonstrate signs and symptoms of jaundice.

3,C    Anemia

**S**    None.

**O**    Conjunctivae pink. No cephalhematoma. No signs or symptoms of inflammation. WBC 13.8 (10/20) Hemoglobin up from 12.9 on 10/18 to 15.1 on 10/19. Active infant. Unable to evaluate for pallor. 10/18 Reticulocytes were 4.1%.

**A**    Anemia is defined as a decrease in hemoglobin content of a given volume of blood, below the level normal for a certain age. Anemia in infancy is a frequent problem. Infants "at risk" are those suspected of sepsis and low birth weight infants. Preterm normal hematologic values are: Hgb, 15-17 (g/dl); hematocrit, 45-55; reticulocytes, up to 10%.* The acute anemia was transient. Physiologic anemia can occur in two or three months. Oral iron given in early infancy could prevent the anemia that usually occurs in the first year of life. Recent studies have shown that preterm infants have good absorption of dietary iron. Infants anemic in the first week after birth will need careful observation for at least the first 6 months of life.

**P**    Obj. 1    The infant should not demonstrate anemia.

10/28/77    **No. 4    Systolic murmur**

**S**    Infant is active.

**O**    No murmur heard 10/28. Record reflects physician heard systolic murmur in pulmonic area 10/17. No sign of peripheral or generalized cyanosis. HR = 140 apically. No dyspnea or tachypnea. Strong and equal femoral pulses.

**A**    Although heart murmurs are normally heard in the first 48 hours of life, these are frequently transient; murmurs persisting beyond the first week should be considered pathologic until properly investigated.

**P**    Obj. 1    The infant should demonstrate adequate circulation and perfusion.

---

*Pierog, S. H., and Ferrara, A.: Medical care of the sick newborn, St. Louis, 1976, The C. V. Mosby Co.

10/28/77   **No. 5   Maternal-infant bonding**                             Case

**S**     Personnel report no calls or visits by parents. A nurse reported that baby's home is approved by PHN but personnel have been unable to contact parents to take baby home. Parents are aware of baby's dismissal personnel believes.

**O**     Chart does not have record of visits or calls. Log on nursery door is negative for visits. Unable to contact parents at home after examining baby. No data reflecting an opportunity for or evidence of maternal-infant attachment. Infant is not easily alerted. He is not actively following with his eyes. There has been no opportunity for fostering an inner competency as with items in trust vs. mistrust.

**A**     Mother and infants separated in the early postpartal hours and days may have difficulty forming an attachment. Mothering disorders such as failure to thrive, child abuse, neglect, may result. There is evidence of a sensitive period in which that special attachment between mother and infant is facilitated. This mother and infant may possibly need facilitation of the bond via professional intervention as decreased maternal attachment persists as long as a month after the reunion. Abused children have a prematurity rate twice that of the general population.

**P**     Obj. 1   The mother and infant should demonstrate behaviors of bonding.

**NURSING ORDERS**

10/28/77  **No. 1  Incomplete data base**

Obj. 1  The family should be available for interview with clinical specialist.

|  |  |
|---|---|
| A.  Phone nursery and identify when parents plan to get baby; meet them at that time. (10/29) | C.S. |
| B.  Prior to baby's homecoming phone and/or visit to parents, concerning feelings and plans for infant. (10/29) | C.S. |
| C.  Contact public health nurse who has screened home as acceptable environment for this baby. (10/29) | C.S. |
| D.  If unable to contact or meet with parents, notify the Child Welfare and Placement Department and make a trip to the home. (10/31) | C.S. |
| E.  If able to talk with parents make an appointment for home visit. (10/31) | C.S. |

10/28/77  **No. 2  Low birth weight (preterm)**

2,A  Gestational maturity

Obj. 1  Jason should demonstrate continued growth and development.

|  |  |
|---|---|
| A.  Plot from birth all vital signs, weights, lengths, head and chest circumferences as a baseline for assessing growth, and function of systems. (Do 10/29) | C.S. |
| B.  Teach mother to keep a record of child's weight and length. (10/31) | C.S.<br>M. |
| C.  Perform regular in-depth neurological exam and compare with baseline data of earlier exams. (Plan for first home visit). | C.S. |
| D.  Administer DDST in conjunction with neurological exam for baseline data of gross neuromotor development. | C.S. |
| E.  Share this information with the parents. | C.S. |

2,B  Nutrition

Obj. 1  The infant should demonstrate adequate nutrition for growth and development.

|  |  |
|---|---|
| A.  Teach personnel and the mother that the cradling position provides an optimum environment for intake of nutrition. (Demonstrate for personnel 10/29, and for mother at time she gets baby for home.) | C.S. |
| B.  Teach mother to monitor and measure the amount of formula and the number of feedings. Teach her about formula types and importance of proper dilution. (Plan for home visit.) | C.S. |
| C.  Teach mother the consequences of diarrhea (dehydration, electrolyte imbalance) and to contact pediatrician if it persists over 12-24 hours. | C.S. |

| | | | PERSONNEL | Case |
|---|---|---|---|---|

10/28/77    **No. 3   Complications following prolonged rupture**

   3,A   Neonatal sepsis

     Obj. 1   The infant should not demonstrate signs and symptoms of neonatal infection.

       A. Move neonatal sepsis to inactive/resolved problem as data is negative for this.     C.S.

     Obj. 2   The infant should not acquire infection post hospitalization.

       A. Teach mother how to protect infant from infection:

         1. Avoid overexposure to cold drafts.     C.S.

         2. Keep infant away from people and places where infant might contract upper respiratory infection (URI) or flu.     C.S.

         3. Teach signs and symptoms of respiratory and GI infection.     C.S.

         4. Instruct mother as to importance of early immunizations. (During home visit)     C.S.

   3,B   Jaundice

     Obj. 1   The infant should not demonstrate signs and symptoms of jaundice.

       A. Transfer problem to inactive/resolved category.     C.S.

   3,C   Anemia

     Obj. 1   The infant should not demonstrate anemia.

       A. Teach mother the necessity of giving infant an iron-enriched formula (home visit) (10/31)     C.S.

       B. Move to the inactive/resolved column.     C.S.

10/28/77    **No. 4   Systolic murmur**

     Obj. 1   The infant should demonstrate adequate circulation and perfusion.

       A. Transfer systolic murmur to inactive/resolved category.     C.S.

       B. Continue to monitor and assess cardiovascular function.     C.S.

10/28/77    **No. 5   Maternal-infant bonding**

     Obj. 1   The mother and infant should demonstrate behaviors of bonding.

       A. Continue to try to contact parents today. (10/28)     C.S.

       B. Make a visit to the home on 10/29 if no word from parents.     C.S.

       C. Notify child welfare agency for assistance with follow-up if necessary. (10/29)     C.S.

       D. Remainder of time that infant is in nursery have infant held and cuddled while eating and whenever possible.     C.S. Personnel of nursery

**265**

**NURSING ORDERS—cont'd**

10/28/77    **No. 5   Maternal-infant bonding—cont'd**

| | |
|---|---|
| E. Start sensory stimulation for visual and auditory following. (10/29) | Nursery staff |
| F. If parents take child home tomorrow, plan home visit 10/31 to collect interactional data. | C.S. |
| G. Observe mother-infant interaction during feeding and after feeding for eye contact, touch, infant alerting, pitch of mother's voice (in nursery before dismissal). | C.S. |
| H. Teach mother the necessity of touching the baby as much as possible for facilitation of development of attachment and love. | C.S. |
| I. Observe father-infant interaction in nursery if possible. | C.S. |

**REFERENCES**

Klaus, M. H., and Kennell, J. H.: Maternal infant bonding, St. Louis, 1976, The C. V. Mosby Co.

Maier, H. W.: Three theories of child development, New York, Evanston, London, 1969, Harper & Row, Publishers.

Pierog, S. H., and Ferrara, A.: Medical care of the sick newborn, St. Louis, 1976, The C. V. Mosby Co.

Vaughn-Wroebel, B. C., and Henderson, B.: The problem oriented system in nursing, St. Louis, 1976, The C. V. Mosby Co.

# Infancy and early childhood

The health care challenge of the infant and young child is indeed a great one. The first five years of life are thought to be the most significant of all the developmental stages, because the foundation is laid for all future development. There are great advances in competency development during these years, and the differences that are achieved in each competency area are more dramatic than at any other time of life. The infant is born with relatively limited competencies. Physical competency is more advanced than any other, and responses to the environment are primarily through physical means. From the early days of life, the child begins to develop significant learning and thought, social, and inner abilities that can be observed and demonstrated. The child learns new ways of relating to the environment and begins to use play as a means of accomplishing learning, thinking, social, and inner tasks. Thus as the infant progresses through these years, play is an important means for relating the inner self to the environment and people who are affecting development.

Health care involves the documentation of development in each of the competency areas and facilitation of the family's own resources in promoting healthy development for the child. The child who is developing adequately inevitably encounters minor health problems, and the health care system becomes a resource for the family in caring for the special needs of their child. In this unit we will consider the basis for documenting the development of the young child in each of the competency areas, and the means by which skilled observations can be accomplished in assessing development and health. In addition, we will consider the common health problems of young children and of health care that is directed toward assisting the child and the family.

The purposes of Chapter 9, "Infancy: The Age of Beginnings," are **267**

(1) to present the scientific bases for development during infancy that have been demonstrated or hypothesized from the biologic and behavioral sciences, (2) to discuss features of the nursing assessment that are particularly relevant to the infant at this stage of development in each area of competency and the health maintenance needs of this period and (3) to discuss nursing management of health promotion and maintenance.

In Chapter 10, "Early Childhood: The Age of Discovery," each of these purposes is expanded in considering the development of the child from 18 months or 2 years of age to the time that he or she enters school. Although it is common to consider toddlerhood (from about 1 to 3 years) as a separate period from preschool (3 through 5 years), we will consider both periods of development in this same chapter, with references to special differences in areas that are significant. For the purposes of this book these periods of development are considered together because health maintenance needs are similar in both periods.

The purposes of Chapter 11, "Acute Health Problems of Infancy and Early Childhood," are to (1) present a means of establishing a nursing diagnosis in relation to acute health care needs, (2) discuss nursing management for young children with specific acute health care problems, (3) consider issues related to special health problems of this period that have far-reaching effects on the child, family, and society, and (4) consider the challenge of integrating care during acute illness with the goals of comprehensive health care.

# CHAPTER 9

# Infancy: the age of beginnings

The first 12 to 24 months after birth are exciting and fascinating both for the child and the family. Changes in body growth and build, behavior, and ability occur in rapid succession, with many important skills appearing for the first time. Mothers and fathers, grandparents, and siblings usually delight in the growing responsiveness and ability of the child. Much has been discovered about the events that occur early during the life cycle to shape and influence the developmental process, but little of this knowledge is understood and skillfully used in guiding those who interact with the growing infant and who provide the environment. A sensitive adult may be aware of signs of development and changes, but the questions and uncertainties that arise in the everyday course of child care are frequent and bothersome. In other instances adults may be relatively insensitive or disinterested. People vary greatly in their acquired and natural ability to respond to an infant and to provide elements that contribute to healthy total development. The challenge for the nurse and others involved in health care is to determine the developmental achievements of the child, assess the adequacy of this level of achievement for this particular child, and respond with the family to needs that are identified for providing an optimal growing environment.

The approach to the nursing process de-scribed in this and later chapters provides a substantial data base from which to (1) derive meaningful, relevant identification of needs and problems and (2) design with the family a realistic plan of care. It must be emphasized that any attempt to closely examine specific areas of development gives an impression of fragmentation of the individual. The interrelationships and interdependency among specific areas of development make it impossible to adequately classify developmental achievements, because the totality of development predominates in reality. For example, the acquisition of speech is a complex interaction of neuromuscular, language, thinking and cognitive, social, and inner development. An attempt is made here to present a systematic, organized approach to the assessment of growth and development during the months of infancy, using the basic conceptual framework presented in Chapter 1. However, references to discussions in other areas of the chapter and the book will occur frequently to emphasize the interrelatedness of the total phenomena of growth and development.

## HEALTH MAINTENANCE DURING INFANCY

Infancy is a period of extremely rapid growth and development. The infant is totally dependent and is susceptible to permanent effects of events during this period. Thus health main-

269

tenance needs are great. Under ideal circumstances, a family can adequately provide most of the environmental components for adequate health maintenance in such a manner that healthy development is encouraged and facilitated. For these families, resources that only the health care system can provide are limited and minimal. Such a family is self-confident, objective in their evaluation of the needs of each member, able to cope adequately with the usual and unusual stresses that occur, and able to independently seek and use various resources in the community when their needs exceed the limits of their own personal resources. This ideal situation is found very seldom in reality, and most young families need some level of assistance from someone outside of the family.

In the past the extended family fulfilled many of the needs and helped with problems as they arose or the young family established lasting relationships with close friends who provided counsel and assistance. Today, community resources are increasingly called upon to help the child-rearing family with stresses and problems of everyday living. In many instances the health care person who is consulted is not the best resource available for counsel and help, but this person often has first contact with the family and their problem or first discovers the existence of a particular need. This is particularly true in infancy and early childhood when the child is not in school. During this period only family and close friends are in regular contact with the child and are familiar with his or her behavior, growth, and development patterns. Intervention and prevention during these years are crucial, since often the effects are lasting.

## SCIENTIFIC BASES OF DEVELOPMENT DURING INFANCY
### Developmental physiology

Development of the physiologic systems proceeds in an almost uninterrupted fashion after birth as a continuous process with development that began during fetal life. While the normal infant is totally capable of sustaining extrauterine life, some physiologic systems remain immature during infancy, and the features of each of these systems account for the nature of much of the infantile patterns of behavior and the

physical and mental capabilities typical of this stage in life.

### Neurologic system

During the months of infancy the nervous system grows and develops functional capacity at the rapid rate that was established before birth. Most of the growth takes place in the cortex of the brain, and the brain reaches about 90% of adult size by the time the child is 2 years of age. During these months the sulci of the lobes in the cortex deepen and become more prominent and increase in number rapidly. The corticospinal tract begins to acquire myelin shortly after birth, and the acquisition of this insulating sheath is closely correlated with the observed neuromotor abilities of the infant. The function of myelin around nervous tissues is to provide protection and insulation, which allows for nerve impulses to travel along the nerve pathway rapidly and without diffusion. Myelination follows the cephalocaudal and proximodistal laws, allowing the infant to bring first the head, trunk, arms, hands, pelvic girdle, and finally the legs under voluntary control. By the age of about 2 years, the major portion of myelination has occurred in all structures of the nervous system. Although coordination, fine movement, strength, and speed are not fully developed, the child can perform most of the motor movements typical of later life.

Reflexive behavior that is normal during the early period of infancy begins to fade away as voluntary control through association pathways begin to develop. Some reflexive reactions never fade completely, such as the knee jerk or the blink. The infantile reflexes that should fade are summarized in Table 9-1, which indicates the ages by which fading should occur completely. The reflexes undergo a gradual change in character over several months preceding the time when they finally disappear.

One important characteristic of the neurologic system is that consistent stimulation is required for development and function to be maintained. During early development this appears to be particularly important, since there seems to be a critical period after which neural function is lost and cannot be regained. If deterioration of nervous tissue or motor or sensory

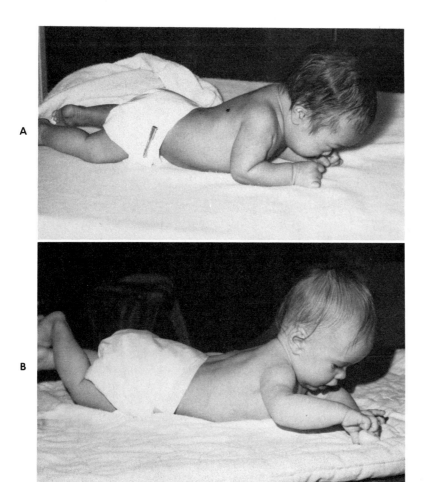

**Fig. 9-1.** Cephalocaudal and proximodistal development of myelination of the neural tracts is observed in motor development. **A,** The 6-week-old infant is beginning to lift his head from the table under voluntary control. **B,** The 5-month-old infant is beginning to bring his arms and hands under voluntary control in reaching for an object. His head is well controlled, and he can visually locate the object. He "rakes" the object at this point, since control of fingers has not yet been achieved.

tissues involved in a particular activity or behavior occurs, regeneration at a later point in life is not possible. Since nervous tissue function is essential for adequate performance of all other systems, stimulation in regard to each system is critical during the early months of life to ensure their continued development. Memory, learning, the ability to conceptualize and form mental structures, and sensory and motor abilities have been identified as being particularly dependent upon early stimulation for maximal development during later periods of human life.

The human infant and child appear to possess more plasticity of neurologic development than

**Table 9-1.** The disappearance of infantile reflexes

| Reflex | Time of disappearance |
|---|---|
| Sucking | Persists throughout infancy; particularly during sleep |
| Rooting | 3 to 4 months while awake; may persist during sleep for 9 to 12 months |
| Palmar grasp | 5 to 6 months |
| Plantar grasp | 9 to 12 months |
| Moro reflex | 4 to 7 months |
| Stepping | 3 to 4 months |
| Placing | 10 to 12 months |
| Incurvation of trunk | 2 to 3 months |

do most animal species. Critical periods of development are not as clearly demarcated, and deprivation or other forms of damage can be more successfully overcome for humans than for animals, but the human infant is not immune to devastating effects of deprivation, lack of stimulation, or damage. The hypothalamus, where instinctive patterns of behavior are laid down, possesses a multiplicity of connections with frontal lobes and all other segments of the nervous system. This renders the infant capable of multiple choices of pathways to accomplish similar tasks. This multiplicity of neural pathways is thought to provide the plasticity observed in human behavior.*

The ability of the infant to receive stimuli from the environment and to integrate them into the perceptual system is dependent upon the development and integrity of the total nervous system as well as certain specialized sensory organs. Impulses originating in the nerve endings of sensory receptors are transmitted along primary neurons to the central nervous system, where integration and association with other stimuli occur. The impulses travel specialized tracts through nerve connections in the thalamus to the parietal lobe of the cortex. On the cortex, sensory impulses are neatly sorted into a geography of localized sensations, and response to the stimulus can be accomplished with voluntary or reflexive action.

The immature infant's inability to localize stimuli results at least partially from the relative lack of myelination in the spinal tracts and the cerebral cortex. This characteristic is observed in the generalized reaction that is stimulated when the infant receives a specific stimulus. For example, if a foot is stroked or pinched, the infant will exhibit withdrawal of the foot, specific reflexive responses of the toes, and generalized body movement and possibly vocalization. The infant can respond to pain stimuli with crying and generalized body movement. Response to tactile touch, to pressure sensations, and to hot and cold is general body movement. As the infant becomes more mature it is possible to respond differentially to stimuli, and the ability to localize the source of the stimulus gradually in-

creases. During the second half of the first year, for example, the infant develops the ability to respond specifically to stimulation of the sole of the foot with a specific withdrawal of the foot, localizing the source of stimulation by looking at or touching his foot with his own hands. Generalized body movement is absent.

The ability to taste and smell is fully developed in the receptor apparatuses of the mouth and nose, but the incomplete myelination of the cortical pathways makes it impossible for the young infant to make associations in the cerebral cortex and to execute voluntary, specific motor activity responses to the stimuli received. Presentation of a noxious odor to a young infant results in a reaction of obvious displeasure, but the reaction is one of generalized body movement and crying. The taste buds for sweet tastes are more abundant during early life than they are later in life, which may account for the preference for sweets that is universally characteristic of the infant and young child.

Hearing is dependent upon intact tissue structures from the external ear to the cortex of the brain. At birth the infant's hearing apparatus is fully matured with the exception of myelination of the cortical auditory pathways beyond the midbrain and complete resorption of connective tissue surrounding the ossicles of the middle ear. The ossicles form from embryonal connective tissue, and as ossification proceeds during fetal life, the connective tissue supporting the ossified bones gradually resorbs, leaving the ossicles suspended in free air by about the second month after birth. The infant can hear sounds and responds to loud noises by crying and to soft soothing sounds by becoming calm and relaxed. The reaction to sound is generalized, in that the infant reacts with the entire body to the stimulus. As myelination proceeds, the infant exhibits the ability to localize the direction of sound and can respond by turning the head in the direction of sound by 2 to 3 months of age. Full development of adultlike hearing behavior, which involves complex cortical function including the ability to listen, to respond with discrimination, to imitate sounds accurately, and to integrate the meanings of sounds, is not complete until about the age of 7 years.[126]

*References 3, 6, 8, 57, 66, 85, 94, 108, 114, 119, 126, 127.

The complex structures of the eye and neural pathways involved in sight are less well developed at birth than are those of the ear. The shape of the eyeball is less spherical than that of the adult, resulting in the normal hyperopic acuity of infancy. The pupils exhibit full maturity in the normal reflex reaction to light intensity at birth. The lens is more spherical than the adult lens, and accommodation is not achieved for several months. The lacrimal glands become functional during the second or third month after birth. The muscles controlling movement of the infant's eyeball are not under voluntary control during the first two or three months after birth because of incomplete myelination of cerebral neural pathways past the midbrain. The eye achieves a significant proportion of total growth in size before birth, reaching about one third of adult size at the time of birth.

The peripheral areas of the retina are almost fully mature at birth, and the infant possesses functionally mature peripheral vision. The macula, or the central area of the retina around the optic disc, provides central vision and is not developed at birth. This structure begins to differentiate and develop during the first month after birth and is well organized by the fourth month of life. This central area of vision provides the infant with the ability to record sharp, clear images and light contrasts and to see colors. By about 8 months of age myelination of the cortical pathways has matured sufficiently, and the macula of the eye has reached a functional capacity that allows the infant to respond differentially to different colors.

Depth perception, a function of integration of the two images received from the macula of each eye, does not begin to develop until about 9 months of age. Full maturity is not reached until about the sixth year. The ability to coordinate movements of each eye is not present at birth but gradually matures by the third month, when the infant begins to develop adequate binocular vision. This coordination is necessary for adequate integration of the separate visual images received from each eye in such a manner that the infant perceives a single object. This cerebral ability reaches full adultlike maturity by the end of the first year (see Appendix, p. 871).

Binocularity illustrates impressively the necessity for consistent stimulation in order for neurologic function to develop adequately. When the infant or young child has persistent imbalance in muscle coordination of the eyes (strabismus), he or she begins to suppress the vision from one eye in order to perceive a single object rather than the impression of double objects as perceived with incoordination. When the suppression lasts for several months, the ability to see with the eye that was suppressed disappears altogether and cannot be reversed. Reversibility may be achieved if the child is forced to use the eye that is being suppressed within a few months of loss of vision. This condition, known as amblyopia, does not involve damage to the retina or other parts of the eye; it is the gradual loss of the ability to see because of lack of stimulation of the neural pathways that provide for vision.[108,126]

### Respiratory system

The significant changes in the respiratory system that occur in fetal life, at birth, and during the neonatal period are discussed in Chapters 7 and 8. By the time that the infant has accomplished adaptation to extrauterine life at the end of the first month of life, the respiratory rate has become relatively stable and has decreased slightly. Throughout infancy the tissues of the respiratory tract remain small and relatively delicate. The dermal layers of the epithelium and mucous membranes gradually thicken, but during infancy they do not provide mature levels of protection from invasion of infectious agents. Trauma to these tissues results in more severe damage than would occur later in life. The proximity of structures, such as the eustachian tube to the throat or the bronchi to the trachea, results in rapid communication of infection from one structure to the other, and thus isolation of infectious processes to a single structure rarely occurs. Further, the anatomic relationship of the eustachian tube, throat, and middle ear renders the infant and young child particularly susceptible to trapping fluid in the ear structures, contributing to the incidence of infection of these structures (see Fig. 11-2).

The lumen of the trachea and bronchi become gradually larger during the first year and remain large compared to total lung size. This allows for relatively low resistance to movement of air in and out of the lungs. The capacity of the airway from the nasal passages through the alveoli to produce mucus is reduced during infancy, resulting in less humidification and warming of air. This contributes to the susceptibility to infection. The amount of dead air space, or that proportion of the airway where air passes but gases are not exchanged, remains large during infancy, requiring proportionately more air to be moved in and out of the lungs per minute than is required in the older child or adult. This accounts for the more rapid respiratory rate. By 1 year the lining of the airway resembles that of the adult.[126]

### Gastrointestinal system

The functions of the mouth and esophagus are relatively immature at birth. The swallow is a reflexive action during the first 3 months of life. It then begins to come under voluntary control so that the infant can hold food in the mouth and swallow it at will or spit it out. The primary teeth begin to erupt by the seventh month after birth, often stimulating increased salivation and facilitating the acquisition of chewing function. The muscular action of the tongue remains related to the swallowing and sucking function typical of early infancy until voluntary control of the tongue slowly develops as neural myelination proceeds. The infant then is able to perform coordinated, smooth chewing and swallowing motions without the forward thrust of the tongue that is typical during sucking.

The ability to secrete saliva increases gradually during the first two or three months of life, and the composition of the saliva changes gradually to contain the immunologic and enzymatic compounds typical of adult saliva. At birth there is a small quantity of the starch-splitting enzyme, ptyalin, present in saliva, but because the food is moved rapidly through the mouth and swallowed, there is little opportunity for enzymatic breakdown of starches to occur.

Rapid movement of food through the entire gastrointestinal system is one of the most predominant functions during infancy. Peristalsis is more rapid than at later periods of life, and during early infancy the immature function of the peristaltic waves results in reverse peristalsis and the occurrence of repeated spitting and vomiting. The severity of this occurrence varies greatly among infants and may persist through the eighth month.

Rapid movement of food through the tract also results in relatively loose stools, which gradually assume a more adultlike character as the composition of the diet changes to contain more solid foods. Stomach emptying time gradually increases from the 2½ to 3 hours typical of the newborn infant to 3 to 6 hours characteristic of the older infant. The stomach begins to accommodate to increasingly larger volumes of food during the first 3 months of life, when the average volume that can be accommodated is about 150 ml.

Gastric digestion in the stomach consists primarily of the action of hydrochloric acid and rennin, which accomplishes the curdling of milk. Protein molecule breakdown, which begins in the stomach later in life, is limited during infancy. In some instances, however, absorption of certain whole proteins through the stomach occurs and a hypersensitive allergic reaction occurs.

As food enters the duodenum, the action of pancreatic juices and bile begins on protein and fat molecules. The infant pancreas is able to secrete trypsin, which breaks whole protein molecules to polypeptides and some polypeptides to amino acids. Pancreatic secretions do not contain amylase, an enzyme necessary for breakdown of starches, until the third month. Thus starch digestion in early infancy is limited. Fat digestion and metabolism in the infant are essentially the same as in the adult.

Normal bacterial flora of the gastrointestinal tract begins to accumulate when the infant begins to ingest food by mouth. The flora changes in composition as dietary components begin to assume the variety of the older child and adult. Stools simultaneously approach adultlike frequency and character.

The gastrointestinal tissues of the infant, like the respiratory system, are relatively undeveloped and delicate, with a decreased ability to secrete the fluids and enzymes typical of later infancy. The delicacy of the tissues and the lack of immunologic characteristics of the mucous linings of the mouth and gastrointestinal tract render this system more susceptible to infection and trauma than is typical during later periods of life. In addition, when irritation or infection of the tract occurs, further increase in movement of food through the tract results. Thus the infant is extremely vulnerable to the development of diarrhea and vomiting.

By the end of the first year the rapid emptying time of the gastrointestinal tract begins to slow. Emptying of fecal material from the rectum remains under involuntary, reflexive control throughout infancy.

The function of the liver remains relatively immature throughout the first year of life. Growth in extrauterine life does not occur until after the third month, and in fact there is some decrease in liver size during the first few weeks of life. The ability of the liver to conjugate bilirubin is achieved during the first few weeks of life, and the ability to secrete bile is mature early in infancy. The capacities of the liver to store vitamins, build glucose into glycogen, form ketones, and deaminize amino acids are relatively immature throughout the first year of life. Hormonal participation in liver function is relatively immature throughout this period and may account for the immaturity of function.

The gastrointestinal tract begins to come under more complete voluntary control throughout infancy, as noted in the processes of swallowing and sucking. In addition, autonomic nervous system control of gastrointestinal function increases gradually, with interconnections between the higher mental functions and autonomic control beginning to develop. The infant's gastrointestinal system has been demonstrated to be responsive to various emotional states, and conditioned control of the reflexive production of saliva and other gastric juices is known to occur during infancy. For example, by the end of the first year the infant will spontaneously salivate at the sight or the anticipation of specific foods that he or she finds particularly palatable.[49,108,126]

### Endocrine system

The function of the endocrine system is probably the most immature of all of the systems at the time of birth. Endocrine function is limited during fetal life and primarily develops during infancy and childhood. Homeostatic hormonal control is largely missing at birth and develops only gradually during infancy. Throughout the first 12 to 18 months of life the infant remains relatively susceptible to ominous effects of imbalances in homeostatic concentrations of fluids, electrolytes, glucose, amino acids, and trace minerals. Endocrine function continues throughout childhood and adulthood to pass through various developmental changes in response to other changes, particularly those related to reproductive function. During infancy the reproductive hormones are relatively nonfunctional, and they exert little influence over the metabolism of the body. Those endocrine functions known to be important during infancy and early childhood are reviewed here.

The hypophysis, or pituitary body, functions in the production of several hormones that are not directly related to reproduction. The anterior pituitary, under neuronal control from the hypothalamus, begins to secrete thyroid-stimulating hormone in limited amounts during fetal life, and this function continues to mature during infancy. Adrenocorticotropins (ACTH), which act synergistically with the adrenal cortex, are limited in function during infancy and do not respond adequately to stress occurring during fluid and electrolyte imbalances.[13,126]

The most important hormone during infancy and early childhood produced by the anterior pituitary is the pituitary growth hormone, or the somatotropic hormone (STH), which appears to play a very important role in the control of skeletal and structural growth during infancy and childhood. This hormone seems to have a direct effect on the metabolism of proteins, fat, and carbohydrates. The effect is widespread, and thus the target is all cells involved in metabolic processes.[13,108,126]

The posterior lobe of the pituitary produces antidiuretic hormone (ADH), or vasopressin, which inhibits water diuresis in the renal tubule. The production and function of ADH during infancy are very limited, and thus this regulatory mechanism during the stress of fluid imbalance is not totally reliable. This factor is probably related to the normally diluted urine that is typical during infancy.[107,126]

The thyroid gland begins to function during fetal life, and deficiencies can result in aberrations of growth, development, and metabolic function. Disorders of thyroid function are the most common endocrine problems encountered during infancy and childhood. Most genetically inherited thyroid disorders result in serious malformations or disease states during fetal life and infancy. Developmental thyroid problems more commonly occur later in childhood. The thyroid gland concentrates iodide from the blood and delivers it to the tissues in a hormonally active form. This hormonal iodine governs the rate of tissue respiration and important cellular metabolic processes concerned with growth and maturation. Thus normal thyroid function is critical at all stages of childhood.[108,122,126]

The adrenal glands decrease in size during infancy, and their function is limited. The adrenal medulla secretes the vital hormones epinephrine and norepinephrine, and it plays a vital role in relation to the autonomic nervous system. Secretion of these hormones is minimal during infancy, increases slightly during childhood, and at puberty increases significantly. Norepinephrine is the transmitter of the sympathetic nervous system and is important in maintaining sympathetic tone throughout the body. Epinephrine is released in great quantity in response to stress, and it mediates the homeostatic balances that occur in response to stress. This function is limited during infancy but not totally absent.[123,126]

The adrenal cortex secretes many hormones, but the function of each has not been fully discovered. Aldosterone and deoxycorticosterone are known to mediate the metabolism of water, sodium, and potassium, particularly under physiologic stress. Cortisol is involved in the metabolism of proteins, fats, and carbohydrates under stressful conditions. Each of these mechanisms is immature during infancy, and it is possible that full potential is not reached until puberty. These functions act synergistically with the hormones produced by the pituitary gland.[75,126]

The islets of Langerhans of the pancreas produce insulin and glucagon, which facilitate the metabolism of glucose. These cells are known to be able to respond to high levels of glucose during fetal life, as occurs when the mother is diabetic and the fetal pancreas responds with overproduction of pancreatic insulin. However, under usual circumstances throughout infancy the blood sugar levels are labile; at one point during the day the infant or young child may be hypoglycemic, while at another point glucose is spilled in the urine. This suggests an immaturity of the regulatory function of insulin and glucagon in the metabolism of glucose, but this mechanism is not confirmed.[108,126]

### Musculoskeletal system

The tissues of the body that provide structure and movement are vitally important during infancy and childhood, for these are the major tissues that provide changes in structural appearance through the growing years. Development of the bony tissue begins during fetal life as densely packed connective tissue, and slowly, in a well-defined sequence of development, cartilage is deposited in the connective tissues and the connective tissue is absorbed. Subsequently, the cartilage is destroyed and replaced by mineral salts, forming rigid bone. The bones of the face and cranium are laid out in a tough membrane and directly ossified during fetal life, but all other bony structures undergo the gradual process of ossification through the stages of connective tissue and cartilage formation. It is believed that skeletal growth is primarily mediated by pituitary growth hormone.

The process of ossification has been most completely studied in the hands, where the major portion of the ossification occurs during the first two years of life. The entire ossification of the skeleton is not completed until after full growth potential is reached toward the end of adolescence. This growth process of bone requires the constant production of new tissue throughout the entire growing period. There is remarkable variation in the timing of the growing process, with periods of relative speed alternating with periods of slower growth.

Muscle tissue, on the other hand, is almost completely formed at the time of birth, and growth is due to increase in size of already existing muscle fibers. As the size of muscles increases, the strength of the individual increases.

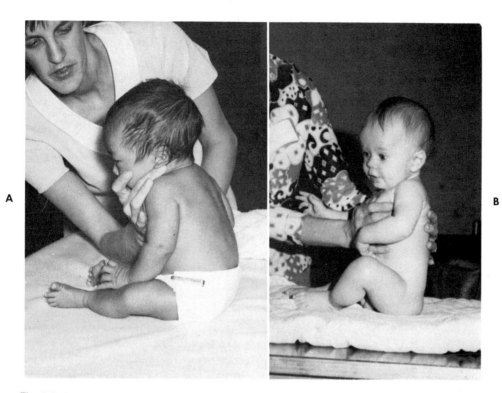

**Fig. 9-2.** Achievement of erect posture begins early during infancy. **A,** The 6-week-old infant cannot reliably support his head in a sitting position, and he is not able to maintain his back in a straight position. **B,** The 5-month-old infant is achieving motor capacities that contribute to the development of erect posture. He now has good control of his head, and in a sitting position his back is maintained in a straight position.

During infancy and childhood, growth in muscle tissue is mediated by growth hormone, thyroxin, and insulin. However, at puberty the male hormone androgen participates most predominantly and accounts for the greater increase in muscle size in boys. Muscle fibers respond to stimulation or lack of stimulation in the same manner as nervous fibers. Stimulation and use result in furthering their function and increasing their capacity and strength. Lack of use and stimulation results in loss of function, which can be reversed only if use and stimulation are resumed before permanent damage occurs.

Changes in posture, which characteristically occur throughout childhood, reflect the growth and maturation of skeletal and muscle tissue, as well as deposition of adipose tissue. The infant gradually achieves erect posture as the skeletal structure and muscle strength reach a point of development allowing support of the body weight in an erect position. Neurologic control of muscles is vital for this task to be accomplished. During this period the postural development of the infant gives a very accurate reflection of the adequacy of the musculoskeletal and nervous systems.[126]

### Integumentary system

At the time of birth the skin of the infant contains all of the structures typical of adult skin, but the functions of the skin are far from mature. This encompassing structure is very important for the infant, because it provides a surface of mediation with the environment, and as such it is vitally important for psychophysiologic development.[77] Furthermore, minor skin disturbances during infancy are common.

The outermost layer of the epidermis provides the major protective function from invasion of materials from the environment. The

**277**

inner layers of the epidermis prevent the escape of materials from the body. The dermis, the innermost layer of the skin structure, provides connective and supportive tissues for the glands, nerves, and blood vessels that supply the epidermis. During infancy the dermis and the epidermis are each very thin and bound loosely to one another. During inflammatory processes these two layers separate and form blisters, whereas in later life the only reaction would be swelling or edema.

The living cells of the epidermis produce the flat, dead cornified cells of the outer layer continuously throughout life. Cells that form melanin and give skin its characteristic pigmentation are present in the lower epidermal layers, and the more active these cells are, the darker the pigmentation of the skin. Impermeability of the layers of the epidermis is greatly underdeveloped during infancy, allowing for a greater degree of loss of fluids from the body through the skin and invasion of material from the outside.

Insensible water loss through the skin is significant during infancy, because the transitional zone between the living and the cornified cells of the epidermis is relatively ineffectual in preventing seepage of fluid into the outermost layers of epidermis. Once water is allowed to enter the outer layer, evaporation occurs to the extent that environmental temperature and humidity promote the process. This loss of body water is independent of the sweat process of the glands (discussed below). As the function of the transitional zone of the epidermis matures during infancy, insensible water loss decreases.

Penetration of the skin by certain substances does occur under ordinary circumstances. Lipids and steroids can be absorbed through the skin, and vitamin D is synthesized in the skin and absorbed in response to the action of light. However, the basic function of the outer layer of skin is to prevent the penetration by substances from the environment. The primary concern in regard to protection is that of bacterial invasion. Bacteria normally exist on the skin surface, and they are prevented from permeating the skin by the action of keratin, sebum, and eccrine sweat. The normal activity and evaporation of these products make the skin slightly acid, which discourages bacterial growth. Dryness of most of

the skin surfaces is the greatest deterrent to bacterial growth. Where the skin is moist, as in the folds and in internal structures such as the stomach and the vagina, the acidity of the skin surface becomes much more crucial for protection. Intactness of the skin surface is essential for the protective functioning of the skin, since once it is damaged or broken, it is unable to provide any protection.

Sebaceous glands, which produce sebum, are distributed over the entire body surface except the palms of the hands and soles of feet. They are most densely distributed on the scalp, face, and genitalia. Production of sebum is constant but is influenced by environmental conditions. These glands are very active during later fetal life and early infancy, and they account for the formation of cradle cap on the scalp and the occurrence of milia on the face. Clogging of the sebaceous glands on the face during the first month of life produces milia, but this condition spontaneously resolves during the first six weeks. As infancy advances, the production of sebum decreases steadily and remains minimal until the onset of puberty. This minimal production of sebum contributes to the relatively dry skin during infancy and childhood, especially when the environmental temperature and humidity are low.

Eccrine glands produce sweat in response to heat and emotional stimuli. These glands are not functional during early infancy, but they begin to assume some function during the first few months of life. The ability to produce sweat remains minimal throughout infancy and childhood, which offers some advantage to the young child in skin fluid loss. Apocrine sweat glands are present during infancy but do not become functional until the onset of puberty.

The ability of the skin to contract and shiver in response to cold or to sweat in response to heat is very limited during infancy, and thus the function of the skin as a thermal regulator is ineffectual. These functions mature gradually throughout infancy and childhood.

The distribution of body hair increases during fetal life and then decreases during the first few months of infancy. Hair growth with permanent forms of hair begins several months after birth. There is great individual difference in the amount and distribution of body hair, and there are great variations in cultural preferences for certain types, colors, and distribution.[108,126]

### Renal system

The immaturity of the renal system has been discussed in relation to prematurity in Chapter 8 and in relation to endocrine function in this chapter. At birth all of the structural components of the kidney are present. The nephrons are the last structural unit to develop during the later weeks of pregnancy, and some development may continue during the early weeks of life. At birth the glomeruli are more fully developed than the tubules, which are short and narrow. By about 5 months of age the tubules approach an adultlike proportional size and shape relative to other functional structures of the kidney. The epithelium of the glomeruli and the tubules is the last structure to attain mature structure. During early infancy this epithelium is composed of tall, columnar cells. By the end of the first 12 to 18 months of life this surface has changed to a very thin pavement epithelium. Absorption and filtration are more efficient in the mature epithelium. Functional limitations in renal capacity after structural maturity occurs are primarily related to the immaturity of the endocrine control mechanisms.[126]

### Cardiovascular system

The immediate postnatal changes in the circulatory system that occur during the first month of life are discussed in Chapters 6 and 7. The complete closure of fetal structures may not occur for several months. Occasionally closure is never completed, with little if any interference in mature function. If these structures continue to allow a significant passage of blood to flow in the fetal direction, there is congenital malformation of the structure, and adequate maintenance of extrauterine life is hampered.

The rate of heart beat falls significantly during infancy from an average of about 130 beats per minute at birth to about 110 beats per minute at the end of the first 18 months (see Appendix, p. 877). Rate is controlled involuntarily by the autonomic nervous system and will respond to emotional states or to states of relative activity or inactivity. Sinus arrhythmia is normal and expected during infancy; in fact, a regular heart rate during rest is an ominous sign. With activity the heart rate increases, and the sinus arrhythmia should largely disappear. The regularity of heart rate seems to be correlated with the rapidity of respiration; when breathing is slow, as during sleep, the heart rate is irregular, but when breathing becomes very rapid, heart rate regularity begins.

One of the important functions of blood flow through the circulatory system is to maintain body temperature. This function is reflected in the close correlation between a higher body temperature during infancy and the rapid heart rate. Elevations of body temperature during fever also are accompanied by a faster heart rate, although there does not seem to be a casual relationship. The typically higher heart rate of girls, which develops during later childhood, is not observed during infancy.

The ability of the capillaries to contract and expand as a regulatory mechanism for blood flow and thermoregulation is absent during the early weeks of infancy and gradually begins to develop during the later months of infancy. Contraction of peripheral capillaries in response to a cold environment serves to conserve body core temperature by concentrating blood flow in the central vessels. This also lessens heat loss by evaporation by limiting the availability of fluid to the body surface. Dilatation of the capillaries in response to environmental heat allows for body heat loss by increased evaporation and insensible water loss, as well as transporting heat to the outer surfaces of the body for conduction, radiation, and convection losses. This phenomenon is mediated by several complex factors, including the autonomic nervous system, endocrine controls, and physical factors.

The many phenomena concerned with blood pressure during infancy have received inadequate study, partly because of the difficulty in measuring these pressures in infants. The systolic pressure following birth is lower than at any other point during life, reflecting the weakness of the left ventricle in being able to pump blood through the extrauterine arterial circulatory pathways. During the first month of life the left ventricle rapidly gains strength, and the systolic blood pressure rises from about 40 mm Hg to 80 mm Hg. The next significant gain in systolic pressure occurs with the onset of puberty. Diastolic pressure also responds with some change and increase during infancy, but the rise is not as great as that occurring in systolic pressure (see Appendix, p. 879).

Fluctuations in blood pressure occur more frequently throughout infancy than at later points during life. The typical systematic pattern of increase in blood pressure toward evening and decrease during the night over a 24-hour period, which is observed during later childhood and adulthood, is not present in infancy. The fluctuations occurring during infancy seem to be more closely correlated with the activity and sleep patterns that are typical of the infancy period.[55,108,126]

### Immunologic system

The complex phenomena that comprise the body's total defense against infection and the presence of foreign material are only partially understood. Most of the known components of these systems are present in the infant, or they demonstrate beginning development during infancy. The antibody immunologic properties of fetal life and prematurity are described in Chapter 8. The skin, which is the body's first line of defense against invasion by a foreign body, has been discussed.

The reticuloendothelial system comprises the second line of defense against infection. The primary process of phagocytosis appears to be fully mature in the infant at birth. This process involves the action of several morphologic types of cells in different organs that recognize, engulf, and destroy foreign material. Cells that exhibit phagocytic capacity include the polymorphonuclear neutrophils, eosinophils, and monocytes of the blood; the histiocytes or fixed microphages of the spleen, liver, and lymph tissues; and microglia of the central nervous system.[111]

Even though phagocytic capacity is present, the inflammatory response of tissues is very immature during the first several months of life. Inflammation processes serve to localize infection, destroy the invading organism, and then repair injured tissue. For reasons that are not

understood the infant is unable to launch a vigorous inflammatory process and thus localize infection. All of the cells that are needed for effective inflammatory processes are present at the time of birth, including the polymorphonuclear neutrophils, mononuclear cells of lymphocytic or monocyte form, eosinophils, lymphoid cells, and the cells involved in the formation of fibrin. It is possible that the sequence of events and the timing of the inflammatory process differ for infants, and thus adequate localization of infection is not possible. There is evidence suggesting that certain bactericidal properties of serum that are at a low level of activity during the first few months of infancy may contribute to the inadequacy of the infant's inflammatory processes.[111]

Complement is a system of protein macromolecules that combine in sequence with an antigen-antibody reaction, but they are not molecule-specific in their reactions. It is clear that complement is necessary for effective antibody reactions to occur, but the exact mode of attachment and the molecular organization required for its varied and physiologically potent action remain obscure. All of the complement components are present at adult levels in the newborn infant; thus, unlike antibodies, specific organism stimuli are not required for formation.[111]

The specific immune response comprises the body's third line of defense against invasion by a foreign body. This is partially dependent upon exposure to specific antigens against which the host forms antibodies. However, the infant's ability to produce antibodies is limited by several developmental factors, and much of antibody protection is derived from those antibodies acquired from the mother during fetal life (see Chapter 8). The immunologic capacity of lymphocytes is probably mature at birth, but the plasma cells, which participate in this reaction, are either absent or present in very immature forms at birth. The spleen, thymus, and lymph nodes participate in the immunologic development of the infant, although the exact mechanisms and roles of each of these organs remain obscure. It is clear that the development of function of these organs is dependent upon the type of environmental challenge that the infant encounters in the form of exposure to infection or invasion by foreign bodies. There is universally a gradual increase in the levels of immunoglobulins present in the system, but the rate of increase is greatly influenced by exposure to foreign organisms.[80,100,112,124]

### Hematologic system

The formed elements of the blood that participate in the defense reactions of the body have been discussed in preceding sections. The occurrence of physiologic anemia during early infancy, along with the prevalence of iron-deficiency anemia, has stimulated increasing study of the red blood cell. The infant's hemoglobin concentration is normally relatively high at birth, and thereafter a normal drop occurs over the first two to three months of life, with a gradual rise thereafter. This drop in hemoglobin level appears to occur independently of the supply of iron available for the infant, and the iron that is released as red blood cells are destroyed in the natural course of this life span is thought to be stored in the liver until erythropoiesis begins to occur more rapidly. This physiologic phenomenon is thought to be regulated at least in part by the hormone erythropoietin, which is released from the kidney or the pituitary in response to anemia or hypoxia. It is thought that the high level of hemoglobin at birth represses the production of erythropoietin, resulting in the period of time when red blood cells are not produced. This period of physiologic anemia then stimulates the production of erythropoietin, with the subsequent stimulation of erythropoiesis. When the supplies of iron are low, erythropoiesis is not sustained adequately when stimulation does occur, and lasting or worsening anemia results. This iron-deficiency anemia becomes obvious by the sixth month of life; by this time the physiologic systems are expected to begin to supply and sustain adequate levels of hemoglobin.[32,68,126] (See Appendix, p. 879.)

## Behavioral and personality development

Theories of behavioral and personality development have contributed much to understanding the interrelationships between environmental influences during infancy and later behavioral patterns in life. Theories are not intended to fully represent reality, and thus most theoretical ideas tend to elicit critique, argument, and challenge from the observer. The primary purpose of any theory is to stimulate empirical investigations that will demonstrate the supposed relationships among the concepts and variables proposed by the theoretical formulations. To the extent that this is accomplished, the theory is useful.

Personality, behavior, learning, and social theories have been greatly limited in stimulating meaningful research because of a lack of means by which the actual events of the personality can be examined. Advances are being accomplished gradually, but most of the ideas to be reviewed here remain speculative and are only partially confirmed by empirical research evidence. This factor bears emphasis, for although theoretical ideas may serve as a useful conceptual framework within which nursing practice may be developed, the discovery of known, predictable relationships will eventually contribute to sound, scientific bases for child nursing practice.

Many of the ideas to be discussed will strike the reader as useful in understanding, observing, and evaluating normal behavior. At the same time, there will be a persistent, accurate impression that something is missing or that reality is somehow misrepresented. This, in fact, is the nature of theoretical formulations, for the complexity of the real world prevents humans from viewing themselves in the totality that is known to exist. The discussions of theories that follow will attempt to introduce the reader to ideas that have significance for the particular developmental stage under consideration, and intensive pursuit of specific theories is urged as they are deemed relevant to the experiences of the nurse.

### Theories of learning and cognitive development

Theories of learning and cognitive development stress one or more of several modes of learning that are known to exist in reality. These may be summarized generally as (1) learning by reinforcement and/or conditioning, (2) learning by insight, (3) learning by natural unfolding of capacity, and (4) learning by identification and imitation. Each of these modes of learning is

**281**

probably important during infancy. Because until recently there was little interest in teaching infants, little attention was given to the learning processes that occur during this critical period of life. Descriptions of behavior during infancy give evidence of the massive learning that does occur, but little is known about the mechanisms by which these tasks are accomplished.[2,7,39]

Many of the changes in ability that occur in conjunction with the changing physiology described in the preceding section interact with the phenomena of learning and cognition, and learning and cognition are certainly dependent upon the physiologic capabilities of the infant's neurologic system. The process of perception is one of the most important phenomena for the infant, since it is from early perceptual experiences that the infant begins to develop cognitive structures and learning processes. The realization that infants are born with fairly well-functioning sensory apparatuses has led to entirely new viewpoints of the learning capacities of infants and to the realization that infants are active, participant, reciprocal individuals in their own learning processes.[39,60,64]

An important idea that has emerged in regard to the learning capacity of infants is that of the vital significance of the person who takes care of the infant. The classic studies by Harlow[52] stimulated interest in the effects of various maternal relationship patterns on several dimensions of infant development, including personality, sexual, social, and learning capacities. These theories and ideas will be discussed in the following sections dealing with personality and socialization theories, but it should be remembered that this factor has great implications for learning. In order for the infant to sustain an active, interested participation in the events available for stimulation, there must be a nurturing relationship with a significant person.[39]

Another most important notion that has developed through research in learning during infancy is the theory that early stimulation is important for the future learning capacity of the individual. While this principle receives some support from the fact that lack of stimulation results in deterioration of the nervous tissue in-

volved, there has been a dearth of psychologic investigation regarding the relative impact of early learning and stimulation. Spitz[114] brought the effects of maternal and stimulation deprivation to the attention of investigators through his observations and work with infants who were kept in hospitals and foundling homes in very austere, sterile, nonstimulating environments. Other investigators have presented impressive evidence supporting the differential effects of early stimulation on future intellectual development.[102] The reasons for this phenomenon remain to be explored, but some theoretical formulations present tentative explanations.

**Neuroassociation theory of Hebb.** The theory of D. O. Hebb[53] contains the most explicit reference to the importance of early learning of any of the associationist or behaviorist theories. This theoretical framework advances the idea that the brain is organized and functions similarly to a computer network of electrical interconnections and associations. During the period of early learning the infant begins to build many alternative connections among cell assemblies that store sensory and perceptual information. The way in which these early patterns of inputs are associated and organized within the brain is critical for future learning and the development of intelligence. According to the Hebb theory, the child's behavior is controlled not only by the environmental inputs that enter the system but also by mediating processes of the system itself in receiving these inputs. These mediating processes are primarily the result of the previous functioning of the system. Thus not only is early learning necessary for later learning to occur, but also the way in which later learning occurs is permanently influenced by the nature of the early learning process. Confirmation of many of these ideas has not been directly possible because of the limitations of the tools available for study. However, clinical and observational study of the development of learning tends to support the general principle that early learning is indeed a critical process in the development of intellectual abilities.

**Piaget's cognitive development theory.** The significant work of Jean Piaget[89] in recent decades has provided exceptional insight into the learning world of the infant and child. In contrast to most other theories dealing with the phenomena of learning and intelligence, Piaget's theories incorporate a developmental point of view and begin with the moment of birth. We will consider some of the basic ideas and conceptualizations that are necessary for understanding all periods of development as identified by Piaget, as well as the stages of the infancy period. In later chapters we will consider the subsequent periods of development.

According to Piaget's theory, intellectual behavior is characterized by function and structure. Function remains invariant throughout life, and the two basic functions, organization and adaptation, operate from the beginning of life and continue throughout intellectual performance. Organization is the process of giving pattern and consistency to every act. Adaptation is the dynamic process that allows for interaction with the environment. There are two basic characteristics of adaptation: accommodation and assimilation.

Assimilation occurs when an organism utilizes something from the environment and incorporates it. Physiologically this process occurs when food is ingested. The intellectual process is similar, in that as perceptual information enters the system, it is incorporated and utilized by the individual. This process brings about a change in the input and in the organism. We learn to perceive an object as being the same even though distance, light, or angle of view may produce striking differences in the visual image that we perceive. At the same time we invest our perceptual impression of an object with certain meanings that develop from our past experiences, such as beauty, ugliness, or desirability. Thus the process of incorporating a perceptual experience changes, to some degree, the nature of that experience.

Simultaneously, the process of accommodation occurs, whereby the perceptual experience itself adds to and changes the basic properties of our internal structure, which then influences differentially all future related experiences. Consider, for example, one's first encounter with fire. Upon visual perception of fire the individual assimilates a certain initial perceptual idea, incorporating this particular visual image of the fire plus whatever properties tend to attract attention, such as bright, red, or pretty. This perception of fire continues to influence the perception of the second fire seen, and regardless of the real properties of the fire, the individual tends to see it as similar to the first fire. If this time the child reaches out to touch the fire and discovers that it is hot, suddenly the perception changes. Through assimilation the child has now received another input, or perception, and through the process of accommodation the mental idea of the properties of fire changes drastically. The fire is thought of as being not only hot, but also ugly and fearsome, although it is still bright and red.

Adaptation, then, is composed of a balance between the two processes of assimilation and accommodation. During most experiences either assimilation or accommodation predominates, but behavior is most adaptive when there is a balance in the accommodation and assimilation processes.

The structural units of Piaget's theory, which change developmentally, are termed schemata. These are the mental frameworks into which incoming sensory data fit. In the illustration above the child's idea of fire after the first experience might be one example of a schema. Piaget has identified several general schemata that occur at each stage of development and that provide a framework for all perceptual data. Piaget's classification of schemata and stages of development has not been accepted universally, and conflicting evidence has led to refinement and further investigation. These studies related to Piaget's work have confirmed several important ideas in relation to his stages, which may be summarized as:

1. Different children pass through the stages of development at different rates, but the sequence remains the same.
2. Each stage is typified by the most recently emerging capability of the individual, but the behaviors and processes that preceded it continue to occur and may even occur with greater intensity and frequency than the new operations.
3. Each stage is the formation of a total structure that includes the predecessor structures and substructures.

Piaget acknowledges that the way in which

each stage emerges for a given child is mediated by environmental influences, but it is believed that environment cannot change the sequential appearance of the schemata.[89]

According to Piaget's theory, play activities are central to the development of the infant and young child. Play serves an important symbolic function, bridging the gap between concrete sensory experience and abstract thought. There are two means by which the young child accomplishes the processes of assimilation and accommodation through play. The first is through imitation, which is almost pure accommodation. Imitation appears very early in infancy and appears to be an effort to accommodate to the environment. The young infant and child mimicks the words and actions of others in the environment and thus learns to speak and behave as they do. The second means is make-believe play, which is almost pure assimilation. The young child engages in an activity for the pure pleasure and fun of it. This type of play emerges later in infancy and begins to predominate the child's activities. When engaging in make-believe play, children form their own cognitive experience out of the objects of play, fantasizing and pretending the experience of objects, people, and actions that are not immediately present. Piaget termed this type of play "ludic symbolism," which refers to the playing-as-if quality that exists in these activities. As the child matures, both means are observed in the child's behavior and form an important means by which the child adapts, through assimilation and accommodation, to the environment.[95]

The period of infancy is termed the period of *sensorimotor development*. The first stage, from birth to 1 month of age, is identified as the stage of exercising the ready-made sensorimotor schemata. These ready-made schemata consists primarily of the reflexes and innate capacities for performance. Because it is clear that infants possess perceptual capacities in each of the modes of sensation, they begin to develop perceptual schemata from the moment of birth and probably before.

The second stage is termed *primary circular reactions* and occurs at about 1 to 4 months of age. This stage is termed "primary" because events are centered on the infant's own body rather than on external objects. For infants at this period there is no existence except their own, and there is no time-space reality. Objects do not exist except as they are in contact with the self. The idea of circular reactions derives from the observation that the infants actively repeat activities they discover accidentally. They begin to achieve perceptual recognition of objects through repeated stimulations and develop coordinated schemata as functional relationships begin to develop between more than one event. For example, infants begin to look toward a sound they hear, to reach toward an object in the line of vision, to smile responsively. This stage is dependent upon the reciprocal effects of assimilation and accommodation, as are all of the subsequent stages.

During this second stage of infancy, imitation begins to emerge. The predominant pattern is sometimes called pseudoimitation, for it usually involves the infant repeating an action in response to an adult doing something that the infant has just done. In other words the infant initiates the behavior as a reflexive or spontaneous action, such as hitting a mobile; the adult repeats the infant's action, and the infant then hits the mobile again in response to the adult's action. However, the child also begins to engage in pure imitation, such as smiling in response to an adult's smile or imitating simple sounds the adult makes.[87,95]

The third stage, from 4 to 8 months of age, is termed *secondary circular reactions*. In building upon the schemata of the first two periods, the infants now perceive objects as more separate from themselves and become more active in causing events to happen. Behavior continues to exhibit the traits of repetition and self-reinforcement, but actions now begin to emerge as intentional, and as such they reflect three characteristics. First, the actions are object-centered. Second, the actions involve intermediate acts (means) that immediately precede the goal act (end). Third, the behavior involves deliberate adaptation (assimilation and accommodation) to a new situation.

These traits of the infant's behavior are only beginning to emerge and may be difficult to detect. Later in infancy they become much more strongly expressed and are easily recognized.

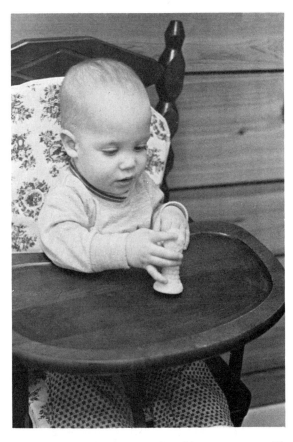

**Fig. 9-3.** This 6-month-old infant is beginning to develop object permanence. The infant's attention is engaged on a block. When the infant throws the block to the floor, he is able to follow its path of movement, and to continue to attend to the object as it is retrieved and placed back on the tray.

During this period, for example, the infants discover that they can cause a musical noise to happen by shaking a mobile hung over the crib. They repeat the act over and over, and are able to follow the movement of the mobile when it is set at different positions around them, always responding by trying to set the mobile in motion by some sort of movement.

During this stage, object permanence begins to develop. When an object that has caught the child's attention (such as the mobile) is removed, the infant actively moves about to follow its disappearance and to search for it in the direction of disappearance. The same behavior merges in regard to the mother or other significant people. When the mother leaves the infant's vision, the infant actively searches for her or anticipates her arrival when she is heard approaching. During this period, in fact, the de-

velopment of "separation anxiety" may be related to the fact that the infant is now able to perceive the presence of the mother when she is not in sight. This ability is not present during the preceding two stages.

During the third stage, imitation predominates in the child's activity, as described above. However, the actions imitated are predominantly those that already exist in the child's repertoire—those that are familiar. Play in the form of pure assimilation begins to emerge, in that the infant begins to repeat actions over and over with visible joy and mastery, taking pleasure in the activity for the sake of the activity itself. For example, the infant will repeatedly move an object, shake a ring of keys, or "play" with mother's hand with obvious enjoyment and pleasure.[87,95]

The fourth stage is the *coordination of sec-*

**285**

*ondary schemata*, from 8 to 12 months of age. During this stage further refinement of the characteristics of the third stage continues, and the infant begins to develop a more mature notion of causality. The infant now begins to perceive clearly that there are causes of events that originate outside of the self and that another person or object can cause something to happen. The infant attacks barriers that prevent or limit a desired activity as if the barrier were the cause of the child's own inability to reach the desired end. This is an important development in the concept of means-end relationships. Before this period, when the intentional behavior toward an end (shaking the mobile to hear it ring) was interrupted by an obstacle (a barrier between him and the mobile), the infant would lose interest in pursuing the original intention. During the fourth stage the infant may attack the barrier and remove it, indicating a strong compelling intention toward the desired end. The concept that the means (shaking) is clearly separate from the end (sound from the mobile) has emerged. When these two concepts are clearly distinguished, the infant is able to engage in play. When they are perceived as separate but continuous relationships, problem-solving develops.

During the fourth stage, imitation abilities of the child are expanded to those behaviors that were not already familiar. The infant begins to develop an interest in novel actions of others and begins to imitate them, which provides an important means of learning and mastery. Play is increasingly evident as the child focuses on engaging in an activity for its own sake. This is often observed as the infant during this period starts to reach a desired goal, but attention is diverted instead to an intermediary action that was necessary to reach the goal.

The fifth stage, that of *tertiary circular reactions*, occurs from 12 to 18 months of age. The child now engages in trial and error experiments in order to discover new characteristics of objects and events. Instead of deliberately repeating the same action or variations of the old theme, the child now begins to repeatedly manipulate an object in increasingly varied ways in order to discover what else can be done. The child also experiments with a variety of means by which the same end can be accomplished.

During the fifth stage imitation behavior becomes more mature, in that the infant's reproduction of the behavior is more precise than before. Ritualistic play emerges during this stage. The infant acquires a focus on certain means associated with attainment of an end and deliberately repeats the means ritualistically. For example, Piaget's daughter at this stage developed a ritual of grasping her hair and then splashing her bath water every time she got into the bath tub.[87,95]

The sixth and last stage of infancy is that of the *invention of new means through mental combination*, which occurs from 18 to 24 months of age. Important change takes place in the infant's intentions and means-end relationships, and it is this feature from which the stage derives its title. The child is now able to intentionally invent new means to an end through reciprocal assimilation of schemata. This achievement is most clearly illustrated through the examination of imitation and play, which have developed out of the preceding stages. Infants at this stage imitate complex new behaviors without the extensive trial and error that was typical for the previous period. They imitate nonhuman and inanimate objects and are able to imitate absent objects and behaviors. This indicates that the pattern of behavior that the child desires to imitate is worked out in the mind before he or she begins to imitate, and the extensive experimentation of the prior period is not always necessary. It should be remembered that each stage in Piaget's theory is named for the most recent ability of the period, and even though this capacity in imitation is present, the infant will continue to experiment as was typical of the preceding period.

Play at this period also takes on the characteristic of being mentally worked out before beginning. Imitation, which is often a part of play, is equivalent to the process of accommodation. Once imitation has accomplished the tasks of making the act or behavior totally familiar, the child begins the assimilation process through play and casually begins to vary behavior and to repeat it with the child's inventions of variations of the theme. "Make-believe" and "pretend" begin to emerge, indicating a symbolic basis for eudic symbolism. Play (assimilation) begins to dominate imitation (accommodation), but they are each fused in the behavior patterns of the infant.[74,87,90,95]

### Theories of speech and language development

Learning to understand and use speech and language is probably the most remarkable and complicated accomplishment of human development.[12,28,125] It involves the development of neuromuscular abilities to control the rhythm and tonal qualities of the voice and complex control of the tongue, lips, and associated facial muscles. Further, it involves the development of complex mental capacities associated with hearing, listening as well as vision, touch and movement. These sensory capacities provide the multitude of sensory inputs that serves as a foundation for cognitive structures around which the child forms concepts and a basis for understanding spoken language. Spoken language, in turn, serves to influence the child's perceptions of the environment.[12,125]

Development of speech and language can be described in terms of norms, but children vary widely in the pattern and style with which these abilities are acquired. Generally accepted norms for speech and language development are presented in the Appendix (see p. 872). Shortly after birth the infant vocalizes in vowels, regardless of the language of the family. For all children, this increases steadily through the first six months of life until the child is vocalizing all 14 of the basic vowel sounds. The first vowel sounds are those made in the front of the mouth, such as the "e" in he, the "i" in hit, the "a" in date, the "e" in met, and the "a" in at. These are followed by sounds made in the middle of the mouth, such as the "er" in her, the "o" in mother, the "u" in hut, and the "a" in about. Those sounds produced in the back of the mouth are usually the last to develop, such as the "oo" in too, the "oo" in book, the "o" in told, the "a" in saw, and the "o" in hot. During the period of time when these sounds become evident as vocalizations during infancy, they have no communicative value, as the child has not developed language ability, which comes

much later. During the second half of the first year, the child begins to utter consonant sounds of "p," "b," and "m," all of which are formed by the lips. These are often combined with one of the vowel sounds, and often the child begins to utter the word "mama" before the first birthday. This is usually not considered to represent acquisition of language, however, because of the probability that the child is simply imitating a commonly heard sound already in the existing repertoire of sounds. (See previous discussion of Piaget's theory of cognitive ability.) By the age of about 12 months, the child can vocalize the consonant sounds formed by the tip of the tongue, such as "n," "t," and "d."

The development of language is described in three dimensions—inner, receptive, and expressive. Inner language is the internal process of associating or assimilating incoming stimuli. During the first year the infant is building a significant repertoire of inner language in response to the sensory experiences in the home. This inner language is difficult to observe and is the least understood of the three language dimensions. The ability of the child to associate a shoe with a foot, a bottle or spoon with eating, or a pillow with sleeping shows some development of an inner language. This should be evident before the end of the first year.

Receptive language is the ability to hear and comprehend the meaning of spoken language. Receptive language precedes the development of expressive language by several months and continues to exceed expressive language in terms of vocabulary throughout childhood. Words first appear to take on meaning for an infant between 6 and 10 months of age. Expressive language does not emerge until between 10 and 18 months of age and should begin no later than 24 months of age. "No" is one of the first words comprehended by many infants in English-speaking Western societies, because of the frequency with which this word is used as a command in this society. Infants generally acquire receptive language comprehension of shorter, less abstract nouns and vowels before understanding of more complicated, multisyllable abstract words. The influence of the quantity and quality of language spoken in the home is a powerful force influencing the development of both receptive and expressive language.[125]

By the age of 18 to 24 months, most infants will be able to use about 20 words with understanding. There is a trait of echolalia present, in that the infant will echo words and phrases used by others in the environment, often without comprehension of meaning. Familiar objects can be named, and the infant can use one or two word phrases to express need or desire. Regardless of the infant's expressive capacity, there should be a definite indication of receptive language, in that the infant can understand and respond appropriately to commands, show recognition of familiar objects and indicate a relationship between the object and its purpose or meaning, such as a spoon for eating or recognition of a favorite toy.[125]

### Theories of personality and social development

Closely related to theories of learning are those theories dealing primarily with the personality and emotional development. In fact, some theories of personality development involve the process of learning to such an extent that they are seen as the same or very similar phenomena, as in stimulus-response theories or operant conditioning theories. However, personality theory is characterized by a consideration of those processes that produce the characteristics of an individual that ultimately identify the person as unique. Each theory of personality stresses some aspects of the life process which, for theorists and their followers, represent a meaningful and reasonable approach to thinking about certain factors of the real world. Theories that are not developmental in nature but concentrate on the description of events that produce variable personality traits contribute to the consideration of healthy development throughout life. Such concepts as operant reinforcement (B. F. Skinner), the creative self (Alfred Adler), or unconditional positive regard (Carl Rogers) might be explored in depth by the reader in relation to the experiences of the infant.[89]

Developmental personality theories have particular significance when considering the infancy period, because these ideas enable us to clearly distinguish those factors that appear to be crucial for later development. The universal factor that emerges as a central theme to all theoretical considerations of the infancy period of personality development is the importance of the relationship of the infant with other people in the environment. There is most often a predominant interest in the infant-mother relationship, and preliminary investigations of relationships between the infant and other persons tend to confirm the idea that the mother-infant relationship, or an equally intense, nurturing relationship with a mother substitute, is indeed a crucial factor during infancy. This is attributable to the infant's total reliance and dependence upon an adult for provision of every need, but this fact does not explain why the nature of the infant-mother relationship has such a significant impact on the personality outcome for the child. Relationships with other persons are identified, but their importance is less clearly understood.*

**Erikson's theory of identity.** Erikson,[38] whose theoretical formulations of the stages of development grew out of the psychoanalytic tradition, identifies the infancy period as the time of the infant's first social achievement—that of basic trust. To the extent that the mother provides for nurturance, familiarity, security, and continuity of experience, the infant is able to develop a basic sense of trust for the world, including the people in it. For Erikson, the infant's behavior reflects the constant testing and exploration of the world in order to discover its predictability or the extent to which it can be trusted. When an adequate mothering relationship is not present, the infant develops a sense of mistrust for the environment and the people in it, and this experience is irrevocable, influencing the way that all subsequent stages evolve. According to this theory, all infants encounter elements of both trustful and mistrustful experience. It is the predominance of one over the other that is important for future personality development.

**Bowlby's theory of attachment.** Bowlby,[14] also of the psychoanalytic tradition, conceptualizes infancy as the crucial period when attachment behavior emerges. The reciprocal behavior of the mother or other significant people is care-taking behavior. The infant's be-

---

*References 9, 14, 31, 38, 50, 52, 59, 64, 77, 106, 129.

havior reflects efforts to maintain proximity to the mother first and then to other family members; they respond by reciprocating the expressed needs for proximity. The ways in which the older infant maintains proximity to the mother and other family members are multitudinous; Bowlby describes five basic patterns of attachment behavior: sucking, clinging, following, crying, and smiling. Some of these behaviors are present at birth, but they do not begin to evolve as the infant's self-directed attachment behavior until about the age of 4 months. Between the ages of 9 and 18 months the infant exhibits sophisticated goal-directed systems of behavior that maintain proximity to mother. Within 1 month after attachment behavior for the mother first appears, some infants begin to exhibit attachment behavior for at least one other person, usually the father. By 18 months of age most infants have established attachment with at least one and usually several other individuals.

Visual and tactile contact is seen as crucial for the development of attachment behavior. The nature of the interactions that occur in these respects gives important indications of the adequacy of attachment formations. The infant uses the mother as a base of security from which to explore the larger world, maintaining visual contact in the process. The child periodically reestablishes tactile contact and then returns to exploration. When the infant is frightened, stressed, or uncomfortable for any reason, contact is established that retains the proximity of mother, such as clinging and following. The phenomena of attachment behavior elicit stronger evidences of internal feeling than any other form of human behavior. In the infant, when the figure of attachment appears in visual contact after an absence, the person is greeted with obvious joy and delight. As long as this figure is in proximity, the infant is secure and comfortable. When loss or the threat of separation occurs, anger, anxiety, and violent distress result. These feelings remain strong and intense throughout infancy.

## NURSING ASSESSMENT OF PHYSICAL COMPETENCY

At birth infants are able to participate in providing their own nutrition by means of sucking.

They are able to cry to make known their basic needs and discomforts. They can move their extremities, but there is no purpose associated with the movement. From this state of physical competency the infant progresses to a stage of physical mobility, purposeful movement, the ability to feed himself or herself when food is provided, and vocalization of differential sounds. The preceding sections provided an introductory basis for nursing assessment and care that contributes toward the maintenance of health during infancy. We now will consider specific aspects of this process.

### Growth and vital signs

Accurate sequential measurements of growth, plotted on a standardized growth grid, are an essential and important dimension of health care during infancy. Because of the acknowledged differences between children of different ethnic groups and different sex, it is recommended that ethnic and sex-specific growth grids be used for the most accurate interpretation of the meanings of growth changes for young children. The length should be measured using a standardized, consistent method, with the infant lying on a flat surface. Body length becomes a more important growth parameter as infancy progresses, for the proportion of body length to body weight aids in interpretation of excessive or insufficient changes in body weight. Each of these growth parameters should fall within a consistent percentile range throughout infancy. If there is a change in the percentile range of body length or body weight or if a wide percentile span persists between the two measurements, a problem in body growth should be considered.[101]

Head circumference remains a vital measurement throughout infancy. A baseline birth head circumference is important, but in any event the head circumference should be recorded and plotted throughout the period of well-child care during infancy. The infant's anterior fontanel should be measured periodically, and the fontanel and suture lines of the head palpated at regular intervals to monitor the degree of calcification and closure of these structures. The anterior fontanel should be fully closed by the fifteenth to eighteenth month of infancy. Symmetry of head growth should be the norm; if

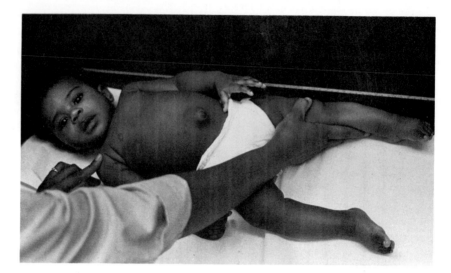

**Fig. 9-4.** The length of an infant is determined by placing the infant's head against a stationary wall and holding the body and knee firmly against a premeasured wall.

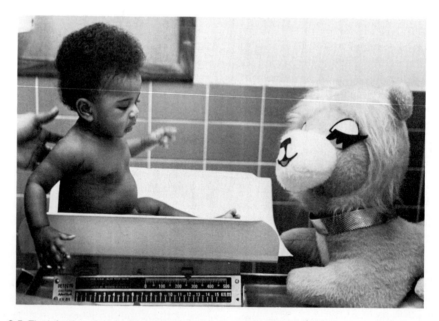

**Fig. 9-5.** The infant's weight is obtained by placing the infant without clothing on a standardized scale. The infant's attention is diverted momentarily by a stuffed animal to minimize movement while the weight is being read.

asymmetry begins to appear during infancy, the parents need to assist in determining the patterns of position that the infant assumes during sleep at home. If the infant consistently assumes a sleeping position that contributes to flattening of the head on one side, the infant needs to be periodically repositioned during sleep to allow for symmetrical head growth. If such measures do not result in development of symmetry, the health care team needs to investigate the possibility of inadequate or early calcification of the suture lines.

Patterns of heart rate and respiration rate should be obtained throughout infancy using auscultation of the chest. These values should fall within the normal ranges for the age of the infancy and reflect a gradual decline in these rates (see Appendix, p. 877). Body temperature should remain stable at approximately 98.1 degrees F (axillary).

Blood pressure during infancy is frequently neglected but should be obtained at regular intervals to monitor adequate development. In Western societies, where salt intake is particularly high, the early development of essential hypertension is an increasing concern, particularly as the infant begins to eat foods prepared for the entire family that contain increased amounts of salt.[103] The flush method of taking blood pressure during infancy (see Chapter 7) is useful as an estimate until it is possible to obtain blood pressure by auscultation.[91]

## Neuromotor function and stimulation

The infant's history of birth and delivery is essential in guiding and interpreting nursing assessment during infancy, particularly in regard to neuromotor function and stimulation. If any unusual events occurred during the prenatal, labor, delivery, or newborn periods, particular attention should be given to sequential assessment of neuromotor function. If the infant received high risk care during the newborn period or for any reason was separated from the family during that period of life, special attention is directed to the stimulation needs of the infant.

In assessing neuromotor function and stimulation, understanding the principles of physiologic development is essential. Through experience with infants, the nurse is able to develop familiarity with details of motor ability as they emerge over the months of infancy. Several resources are available that provide detailed descriptions week by week or month by month of the expected motor development sequence.[39,109,117] The Denver Developmental Screening Test,[44] which appears in the Appendix (p. 902), provides the most useful tool presently available for most nurses in screening variations in gross neuromotor development. It should be remembered that the DDST is sim-

ply a screening tool, and additional information should be obtained by more detailed assessment of the infant's motor, language, and social development.

Language and social development of the infant provide important indications of the quality of stimulation that the infant receives in the environment. While conclusions cannot be drawn based solely on the language and social development of the infant, if these appear to be delayed, further observation of the actual family-child interactions would be indicated. The infant should respond to verbal interactions as indicated in the Table, "Landmarks for Speech, Language and Hearing Development" (see Appendix, p. 872). Receptive language is particularly important during infancy, for a wide variation in normal expressive ability of infants exists during this age period.

The phenomenon of separation anxiety, while providing an important social and inner parameter, also indicates the development of critical cognitive skills in the infant. This event should occur at about the age of 7 months, and a delay beyond the age of 8 months should alert the nurse to obtain further information regarding the child's cognitive and social development.

The neurologic assessment of the infant provides useful information regarding the adequacy of physiologic development of the neuromotor system. This evaluation resembles the assessment described for the newborn (see Chapter 7). The nurse is interested in the fading and disappearance of reflexes that were present in the newborn period (see Table 9-1). Several reflexes and motor capabilities that were not present in the newborn period are evaluated as they are expected to appear and then disappear. These reflect the level of maturation of the central nervous system. The Landau reflex appears at 3 months of age and persists until 12 to 24 months of age. This reflex is elicited by suspending the infant in a horizontal prone position and depressing the head against the trunk. The infant's legs flex and are drawn up against the trunk in response to flexion of the head.

The parachute reflex appears at about 7 to 9 months and persists indefinitely. The infant is suspended in a horizontal prone position as for the Landau reflex and is suddenly thrust down-

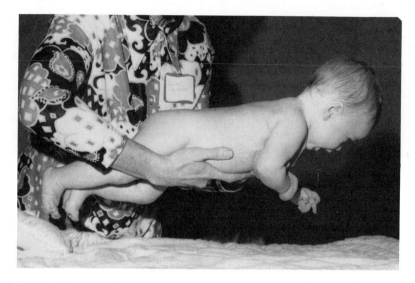

**Fig. 9-6.** The infant is suspended in a horizontal prone position. At 5 months of age the infant assumes nearly horizontal posture, with the head slightly elevated. The Landau reflex is elicited by flexing the head against the trunk, and the legs reflexly draw up against the trunk in response to the passive flexion of the head.

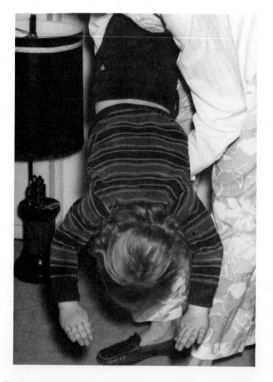

**Fig. 9-7.** The parachute reflex is elicited by suddenly thrusting the infant downward from a horizontal position. His hands and fingers extend forward and spread as if to protect against a fall.

**Table 9-2.** Expected hearing responses in infancy*

| Age | Response |
| --- | --- |
| 4 months | Widening of the eyes |
|  | Slight turning of the head in the direction of the sound |
|  | Quieting, listening attitude |
| 6 months | Turning of the head toward the sound but need not recognize that the sound source is below or above him |
| 8 months or older | Turns head 45 degrees or more in direction of the sound |
|  | Usually determines whether sound source is above or below him |

*From Down, M. P., and Silver, H. K.: The A.B.C.D.'s to H.E.A.R.; Early identification in nursery, office, and clinic of the infant who is deaf, Clin. Pediatr. **11**:563, 1972.

ward. The infant's hands and fingers extend forward and spread as if to protect against the fall.[83]

Evaluation of each of the sensory modalities is assessed as the infant grows older. The infant should respond to smell and taste, and touch sensations should be obvious over the entire body. Until the child can verbally report the differential sensations of cold or hot, these touch modalities are difficult to evaluate.

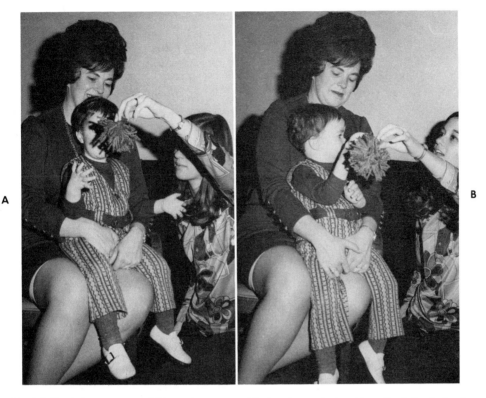

**Fig. 9-8.** The infant or young child may be screened for hearing seated on his mother's lap facing the same direction as mother. **A,** His attention is engaged with an object held in front of him by the tester. **B,** When this is accomplished, a sound is made with a bell, rattle, or squeeze toy held to the side of the infant, and his responses are noted.

Downs and Silver[34] have described a screening test for hearing in infancy. Hearing in the young infant may be evaluated by observing the developmental responses to soft sounds that usually attract attention. There should be little distraction from other noises. With the infant seated on the mother's lap facing the same direction as mother, the tester kneels beside the mother and infant. The infant's attention is engaged with a toy or doll held in the child's line of vision by the tester. When this is accomplished, a sound is made with a bell, rattle, or squeeze toy to the side of the infant, and the child's responses are noted. The sound must be repeated on each side in order to determine adequate hearing. The responses expected for each age are indicated in Table 9-2. In addition, the history of the infant's newborn experience and development since birth indicate important factors that increase the likelihood of a hearing loss, and thorough audiometric evaluation must

be obtained. The important points in the history that may be indicative of hearing loss are arranged by Downs and Silver as follows:

Affected family or the presence of hearing loss in any family member prior to 50 years of age

Bilirubin level elevated above 20 mg/100 ml of serum during the newborn period

Congenital rubella syndrome, which may be suspected if rubella infection occurred at any time during pregnancy

Defects of the ear, nose, or throat

Small size at birth, particularly under 1,500 g

In regard to development during the period since birth, the following concerns indicate a need for further audiometric testing:

Hearing concern? If the child has a hearing loss, the mother is often concerned by the time the child is 6 months of age.

Ear test results? The test described above may reveal a hearing loss.

**293**

Awakens to sound? An infant is expected to stir or awaken in response to nearby sounds while asleep. The sound may be loud or moderately loud but should not be accompanied by vibrations, such as with a slamming door. Mother may need to deliberately observe this reaction.

Responses in communication development? The infant's verbalization and linguistic skills should be consistent with that expected for his or her age. Delays in language and verbalizations accompany hearing loss.

Lack of hearing stimulation results in further loss of hearing ability, following the physiologic principle that stimulation is necessary to prevent deterioration of a particular neurologic pathway. Thus it is particularly important to detect an infant's inability to hear ordinary sounds in the environment, since amplification and therapy may prevent further deterioration of existing hearing ability. Further, there is indication that language development depends critically upon auditory experiences of sound during the first two years of life. If an infant does not experience the sounds of the cultural language during this time, there may be permanent disadvantage in the ability to vocalize, even if the sounds are made available by amplification at a later point in development.[50,70,118]

Vision testing during infancy involves the observation of each of the neurologic capabilities of the infant's eyes that can be identified as appropriate for his or her age (see Appendix, p. 871). Pupillary reaction to light, blink response stimulated either by light or by touching the eyelashes or cornea, coordination of eye movements, and the ability to fixate and follow a moving object are readily observed during the early months of infancy. As the infant approaches the fourth month, it is possible to identify various levels of development in head-eye coordination and the ability to fixate on an object at some distance. During the second year the child should be able to discriminate simple geometric forms and associate with visual experiences. The Denver Eye Screening Test[4] provides a suitable

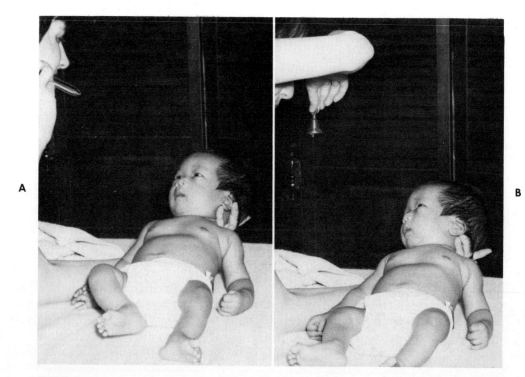

**Fig. 9-9.** The infant's eye responses are noted. **A,** Pupillary response is observed when a light is directed into his eyes. Pupillary light reflex may also be noted. **B,** The infant's ability to fixate and follow a moving object is observed.

standardized approach for vision evaluation of infants.

The principle of stimulation remains one of the most important aspects of nursing assessment and care during infancy. Careful interviewing and history-taking and developmental assessment may reveal clues of adequacy or inadequacies in physical competency, as well as in the environmental and interpersonal world of the child. This assessment must include and integrate all that is known about the family and their style of life and social and cultural patterns, since the cultural expectations for behavior may produce behavior or personality traits that, from the nurse's own frame of reference, might suggest some deficiency in the environment. For example, the mother and infant may be noted to always behave very somberly, to seldom smile, or to not engage in motor activities in the clinic setting. When seen in their home, there may be a similar reaction in the room where the nurse is present, but activity in other parts of the house, plus a more relaxed interaction between the mother and child, would suggest that the behavior is closely related to cultural or life style patterns of this particular family. Often several contacts are necessary before an accurate evaluation of the adequacy of environmental stimulation can be achieved.

## Evaluation of remaining physical systems

Assessment of respiratory and gastrointestinal systems during infancy is concerned with the monitoring of normal function and identification of signs of infection or illness. The parents' report of events that occur regularly at home, such as eliminative function, the present diet, or communicable illness present in the home, helps to direct the nurse's attention to detailed physical evaluation of a specific system. If the parents report that the infant consistently cries or strains with bowel movements, the infant's rectum should be examined for fissures or for a congenital stricture of the anorectal segment. Visual examination of the anus and palpation of the rectum with a small finger reveals either of these minor problems.[47]

As the infant's teeth begin to erupt, they are inspected for uniformity of shape and appropriate placement. If a tooth erupts in areas of the mouth other than that of the normal gumline, a dental consultation may be indicated. Parents should be counseled regarding the most common cause of dental caries in infants—slow sucking on a bottle of milk after the infant goes to sleep, which results in the infant retaining small amounts of milk in the mouth while sleeping. Further discussion regarding counseling related to nutrition and dental caries prevention is found later in this chapter.

Assessment of the heart includes observation of the rate and rhythm, estimation of the size and shape of the heart, auscultation of the quality of heart sounds, determination of the quality of femoral and other pulses, and measurement of the blood pressure. Inspection of the chest should reveal a symmetrical shape and the presence and location of a visible cardiac impulse. A visible cardiac impulse usually corresponds to the location of the apex of the heart and may be normal, but if it is diffuse and predominant, it may indicate cardiac enlargement or failure. A normal visible cardiac impulse is apparent frequently in children who are hyperactive, thin, or excited.[5]

Estimation of the size of the heart is accomplished by palpation to locate the point of maximum impulse (PMI). The PMI usually indicates the location of the apex of the heart, although a more reliable landmark for the location of the apex is the apex beat. The apex beat is the point farthest toward the axilla and toward the lower left costal margin, where the heart beat can be easily palpated. During infancy the apex beat is normally felt in the fourth interspace just to the left of the midclavicular line. Further estimate of heart size and location is accomplished by percussion of the chest, combined with auscultation. With the stethoscope placed just to the right of the sternum, the chest wall along an intercostal space is tapped lightly with the index finger, beginning in the axillary line and moving medially. As the finger percusses over the heart, an immediate intensification of sound will be heard. The heart is usually percussed as a triangular area with one side of the triangle extending along the right sternal border from the second to the fourth rib, one side being from the

**295**

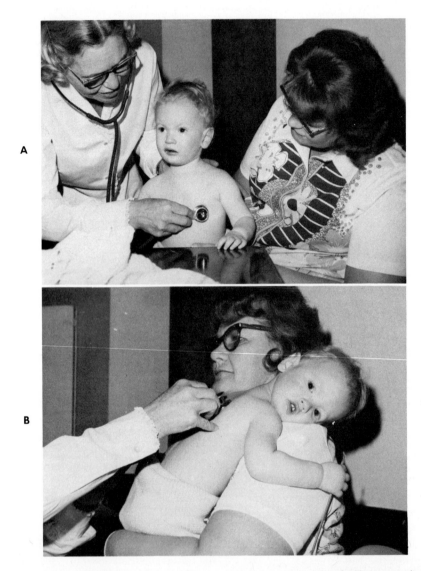

**Fig. 9-10.** Approaches appropriate to the developmental stage of the infant facilitate auscultation and visualization of specific areas. **A,** The infant is seated on mother's lap while the nurse auscultates his chest. **B,** He is held over her shoulder while auscultation of his back is accomplished, providing needed security and quieting. **C,** Immobilization to protect from accidental injury during visualization of the mouth and throat is accomplished with the infant on his back, arms held to the side of his head, and his trunk immobilized by another adult. **D,** Maximal immobilization for visualization of ears is accomplished with two adults restraining the infant's head and trunk. He is in a prone position with his arms held to his side.

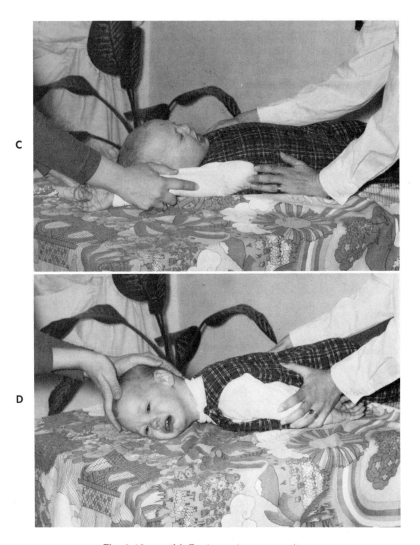

**Fig. 9-10, cont'd.** For legend see opposite page.

right sternal border along the fourth rib to a point just to the left of the left nipple, and the third side being from the right sternal border at the second rib to the point just beyond the left nipple at the fourth rib.[5]

Auscultation of heart sounds requires experience and astute judgment. The following guidelines are intended to assist the beginning practitioner in developing listening capacity but should not serve as guidelines for interpretation. The sounds heard should always be described as accurately as possible, and any unusual or questionable sounds referred to an experienced practitioner for evaluation. Fig. 9-12 indicates the positions on the chest where the

stethoscope should be placed for auscultation, although for the young infant the fourth position will be located in the fourth interspace and the fifth position more to the right of the sternal border. The first heart sound is best heard with the bell and the second with the diaphragm of the stethoscope.

The first heart sound is due to mitral and atrioventricular valve closure. This is the systolic part of the cardiac cycle and is heard as the louder of the two heart sounds in the apical area. The second heart sound is due to aortic and pulmonic valve closure. It is the diastolic portion of the cardiac cycle and is heard as the louder of the two sounds in the aortic and pulmonic area. Third and fourth sounds can sometimes be detected and are associated with the diastolic portion of the cardiac cycle. These sounds must be distinguished as normal by specialists. Splitting of the second sound is often heard in young children and infants and is normal during this developmental period. The split can be detected as such in that it widens on inspiration, indicating that the split sound is caused by pulmonic valve closure, which is delayed by deep inspiration. The heart sounds should be systematically heard in at least the five areas identified in Fig. 9-12, with any unusual characteristic described as accurately as possible. The areas indicated are the sites where maximum auscultation of the particular valve sound is possible and not the anatomic site of the valve.[5,20,45,130]

Functional or innocent murmurs are not un-common in young children, but all unusual heart sounds should be referred to a specialist for full evaluation. Functional murmurs may be characteristically described as beginning within a very brief interval after the first heart sound and ending well in advance of the second heart sound. The heart sounds themselves are normal. The murmur is usually low-pitched, coarsely vibratory, and somewhat decrescendo. It is usually heard best at or near the upper left sternal border in the second or third interspace.[5,45,130]

Laboratory testing is needed to determine the adequate functioning of the blood and the renal system. The prevalence of iron deficiency anemia during infancy and the particular pattern of development of iron deficiency anemia (described in preceding sections) indicate the necessity of determining the hemoglobin level of the infant at about 6 months of age. Dietary or therapeutic response to iron administration in the face of inadequate hemoglobin levels rules out the possibility of serious disease states of the blood.

Testing of the urine should be done by the

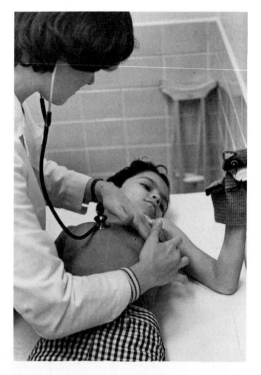

**Fig. 9-11.** Estimation of heart size and location is accomplished by percussion of the chest combined with auscultation. With the stethoscope placed just to the right of the sternum, the chest wall is tapped lightly along an intercostal space beginning in the axillary line and moving medially. As the finger percusses over the heart, an immediate intensification of sound will be heard.

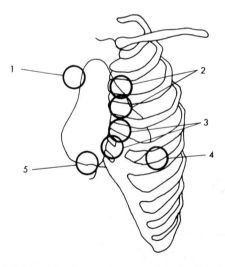

**Fig. 9-12.** The heart sounds are systematically auscultated in the five areas identified. These are the sites where maximum auscultation of the particular valve sound is possible, not the anatomic site of the valve. *1,* Aortic; *2,* pulmonic; *3,* right ventricular; *4,* mitral or apical; *5,* xiphoid.

time that the infant is 1 year of age in order to establish knowledge of adequate functioning of the renal system. The infant's urinary stream should also be observed to determine strength and direction of flow.

The skin is of particular concern during infancy because of the particular physiologic hazards that dispose the infant to serious effects of infection or damage to the skin. The aesthetic impact of skin disorders on the face and visible body areas is serious for the parents, regardless of the seriousness of the skin problem. A diaper rash likewise creates particular problems for the parents in relation to their care-taking ability, and often insightful nursing counsel is needed to help with a persistent problem. Specific recommendations for prevention of minor skin prob-

lems of infancy may be helpful for young, inexperienced parents. These should include information about cleansing and hygiene practices to be used at each diaper change, the need for frequent changing and judicious use of plastic pants, and laundering techniques.

## Feeding and nutrition

Assessment of nutrition includes the diet history of the infant, determination of the medical and socioeconomic history of the family, physical evaluation of the infant, and laboratory evaluation of the blood and urine. Table 9-3 indicates the specific parameters that must be assessed for adequate determination of nutritional status in infants up to 24 months of age. The minimal level of assessment should be obtained

**Table 9-3.** Levels of nutritional assessment for infants and children (birth to 24 months)*

| Level of approach† | History | | Clinical evaluation | Laboratory evaluation |
|---|---|---|---|---|
| | **Dietary** | **Medical and socioeconomic** | | |
| Minimal | 1. Source of iron<br>2. Vitamin supplement<br>3. Milk intake (type and amount) | 1. Birth weight<br>2. Length of gestation<br>3. Serious or chronic illness<br>4. Use of medicines | 1. Body weight and length<br>2. Gross defects | 1. Hematocrit<br>2. Hemoglobin<br>3. Urine protein and sugar |
| Mid-level | 1. Semi-quantitative<br>  a. Iron-cereal, meat, egg yolks, supplement<br>  b. Energy nutrients<br>  c. Micronutrients—calcium, niacin, riboflavin, vitamin C<br>  d. Protein<br>2. Food intolerances<br>3. Baby foods—processed commercially; home cooked | 1. Family history: diabetes tuberculosis<br>2. Maternal: Height Prenatal care<br>3. Infant: Immunizations Tuberculin test | 1. Head circumference<br>2. Skin color, pallor, turgor<br>3. Subcutaneous tissue paucity, excess | 1. RBC morphology<br>2. Serum iron<br>3. Total iron binding capacity<br>4. Sickle cell testing |
| In-depth level | 1. Quantitative 24-hour recall<br>2. Dietary history | 1. Prenatal details<br>2. Complications of delivery<br>3. Regular health supervision | 1. Cranial bossing<br>2. Epyphyseal enlargement<br>3. Costochondral beading<br>4. Ecchymoses | Same as above, plus vitamin and appropriate enzyme assays; protein and amino acids; hydroxyproline, etc., should be available |

*From Christakis, G., editor: Nutritional assessment in health programs, Am. J. Public Health, (suppl). vol. 63, Nov., 1973, p. 46.
†It is understood that what is included at a minimal level would also be included or represented at successively more sophisticated levels of approach. However, it may be entirely appropriate to use a minimal level of approach to clinical evaluations and a maximal approach to laboratory evaluations.

for all infants at regular intervals during infancy. Midlevel and in-depth level assessment is pursued for infants who show some sign of nutritional deficit or are known to be at risk for developing a nutritional deficit.[29,37]

Iron-fortified milk with vitamin C supplementation provides all nutritional requirements for infants throughout the first year of life. However, most families in Western societies add foods during the first year. The diet history of the infant is evaluated using the guidelines of the basic four food groups and the recommended minimum daily requirements (see Appendix, pp. 882 to 883). Estimating the actual nutritive value of various foods in the infant's diet is difficult, and a nutritionist should be consulted if there is any doubt as to its adequacy.[72,98,119]

Nutritional requirements remain similar throughout the period of infancy, although slight increases in minerals and some vitamins are recommended, and substantial increases are needed in caloric intake. The increase in caloric needs with nutrition-rich foods, rather than empty carbohydrates, supplies the slight increase needed in some of the vitamins and min-

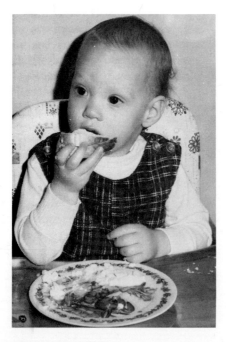

**Fig. 9-13.** Addition of foods to the infant's diet is determined by developmental achievements such as eye-hand-mouth coordination and fine pincer grasp.

erals. Thus the infant's diet may remain relatively simple throughout the first several months. Different foods will be added according to the needs of the infant to experience differences in food, to begin to eat solid foods, to manipulate foods, and to participate as a social member of the family. When whole or evaporated milk is used rather than a fortified commercial formula, the infant must receive some source of iron and vitamin C. One source of iron is infant enriched cereal; orange juice or commercial vitamin preparations provide vitamin C. Fluoride should be provided from some natural or artificial source.[1] Such a diet, with increasing amounts of milk to provide needed calories and minerals might suffice for the first 12 months.[41]

The feeding behavior of infants is highly variant, depending upon the usual attitudes and circumstances surrounding the feeding and upon their own basic temperamental inclinations. Most infants develop early traits of behavior indicating hunger, responses during the feeding period, and responses indicating satiety. These behaviors reflect the general developmental stage of the infant; they also give an indication of the adequacy of care-taking capabilities of the mother and of the mother-infant relationship. Typical behaviors expected for various periods during infancy with a description of the variations that may normally occur for some infants are presented in Table 9-4.

### Sleep and activity

The organization of sleeping and waking states is a primary indicator of the infant's developing neurologic capacity, learning and thought potential, and potential for social and inner development. Developing a sleep-wake pattern that is congruent with family life is a major concern for the family and a catalyst for the important family interactions that occur with the infant.

By about the age of 3 to 4 months, the infant should be sleeping primarily at night, averaging about a total of 10 hours of sleep during the evening, night and early morning hours, although there may still be the need for feeding during this time span. During the day the infant at this age will continue to sleep about four to five hours total, but the periods of sleep will be

**Table 9-4.** Feeding behavior development

| Age | Hunger behavior | Feeding behavior | Satiety behavior | Normal variations |
|---|---|---|---|---|
| Birth to 13 weeks | Cries to express hunger every 3 to 4 hours<br>Begins to regard bottle<br>Hands fisted, body tense, movement intense<br>Hunger gradually begins to occur less frequently | May need help in securing nipple<br>Tongue surrounds lower half of nipple<br>Strong suck reflex<br>Strong suck demands<br>Regards mother's face while feeding<br>Sucks solid foods off of spoons, thrusts solid foods back out of mouth due to sucking mode of manipulation foods and immature swallow<br>Gags easily<br>Needs "burping" to expel air from stomach | Withdraws head from nipple<br>Falls asleep<br>When nipple reinserted, closes lips tightly<br>Bites nipple, purses lips, or smiles and lets milk run out of mouth | Some infants are not particularly interested in food; mother needs to heed hunger signals, which may be subtle<br>Some infants do not give strong indications of satiety; mother may need to heed subtle signs<br>Great variations in self-patterning of eating occurs |
| 14 to 24 weeks | Eagerly anticipates food being prepared<br>Has some ability to wait for food<br>Mouth poises to receive nipple<br>Secures nipple easily<br>Grasps and draws bottle to mouth but releases hold<br>Reaches to cup with open mouth | Able to sleep through night<br>Appetite for milk may decrease<br>Tongue holds nipple firmly<br>May shift regard for mother's face to surroundings<br>Coughs and chokes easily<br>Sucking demand strong<br>Enjoys a variety of strained foods<br>Swallow becomes more mature<br>Preference for tastes emerges<br>Sucks on finger foods<br>Makes smacking noises with lips | Throws head back<br>Fusses or cries<br>Obstructs mouth with hands<br>Plays with nipple<br>Increased attention to surroundings<br>Ejects food with tongue projection | May be so easily distracted that quiet surroundings are needed to eat well<br>Objects to changes in routine<br>Extreme preferences for taste |
| 28 to 36 weeks | Impatient and eager as meal is prepared<br>Vocalizes desire to eat<br>Reaches toward bottle, spoon, cup | Holds bottle during feeding<br>Withdraws and inserts nipple himself<br>Grasps spoon<br>Sucking demands decrease<br>Mature swallow<br>Grasps food off spoon easily<br>Lateral jaw and tongue movements begin<br>Finger feeding begins | Changes posture<br>Keeps mouth tightly closed<br>Shakes head as if to say "no"<br>Plays with utensils<br>Hands become more active<br>Throws bottle or utensils | May be ready to wean during this period |
| 40 to 52 weeks | Vocalizes eagerness<br>Grasps bottle or spoon | Able to chew with appearance of teeth<br><br>Draws in lower lip when spoon is removed from mouth<br>Lateral chewing movements more mature<br>Finger feeds well<br>Tongue licks food from lower lip<br>Approximates lip to edge of cup<br>Drinks from cup with spills from sides<br>Weaning begins<br>Changes to table foods<br>Demands to help feed self | Behaviors of above period typical<br><br>Sputters with tongue and lips<br>Shakes head "no"<br>Hands bottle to mother | Slow to accept changes in texture<br><br>Not interested in feeding self<br>Begins to develop rituals and routines<br>Refuses milk completely when weaned |

shorter than those during the night hours. More time will be spent during the day in waking states, and the frequency and quantity of food intake will be greater during the day than at night. The quality of the infant's sleep will have also changed markedly, with a greater proportion of sleep being in active, no-rapid-eye-movement sleep. The parents will observe that the infant sleeps more soundly and is less prone to being awakened, particularly at night. The infant will spend a portion of the waking time crying vigorously, but there should not be undue difficulty in the family's ability to quiet the infant by responding to needs for feeding, diaper changes, or holding and rocking. There is usually a period of time during the first three months of infancy when the infant is "fussy" beyond the family's tolerance and ability to respond, but this period should be satisfactorily resolved as the fifth and sixth month are approached. During the infant's waking states, there should be an increasing amount of time spent in states of relative inactivity and relative activity, without crying. During this period the infant should be observed to be attentive to events in the environment and able to focus attention briefly on objects or people. The parents should be able to describe activities that the infant engages in during periods of alert activity and inactivity, particularly those that draw attention from those in the environment.

During the second half of the first year, the infant begins to be mobile and becomes increasingly involved in activity that demands the attention of the family and care-takers. A well-established diurnal pattern of sleeping evolves, and night-time feedings are discarded. One or two naps may be needed during the day, and each of the periods of sleep is relatively inactive, no-rapid-eye-movement sleep. The infant should have established well-recognized signals indicating the need for sleep, which tends to occur at predictable time intervals. Active alert states predominate during the periods of waking, with very little time spent crying and fussing. This pattern of sleep-waking activity lasts well into the toddler period, with gradual decreases in the amount of time needed for daytime naps.[37,105]

Assessment of learning and thought compe-tency during infancy is accomplished by sequential evaluation of the neuromotor development of the infant, the quantity and quality of the stimulation provided the infant, and the infant's response to stimulation. Several useful tools have been developed for screening and testing of the infant's learning and thought competency, recognizing the fact that the infant does have significant thinking ability and that early experiences are crucial for later development of thinking ability. The general parameters included in such testing are described in the following section.*

The assessment of the quantity and quality of stimulation in the infant's environment is essential for evaluation of the dynamic interrelationship between the environment and the infant's actual response.[37] The elements of assessment of the stimulation environment are described in this section, while the infant's developmental response is discussed in the sections that follow.

Table 9-5 presents the essential elements of assessment of care-giver behaviors that most directly stimulate or fail to stimulate the infant's learning and thought competency. These behaviors should be observed directly for all primary care-givers, including the parents, day-care workers, and baby sitters. An indication of the quantity and quality of stimulation may be obtained by interview and observation of interactions in the health care setting, as well as by observation of the infant's actual development. However, for any infant whose development is delayed or incomplete or who is known to be at risk for developmental delay, abuse, or neglect, direct observation of the infant's usual environment is essential.

### Infant's sensory development

The infant's sensory development is assessed by sequential evaluation of the neuromotor competency of the infant at regular intervals throughout infancy and observation of the infant's responses to the care-giver behaviors listed in Table 9-5. The neuromotor developmental landmarks have been described previously in this chapter and are available in other sources included in the references. Repeated

---

*References 17, 56, 61, 73, 105, 121.

**Table 9-5.** Assessment of care-giver behaviors that stimulate learning and thought competency during infancy*

| | |
|---|---|
| 1. Language facilitation<br>  a. Elicits vocalization (through initiation and contingent responses)<br>  b. Converses; chats to infant<br>  c. Praises or encourages infant<br>  d. Offers help or solicitous remarks<br>  e. Inquires of child; requests<br>  f. Gives explanation, information, cultural rules<br>  g. Labels sensory experiences<br>  h. Reads to or shows pictures<br>  i. Sings to or plays music for<br>2. Social-emotional positive inputs<br>  a. Smiles at infant<br>  b. Uses loving or reassuring tones<br>  c. Provides loving physical contact<br>  d. Plays social games with infant<br>  e. Uses eye contact to arouse, orient, or sustain infant's attention<br>3. Social-emotional negative inputs<br>  a. Criticizes verbally, scolds<br>  b. Forbids; negative commands<br>  c. Acts angry; is physically impatient; frowns; restrains infant<br>  d. Punishes physically<br>  e. Isolates child for unacceptable behaviors<br>  f. Ignores child when child shows need for attention | 4. Presents planned learning games<br>  a. "Things don't disappear" games<br>  b. "Using a tool" games<br>  c. Imitation<br>  d. "Cause it to happen" games<br>  e. Handling and pickup games<br>  f. The use of space, such as resting and stacking games and detour games<br>  g. Introduces new games appropriate to developmental changes<br>5. Care-giving routines with child<br>  a. Feeds<br>  b. Diapers; toilets<br>  c. Dresses; undresses<br>  d. Washes; cleans<br>  e. Prepares infant for sleep<br>  f. Physical shepherding<br>  g. Eye checks on infant's well-being<br>6. Care-giving routines with environment<br>  a. Prepares food<br>  b. Tidies room or environment<br>  c. Helps other care-givers<br>7. Physical development<br>  a. Provides kinesthetic stimulation<br>  b. Provides large-muscle play |

*Adapted from Honig, A. S., and Lally, J. R.: Assessing teacher behaviors with infants in day care. In Friedlander, B. Z., Sterritt, G. M., and Kirk, G. E., editors: Exceptional infant, vol. 3, New York, 1975, Brunner/Mazel, p. 533.

assessment sequentially throughout infancy is essential in order to obtain an accurate judgment of the infant's learning and thought competency because of the variation that exists among infants in development and the fact that an infant's temperament on any one day may affect or change the usual pattern of behavior, giving an erroneous impression of the usual pattern of response.

The infant's development of receptive and expressive language, presented on p. 872 of the Appendix, provides a useful guide for evaluation of the development of speech and language. Changes in neurologic capacity and social response should be documented, with particular attention to expected developmental landmarks throughout infancy.

## Play

The review of Piaget's theory offered some theoretical notions regarding the early development of play during infancy. Other theorists and researchers have explored this childhood phenomenon and attach varying interpretations and meanings. The early fascination of children with their surroundings and their spontaneous ability to manipulate and use objects and their own bodies to form symbolic representations of inner experiences of the world through play are important parts of development. Symbolic play should appear by about 15 months of age, and the infant should then be capable of entertaining himself or herself for brief periods of time without adult interaction. The ability of infants at this period of life to play interactively is very limited, although infants in constant contact with older children learn very early to depend upon the play stimulation offered by the older children. During infancy most play is parallel, with the infant pursuing individual play interests alongside another child. Squabbles over toys occur, and the ability to give and take, to cooperate, or to share is not present.[54]

As the infant enters the second half of the first

year and becomes mobile, the family or care-giver should provide the infant with increasing opportunities for spontaneous play and exploration. There needs to be a planned period of time in an environment that is safe and suitable for the infant for unrestricted activity and objects that can be manipulated at will by the infant. The adult does not deliberately initiate, directly stimulate, or interfere with the infant's play during such periods but maintains attentiveness to the needs of the infant and responds appropriately. Such periods of play are increasingly important for adequate development of learning and thought.

## NURSING ASSESSMENT OF SOCIAL AND INNER COMPETENCIES

Because of the extremely close relationship between social and inner competencies during infancy, we shall consider assessment of each simultaneously.

### Relationships with mother and other significant people

The theoretical formulations of Erikson and Bowlby and Klaus and Kennell provide guidelines for assessment of the adequacy of the infant-mother relationship (Fig. 9-14). Bowlby provided further indications of the development of attachment behavior for father, siblings, and other family members. These relationships represent the infant's first socialization experiences, as well as the foundation upon which infants begin to build a sense of self (Fig. 9-15). The development of the expected separation anxiety between 6 and 10 months of age, as well as observation of behaviors between mother and infant at all stages, gives sound evidence of this important relationship.

The mental health of the mother and any other primary care-giver needs to be determined, as this factor is a critical variable influencing the quality of the early relationships experienced by the infant. The family assessment, presented in Chapter 3, provides a basis for evaluating the mental health of the family. Of particular importance are the family's pattern of response to stress and how they identify stressors. If the family seems overwhelmed by events that tend to occur during the usual course of living and use immature means of coping, their ability to form a caring relationship with the infant will be in jeopardy. The response of the family to unusual stress events or the chronic stress of economic inadequacy or long-term illness should be carefully evaluated, and the effect of these factors considered for the infant. Individual psychologic assessment of individual family members may also be needed to determine particular individual dynamics that may affect the family relationships and the infant's development.[113] Of particular importance to the infant relationship is the individual adult's experience as a young child. Their recollections of their own early experience and the nature of these memories as good or bad, satisfying or distressing should be explored and documented.

The relationship between the infant and primary care-givers should be one of interpersonal synchrony.[105] Both the infant and the care-giver have needs, motives, or goals for interaction and for themselves alone. Their ability to establish an interactive balance and synchrony is the basis for the early relationship. During the first half of the first year of infancy, the infant should demonstrate the ability to focus attention on people in the environment and provide signals regarding wants and needs. There is no regard for the needs or intentions of others in the environment, and there is little indication of the infant's ability to respond differently to various people in the environment. The mother and other primary care-givers, on the other hand, exhibit numerous behaviors that attend to the needs of the infant according to the infant's signals, provide appropriate stimuli for the establishment of diurnal patterns, and attend to their own individual needs during periods of time when the infant is sleeping or not signaling a need or desire for direct interaction.

During the second half of the first year, as the infant becomes mobile and begins to discriminate between different people in the environment, there is an increasing tendency for the infant to direct signals for attention and care specifically to the primary care-giver. The infant cries, smiles, babbles with the clear intention of engaging that person's attention, and rejects, on occasion, efforts of others in the environment to

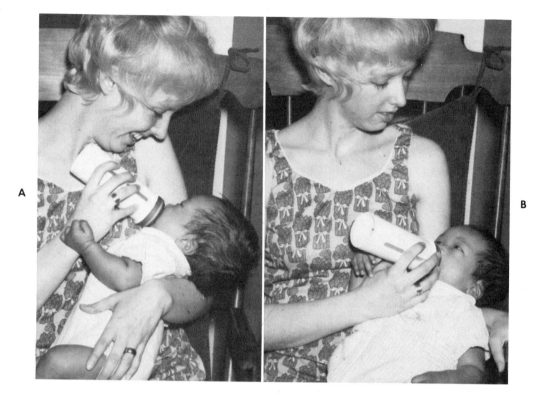

**Fig. 9-14.** Mother-infant contacts that demonstrate maximal physical involvement and eye-to-eye contact are demonstrated. **A,** The infant is held close to mother's body, with optimal alignment of her face with the infant's to achieve direct eye-to-eye contact. **B,** The infant is held away from mother's body, with less adequate alignment for achieving eye-to-eye contact, even though the infant seeks mother's face. (See discussion on Bowlby's theory earlier in this chapter.)

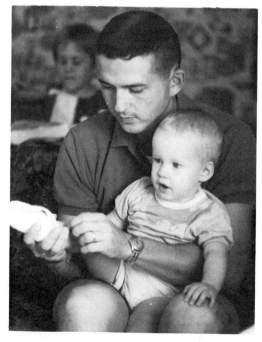

**Fig. 9-15.** Attachment and socialization with each member of the family develop during infancy.

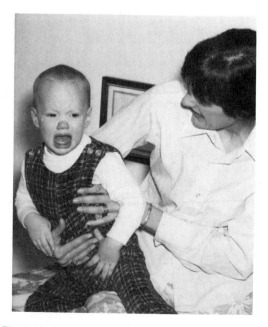

**Fig. 9-16.** Separation anxiety is demonstrated by the infant's desperate attempts to remain in close proximity to mother, giving evidence of the development of attachment formation.

provide attention and care. Separation anxiety emerges, and the infant actively protests separation from the primary care-giver. As the infant becomes mobile, the infant will maintain proximity with the primary care-giver by following that person and maintaining the ability to see and touch that person. Toward the end of the first year, the infant increasingly regards strangers with caution, but at the same time the infant is able to develop regard for subsidiary care-givers and often develops strong attachments with several people in the environment, including extended family members, friends, and regular baby-sitters. The infant continues to show primary regard for the mother or primary care-giver and will continue to protest separation from that figure even when left in the presence of a subsidiary care-giver. In such an instance the infant's protest against separation is brief and temporary, and the infant ends the protest with a period of crying rather than continuing the protest with despair and denial (see Chapter 16, p. 665).

During the second year, another significant change occurs in the nature of the relationship between the infant and the primary care-giver, in that the infant exhibits the ability to sense, anticipate, and behave in accord with the needs and desires of the care-giver. While the infant does not behave out of consideration for the care-giver's needs and desires, the relationship becomes more complex and the ability of the infant to infer the intentions of the care-giver does affect the behavior. The infant continues to maintain proximity with the primary care-giver and directs signals for attention and care primarily to that person. However, the infant explores the environment with increasing confidence at distances further removed from the proximic figure and increasingly uses eye contact, rather than touch, to maintain attention. The mother is increasingly facilitative of the infant's needs for manipulation and exploration and encourages the infant's interactions with other people. At the same time the mother begins to use various means of controlling and directing the infant's behavior, such as voice commands, eye contact, praise, reprimands, and physical restraint. Styles in achieving control and discipline for the infant vary greatly among

mothers, and there is a wide range of acceptable or healthy approaches that can be used. The risk of early neglect and child abuse is great during this period, and therefore the assessment of the early relationship should include determination of the presence of such approaches. Physical restraint, hitting, abusive voice tones and language should not occur. The mother should express anger in the presence of the infant but in a manner that is not abusive or harmful to the infant directly nor to other people or objects in the environment. A positive approach includes direct manipulation and control of the environment to minimize the need for control or restraint of the infant directly. In addition, the care-giver initiates and facilitates the infant's engagement in acceptable activities, such as those presented in Table 9-5. Positive reinforcement and praise for desired behaviors should predominate.[11,14,105,116]

### Assessment of temperament and personality

Objective assessment of the infant's unique temperament provides some clues as to important areas of health care management. Table 9-3 indicates a few temperamental differences in infants that differentially affect their feeding behavior. Very active, persistent, or exploratory infants tend to encounter more accidents than do quiet, sedate infants. The interaction between the mother's temperament and the infant's temperament is important in their developing satisfying relationships. Most mothers experience periods when they are not in harmony with their infants, but some mothers experience more disharmony with a certain infant than they would with another child because of temperamental differences. Mothers vary in their ability to tolerate various temperaments among infants. Understanding these differences assists in offering relevant, insightful nursing guidance during this period.[16,23,27,37,120]

### HEALTH MAINTENANCE, PROMOTION, AND PREVENTION OF ILLNESS

The health care system in the United States has provided for health maintenance needs of infants in a manner that is not generally available for other groups in society. Well-baby visits and clinics are an integral component of private medical practice as well as community health programs. However, these services are often limited to prevention of illness through immunizations and cursory monitoring of growth and development, and the services have limited accessibility to many high-risk groups in society. Vast improvements are needed in the comprehensiveness of these services and their accessibility to underserved groups if the foundations for an improved quality of life are to be laid. The following section presents the primary health maintenance needs for all infants and describes the nursing measures that may be used in the maintenance of health and prevention of lifelong health problems during this critical period of development.

### Feeding and nutrition

Central to health maintenance during infancy is concern for the adequacy of nutrition. The family's socioeconomic level does not ensure adequate or inadequate nutrition for a family or an infant, and skill must be developed in working with all families to make determinations of the adequacy of nutrition. Further, it is not sufficient just to tell parents what they should be feeding their infant from month to month, because they receive information and advice regarding food from many sources. The goal of adequate health care is to convey to the parents some understanding of the basic principles of adequate nutrition, along with an understanding of all the physical and emotional factors that contribute to healthy feeding and nutrition. There is a vast variation in findings related to these concerns among families and individual infants, but some guidelines help in making a sound evaluation of the factors that contribute to good nutrition.[10,28,33,37]

By the age of 12 months and usually much sooner, the parents, the infant, or both desire to expand the number of foods in the diet. The choice of which foods to add to the diet is guided more by the expanding chewing and motor capabilities of the infant (such as hand-eye coordination and fine pincer grasp) than by actual nutritional needs. Family and cultural preferences are also relevant determinants.

As calorie sources are met with foods other than milk, greater attention must be directed toward the adequacy of these foods to promote growth and development. Recommended daily dietary allowances provide a sound guideline for evaluating the adequacy of the diet and for recommending additions to the diet. In addition, it is necessary to determine, when possible, the nutritional content of foods being consumed. This is a difficult and complex task and requires knowledge of the effects of various methods of preparation. A nutritional consultant is an essential component of the health care team, because the information and skills needed for unusual or difficult situations usually exceed those of the nurse or physician.[37]

There is often a specific regimen established by a health care team in recommending dietary changes to the parents. These standard recommendations may be used, but the important component of health care responsibility is helping the parents to understand basic principles of nutrition, which they can then apply using their own judgment and creativity to prepare healthy foods for the family.[58]

Food money management is often a problem, both for lower and higher income families. Expensive special foods are not necessary for the infant; very early in life children may be given the usual diet of the family with a minimum of expense. Regardless of approach, however, the responsibility of the nurse remains to help the parents understand what they are feeding the infant and what food requirements are being met.

The usual circumstances surrounding the infant's meals are important as a measure of the adequacy of developing eating habits. Actual amounts of intake, the absorption and utilization of the foods eaten, and the infant's developing attitudes toward the eating occasion are all thought to be influenced by the situation that surrounds the family during meals. The parents' attitudes and emotional state significantly alter feeding behaviors. The atmosphere should be one of relaxation and acceptance, but the specific effects of differential attitudes toward eating are not known. The infant's behavior and adequate physical growth provide some estimate of the total adequacy of the feeding situation.[81]

## Body hygiene

Parents bring many concerns to health care workers regarding daily care, such as questions regarding proper dressing, travel, and the use of various lotions and creams. Insightful judgment is required, since few scientific guidelines specifically apply to these ordinary, but important, concerns.[35]

While hygiene standards vary greatly among cultures and subcultures, certain aspects of hygiene remain consistently important for health maintenance and should be encouraged for all families. The predominant concern in relation to the infant is the importance of skin care, because as discussed earlier, the skin of the infant is particularly susceptible to infection and damage. The diaper area and scalp are particularly prone during early infancy to development of minor problems of rash and cradle cap. Adequate cleansing of the diaper area, frequent changes, and adequate laundering may intervene for a diaper rash.[65] Cradle cap may be prevented with daily thorough scrubbing of the scalp. Once this problem develops, the parent needs to shampoo vigorously with a soft toothbrush at least once a day until the condition clears. Without generating undue concern about scrubbing and grooming an active, healthy, exploring infant, parents should be aware of the hygiene needs of their infant.

## Prevention of illness

Immunizations have become one of the most important preventative means ever developed in health science. The eradication of serious communicable disease has significantly altered the life and health expectancy for children and families, and continuing attention to adequate immunizations is vital for adequate health maintenance. Immunization against diphtheria, tetanus, pertussis, polio, rubella, rubeola, mumps, and smallpox is available for the infant. Recommendations on dosage and frequency of dosages are available from the American Academy of Pediatrics (Table 9-6). Continuing investigation in response to the epidemiology of the world and the nature of the immune reactions in pregnancy, fetal life, and infancy requires continuing reevaluation of immunization practices.[43,76] For example, the use of the small-

**Table 9-6.** American Academy of Pediatrics recommended immunization schedule for infants (1974)*

| Age | Immunizations |
|---|---|
| 2 months | Diphtheria, tetanus, pertussis (DTP) Trivalent oral polio vaccine (TOPV) |
| 4 months | DTP, TOPV |
| 6 months | DTP, TOPV |
| 15 months | Measles, rubella, mumps Tuberculin skin test |
| 18 months | DTP, TOPV |
| 4-6 years | DTP, TOPV |
| 14-16 years | Diphtheria, tetanus (repeat every 10 years thereafter) |

*Current recommendations and information available from the American Academy of Pediatrics, P.O. Box 1034, Evanston, Ill. 60204. Also refer to Powell, K. R.: Basic principles of immunization, Pediatr. Nurs. **3:**7, Sept./Oct., 1977.

pox vaccine came under close scrutiny early in the 1970s because of the virtual irradication of the disease in the United States and Western European countries and the comparative risk of serious reaction and illness from administration of the vaccine. This led to the recommendation that children in the United States no longer receive this protection as a routine procedure and that it remain available for children and adults anticipating travel to another country only.*

Skin testing for determination of exposure to tuberculosis is widely and routinely administered during infancy. Identification of infants who may be exposed leads to careful evaluation for possible infection; thus institution of early treatment of the disease during childhood becomes possible.

Most immunization programs should be completed during infancy with the exception of booster dosages, which are administered at ages 4 to 6 years or later in life, as recommended by the American Academy of Pediatrics. Should an infant not complete the recommended immunization routine, this protection may be offered at the earliest age that incomplete immunization is discovered.

Adequate technique of administering immunizations to infants involves choosing an appropriate route and site, sound administration tech-

*References 18, 19, 62, 67, 86, 93, 110.

niques, and adequate approach to the infant before and after immunization. The mother should be encouraged to comfort the infant immediately after an injection.

Prevention of iron deficiency anemia is a major component of prevention of illness. The infant should be screened for hemoglobin level at the sixth month of age, as this is the period when iron deficiency is most likely to occur because of the shift that has just occurred in the infant's dependence upon his or her own ability to produce red blood cells (see p. 239). An infant whose hemoglobin is at a borderline level (10-12 g/100 ml) should be given additional oral supplements of iron, and the adequacy of existing dietary intake should be studied carefully. In addition, the parents may need teaching and counseling regarding diet and feeding. Such an infant should be periodically reevaluated for adequacy of hemoglobin level to assure prevention of iron deficiency. All infants whose hemoglobin level is clearly deficient should receive parenteral iron, regular evaluation of hemoglobin level, and teaching of the family with regard to nutrition and diet.

Prevention of dental caries is another concern in health maintenance for the infant. Many communities provide fluoridation of the community water supply, which is sufficient in amount to provide prophylaxis against caries for infants and young children. If fluoridation of the water is not available, fluoride may be given orally to the infant in daily doses. The recommended dose for infants up to 2 years of age is 0.25 mg/day.[40]

Other dietary and feeding practices are of concern in the prevention of dental caries, such as offering sweets frequently to the infant as a reward for desired behavior and allowing the infant to go to sleep with a bottle. Retaining milk in the mouth while sleeping with a bottle contributes to significant dental decay early in infancy, and the parents need to understand this problem and use other means of encouraging her infant to go to sleep. Counseling regarding this problem, as well as alternate means for rewarding desired behavior, may be needed.[96,99]

Counseling with the family in regard to protection of the infant from common communicable disease is often needed. Parents need to understand the basic principles of sound hygiene in preparation of formula, body hygiene, and transfer of communicable disease from person to person. When another member of the family is ill with a communicable illness, the family needs to understand measures that may be taken to provide the infant with as much protection as possible, such as relative isolation from the ill person, care in handling of food and dishes, and careful hand-washing when handling the infant.[51]

## Prevention of accidents

Accident prevention is of particular concern as the infant becomes increasingly mobile. This very serious hazard to the life and well-being of the infant is totally vulnerable to intervention through careful anticipatory guidance for the mother or care-giver. The newborn may be capable of rolling off an unguarded table. The infant rapidly gains the capacity to move his or her body about through sequential rolling and then crawling and creeping. Physiologic and cognitive needs to explore the environment should not be curtailed because of the possibility of dangers in the environment; rather the dangers should be removed.

Toxic cleaning and home care agents should be placed out of reach. Hot appliances should be guarded during use, and the infant's activity and mobility should possibly be limited when the appliance is in use. Dangling electric cords from coffee pots and irons are particularly hazardous for the infant who crawls freely and automatically mouths all objects he or she can find. In addition, an infant can easily pull the appliance down by the cord, causing severe injury and burns. Small objects that might be mouthed present potential choking hazards. The parents should be taught and encouraged to make a thorough assessment of their home for possible hazards and should know the precautions that may be taken when leaving the infant with a babysitter. They may need specific assistance in their home.

Guidance in selecting safe toys is also helpful. Appropriate toys for the infant's interest and capability may have hidden dangers, such as flammability, sharp internal nails and wires, or easily detachable button eyes.

**309**

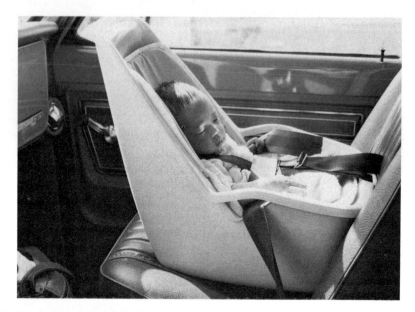

**Fig. 9-17.** A special car carrier provides maximal automotive protection for the infant at a minimal cost. The infant faces the seat, and the car belt secures the seat and infant into the seat.

Automobile safety is too often neglected for infants. The family should understand the need to securely and safely fasten the infant to the car's seat. This is most effectively accomplished by placing the infant on an infant carrier and securely fastening the carrier with the adult seat belt (Fig. 9-17). When the infant can sit erect, an approved car seat that provides adequate seat belt protection may be used.[30,71]

### Stimulation and play

The assessment of the infant's stimulation and play experiences described previously in this chapter provides the basis for nursing management and intervention. If there are any deficits in the infant's stimulation, specific teaching and counseling of the infant's care-givers are needed, and it may be desirable to provide planned infant stimulation programs through the health care setting or a day-care facility. The program planned for the infant is individualized according to the resources of the family, the deficits that exist, and the infant's developmental capacity.*

When stimulation needs are not being met,

the nurse may give guidance in relation to specific recommendations for increase of stimulation. Ideas for stimulation are introduced gradually. Judgments must be made regarding the family's ability to follow recommendations and the infant's priority of need. A planned sequence of events may then be prescribed for the mother or care-giver to apply with the infant.

All six perceptual systems must be stimulated. One perceptual system at a time may be involved in stimulation instructions that are made on one occasion in order to achieve clarity and specificity for the mother. At some point, each of the senses of vision, hearing, touch, kinesthetic movement, smell, and taste are stimulated in the various space sectors—near and far. Thus parents may be instructed to bang a particular pot in the kitchen with a spoon near the infant or to rattle a toy and to present as many hearing stimuli as they can think of to attract the infant's attention. As the infant responds, other perceptual systems may be stimulated, and then these same stimuli are repeated but at changing distances away from the infant. The infant is next engaged in active participation in the stimulation program. The child is encouraged to hold the sound-producing spoon,

*References 25, 36, 48, 78, 92, 115, 128.

to move the rattle, to manipulate the soft cotton and the hard rock, and so forth.[6,48] It is clear that the infant who receives adequate interaction with significant adults and who is not handicapped by neurologic or motor deficits participates early in infancy in each of the perceptual stimulation modalities available. Yet the deprivation in poverty-stricken, isolated, or intellectually limited families continues, rendering the infant's world relatively sterile and nonstimulating, and producing permanent, damaging effects.[21,102]

Parents often need assistance in understanding the play capabilities of infants. The short attention span, the inability of the infant to play with other children, and the frequent need to return to mother are frustrating to some. Active listening, guidance in relation to the anticipated developmental changes that naturally evolve, and teaching in regard to some play approaches in infancy can be helpful to inexperienced parents.

## Social interactions: attachment and separation

Even in the most healthy of families, social integration and interaction with the new infant and the development of parenting competency are primary concerns. Many of the questions of parents in the well-baby supervision setting involve problems in managing the daily routine for the infant, responding to the infant's needs and developmental changes, and achieving a balance between the needs of the infant and the needs of other members of the family. In addition to such expressed concerns by the parents, the nurse's assessment of the infant provides guidelines in planning and implementing strategies to assist the family in establishing satisfactory social interactions.

Establishing and maintaining a suitable diurnal behavioral pattern is essential for the physical and emotional well-being of the family. Many infants have brief periods when they experience waking up at night for no apparent reason and are either in a fussy and distressed mood or attempt to engage some member of the family in social interaction. The parents quickly become tired and irritable because of the interruption in their own sleep pattern.

Their response to the infant during such periods may cause the infant to continue to awaken at night, or it may influence reestablishment of sleeping through the night. The temperament and daily activity pattern of the family must be evaluated and used sensitively in helping the family find a suitable strategy to meet their needs. If the infant appears to become increasingly agitated and excited toward bedtime and has difficulty getting to sleep, the family might try planning for a change in routine and activity during the evening and for establishment of bedtime rituals that assist the infant in preparing for going to sleep. If the infant begins to sleep more than usual in the daytime, the parents may need to spend several days in deliberately keeping the infant awake and active during the day to facilitate sleep at night. They may need to enlist the assistance of day-time caregivers in order to achieve this goal.[24,37]

Sibling rivalry and adjustment to the changing development of an infant also constitutes a problem in many families. This problem should be anticipated by the health care worker early during infancy, and guidance and counseling should be offered the family in regard to giving particular attention to older children in the family. The older child may be expected to exhibit some form of sibling rivalry during the period of infancy, even though early responses to the infant may seem positive. Early measures to give particular attention to an older child as an individual, and without the interference of the new infant, should be made by the family.[82]

The descriptions of parenting behaviors that facilitate learning and thought and social and inner competency may be used as guidelines in teaching parents how to interact with their infant. Means of facilitating language development, use of positive social-emotional inputs, and presentation of planned learning games, as outlined in Table 9-5, provide specific activities that can be suggested or taught to the family. The family may need particular teaching regarding the temperament of their infant and appropriate responses during periods of active waking states. They may also need assistance in finding ways to calm the infant during periods of crying and in understanding ways to discriminate between the various signals that the infant

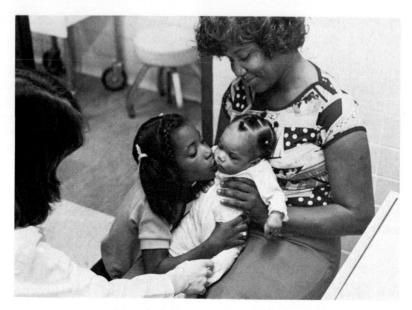

**Fig. 9-18.** Older siblings may be expected to experience some form of sibling rivalry, even though early responses to the infant may seem positive. Nursing counseling and guidance can help a family anticipate the needs of the older child for individual attention.

intends when crying occurs. The common myth that the infant will be spoiled by attention when he or she cries should be dispelled and the family led to understand the crying behavior as a primary means of communication during infancy. Means of minimizing the infant's crying behavior through adequate physical care, feeding, holding and cuddling, and age-appropriate activities should be discussed with the family.[79]

When definite inadequacies are detected in the infant-mother relationship, serious consideration must be given to providing intensive help and resources for the family; otherwise, the infant's well-being and safety may be in jeopardy. The family that does not provide an adequate relationship for the infant may be prone to inflict neglect or harm. Removal of an infant from such a home is a difficult decision to reach, and in our society it is even more difficult to effect. There is some indication from intensive experience with families who are known to neglect or inflict harm on infants and children that meaningful intervention can be effective in protecting the infant.[63]

Helping a parent with a stimulation program when the situation seems to be borderline or is difficult to evaluate often gives a means by which he or she can establish a relationship and achieve satisfactory interaction with the infant. The inner resources to do the things that many parents do naturally in interacting with their infant are simply limited, and the specific instruction and help offered provide the means by which to accomplish this.[84,91,104]

**Day-care**

The role of the nurse in day-care for infants is apparent when one enters many day care facilities. When the nurse is providing health maintenance for an individual infant and family, attention must be given to the quality of day care received outside the home. In working within a community, facilities that give day-care for infants need particular attention. Often, such facilities lack appropriate hygienic measures for the protection of infants against illness, provide inadequate physical care, inadequate nutrition, and give little attention to the learning and social-emotional needs of infants, even though state licensing requirements may be fulfilled. Such facilities need to be evaluated for each dimension of infant care described in this chapter, and the nurse can provide an invaluable service in assisting the day-care workers to

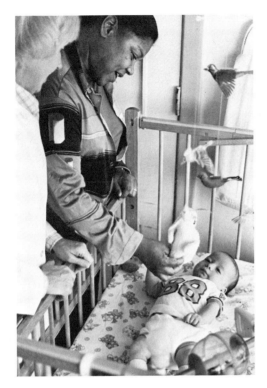

**Fig. 9-19.** The nurse provides assistance to a day-care worker in learning to offer learning games and stimulation for infants.

attain adequate standards of care. The nurse can plan programs for teaching day-care workers the basic principles of infant care, hygienic measures in caring for infants, infant development principles, learning games for infants, and methods of positive social interactions. Attention must be given to providing for the needs of the infant-care worker for periodic relief from the demands of infant care and planned ways of restoring physical and emotional energy needed for caring for groups of infants. Assistance in actual application of these principles is often needed, as is encouragement in altering former practices.[42,69]

## STUDY QUESTIONS

1. Relate the behaviors that Bowlby describes to each of the following areas of development:
   a. Physiologic system development
   b. Piaget's period of cognitive development
2. Observe an infant whose exact age is not known to you for at least an hour during a waking period. Estimate his age based on his behavior capabilities, giving a thorough description of each observation you make. Confirm his actual age and discuss the accuracy or inaccuracy of your estimate.
3. Describe ways in which you might offer creative nursing care for a hospitalized infant. What would be the components of an adequate data base upon which to plan care, and what specific concerns would you consider in identifying needs and a plan of care. Relate your ideas to the physiologic and behavioral principles involved.
4. Observe an infant in a feeding situation. Describe the behavior you see and relate this to the feeding behavior development. Also indicate behaviors of the mother and the infant that reveal the nature of the mother-infant relationship.
5. Assess your own living area for factors that might result in injury for a crawling or walking infant. Determine how you might rearrange dangerous objects, and what precautions you could take to increase the safety of your home for an infant.
6. Determine specific aspects of a stimulation program which you might prescribe for a mother with existing resources in the home similar to your own. Include specific instructions that you might make for stimulating each of the sensory modalities, and how you would introduce active participation for the infant.
7. Administer a hearing evaluation for an infant, and describe your results. Also administer the Denver Developmental Screening test and the Denver Eye Screening Test. Describe your experience with each of these instruments.
8. Keep a record of your diet for a day. Describe how you might have used this same diet for an infant who was just beginning to table feed, and determine how adequate the diet would be. Describe what special preparation would be needed for each component.

## REFERENCES

1. American Academy of Pediatrics: Fluoride as a nutrient, report of the Committee on Nutrition, Pediatrics **49:**456-459, 1972.
2. Ames, L. B.: Predictive value of infant behavior examinations. In Hellmuth, J., editor: Exceptional infant, vol. 1, The normal infant, New York, 1967, Brunnel/Mazel, p. 207.
3. Ames, L. B., and Igl, F. L.: The developmental point of view with special references to the principle of reciprocal neuromotor interweaving, J. Genet. Psychol. **105:**195, 1964.
4. Barker, J., Goldstein, A., and Frankenburg, W. K.: Denver eye screening test manual, Denver, 1972, University of Colorado Medical Center.
5. Barness, L. A.: Manual of pediatric physical diagnosis, ed. 4, Chicago, 1972, Year Book Medical Publishers, Inc.
6. Barsch, R. H.: The infant curriculum—a concept for tomorrow. In Hellmuth, J., editor: Exceptional infant, vol. 12, The normal infant, New York, 1967, Brunner/Mazel, p. 543.
7. Bayley, N.: Bayley scales of infant development, New York, 1969, The Psychological Corporation.

8. Beach, F. A.: The individual from conception to conceptualization. In Rosenblith, J. F., and Allinsmith, W., editors: The causes of behavior; readings in child development and educational psychology, ed. 2, Boston, 1966, Allyn & Bacon, Inc.

9. Benedek, T.: Motherhood and nurturing. In Anthony, E. J., and Benedek, T., editors: Parenthood, its psychology and psychopathology, Boston, 1970, Little, Brown and Co., p. 153.

10. Berkelhamer, J. E., Whitham, R. H., and North, J. J.: Distorted conceptions of infant nutrition among urban mothers; an illustration of the great need for well-baby health supervision, Clin. Pediatr. 16:986, Nov., 1977.

11. Bishop, B. E.: A guide to assessing parenting capabilities, Am. J. Nurs. 76:1784, Nov., 1976.

12. Blank, M.: Mastering the intangible through language, Annals of the New York Academy of Sciences 263:44, Sept. 19, 1975.

13. Blizzard, R. M.: Anterior pituitary, In Kudolf, A. M., editor: Pediatrics, ed. 16, New York, 1977, Appleton-Century-Crofts, p. 1601.

14. Bowlby, J.: Attachment and loss, vol. 1, Attachment, New York, 1969, Basic Books, Inc., Publishers.

15. Brandt, P. A., and others: Intramuscular injections in children, Am. J. Nurs. 72:1402, Aug., 1972.

16. Brazelton, T. B.: Infants and mothers; differences in development, New York, 1969, Dell Publishing Co.

17. Brazelton, T. B.: Neonatal behavioral assessment scale, National Spastics Society Monographs, London, 1973, Wm. Heineman Ltd.

18. Brown, M. S.: What you should know about communicable diseases and their immunization. I. Nursing '75 5:70, Sept., 1975.

19. Brown, M. S.: What you should know about communicable diseases and their immunization, Nursing '75 5:56, Oct., 1975.

20. Brown, M. S., and Alexander, M.: Physical examination. II. Examining the heart, Nursing '74 4:41, Dec., 1974.

21. Caldwell, B. M., and Richmond, J. B.: Social class level and stimulation potential of the home. In Hellmuth, J.: Exceptional infant, vol. 1, The normal infant, New York, 1967, Brunner/Mazel.

22. Capute, A. J., and Biehl, R. F.: Functional developmental evaluation, Pediatr. Clin. North Am. 20:3, Feb., 1973.

23. Carey, W. B.: Clinical applications of infant temperament measurements, J. Pediatr. 81:823-828, Oct., 1972.

24. Carey, W. B.: Night waking and temperament in infancy, J. Pediatr. 84:756, May, 1974.

25. Charnley, L., and Myre, G.: Parent-infant education, Children Today 6:18, March-April, 1977.

26. Chess, S., and others: Your child is a person, New York, 1965, The Viking Press.

27. Chess, S.: Temperament in the normal infant. In Hellmuth, J., editor: Exceptional infant, vol. 1, The normal infant, New York, 1967, Brunner/Mazel, p. 143.

28. Chomsky, N.: Reflections on language, New York, 1975, Random House.

29. Christakis, G.: Nutritional assessment in health programs, Am. J. Public Health (suppl.), vol. 63, Nov., 1973.

30. Cooney, C. E., and Kummerow, S.: Childsafe; when children travel by car, Children Today 6:11, July-Aug., 1977.

31. Coopersmith, S.: The antecedents of self-esteem, San Francisco, 1967, W. H. Freeman and Co.

32. Dallman, P. R.: The red cell. In Rudolf, A. M., editor: Pediatrics, ed. 16, New York, 1977, Appleton-Century-Crofts, p. 1109.

33. Dansky, K. H.: Assessing children's nutrition, Am. J. Nurs. 77:1610, Oct., 1977.

34. Downs, M. P., and Silver, H. K.: The A.B.C.D.'s to H.E.A.R.; early identification in nursery, office and clinic of the infant who is deaf, Clin. Pediatr. 11:563, Oct., 1972.

35. Dyment, P. G., and Bogan, P. M.: Pediatricians' attitudes concerning infant's shoes, Pediatrics 50:655, Oct., 1972.

36. Engelhardt, K.: Piaget; a prescriptive theory for parents, Maternal-child Nurs. J. 3:1, Spring 1974.

37. Erickson, M. L.: Assessment and management of developmental changes in children, St. Louis, 1976, The C. V. Mosby Co.

38. Erikson, E. H.: Identity, youth and crisis, New York, 1968, W. W. Norton & Co., Inc.

39. Escalona, S. K.: The roots of individuality; normal patterns of development in infancy, Chicago, 1968, Aldine Publishing Co.

40. Fey, M. R.: Fluoride therapy, Nurse Pract. 2:26, Sept.-Oct., 1977.

41. Fomon, S. J.: What are infants fed in the United States? Pediatrics 56:350, Sept., 1975.

42. Fowler, W.: A developmental learning approach to infant care in a group setting. In Friedlander, B. Z., Sterritt, G. M., and Kirk, G. E., editors: Exceptional infant, vol. 3, Assessment and intervention, New York, 1975, Brunner/Mazel, p. 341.

43. Francis, B. J.: Current concepts in immunization, Am. J. Nurs. 73:646, April, 1973.

44. Frankenburg, W., and Dodds, J.: Denver Developmental Screening Test Manual, Denver, 1968, University of Colorado Medical Center and Mead Johnson.

45. Friedman, S.: Some thoughts about functional or innocent murmurs, Clin. Pediatr. 12:678, Dec., 1973.

46. Grant, W. W., Street, L., and Fearnow, R. G.: Diaper rashes in infancy; studies on the effect of various methods of laundering, Clin. Pediatr. 12:714, Dec., 1973.

47. Greenberg, L. W.: The rectal examination; a reminder of its importance, Clin. Pediatr. 13:1029, Dec., 1974.

48. Gutelius, M. F., and Kirsch, A. D.: Factors promoting success in infant education, Am. J. Public Health 65:384, April, 1975.

49. Guyton, A. C.: Textbook of medical physiology, ed. 5, Philadelphia, 1976, W. B. Saunders Co.

50. Hall, C. S., and Lindzey, G.: Theories of personality, ed. 2, New York, 1970, John Wiley & Sons, Inc.

51. Hargrove, C. B., Temple, A. R., and Chinn, P.: For-

mula preparation and infant illness, Clin. Pediatr. **13:** 1057, Dec., 1974.

52. Harlow, H. F., and Harlow, M. I.: The effect of rearing conditions on behavior, Bull. Menninger Clin. **26:**213, 1962.

53. Hebb, D. O.: The organization of behavior, New York, 1949, John Wiley & Sons, Inc.

54. Herron, R. E., and Sutton-Smith, B.: Child's play, New York, 1971, John Wiley & Sons, Inc.

55. Hoffman, J. I. E., and Stranger, P.: Systemic arterial hypertension. In Rudolf, A. M., editor: Pediatrics, ed. 16, New York, 1977, Appleton-Century-Crofts, p. 1484.

56. Honig, A. S., and Lally, J. R.: Assessing teacher behaviors with infants in day care. In Friedlander, B. Z., Sterritt, G. M., and Kirk, G. E., editors: Exceptional infant, vol. 3, Assessment and intervention, New York, 1975, Brunner/Mazel, p. 528.

57. Hunt, J. M.: Where education begins, Am. Educ. **4:**15, Oct., 1968.

58. Ishida, M. C., Ewers, Sr. V., and Ishida, Y.: Introducing solid foods to infants, J. Obstet. Gynecol. Neonatal Nurs. **2:**27, Sept.-Oct. 1973.

59. Jessner, L., Weigert, E., and Foy, J. L.: The development of parental attitudes during pregnancy. In Anthony, E. J., and Benedek, T., editors: Parenthood, its psychology and psychopathology, Boston, 1970, Little, Brown and Co., p. 209.

60. Kagan, J.: The growth of the "face" schema; Theoretical significance and methodological issues. In Hellmuth, J., editor: Exceptional infant, vol. 1, Normal infant, New York, 1967, Brunnel/Mazel, p. 335.

61. Kagan, J.: Do infants think? Sci. Am. **227:**74, March, 1972.

62. Kempe, C. H.: The end of routine smallpox vaccination in the United States, Pediatrics **49:**489-492, April, 1972.

63. Kempe, C. H., and Helfer, R. E., editors: Helping the battered child and his family, Philadelphia, 1971, J. B. Lippincott Co.

64. Kessen, W.: Research in the psychological development of infants; an overview. In Bernard, H. W., and Huckins, W. C., editors: Exploring human development; interdisciplinary readings, Boston, 1972, Allyn & Bacon, Inc., p. 216.

65. Koblenzer, P. J.: Diaper dermatitis—an overview with emphasis on rational therapy based on etiology and pathodynamics, Clin. Pediatr. **12:**386, July, 1973.

66. Krech, D.: Psychoneurobiochemeducation. In Bernard, H. W., and Huckins, W. C., editors: Exploring human development; interdisciplinary readings, Boston, 1972, Allyn & Bacon, Inc., p. 160.

67. Krugman, R. D.: Immunization "dyspractice," Pediatrics **56:**159, Aug., 1975.

68. Lahey, M. E.: The erythrocyte; physiologic considerations. In Cooke, R. E., editor: The biologic basis of pediatric practice, New York, 1968, McGraw-Hill Book Co., p. 421.

69. Lambie, D. Z., Bond, J. T., and Weikart, D. P.: Framework for infant education. In Friedlander, B. Z., Sterritt, G. M., and Kirk, G. E., editors: Excep-

tional infant, vol. 3, Assessment and intervention, New York, 1975, Brunner/Mazel, p. 263.

70. Lenneberg, E. H.: Biological foundations of language, New York, 1967, John Wiley & Sons, Inc.

71. McDonald, Q. H.: Safety of infants in automobiles, Pediatrics **52:**463, Sept., 1973.

72. McLaren, D. S., and Burman, D., editors: Textbook of pediatric nutrition, New York, 1976, Churchill Livingstone.

73. Meier, J. H.: Screening, assessment, and intervention for young children at developmental risk. In Friedlander, B. Z., Sterritt, G. M., and Kirk, G. E., editors: Exceptional infant, vol. 3, Assessment and intervention, New York, 1975, Brunner/Mazel, p. 605.

74. Melnick, S. D.: Piaget and the pediatrician, Clin. Pediatr. **13:**913, Nov., 1974.

75. Migeon, C. J.: Adrenal cortex. In Rudolf, A. M., editor: Pediatrics, ed. 16, New York, 1977, Appleton-Century-Crofts, p. 1619.

76. Miller, L. W., McGowan, J. E., and Leffingwell, L. M.: Poliomyelitis in a high risk population; do we need to immunize the newborn? Pediatrics **49:**532, 1972.

77. Montagu, A.: Touching; the human significance of the skin, New York, 1971, Columbia University Press.

78. Morris, A. G.: The use of the well-baby clinic to promote early intellectual development via parent education, Am. J. Public Health **66:**73, Jan., 1976.

79. Murphy, M. A.: The crying infant, Pediatr. Nurs. **1:** 15, Jan.-Feb. 1975.

80. Nysather, J. O., Katz, A. E., and Lenth, J. L.: The immune system; its development and functions, Am. J. Nurs. **76:**1614, Oct., 1976.

81. O'Grady, R. J.: Feeding behavior in infants, Am. J. Nurs. **71:**736-739, April, 1971.

82. Ostrovsky, E.: Sibling rivalry, New York, 1970, Cornerstone Library Publications.

83. Paine, R. S.: Neurologic examination of infants and children, Pediatr. Clin. North Am. **7:**471, Nov., 1960.

84. Parens, H.: Indices of the child's earliest attachment to his mother, applicable in routine pediatric examination, Pediatrics **49:**600-603, April, 1972.

85. Penfield, W.: The uncommitted cortex, the child's changing brain. In Bernard, H. W., and Huckins, W. C., editors: Exploring human development; interdisciplinary readings, Boston, 1972, Allyn & Bacon, Inc., p. 189.

86. Phillips, C. F.: Children out of step with immunization, Pediatrics **55:**877, June, 1975.

87. Phillips, J. L., Jr.: The origins of intellect; Piaget's theory, San Francisco, 1969, W. H. Freeman and Co.

88. Piaget, J.: The language and the thought of the child, New York, 1965, The World Publishing Co.

89. Piaget, J.: The theory of stages in cognitive development, New York, 1969, McGraw-Hill Book Co.

90. Piaget, J., and Inhelder, B.: The psychology of the child, New York, 1969, Basic Books Inc., Publishers.

91. Porter, L. S.: The impact of physical-physiological activity on infant's growth and development, Nurs. Res. **21:**210, May-June 1972.

92. Porter, L. S.: On the importance of activity, Maternal-Child Nurs. J. **2**:85, Summer 1973.

93. Powell, K. R.: Basic principles of immunization, Pediatr. Nurs. **3**:7, Sept.-Oct., 1977.

94. Provence, S.: Some determinants of relevance of stimuli in an infant's development. In Hellmuth, J., editor: Exceptional infant, vol. 1, The normal infant, New York, 1967, Brunner/Mazel, p. 443.

95. Pulaski, M. A.: Understanding Piaget—an introduction to children's cognitive development, New York, 1971, Harper & Row, Publishers.

96. Rabinowitz, M.: Why didn't anyone tell me about bottle mouth cavities? Children Today **3**:18, March-April, 1974.

97. Rance, C. P., Argus, G. S., Balfe, J. W., and Kooh, S. W.: Persistent systemic hypertension in infants and children, Pediatr. Clin. North Am. **21**:801, Nov., 1974.

98. Rios, E., and others: The absorption of iron as supplements in infant cereal and infant formulas, Pediatrics **55**:686, May, 1975.

99. Ripa, L. W.: The role of the pediatrician in dental caries detection and prevention, Pediatrics **54**:176, Aug., 1974.

100. Robbins, J. B., and Smith, R. T.: The specific immune response. In Cooke, R. E., editor: The biologic basis of pediatric practice, New York, 1968, McGraw-Hill Book Co., p. 507.

101. Robson, J. R. K., and others: Growth standards for infants and children, Pediatrics **56**:1014, Dec., 1975.

102. Rubenstein, L., Pedersen, F. A., and Jankowski, J.: Dimensions of early stimulation and their differential effects in infant development. In Stone, L. T., Smith, H. T., and Murphy, L. B., editors: The competent infant; research and commentary, New York, 1973, Basic Books, Inc., Publishers, p. 967.

103. Salt intake and eating patterns of infants and children in relation to blood pressure; report of the Committee on Nutrition, AAP, Pediatrics **53**:115, Jan., 1974.

104. Scarr-Salapatek, S., and Williams, M. L.: A stimulation program for low birth weight infants, Am. J. Public Health, **62**:662-667, May, 1972.

105. Schaffer, R.: Mothering, Cambridge, Mass., 1977, Harvard University Press.

106. Sears, R. R.: A theoretical framework for personality and social behavior, Am. Psychol. **6**:476, 1951.

107. Segar, W. E.: Primary disturbances of water homeostasis. In Rudolf, A. M., editor: Pediatrics, ed. 16, New York, 1977, Appleton-Century-Crofts, p. 1614.

108. Selkurt, E. E., editor: Physiology, ed. 4, Boston, 1976, Little, Brown and Co.

109. Sheppard, W. C., and Willoughby, R. H.: Child behavior; learning and development, Chicago, 1975, Rand McNally College Publishing Co.

110. Smallpox vaccination in the United States; the end of an era, J. Pediatr. **81**:600-608, Sept., 1972.

111. Smith, R. T., and Robbins, J. B.: The defense systems; general physiology. In Cooke, R. E., editor: The biologic basis of pediatric practice, New York, 1968, McGraw-Hill Book Co., p. 495.

112. Smith, R. T., and Robbins, J. B.: Developmental aspects of immunity. In Cooke, R. E., editor: The biologic basis of pediatric practice, New York, 1968, McGraw-Hill Book Co., p. 521.

113. Snyder, J. C., and Wilson, M. F.: Elements of a psychological assessment, Am. J. Nurs. **77**:235, Feb., 1977.

114. Spitz, R. A.: The psychogenic diseases in infancy; an attempt at their etiological classification. In Psychoanalytic study of the child, vol. 6, New York, 1951, International Universities Press, Inc., p. 255.

115. Stein, M. T.: The providing of well-baby care within parent-infant groups, Clin. Pediatr. **16**:825, Sept., 1977.

116. Stern, D.: The first relationship; infant and mother, Cambridge, Mass., 1977, Harvard University Press.

117. Taft, L. T., and Cohen, H.: Neonatal and infant reflexology. In Hellmuth, J., editor: Exceptional infant, vol. 1, The normal infant, New York, 1967, Brunner/Mazel.

118. Tervoort, B.: Development of languages and the critical period. The young deaf child; identification and management, Acta Otolaryngol. (suppl.) **206**:247, 1964.

119. Theurer, R. C.: Iron undernutrition in infancy, Clin. Pediatr. **13**:522, 1974.

120. Thomas, A., and Chess, Stella: Temperament and development New York, 1977, Brunner/Mazel.

121. Uzgiris, I. C., and Hunt, J. McV.: Assessment in infancy; ordinal scales of psychological development, Urbana, 1974, University of Illinois Press.

122. Van Wyk. J. J., and Fisher, D. A.: Thyroid. In Rudolf, A. M., editor: Pediatrics, ed. 16, New York, 1977, Appleton-Century-Crofts, p. 1663.

123. Voorhees, M. L.: Adrenal medulla and sympathetic nervous tissue. In Rudolf, A. M., editor: Pediatrics, ed. 16, New York, 1977, Appleton-Century-Crofts, p. 1655.

124. Wara, D. W., and Ammann, A. J.: Immunologic disorders of childhood. In Rudolf, A. M., editor: Pediatrics, ed. 16, New York, 1977, Appleton-Century-Crofts, p. 299.

125. Weiss, C. E., and Lillywhite, H. S.: Communicative disorders, St. Louis, 1976, The C. V. Mosby Co.

126. Whipple, D. V.: Dynamics of development; euthenic pediatrics, New York, 1966, McGraw-Hill Book Co.

127. White, B. L., and Held, R.: Plasticity of sensorimotor development in the human infant. In Rosenblith, J. F., and Allinsmith, W., editors: The causes of behavior; readings in child development and educational psychology, Boston, 1966, Allyn & Bacon, Inc.

128. Williams, J.: Learning needs of new parents, Am. J. Nurs. **77**:1173, July, 1977.

129. Winnicott, D. W.: The mother-infant experience of mutuality. In Anthony, E. J., and Benedek, T., editors: Parenthood, its psychology and psychopathology, Boston, 1970, Little, Brown and Co., p. 245.

130. Ziegler, R. F.: Cardiac evaluation in normal infants, St. Louis, 1965, The C. V. Mosby Co.

# Toddlerhood and early childhood

## THE AGE OF DISCOVERY

The continuum of development considered in the previous chapter progresses gradually into the period of toddlerhood and early childhood. As with infancy the exact points of beginning for each of these periods are impossible to identify, even for an individual child. The beginning of toddlerhood is characterized by the child's security in the ability to walk and run and in the achievement of language ability sufficient to express most needs and desires. During this period the child's body structure continues to resemble that of the infant more than that of the adult, and the child is primarily involved in developing a separate sense of self. These characteristics tend to emerge between 18 and 24 months of age. The period of early childhood, on the other hand, is characterized by a more mature body structure, ability to control and use the body, and facility with language that more closely resembles that of the adult. The major psychologic thrust of this period of development is mastery of the self as an independent human being, with willingness to extend experiences beyond that of the family.[31] The end of early childhood is marked in most families of the Western world with entrance into formalized educational systems. At some point close to 5 or 6 years of age, the child's interests and developmental traits begin to center increasing-ly outside the family unit, and interactions with peers begin to occupy a more central role.

These two periods of development during early childhood are considered together in this chapter because of the basic similarity of health problems that occur. The young child continues to be vulnerable to numerous health problems and environmental influences that can have life-long effects. Further, the toddler and preschool age child are usually more isolated from the health care system than at any other point during childhood and from other resources that provide evaluation of growth and development or that might detect developmental delays or hazards. The fact that in Western societies the child remains almost exclusively within the family circle or in day-care settings that are predominantly an extension of the family has great implications for health during the early childhood years. Detection of health and developmental problems is vitally important during these years, since these problems may be subject to successful intervention during this period. At a later period such intervention may be relatively ineffective. Unfortunately, with the major forms of health care available to families today, the child during this period is likely not to receive adequate health supervision. Many families are convinced of the benefits of routine

**317**

immunizations during infancy and are therefore motivated to seek health care for their infants. Once the immunization program is complete, however, the child is not brought into the health care system unless disturbing illness occurs; health maintenance problems are therefore neglected.

A highly resourceful family may find this pattern of health care desirable and useful in meeting the needs of the child. They are able to accurately monitor for themselves the normal developmental adequacy of their children and to seek direct assistance when a matter of concern arises. They usually recognize the limitations of their own observational and assessment abilities, and they seek periodic assessment by the health care system of those areas not readily available to their own observation, such as laboratory testing of blood and urine or evaluation of vision and hearing capacity.

This description represents optimal use of health care resources during this period of life. Unfortunately, many families who need health care services do not recognize their own needs or the needs of their young children. The children suffer the consequences of poor health maintenance without being known to the health care system. We will attempt to discuss the features of total health maintenance during the early childhood years, with the understanding that the family's ability to provide for their own needs must be constantly evaluated and encouraged by the health care worker.

## SCIENTIFIC BASES FOR DEVELOPMENT DURING TODDLERHOOD AND EARLY CHILDHOOD
### Developmental physiology

The foundations of developmental physiology are described in detail in Chapter 9. In this chapter we will briefly review the continuation of these processes during toddlerhood and early childhood.

#### Neurologic system

Full development of voluntary motor movement during early childhood is not presently understood. Myelination of the corticospinal tract is functionally advanced enough to support most movement, but achievement of full control

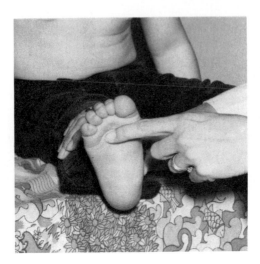

**Fig. 10-1.** Advancing myelination of the corticospinal tracts and cortex is indicated by the mature Babinski reflex (see Fig. 7-12).

does not occur until much later in life (Fig. 10-1). Throughout early childhood voluntary motor movement is often accompanied by involuntary movements on the other side of the body. This mirroring of action is more pronounced in children who suffer some damage of the central nervous system, but the mechanisms by which this occurs are unknown. Predominance of one-sided function of the body is fully established by about 4 years of age.[70]

Practice, gains in muscle size, continuing organization of associations between established neural pathways, and the establishment of new pathways for already accomplished tasks are a few of the many complex factors that probably contribute to the advances in functioning observed during early childhood. The ability to maintain focal attention emerges as the hallmark of the age of early childhood (Fig. 10-2). Multiple stimuli attract the young child's attention, causing exploration and discovery of new experience. Great gains are made in cognitive and intellectual functioning, memory, consciousness, and thought, as described in later sections. These functions are primarily performed through the cerebral cortex, with essential connections to the thalamus. Areas specific to the various functions of the cerebral cortex have been mapped. The bases for the higher intellec-

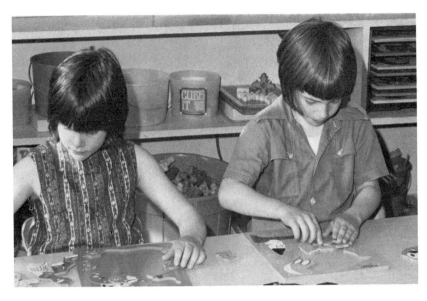

**Fig. 10-2.** The ability to maintain focal attention emerges as a hallmark of early childhood.

tual functioning of humans, for memory, and for learning processes remain speculative, and multiple theories are under investigation.

The limbic system that surrounds the hypothalamus functions specifically in mediating temperamental and emotional aspects of behavior. Such sensations as pleasure and discomfort and the meaning that such experiences develop for the individual originate and are "stored" in this system. Sleep, wakefulness, excitement, anger, and fear are known to be related to these areas of functioning. Each of these functions becomes progressively more sophicticated as young children begin to experience a wider range of stimuli and are able to control their own behavior and the behavior of those about them. During early childhood the feeling response is dominant in determining behavior, indicating that the limbic system is functioning and that associations with voluntary motor areas have been made. However, the complex associations that allow children to effectively "cover up" or control the emotional component of their behavior are not fully developed during early childhood.[39,116]

Vision capabilities, which are well developed by 2 years of age, continue to undergo refinement during the early childhood period; by about 6 years of age the child should approach a 20/20 visual acuity level. The possibility of development of amblyopia is maximal from infancy through about the fourth year. Depth perception and color vision are fully established; the child is able to recognize subtle differences in color shading by the sixth year. Maximal visual capability is usually achieved by the end of the early childhood years (see Appendix, p. 871).

Changes in visual capacity throughout the remaining period of life are in the direction of deterioration of function rather than increase of function. This phenomenon is partially due to the refractive power of the lens and developmental changes that occur in the shape of the eyeball. In the normal sequence of growth the eyeball becomes increasingly more spherical, losing the short shape typical of infancy and progressing to the point where light converges accurately on the surface of the retina. This occurs at about 6 years of age. When this sequence occurs before the sixth year, continuation evolves past the point of ideal light conversion, lengthening of the eyeball occurs, and the child may develop early myopic vision, which will progress with age. Glasses are always indicated for the young child who develops myopia before the age of about 8 years.[39,116]

The capacities to taste and smell, which have reached an optimal level of functioning during

**319**

infancy, come under the influence of voluntary control and association with other sensory and motor areas. Thus young children are able to refuse to taste something that looks displeasing to them. They are able to react accurately to the sensation that a taste or smell arouses within them and begin to learn conditioned associations between certain smells and culturally acceptable values. The foods of the culture become palatable, and the foods that are not acceptable become displeasing. For example, children who are raised in a family who does not eat a certain meat will learn that this meat tastes bad; they may even be unable to develop a pleasurable association with such a taste later in life. Odors of body processes such as sweating and elimination become extremely offensive for children in some cultures, while in others they are not considered unpleasant.

### Respiratory system

Growth and development in the respiratory tissues continue as noted during infancy. Respiratory rate gradually decreases, and the volume of the lungs increases with the child's growth (Fig. 10-3). The proximity of respiratory structures gradually begins to become less of a factor in respiratory infection as early childhood progresses. The anatomy of the ear and the throat continues to resemble that of the infant more closely than that of the adult (see Fig. 11-2), but gradual increases in the size of the structures lessen the probability of communicating infection from one area to another. The tonsils and adenoids remain relatively large during early childhood—another factor that contributes to the particular pattern of respiratory illness during this stage.[39,116]

### Gastrointestinal system

Primary dentition is complete by the end of early childhood (see Appendix, p. 876), but the rate at which teeth appear and begin to loosen as permanent teeth near the surface varies greatly among children. As with other aspects of development, the sequence with which teeth appear is usually the same, although variations do occur. A mature swallowing pattern without a forward tongue thrust and permanent lip and tongue habits, which influence the occlusion and development of arch and jaw relationships, are formed during the second and third year.

Food begins to move through the gastrointestinal system less rapidly. The glands that participate in digestion approach adult maturity. The salivary glands have reached full size and function by the end of the second year of life. The acidity of gastric secretions continues to in-

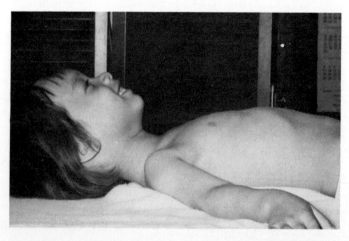

**Fig. 10-3.** The child's respiratory movements are observed for symmetry and adequate chest expansion. The abdominal muscle involvement in breathing typical of the toddler disappears as early childhood advances. There is a slight lower costal margin flare remaining throughout early childhood; however, the lower diameter of the chest is not increased.

crease during early childhood but does not approach adultlike levels until puberty. The secretions of the liver and pancreas that participate in digestive processes are functionally mature during early childhood (see Gastrointestinal development during infancy, Chapter 9).

Control of eliminative function of the bowel develops during the second or third year. This ability develops spontaneously without deliberate teaching, as is demonstrated in cultures where deliberate toilet training does not occur. The child learns whatever provisions for elimination are available in his or her culture. The child may learn by imitation when voluntary control capacity develops or may be deliberately taught and encouraged to use a particular means. The capacity to control the anal sphincter probably emerges toward the end of the second year, but there is great variability in the time of appearance. Teaching may successfully achieve sphincter control earlier than would occur spontaneously after full neurologic voluntary capacity is reached. Emotional factors are significant in the development of this function, and indeed they influence the function of the entire gastrointestinal system. By the onset of early childhood, secretion of saliva and gastric juices responds to those stimuli that indicate that food is forthcoming; secretion is inhibited by emotional upset and trauma.[39,116]

### Endocrine system

Understanding of the endocrine system during early childhood is primarily in relation to abnormalities of function; normal function has not been fully determined or understood. With the exception of reproductive endocrine functions, most of the endocrine factors discussed in Chapter 9 become functionally mature during early childhood, although function continues at a minimal level. The production of glucagon and insulin may be limited or labile, producing variations in blood sugar levels that may be demonstrated throughout early childhood. The production of corticol, aldosterone, and deoxycorticosterone by the adrenal cortex probably remains somewhat limited but seems to function more effectively in protecting the young child against the hazards of fluid and electrolyte imbalance than during infancy. Secretions of epinephrine and norepinephrine from the adrenal medulla increase sufficiently to perform homeostatic functions in relation to autonomic nervous system function and in mediating certain aspects of increased emotional components of behavior. Regulation of growth during early childhood remains one of the most important functions of the endocrine system. Growth hormone, thyroid, insulin, and corticoids probably are the most vital hormones for normal growth and development during this period.[39,109,116,118]

### Musculoskeletal system

Changes in the proportion of body size continue at slower but significant rates during early childhood. By about 6 years of age the body proportions more closely approximate those of the adult. The head reaches about one sixth of total body length; in adulthood it is about one eighth of total body length. This change in proportion occurs because of relatively large increments of growth in the trunk and legs, with the head slowing in growth rate. Ossification gradually declines as this process becomes more advanced in many areas of the body, but it continues until full stature is reached.

Increases in the size and strength of muscle fibers continue. During this period, as during infancy, use of muscle tissues is the primary stimulus for increases in size and strength. Children who tend to develop a significant amount of muscle mass during early childhood do so in response to a combination of genetic inheritance and stimulation through use. Boys demonstrate this pattern more often than do girls, but this is not a true sex difference, since differential hormonal control of body growth and development is not operative during early childhood.[109,116,118]

### Integumentary system

As early childhood progresses, the skin achieves a significantly advanced level of maturity in protecting from outer invasion and loss of fluids. The ability of the defense function of the skin in localizing infection increases but remains less than mature. Sebum is secreted in very minimal amounts throughout early childhood, rendering the skin particularly dry. Hair develops into the more mature, coarse type that is typical of the child's genetic inheritance. Changes occur in both color and curliness of the hair. It usually becomes darker and straighter than it was during infancy. The function of the eccrine sweat glands gradually increases, but the quantity of eccrine sweat produced in response to heat or emotion remains minimal. Apocrine sweat glands remain nonsecretory during this period.

Adipose tissue accumulation continues to decline or ceases altogether during early childhood. This results in the "thinning out" appearance that occurs during the transition from infancy to early childhood. This continues until about the sixth year, when adipose tissue accumulation again begins to increase gradually. Children who genetically seem to carry a consistently greater portion of adipose tissue thin out somewhat during early childhood. They gain length rapidly, with no increase (or perhaps even a loss) in girth and relatively little weight gain. Caloric intake does not seem to influence this pattern of adipose tissue accumulation, and there may be a differential metabolic utilization of calories that is not understood at the present time. The extreme activity level of young children is probably a contributing factor, but activity level does not seem to be as closely correlated with the amount of tissue accumulation as it is during other periods of life.[39,116]

### Renal system

Anatomic structure of the kidney reaches full adult maturity by the end of infancy. Therefore, the kidney's ability to function is determined solely by endocrine control functions of the body. Functional maturity is quite advanced under normal homeostatic conditions; the renal system is able to conserve water and concentrate urine on a level that approximates adult abilities. However, under conditions of stress, this ability is still decreased, and the reaction of the renal system in the establishment of homeostatic balance is probably slower than that of the adult system.[109,116,118]

### Circulatory system

Permanent circulatory pathways are fully established by the time the child reaches later infancy or early childhood. Changes in the nature

of function of the system, including decreases in heart rate, increases in blood pressure, and changes in vascular resistance of varying areas of the body in response to growth in the size of the vessel lumen, continue gradually. The capillary beds gradually increase their capacity to respond to heat or cold in the environment and thus to participate more effectively in thermoregulation. Autonomic control of this function becomes more fully integrated into the total functioning of the central nervous system, so that the child can now begin to take voluntary measures to relieve the discomfort of heat or cold. For example, the child can put on clothing or move to warmer or cooler areas of the environment and assist physiologic efforts to maintain a constant internal thermal environment.[39,106,116]

### Immunologic system

The skin, as noted earlier, achieves a progressively more mature level of function in defense against infection, and the processes of phagocytosis continue to function at a mature level during early childhood.

The immune system of specific antibodies becomes quite well established. By this time, most of the common organisms of the environment have been encountered and immune responses have begun to function adequately. When children enter the world of nurseries and preschools, exposure to new and different organisms is greatly increased, and they may experience a period of time when they seem to succumb to many minor respiratory and gastrointestinal infections. As immunity begins to develop against the organisms of the new environment, their resistance likewise increases. Despite environmental exposure, however, increases in immunoglobulin levels have been demonstrated to follow a well-defined pattern during early childhood. IgG continues to rise sharply. IgM reaches an adult level during later infancy or the early part of childhood. IgA demonstrates a gradual increase during this same period, with the most dramatic rise occurring during later childhood. The basis for these developmental patterns remains uncertain.[109]

The tonsils have been recently demonstrated to participate in local cell-mediated immunity at the mucosal surfaces. Most localized and systemic viral infections have as their portal of entry the respiratory route, and the tonsils are frequently involved in infections during early childhood. However, secretory antibodies have been shown to increase in response to localized infections when the tonsils are present, indicating that this tissue participates in some manner in the development of immunity to such infections.[147]

Passive immunity to communicable disease acquired through transfer of maternal antibodies during fetal life has disappeared by this time, but active immunity to certain communicable diseases through modern immunization techniques should be completed to offer full protection during this period of life. Booster doses of immunizations are recommended near the end of early childhood to ensure continued protection throughout later childhood and adolescence.[39,109,111,116]

### Hematologic system

The young child is capable of maintaining adequate levels of hemoglobin provided that dietary intake of iron is sufficient to meet the demands of formation. The bone marrow of the ribs, sternum, and vertebrae is fully established as the main site for formation of red blood cells, but the liver and spleen maintain the capacity to form erythrocytes and granulocytes during hematopoietic stress.[39,61,116]

## Behavioral and personality development

Behavior of the young child has stimulated a great deal of speculation, theory building, and empirical research. A few of the many theories available have been chosen for discussion because of their particular relevance to this period. Reference will be made to many individual theorists who have developed variations of similar ideas, and the reader is encouraged to seek further study of those ideas that are of particular interest.

### Theories of learning

Four general modes of learning are known to operate throughout early childhood; however, some are more completely understood than others. First, learning by reinforcement and/or conditioning is a powerful force for learning and behavior control during this period of life. Because the child has not yet developed means beyond the emotional level for internal control of behavior, the environment exerts a strong controlling influence. An important aspect of this control is in the use or misuse of the principles of reinforcement and conditioning.

The second major means of learning is through insight. This may be referred to as the "Aha" reaction, and young children are often observed to experience this. It comes about through secondary means of learning, such as play, experimentation, exploration, or repeated manipulation of the object world (Fig. 10-4).

Third, the child learns by the natural unfolding of capacity. Physiologic principles of development offer some understanding of the basis of this phenomenon, but capacity is not universally accepted as limiting behavior or causing certain behavior to occur. Nevertheless, we can observe certain behaviors that seem to unfold naturally, such as the child's means of climbing up and down stairs before the time that full stair-walking capacity is present. There is usually not someone else to imitate creeping or sliding up and down the stairs; the ability seems to develop in concert with his or her physiologic capacity at the moment.

Fourth, the child learns by identification and imitation. This powerful means of learning is discussed in more detail on p. 284.

Learning is thought of as the central responsibility of the family during the early childhood years, and the end result for the child is socialization. Increasingly, the family in Western societies is becoming dependent upon the services of daytime sitters, day-care facilities, and preschools to share this responsibility. Learning phenomena are critically important for adequate cognitive, intellectual, and inner development. Even when a child's innate capacity for learning is restricted because of mental retardation, learning that occurs during this time lays the foundation for development in each of the major competencies and is built upon the earlier learning of the infancy period.

The learning theories that will be reviewed here are those incorporating the ideas of reinforcement and conditioning, because the impli-

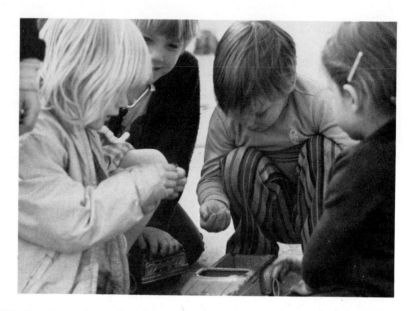

**Fig. 10-4.** Experimentation, exploration, and manipulation provide important discoveries for young children.

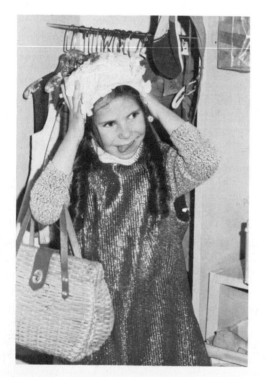

**Fig. 10-5.** Identification and imitation of significant adults provide learning experiences.

cations for control of behavior are great. Used as tools for behavior therapy for several decades, these theories have provided great insights into human nature and possibilities for fulfilling the human potential. Whether or not the propositions are adopted or desired for application in nursing, many have been demonstrated reliably to be a part of the learning experience of every human being throughout life. A few behavioral scientists[72,98,114] propose that these principles govern almost all behavior, but most maintain a more moderate view that behavior is mediated through a wider range of factors.[54,71,93]

Behaviors that bring approval and pleasure tend to be repeated, learned, and incorporated into the behavior patterns of the individual. Those behaviors that bring disapproval, pain, displeasure, or no reaction at all tend to be forsaken and forgotten. The young child engages in a vast amount of experimentation with every conceivable behavior that is available. The reactions of other people determine which of these behaviors tend to be learned.[95]

**Learning theory of Robert Sears.** The learning theory of Robert R. Sears[67,94] is useful in bringing some understanding and insight related to reinforcement and behavioristic theory.

Sears also attempts to reconcile psychoanalytic theory and behaviorist theory, but we will concentrate on the reinforcement ideas he proposes.

Personality and learning may be measured by monadic action of the individual and by dyadic interaction between the individual and other significant people.[67,94] For Sears, parents are the most important reinforcing agents of behavior, and their child-rearing practices are crucial determinants of behavior. Developmental stages are viewed as existing because they are dictated by social expectations; in other words the child does not follow developmental patterns of behavior as a result of the natural unfolding of capacity but rather because of the age-appropriate expectations placed upon behavior by the parents. Sears deals briefly with readiness to perform a given behavior, but he views emergence of behavior as a result of parental expectancy and anticipation of the child's readiness, resulting in reinforcement of all behaviors that approximate the desired expected behavior.

Learning during early childhood consists of three phases for Sears. The first is during the early stages of infancy when the child's rudimentary behavior is primarily directed by inner drives for basic physical needs; gradually, as the relationship with the mother begins to develop, these need-centered actions become replaced with socially centered behavior. This results in the learning pattern typical of early childhood, which Sears calls *secondary motivational systems: family-centered learning*. The third stage begins when the child enters school, and it involves the increasing importance of peer groups in determining behavior.

For Sears, reinforcement is any event, behavior, or satisfactory result that causes a certain behavior to be repeated. When the behavior is reinforced constantly and specifically, the behavior is learned with such force that it becomes a learned, or secondary, drive equivalent. For example, the young child initially eats because he or she is hungry (primary drive) but learns through consistent reinforcement that eating upon a time schedule produces satisfaction from the parent. Therefore, the behavior of eating becomes motivated by the desire to please

the parent, and it is said to possess reinforcing properties.

The above illustration also indicates what Sears means by action-oriented dyadic units of behavior, upon which he centers his theory and research. The eating behavior of the infant is an adaptive response that has been reinforced, but it would not persist in the pattern of the culture were it not for the actual or anticipated response of the mother. Eventually the child's behavior becomes self-motivated, a natural growth from the period of incorporating those behaviors that cause desirable responses from parents.

Sears deals with punishment during this stage, since the use of punishment in child-rearing usually begins at some point during early childhood, when the child's experimentation with many behavior patterns produces occasional behavior that is not acceptable to parents. In his major study of punishment, Sears concluded that punishment has no reinforcement effect and does not tend to extinguish behavior.[96] Punishment does produce a reaction by the child to the administering adult. Rather than the child connecting the adult's actions with the undesired behavior, the child experiences the adult's behavior as an expression of anger and learns to avoid this anger. Genuine social learning occurs when the child replaces previous behaviors that are not desirable with new, more appropriate behaviors that bring satisfaction. Punishment does not usually allow for this kind of learning experience.

During the early stages of learning the motivating factor for the child's behavior, or a secondary drive that causes certain behaviors to recur, is the desire to remain dependent upon the mother or other significant people in the family. As early childhood progresses, Sears sees this drive as becoming undesirable for the mother, and other means of satisfying the child's dependency drive are reinforced. One of the behaviors that begins to emerge is imitation, whereby the child seeks to secure certain satisfying goals by imitating the adult behavior that leads to fulfillment of the goal. Gradually the child learns to achieve goals that formerly required action from the mother or father. Dependency drives continue to operate to a very real extent, however, and they are particularly obvious when the child fears the loss of dependency-maintaining activities of the adult. This threat means to the child that the adult no longer is caring or loving and the child immediately reverts to behavior that is perceived to again secure the dependency function. For Sears, this mechanism is the most powerful alternative to reinforcement in shaping desirable behavior. Other behavioral theorists would interpret this type of withdrawal as negative reinforcement and the behavior sequences involved as operants.[98] For example, the child may engage in temper tantrums, which operate upon the parents' behavior and cause them to pay undue attention, which causes temper tantrums to persist. Withdrawal of parental attention may be seen as causing an abrupt change in the child's tantrum behavior to behavior that the child anticipates will restore dependency functions of the parents. The restoration of the adult behavior of giving attention to the tantrum is a return to positive reinforcement.

Aggression grows out of the child's inevitable encounters with frustration. Permissiveness toward displays of aggression fails to reinforce the behavior pattern (as in the example cited above), but it leaves the child with unchanneled aggression (Fig. 10-6). Sears believes that the child must learn to channel aggressive drives in socially acceptable ways and that control by parents over such channeling behavior results in the eventual capacity to control aggression. Thus parents must maintain a very delicate balance between permissiveness and restraint in reacting to the child's aggression. In each of Sear's motivational systems—dependency, feeding, toileting, sex education, and aggression—he tends to identify success with finding a middle ground that fosters a fine balance between the extremes of the behavior that might be exhibited by the child and the extremes of reactions that the parents tend to develop.[67,94,95,96]

**Cognitive learning theory of Piaget.** As early childhood progresses, the child makes great gains in conceptual and cognitive capacity. Concepts of time emerge, so that the child gradually is able to differentiate today from yesterday and to think of tomorrow and the future. The child becomes more fully oriented in space and develops awareness of the location of home within the neighborhood. Structure and value order begin to be recognized to the extent that the child be-

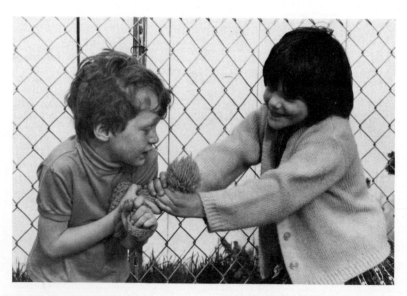

**Fig. 10-6.** Aggression and conflict grow out of the child's inevitable encounters with frustration. Learning to channel aggressive drives in a socially acceptable way grows out of early childhood experiences with parents and peers.

gins to take measures to provide a structure for daily activities and values certain activities, objects, and people above others. Ritual behavior continues during toddlerhood with events such as meals, bedtime, or bathing. By establishing such rituals, the child repeats experiences that are unique to the self and provide a means of knowing the self as an individual (Fig. 10-7).

The cognitive learning theory of Jean Piaget[67,78] will be continued from the discussion of his theory of infancy in Chapter 9. The early childhood period, which for Piaget extends from the ages of 2 to 7 years, is termed the *preoperational subperiod of concrete operations*. Many of the ideas discussed by Piaget and the behaviors that he describes as typical of early childhood are not unlike those described by Sears and other developmental theorists. The unique quality of Piaget's work is his concentration upon the inner, step-by-step acquisition of patterns of thought, which in turn shape and determine the behavior patterns. Piaget does not deny the influence of the environment in determining behavior, but he believes that the natural evolution of the individual's thought capacity represents a major cause for behavior.

The preoperational subperiod may be differentiated from the sensorimotor period of infancy by the child's increasing ability to use symbols to represent the environment. This ability began to develop in rudimentary forms during the sensorimotor period in that certain events began to take on specific meanings for the child, and the child began to imitate, play, and work out behavior in his or her mind before acting. However, the child now begins to differentiate between the "signifier," or the symbol of an object or an event, and the "significate," the actual object or event in its totality. For example, the child may have previously formed an association between a pillow and sleep, so that the signifier (pillow) was thought of as synonymous with the meaning of the significate (sleep). During the preoperational subperiod the child begins to recognize the pillow as something that has a meaning that is different from, but sometimes related to, sleep.

The development of language plays a vital role in the cognitive development of symbolic representation. For Piaget this type of symbolic act greatly enhances the act of internalizing, or mediating, the symbolic functions of the intellect. Language is not the full representation of the thought processes of human beings; language does not fully express the full richness or symbolic possibilities in thinking capacity. Signifiers become formed before there is a linguistic sign for the child. The ability to think about the relationship between the signifier and the significate exists before the ability to repre-

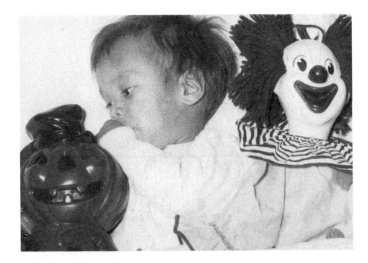

**Fig. 10-7.** Ritualization of events such as bedtime provides constancy for the child and incorporates objects that are associated with comfort and security.

sent each of them in the form of language. The signifiers become internalized as images, and then a word is found that represents the meaning already acquired. The child's language often reflects the meanings that have been acquired. For example, the word "Mommy" may be used to represent a very wide range of behaviors and actions in addition to its noun sense (mother). The context and differential vocalization inflection give it the intended meaning. "Mommy" may mean "help me" on one occasion and "pick me up" on another. The continuing adaptive functions of assimilation and accommodation provide the child with the means by which to gradually acquire internalized, differentiated, and more precise meanings between signifiers and significates.

It is helpful to consider the limitations of preoperational thought in order to understand its nature. The cardinal trait of this period and the one that follows is the concreteness of the thought processes in comparison with thinking of the adult. The child who is beginning to experience symbolic mental representations simply runs through all of the mental symbols as they would occur if he or she were actually participating in the real event. The adult is capable of analyzing and synthesizing symbolic information, and mental connection with the real event is not necessary. The child is not able to perform mental gymnastics such as skipping from one part of an operation to another, of reversing the operation mentally, or of thinking of the whole in relation to the parts.

Concreteness is further characterized by the limitation of egocentrism. At this stage children are unable to conceptualize another person's point of view. They can only think about meanings from the point of view of their own attached meanings and symbols and cannot understand why another person fails to follow these idiosyncratic communications.

Further, the child is unable to shift attention from one part or detail of an event to another once attention is centered on one particular aspect. This is termed "centering" by Piaget and is illustrated by the child's inability to take into account more than one factor in solving a simple problem. For example, a child is given two identical cups containing equal amounts of water and is asked which cup contains the greater amount of water. During the preoperational period, the child would respond that they contain the same amount of water. The child is then asked to pour the water from each cup into two different containers, one that is flat and wide and another that is tall and narrow. When asked which container now has more water, the child always identified one, usually the taller and narrower one where the water reaches a higher level. When the water is again transferred to the equal cups and the experiment is repeated, the child continues to respond in exactly the same manner as before.

This experiment also illustrates the trait of irreversibility. The child is not able to connect the reversible operation, which is observed in the transfer of the water back into the original cup, and make the logical conclusion that the differently shaped containers hold the same amount of water. The child is not able to mentally associate the fact that the transformation that takes place between one state to another is not a function of the amount of water but of the shape of the container. The ability to mentally conceive the transformation that takes place in the shape of water does not exist.

Finally, Piaget describes the preoperational period of thinking as utilizing transductive reasoning. The child is not able to proceed from general to particular (deduction) or from particular to general (induction); rather the child moves only from particular to particular in making associations and solving problems. For example, Piaget relates an association made by one of his children between being hunchbacked and being ill. When a neighbor who was hunchbacked was not able to visit on a certain day because he had a communicable illness, the child was able to understand that the neighbor was ill. However, when the child was told later that the neighbor was better and that she could go to see him, her conclusion was that now his hunched back was straight and well. She was able to think in terms of being well or ill, but she placed the man in one or the other category and assumed he possessed all of the attributes and meanings that she linked symbolically with either trait.[67,78]

During the period between about 18 and 24

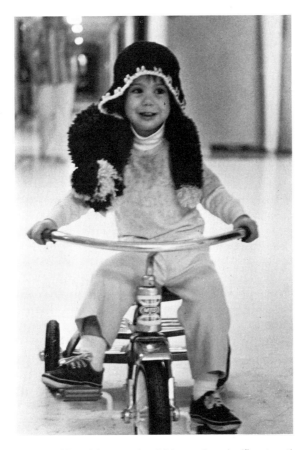

**Fig. 10-8.** Between the ages of 2 and 4 years, the child spends a significant portion of time acting out imagined events. Here the child imagines dressing up in her hat and "fur" and driving to the store.

months, the young child experiences a major transition in imitation and play. Piaget has labeled this stage the invention of new means through mental combinations. The child develops the capacity to imitate models that are not immediately present without extensive trial and error. There is imitation of nonhuman and nonliving objects, which serves the important function of direct experience with object events in the world that are difficult for the child to understand. The relative absence of trial and error in imitation is indicative of the fact that the child has developed the ability to work out the pattern of experience before engaging in the activity. Play takes on increasingly symbolic functions and meanings. The child engages in repeating actions over and over for fun and pleasure as previously, but now there is increasing

symbolic meaning in the activity for the child. An object such as a stone or a block of wood can now symbolize, in the child's mind, a person, animal, or any other object that is conceptualized. In play the child manipulates the object to go through patterns of activity that are imagined for the symbolized object.

This make-believe form of play, or ludic symbolism, predominates throughout early childhood. Between the ages of 2 and 4 years, the child spends a significant portion of time acting out whole scenes of imagined events. Imaginary companions are frequently present for the child; these serve the important function of a mirror for the child's self or a sympathetic audience for the child as the self is allowed full and unrestrained expression and experimentation through play. During this period the child uses

**329**

play to act out what is forbidden in reality, providing important trial experiences with behaviors that are otherwise not allowed and providing an important means of expression of parts of the self that are not socially acceptable but that need some form of acceptable outlet. For example, the young child may pretend to eat an infant sibling for dinner, expressing a dimension of ambivalent feelings toward the infant in a manner that is not punished and that provides discharge of hostile or angry feelings.[78,80]

At about the age of 4 years, symbolic games become much more orderly and representative of reality as the child begins to emerge from the egocentric world of earlier childhood and begins to incorporate the reality of the world as it exists outside the self. The child increasingly seeks play objects that are models of authentic objects in the environment and increasingly models the social rules of society. Social interactive play becomes more predominant as the child develops a more secure sense of the self.[78,80]

**Theories of speech and language development.** By the time the child reaches the end of the preschool period, expressive language may be very similar to that of adults in the environment except for minor deficiencies in refinement, vocabulary, and structure. The degree to which a child fulfills this ability is dependent upon the child's aptitude for language, opportunity for using the language, the quality and quantity of language used at home, and the range of experiences to which the child is exposed outside the home. Regardless of the child's expressive capacity, the development of receptive language during the preschool years is deemed to be of vital importance, as this ability provides the foundation for later expressive ability. Throughout early childhood the receptive capacity of the child exceeds that of expressive capacity, in that the child comprehends the meaning of words and phrases that are not a part of the expressive vocabulary, and the child can make associations between concepts even though there is not the ability to explain these concepts. The table, "Landmarks of Speech, Language, and Hearing Development" in the Appendix, p. 872, provides a general description of expected receptive and expressive language capacity during the early childhood years.

During the early childhood years the development of rhythm is an important dimension in the development of speech capacity. By about the age of 3 years, the child has a desire to speak in sentences but lacks sufficient neuromotor coordination for connected, rhythmic speech and lacks sufficient vocabulary to speak in sentences. Between the ages of 3 and 5 years the child begins to practice talking like an adult, which serves to develop neuromotor capacities for the language of adults and stimulates verbal interaction that develops the vocabulary and a sense of the rules of grammatical structure that govern the use of language. These attempts are characterized by hesitations, repetitions, and frequent revisions in speech, which may be labeled by adults as stuttering but which actually represent the normal immaturity of speech. It is believed that actual stuttering has its origins during this period of development, arising not from an inadequacy in the child but from the response of adults to this normal broken pattern of speech. Such reactions are thought to include impatience in waiting to listen to the child's lengthy attempts to express his or her thoughts, which decreases the child's opportunities to use language, and the insistence that the child correct this pattern of speech before the capacity for fluent speech is developed.[89,115]

The development of hearing capacity, which is critical for the development of speech and language, reaches essential maturity by the age of 3 or 4 years. However, during this period the child begins the life-long process of learning to listen and comprehend. It is estimated that all humans listen to about 50% of what they hear and comprehend only about 25%. Listening ability includes attending to what is heard, discriminating between the various qualities of sound, making cognitive associations with what is heard and previously learned experiences, and remembering that which is heard. The quantity and quality of language used in the home is thought to be even more important for the development of listening ability, and therefore receptive language, than for the development of expressive language. The increased availability of television and other mass-media sound stimuli may have an effect on this dimension of language development, but because the child is not required to respond and receive language feedback and interaction, the extent to which these forms of passive stimuli are effective is not known.[84,115]

### Social development

Social development within the family was considered at length in the discussion of Sears' theory and is considered from other points of view in other chapters. Socialization in relation to peers during early childhood has been less specifically explored in theory or empirical research. Sibling relationships and ordinal position in the family have received some attention,[1,4,92] but the evidence that has accumulated remains scanty and of questionable reliability. It is generally agreed that ordinal position in the family, peer relationships, and experiences with children as opposed to predominant experiences with adults have differential effects on the child's developing personality and social skills, but this belief and the values that are given to different practices tend to remain a matter of personal preference.[20,24,112]

The dramatic shift in family life and early experiences for young children in Western societies calls into question the adequacy of many social theories to explain the effects of early socialization experiences for children. For example, the widely accepted theory of Parsons and Bales[77] described the emergence of acceptable social behavior in children as arising from a family experience in which the parents each have mutually recognized areas of responsibility, each is trusted and supported by the spouse in their respective socially defined role-appropriate areas, children know and accept the differential parental authority and during early years of development do not seriously question or challenge parental roles or responsibilities. The vast changes in society that have resulted in changes in these dimensions of family life were discussed in Chapter 3, and the effects of these changes on the social competence of young children are not yet known.[5,57,65] Solnit has presented criteria for healthy development that transcend variations in cultural and social setting and expectations, but the problem remains as to what conditions, given the vast changes in society, will increase the child's attainment of these criteria. Those criteria that are particularly relevant to the experiences of early childhood include:[100]

1. Attainment of neuromotor capacity in locomotion, speech, coordination, and social responsiveness
2. Capacity to move toward active mastery of situations that formerly required full-time

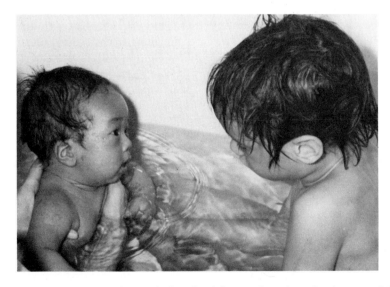

**Fig. 10-9.** Early sibling relationships are believed to influence the unique development of the child.

adult attendance, such as eating, dressing and undressing, toileting, and other skills appropriate to the life-style of the family

3. Capacity to postpone impulsive behavior when it is not suitable for the social setting
4. Achieving a balance between adapting to the social environment and having an influence on modifying that environment in the service of the self and those to whom one is attached
5. Achieving a capacity to accept gratification or experiences according to family and cultural patterns that may not be the same as those the child would seek
6. Acquiring a sense of self as worthy of respect and affection according to the values of the society
7. Achieving the ability to respond to expectations of the family and society with satisfaction and without losing a sense of one's inner self and inclination

Haggard[40] has presented a theory of adaptation and risk of trauma that provides some insight into the meaning of early experiences that facilitate adequate adaptation and social behavior later in life. According to this theory, the innate and acquired structures that regulate behavior are formed out of the inner motivation of the self and the environmental context in which the behavior occurs. The infant is born with the capacity to develop the structures that regulate behavior and during early life is extremely plastic and adaptable but gradually looses plasticity over the life span. Early learning may provide a foundation that facilitates adaptable adult behavior, or it may interfere with or restrict later adaptation. One way in which early learning interferes with later adaptation lies in the incompatibility between what one is taught as a young child and that which is valued and required as an adult. For example, many young children in Western societies are expected to be nonagressive and nonsexual as young children but then expected to be agressive and sexual as adults. Another way in which early learning interferes with later adaptation is when the early learnings themselves are maladaptive. Young children who identify with unstable and immature adults experience strong feelings of rejection, develop strong antago-

nisms toward their families and other social experiences, and tend to carry these early learnings into adulthood and exhibit the same types of social behaviors. Because of the loss of plasticity in the behavioral system, change in this maladaptive behavior becomes extremely difficult, if not impossible.[40]

The experience of early trauma in the life of the young child has been explored and is relevant in considering the health of children because of the increasing incidence of traumatic family disorganization during the early childhood years.[7,57] The developmental age of the child is considered to be one of the major factors that determine the extent to which the family's disruption will indeed become traumatic for the child. Anthony[7] dispells the myth that absence of a parental figure with whom the child can identify causes the source of trauma. Rather, trauma to the child's development arises out of the way in which the remaining parent is manipulated by the child into the role of the absent parent. During early childhood the dynamics of family disruption initiates a strong separation anxiety and fear of losing the remaining parent, which results in excessive dependency of the child, regression to earlier forms of behavior, and loss of previously established feelings of self-esteem.[7]

Early childhood education has proliferated in response to evidence that socially disadvantaged children were permanently encumbered intellectually and socially. Efforts to erase this disadvantage and cultural difference took the form of governmentally supported preschool and nursery programs across the United States. The full impact of these programs has not been subject to full evaluation, and the relative merits of this sort of experience remain uncertain. The goals of such education remain debatable and highly variable from one program to another, and the effects seem to vary likewise.[53,90,102,121] Thus this issue remains unsettled, but more children are being cared for in the group nursery setting than has previously been the case in the United States.

The kibbutz system of child-rearing in Israel provides one means of evaluating the effects of peer relationships during early childhood when these relationships are culturally expected to

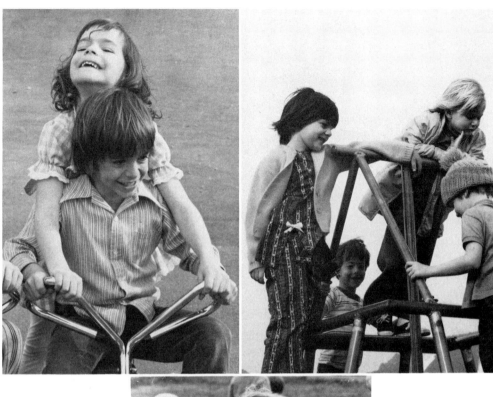

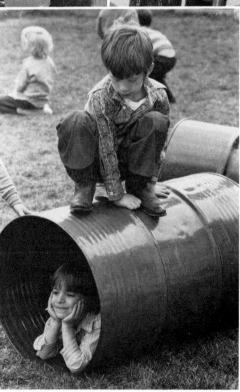

**Fig. 10-10.** Early childhood education programs provide opportunities for stimulation, play, development of muscle coordination, and socialization.

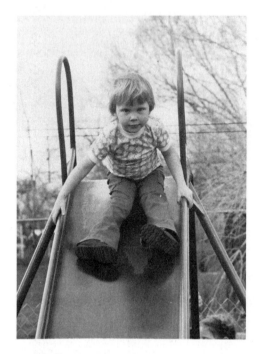

**Fig. 10-11.** Gaining autonomy and initiative are developmental challenges accomplished through play, mastery of new skills, and independent experiences.

gradually take over many of the functions of the Western family.[32,83] Transfer of these effects to the experience of a child growing up in a family-centered culture is not, however, possible.

### Emotional development

Each of the theories discussed thus far has far-reaching implications for the emotional development of the child. Theories that center upon phenomena that most directly involve emotional or inner development during toddlerhood and early childhood provide yet another channel through which we may examine and seek understanding of the young child's life experiences.

Erikson's[30,31] description of emotional development during early childhood encompasses two stages of development, which are intimately related. The first is the stage that is typified by the struggle to attain autonomy, a sense of one's self, and of separateness. Simultaneously the child must overcome the hazards of doubt

and shame. During this toddler period, according to Erikson, the child learns to exercise control of the modalities of having and of letting go, and the environment of the family offers restraint and freedom in appropriate balance to allow the young child to experiment without becoming the victim of indiscriminant use of the abilities to hold on and let go. As the child is able to possess the self, the experience of a sense of self, or autonomy, emerges.

Erikson's second stage of early childhood begins at about the end of the third year and involves the struggle to gain a sense of initiative and to overcome the hazards of guilt. Erikson describes the difference between this stage and the one preceding it as the difference between knowing one's self and knowing one's potential. In this process the child develops a sense of conscience—the super-ego, or regulative, control function of the personality. Overdevelopment of this function results in tendencies toward self-destruction rather than toward creativity and initiative. As with all stages of development, the goal is toward a dominance of the positive task accomplishment and overcoming the hazards of the stage.[10]

Social factors influencing the emergent awareness of self among preschool black children have been investigated with particular attention to the influence of racial identity formation and the social consequences of belonging to this particular minority group. Such studies have supported the notion that a healthy personality depends upon a healthy, adequate social and cultural climate. Where black preschool children tend to be exposed to a great deal of participation in their particular culture and environment and this environment provides resources for physical and emotional needs and promotes favorable attitudes toward the self, the children tend to develop adequate mental health and emotional security.[23,82,85]

Behavioral theories have provided a concept that has been useful in understanding some of the irrational fears and emotions that are commonly experienced during early childhood. Conditioning occurs as a result of associations between two separate events that occur simultaneously. This phenomenon may be illustrated by the experience of young children when they receive an injection. The injection, a fearful and painful experience, is associated with the location, with the particular person who administered it, or with the white uniform or laboratory coat. Thereafter, the room, clinic, person, or white coat is capable of producing the same or similar fears and pains. Once a conditioned response is acquired, overcoming it is a slow and tedious process. The fact that this phenomenon occurs with greater frequency and intensity during early childhood has stimulated speculation and investigation but is still not understood. Immature cognitive abilities probably contribute to the development of such fears, because the children are not able to assess a situation from more than their own point of view or to understand the reasons for an event that may, to them, seem quite unrelated. Further, children's imitation and play (imaginative) skills are beginning to develop. They "rehearse" in their minds events as they perceive them, with all of the distorted perceptions or inaccurate understandings; the meaning of the situation for them is often entirely different from what is experienced by adults. The child's reality of the situation is indeed often frightening, but the adult may be unable to make the connection that occurred for the child.[46] For further exploration of the concepts of conditioning, the reader is referred to specific theorists.[72,98]

Murphy[73,74] examined in detail the pre-school age child's developing ability to cope with stress, and from this has proposed ideas relating to the child's inner development and mastery of the world. For Murphy, coping involves the young child's ability to use developing resources (e.g., reflexes, language, social relationships, inner control) to master individual problems encountered with the environment. Several positive resources for coping that evolve during early childhood are identified as (1) interest and warmth in social relationships, (2) a positive, outgoing attitude toward life, (3) a range and flexibility in reflexes such as withdrawal from painful stimuli or crying in distress, (4) the capacity to regress or relax in the face of overwhelming pressure, (5) resilience and flexibility in mobilizing resources currently available under stressful situations, (6) the inner control of impulses, and (7) the ability to accept limits imposed from the environment. While use of each of these mechanisms is indicative of healthy emotional development, when the child uses one exclusively, when they are used to an extreme, or when the child resorts to them in the face of very mild stress or discomfort, emotional disturbance is suspected.[73,74]

Another important aspect of inner development is the development of concepts of right and wrong—of morality as defined by the child's culture.[10] Again, many of the learning mechanisms enter into this developmental process, and Erikson provides a way of viewing such development from a psychoanalytic framework. Piaget has also studied this developmental process from his particular frame of reference. A sense of ethics and justice, for Piaget, is anchored first in complete adherence to adult authority, to be replaced by a relationship of mutuality, then social reciprocity, and finally to adherence to the child's own social integrity.[79]

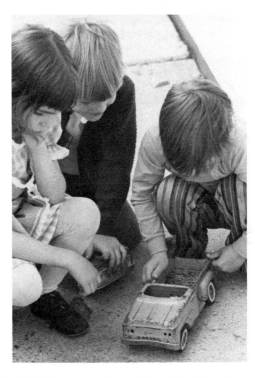

**Fig. 10-12.** Interest and warmth in social relationships are resources the child develops to learn to cope with problems and achieve mastery of the world.

**335**

## NURSING ASSESSMENT OF PHYSICAL COMPETENCY
### Approaching the child

The early childhood period presents one of the most interesting challenges in relation to approaching and relating to the child as an individual. Children's reactions to health care workers often become conditioned as feelings of fear and apprehension and their limitations in experiences with people outside of their own family render them doubtful and uncertain of encounters with strangers. An effective approach to a child of this age requires knowledge of the developmental characteristics of the child and the incorporation of behaviors by the nurse that are personally comfortable and successful in establishing rapport.[22,104]

Each of these factors influences the manner and order in which the nurse conducts the health assessment of the child. Such an assessment rarely follows a predetermined pattern by the nurse; rather, each component of the assessment must be approached in accord with readiness cues from the young child. Often, developmental screening that involves play activities and motor movement is used initially to promote the child's familiarity with the environment and to help establish interaction with the nurse. Assessment procedures that require restraint or discomfort should be planned to be integrated into the assessment period after the child is at ease and has established a sense of confidence. Activities that restore the child's comfort and sense of security should be planned to follow such procedures so that the child does not leave the encounter with a negative feeling of being manipulated into a frightening or uncomfortable situation.

The child's imaginative abilities may be used effectively when the nurse approaches the child with an age-appropriate toy, book, or game. Speaking in language that is appropriate, but not demeaning, helps in establishing contact. The overwhelming size difference between a nurse and a young child may be overcome by kneeling beside the child and approaching the child at eye level. Colors in the nurse's clothing and pictures and toys in the setting all contribute to providing a sense of familiarity that may be missing from the white, polished environ-

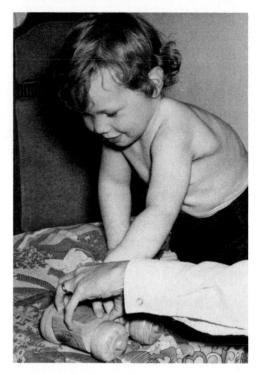

**Fig. 10-13.** Approaching a young child with an appropriate toy helps him to feel comfortable in new surroundings.

ment of the hospital or clinic. Children of this age need time to explore, to become familiar, and to "settle in" to a new environment. Having time to play with toys, listening to the mother interacting with those who are unfamiliar, and becoming accustomed to the smells and feels of the environment are very important to children. In addition, they need evidence of whether or not they can trust this new environment and the people in it. When painful, discomforting, or threatening procedures must be done, time must be devoted to establishing a sense of trust and confidence. When children are warned immediately in advance that a particular procedure will hurt, they will learn to trust the nurse. Warnings that come too far in advance of painful procedures, on the other hand, produce undue anxiety and fear to the point that the safe and adequate administration of the procedure is hampered by the child's resistance.

By the end of infancy, children have reached a significant proportion of the total physical competency potential with which they were

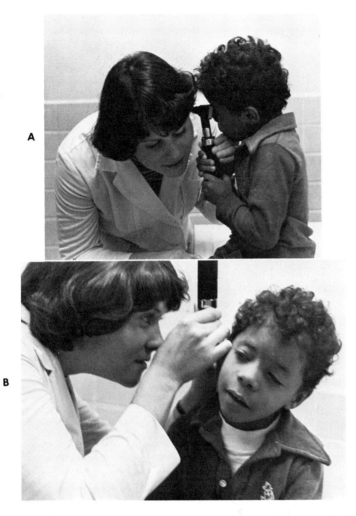

**Fig. 10-14. A,** The child needs to explore and establish familiarity with strange objects in the health care setting. He learns the feel and function of the otoscope before it is used to visualize his ear. **B,** Note the position in which the nurse holds the otoscope in order to steady the instrument against the child's head, this guarding the child from injury.

born. Practice in motor and physical functions provides further refinement of their capabilities, and thus the age of early childhood is important for their discovery of exactly what capacities they have. The use of physical capabilities now awaits the further development of mental capacity so that the child may direct, control, and use maximally all capacities for physical performance.

## Assessment of physical systems

Assessment of the young child begins with a history of the child's physical, learning and thought, social and inner development. The parent's recall of specific developmental events should be obtained and recorded, for even though their memory of exact detail may be lacking, their reports of the child's development provides an indication of their attitude, feelings, and perception of the child. Accurate details of development are most reliably obtained from a comprehensive health record and should include all dimensions of health assessment and supervision during the prenatal, newborn, and infancy periods.[45]

Continuous monitoring of the child's body

337

growth, including weight, height, and head and chest circumferences, should be obtained and entered on a growth grid. The grid provides comparison of changes in these dimensions over a period of time and allows quick recognition of any apparent deviation from the expected growth pattern.

Progressive monitoring of developmental changes in pulse and respiratory rates, blood pressure, and temperature also indicates adequate physiologic development. The blood pressure should be taken using the auscultation method during early childhood. An appropriate cuff size is imperative in achieving accurate blood pressure measurements in children, and because of the wide range of arm diameters in children, cuffs of 3, 5, 8, 12 and, 18 cm should be available. The cuff selected should be that which is closest to 20% greater in width than the diameter of the arm.[76] A cuff that is too narrow or too close to the diameter of the arm, will yield a false high blood pressure; one that is too wide (over 30% wider than the arm diameter) will yield a false low blood pressure measurement. The child should be lying down and calm, and a simple explanation given as to what the blood pressure cuff will feel like. For a child who is particularly apprehensive, the nurse might demonstrate the procedure on a life-sized doll or have the child pump the bulb into a cuff applied to the mother's or the nurse's arm.

Laboratory testing for kidney and blood functions is repeated as indicated. A yearly determination of the function of each of these systems provides evidence of adequate development. Of particular concern during early childhood is the continued risk for iron deficiency anemia, and periodic evaluation of hemoglobin and hematocrit levels provides useful information in this regard.

Various screening approaches have been developed to facilitate identification of children who need more detailed and comprehensive assessment of development. Several of these will be discussed in the following section and in later chapters. The Minnesota Child Development Inventory* provides a standardized ques-

*Interpretive Scoring Systems, 4401 West 76th St., Minneapolis, Minn. 55435

tionnaire that has been demonstrated to be useful and reliable in screening the child's current developmental status. The tool facilitates reliable responses from the parent regarding current behaviors observed in the child, and the results can be plotted on a graph that gives a general interpretation of the child's development. Possible areas of developmental lag can be ascertained, and further evaluation conducted.[49]

The Denver Developmental Screening Test provides one means of screening for physical developmental problems.[35] This tool provides an estimate for the adequacy of motor skills that the child should be able to perform by a given age, but its usefulness decreases during the fourth and fifth years. There may be some difficulty encountered when the tool is used with children who are bilingual or members of a minority subculture, since some of the items appear to be culture-biased. Insightful nursing judgment and further assessment may be needed to determine the accuracy of the test for a given child (see Appendix).

In using any developmental screening tool, the nurse needs to be fully prepared in the standardized techniques for administration, appropriate approaches to the child, and scoring and interpretation of results. The usefulness of the tool is lacking when inappropriate methods are used in administration, when the child's behavior is adversely affected by the approach of the nurse, or when the tool is scored incorrectly. Mead Johnson Laboratories provide Denver Developmental Screening Test kits and manuals, but anyone who anticipates using the tool for clinical practice needs to study the standardized methods, practice with supervision, and have their initial scoring validated by an experienced user of the tool.[107]

Vision, hearing, and articulation skills may be evaluated by a number of screening methods.[2,14,69] By the age of about 5 years, the child should be able to speak the primary language of his or her culture with 90% fluency.[115] The Denver Articulation Screening Test is an easily administered tool for determining the adequacy of the English-speaking child's articulation abilities, and it may contribute to detecting hearing loss.[28] (See Appendix.)

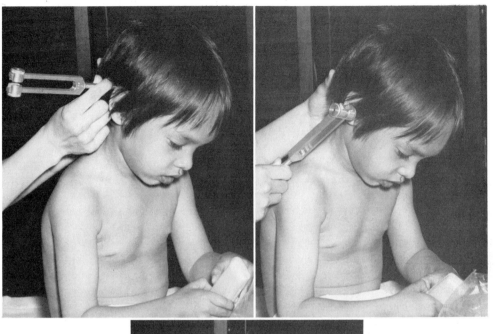

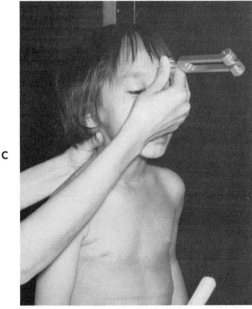

**Fig. 10-15.** The child's hearing ability is screened using the tuning fork. **A,** After the examiner strikes the fork, the handle is placed on the bony prominence behind the ear. The child is asked to indicate when the sound goes away. **B,** When he reports that he can no longer hear the sound, the fork is transferred in proximity to the external ear without interfering with the sound to test for air conduction. The child is again asked to indicate when the sound disappears, at which time the examiner compares the presence of sound with his own ability to hear remaining sound (Rinne test). **C,** The Weber test is used to screen for either conductive or sensorineural loss. After the examiner strikes, the handle of the fork is placed on the center of the child's forehead. He is then asked to indicate where he hears the sound. He should hear sound equally in both ears.

The child's ability to hear is most accurately determined by audiometric methods, but the nurse may estimate hearing capacity by whispering instructions when the child's back is turned and observing the ability to hear and respond accurately. The child may be asked to listen to a radio volume gradually increased and to report when the sound is first heard. Use of a tuning fork offers the advantage of testing for both bone and air conduction (Fig. 10-15). The limitation of each of these methods is that they depend upon the nurse's own ability to hear, and a comparison is made with this ability in order to estimate the child's ability. A history giving factors that indicate risk of hearing loss should be obtained if this has not previously been a part of the child's data base (see Chapter 9, p. 293).

Visual abilities may be estimated by using the Denver Eye Screening Test or the Snellen Screening Test. The Denver Eye Screening Test is designed particularly for preschool chil-

dren and includes detection of the commonly occurring visual problems such as refractive errors, strabismus, and amblyopia.[8]

Snellen Screening, when administered under standardized procedures, has the advantage of rendering a reliable estimate of the actual visual acuity of the child. The child must be able to understand the test requirements of either pointing in the direction of the Es or naming the letters.[59]

The Snellen E chart is usually used for preschool children, and a version for testing by the mother at home is available from the National Society for Prevention of Blindness. Such home testing has been demonstrated to be very reliable and offers the advantage of obtaining an estimate for young children who might not cooperate with such testing in a strange environment. The Snellen test for preschool children provides the important function of detecting a child with amblyopia and is intended for the child who cannot see adequately out of one eye

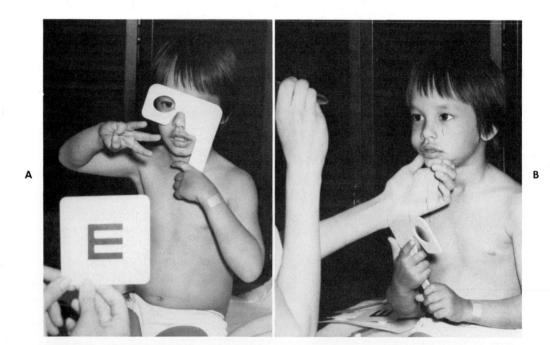

**Fig. 10-16.** The Denver Eye Screening Test is useful in estimating acuity and function during the preschool period. **A,** The child is asked to indicate, under standardized conditions, the direction of the "E." **B,** Pupillary light reflex and pupil light reflection are determined by shining a pen light into the child's eyes and noting the reflexive constriction of the pupils in each eye and the light reflection on the pupils.

cannot respond to the testing of that eye. Details of standardized screening procedures and requirements are found in Chinn and Leitch, *Child Health Maintenance: A Guide to Clinical Assessment.*

The pupillary light reflex provides a screening approach for heterotropia, a condition in which the child's eyes do not focus together in such a way as to transmit good coordinated binocular vision (Fig. 10-16, *B*). If the child has developed heterotropia, the light from a penlight held about 20 inches from the child's eyes will reflect off the pupil slightly off center. There may be consistent and observable crossing of the eyes (strabismus). The cover test provides further evidence of a tendency for the child's eyes to cross (heterophoria). The child focuses on a spot first 14 inches away, then 20 feet away. While the child gazes at the designated spot, one eye is blocked completely for 10 seconds (the eye and eye lashes must not be touched) and then removed abruptly. If the covered eye moves from the line of vision of the uncovered eye, that eye has a tendency toward muscle imbalance and must be further evaluated.[15]

Color blindness presents a particular prob-

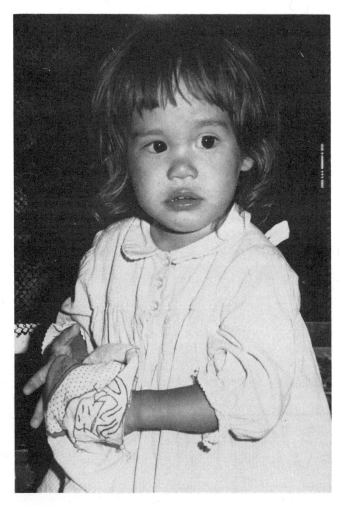

**Fig. 10-17.** The light reflection on the child's pupils confirms appropriate balance of the eye muscles. Here the light reflection is equal in both pupils, indicating adequate muscle balance, in spite of the subjective impression of slight crossing of the eyes created by the epicanthal fold.

lem for young children, particularly in relation to school, because many of the cues encountered in the academic setting depend upon the ability to distinguish colors. Early detection can result in the child receiving some assistance with learning to interpret visual perceptions in such a way that the disadvantage is minimized. Screening for certain types of color discrimination difficulties may be conducted by asking the child to respond to various colors in the environment; however, adequate testing for all color blindness types requires the use of a specialized test, such as the Ishihara test.[108]

The ears are inspected for size, shape, and placement in relation to the outer canthus of the eye. Any drainage or accumulation of cerumen around the external meatus should be noted. The canal and tympanic membrane should be visualized; if cerumen inhibits visualization and the child has no other signs of possible infection, visualization of the tympanic membrane may be deferred. It may be desirable to remove thick, tenacious, or excessive cerumen that might be interfering with the child's hearing. The largest otoscopic speculum that can fit comfortably into the external canal is used. For the young child the auricle is pulled downward and outward to straighten the canal (see Chapter 11). The color, luster, transparency, curvature, and vascularity of the membrane is noted.[105]

Neuromotor assessment of the child gives detailed evidence of physical capacities and development during the preschool years. Reflexes that are expected to persist indefinitely include the knee jerk, the Achilles tendon jerk, the biceps and triceps reflexes of the arms, pupil reaction to light, and the blink reflex. Screening should also be done for reflexes that should have disappeared or changed, such as the Babinski and other infantile reflexes (see Chapter 9).

Screening for function of each of the cranial nerves becomes possible as the child is able to follow verbal instructions or imitate certain actions by the nurse. The following abilities should be present by the onset of early childhood (Roman numerals refer to the nerves involved):

I. *Olfactory:* The child should be able to identify familiar odors such as chocolate, alcohol, or peanut butter.

II. *Optic:* Screening for visual function identifies intact function of this nerve.

III, IV, and VI. *Oculomotor, trochlear, and abducens:* The child's ability to coordinate eye movements, symmetry of the blink reflex with no ptosis of the lids, pupillary reactions, and the absence of nystagmus indicate adequate function of each of these nerves.

V. *Trigeminal:* The child's ability to feel light touch sensations on the face and to blink reflexly in response to a light touch of the cornea indicates intact neural pathway of this nerve.

VII. *Facial:* The child is able to wrinkle the forehead, frown, smile, or squint both eyes symmetrically and discriminate tastes such as salt and sugar on the anterior portion of the tongue.

VIII. *Acoustic:* The child's ability to hear indicates intact function of this nerve. Also, the ability to balance on one foot, to walk a straight line, or to balance with eyes closed indicates adequate function of the acoustic nerve.

IX and X. *Glossopharyngeal and vagus:* Evidence of adequate salivation; the ability to form speech sounds with the pharynx, larynx, and soft palate; and sensations of these structures indicate intact nerve function. Further, the presence of the gag reflex when the throat is visualized or swabbed gives evidence of function.

XI. *Accessory:* Symmetry and strength of the trapezius and sternocleidomastoid muscles are assessed by having the child turn the head against opposing pressure on either side by the nurse and then lifting the shoulders simultaneously against opposing pressure by the nurse. The ability to perform these tasks symmetrically indicates intact function of the nerve.

XII. *Hypoglossal:* The function of the tongue indicates the intact function of this nerve. The child may be asked to stick out the tongue, to move it around from side to side, and to press the tongue against the cheek with the

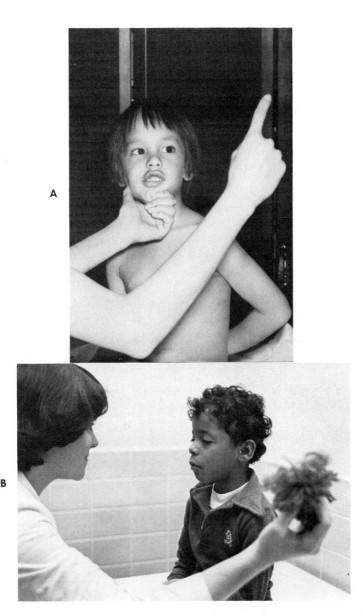

**Fig. 10-18.** Further evidence of visual function is obtained. **A,** With the child's chin anchored, he is asked to follow the movement of the examiner's finger through all hemispheres. The adequacy of coordination and eye movement and symmetry of movement are noted. **B,** Peripheral vision is estimated by asking the child to report when he first sees the ball of yarn approaching from the side. When he is focused on an object straight ahead, he should be able to detect movement at about a 90-degree angle.

nurse feeling each side to determine symmetry of strength of each side.[56]

Asymmetry of function or strength deserves further attention. The development of handedness near the end of the preschool period may result in a slight increase in strength of the preferred hand, but gross weakness of the opposing side is not present.

Indications of cerebral function may be elicited by asking the child to recall memorable past

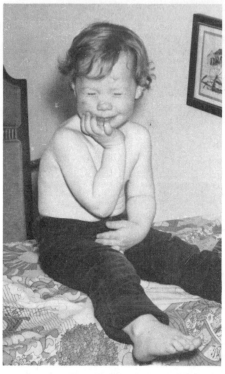

**Fig. 10-19.** Adequate function of the seventh cranial nerve (facial) is required in order for the child to be able to squint symmetrically.

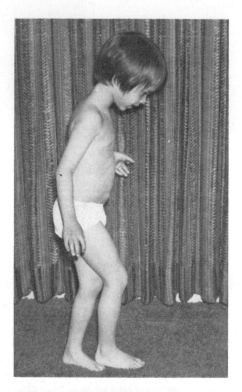

**Fig. 10-20.** The ability to walk heel-to-toe requires adequate function of the eighth cranial nerve (acoustic).

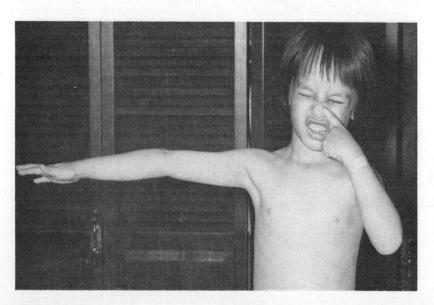

**Fig. 10-21.** Coordination in touching the tip of the nose with the index finger while keeping eyes closed requires several neurologic functions, including acoustic balance.

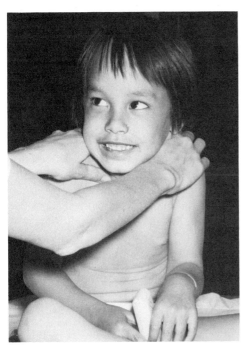

**Fig. 10-22.** Symmetry and strength of the trapezius and sternocleidomastoid muscles and function of the ninth cranial nerve (accessory) are estimated by observing the ability of the child to lift his shoulders simultaneously against opposing pressure by the examiner.

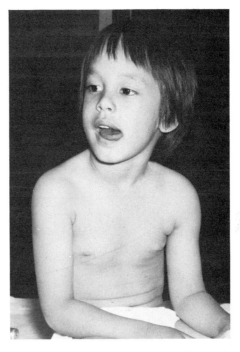

**Fig. 10-23.** The function of the twelfth cranial nerve (hypoglossal) is demonstrated by the symmetrical movement of the tongue and the strength of muscle function.

events, such as a birthday party or visiting grandmother. The accurateness of the story may be confirmed to differentiate imaginative from real responses. The child's ability to draw, copy geometric figures, and write and the ability to perform a number of skilled motor acts such as working a puzzle indicate cerebral function, regardless of the intelligence capacity of the child.[9,56,75] Memory may be tested by asking the child to repeat an arbitrary sequence of numbers. By the time children are about 5 years of age (or ready to start kindergarten) they should be able to easily repeat four consecutively named numbers. By this time also their fine motor coordination should be well integrated so that they can draw a figure of a man with three to six parts that they can identify and that bear some resemblance to the part identified by virtue of its location in relation to the other body parts.

The child's external appearance is observed. Dry skin is expected during this period of life,

but when the environment is cold or arid, the child may be uncomfortable or the skin may begin to crack and peel. Intervention is indicated to relieve these discomforts and hazards.

Hygiene is estimated by the condition of the skin, scalp, and teeth. Teaching and guidance may be directed toward the child as the early childhood period progresses; including the family encourages the child's cooperation and involvement in his own health care.

Examination of the genitalia of young children is an important component of the physical assessment. This part of the examination should be approached in a matter-of-fact manner, explaining to the child and the adult present what is being done just as the examination is approached. The findings are discussed with the young child and the adult in terms that can be understood, and any possible concerns are approached by the nurse. The labia of the young girl should be separated gently, and all tissues examined for ulcerations, masses, abnormal

**345**

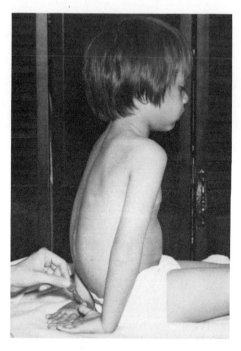

**Fig. 10-24.** The child is asked to identify small objects placed in his hands behind his back. His ability to recognize objects by feel gives an indication of sensory integrity, past tactile experiences, and cerebral function.

structure, and discharge. Of particular concern are signs of infection, venereal disease, or sexual abuse. Signs of scarring, sores or ulcerations, or discharge are matters of concern, and further evaluation is needed. A vaginal examination should not be done on preschool girls unless there is the possibility of serious vaginal infection, venereal disease, sexual abuse, or a foreign body in the vagina.[17,81] The testes and inguinal canal of the preschool boy are palpated to determine adequate descent of each testes and the absence of masses or herniations. The penis is inspected for adequacy of the urinary meatus, ulcerations, and masses.[3]

The adequacy of immunologic mechanisms is indicated by the absence of frequent communicable disease. However, when a young child experiences frequent infections, particularly of the upper respiratory tract, factors other than inadequacy of the immunologic system need to be explored first. If the young child has encountered new playmates since the infections began, immunologic competency may still be de-

veloping; within four to eight months the child should begin to demonstrate some resistance. The winter months bring greater exposure to respiratory and gastrointestinal illness, and the epidemiology of the family and the community need to be known in order to judge the nature of the many nonspecific illnesses that a child develops. Under usual circumstances, a young child from 2 to 6 years of age may experience as many as four to eight colds yearly. It is speculated that each of these infections represents exposure to a new and different infectious agent; therefore, the child's immunologic capacity has not yet developed. When complications of the common cold occur with this frequency, however, other factors must be explored.[50,64] These are described in Chapter 11.

## Daily activities

Knowledge of a typical 24-hour period in the life of a young child is helpful in determining the adequacy of the child's exercise and rest patterns. There is usually little question of the adequacy of large muscle activity. Activities involving all of the senses and exercising all muscles should be occurring with sufficient balance to provide stimulation of each function. Sleep presents a matter of concern more frequently during the early childhood years. Children vary greatly in their needs for sleep and in how well they sleep. If a child has stamina and energy to last throughout the waking hours of the day and if temperament and disposition remain fairly constant and reasonably harmonious with others, sleep and rest are probably adequate regardless of the amount of time of sleep or the qualitative nature of the sleep. When restlessness, nightmares, or resistance to bedtime begin to result in symptoms of inadequate rest, adjustment in sleeping arrangements or bedtime practices may help the child to overcome a temporary difficulty.[30,42,48]

## Feeding and nutrition

By the beginning of toddlerhood, weaning from breast or bottle has usually occurred, and milk intake has decreased in proportion to the amounts of food taken as solids or table foods.

Essential features of nutritional assessment for toddlers and preschool children are present-

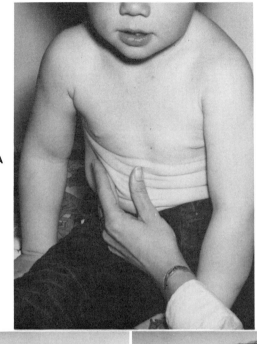

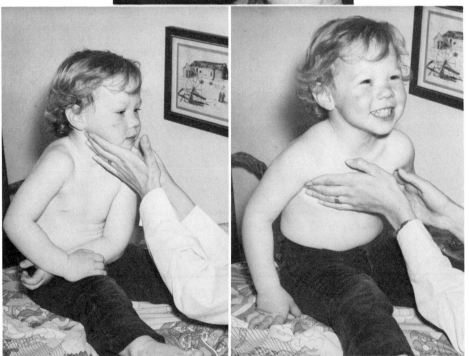

**Fig. 10-25. A,** Inspection of the child's skin indicates adequacy of hydration as well as condition of the skin itself. **B,** Enlarged lymph nodes may accompany other signs of infection. The nodes of the neck and throat are palpated. **C,** Nodes in the axillary region are palpated.

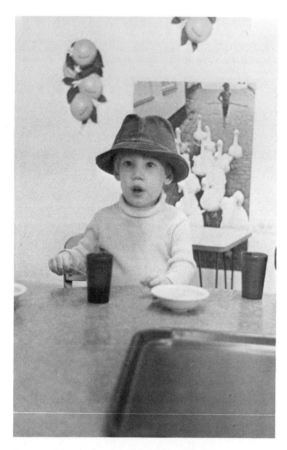

**Fig. 10-26.** During early childhood, ritual behaviors related to mealtime are important to the child.

ed in Table 10-1. Toddler and preschool children frequently develop ritual behaviors related to feeding and begin to express strong food preferences. Their individual habits and behaviors related to feeding need to be explored with the family, and the extent to which the child's behavior is congruent with the family's life style should be determined. The effect of this interaction on the nutritional status of the child may be significant, and these dynamics also exert an important influence on the child's and family's mental status.

## ASSESSMENT OF LEARNING AND THOUGHT COMPETENCY

As early childhood progresses, parents become increasingly more aware of and concerned about the intellectual development of their children. In assessing learning and thought compe-

tency, the nurse is concerned with intellectual capacity, but more comprehensively with all functions contributing to the child's ability to think, learn, reason, communicate, solve problems, and form abstractions regardless of innate intellectual capacity. Tools for determining intellectual capacity are not usually available for use by the nurse, but upon occasion such evaluation may be sought from psychologists in determining a particular problem that a child may be experiencing.

### Estimating learning and thought competency

Many of the behaviors observed in the course of assessment related to physical competency also indicate development of learning and thought capacity. Children's ability to draw a person in a manner that is appropriate for their age, their speech and related language capacity, and their ability to learn and participate in their own health care are indicators of maturing learning and thinking capacities. Because the variations in the level of learning and thought capacities are great and the rate of development is highly differential during early childhood, it is difficult to estimate definitive age-appropriate tasks during the preschool years unless professionally administered psychologic tests are used. The nurse may participate in screening for difficulties in this area and, when a problem is suspected, refer the child for more definitive evaluation of learning and thought capacity. The child's ability to hear, see, perform appropriate motor tasks, follow instructions, speak and communicate, relate to others socially, and to relate a self concept are all indicators of the child's learning and thought competency. The Denver Developmental Screening Test provides screening for some of these interrelated areas of development for months and years of early childhood, but this test is not to be confused with an intelligence test.

The child's level of development of receptive and expressive language should be assessed at regular intervals throughout early childhood. The earlier a speech, language, or hearing lag is identified, the more effective will be the outcome of intervention. Detailed guidelines of expected abilities are presented in the table

**Table 10-1.** Levels of nutritional assessment for infants and children (ages 2 to 5 years)*

| Level of approach† | History | | Clinical evaluation | Laboratory evaluation |
| | Dietary | Medical and socioeconomic | | |
| --- | --- | --- | --- | --- |
| Minimal | 1. Source of iron<br>2. Vitamin supplement<br>3. Milk intake (type and amount)<br>4. Eating habits, patterns | 1. Birth weight<br>2. Length of gestation<br>3. Serious or chronic illness<br>4. Use of medicines<br>5. Probe about pica | 1. Body weight and height<br>2. Gross defects | 1. Hematocrit<br>2. Hemoglobin<br>3. Urine protein and sugar |
| Midlevel | 1. Semiquantitative<br>  a. Iron-cereal, meat, egg yolks, supplement<br>  b. Energy nutrients<br>  c. Micronutrients—calcium, niacin, riboflavin, vitamin C<br>  d. Protein<br>2. Food intolerances | 1. Family history: diabetes tuberculosis<br>2. Maternal height Prenatal care<br>3. Infant Immunizations Tuberculin test | 1. Head circumference<br>2. Skin color, pallor, turgor<br>3. Subcutaneous tissue paucity, excess | 1. RBC morphology<br>2. Serum iron<br>3. Total iron binding capacity<br>4. Sickle cell testing<br>5. Serum lead |
| In-depth level | 1. Quantitative 24-hour recall<br>2. Dietary history | 1. Prenatal details<br>2. Complications of delivery<br>3. Regular health supervision | 1. Cranial bossing<br>2. Epyphyseal enlargement<br>3. Costochondral beading<br>4. Ecchymoses<br>5. Triceps skinfolds | Same as above, plus vitamin and appropriate enzyme assays; protein and amino acids; hydroxyproline, etc., should be available; serum micronutrients (vitamins A, C, folate) |

*Adapted from Christakis, G., editor: Nutritional assessment in health programs, Am. J. Public Health **63**(suppl.):46, 1973.
†It is understood that what is included at a minimal level would also be included or represented at successively more sophisticated levels of approach. However, it may be entirely appropriate to use a minimal level of approach to clinical evaluations and a maximal approach to laboratory evaluations.

"Landmarks of Speech, Language, and Hearing Development" in the Appendix, p. 872. Table 10-2 presents a summary of screening items that can be used for the preschool child of 4 or 5 years who is ready to enter school, a milestone that frequently brings the child to the health care system. The nurse's assessment of neuromotor capacity, quantity and quality of stimulation in the child's environment, and quality of the relationship between the family and the child are critical in interpreting speech and language ability.[36,89]

### Readiness for academic learning

Another tool that is useful during the later months of early childhood has been developed by Rogers and Rogers.[86,87] and is known as the PRESS (Preschool Readiness Experimental Screening Scale). Determinations of its validity and reliability indicate that it is reliable in assessing school readiness. It is easily administered during the course of a health assessment. This screening tool is shown on pp. 351-353. The central concern is not measurement of intellectual level but screening for developmental lags or abnormalities that would interfere with the child's ability to succeed in the academic and social world of school. The tool was constructed for the average capabilities of 5-year-old children, but it may be useful in estimating readiness in children slightly older or younger.

### Scores of intelligence and mental age

When it is desirable to obtain scores of intelligence or mental age during early childhood, it

**Table 10-2.** Language screening of preschool child*

| Language area | Expected behavior |
|---|---|
| **Receptive language** | |
| Understanding of spoken language | Carries out 3-item commands by fourth year (give me the doll, pick up the block, and sit down) |
| | Responds appropriately to stories; laughs when appropriate; imitates action of characters in story |
| | Responds to questions, such as where is the doll, which color is red, which book is bigger |
| Concept formation | Identifies big and little |
| | Identifies objects that are alike and different |
| | Completes opposite analogies, such as brother is a boy, sister is a _____ |
| **Expressive language** | |
| Speech development | First words uttered before second birthday |
| | First sentences uttered before third birthday |
| | Speech 95% intelligible before fourth birthday |
| Grammatical form | Uses 5 or 6 word sentences by fourth birthday, including nouns, verbs, pronouns, adverbs, adjectives |
| | Uses plurals appropriately; can distinguish between one and several |
| | Uses verb forms accurately, such as is/are, be/been, can/could, do/done |
| | Uses possession words accurately, such as mine, yours, ours |
| Use of concepts | Counts to three by fourth birthday, five by fifth birthday |
| | Accurately names the primary colors by fourth birthday |
| | Asks questions to find out how things work, what things are for, and why |
| | Assigns value to objects and behavior, such as that is good, pretty, funny; I am good, little, tall, strong |

*For additional information, see references 16, 60, 91, 115.

must be remembered that such measurements do not reliably represent the child's actual capacity during this age period. An estimate may be made, and extreme cases of retardation or giftedness may be reliably identified.

The intelligence test score, which is most commonly derived from a Stanford-Binet Intelligence Scale or a Wechsler Preschool and Primary Scale of Intelligence, indicates both verbal and nonverbal capacities including the, child's ability to think abstractly, to adapt, to solve problems of concrete and abstract nature, and to provide definitive self-direction in thought processes.[25,88] The fact that preschool children are in transition in developing these abilities and that they tend to use these skills in combination with less mature patterns of behavior contributes to the difficulty in obtaining a satisfactory and adequate score.

When the intelligence score is obtained, it is possible to convert this score to a mental age score or to estimate the age at which an average child would be able to perform similarly to the performance of the child who is tested. This score is useful in providing some insight into the expectations that are reasonable for the child, and it holds more meaning for parents and those not acquainted with the many ramifications of the I.Q. score. However, knowledge of this score tends to place the child in a "labeled" category, and expectations of behavior in all areas of functioning tend to be set at the mental age level. This may not accurately represent a child's level of functioning in other areas.[25] For example, an intellectually gifted child may tend to appear advanced in many areas of functioning, but his or her emotional reactions to social situations may be typical of the chronological age group. Pressure to behave more maturely than the actual capacity allows presents significant problems for the child.

Screening for intellectual capacity can be

## Administration and scoring of the
## Preschool Readiness Experimental Screening Scale (PRESS)*

**Introduction.** As the child is placed on the examining table and the records and equipment are organized, the following is said:
1. "Mrs. Smith, as I examine Johnny I will be asking him a few questions, so please don't talk to him for a few minutes." I smile and ask: "O.K.?"
2. "Johnny, I hear you're going to start kindergarten soon. Do you think you'll like that?"

**Knowledge of colors.** These questions are asked during the EENT exam.
1. "I hear your teacher will want you to know colors. Do you know any colors yet?"
2. "If she asks you to color a house, *what color should you make the grass?*"
3. "*And what color should you make the sky if there are no clouds?*"

---

NAME _____     BIRTHDATE _____

SCHOOL _____     DATE _____

1. a. What color is grass:                                          _____
   b. What color is the sky if there are no clouds?                 _____

2. a. Repeat four numbers (one success in two tries). 4-1-7-3 or 3-8-6-4   _____
   b. Recognize four tongue blades.                                 _____

3. a. Does Christmas come in the winter or the summer?             _____
   b. Where is your heel?                                           _____

4. Draw a square (best success in two tries).                      _____

5. a. Comprehension and performance                                _____
   b. Personal-social maturity                                     _____
                                                    TOTAL           _____

**Comments**

PRESS General Outline and Record Form. The children were asked to reproduce a standard 1-inch square.

---

*From Rogers, W. B., Jr., and Rogers, R. A.: A new simplified preschool readiness experimental screening scale (The PRESS), Clin. Pediatr. **11:**10, Oct., 1972; and Rogers, W. B., Jr., and Rogers, R. A.: A follow-up study of the Preschool Readiness Experimental Screening Scale (the PRESS), Clin. Pediatr. **14:**253, March, 1975.

## Administration and scoring of the
## Preschool Readiness Experimental Screening Scale (PRESS)—cont'd

**Knowledge of numbers.** Asked during the heart and lung exam.
1. "If the teacher tells you some numbers, could you remember them and repeat them back to her?"
2. *"I'm going to tell you some numbers. Now you remember them and say the same numbers right back to me."* (4-1-7-3 and 3-8-6-4)
3. "If the teacher asks you to count, could you do that?"
4. *"Tell me, how many tongue blades are there?"* At this point place four tongue blades on the table beside the patient.

**General knowledge.** As the abdomen, genitalia, and extremities are examined.
1. "I'm going to examine your tummy. You know where your tummy is, don't you?" or "Do you have a tickly tummy?"
2. *"Tell me, does Christmas come in the winter or the summer?"*
3. *"Can you show me where your heel is?"*

**Drawing coordination.** This is usually done at the end of the exam.
1. "If the teacher asked you to draw a square like this one (indicate the sample square), *let's see you draw one just like it right beside mine.* Take your time and make a good one."

**General assessment: performance and maturity.** These are best evaluated following the hearing and visual acuity tests when everything else is finished.

### Scoring

COLORS. 1 point for knowing grass is green. 1 point for knowing the sky is blue. Any other answer, such as white, blue and white, or black gets no point.

NUMBERS. 1 point for repeating the four numbers in the same sequence. If the child misses the first set of numbers, try the second set. Score 1 point for *either* set of numbers repeated back correctly. 1 point for answering the correct number of tongue blades as four. If the child only counts "one, two, three, four," this is not given a point. You may then ask the child *one time only,* "Yes, but how many are there all together?" If the child does not answer four at this time, score 0.

GENERAL KNOWLEDGE. 1 point for answering *winter.* It is important to suggest winter first. Most children will give the second of two choices if they do not know the correct answer. 1 point for knowing the heel. The child must point to the heel or the Achilles tendon, not to the malleolus.

DRAWING COORDINATION. Allow the child to draw a second square if the first one is poorly done. Encourage him or her to make the second more like the sample. Choosing the best square, score in the following manner:

2 points for drawing a good, readily recognizable square
1 point for drawing a fairly recognizable square
0 points for drawing a poor, unrecognizable square

COMPREHENSION AND PERFORMANCE. 1 point for those who reply promptly and follow instructions well (e.g., during the hearing and visual acuity tests). 0 points for those who have to be coaxed, need frequent repetition of instructions, or need repeated clarification of what you ask.

PERSONAL-SOCIAL MATURITY. 1 point if the child seems reasonably mature and self-confident. 0 points for:
Excessive silliness or playing around
Overtalkative or hyperactive
Uncooperative, evasive, no interest
Unduly attached to mother
Generally immature compared with most 5-year-olds you see

It should be evident that the PRESS is not so much a standardized test with strict rules of administration as it is a set of standardized questions that can be blended into a physical examination. One should note that it includes a few questions that are asked but not scored. These questions establish rapport and put the child at ease. They also serve as a lead-in to the test questions and serve indirectly in assessing the child's general maturity. The physician [or nurse] may intersperse or substitute other lead-in questions if he feels they would better express his method of dealing with children. It is important to ask the parent not to speak, else an oversolicitous parent may interfere by offering help and encouragement.

---

**Administration and scoring of the
Preschool Readiness Experimental Screening Scale (PRESS)—cont'd**

**Rating system**

1. *A score of 9 or 10 indicates high average to above average school readiness.* A child in this score range should have no difficulty doing average or above average school work.
2. *A score of 7 or 8 indicates average school readiness.* A child in this score range should have little difficulty doing average school work.
3. *A score of 6 indicates borderline school readiness.* About half of the males and about a fourth of the females with this score may have difficulty in school. It is recommended that close liaison be maintained with the teacher. If at any time the child is not functioning at class level, further study should be made at once.
4. *A score of 5 or less indicates insufficient school readiness.* Such children should be referred to a school psychologist or diagnostic center for further psychologic evaluation.

---

done by the nurse, using several screening tools available for use with preschool children. Such screening tools provide only a rough estimate of ability but may be useful in identifying those children who need more extensive evaluation of intellectual capacity.

The *Bender Copy Forms* give an estimate of the child's visual-motor perception. Standard figures are presented to the child, and attempts to reproduce the figures are timed and scored against normative data supplied with the test. This test is considered to be culture-free, in that it is not dependent upon concepts or language peculiar to any cultural group but rather depends upon visual and motor perception of figures common to the experience of children in all cultural groups.[58]

The *Peabody Picture Vocabulary Test* is an easily administered test of verbal intelligence, but its use is limited to middle-class children who have acquired standard English-speaking ability. The score obtained is a reliable estimate of verbal intelligence ability, provided the child fits into the middle-class, English-speaking cultural group. For children who have received insufficient language stimulation or who come from another cultural group, the score obtained is likely to be a false low score.[29]

Draw-a-person and draw-a-family tests can be graded to give estimates of intelligence, as well as interpreted in relation to emotional develop-

ment; however scoring of figure drawings requires administration of the test under standardized conditions and scoring by a qualified psychometrist. Such drawings can be obtained by the nurse and assessed for general developmental expectations, fine motor control, and evidence of concept formation and of the child's perceptions of family relationships. The 4-year-old child should be able to draw a person with at least six body parts that are placed in proximity to one another and in the appropriate locations. The child should be able to name the parts appropriately. The parts need not be accurate renditions but should bear some resemblance to the actual body part and be rendered with strong, evenly flowing lines. The family drawing may or may not include all family members, and the drawing of each figure may not be as sophisticated as the child's actual figure-drawing capacity. The child should be able to name the family members shown and describe any unique characteristics about the individuals that the picture portrays from the child's point of view. The child should be able to identify which figures are big or little as drawn on the sheet of paper. In using the test clinically, the nurse provides a pencil and plain sheet of paper and asks the child to draw the very best picture he or she can draw. The child is informed that the nurse will keep the picture, but that another may be drawn to take home.[37,41]

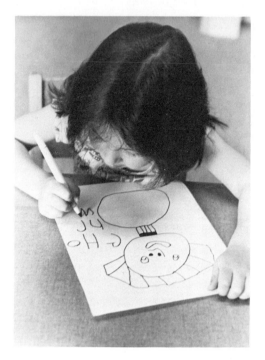

**Fig. 10-27.** At 4 years of age the child should be able to draw a person with at least six body parts and name the parts drawn.

## ASSESSMENT OF SOCIAL COMPETENCY

The approach that the nurse uses in relating to the child and family results in social interaction that either enhances or distracts from the nurse's ability to assess social skills and development and to use social interaction as a therapeutic tool. Careful and considerate critique and validation of nursing social skills are imperative for ongoing professional development.

### Assessment of social behavior

Throughout the nursing process, behavioral evidence evolves of the child's level of social interaction with the mother and other significant adults and with the nurse, who represents either a friend or a stranger. The child of 2 or 3 years is still predominantly involved in attachment and dependency processes. The modes that are used for these processes should be documented, along with an indication of the frequency of occurrence. For example, one child

may seek physical contact with the mother almost continuously, and not wander more than 10 feet from her side without establishing frequent visual contact. Another child may be comfortable with occasional visual contact only. As the child progresses into the later stages of early childhood, he or she is expected to change in social capacities, to widen his or her world of interest, and to show signs of decrease in dependency behavior. Documentation of modes of social behavior provides an estimate of individualized social development just as graphing of measurements provides a comparative estimate of physical growth. The child's comparison with his or her own previous behavior is significant, and in most cases this outweighs comparison with other children of the same age, because the wide variations that normally occur among children tend to lead to undue concern for extreme behaviors that may be within normal limits. For example, a child who is temperamentally quiet, introverted, and subdued may appear to be quite attached to mother as school age approaches in comparison to other children the same age. However, when comparing the child's social behavior with that of earlier years, it may be noted that there has been a great deal of progress toward independence and that when mother is not available the child makes sufficient adaptations to remain comfortable and secure.

Evidence of the preschool child's social competency can be obtained by discussion and evaluation of the child's drawing of his or her family. The child is asked to draw a picture of the family and given the materials for drawing. The nurse observes the drawing and responds to any comments or questions volunteered by the child. If the child asks for advice or assistance, the nurse encourages the child to proceed with the drawing just as he or she would like to do it. Positive encouragement and praise for the child's efforts may be made, particularly if the child becomes disinterested or is reticent to draw. After the drawing is completed, the nurse asks the child to identify the persons drawn and to describe individual characteristics of each family member. The names of each family member are written on the drawing, as well as any specific perceptions of the person that the child

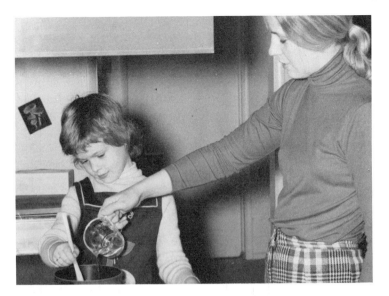

**Fig. 10-28.** "Helping" mother provides a play experience that allows the child to experiment with possible future roles.

relates. Other questions, such as what do you like best about your brother or when do you get angry with your sister, may be posed to encourage the child to describe the nature of family interactions. If an adult family member is present, the purposes of the drawing and interview of the child need to be explained and the adult requested not to participate until after the completion of the drawing and interview. Any areas of concern or questions that arise in relation to the child's drawing or verbal reports need to be discussed, and the parent reassured of the confidentiality of the interview. The child's perceptions may be verified with the adult at the conclusion of the interview or further information sought to clarify the child's perceptions.

The *Vineland Social Maturity Scale* provides an objective, standardized estimate of social maturity. The tool provides a profile of the child's self-help skills, self-direction, locomotion, occupation, communication, and social relations. It is designed to measure the child's progression toward independence. The data is obtained by observation of the child's behavior and by interview of the mother or primary caretaker. The tool may be used by interview data alone if needed, but direct observation of the child's behavior is preferred.[27]

## Play

Play for young children constitutes an important role in their social and inner development. It is a vehicle for children's exploring and experimenting with the ways of the world, with who they are, with who they might become, and with how they relate to others socially. The drama of play allows them to get outside of themselves and to comprehend themselves momentarily from some other perspective. Play often reveals the child's inner reality and perception of the world. Children "act out" the behaviors of those who are familiar to them, and in so doing they rehearse what has been demonstrated to them as appropriate behavior. The role of play in helping them to identify a role in society is accentuated by the fact that they seldom, if ever, take on a role that is not consistent with what they see as desirable. Young children seldom assume the role of a younger child or infant in playing "house"; they more often assume the roles of mother or daddy and use a doll for the younger child. Through play they learn to exert control over their own behavior; in voluntarily assuming an adultlike role, children consciously adopt, for the moment, a more mature form of behavior than is typical for their own age. Thus children may be seen to practice

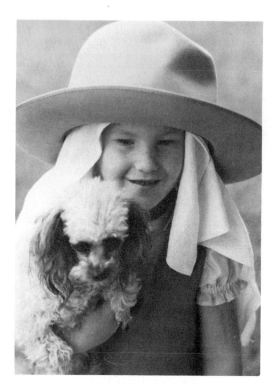

**Fig. 10-29.** In the child's perception of her play drama, she has long "hair" and a "baby" like Mommy. She has momentarily adopted a role and behavior that are more mature than her own stage of development.

expressing displeasure and anger in a play situation by vocalizing their distress, scolding the offending party, or using withdrawal of attention. Were they confronted with a similar but real anger-provoking situation, they would more likely respond with aggression, crying, or tantrum behavior. Observation of a child's play reveals many physical developmental capacities in a more natural setting than that of the examination or testing occasion and gives further evidence of the child's social and inner development.

Social competency can be estimated by observing a child's play in peer groups or through observing imitation play. In a peer group in which the child is a stranger the young child may be expected to stand back and simply observe other children for a while and then approach a toy object to begin manipulating the toy. During toddlerhood, conflict may arise over possession of a particular toy; the toddler may either passively hand over the toy, protest briefly and then divert attention to another toy, or protest intensely. During the course of play the child will be observed to attend to the other children in the group frequently, mimic behaviors of other children, or approach them with comments or questions. Their activity remains centered on manipulation of toys and active body movement, with attention changing at frequent intervals. During the preschool period the child engages in more interactive play, particularly make-believe play. Two or more children may become involved in a make-believe plot, particularly if toys and equipment are present that suggest a particular plot to the children, such as toy kitchen equipment.

Imitation may be elicited in a young child by presenting a toy model of a frequently used adult object and asking the child to show or demonstrate what someone does with the object. For example, the child may be given a toy telephone and asked to demonstrate how mother talks on the phone. Or the child might be given a few coins and asked to "purchase" something from the nurse, such as a crayon or a piece of paper. These types of play activities planned by the nurse reveal the extent to which the child has been exposed to cultural activities and standards and the use of materials such as coins and telephones.

## ASSESSMENT OF INNER COMPETENCY
### Evaluation of inner competency

Nursing assessment of inner competency depends upon many of the observations that have already been described, particularly those related to social capacities of the young child. During early childhood many behaviors normally emerge that are disturbing to those around the child and that would indicate emotional and inner distress at other points in life. Temper tantrums, nightmares, fears (of dark, night, or of being alone), or regression to infantile forms of behavior all occur periodically during toddlerhood and early childhood. When such behavior persists and predominates over a period of several months, serious disturbance must be considered. However, with the occasional, transient occurrence of such behaviors, the family helps the child to cope and to learn

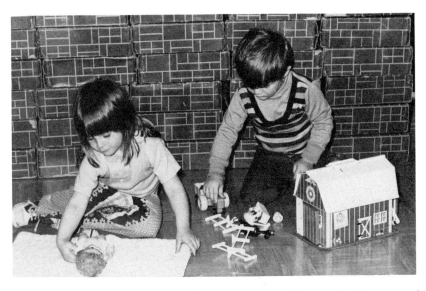

**Fig. 10-30.** The play of 3-year-olds is often centered on their own interests with little concern for the other child's activity.

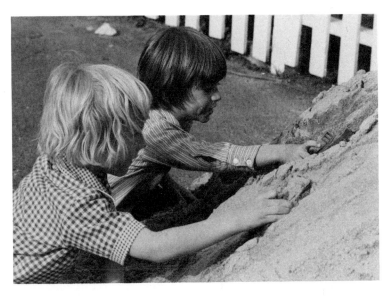

**Fig. 10-31.** Six-year-olds achieve a greater degree of cooperation and mutuality in play. They use fantasy in setting up a play-drama situation that both children enjoy together.

what is socially desirable and what is not. The child learns the difference between reality and what is imagined as other persons validate the presence or absence of frightening stimuli. Thus important tasks of childhood are accomplished through these discomforting occurrences, and more mature coping can be learned. Parents may seek advice and support from health care workers in relation to these problems. Counseling, listening, active support, and reinforcement for parental attitudes and approaches that promote healthy inner and social development may provide an important source of help.[6,38,62,66,120]

The appearance of questions related to sexual function of human beings emerges as children begin to recognize both their own sex and the differences between their endowment and that of children of the opposite sex. Their developing mental image of their own bodies is integrally involved in this task of development. During early childhood there are alternating periods of extreme curiosity and exploration of the body with periods of relative unconcern.

## Play for assessment of inner competency

Various play approaches are useful in eliciting behavior indicative of the child's sense of self and self-esteem, the child's prediction of success or failure, sense of acceptance and competence. These dimensions will emerge in conjunction with the draw-a-family approach described earlier in this chapter, often as a part of play approaches used to assess social competency. Specific approaches designed to assess self-esteem are described in the following section.

Doll play is often useful in observing a child's sense of self, although it may be difficult to elicit doll play from a young child in a clinic setting. A "family" of dolls, including a doll representing a young child of the same sex as the child, should be the only toy objects available to the child when doll play is desired. The child is presented with the family of dolls, and a few comments regarding who they might represent are made. If the child spontaneously begins to engage the doll family in make-believe activity, no further guidance should be given to the child. If the child seems reluctant to begin play with the dolls, the nurse begins a make-believe situation, moving the dolls through various activities related to the situation. For example, the nurse might begin by having the mother doll ask the young child doll if she or he would like to go to the store, hand the child doll to the child, and ask the child what the doll would like to do. Often, a young child will then continue the scenario for a period of time.

A related technique is the use of mutual story-telling. The child is instructed that the nurse will begin a story and that he or she will finish the story. The nurse then begins a story with a standard line, such as "Once upon a time there lived a (girl, boy, cow, monkey, etc.) who. . . ." The nurse then pauses to indicate that the child can pick up on the story. If the child is reluctant to participate, the nurse **might** continue the story for another sentence or two or ask the child what the figure in the story might be doing. As the child begins to supply details of the story, the nurse asks questions that encourage the child to fill in details or continue with the story, such as "And then what happened?" or "Was the little boy frightened?" The child's story is then evaluated for several dimensions that indicate the child's inner nature. First, the emotional theme of the story should be noted and should be congruent with the child's tone and expression. For example, if the child focuses on a theme of aggression and destruction but describes anger expressed by one of the characters in a monotone, emotionless manner, incongruence of content and expression exists, which suggests that the child has difficulty in expressing his or her own feelings. Second, the possible meaning of the characters in the story may be suggested by asking the child if he or she is like one of the characters at the conclusion of the story.

Puppet play is often helpful in engaging a child in mutual story-telling or make-believe role-playing. The child is given a puppet selected from a group of puppets. The nurse selects a puppet and then begins a dialogue or make-believe story plot enacted by the puppets. The child speaks and acts on behalf of his or her puppet.

Interpretation of the child's behavior and responses in such play situations is highly speculative and several encounters at different times may be needed to determine themes that may be present or to obtain an estimate of the child's self-esteem. In addition, it should be remembered that the nurse's personality and approach to the child has a significant effect on the child's ability to tell a story and on the spontaneity with which the child responds. The actual observed behavior and responses of the child should be recorded for future reference and interpretations avoided until experience and validation from an experienced child health worker have been established.

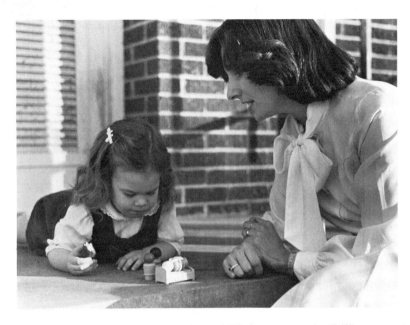

**Fig. 10-32.** Doll play is often useful for observing a child's inner sense of self. When presented with the doll family, this child began to act out a typical family scene, portraying herself as a loved member of the family.

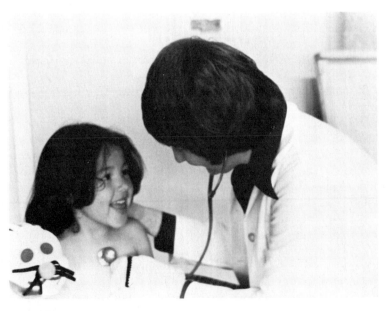

**Fig. 10-33.** The nurse is using puppet play to engage the child in a mutual story of a visit to the hospital. The child's puppet "tells" her feelings about the planned experience.

## HEALTH MAINTENANCE, PROMOTION, AND THE PREVENTION OF ILLNESS

The toddler and preschool periods are relatively healthy ones for most children. Accidents remain the primary cause of death during this period, and the normal young child is likely to have several episodes of minor respiratory and gastrointestinal illnesses until more mature immunologic competence is achieved (see Chapter 11). The health maintenance problems discussed in the following section represent the primary concerns of most families with young children.

### Feeding and nutrition

The assessment of the child's nutrition status, as outlined in Table 10-1 (p. 349) provides the basis for counseling and guidance regarding nutrition. The primary concern in American society is prevention of iron-deficiency anemia and some means of assuring adequate iron intake needs to be provided, particularly as the toddler changes from iron-fortified milk formula to whole milk. Other food sources of iron, such as meat, may be avoided or rejected by the toddler, and the family's resources may limit provision of this expensive food. Eggs (specifically the egg yolk) offer a valuable source of iron that is relatively easily incorporated into the toddler and preschooler's diet, particularly if the family is aware of the child's need for this important nutrient. As during other periods of life the basic four food groups should be used as a guide in estimating the adequacy of intake of all essential nutrients, and the family counseled with regard to means of providing each food groups for the toddler and preschooler.

The eating behavior and habits of the young child present one of the major barriers in providing adequate nutrition. The young child often begins to use the meal event as an occasion to assert individuality, control of the environment, and for simple exploration of food textures and qualities. Definite food preferences and food fads emerge. The basic life-style of the family should be used as a basis for offering counseling and guidance related to feeding, for families vary greatly in their expectations for feeding behavior and mealtime routines. For example, if the adults in the family consistently eat a wide variety of foods and enjoy mealtime together, their expectations of the young child will differ greatly from those of the family that eats meals individually or that has a limited variety in the foods selected. The family needs to explore their fundamental expectations of meal-time behavior for the young child and to determine which expectations are appropriate in guiding the young child at different developmental levels. The young toddler who is just beginning to learn to use a spoon or fork, for example, may be encouraged to use these utensils but will also need to continue to finger-feed until sufficient motor skill is gained to use utensils consistently. If it is important to the family for the child to learn to eat the foods served at each meal and to eat during the family meal time, they may need assistance in anticipating the adjustments that are needed to assist the young toddler to acquire feeding behaviors congruent with this expectation. If the family finds that the young toddler is disruptive of other family interaction during meal time, they may prefer to continue feeding the young toddler apart from the rest of the family for a period of time and delay integrating the youngster into the family experience until later but concentrate on setting the expectation that the child eat what is served. Within the limits of the family resources, the family should understand the need to provide sufficient variety of foods for the young child to assure adequate nutrition. The family may need specific directions and assistance in selecting such a variety and in preparing these foods in such a manner that the young child will accept the foods and be able to chew and swallow them adequately.

During these years parents often need a great deal of sound, reasonable counseling in regard to feeding their young children. Understanding the basic four food groups is a great asset, but other kinds of guides for good nutrition may be needed by parents in a different culture or with limited resources. The use of prepared toddler foods during the transition from infancy to early childhood presents a special concern, since these products may not provide optimal nutrition or range of food experiences needed by the child. Helping parents to understand the information on the labels of all prepared foods is a valuable way in which to convey both some principles of nutrition and a sense of sound marketing and consumer protection. When the parent chooses to give the child prepared toddler foods, the choice should be made with some awareness of the nature of the product. Further, the expense of such foods may not be understood by the family, and when convenience in preparation of foods for a young child is a minimal requirement, the child may be fed more economically and nutritionally with the regular family diet. Very little extra preparation is needed by the time that the child's first molar teeth appear.

As early childhood progresses, intense expressions of food preferences tend to emerge. This behavior is a natural outgrowth of the increased physical capacity to react to the taste and textures of foods and the realization that it is possible to control the environment by expressing an opinion. Families vary in their tolerance of expressed individual food preferences, and children vary in their tendency to develop strong likes and dislikes. When a family and a child reach extreme differences over this matter, major conflict arises, and insightful counsel and support may be needed until some solution is discovered that satisfies both the child and the family. The challenge for the nurse is (1) to provide assessment of the nutritional adequacy of the foods liked, disliked, and needed by the child, (2) to help the family reach a comfortable approach in handling the situation, and (3) to maintain a receptiveness to the wide range of possibilities that exist for all families in providing the essential nutrients needed for growth and development.[12,51,119]

### Toilet training and body hygiene

Toilet training is often a major family concern as the infant grows into toddlerhood. For the family who has never experienced this challenge before, it can be a major dilemma, and yet most families are reluctant to seek advice and assistance. The nurse should anticipate this developmental task toward the end of infancy and initiate discussion with the parents to determine their understanding of the child's developmental signs of readiness for toilet training and discuss their attitudes and plans well in advance of their early trials.

The child's ability with regard to toilet training is dependent upon sufficient neurologic and psychologic maturation, including local conditioning of reflex sphincter control (about 9 months of age), completion of myelination of pyramidal tracts (12 to 18 months of age), and the ability to cooperate voluntarily (12 to 15 months of age). Psychologic readiness and desire to control urination and defecation does not usually develop until between 18 and 30 months of age and is significantly affected by parental expectations and attitudes. Often, parents begin toilet training in advance of their child's readiness, resulting in months of frustration. The nurse should respond to the parent's desire to begin early toilet training by discussing the usual periods of readiness and assist them in planning for approaches that they will use in relating to the child if their efforts are not successful. If the child responds favorably to the fam-

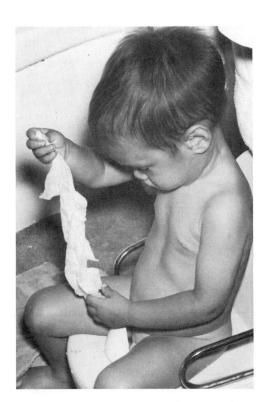

**Fig. 10-34.** The child is able to achieve toileting capacities appropriate to his culture in an atmosphere of warm, secure acceptance.

ily's plan for toilet training, they should be encouraged to continue with the established routine and encourage those responses in the child that are desired. If the child does not respond as desired, they may either choose to abandon efforts for a few weeks and resume toilet training later or they may prefer to continue with the established routine. If this is their preference, the nurse should help them identify behaviors in their child that they will encourage and praise and plan for ways to discharge their frustrations other than direct them to the child. The need to understand that as long as they communicate a warm, accepting atmosphere, the exact manner in which they accomplish toilet training is of little consequence.[19,103]

Specific needs of the young child with regard to body hygiene are also approached according to the needs and desires of the family. If hygienic practices of the family are minimal to the point that the child suffers repeated skin infections such as impetigo, attention needs to be di-

rected to specific teaching and counseling with regard to bathing and skin care. Many families, regardless of their level of care with regard to body hygiene, need guidance with regard to bathing the young child's genitalia, for there is often an emotional prohibition against touching this area of the body once the child no longer uses diapers. The family and the child, as bathing of the self begins, need to understand the need for regular bathing of the genitalia.

### Prevention of illness

Ongoing health supervision provides one means by which illness prevention may be accomplished. The family may need assistance in understanding typical patterns of illness during early childhood and in learning to cope independently with the frequent colds, skin irritations, cuts and scratches that inevitably occur during this period of life. Therefore, the goals of health maintenance are to assist the family in their ability to care for minor illnesses and acci-

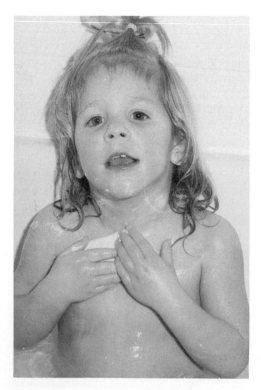

**Fig. 10-35.** The young child begins to acquire skills in providing for her own body hygiene needs.

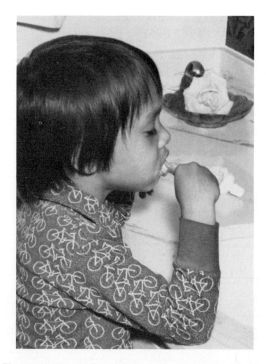

**Fig. 10-36.** The ability to brush one's own teeth requires advanced motor coordination and provides independence and learning.

dents which occur in the normal course of life, to understand prevention of progression to a more serious illness state, and to recognize and differentiate serious illness from the common, minor illnesses typical of early childhood.

The program of immunizations begun during infancy should be continued during early childhood as outlined in Chapter 9, p. 308. Table 10-3 presents the recommendations (1974) of the American Academy of Pediatrics for immunization of children who did not begin immunizations during infancy.

Prevention of dental caries is a major concern during early childhood, for the diet of the young child changes dramatically and often begins to include frequent snacks, and the child acquires a full first set of teeth requiring the need for beginning oral hygiene. The dangers of prolonged sucking on a bottle, discussed in Chapter 9, should be discussed with the parent if bottle-feeding at bedtime or naptime continues during toddlerhood. The nutrition assessment provides information regarding the frequency and amount of carbohydrate intake. The family should be counseled in accord with this assessment and encouraged to use snacks that do not promote tooth decay, such as fresh fruit, vegetables, nuts, cheese, popcorn, milk, pretzels, and sugar-free drinks and candy. By about the age of 3 years, the child should begin to acquire a habit of regular toothbrushing. The family should encourage the child in assuming this responsibility with supervision, in that the child brushes his or her teeth for the experience of handling the brush for a brief period, with the parent completing the cleaning process with thorough brushing of all tooth and gum surfaces. The use of disclosing tablets, a harmless food dye available without prescription, should be demonstrated for the child and family to assist them in determining the extent to which brushing has been effective in removing harmful plaque and food particles.[52,99]

Young children who do not receive fluoride in their drinking water should continue to receive fluoride supplements during early childhood to protect the primary teeth and the permanent teeth that are forming. The recommended dose for children 2 to 3 years of age is 0.5 mg/day; for children 3 years and older the recommended dosage is 1.0 mg/day.[33]

Another problem related to dental health is that of prolonged thumb or finger sucking. Before the age of 3 years, pacifier, thumb, and finger sucking is expected in a large number of children, and most of these voluntarily forsake the habit by the fourth year. Sucking habits during this period do not usually contribute significantly to malocclusion problems, and the family should be counseled to ignore the habit entirely and not focus attention on it, which may contribute to the child prolonging the habit. If the habit persists beyond the age of 4 years, particularly during the day, orthodontic consultation should be sought. If the orthodontist feels that the habit is contributing to malocclusion problems, preventive early intervention may be taken in order to assist the child in breaking the sucking habit and to prevent further development of malocclusion.[26]

## Prevention of accidents

The family should be counseled regarding the selection of toys that are safe for the toddler and preschool age child. Of particular concern during toddlerhood are toys with sharp edges and hazardous points or internal rods and wires, which are a source of injury, particularly if the child falls while carrying the toy. Another frequent source of injury is the ingestion of small

**Table 10-3.** Recommendations of the American Academy of Pediatrics for immunization of children not immunized during infancy*

| Time interval | Immunization |
|---|---|
| First visit | Diphtheria, tetanus, pertussis (DTP) Trivalent oral polio vaccine (TOPV) Tuberculin skin test |
| 1 month later | Measles, rubella, mumps |
| 2 months later | DTP, TOPV |
| 4 months later | DTP, TOPV |
| 6-12 months later | DTP, TOPV |
| Age 14-16 years | Tetanus, diphtheria (every 10 years thereafter) |

*Report of the Committee on Infectious Disease, American Academy of Pediatrics, 1974. For current recommendations, contact the American Academy of Pediatrics, P.O. Box 1034, Evanston, Ill. 60204.

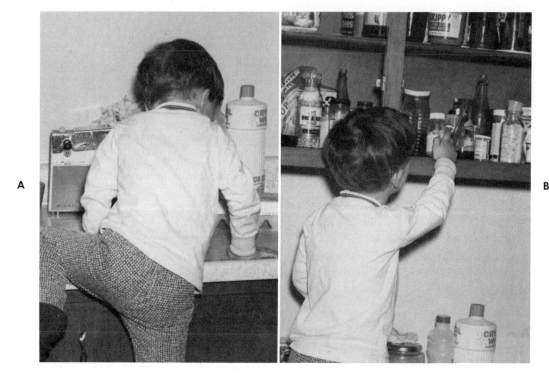

A

B

**Fig. 10-37.** Anticipated accidents can be avoided with attention to special household hazards. **A,** The young child gaining new motor skills easily pulls a chair to the kitchen counter, climbs up, and has easy access to fatal hazards in attractive medicine jars, **B.**

wheels, buttons, or rods that can be manipulated loose from a toy. The family needs to be aware of the possibility of flammability hazards of many toys and look for labeling that indicates that the toy has passed minimum flammability standards.[48,101]

Accidents comprise the most serious threat to the well-being of a young child. Ingestion of poisonous substances, such as medicines, vitamin and iron preparations, cleaning fluids, or household poisons, becomes an increasing hazard as the child is able to walk and climb. The family should anticipate this period of development before its arrival. They should carefully assess the hazards that still exist after implementing measures designed to protect the infant, and they should faithfully lock up every substance that might present a hazard to the exploring, climbing child. Placing items out of reach may be sufficient for a child who temporarily is less active or exploratory than the average child, but this is not a sufficient safeguard

for most young children, and it does not provide the kind of guarantee that most children need.[63,68,110,113]

The increased ability of the young child to climb and wander away from the immediate surroundings of home or preschool and the inability to exercise judgment in anticipating potential dangers make him or her particularly susceptible to injuries and accidents that may result in tragedy. While the child desires and needs to experience increasing freedom, autonomy, and exploration, constant supervision is required to assure continued safety. Even toward the end of early childhood, the child's judgment and reasoning abilities are not developed to the point that he or she can fully protect himself from the multiple hazards of the larger world.

Automobile safety, which extends to the pedestrian problem for the young child, becomes increasingly a challenge for the family as the child is more active and mobile, especially

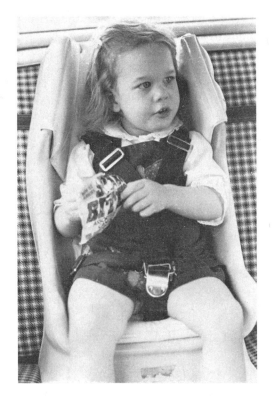

**Fig. 10-38.** Appropriate automobile restraint for the pre-schooler includes a special seat that is anchored by the car seat belt.

when confined to a car. A regular habit of re-straining all passengers when the car is in mo-tion may become a sacred ritual for the child, and it is imperative in providing maximum pro-tection against automobile injuries.[97]

Accepting invitations of strangers is a less commonly encountered, but critical, hazard during early childhood. In the face of many fears and imagined dangers of goblins, ghosts, and boogeymen, the young child is easily cajoled into accepting treats in return for joining a stranger in a "ride home."

Fires inadvertently started by a young child playing with matches occur with sufficient fre-quency that families need to investigate and re-move all accessible fire hazards. In addition the family might consider ways in which they can begin to introduce the young child to such haz-ards. Without instilling fear, the child may be led to develop a healthy respect for dangers that do exist in the environment. While reliability

in adhering to the lessons taught may not de-velop during this period of life, the child's early exposure and learning may result in the pre-vention of similar accidents during later child-hood.

Local fire and law enforcement agencies can often provide safety instructions for families and children related to fire, poisons, and automobile hazards. Lessons instilled by these community helpers may have a meaningful impact for the preschool child whose hero is the fireman or policeman.

**Stimulation and daily routine**

The use of stimulation techniques, which were described in Chapter 9, may be useful during early childhood, particularly if lack of a stimulating environment is suspected. There is evidence that a child may accomplish significant gains in abilities or overcome developmental lags through purposive, deliberate stimulation. Attention to the totality of the child's needs must be considered, so that emotional, cogni-tive, and physical needs are met at the same time.[53,102]

Normally, the toddler and preschool age child is extremely active and self-stimulating and highly inquisitive, often beyond the family's ability to cope. They may need assistance in finding effective ways to calm the child, par-ticularly at bedtime or during periods when the child is confined inside, such as when bad weather interferes with outdoor play. The fam-ily's own life-style patterns need to be discussed and this used in counseling with the family to plan for provision of direct interaction with the child, including activities that allow the child to use large muscles. Planned periods for ball play, running or chasing, and friendly "wrestling" may help to discharge some of the young child's energy and satisfy the need for personal atten-tion, which may help to decrease undesirable aggressive or nondirected physical activity. In-teraction that serves to calm the child should also be planned for periods of time when the child needs to settle down, such as story-tell-ing, listening to music, drawing, or working puzzles. The importance of rituals should be discussed as an effective way to provide the child with a structure that assists in making a transition from one form of activity to another, such as at bedtime.

Disturbances in sleep frequently occur during the early childhood years, in the form of nightmares or waking to play. The family needs to respond to such events in a reassuring fashion and gently but firmly assist the child in returning to sleep. They need to be reassured that most often such periods of disturbance are temporary and usually do not persist. If the child continues to awaken in a cheerful mood to play, the day-time nap pattern should be reevaluated and the child encouraged to stay awake during the day to determine if this brings about a more prolonged pattern of nighttime sleep.

### Limit setting and parent-child communication

Setting of limits becomes paramount during the active toddler and preschool years. Assessment of the family's beliefs, attitudes, and lifestyle and a profile of their own early childhood experience must be used as a foundation for providing counseling and teaching. Adults are most likely to respond to their own child as they were treated during childhood, and any parent who has negative feelings about their own childhood or who reports that undue physical punishment was inflicted on them as children should be particularly counseled with regard to effective means of setting limits and of handling their own anger and frustration with the child. The fact that all parents experience anger and frustration with their child, to the point of feeling like slapping or hitting their child out of anger, should be frankly discussed by the nurse. If the parents express the belief that children should not be physically punished or spanked, the nurse should explore with them effective ways of accomplishing limit-setting and of using positive means of reinforcing desired behavior as well as expressing authentic feelings of displeasure with the child.[13,21] They need to anticipate the effects of fatigue and outside pressures on their ability to cope with the active youngster. If they express a belief that children should be spanked or physically punished in some way, these alternate means of behavior control need to be discussed, as well as guidelines for the use of spanking. For example, the spanking should not involve parts of the body that would be easily injured, objects for spanking should not be used, and a spanking should not be rendered out of uncontrolled anger directed to the child. The parents may need to discuss their feelings at length and have available a parent "hot-line" or telephone resource that they can call on when they feel that their limits of coping are reaching the point of being uncontrolled. Such approaches to counseling and support for adults have been demonstrated to be effective in preventing child abuse, for most adults do not intend to harm the young child and will draw upon supportive resources to assist them through a crisis if they sense that the helping person is understanding, accepting, and supportive.[11,30,43,48]

Establishing an effective means of communication with the child during early childhood will serve the parents in good stead during later years of development. Role-playing with the parent the use of open, direct, and authentic communication often assists them in achieving such a pattern of communication with the young child. They need to anticipate and practice means of providing reasonable choices for the young child, according to the developmental capability of the child. For the toddler whose level of understanding is incomplete and ability to reason is lacking, the parents need to limit the number and complexity of choices provided the child but provide some situations in which the child can begin to make choices, such as selecting which shoes to wear. As more mature reasoning develops, the child can begin to understand reasons for making choices, such as if you stay up too late at night, you will feel tired tomorrow. Counseling with regard to firm consistency in helping the child anticipate the outcome of his or her actions and then adhering to the predicted outcome is important in developing a basis for trustworthy communication within the family.

As the young child develops interest in sexuality, questions begin to emerge that may be uncomfortable or unanticipated by the parents. Anticipating this developmental trait, the parents can be counseled with regard to their own feelings and attitudes and plan for simple, direct and honest responses to the young child's questions and comments. The family's reactions to questions and physical exploration influence to a significant extent the attitudes and images formed by the child. Literature may help parents to deal with their own reactions and feelings, but the example of the health care worker in presenting a frank, open, and accepting attitude conveys a strong message of the kind of adult behaviors that will enhance healthy childhood development. While families cannot be expected to forsake well-learned habits of modesty, propriety, or emotionality associated with sex, they can be assisted in realizing the real needs of the child, in separating his or her questions and exploration from moral implications and issues and in seeking ways in which to satisfy the child's needs when they are not able to do so themselves.[34,117]

## Day-care and preparation for entering school

Parents of toddlers and preschool children often need or want to make provisions for full-time or part-time day-care for their child outside of the home. Counseling should include the following areas of concern:

1. *Feelings of ambivalence or guilt related to placing the child in day-care settings outside of the home.* Regardless of the reasons for the family wanting or needing day care for the child, the traditional expectation of caring for the young child at home continues to influence the parents' concept of what they "should" do for their child (see Chapter 3). They need to be reassured regarding the fact that a day-care environment that is congruent with the family environment is not detrimental to the child, that they are not neglecting their duty as a parent, and that their choice or necessity arises out of achieving goals that will ultimately benefit the child. For example, if the parent must work to earn an income or needs to obtain job training or education or simply needs outside activity and stimulation for self-development, the child will benefit.

2. *Selection of the day-care setting.* Several factors must be considered in selecting the day-care setting. The economic factor is often the determining variable, but if possible the family needs to also include such factors as convenience of location, range and flexibility of hours and services available, quality of the day-care facility, and congruence of the philosophy of child care with that of the family. The parent may need assistance in determining the quality of day care and in estimating whether the day-care service is congruent with their own philosophy of child care. If a child has been placed in a setting that is detrimental to physical or emotional development, the parent may need assistance in selecting an alternate setting, and community action must be taken to intervene at the setting to protect the health of all other children involved.

3. *Anticipatory provisions for care of the child during episodes of illness.* When young children first enter a day-care setting where other children are present, the frequency of episodic illness usually increases dramatically until the child develops immunologic defenses against the infectious organisms encountered. The family needs to anticipate this probability and know what provisions will be made under such circumstances. If this will place an additional financial burden on the family because of loss of income if the parent remains home from work to care for the child or employs another adult to care for the child, planning for this added expense may ease the financial burden.

4. *Planning for regulating and controlling the parents' physical and emotional resources.* Often when parents work and then return home to the demands of caring for an active, dependent young child, their own physical and emotional capacity is rapidly depleted, and their ability to cope with the young child's demands wanes. The nurse should guide parents in recognizing their own limits of energy and help them identify ways in which they can conserve energy, obtain relief during difficult periods of time, and plan for their own restoration needs.

5. *Anticipation of separation protest.* If the child is in the toddler period, and often during the preschool period, an initial or transient reoccurring separation protest can be anticipated. The parent needs to understand that this is a normal reaction and that they should plan to firmly leave the child soon after arriving at the day-care setting and clearly inform the child that he or she is leaving now but will return

later in the day. The parent will need reassurance that the child will settle down soon and become involved in the activities of the day-care setting and that the early repeated episodes of protest will gradually decline.[55]

## STUDY QUESTIONS

1. Identify specific health maintenance problems that would appropriately be listed on the problem list of children in the early childhood period. Describe the data base that would be needed to formulate a plan.

2. Read and study further one of the theoretical ideas presented in this chapter or a related one that you identify. Expand upon the ideas the theory offers in understanding the child during these years and the effect that these propositions could have on nursing care and relationships.

3. Observe young children in each of three settings. First, observe what kinds of behavior emerge when the child is in a setting where no provisions are made for special needs and interests, such as a clinic waiting room or a public business. Second, observe the child's behavior in a setting where provision for his or her needs is made, but where the setting is not necessarily specifically created for the child. Such settings would be a clinic waiting room, a hospital ward, or a home. Third, observe young children in a setting that is created especially for them, such as a nursery school or day care center. Describe the differences in the behavior of the children.

4. Plan an approach that you would like to try with a young child who is a stranger to you in establishing a relationship. Plan the activities that you will pursue during the interaction and how you will terminate the interaction. Find a child you do not know of appropriate age and implement your plans. Describe what happens and how you might have been more effective with the child.

5. Observe the mother-child interactions of a 2-year-old child and a 5-year-old child. Describe in detail the differences that you observe, and draw application of some of the theoretical notions that were discussed in this chapter.

6. Formulate your personal ideas regarding how toilet training, feeding, discipline, and sex education should be accomplished during this period. Describe how you might accomplish the task of laying these ideas aside, and indicate which behaviors on the part of parents might most interfere with your ability to help the family.

## REFERENCES

1. Adler, A.: Problems of neurosis, New York, 1930, Cosmopolitan Book Corp.
2. Alexander, M., and Brown, M. S.: Physical examination. VIII. Hearing acuity, Nursing '74 4:61, April, 1974.
3. Alexander, M. M., and Brown, M. S.: Physical examination. XIV. Examining male genitalia, Nursing '76 6:39, Feb., 1976.
4. Altus, W. D.: Birth order and its sequelae, Science 151:44, 1966.
5. American Medical Association: Quality of life; the early years, Acton, Mass., 1974, Publishing Sciences Group, Inc.
6. Anthony, E. J.: The reactions of parents to the oedipal child. In Anthony, E. J., and Benedek, T., editors: Parenthood, its psychology and psychopathology, Boston, 1970, Little, Brown and Co., p. 275.
7. Anthony, E. J.: Children at risk from divorce; a review. In Anthony, E. J., and Koupernik, C., editors: The child in his family; children at psychiatric risk, vol. 3, New York, 1974, John Wiley & Sons, p. 461.
8. Barker, J., Goldstein, A., and Frankenburg, W. K.: Denver eye screening test manual, 1972, W. K. Frankenburg.
9. Barness, L. A.: Manual of pediatric physical diagnosis, ed. 4, Chicago, 1972, Year Book Medical Publishers, Inc.
10. Bernard, H. W.: Human development in Western culture, ed. 4, Boston, 1975, Allyn & Bacon, Inc.
11. Besharov, D. J.: Building a community response to child abuse and maltreatment, Children Today 4:2, Sept.-Oct., 1975.
12. Birch, H. C., and Gussow, J. D.: Disadvantaged children; health, nutrition and school failure, New York, 1970, Harcourt, Brace and World.
13. Brennan, E. C.: Meeting the affective needs of young children, Children Today 3:22, July-Aug., 1974.
14. Brown, M. S.: Approaches to hearing testing of children in the office, Clinical Pediatr. 14:639, July, 1975.
15. Brown, M. S.: Vision screening of preschool children; how to check on visual acuity and heterophoria as part of a routine physical examination, Clin. Pediatr. 14: 968, Oct., 1975.
16. Brown, M. S.: Testing of a young child for articulation skills, detecting early danger signs, Clin. Pediatr. 15:639, July, 1976.
17. Brown, M. S., and Alexander, M. N.: Physical examination. XV. Examining female genitalia, Nursing '76 6:39, March, 1976.
18. Campbell, J. D.: Peer relations in childhood. In Hoffmon, M. L., and Hoffmon, L. W., editors: Review of child development research, vol. 1, New York, 1964, Russell Sage Foundation, p. 289.
19. Carlson, S. S., and Asnes, R. S.: Maternal expectations and attitudes toward toilet training; a comparison between clinic mothers and private practice mothers, J. Pediatr. 84:148, Jan., 1974.
20. Chamberlin, R. W.: Authoritarian and accommodative child-rearing styles; their relationships with the behavior patterns of 2-year-old children and other variables, J. Pediatr. 84:287, Feb., 1974.
21. Chamberlin, R. W.: Parental use of "positive contact" in child-rearing, Pediatrics 56:768, Nov., 1975.
22. Chopoorian, T.: Communication beyond the assessment process. In Brandt, P. A., and others, editors: Current practice in pediatric nursing, vol. 2, St. Louis, 1978, The C. V. Mosby Co., p. 3.
23. Clark, K. B., and Clark, M. K.: The development of

consciousness of self and emergence of racial identification in Negro preschool children. In Wilcox, L. C., editor: The psychological consequences of being a Black American; a collection of research by Black psychologists, New York, 1971, John Wiley & Sons, Inc., p. 323.

24. Coopersmith, S.: The antecedents of self-esteem, San Francisco, 1967, W. H. Freeman and Co.

25. Cronbach, L. J.: Essentials of psychological testing, ed. 3, New York, 1970, Harper & Row, Publishers.

26. Cruzon, M. E. J.: Dental implications of thumb-sucking, Pediatrics 54:196, Aug., 1974.

27. Doll, I. A.: Vineland social maturity scales, Circle Pines, Minn., 1965, American Guidance Service, Inc.

28. Drumwright, A. F.: The Denver articulation screening exam, Denver, 1971, University of Colorado Medical School.

29. Dunn, L. M.: Peabody picture vocabulary test, Minneapolis, 1965, American Guidance Service, Inc.

30. Erikson, M. L.: Assessment and management of developmental changes in children, St. Louis, 1976, The C. V. Mosby Co.

31. Erikson, E. H.: Childhood and society, ed. 2, New York, 1963, W. W. Norton & Co., Inc.

32. Faigin, H.: Social behavior of young children in the kibbuta. In Rosenblith, J. F., and Allinsmith, W., editors: The causes of behavior, Boston, 1966, Allyn & Bacon, Inc., p. 245.

33. Fey, M. R.: Fluoride therapy, Nurse Practitioner 2: 26, Sept.-Oct., 1977.

34. Field, W. E.: Watch your message, Am. J. Nurs. 72: 1278-1280, July, 1972.

35. Frankenburg, W. K., and Dodds, J. B.: Denver developmental screening test manual, 1972, W. K. Frankenburg.

36. Friedman, R. J.: The young child who does not talk; observations on causes and management, Clin. Pediatr. 14:403, April, 1975.

37. Goodenough, F.: The measurement of intelligence by drawings, Yonkers, 1926, World Book Company.

38. Gordon, T.: Parent effectiveness training, New York, 1970, Peter H. Wyden, Inc.

39. Guyton, A. C.: Textbook of medical physiology, ed. 5, Philadelphia, 1976, W. B. Saunders Co.

40. Haggard, E. A.: A theory of adaptation and the risk of trauma. In Anthony, E. J., and Loupernik, C., editors: The child in his family; children at psychiatric risk, vol. 3, New York, 1974, John Wiley & Sons, p. 47.

41. Harris, D. B.: Children's drawings as measures of intellectual maturity, New York, 1963, Harcourt, Brace & World.

42. Healy, A.: The sleep patterns of preschool children; general principles and current knowledge, Clin. Pediatr. 11:174, March, 1972.

43. Helfer, R. E., and Kempe, C. H., editors: The battered child, ed. 2, Chicago, 1974, The University of Chicago Press.

44. Herron, R. E., and Sutton-Smith, B.: Child's play, New York, 1971, John Wiley & Sons, Inc.

45. Hoekelman, R. A., Kelly, J., and Zimmer, A. W., The reliability of maternal recall; mother's remembrance of the infant's health and illness, Clin. Pediatr. 15:261, March, 1976.

46. Hurlock, E. B.: Child development, ed. 5, New York, 1972, McGraw-Hill Book Co.

47. Hurtado, R. C., and others: Immunologic role of tonsillar tissues in local call-mediated immune responses, J. Pediatr. 86:405, March, 1975.

48. Illingworth, R. S.: The normal child; some problems of the early years and their treatment, ed. 6, New York, 1975, Churchill Livingstone.

49. Ireton, H., and Thwing, E.: Appraising the development of a preschool child by means of a standardized report prepared by the mother; the Minnesota child development inventory, Clin. Pediatr. 15:875, Oct., 1976.

50. Janeway, C. A.: Recurrent infections. In Green, M., and Haggerty, R. J., editors: Ambulatory pediatrics. II. Philadelphia, 1977, W. B. Saunders Co., p. 73.

51. Jelliffe, D. B., and Jelliffe, E. F. P.: The at-risk concept as related to young child nutrition programs, Clin. Pediatr. 12:65, Feb., 1973.

52. Jenny, J.: Preventing dental disease in children; an ecological approach, Am. J. Public Health 64:1147, Dec., 1974.

53. Jones, R. J., Terrell, D. L., and DeShields, J. L.: Intellectual and psychomotor performance of pre-school children from low-income families. In Wilcox, R., editor: The psychological consequences of being a Black American; a sourcebook of research by Black psychologists, New York, 1971, John Wiley & Sons, Inc., p. 20.

54. Kagan, J.: Understanding children; behavior, motives, and thought, New York, 1971, Harcourt, Brace, Jovanovich.

55. Kearley, R. B., and others: Separation protest, Pediatrics 55:171, Feb., 1975.

56. Kempe, C. H., Silver, H. C., and O'Brien, D.: Current pediatric diagnosis and treatment, ed. 4, Los Altos, Calif., 1976, Lange Medical Publications.

57. Keniston, K., and the Carnegie Council on Children: All our children; the American family under pressure, New York, 1977, Harcourt, Brace, Jovanovich.

58. Koppitz, E. M.: The Bender Gestalt test for young children, New York, 1971, Grune & Stratton, Inc.

59. Kugel, R., editor: Vision screening of pre-school children; report of the Committee on Children with Handicaps, American Academy of Pediatrics, Pediatrics 50:966, Dec., 1972.

60. Kulig, S. G., and Baker, K. A.: Preliminary field testing of the physician's developmental quick screen for speech disorders ("PDQ"), Clin. Pediatr. 15:1146, Dec., 1976.

61. Lahey, M. E.: The erythrocyte; physiologic considerations. In Cooke, R. E., editor: The biologic basis of pediatric practice, New York, 1968, McGraw-Hill Book Co., p. 421.

62. LeMasters, E. E.: Parents in modern America; a sociological analysis, Homewood, Ill., 1970, The Dorsey Press.

63. Lillibridge, C. B.: A simple system to block toddlers from reaching toxic ingestibles; add a spring and two latches to all doors where danger lurks, Clin. Pediatr. **12**:441, July, 1973.

64. Loda, F. A., and others, editors: Respiratory disease in group day care, Pediatrics **49**:428-437, March, 1972.

65. Love, L. R., and Kaswan, J. W.: Troubled children; their families, schools and treatments, New York, 1974, John Wiley and Sons.

66. Mahler, M. S., Pine, F., and Bergman, A.: The mother's reaction to her toddler's drive for individuation. In Anthony, E. J., and Benedek, T., editors: Parenthood, its psychology and psychopathology, Boston, 1970, Little, Brown and Co., p. 257.

67. Maier, H. W.: Three theories of child development; the contributions of Erik H. Erikson, Jean Piaget, and Robert R. Sears, and their application, New York, 1965, Harper & Row, Publishers.

68. Matheny, A. P., and others, editors: Assessment of children's behavioral characteristic; a tool in accident prevention, Clin. Pediatr. **11**:437, Aug., 1972.

69. McCurdy, J. A., Goldstein, J. L., and Gorski, D.: Auditory screening of preschool children with impedance audiometry—a comparison with pure tone audiometry, Clin. Pediatr. **15**:436, May, 1977.

70. Menkes, J. H.: The neuromotor mechanism. In Cooke, R. E., editor: The biologic basis of pediatric practice, New York, 1968, McGraw-Hill Book Co., p. 254.

71. Miller, N. E.: Extensions of liberalized S-R-theory. In Koch, S., editor: Psychology; a study of science, vol. 2, New York, 1959, McGraw-Hill Book Co., p. 196.

72. Mowrer, O. H.: Learning theory and behavior, New York, 1960, John Wiley & Sons.

73. Murphy, L. B.: Preventive implications of development in the preschool years. In Caplon, G., editor: Prevention of mental disorders in children, New York, 1961, Basic Books, Inc., Publishers.

74. Murphy, L. B.: The widening world of childhood; paths toward mastery, New York, 1962, Basic Books, Inc., Publishers.

75. Paine, R. S.: Neurologic examination of infants and children, Pediatr. Clin. North Am. **7**:471, 1960.

76. Park, M. K., and others: Need for an improved standard for blood pressure cuff size; the size should be related to the diameter of the arm, Clin. Pediatr. **15**: 784, Sept., 1976.

77. Parsons, T., and Bales, R. F., editors: Family, socialization, and interaction process, Glencoe, Ill., 1955, Free Press.

78. Phillips, J. L., Jr.: The origins of intellect; Piaget's theory, San Francisco, 1969, W. H. Freeman Co.

79. Piaget, J.: The moral judgment of the child, New York, 1932, Harcourt, Brace.

80. Pulaski, M. A.: Play symbolism in cognitive development. In Schaefer, C., editor: The therapeutic use of child's play, New York, 1976, Jason Aronson, Inc.

81. Redman, J. F., and Bissada, N. K.: How to make a good examination of the genitalia of young girls, Clin. Pediatr. **15**:907, Oct., 1976.

82. Reece, B.: Black self-concept, Children Today **3**:24, Mar.-April, 1974.

83. Rich, A.: Of woman born; motherhood as experience and institution, New York, 1976, W. W. Norton and Co., Inc.

84. Ringler, N. M., and others: Mother-to-child speech at 2 years—effects of early postnatal contact, J. Pediatr. **86**:141, Jan., 1975.

85. Roberts, S. O.: Some mental and emotional health needs of Negro children and youth. In Wilcox, R. C., editor: The psychological consequences of being a Black American; a collection of research by Black psychologists, New York, 1971, John Wiley & Sons, Inc., p. 332.

86. Rogers, W. B., and Rogers, R. A.: A new simplified preschool readiness experimental screening scale (the PRESS); a preliminary report, Clin. Pediatr. **11**: 558, Oct., 1972.

87. Rogers, W. B., Jr., and Rogers, R. A.: A follow-up study of the preschool readiness experimental screening scale (the PRESS), Clin. Pediatr. **14**:253, March, 1975.

88. Rosenburg, L. A.: Psychological examination of the handicapped child, Pediatr. Clin. North Am. **20**:61, Feb., 1973.

89. Rubin, H., and Culatta, R.: Stuttering as an after-effect of normal developmental disfluency; advice from speech professionals on how to recognize this process and take preventive steps, Clin. Pediatr. **13**:172, Feb., 1974.

90. Sale, J. S.: Family day care—potential child development service, Am. J. Public Health **62**:668-670, May, 1972.

91. Schwartz, A. H., and Murphy, M. W.: Cues for screening language disorders in preschool children, Pediatrics **55**:717, May, 1975.

92. Sears, P. S.: Doll play aggression in normal children; influence of sex, age, sibling status, father's absence, Psychol. Monograph **56**:6, 1961.

93. Sears, R. R.: Experimental analysis of psychoanalytic phenomena. In Hunt, J. M., editor: Personality and the behavior disorders, vol. 1, New York, 1944, The Ronald Press Co., pp. 306-332.

94. Sears, R. R.: A theoretical framework for personality and social behavior, Am. Psychol. **6**:476, 1951.

95. Sears, R. R.: Social behavior and personality development. In Parsons, T., and Shils, E. A., editors: Toward a general theory of action, Cambridge, 1951, Harvard University Press, p. 465.

96. Sears, R. R., and others: Patterns of child-rearing, Evanston, Ill., 1957, Row, Peterson, and Co.

97. Shelness, A., and Charles, S.: Children as passengers in automobiles, Pediatrics **56**:271, Aug., 1975.

98. Skinner, B. F.: Science and human behavior, New York, 1953, Macmillan Publishing Co., Inc.

99. Slattery, J.: Dental health in children, Am. J. Nurs. **76**:1159, July, 1976.

100. Solnit, A. A.: A summing up of the Dakar Conference; "Care for your children as you wish them to care for your grandchildren"; Risk and mastery—sociopsycho-

logical aspects of the vulnerable child. In Anthony, E. J., and Loupernik, C., editors: The child in his family; children at psychiatric risk, vol. 3, New York, 1974, John Wiley & Sons, p. 405.

101. Southard, S. C.: A comprehensive protocol for evaluating the safety of toys for preschool children. Clin. Pediatr. **15**:1107, Dec., 1976.

102. Stendler-Lavatelli, C. B.: Environmental intervention in infancy and early childhood. In Deutsch, M., Katz, I., and Jensen, A. R., editors: Social class, race, and psychological development, New York, 1968, Holt, Rinehart and Winston, Inc., p. 347.

103. Stephens, J. A., and Silber, D. L.: Parental expectations vs. outcomes in toilet training, Pediatrics **54**:493, Oct., 1974.

104. Stollak, G. E.: Learning to communicate with children, Children Today **4**:12, March-April, 1975.

105. Stool, S. E., and Anticaglia, J.: Electric otoscopy—a basic pediatric skill; notes on the essentials of otoscopic examination and on the evaluation of otoscopes, Clin. Pediatr. **12**:420, July, 1973.

106. Thompson, W. M., and Dammann, J. F., Jr.: Systemic circulation. In Cooke, R. E., editor: The biologic basis of pediatric practice, New York, 1968, McGraw-Hill Book Co., p. 413.

107. Thorpe, H. S., and Werner, E. E.: Developmental screening of preschool children; a critical review of inventories used in health and educational programs, Pediatrics **53**:362, March, 1974.

108. Thuline, H. C.: Color blindness in children; the importance and feasibility of early recognition, Clin. Pediatr. **11**:295, May, 1972.

109. Timiras, P. S.: Developmental physiology and aging, New York, 1972, Macmillan Publishing Co., Inc.

110. Turbeville, D. F., and Fearnow, R. G.: Is it possible to identify the child who is a "high risk" candidate for the accidental ingestion of a poison? Comparison of oral gratification habits between 100 poison ingestors and 100 controls, Clin. Pediatr. **15**:918, Oct., 1976.

111. Vessal, S., and Kravis, L. P.: Immunologic mechanisms responsible for adverse reactions to routine immunization in children, Clin. Pediatr. **15**:688, Aug., 1976.

112. Wahler, R. G.: Child-child interactions in free field settings; some experimental analyses, J. Exp. Child Psychol. **5**:278, 1967.

113. Waldman, J., Mofenson, H. C., and Greensher, J.: Evaluating the functioning of a poison control center; suggestions on how to protect children from toxic accidents, Clin. Pediatr. **15**:75, Jan. 1976.

114. Watson, J. B.: Behaviorism, New York, 1924, People's Institute.

115. Weiss, C. E., and Lillywhite, H. S.: Communicative disorders, St. Louis, 1976, The C. V. Mosby Co.

116. Whipple, D. V.: Dynamics of development; euthenic pediatrics, New York, 1966, McGraw-Hill Book Co.

117. Wilbur, C., and Aug, R.: Sex education, Am. J. Nurs. **73**:88, Jan., 1973.

118. Wilkins, L., and Najjar, S.: Developmental interrelationships of the endocrine glands. In Cooke, R. E., editor: The biologic basis of pediatric practice, New York, 1968, McGraw-Hill Book Co., p. 1104.

119. Wolman, I. J.: Some prominent developments in childhood nutrition, 1972, Clin. Pediatr. **12**:72, Feb., 1973.

120. Zager, R.: The pediatrician and preventive child psychiatry; four approaches to the recognition of parents' and children's responses to stress, Clin. Pediatr. **14**:1161, Dec., 1975.

121. Zigler, E. F.: Project Head Start; success or failure? Children Today **2**:2, Nov.-Dec., 1973.

# CHAPTER 11

# Health problems of infancy and early childhood

In the course of normal growth and development we all encounter injuries and illness that temporarily interfere with maximal healthy functioning. Such encounters during infancy and early childhood are particularly disturbing. Parents and others caring for the child become anxious and distressed, and often they would rather bear the suffering themselves than watch the child suffer. When the problems might have been prevented, the distress is even greater. The child, furthermore, is not able to relate many of the symptoms or to explain the nature of the discomforts. Therefore, detecting the exact nature of an illness may be difficult.

In Chapters 9 and 10 we considered health maintenance needs and prevention of illness. In this chapter we will consider problems of minor illness and injury that most commonly occur for infants and young children in technological, Western societies at this point in their lives. The list is not intended to be comprehensive, but it is representative of the kind of data base and sound nursing judgment that are indicated for health problems occurring during this period of life. Sound nursing judgment and skill are developed through understanding of multiple factors involved in each problem that is encountered. Knowledge must be acquired through the literature and through experience and prac-

tice in nursing care of the child with health problems.

## NURSING DIAGNOSIS AND CARE OF THE CHILD WITH ACUTE HEALTH PROBLEMS

Many acute problems of infancy and early childhood are subject to nursing diagnosis and care. The reader is referred to the discussion of nursing assessment and management presented in Chapter 2 as a background for considering nursing diagnosis and intervention for the child who is suffering an acute health problem.

### Nursing diagnosis
#### *Definition*

In the previous chapters of this unit, health needs of infants and children and related nursing intervention were discussed. This chapter will focus on problems and diagnoses that involve a health deficit and are subject to direct nursing intervention. Often a differentiation between a "problem" and a "diagnosis" is not necessary or desirable, but for clarification these related concepts are each defined as follows:

**nursing problem** A statement of a child/adult health status derived from the nursing assessment process reflecting an actual or potential health deficit and the primary related factors that are possible or probable causes and that is subject to direct nursing intervention.

**nursing diagnosis** A statement of a child/adult health status derived from the nursing assessment process reflecting an actual or potential health deficit and the documented cause, which is subject to direct nursing intervention.

The concept of direct nursing intervention in these definitions refers to legally sanctioned nursing actions that can be enacted by the nurse. The process of the nursing assessment often reveals client problems that require referral to another health care provider and therefore are not nursing problems. Often, a client problem requires intervention by the nurse and another health care provider, with the focus of the different professionals being directed to different but related dimensions of the problem. The statement of the nursing problem or diagnosis reflects the dimension of the problem addressed by nursing intervention. The relationship between nursing and medical diagnoses is often complementary, and the choice of problem or diagnostic statements reflects this interrelationship and the focus of nursing and medical intervention. For example, the nursing diagnosis of *inadequate exchange of gases related to obstruction of air flow* may be a sign of the medical diagnosis *epiglottitis.* Nursing intervention is directed toward physical and psychosocial means of optimizing gas exchange and reducing obstruction of air flow. Medical intervention is directed toward treatment of the underlying infection. Conversely, a medical diagnosis may be a sign of a nursing diagnosis. The medical diagnosis of *lead poisoning* may be a sign of the nursing diagnosis of *environmental hazard related to peeling paint and plaster.* Medical intervention is directed toward alleviating the physical sequelae of lead intoxication, while nursing intervention is directed toward removing or controlling the environmental hazard.[7,97,154]

Consistent and accurate labeling and classification of nursing problems and diagnoses are essential for complete evaluation and audit of the quality of nursing care and for refinement of nursing intervention and approaches that achieve health care goals. Classification allows for systematic study of criteria used in establishing a statement of nursing problems or diagnoses and of the effectiveness of alternative approaches used in nursing intervention. Systems for labeling and classifying nursing diagnoses have begun to be developed that will ultimately provide for comprehensive and systematic study of nursing practice.[80,164] The Minnesota Nursing Problem Classification (MNPC) for children and youth is presented in the Appendix, pp. 884-895 to provide the reader one means of conceptualizing and classifying nursing problems. Reference to these categories is made throughout this text, although in some instances the labels used may differ from those found in this system.

### Using an adequate data base

The importance of obtaining a comprehensive data base cannot be overemphasized. From this base of information, which includes factors provided by the child, family, and professional team members, the criteria upon which the nursing diagnosis or statement of the problem is based are derived. In addition the data base provides information that helps to determine the relevance of an intervention plan for a particular child and family, For example, intervention plans for a family who does not have refrigeration in the home may be differentially affected by this social and mechanical factor.

In addition to giving complete evidence of all criteria that have been established as essential for making a nursing diagnosis or problem statement, the data base provides evidence that all related possibilities have been thoroughly considered and are not objectively present. For example, in making the nursing diagnosis *acute febrile state* (MNPC no. 350.0) the data base contains evidence of all criteria needed for making this diagnosis, as described in a following section. In addition the data base contains objective evidence that the possible diagnoses of disturbance of fluid and electrolytes, acute gastrointestinal problems, or upper respiratory problems are not applicable, since each would require an altered or different approach to intervention.

### Establishing sound criteria

To achieve precision, reliability, and validity in nursing diagnoses and problem statements, criteria must be established that define specifically the conditions under which a given diagnosis or problem may be assigned. Ideally, these criteria are determined in advance by a team of health workers who will be concerned with diagnosis, care and intervention, and follow-through. These standing criteria then become the basis upon which all members of the team make decisions, and they must be demonstrated or observed in order to make the particular diagnosis or problem statement. Diagnostic criteria are suggested here, but revisions and modifications may be made according to the judgment of members of a particular health team.[64,217,231]

In establishing criteria for nursing diagnoses and problem statements, each of the following factors are considered and are reflected in the established criteria:

1. *Exact etiology or probable related factors that must be documented in the data base.* For example, to make the nursing diagnosis of *headaches associated with emotional problems*, the data base must include documentation of the exact nature of the child's emotional problem. In establishing criteria the health care team designates the precise objective documentation that can be used to substantiate this diagnosis, such as conflict between parents or school, objective measures of anxiety, fear, etc. In addition the criteria must include the necessary rival etiologies that must be ruled out to make the diagnosis and the evidence needed to support this conclusion. The criteria for the diagnosis related to headaches might then include objective evidence of intact neurologic function appropriate to the developmental age, evidence of adequate nutrition, and adequate cardiovascular function.

2. *Essential signs and symptoms associated with the diagnosis or problem.* The criteria should specify the signs and symptoms that are essential and that are sufficient to justify making the diagnosis or problem statement. This includes those signs and symptoms that must be objectively present and those that must be absent to make the diagnostic or problem statement. For example, the criteria for the nursing diagnosis of the common cold, presented later in this chapter, includes the symptoms and signs that occur as well as signs and symptoms that must be absent, such as evidence of infection of the tympanic membrane.

3. *Limiting factors associated with the scope of nursing practice.* Factors that define a problem as subject to direct nursing intervention are explored and incorporated within the criteria for the diagnosis or problem statement. Sometimes the etiology or essential signs and symptoms sufficiently delineate the nature of the problem as being clearly within the scope of nursing practice, as might be the case with the nursing diagnosis of *inadequate gas exchange related to obstruction of air flow*. Often, however, the diagnostic label, etiology, and signs and symptoms do not sufficiently imply the range and scope of nursing responsibility and specific criteria must be included and documented that further define the scope of responsibility. For example, the *common cold* might be designated as a problem within the scope of nursing practice and intervention, given documentation of related factors, signs and symptoms, provided these signs and symptoms are confined to a one-week duration. If the duration of the signs and symptoms (without the development of other signs and symptoms) exceeds this time span, the health care team may judge that competing diagnoses should be considered (such as allergy) or that a medical diagnosis and management is required.

## Tools for nursing intervention

An old folk saying aptly summarizes the purpose toward which nursing intervention during a young child's illness is directed: "To cure sometimes, to relieve often, to comfort always."[221]

Nursing intervention approaches are specified in a management protocol that accompanies the diagnostic criteria. Measures are included for cure or elimination of the causative or related factor, for relief of signs and symptoms, and for the total comfort of the child/adult physically, emotionally and socially, including measures to prevent worsening or complication of the problem. The management protocol is often developed and approved by all members of a health care team and includes specification of instances in which interdisciplinary action is indicated. The following section presents a summary of tools for nursing management that are commonly used in the care of young children with short-term, acute health problems.

### Measures for comfort and symptomatic relief

During infancy and early childhood, effecting relief and comfort may be difficult because the young child cannot specifically identify the source of discomfort. The child's skin may be itchy, but the only symptoms may be irritability and generalized distress. The child may have a sore, painful throat but not be able to identify the source of the pain. The child may feel hot and miserable with fever but not express this misery. The nurse can make an objective observation of a rash, an inflamed throat, or elevated temperature, and make the logical assumption based on our own experience with such conditions that the child is feeling itchy, sore, or miserable. However, the objective signs of discomfort may escape notice, or they may not be available to observation. Hunger, fatigue, nausea, abdominal pain, joint pain, or headache may be felt, but the young child has limited means of communicating such feelings to others. When a child expresses behavior symptomatic of discomfort, a trial and error approach to finding something that brings relief may be needed.

Physical measures for relief of specific nursing diagnoses are described in relation to each problem in the following sections. In general the nurse employs several therapeutically useful modalities. The sense of touch provides a powerful therapeutic tool for a child in disstress. Holding, rubbing, stroking, bathing, and massaging all have significant effects for most children. They provide feelings of being cared for, of being secure, of someone offering comfort. Touch from those who are significant, such as mother or father, usually provides the most effective comfort, but the nurse may also provide important relief and comfort with touch.

Warmth and cold may be used therapeutically by the nurse. Understanding of the physical dynamics that are produced by warmth and cold is essential in order to use these tools therapeutically. Water that is cooler than body temperature on or around the body provides for heat loss by conduction, convection, or evaporation. Heat applied to an area of the body causes vasodilation and increased blood flow to the area. Cold applied to an area causes vasoconstriction and decreased blood flow to the area.

Other principles derived from a knowledge of physics are applied therapeutically in providing relief and comfort. Positional adjustments and changes in parts of the body provide for the forces of gravity to act upon certain dynamic body processes. External forces that aid in the action of gravity are also applied, such as positive or negative pressure.

Fluid dynamics of the body may be influenced therapeutically by nursing intervention. For example, the child may be given extra amounts of plain water to drink for a specific reason, or the water may contain solutes that are specifically known to exert a certain influence on fluid dynamics. Control of the humidity in the air and measures for control of body temperature affect the amount of insensible water loss.

Changes in the environment may be used to accomplish a therapeutic effect. Humidity or mist may be added to environmental air. Therapeutic light or air exposure may be used. Changes in objects or compounds in the environment may effect a change in a child's health. Laundry compounds and bathing agents, for example, may influence the health of an infant's skin. Pets, the composition of rugs or blankets, dust, or microorganisms in the environment may affect the health of the child.

The therapeutic use of rest and exercise may be required during infancy and early childhood. It is difficult to encourage children to sleep when they are feeling well, but when they are not well, they may sleep a great deal. Understanding increased needs for rest may help a parent to let a child sleep the extra hours rather than to yield to the desire to "do something" for the child. Passive and active exercises may be needed to restore full function to a limb after an injury.

Food is also used therapeutically by the nurse. By understanding the basic nutritional composition of foods and the needs if the child for maintenance plus restorative functions, dietary changes may be made to provide the additional dietary components needed.

### Play

The needs and responses of the infant and child for play and fantasy change during periods of acute illness and stress. Often the infant or young child appears indifferent to play because of the states of irritability and lethargy that arise from the altered health state. However, play and fantasy remain a primary means by which the adult health care worker can effectively relate to the young child and provide a source of learning, comfort, and familiarity for the child.

During the acute phase of an illness, active play is rejected by young children, but they quickly resume active play as soon as symptomatic relief is achieved. While the child is not responsive to active play, diversional play activities can be planned that promote the child's ability to rest and provide relief and comfort. Storytelling and reading to the young child provides adult companionship and comfort, and the story provides the child an opportunity to work through emotions and feelings through fantasy. Stories that involve children or animals who are not well, who are experiencing visits to a physician, or who cope with painful or uncomfortable experiences are particularly helpful to the young child.

In working with the infant and young child during the nursing assessment, play and fantasy provide a valuable tool for establishing a relationship and for teaching. The use of puppets helps to divert the child's attention momentarily away from their own physical and emotional misery and gives the nurse an opportunity to obtain thorough and accurate information from the child. For example, a child who might otherwise be irritable and fussy when the nurse attempts to auscultate the chest, might remain quiet and still if attention is diverted to a puppet who participates in the procedure. The puppet is introduced to the child and "tells" the child about the procedure, asking permission to listen. The puppet might volunteer to let the child listen first if the child appears to be responsive and alert enough to participate to this extent. The nurse then uses the puppet to hold the

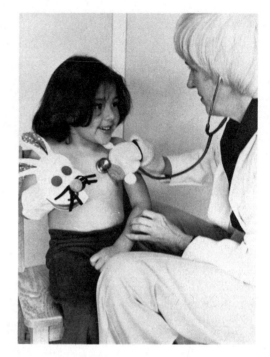

**Fig. 11-1.** The nurse uses a puppet to auscultate the child's chest and thus gains the child's cooperation and involvement in the procedure.

stethoscope, and the puppet consequently praises the young child for his or her cooperation and comments on the sound of the chest. If the young child does not respond to such a play approach, it is abandoned and the nurse proceeds to obtain the needed observations as quickly and efficiently as possible.

A child can also be guided and assisted with other components of the assessment by active participation and with gaining familiarity by handling strange equipment and trying it out on a doll. For example, a child may be given the otoscope to handle and look at and pretend to examine a doll's mouth or ears. Brief games can be designed to elicit needed assessment behavior. For example, the child can be asked to blow out the otoscope light to assess the ability to follow directions and to watch for the ability to form a symmetrical "o" shape with the mouth. The child can be instructed to take a very deep breath and then make the "choo-choo" sounds of a train as he or she lets out the air. Detailed observation of breath sounds can be obtained while the child is playing this type of game.

The child's ability to respond to play and games during the assessment is also an indication of the extent of debilitation the child has experienced. This judgment is best made based on prior experiences with the child during states of optimal health, but when the nurse has not had previous contact, an adult's description of usual behavior, combined with developmental expectations for performance, can be used in making such a judgment.

### Preparation for painful procedures

Whenever the infant or young child must be subjected to a painful procedure, a simple, direct, and honest explanation should be given immediately before the procedure. Even when the infant appears too young to be able to comprehend an explanation, the explanation should be offered, the procedure completed with efficiency, and the infant or young child immediately comforted and reassured. The explanation prior to such procedures should include a direct statement of what will hurt, what the child needs to do during the procedure, how long it is expected to hurt, and reassurance as to who will comfort him or her. Adequate provisions for restraint are essential to minimize pain and prevent inadvertent injury to the child. If additional adult assistance is needed in restraining the child, a person needs to be located and present before introducing the child to the painful procedure. The trauma of the event is greatly increased when an attempt is made to complete a procedure that is interrupted by failure to provide adequate restraint. If at all possible, the child's parent or the adult accompanying the child should not be used to assist with providing restraint but should be encouraged to provide the source of comfort and reassurance so that the young child does not associate the significant adult with the inflicting of pain. If the adult is known to have prepared the child for a painful procedure such as a shot, building a foundation for trust with regard to the experience, the child may receive security and comfort in being held or restrained by the adult, as well as in receiving reassurance and comfort after the procedure. In such a circumstance,

even a very young child will often be observed to exert a great deal of self-control and ability to cooperate during the procedure.

When a child comes into the health care setting expressing fears and asking for information regarding painful procedures, the nurse needs to determine what the child has previously been told. If the child has been threatened with a shot in return for poor behavior, the nurse needs to acknowledge frankly that a shot may be needed but that if it is, it will be given for the bad germs that are in the child's body. If the child has been told that a shot will not be given, the nurse needs to explain that while nobody wants or likes shots, sometimes they are needed and the child will be told about it when the assessment is completed. Such situations are extremely delicate, for the integrity and trustworthiness of the parent, as well as the health care worker, are at stake, and the child's own self-concept may be damaged. Attention needs to be directed to counseling the adult who is with the child, acknowledging their feelings and desires for protecting the child, controlling desired behavior in the child, or wanting to provide some sort of assurance. The parent needs to be encouraged to provide positive reinforcement for those aspects of the child's behavior that are desired and given guidelines for future information to give the child concerning visits to the health care setting. If the parent's response indicates a persistent focus on threatening the child, on negative behaviors, or if the parent seems uncertain and confused as to how to relate to the child, more detailed family assessment and nursing intervention should be planned for the near future.

### Use of drugs

While drugs have not been traditionally used by the nurse except in the sense of administering agents prescribed by the physician, it has become increasingly necessary and desirable for all aspects of drug administration to be more completely assimilated into nursing practice. Legal concerns limit to some extent the use of drugs by the nurse, but most settings, notably hospitals, have made use of the "P.R.N." or "standing" physician's order to cover the discriminating use of drugs by nurses. Thus the nurse is intimately involved in the responsibility making a sound judgment as to the justification for administering or not administering a specific drug for a specific reason. Further, the fantastic availability of an ever increasing number of agents produced for over-the-counter sale brings many drug administration concerns to the attention of all health care workers. Rather than abdicating all responsibility for the use of all drugs, nurses should use their knowledge, background, and understanding to make sound judgments in cases of drug use, and they should seek collaboration from pharmacists, pharmacologists, or physicians when choices and judgments extend beyond this basic understanding. Responsibility and accountability for the use and administration of drugs may initially be limited to a few drugs, but as experience and understanding expand in regard to composition, action, dosage, reactions, interactions, side effects, and related issues surrounding the use of additional agents, the nurse assumes a wider range of function. Memorization of facts involved does not suffice. Intimate familiarity and knowledge are required for safe, sound judgment.

In evaluating drugs used by the parent at home and drugs that might be recommended or prescribed in the health care setting, each drug needs to be considered in relation to each of the principles for drug use with children, as discussed in Chapter 2, p. 44. These factors include:

Age of the child

Body weight, blood volume, and body surface area

Route of administration

Rate of metabolism and excretion, time of administration

Tolerance pattern usually exhibited in children

Pathologic state of the child

Form in which the drug is administered

The possibility for drug incompatibility or inadvertent overdoses that occur when several different drugs are used, should be carefully considered. The adult needs to participate in discussion regarding the best manner in which to administer the drug to assure that the child receives accurate doses. Clearly stated, written instructions should be given to the adult in the health care setting, providing specific instructions as to the times and means of administration of the drug. If over-the-counter drugs are used, clearly written instructions for administration of these drugs should also be given to the parent, with particular instructions as to which drug is to be administered when. The pharmaceutical label or the parent's ability to remember verbal instructions should *never* be relied on; regardless of the adult's intellectual capacity or familiarity with drug terminology, the ability to remember and adequately carry out drug administration instructions may be limited during the stress of the child's illness, and the parent needs the written instructions for later reference and assurance.

Parents need to be fully informed of any reaction that might occur when the child takes the drug. Serious hazards need to be discussed thoroughly, particularly those that might occur if the drug is given in combination with another drug. For example, when parents are using aspirin for the child at home, they need to be aware of the possibility of a toxic accumulation of the drug in the young child's system and warned to limit its use or discontinue use as soon as possible.[6,17,43,240]

### Teaching the child and family

A very important aspect of nursing care during episodes of acute illness is the teaching and counseling that transpire between the nurse and family. As childhood progresses, the child should become increasingly involved in this process. Acute minor illnesses are likely to be repeated during the span of a family's experience, and thus the health care foundation that is laid during the first encounter for a family has great implications for helping the family to assume increasing independence and initiative in their own health care needs. They should learn as much about the illness or injury as they can, including which aspects need professional health care and which aspects deserve and require their own intervention and care. Each of the measures used for relief and comfort by the nurse should be understood by the family in relation to a particular illness or symptom, and their own use of many of these measures should be encouraged whether in a hospital or at home. When the family members are capable of understanding part or all of the rationale for a specific intervention, their ability to make sound judgments in applying similar measures under similar circumstances will be enhanced. Each of the alternatives in making a health care decision should be shared with the entire family when circumstances allow and their participation in the decision is encouraged. Thus relevant learning is facilitated, and the family assumes a more integral participation in its own health care.

Often parents profit and learn by participating in some of the nursing assessment or in sharing some of the observations of the nurse. When the parents see the child's sore throat or red ear, hear congestion in the lung fields, or feel the enlarged nodes in the child's throat, their involvement helps to focus attention on the problem. Thus understanding of the explanations and their motivation to participate in the child's care may be enhanced. The nurse is also teaching the parents that their participation, understanding, and involvement in health care of their own child are their right and responsibility and not the exclusive domain of the nurse or physician.[35,90]

## Evaluation of care

Ongoing evaluation of care and management provides the means for improvement of nursing care and for the nurse's own learning from each situation. Evaluation begins at the initial contact, where the nurse engages in obtaining and giving the feedback and validation messages that are an essential component of the nursing process (see Fig. 2-1). This aspect of nursing care allows for immediate adjustments and improvement of nursing care by obtaining more accurate information. This process indicates that the nurse understands the family, that the family understands the nurse, and that the health care process is relevant and meaningful.

Further, there must be provision for evaluating the more long-term effects of the health care process. The nature of most illness during early childhood requires further assessment of the child after the initial therapy is instituted, and some follow-through care for certain aspects of the illness is often necessary. When specific therapy is required in order for improvement to occur, the success of therapy may be measured by the disappearance of the illness. However, many of the acute problems that occur during infancy are self-limiting and may not require therapy in order for the illness to disappear. The child's comfort may be enhanced by the use of therapeutic measures, or resolution of the illness may be brought about more rapidly; therefore, one measure of the effectiveness of treatment may be the readiness with which the child's symptoms respond to therapeutic efforts. This response is often confused with curing the illness which, in fact, may not be the only significant factor. In addition, many childhood illnesses are accompanied by a significant risk of serious complications, such as the risk of mastoiditis or hearing loss when otitis media is not treated. The bacterial or viral infection itself may be self-limiting, but without treatment the organism's strength and virulence for the particular host may grow to a dangerous point during the natural life span of its disease effect. Thus the absence of complications and serious progression of an initially minor illness may be attributed, with some reservation, to the effects of therapy.

Another important aspect of evaluation is the long-range evidence of effectiveness of learning incorporated by the child and the family. If, over a period of time, a family becomes increasingly dependent upon the health care system for an increasing range of health care problems, with very little demonstration of independence and confidence in providing for their own health care, the learning that has occurred may not be what was intended by the health care worker. If, on the other hand, the family demonstrates an increasingly independent ability to judge accurately their health care needs in relation to the health care system, the goal of teaching and helping them to incorporate their own efforts to care for acute minor illness may be judged successful.

The tool by which this kind of information is accumulated and made available for evaluation is, again, the detailed health care record. The problem-oriented system proposed by Weed and discussed in Chapter 2 provides an efficient, deliberate way in which such data may be gathered.

The quality of nursing care is evaluated using the Standards of Maternal-Child Health Nursing practice presented in Chapter 2. Evidence of attainment of each of the standards should appear in the child's record. The assessment factors that appear with each standard provide general guidelines for quality of care. Specific diagnostic criteria and protocols for management that are developed by the local health care team provide more specific factors against which to evaluate the quality of care. A framework for nursing practice, such as the competency framework used in this text, provides a means of assuring comprehensive care and should be reflected in the child's record.

## NURSING PROBLEMS RELATED TO PHYSICAL COMPETENCY

The physical immaturity of the infant's and young child's body structure and function creates a high level of vulnerability to frequent episodes of physical illness (see Chapters 9 and 10). The following section presents a discussion of nursing problems and diagnosis that occur frequently during these stages of development. Related pathophysiology and medical diagnoses, where appropriate, are presented. Suggested criteria for nursing diagnosis and problem statements are given along with recommended management approaches that might be incorporated into a management protocol. The Minnesota Nursing Problem Classification number (MNPC) is given for each problem or group of problems, and the reader is referred to the Appendix (p. 884) for the complete listing of problems.

### Acute febrile states (MNPC no. 350.0)

During infancy and early childhood, acute febrile states occur in the absence of other signs of illness and without serious complication. The appearance of an elevated body temperature is indicative and symptomatic of an underlying pathologic condition, but it is often not practical nor desirable to attempt to determine the underlying pathology for a child whose febrile state is brief and is not accompanied by other signs of illness. Given specific criteria for diag-

nosis, acute febrile states are subject to direct nursing intervention. A related medical diagnosis may be desirable and is necessary if the criteria for nursing diagnosis are not clearly obtained.

### Pathophysiology of fever

The exact mechanism by which fever occurs is not known. It does not offer the body any advantage during disease states and, in fact, presents a serious hazard. This phenomenon seems inconsistent with the body's tendency to attempt to maintain homeostasis under other severe, stressful conditions. Fever is important in signaling disease states, but it actually interferes with the body's capacity to recover and resist the effects of most associated diseases.

The center for temperature control is in the hypothalamus. This area of the brain center seems to operate in response to environmental changes in heat and cold in a manner similar to a room thermostat. It keeps the core body temperature within a neutral zone. This normally neutral zone, as measured orally, has a very wide range of 96° to 101° F. Within these limits individuals tend to exhibit a lesser variation, maintaining a constant body temperature range more limited than this general range. The young child seems to respond sensitively to exercise, stress, and other causes of increased or decreased temperature, but under conditions of health his or her temperature usually does not vary beyond this range unless a pyrogenic agent is present.

Pyrogenic agents associated with disease states, such as endotoxin from gram-negative bacilli, apparently interact with a host product, which has been termed "endogenous pyrogen" and which seems to be produced by leukocytes. The endogenous pyrogen apparently acts directly upon the hypothalamus to cause fever, and it has been described as an effect that is similar to raising a thermostat to a higher level. Some tolerance seems to be built up in the febrile response when certain pyrogenic agents are repeatedly encountered. This tendency may account for the fact that young children react with very high, severe fever to a relatively small, localized infection such as otitis media. On the other hand, a severe, generalized infection during infancy may not result in any febrile response, suggesting that certain properties of the offending organism may interact differently with endogenous pyrogen at different stages in life.

Fever in infancy and early childhood seems to be a much different response than that of the older child or adult. Brisk rises are not usually typical of febrile responses in early childhood, although they do occur and may be a factor in febrile convulsions. Chills, headache, and skin sensitivity do not seem to be typical of the young child's febrile reaction. However, as with adults, the physiologic response of vasoconstriction, which inhibits heat loss, appears to be the main mechanism by which core body temperature is raised in response to the febrile stimulation of the hypothalamus. This vasoconstriction affects heat loss from the skin by evaporation as well as from the lungs by convection. These mechanisms occur in the young child, but the accompanying decrease in sweating (which normally is only minimal) and the chilling sensation are not present. In fact, young children may suffer from a relatively high fever and exhibit almost no other signs of illness, nor do they appear uncomfortable. When the child does appear lethargic, miserable, and ill, acute infectious disease is probably involved.

When the agent responsible for the fever is no longer effective, the body reacts as to a warm thermal environment. Vasodilation and increased sweating, which allow for rapid and effective heat loss, occur rapidly, and the body temperature is restored to normal ranges.[114,150]

Acute febrile states during childhood are most commonly caused by viral or mycoplasmal infections, which frequently are not accompanied by other signs or symptoms of illness. The infection is usually of short duration (three days or less), and self-limiting. Occasionally these infections are accompanied by mild respiratory symptoms of coryza, exanthema, or gastrointestinal disturbance. More serious and specifically treatable bacterial infections give rise to specific signs and symptoms of inflammation of the upper respiratory tract, the middle ear, the genitourinary tract, or central nervous system.[75]

## Assessment and criteria for nursing diagnosis of acute febrile states

The assessment that leads to the diagnosis of fever is accomplished with measurement of body temperature. However, identifying the excessive body temperature observation as a nursing diagnosis requires a very skilled, careful diagnostic approach. The symptom of fever occurs with a wide range of conditions that vary in severity and risk. Fever cannot exist as a single entity or disease state; thus the initial assessment task in determining a nursing diagnosis and treatment of fever is in relation to the condition related to the fever.

Most illnesses producing acute fever in children are relatively benign, self-limiting, and carry little risk of complication. Fevers seldom rise above 104° F, the area of critical risk of febrile convulsions. Such disorders include minor viral infections, some bacterial illnesses, reactions to immunizations, and some allergies. It may not be feasible or desirable to identify the exact etiology involved in an infectious process, but factors indicating an infection rather than a chronic disease state, trauma, endocrine disorder, or reaction to drugs may be determined with reasonable certainty. The epidemiology of the family and the community provides helpful clues, and the child may exhibit specific signs of infection in a discrete area of the body, such as the ear, throat, or gastrointestinal tract. In spite of reasonable certainty that the cause of fever is related to a transient communicable illness, occasionally a more serious cause may be present. In such a case, fever will persist after treatment is instituted and after the symptoms of the infectious illness have subsided.[67,75,132]

Criteria recommended for a nursing diagnosis of an acute febrile state are:
1. The infant is over 6 months of age.
   **RATIONALE:** A young infant is prone to serious pathologic consequences of an illness where fever is present, due to the immaturity of homeostatic mechanisms; therefore all instances of fever in young infants should be medically managed.[143]
2. There are no signs or symptoms of acute or chronic illness involving the respiratory tract, gastrointestinal tract, blood, or urine

other than mild, brief-duration signs of the common cold.

RATIONALE: When other signs of illness are present, either a different nursing diagnosis or a medical diagnosis that accounts for the meaning of these symptoms and signs is indicated.[67]

3. The fever is of relatively brief duration before the diagnostic encounter; the history of fever should not exceed 24 hours.

RATIONALE: An acute febrile state that has persisted previously and not responded to the family's intervention or resolved spontaneously may be indicative of a condition requiring medical diagnosis.[67,135,178]

4. The fever does not exceed 104° F.

RATIONALE: Complications of fever, such as dehydration or febrile convulsions, occur with excessive fever above this point. Further, excessive fever may be indicative of a pathologic condition requiring medical diagnosis.[67,168]

5. The acute febrile state is resolved within 72 hours with no complication.

RATIONALE: An acute febrile state that responds to symptomatic management and yields no complications within this period of time is likely related to a transient viral infection requiring no further diagnosis or treatment.[67,178]

6. The child's family demonstrates the capacity to understand and implement the care required, to administer drugs safely, and to recognize signs and symptoms of complications.

RATIONALE: If there is doubt of the family's ability to care for the child, health care team collaboration is needed to determine the approach needed to assure adequate care for the child and prevent complications arising from the possible inadequate care.

The health record must contain documentation of each of these criteria, as defined by the local health care team. The management protocol, which is closely related to the diagnostic criteria, often includes actions that help to assure that the acute febrile state remains within these diagnostic limits. For example, the family is taught how to use antipyretic drugs, frequent cool sponge or tub bathing, and environmental measures to prevent the fever from reaching excessive limits. Further, the management protocol might include providing explicit written instructions in administering recommended drugs in order to augment their ability to provide safe administration of the drug.

In some settings the health care team may alter these recommended criteria to meet particular legal or situational circumstances. Once the criteria are determined by an individual nurse, the total health care team, or both, the record can reflect clear standards of practice.

*Nursing intervention*

Nursing management for a child with an acute febrile state is based upon an established management protocol and the particular needs of the family. The management protocol includes the components of management that are essential for all children with this nursing diagnosis and specific approaches that are to be used with all families. The family's own needs and circumstances provide the basis for augmentation of these necessary management approaches to assure comprehensive quality care. For example, the management protocol might specify that all parents are to be instructed to use acetaminophen in doses determined by the age of the child and are to be given explicit written instructions for use of this drug. If there is doubt as to the family's ability to measure the dose accurately or gain sufficient cooperation from the child in administering the drug, the nurse may, in addition, have the parent demonstrate measuring the dose of the drug in a pediatric oral drug-dispensing syringe and assist the parent in administering a dose while the nurse is present and can assist in gaining the child's cooperation.

**Environmental measures.** Environmental measures to increase body heat loss may include lowering the room temperature, dressing the child in light clothing, and giving a sponge or tub bath in water that is equal to or cooler than body temperature. Alcohol sponge bathing and cold water baths have been demonstrated to be most effective in bringing excessive temperature under very rapid control, but discomfort for the child under these conditions usually contraindicates these more extreme measures.

When the temperature is spiking and there is known danger of febrile convulsion, extreme, rapid measures may be essential. The use of a water mattress with circulating cold or cool water may be desirable in a hospital setting if the child is suffering from continuing high fever. Likewise, at home an ice pack or cold water bottle is effective in helping to control the fever.

The mechanism by which these measures operate is to induce heat loss by convection, conduction, and evaporation in the face of vasoconstriction brought about by the febrile condition. Such intervention can be repeated as often as necessary to keep the fever under control, thus preventing the continuance of spiking and unreasonably high temperature elevations over a period of time. These measures increase the comfort of the child and often allow for rest or sleep.

**Drugs.** Drugs used in the control of fever also act by inducing body heat loss primarily through sweating, but the effect is not as rapid as environmental measures. An interesting property of the action of these drugs is that they do not lower body temperature when it is within normal limits. These drugs also have an analgesic effect, which operates regardless of body temperature.[75,150]

*Aspirin* (acetylsalicylic acid) has a long history of use and continues to be widely used in the control of fever and pain in children. Its properties are antipyrogenic, analgesic, and anti-inflammatory. It is supplied in tablet and rectal suppository forms and is available freely over the counter. Tablet forms for children are available in doses of 100 mg (1½ gr). Aspirin in liquid form is not available because it is extremely unstable at room temperature. For a young child who is not able to swallow a whole tablet, flavored tablets may be crushed and given directly or mixed with jelly, honey, or gelatin.

Children's dosage for aspirin may be calculated by weight or surface area as follows:

Weight: 65 mg (1 gr)/kg/24 hours
Surface area: 1.5 g/m²/24 hours

The total dosage of aspirin per 24-hour period, for any child regardless of size or age, *should not exceed 3.6 g.* The dosage is divided into four or six single doses for the 24-hour period but should not be given more frequently than every four to six hours.

Particular caution must be given to the administration of aspirin to children under 2 years of age, since toxic accumulation of the drug in the system is a real hazard. Aspirin is degraded and excreted by the kidney, and the infant's renal mechanisms for excretion may not be reliable in preventing accumulation of the drug in the face of repeated administration. A one-time dose of the drug is usually safe, as when the infant receives an immunization and suffers a temporary febrile reaction.

Unintentional therapeutic salicylate intoxication may occur when aspirin is used in combination with other pediatric preparations intended to control symptoms and related illness. Many cough preparations, for example, contain aspirin, and this fact may not be apparent without careful reading of the label and understanding the terminology that is used in reporting drug composition. A mother may give her child such a cough preparation in addition to giving aspirin and not realize that the child is receiving a double dose of aspirin. The high dosage, plus the accumulative tendency in young children, leads to an eventual toxic effect which may be life threatening. The usual course of child-health maintenance must include teaching regarding the use of such drugs, because the ready availability of these drugs to mothers may result in tragic misuse before a health care worker becomes aware of the problem.[35,90]

Aspirin is absorbed in the gastrointestinal tract and, in most forms available for children, causes gastric irritation and some bleeding. Over a prolonged period of time this may result in iron-deficiency anemia, but the limits of time have not been adequately determined. The most common signs of aspirin toxicity are mild tinnitis and nausea, progressing to pulmonary edema, hemorrhage, renal failure, hyperventilation, hyperthermia, convulsions, and coma. Allergic reactions to aspirin during early childhood are extremely rare, but the use of aspirin during this period may contribute to the development of an allergic condition later in life. In comparison with the widespread use of the drug in children, the adverse effects are extremely few when the drug is used within the limits of sound, considerate judgment.[21,28,92,191] In infants and preschool children, the safest guide for usage is the smallest dose possible over the briefest amount of time, and the time span probably should not exceed three days without medical attention.

*Acetaminophen* (Tylenol, Tempra, Liquiprin) has come into popular use for young children because it is available in liquid form. This drug has antipyretic and analgesic, but no anti-inflammatory, properties. Degradation of the drug occurs primarily in the liver and requires conjugation with glucuronic or sulfuric acid. Excretion is accomplished by the kidney. Therefore, limited function of either of these organs leads to incomplete clearance and possible accumulative toxicity similar to that of aspirin. Toxic and adverse effects of these preparations are not understood as well as those for aspirin, but allergic reactions and possible interference with blood-forming processes and renal function may be associated with prolonged use. Initial experience has indicated that these are relatively safe drugs for children, and they do not have the gastric irritation property of aspirin.

The signs and symptoms of acetaminophen toxicity include gastrointestinal irritability, anorexia, nausea, and vomiting. When toxic levels have persisted, diaphoresis followed by drowsiness occurs. After 24 to 36 hours, hepatic symptoms appear, as well as central nervous system depression, cardiac function damage, and renal damage.[84,191,198,222]

The dosage may be calculated by age or by surface area as follows:

| Age | Dose |
|---|---|
| Under 1 year | 60 mg |
| 1-3 years | 60 to 120 mg |
| 3-6 years | 120 mg |
| Over 6 years | 240 mg |

These single doses are repeated every 4 to 6 hours.

**Body surface area**
$0.7$ g/m$^2$/24 hours, divided into four to six doses

When using these preparations with infants, it is advisable that a one-time dose only be used, or that there be a specific prescription for a limited number of doses widely spaced over one or two days. For example, the parent may be instructed to give the infant the appropriate single dose of the drug at 6 o'clock this evening, midnight, 6 o'clock in the morning, noon tomorrow, and then to call during the afternoon to report the child's progress. At that time a judgment may be made regarding continuing the drug.[92]

### Potential complications

The first and foremost potential complication of fever is *dehydration from fluid loss*. The increased body temperature and the therapeutic effects of drugs that enhance the mechanism of sweating may lead to rapid body fluid depletion. The young child who is particularly vulnerable to the effects of water and electrolyte imbalance will demonstrate a pathologic condition resulting from this imbalance much faster than will an adult. This problem is discussed in detail in the following section on gastrointestinal problems. However, it should be mentioned here that this complication is preventable and that every effort should be made to prevent the development of dehydration in the face of fever. It is essential to offer oral fluids frequently.

Another major complication resulting from high temperatures (usually over 104° F) is febrile convulsions. Such seizures occur almost exclusively in children under 7 years of age, and they occur without primary disease of the nervous system. Febrile seizures may occur with lower body temperatures, and children seem to vary in the threshold at which they will experience a seizure. The rapidity with which the temperature rises, the nature of the accompanying infection, allergy, and electrolyte imbalance have been associated with the occurrence of febrile seizures, but the exact nature of the problem is not clearly understood. The seizures themselves range in severity and duration from mild focal or generalized involvement lasting only a few seconds to severe generalized involvement lasting as long as 15 minutes. It is estimated that 50% to 60% of all children experience febrile convulsions at least once, but only 10% to 20% of all children suffer more than four such seizures during childhood. A careful assessment of the nature of the febrile seizure is vitally important in determining the prognosis for the particular child in relation to the development of lasting brain involvement. Such involvement may result from the febrile episode, or it may have been present as a factor causing the episode. The diagnosis of brain involvement requires the medical use of electroencephalogram studies. Because of the high incidence of single occurrences of febrile convulsions among young children, full medical diagnosis of the problem is often deferred until a second convulsive episode has occurred, unless the severity of the first episode or the desires of the family indicate that medical diagnosis would be valuable after the first occurrence.

The primary concern, once a febrile seizure has occurred, is to prevent recurrence. Measures to control recurrence primarily involve nursing intervention for fever, and the parents must be acutely aware of ways in which they can safely begin these interventions as soon as the child shows sign of fever. Occasionally, when the initial seizure was particularly disturbing or when there have been several recurrences, anticonvulsant drugs during a febrile illness are employed.[118,150]

Management of febrile seizures during childhood illustrates the benefits of collaborative nursing and medical efforts in health care. Management is primarily a medical responsibility, but the child and family may profit from collaborative use of nursing intervention, support, and teaching, as well as medical diagnosis, control, and intervention.[71,150,168]

## Respiratory problems (MNPC no. 350.5)

Upper respiratory infections (URIs) are the most common cause of illness in infancy and early childhood. Some of these disorders are relatively minor and cause minimal interference with the child's functioning.[120,207] Others become serious and life threatening, particularly in the absence of adequate treatment. Infections of the lower tract usually arise as a complication of infections of the upper tract and will be considered in this section as such a complication. Often the rapidity with which infection spreads from one area of the respiratory tract to another in early childhood makes it impossible to differentiate the initial site of infection or isolate the most severe effect to one particular structure. Thus upper respiratory infection in general is considered as a single entity, with reference to particular aspects involving a particular structure.

### Pathophysiologic considerations

Several of the physiologic characteristics of the respiratory tract of the infant and child have been presented in previous chapters. The physiologic protective mechanisms typical of the respiratory tract must be understood before the nurse can understand the particular susceptibility of these structures to infection and the nature of respiratory illness during early childhood.

First there is a ring of lymphoid tissue conveniently located around the entrance to the pharynx that helps to localize foreign infectious agents and holds them trapped for destruction. These tissues include the faucial tonsils, lingual tonsils, nasopharyngeal tonsil (adenoid), and pharyngeal lymphoid tissue.

Second, ciliated columnar epithelium throughout most of the respiratory tract produces mucus that is kept flowing over the membrane by the action of the cilia. Foreign agents are swept along on the current to be swallowed or swept out of the respiratory system. The lowered production of mucus by this membrane under normal conditions during infancy and early childhood may interfere with the effectiveness of this defense.

Third, the tracheobronchial tree tends to elongate and dilate on inspiration and shorten and contract on expiration. This dynamic activity aids in the movement of air while at the same time trapping foreign invading organisms in the tissue, preventing further transport to the lower portions of the tract.

Fourth, the reflexive, forceful cough that occurs in response to the presence of foreign material operates to move material and organisms further upward in the tract rather than trapping them in the lower portions. The young child is disadvantaged in coughing, because the force and strength of his or her cough are not as effective as in the adult's. In addition the smaller diameter of the airway passages increases resistance during coughing. Once an infectious process has begun, the lumen is further constricted.

Fifth, the epiglottis acts as a trap door to prevent the passage of a portion of materials and agents into the lung structures. Many agents that would otherwise enter the lung fields are swallowed and more effectively destroyed in the gastrointestinal tract.

Sixth, the changes in position of the human body that occur throughout the ordinary course of 24 hours help to bring agents out of the lower tract and into the upper tract. This factor becomes an important therapeutic tool for children in the use of postural drainage.

Seventh, there are regional lymph nodes throughout the respiratory tract that serve as a site for destruction of invading organisms. These nodes may have limited function during infancy and early childhood.

Finally, related to the presence of the lymph nodes in the respiratory tract, the mechanisms of phagocytosis, enzymatic processes, and immune responses (particularly IgA) are activated in the presence of invading organisms. This pro-

tection becomes more effective as early childhood progresses.[99,181,200]

The communicating passages that enter into the pharynx are important in the nature of respiratory illness of the young child. The paranasal sinuses are often involved in inflammatory processes during infancy or early childhood, even though they are not completely formed until later in childhood.[134] The eustachian tube is frequently involved in infections, and blockage of this orifice by adenoidal tissue often results in serous otitis. Bacterial infection of the middle ear results from passage of the organism from the nasopharynx through the eustachian tube. Normally, ventilation of the eustachian tube occurs as a result of opening the tubes during swallowing, chewing, yawning, or as a result of a slight positive pressure gradient in the nasopharynx. Enlarged adenoids prevent this ventilation, and the resulting susceptibility to middle ear infection is a real hazard. Further, once fluid

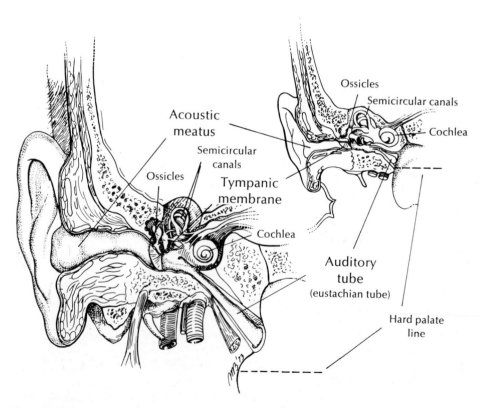

**Fig. 11-2.** Comparison of the anatomy of the ear of the adult and the young child. Notice that the ossicles, semicircular canals, and cochlea are almost fully grown in the young child.

accumulates in the middle ear, drainage into the nasopharynx is inhibited both by enlarged adenoidal tissue and by the relative anatomic angle of the tube in the infant and young child. Fig. 11-2 illustrates the relative horizontal relationship of this structure as compared to the angle in the adult that facilitates drainage. The trapped fluid directly behind the tympanic membrane provides a rich medium for growth of infectious organisms.[99]

### Drugs used for respiratory problems in children

The use of drugs for respiratory problems in children requires astute judgment based on knowledge of the action of drug agents, the probable etiology of the problem, specific age-dependent factors involved in the use of each specific drug, and an accurate diagnosis of the problem. Drugs are frequently misused in the treatment of children's respiratory problems, both by health care practitioners and by parents who are eager to provide rapid and effective alleviation of signs and symptoms and to prevent undesired complications from the initial problem. Specific recommendations for the use of drugs for each condition discussed in the following sections are included in those sections. The general classifications of drugs used for treatment of respiratory problems are presented here, with their particular use in children and cautions to be taken in their use.

Antibiotics are frequently used with respiratory infections. Ideally, an antibiotic should only be used when the specific causative organism is identified by culture. However, a few conditions have been studied sufficiently to warrant the use of antibiotics based on the general knowledge of the usual invading organism. For example, the most frequent causative organisms of otitis media in young children have been identified sufficiently to justify the use of antibiotics, a factor combined with the difficulty of obtaining an accurate culture of the infection site and the hazards of serious complications from untreated or undertreated infections of the middle ear (see p. 400). However, antibiotics are seldom indicated in the treatment of upper respiratory infections in children, as the majority of such infections are caused by virus infec-

tions. Further, indiscriminant use of antibiotics increases the opportunity for developing allergic responses later in life and resistance of organisms to the drug used.[*]

Analgesics are often used to relieve discomfort and/or fever associated with the respiratory problem. The use of these drugs was discussed in relation to management of acute febrile states (see p. 383). Particular caution must be used when these drugs are used in combination with various cold remedies, for often these remedies contain an analgesic and combined use may result in overdoses.

Decongestants are frequently used for upper respiratory problems in children. Most decongestant drugs act on the sympathetic division of the autonomic nervous system by stimulating the alpha adrenergic receptors of vascular smooth muscle, resulting in constriction of the arterioles, reducing blood flow to the mucosa of the respiratory tract, and producing a decrease in secretions. Adverse reactions include general vasoconstriction, elevation of blood pressure, and cardiac stimulation.

Antihistamines are included in many cold remedies available over the counter as well as in many prescription drugs containing decongestants. These drugs inhibit histamines that are released in response to an allergic reaction and are of questionable value in respiratory problems that do not involve an allergic reaction. Their widespread use in various remedies is based on the drying effect that results from action on the capillaries to reduce their permeability. Antihistamines can be detrimental for young children who have a dry, tenacious cough, wheezing, or bronchial asthma, because the drying effect of the drug interferes with effective coughing and clearing of the airway.

Antitussives are another class of drugs frequently found in nonprescription cold remedies for children. These drugs are often selected by parents in a desire to lessen a child's cough, without the realization that the cough is an important defense mechanism that is needed to keep the respiratory tract clear. Antitussives may be recommended to decrease an overactive cough reflex, but other measures should be

*References 10, 26, 47, 79, 179, 180, 216.

used to loosen bronchial secretions and assist the child in clearing the airway. Cough depressants or suppressants act on the central nervous system to raise the threshold of the cough control center; expectorants increase the productivity of the cough by thinning respiratory tract secretions and by increasing the fluid production of the glands lining the lower respiratory tract.[26]

### Nursing diagnosis and intervention for the common cold (MNPC no. 350.5)

The common cold, also termed acute coryza, rhinitis, and acute nasopharyngitis, is primarily identified by the presence of typical symptoms without complicating or more serious respiratory infections. The frequency of colds in young children (up to eight per year) illustrates the relative innocuous nature of the problem; nevertheless, adequate care and intervention by the family during episodes of colds may be important in the prevention of complicating problems.

Even though the invading organism causing the common cold is viral (most commonly the rhinoviruses), young children are particularly prone to bacterial complications of colds. Change in the flow of the mucus of the epithelium is thought to be primarily responsible for this susceptibility. Once viral agents invade the ciliated columnar epithelium in young children, function comes to a halt and the tissue is particularly vulnerable to further invasion. Adult tissues seem to have more resilience in this regard.

Nursing diagnosis of the common cold rests on the following criteria:

1. The objective presence of a combination of any of the following symptoms:
   a. Nasal congestion
   b. Sore or "scratchy" throat
   c. Cough
   d. Sneezing
   e. Minimal degree of fever
   RATIONALE: These symptoms are often associated with the common cold even in the absence of other forms of respiratory illness.[33,108,134]
2. The documented absence of definitive signs of infection of related structures:
   a. Ears: tympanic membranes appear normal
   b. Lungs: breath sounds are normal; no congestion, and breathing is not distressed
   c. Throat: no evidence of purulent drainage or excoriated lesions; swallowing is not impaired; negative throat culture
   d. Mouth: no signs of Koplik spots on the buccal membranes (indicative of measles)
   e. Nose: no sign of foreign body
   f. Neurologic: no signs of meningeal irritation
   RATIONALE: Absence of these signs and symptoms indicates the probable absence of other forms of respiratory illness.[33,108,134]
3. Symptoms do not last longer than one week.
   RATIONALE: The clinical course of the common cold resolves spontaneously within four to seven days. If the signs and symptoms persist beyond this period of time, another form of respiratory illness must be considered.[134]
4. The child is over 6 months of age.
   RATIONALE: Infants under 6 months of age may exhibit symptoms typical of the common cold with more serious forms of illness. Medical judgment and management is required for this age group.

The common cold has an incubation period of 48 to 72 hours, regardless of the specific virus responsible for the infection. The related viruses that cause similar clinical symptoms require very specific immunologic response of the host, and the length of immunity to each specific agent is not known.[99,108]

Often when a child first comes to the health care setting with a common cold, the infection has been in progress for several days; the parents have become worried about some complication or worsening of the condition, or they feel that the condition is not resolving rapidly enough. It is important to learn about each measure they have employed in treating the illness. Some measures may be unfamiliar to the nurse, but as long as no harm can come to the child, the parents' care efforts should be reinforced and supported. The chances of obtaining totally accurate information about the self-care abilities of the family are enhanced, and the nurse strengthens the family's confidence in their own ability to make health care decisions.[33,192]

When the cold has persisted for several days, it is particularly important to determine the presence of any complicating conditions. Reassurance for the parents regarding signs of serious illness, information about the ordinary progression of the common cold, and recommendations for measures that will make the child more comfortable and will increase the parents' ability to cope with the illness are important aspects of care. Care should be taken to offer real reassurance and not to arouse undue concern over an illness that is understandably distressing but is part of the usual course of early childhood.

Allergy should be considered a possible cause of coldlike symptoms when community and family epidemiologic evidence suggest that the illness may not be a viral cold or when the symptoms are of prolonged duration. This problem is discussed later in this chapter.

Nursing intervention for the common cold is focused on symptomatic relief and comfort and to teaching and counseling with the family. Frequent occurrence of colds is often distressing for young families; they may profit from a discussion of the many factors involved. Such a discussion may enhance their ability to cope with the problem and may help them to understand the circumstances under which they should become concerned for the well-being of their young child.

The use of drugs for fever has been discussed; often environmental intervention will suffice without prolonged use of antipyretic drugs. There is disagreement concerning the use of decongestants, cough suppressants, expectorants, nose drops, antihistamines, and ephedrines to shrink mucous membranes.[26,126,234]

A single drug that is not combined with other agents is most desirable for young children. Using a single agent aids in teaching the mother specific actions and interactions of drugs, promotes a conservatism in relation to drug usage in young children, and enhances identification of the agent causing an adverse reaction. The nurse can gain familiarity and discrimination in use of several specific agents among the many drugs available over the counter and through prescription. A simple bronchodilator, such as pseudoephedrine hydrochloride, yields some relief from constant nasal drainage and eases passage of air through the upper airway.

Nasal decongestant sprays and drops should be discouraged for infants and young children because of the dangers of their causing pathologic changes in the mucosa, particularly a rebound congestion that leads to habitual use of the spray or drops. Saline nose drops prepared by the mother are, on the other hand, most useful in loosening excessive nasal secretions. These drops offer the advantage of being administered as frequently as needed, and they stimulate the infant and young child to swallow, which helps to ventilate the eustachian tube. The drops are made by mixing ¼ teaspoon of salt in 1 cup of water. The mother is instructed to use a bulb syringe to suction the excessive fluid and nasal secretions from the nasal passages after instillation of the drops.[26]

Steam or cool mist added to environmental air may aid in symptomatic relief of the common cold. The use of mist rather than steam obviates the hazard of accidental burns and is more effective in penetrating the alveoli. Electrical devices always present some danger, and this should be considered by the adult members of the family. Such environmental intervention has come under scrutiny and debate in recent literature, but many practitioners and families believe that mist aids in relief of cough and congestion. Others feel that its use is justified at least on the basis of the psychologic advantage of doing something as a means of relief.[9,230]

### Respiratory problems requiring nurse-physician collaboration

In providing for the needs of young families with infants and children frequently prone to respiratory infections, the health care team must analyze the specific needs of their client group, the professional expertise of each member of the health care team, and the legal implications of each member's practice. Many minor forms of respiratory illness during early childhood can be handled by the family themselves, with occasional support from the nurse. The local health care team may choose to establish

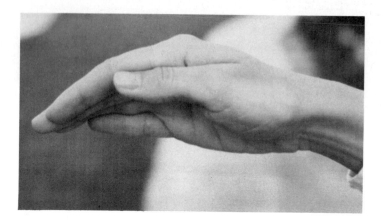

**Fig. 11-3.** The therapist's or mother's hand is cupped for percussion, which produces a hollow sound and causes vibrations throughout the lung. This loosens secretions lodged in the air passages. Percussion is not done over the stomach, sternum, kidneys, or on bare skin, but only over the rib cage. The child's color and respiratory pattern are observed and treatment is adjusted to his or her condition.

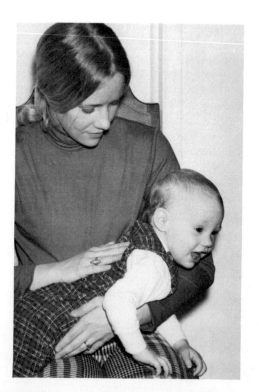

**Fig. 11-4.** The child is lying prone with his right shoulder elevated on his mother's arm. The posterior segment of the right upper lobe is percussed and drained.

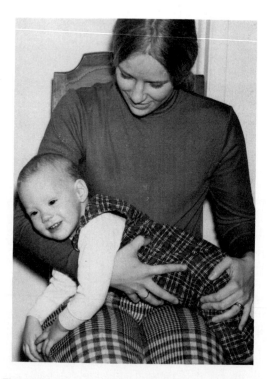

**Fig. 11-5.** The child is lying prone with his left shoulder elevated on his mother's arm. The posterior segment of the left upper lobe is percussed and drained.

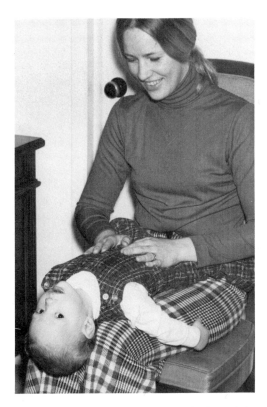

**Fig. 11-6.** The child is lying supine in a horizontal plane. The anterior segments of the left and right upper lobes are percussed and drained.

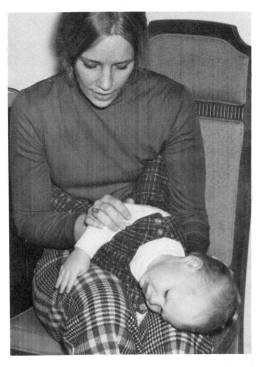

**Fig. 11-7.** The child lies on his right side rotated back one-quarter turn and tipped with his head down about 30 degrees. The lingular lobe of his left lung is percussed and drained.

specific criteria for independent nursing diagnosis and management of transient, mild forms of such problems as otitis media, tonsillitis, or streptococcal throat infections. Because these problems usually require medically prescribed drugs, carefully planned nurse-physician collaboration is essential.

Nursing management for respiratory problems is directed to physical and environmental measures for relief of symptoms and to the teaching needs of the family and child. The measures described in the previous section on the common cold may be implemented for children who have more serious forms of respiratory illness.

Infants and young children who suffer from respiratory illness involving the mechanism of the cough often profit from therapeutic use of postural drainage. When nursing intervention for lower respiratory illness is indicated in con-

junction with medical therapy, this procedure may be employed by the nurse and taught to the parents for application in hospital or home. The procedure is illustrated in Figs. 11-3 through 11-13. It involves positioning and percussion to loosen tenacious, trapped secretions of the lower respiratory tract and encouraging the infant to cough up the loosened secretions. The amount of time spent in percussion and the variety of positions that are used depend upon the infant's particular condition and lung involvement.

This approach is also presented to illustrate an important modification of a therapy that is often used on older children and adults. Note that the infant is positioned directly on the mother's lap rather than on a bed with pillows. This achieves maximal control of the active young child and effects greater familiarity and comfort through direct contact with the moth-

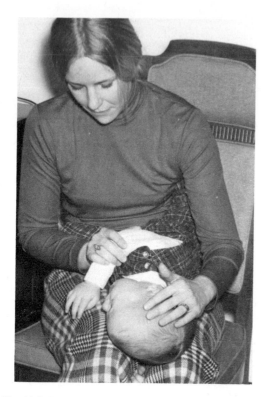

**Fig. 11-8.** The child lies on his left side rotated back one-quarter turn and head tipped downward about 30 degrees. The middle lobe of his right lung is percussed and drained.

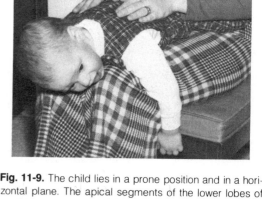

**Fig. 11-9.** The child lies in a prone position and in a horizontal plane. The apical segments of the lower lobes of each lung are percussed and drained.

er's body. The head-down position may produce fear and crying during the first few attempts, but this fear is gradually overcome through familiarity. Crying produces contraction of the diaphragm, which aids in producing the cough needed to bring up loosened secretions; after familiarity is established and crying does not occur, the infant can be stimulated to laugh to produce the same results.[176]

**Otitis media.** Otitis media and serous otitis result from obstruction and bacterial infection of the middle ear. Fig. 11-2 illustrates how fluid can easily become trapped behind the tympanic membrane in the young child, thus encouraging the growth and proliferation of bacterial and viral infection in a space that normally contains air. The pathogenesis of otitis media involves a dysfunction of the eustachian tube to which the young child is particularly prone. The eustachian tube serves three physiologic functions.

The first is *protection* from nasopharyngeal secretions for the structures of the middle ear. The second is *drainage* of secretions produced in the middle ear to the nasopharynx. The third is *ventilation* of the middle ear to establish equilibrium of air pressure between the middle ear and the atmosphere. These functions are substantially reduced for the infant and young child due to the relative horizontal position of the tube, and the proximity of the tube with the hard palate line. Ventilation of the middle ear normally occurs with swallowing and yawning, and these mechanisms cannot be used voluntarily by the infant or young child to relieve a sensed disequilibrium of pressure. In the face of an infection the tissues of the middle ear increase production of secretions, the lumen of the tube is decreased with swelling and irritation, and the normal physiologic functions of the tube are decreased.[18]

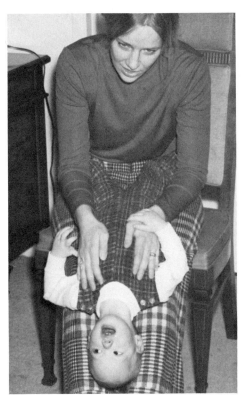

**Fig. 11-10.** The child lies in a supine position on his mother's lap and legs with his head tipped downward at about 45 degrees. The anterior basal segments of the lower lobes of each lung are percussed and drained.

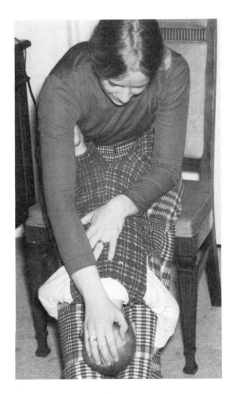

**Fig. 11-11.** The child lies in a prone position tipped as in Fig. 11-10. The posterior basal segments of the lower lobes are percussed and drained.

In infants the most common causative agents of otitis media are pneumococcus and *Haemophilus influenzae.* When diagnosis does not specifically identify the causative agent, antibiotic treatment with a broad-spectrum agent is begun. In school-age children group A beta hemolytic streptococci rather than *H. influenzae* more frequently cause otitis media.[18]

A positive nursing or medical diagnosis of otitis media may be made on the basis of culture results of aspirate of fluid from the middle ear (accomplished by needle aspiration through the tympanic membrane). An indirect and less reliable diagnosis is made by objective visualization of signs of infection in the tympanic membrane. In practice the latter approach offers sufficient reliability and avoids the hazards and trauma of entering the middle ear directly.

Adequate visualization of the tympanic membrane is essential. Often when a young child has symptoms of illness involving the ear, the external canal is obstructed by a buildup of wax or a foreign body. These obstructions must be carefully removed, using a small curet or wire loop. Instillation of water or oil is contraindicated because of the possibility of the membrane having ruptured, allowing the fluid to enter the middle and inner ear. The use of a cotton swab is likewise contraindicated, because additional impaction with strands of cotton further complicates the situation. The young child must be firmly restrained, preferably lying prone on a firm table, with the hands held to the side of the body and the head immobilized to one side. When the canal is cleared, visualization may be quickly accomplished while the child is safely restrained, minimizing the possibility of damage to the canal by the insertion of the canula and sudden movement of the child. In order to fully visualize the young child's tympanic membrane,

**393**

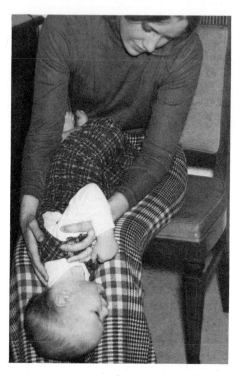

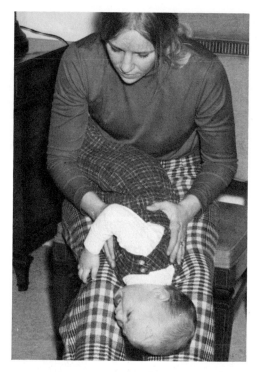

**Fig. 11-12.** The child is on his right side with his head tipped downward at about a 45-degree angle. The lateral basal segments of the left lower lobe are percussed and drained.

**Fig. 11-13.** The child is on his left side in a position similar to that shown in Fig. 11-11. The lateral basal segment of the right lower lobe is percussed and drained.

the external ear is pulled down and back, as illustrated in Fig. 11-14.

The criteria that may be accepted as sufficient and necessary for probable otitis media include three of the following conditions:

1. Injection, redness, and induration of the tympanic membrane
2. Disappearance of the bony landmarks
3. Absence of the light reflex
4. Bulging of the membrane

In addition, the child will often have a fever, but the absence or presence of fever is unrelated to the diagnosis of probable otitis media.*

Medical intervention involves the use of antibiotics chosen on the basis of broad-spectrum attack on the common organisms involved in most instances of otitis media. Ampicillin is effective as such an agent, but other agents may be chosen, such as penicillin G or erythromycin. Antibiotic therapy is thought to be neces-

sary for ten days or longer for young infants and children.[201] The rationale for choice of each drug must be fully understood by the practitioner and includes evidence of the possible offending organisms, the child's past tolerance or allergic reaction to antibiotic drugs, and socioeconomic factors.

Decongestant drugs may be a valuable adjunct in the treatment of otitis media; there is some evidence that these agents promote drainage and clearance of the eustachian tube and thus allow the body's natural defenses to effectively destroy and combat the infection. There is limited evidence that this approach alone may suffice in some middle ear infections, which are, indeed, self-limiting.[137,201] Analgesic drugs are used for symptomatic relief of ear pain and to reduce any fever present.

Associated measures to relieve ear pain include the application of ear drops, saline nose drops, or cold packs. These measures seldom bring sufficient relief for the child who is expe-

**394**  *References 134, 137, 138, 140, 196, 224.

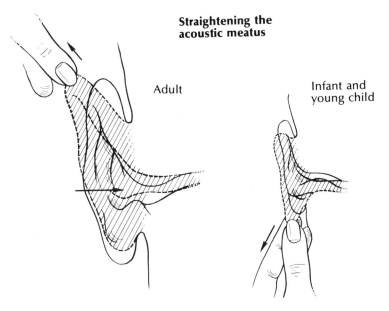

**Straightening the
acoustic meatus**

Adult

Infant and
young child

**Fig. 11-14.** Comparison of the maneuver required to alter the contour of the external canal for visualization of the adult tympanic membrane and the young child's tympanic membrane.

riencing excruciating ear pain, and the parent experiences extreme frustration in trying to comfort the frantic child. It is possible to avoid the crisis of pain in the middle of the night if the parents are sensitive to the early signs of ear infection and distress in infancy and early childhood. The only means of determining whether ear disease is present is to visualize the tympanic membrane; therefore, the parents should remain confident in their desire to have the child evaluated at the earliest possible time. Infants and young children often tug at the affected ear for 24 to 48 hours before onset of acute ear pain, or they may simply become lethargic, irritable, tired, and restless, and they may exhibit signs of upper respiratory infection. Once a child has experienced an ear infection, the usual pattern of early response is known, and the parents can often reliably predict recurrence with great accuracy.

When otitis media recurs within several weeks or months, complete medical evaluation of the child should be obtained. Repeated attacks of otitis media that involve infection of the structures of the throat may result in permanent damage to the defense functions of the tonsils and/or adenoids; in addition, complications of

the ear and surrounding structures can lead to hearing loss. Prevention of these complications is imperative, and intervention may involve surgical removal of the adenoids and/or tonsils and/or insertion of a tympanostomy tube into one or both membranes to provide for prolonged drainage of fluid into the outer ear canal while the structures of the throat, eustachian tubes, and middle ear recover and gain maturity in resisting further infection. The decision to surgically intervene is often a difficult one, and evidence regarding the relative merits of surgery as opposed to repeated medical management of infection throughout the early childhood years remains highly controversial.[106,134,169,181,187]

**Streptococcal throat infections and viral pharyngotonsillitis.** When a young child develops symptoms of an infection of the throat, the initial concern is differentiating between a bacterial, group A beta-hemolytic streptococcal infection and a viral infection. Often the clinical signs and symptoms are similar for both types of infection, and in infants a streptococcal infection of the throat causes mere symptoms of a common cold. All infants with common cold symptoms and young children with possible in-

**395**

volvement of the throat with an upper respiratory infection should be cultured for presence of the streptococcal organism in the throat. The importance of making the differentiation between these etiologic organisms rests on the fact that adequate treatment with antibiotics is essential to prevent the long-term cardiac and renal sequelae of a streptococcal infection, whereas if the bacterial organism is not present, antibiotic treatment is not necessary and may lead to undesirable consequences including increased risk of allergy, resistance of organisms to the drug, and increase in susceptibility for later bacterial infection.[33,34,99,108,134]

A child whose symptoms are sudden in onset and include a high fever (102° to 105° F), abdominal pain, vomiting, headache, and red swollen tonsils with yellowish exudate is likely to yield a positive culture for group A beta hemolytic streptococci. Antibiotic therapy is usually initiated before the results of the throat culture are available and are continued regardless of the outcome of the culture. Children who have a more gradual onset of illness or whose clinical signs and symptoms are less typical of this usual course of illness should receive symptomatic treatment only until the results of the throat culture are obtained.[33,34,60,108,134]

A particular concern for nursing management is teaching the parents how to administer the drugs indicated for the child's illness and the importance of maintaining adequate use of oral antibiotic drugs for a full course of ten days. If the family's ability to maintain adequate oral antibiotic therapy is doubtful, a single injection of benzathine penicillin G might be used instead of the oral preparations. Parenteral antibiotic therapy is also preferred when the child is very ill with a typical clinical pattern of acute streptococcal infection.

Penicillin remains the drug of choice for treatment of streptococcal infections, as it offers the greatest protection against undesired long-term sequelae. Amoxicillin is a form of penicillin with few side effects but is more expensive than penicillin G or penicillin V. Erythromycin may be used for a child who has a known or suspected sensitivity to penicillin but does not provide the level of protection against long-term sequelae as that offered by penicillin. The appro-

**Table 11-1.** Antibiotic dosage for group A beta hemolytic streptococcal infections of the throat

| Drug | Dose | Duration |
|------|------|----------|
| Oral penicillin G or penicillin V (phenoxymethyl penicillin) | Total of 500 mg/day (800,000 U/day) divided into 2, 3, or 4 doses* | Full 10 days |
| Amoxicillin (oral) | Body weight <20 kg: 20 mg/kg/24 hrs divided into 3 doses† | Full 10 days |
| | Body weight >20 kg: 750 mg/24 hrs divided into 3 doses† | Full 10 days |
| Intramuscular Benzathine Penicillin G | Body weight <25 kg: 600,000 μm* | 1 dose only |
| | Body weight >25 kg: 1,200,000 μm* | 1 dose only |
| Oral erythromycin (if child is allergic to penicillin) | 40 mg/kg/day up to a total dose of 1 gm/day, divided into 4 doses* | Full 10 days |

*Doses from Lipow, H. W.: Respiratory tract infections. In Green, M., and Haggerty, R. J., editors: Ambulatory pediatrics II, Philadelphia, 1977, W. B. Saunders Co., p. 46.
†Doses from Shirkey, H. C., editor: Pediatric therapy, St. Louis, 1975, The C. V. Mosby Co., p. 1218.

priate doses of these antibiotics are presented in Table 11-1.*

**Croup syndromes.** The fearsome symptoms that accompany the onset of "croup" in its many forms are easily identified and should be rapidly brought under therapeutic management. The child usually suffers from viral infection involving a combination of sites, including the epiglottis, larynx, trachea, and bronchi. Inflammation, swelling of the walls of the airway, and the narrowing of the lumen of the passages result in (1) a hoarse "barking" cough that is urgent and persistent, (2) trapping of air in the lungs, (3) some degree of respiratory distress, and (4) some degree of oxygen hunger. Immediate intervention with high humidity levels and oxygen brings some relief, and the nurse need not await medical collaboration before instituting these measures. When the epiglottis is involved, the illness is extremely serious and surgical intervention to provide an adequate airway may be im-

*References 20, 34, 60, 134, 180, 183.

**Table 11-2.** The croup syndromes—clinical patterns*

| | Epiglottitis (acute) | Spasmodic croup | Laryngotracheitis (acute) |
|---|---|---|---|
| Synonyms | Epiglottitis<br>Supraglottitis<br>Obstructive supraglottic laryngitis | Acute spasmodic croup<br>"Midnight croup"<br>Allergic croup<br>Spasmodic laryngitis | Laryngotracheitis<br>Viral croup<br>Laryngotracheobronchitis<br>Obstructive subglottic laryngitis |
| Maximum obstruction | Above the vocal cords (supraglottic) | At the vocal cords (glottic) | Below the vocal cords (subglottic) |
| Age | Any age, maximum from 2 to 8 years | Usually 1 to 4 years, with tendency to recur | Usually 6 months to 3 years |
| Etiology | Almost always due to *Haemophilus influenzae* type B, occasionally pneumococci or viruses | Unknown; suspected mild viral infections or allergy | Parainfluenzae virus, 1,2,3; respiratory syncytial virus; influenzae virus $A_2$, B |
| Onset | Usually rapid, over a period of 4 to 12 hours | Very sudden; typically late at night | Gradual; frequently in the course of a viral upper respiratory illness. May become progressively more severe over a 24 hour period of time. |
| Initial clinical picture | Rapidly increasing inspiratory stridor in toxic child with high fever. Sore throat with pain on swallowing, and muffled voice. | Severe inspiratory stridor, without fever, but with "barking" or "brassy" cough. | Gradually increasing inspiratory (and at times expiratory) stridor; frequently hoarse voice. "Barking" or "brassy" cough, and fever which may be low or absent. |
| Examination of posterior pharynx† | Grossly swollen epiglottis—fiery red color, but irregular swollen appearance (like a raspberry) | Epiglottis normal or mildly reddened | Mildly reddened and mild to moderately swollen epiglottis |
| X-ray of neck | Lateral neck films show swollen epiglottis, ballooning hypopharynx, but normal subglottic area. | Probably normal | Normal supraglottic area on lateral view; posteroanterior view: concave medial swelling in subglottic region. |
| Clinical course | Tendency to rapid total airway obstruction within first 6 to 12 hours. | May last several hours if untreated; may be entirely well the following morning, with recurrence of symptoms the following night. | Persistent moderate airway obstruction (rarely complete), but may tire and then rapidly develop respiratory failure. |
| Treatment | Intensive intravenous antibiotic therapy for *H. influenzae;* careful management in intensive care unit; cold mist and oxygen; early passage of small endotracheal tube or tracheostomy. | Warm or cold mist; reassurance; rapid relief by racemic epinephrine delivered by IPP machine | Cold mist and oxygen. Stridor usually rapidly improved by racemic epinephrine administered with oxygen by IPPB apparatus; occasionally, may require endotracheal tube or tracheostomy. |

*From Lipow, H. W.: Respiratory tract infections. In Green, M., and Haggerty, R. J., editors: Ambulatory pediatrics, II. Philadelphia, 1977, W. B. Saunders Co., p. 55.
†Caution: Examination of the posterior pharynx should be gentle and completed quickly. Total airway obstruction may result from vigorous examination.

mediately indicated. Children who have the "croup" syndrome should be evaluated by visualization of the epiglottis, since this is the only reliable way to determine the extent of involvement. The swelling and rapid progressive induration of the epiglottis (which invariably accompany infection) cause, within a matter of two to three hours, complete obstruction of the air passage below the level of the epiglottis and imminent death. Table 11-2 summarizes the clinical patterns of the three major forms of croup.

A sufficient airway must be assured immediately, and the child should then be placed in a cold mist and oxygen tent, which often brings significant relief. Racemic epinephrine (2.25%) nebulized with 100% oxygen is administered

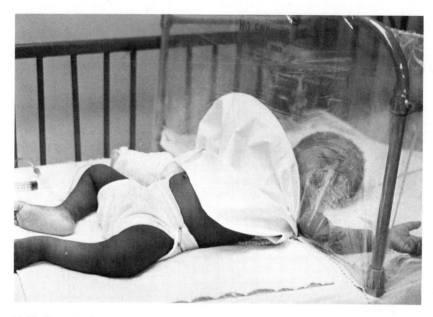

**Fig. 11-15.** The child is placed in a cold mist and oxygen tent; which often brings dramatic relief, in addition to assuring a sufficient airway.

with intermittent positive pressure, gradually increasing the pressure to 20 to 25 cm $H_2O$. The child may be treated for a few hours in the emergency room or may be hospitalized for a brief period of time until the symptoms have resolved.[108,134] The dramatic nature of the croup syndromes is a frightening experience for the child and the family, and nursing intervention must include support, reassurance, and teaching to help the family understand the illness and the treatment involved (see Chapter 16).

Foreign bodies in the airway may result in symptoms that resemble croup, since the effect of blockage of the airway is similar. The child will not respond at all to high humidity and oxygen, and visualization of the larynx and epiglottis does not reveal signs of infection. The obstruction may be discovered with visualization, or radiologic or surgical procedures may be needed to uncover the source of distress.[25,134,182]

**Bronchiolitis and asthma.** Bronchiolitis and asthma produce very similar clinical symptoms during infancy and early childhood. Bronchiolitis is a viral infection of the small distal bronchioles, resulting in marked expiratory airway obstruction and respiratory distress. Respira-

tory syncytial virus causes the majority of such infections, but other viruses are sometimes involved. Edema, inflammation, and thickening of the small bronchi and bronchioles causes trapping of air with marked impairment of gas exchange. The child often has a mild coldlike illness for one or two days before developing symptoms of bronchiolitis, which include expiratory wheezing, increased respiratory rate, intercostal and subcostal retractions, flaring of the alae nasi, and cyanosis. The child has an anxious appearance and rejects feedings, with all energy concentrated on the work of breathing. Support of gas exchange may require administration of oxygen and mechanical ventilation. Mist therapy is usually not helpful and may cause bronchospasm. Fluid and electrolyte management is essential if the child has developed hypoxemia. Prevention of fluid and electrolyte imbalance is a major concern, for the child rapidly develops metabolic acidosis in the face of the respiratory distress (see Chapter 16).

Asthma, on the other hand, is a condition of allergic origin that may be triggered by any number of stimuli, including specific allergens, a mild respiratory illness similar to a common cold, or emotional factors. The history of the illness is usually similar to that described above for bronchiolitis, and the symptoms appear very similar. Asthmatic symptoms usually do not involve the severe degree of respiratory distress that can occur in bronchiolitis but resemble a mild form of the infectious illness. Symptomatic support is essentially the same as that given for bronchiolitis. Ephedrine or an ephedrinelike drug is given in a dose of 2.5 to 3 mg/kg/24 hours, which provides dramatic relief for the child with asthma. Ephedrine may be combined with theophylline derivatives in a dose of 5 mg/kg/every six hours.[62,129,134,141,202]

The similarity between bronchitis or bronchiolitis and asthma during early childhood requires astute diagnostic judgment. Asthma does not occur before age 2 years, probably because of the nature of the allergic response during infancy. Bronchiolitis, on the other hand, tends not to occur after the age of 5 years because of the greater maturity of the respiratory tissues in trapping infection in the upper parts of the respiratory tract. Thus the differential challenge exists between the ages of 2 and 5 years when either the infectious process or the allergic problem could produce the same symptomatology. An adequate prior data base is of infinite value when such a decision is needed; a family history for respiratory allergies supports the possibility of allergic involvement. The eosinophil count of the blood is elevated in allergic asthma, and this condition responds within 20 minutes to a clinical test dose of epinephrine 1:1,000, 0.01 ml/kg of body weight. If the child is suffering from an infectious process, the symptoms of wheezing (primarily expiratory but possibly inspiratory), increased respiratory and heart rates, respiratory distress, and decreased gas exchange will not be immediately relieved by the epinephrine.[8,226]

**Acute sinusitis.** Acute bacterial sinusitis occurs fairly frequently in young children as a complication of the viral common cold. If the swollen infected mucous membranes occlude the ostea, the communicating passage allowing for drainage of the sinus cavities into the nasopharynx, the fluid in the sinuses is trapped and results in a secondary bacterial infection. The child begins to develop increased mucopurulent discharge draining into the anterior nares or nasopharynx, initiating a period of coughing just when the child would be expected to be recovered from the initial cold. The usual adult symptoms of sinusitis, such as local sinus pain, headache, and fever, are not present in young children. A culture of the posterior nasal cavity is desirable to determine the organism involved. The most frequently involved organisms are pneumococcus, streptococcus, staphylococcus and *H. influenzae.* Ampicillin is usually the drug of choice, in a dose of 100 to 150 mg/kg/day. Symptomatic relief of congestion may be achieved as described for the common cold (see p. 389).[96,123,134]

**Acute tracheobronchitis and pertussis.** Infections of the lower trachea and larger bronchi often occur in conjunction with a viral upper respiratory infection but may occur as an isolated infection. Rhinoviruses, respiratory syncytial virus, adenovirus, and Coxsackie virus are the most common organisms involved. Rubeola causes a diffuse tracheobronchitis. The most serious form of tracheobronchitis is that caused by the bacteria gram-negative rod, *Bordetella pertussis.* Pertussis continues to occur in the United States and Canada, with the majority of children affected being those who have not been immunized or have not completed the immunization program, although the illness occasionally occurs in children who have been immunized. In 1974, there were 2400 reported cases of pertussis in the United States.[134]

Acute tracheobronchitis begins with a persistent, dry hacking cough, and there is usually a fever. As the illness progresses, the inflamed tracheobronchial tissues produce a thick yellowish mucus, and course rales and low-pitched rhonchi can be heard over the lungs. The fever subsides within three or four days and the cough within seven to ten days. Treatment includes measures to control the body temperature and symptomatic relief. The persistent coughing of the child is tiring and distressing for the child and the family, and the desire to control the cough may lead them to obtain over-the-counter drugs for this purpose. Nursing care is directed to assisting the family to understand the nature of the illness, the value of the child's cough in clearing the air passages, and ways in

**399**

which they can assist the child to achieve this and provide relief from the discomfort. Postural drainage and percussion of the chest are useful and should be taught to the family. Steam or cool mist provides a soothing effect and promotes loosening of the thick mucus. Plain syrups, such as wild cherry syrup or a mixture of honey and lemon juice, provide a soothing effect on the throat and may reduce coughing when the child needs to rest. Antihistamines are contraindicated, as the atropinelike action will thicken the mucus and make it more difficult for the child to clear the airway. Cough suppressants should be avoided and if used at all should be used at night when the child needs sufficient relief to sleep.[134]

Pertussis has an incubation period of 10 to 14 days after exposure to the organism. The first symptom is a dry cough with a watery nasal discharge. The catarrhal phase of the illness lasts from one to two weeks, during which time the disease is highly contagious if the child is not treated with appropriate antibiotic therapy. The cough gradually becomes more severe, occurring in paroxysms consisting of short repetitive harsh expiratory coughs of such severity that the infant or child is not able to obtain an inspiratory breath. When the paroxysm abates, the child makes a violent inspiratory effort to combat the air hunger that has developed, producing the typical whoop. The infant or child develops cyanosis and hypoxemia and becomes exhausted. The paroxysmal phase of the illness lasts from four to eight weeks, even when the child is treated with appropriate antibiotics. Gradually the coughing subsides, and the child begins a period of several weeks of convalescence.

Antibiotic therapy is based upon the results of the cultures that reveal the exact nature of the organism and its sensitivity. Erythromycin usually produces the most rapid results in terms of rendering the disease noninfectious and preventing bacterial complications of the illness. Other dimensions of treatment consist of respiratory and fluid and electrolyte support and the measures described above for symptomatic relief and comfort.[107,133,134,165]

**Serious complications of respiratory problems.** Untreated respiratory infections during infancy may result in a wide variety of serious effects, including those of complicated otitis media. In addition the most serious threats to infants and young children are the dangers of pneumonia and meningitis, which develop as sequelae to upper respiratory infection. Children who suffer from these problems tend to be undernourished and suffer from iron deficiency anemia,[8,39] but these complications can arise in any child. There appears to be an individual susceptibility, or vulnerability, to the development of one sort of complication or another. Both problems may exist simultaneously.

Viral and bacterial infections are thought to occur simultaneously in many instances. The organisms usually responsible for pneumonia and meningitis in early childhood are those that most frequently cause the minor respiratory illnesses—*H. influenzae* and pneumococci. Meningococcus is also frequently responsible for meningitis, and the gram-negative pathogens are frequently implicated in pneumonia during infancy.

Children who have developed pneumonia usually have a high fever, which rises after the initial fever of a minor respiratory illness has subsided. They begin to have a dry, very painful cough, and they are not able to bring up secretions with coughing. Auscultation of the lungs in the early stages reveals fine, crepitant, dry rales that are localized to the affected area and lobe of the lung. These sound like the crunching of footsteps on fresh snow. A pleural friction rub may be distinguished, which sounds like rubbing one's finger against the face just anterior to the external ear. Rhonchi, which are heard in diseases of the bronchus and are not usually present with pneumonia, produce wet, loose sounds similar to those produced by sucking through a straw when a glass is being emptied. During the course of pneumonia, the rales disappear as consolidation progresses and than reappear as the infiltrate begins to loosen.

X-ray studies of the chest are most helpful in determining the exact nature of the disease in infants and young children, because the clinical symptoms and signs may be nonspecific enough to cause confusion in medical diagnosis. The infant may have minimal auscultatory sound indicating pneumonia and may exhibit respiratory distress similar to lower airway blockage as might occur in bronchiolitis.*

Children with pneumonia may be treated at home if circumstances permit and if the child does not have an electrolyte imbalance requiring parenteral therapy. Broad-spectrum antibiotics are given in either long-acting forms or in repeated doses for 10 to 14 days or until the illness disappears. Rest in bed is important for young children. Although this presents little problem in the early acute stages of the illness, when the child begins to feel better, his or her energy level returns and some allowance must be made for providing outlets for the urge to move about. Hydration is essential in maintaining fluid balance of the body and in promoting liquefication of secretions in the lungs. Fever is treated symptomatically, with particular attention to the child who may be prone to febrile convulsions.

During episodes of pneumonia young children should be encouraged to cough and produce sputum, even though they usually immediately swallow it. Cough suppressants are therefore contraindicated, and postural drainage is highly desirable to promote the movement of secretions out of the lungs and to promote the coughing reflex.

Humidity added to the air may assist in liquefication of secretions and in promoting comfort. Nebulization is required to produce droplets small enough to enter the lower respiratory tract, where the secretions are thick and dry and tend to remain static.

Complications of any sort, including failure of the child to begin to improve within 48 hours, indicate the need for hospitalization.[65,103,134,185]

Meningitis, which may arise as a complication, occur concomitantly, or exist alone, may be detected by observation for rigidity of the neck, complaints of headache, extremely ill appearance and behavior of the child, and positive Kernig's and Brudzinski's signs. Kernig's sign is elicited by bending the thigh at the hip with the child in a supine position and attempting to extend the leg at the knee. Meningeal irritation prevents this maneuver without a great deal of pain and an effort to protect by the child. Brudzinski's sign is elicited by bending the child's neck in an effort to have the chin touch the chest while in the supine position. With meningeal irritation, the child's knees will spontaneously flex, and pain will be present. These signs may indicate meningismus, which may occur in young children without pathologic involvement of the central nervous system, but thorough medical evaluation, including examination of the spinal fluid, is indicated to determine the exact nature of the child's problem.[3,124,155,232]

It is estimated that few children escape an encounter of bacterial meningitis without serious, permanent effects on the function of the central nervous system. The prevalence of this disease in relation to respiratory illness in early childhood and the rising incidence of *H. influenzae* meningitis among children in this age group point to the increasing importance of prevention through adequate treatment of minor respiratory illness that involve or may involve organisms capable of producing meningeal infection.[205,206]

## Gastrointestinal problems

The frequency of minor illness in early childhood involving vomiting and diarrhea probably approaches that of respiratory infections, and these problems may accompany such infections. In most cases it is not practical to determine the etiology of the disorder, but some indication of community and family epidemiology is helpful in making an early determination that a minor communicable disorder is probably the cause.

### Pathophysiologic considerations

As discussed in Chapter 9, the gastrointestinal tract of the infant is characterized normally by more rapid movement of food through the system than is typical for the older child or adult. This gradually declines, and at some point during early childhood the motility of the bowel begins to resemble that of the adult. The absorptive capacity of each section of the bowel assumes adultlike function.

When viral infection strikes the gastrointestinal tract, absorptive function decreases or ceases, and motility is greatly increased. This

*References 8, 118, 124, 134.

causes the resulting symptoms of vomiting and/or diarrhea. Absorption of the fluid products of digestion in the upper tract is not accomplished, and the contents are moved quickly out of the system. Although such an occurrence is relatively common and is usually brief during early childhood, the consequences of this rapid loss may be grave for the infant and young child.

Bacterial infections of the bowel, on the other hand, generally involve more serious signs of illness and there are typical clinical traits that can lead to differential diagnosis of the specific causative organism. *Salmonella* and *Shigella* infections produce severe abdominal pain and watery green or greenish yellow stool that contains pus, mucus, and blood. The normal course of the disease lasts as long as ten days to two weeks. The odor of the stool is characteristic for each offending organism, and although this is not a diagnostic tool, it may be useful in differentiating the incidence of viral infection in which the odor is not as strong or offensive.

In addition to the dangers of loss of fluids, the accompanying loss of electrolytes presents a serious hazard for the infant and young child. The increased percentage of fluid in the extracellular spaces renders fluid losses more readily vulnerable, and the resulting imbalance in fluid and electrolyte composition of interstitial and intracellular spaces presents a serious threat. When the loss of solutes (particularly sodium, potassium, and chloride) is in proportion to the net loss of water, the loss is considered isotonic and the replacement needs for both components equal the proportions normally found in body extracellular fluids. When the proportion of solute loss exceeds the proportion of water loss, the dehydration is termed hypotonic. When the loss of water exceeds the proportion of net loss of solutes, the dehydration is termed hypertonic. In infants and young children the loss from diarrhea and vomiting is initially assumed to be isotonic for purposes of instituting immediate therapy. Further medical diagnosis of the losses is then pursued to determine the exact range of net replacement of fluid and solutes that is needed (see Chapter 16).

The electrolyte composition of the extracellular spaces of the infant and young child differs significantly from that of the older child and adult, and this fact is important in estimating replacement needs. In comparison to the adult, these spaces in the young child contain *more* phosphorus and chloride, *less* bicarbonate and protein, and the *same* amount of potassium and sodium. Metabolic acidosis that results from water and electrolyte losses in vomiting and diarrhea yields increased hydrogen ion activity in the body. This results primarily from the losses of metabolic components that ordinarily participate in the buffering of $H^+$ activity. Respiratory, blood, and renal mechanisms to establish homeostasis and balance in the system may not be able to keep up with the losses that are occurring without therapeutic intervention. Hydrogen and sodium ions enter the cells from the extracellular spaces, and potassium leaves the cells under conditions of acidosis, causing an increase in extracellular potassium and a condition of hyperkalemia.

There are four major reasons for the young infant's and child's increased susceptibility to dangerous effects of changes in water and electrolytes compared with the older child and adult. These may be summarized as:

1. The already existing higher metabolic rate placed a greater stress on the system during times of imbalance; the energy needed to restore homeostasis above the ordinary maintenance requirements is quickly depleted.
2. There is decreased glomerular filtration, and the renal-hormonal axis involving the parathyroid, adrenal cortex, and pituitary is not able to respond reliably under stress. Thus electrolyte balance and water conservation or elimination in response to changes in the system do not occur with the same facility as in the older person.
3. The buffer system of the intracellular spaces involving the glutamine and carbonic anhydrase systems is thought to be inefficient in the young child, particularly in the renal epithelium.
4. The presence of a larger volume of water within the extracellular spaces places water and extracellular electrolytes in a position for ready loss.[137,147,148,209,242]

Rehydration of the young child must be done with great care, particularly when the degree of dehydration is severe. Medical intervention is imperative in judicious use of parenteral fluids to replace losses. Nursing and medical management together assure that overhydration does not occur when the losses have been compensated. In addition the type of dehydration that has occurred is important in determining the proportion of electrolytes to administer (see Chapter 16).

### Nursing criteria for diagnosis of vomiting and diarrhea (MNPC no. 350.4)

As in the case of nursing diagnosis of the common cold, the presence of subjective symptoms of illness does not suffice in formulating a sound, definitive statement of the problem. Several factors are determined in the process of ruling out the presence of serious, complex disease processes and dangerous states of dehydration. When the limitations of all aspects of the nursing diagnosis are demonstrated, nursing management of the problem is safely indicated. The criteria that must be demonstrated include:

1. Subjective presence of vomiting and diarrhea of prior duration not longer than 24 hours.

    RATIONALE: Vomiting and diarrhea that have persisted longer than 24 hours in an infant or young child may have produced fluid and electrolyte hazards requiring medical evaluation.

2. Documentation of absence of definitive signs of serious illness, including:

    a. Abdomen: No masses palpated. no abdominal enlargement, absence of localized pain, abdominal palpation does not produce signs of pain, although some tenderness may be present.

    b. Chest and respiratory system: no evidence of serious respiratory infection.

    c. Neurologic: no signs of meningeal irritation.

    d. Urine: results of screening for protein and sugar and blood cells are normal.

    e. Characteristics of stool and/or vomitus: no evidence of blood in stool or vomitus, absence of bile staining or fecal odor in vomitus.

    RATIONALE: Presence of these signs and symptoms suggests the possibility of serious problems requiring medical evaluation.

3. Documentation of estimated urinary output over the past 24 hours; specific gravity of a current sample of urine to approximate 1.015 and not to exceed 0.1030.

    RATIONALE: Decreased urinary output and concentration of urine reflects a physiologic response to conserve water in the face of dehydration.

4. Documentation of today's weight and, if possible, a percentage estimate of any weight loss that may have occurred since the onset of illness (weight loss not to exceed 5% of initial body weight).

    RATIONALE: A weight loss that remains under 5% of initial body weight represents mild dehydration that can be controlled with management of oral fluids if the child continues to retain sufficient intake.

5. Documentation of body temperature; not to exceed 24 hours prior duration or 104° F.

    RATIONALE: Accompanying fever may indicate serious illness or place the child in a situation of risk for rapid dehydration; medical evaluation may be required.

6. Documentation of other signs of adequate hydration:

    a. Fontanel retains normal tension and is not depressed.

    b. Skin turgor is normal.

    c. Mucous membranes are moist.

    d. Tearing is normal.

    RATIONALE: These signs of adequate hydration support the estimates of adequate hydration as determined by body weight estimate and urinary output estimate.[50,130]

Clinical signs of the state of hydration of the young infant may be nonspecific and difficult to determine, but every effort should be made to determine possible dehydration or overhydration. These signs are reflected in the criteria for nursing diagnosis and as such serve as a reliable and useful guide in estimating hydration level of a young child in any setting. For example, the young child who is receiving parenteral therapy in the hospital may be periodically evaluated on the basis of these criteria (criterion numbers 3 to 6, particularly) in order to provide a comparative documentation of the level of hydration achieved from one time to another.

Specific signs of dehydration in an infant and young child include:

1. Dry skin, parched tongue, sunken eyeballs, sunken fontanel
2. Decreased urinary output
3. Specific gravity of the urine greater than 1.030
4. Recent weight loss of over 5% of initial body weight

Overhydration, on the other hand, is signaled by the following signs:

1. Increased urinary output
2. Weakness, lethargy, drowsiness
3. Vomiting
4. Edema, sudden weight gain
5. Coma and delirium (resulting from intracellular edema)
6. Convulsions

### Nursing intervention

Specific management of vomiting and diarrhea is open to challenge and controversy, because sound scientific evidence is not presently available upon which to base rational therapeutic approaches. The following recommendations appear to represent a consensus expressed in the literature and provide for clinical evaluation of effects of therapy.

Interventions for vomiting and diarrhea are essentially the same and thus are considered together. When the child has difficulty retaining fluids because of nausea and vomiting, some intervention can be attempted without the use of drugs, but medical attention must be sought when these measures are not effective.

The first objectives of therapy are to give the gastrointestinal tissues a rest, to replace minimal deficits of fluids and electrolytes, to keep up with losses, and to provide for continuing maintenance needs. Thus the ordinary diet of the child is halted, and only clear isotonic liquids are given. Infants on formula only may be given an isotonic electrolyte solution prepared commercially (Lytren, Pedialyte) or a homemade solution that meets the basic electrolyte requirements of the body. Homemade solutions present specific hazards, in that they must be cautiously prepared to meet isotonic require-

ments. Accidental hypertonic or hypotonic solutions can render more damage to the young child and create a major medical problem. Therefore, homemade solutions must be carefully and judiciously used, if used at all. A standard prescription calls for 3 tablespoons of sugar, ½ level teaspoon of salt (not to exceed), and 1 quart of water.[52,68] In many instances, clear apple juice, soda pop, or Jello water is readily available. This provides a suitable solution for the infant or young child and avoids the hazard of error in the preparation of a homemade solution.

Children of preschool age may be placed on the same type of clear liquid diet; soda crackers may be taken as the appetite allows; they provide a suitable source of sodium and chloride. This diet is maintained for at least 24 hours. The liquids are offered frequently in small amounts so that retention of about 150 ml/kg/24 hours is assured. If the symptoms have not subsided within 24 hours, reevaluation of the condition of the child is imperative, especially to determine any changes in body weight, urinary output and specific gravity, and body temperature. As the child improves, half-strength formula may be instituted and continued for an additional 24 hours. Subsequently a soft diet may be given. These measures may be continued and progressively advanced to include the regular diet unless symptoms recur.[16,24,102,199]

Loss of body fluids through insensible losses may be diminished by providing a high ambient humidity and cool ambient temperature. Controlling excessive body temperature when fever is present also prevents excessive body fluid loss resulting from the mechanisms needed to bring high body temperature into normal ranger.[53,69,197,214]

When nausea and vomiting interfere with the ability of the young child to retain fluids, several measures may be attempted to promote retention of the needed amounts of fluid. Offering very small amounts of fluid may provide enough retained fluid to meet intake needs until the nausea subsides and the child is able to take greater amounts. Coca-cola has antiemetic properties, and the plain syrup base may be used; however, Coca-cola has a high concentration of potassium and may lead to a dangerous level of hyperkalemia, particularly in the presence of metabolic acidosis. A single dose of 1 teaspoon of Coke syrup usually suffices in minor episodes of nausea in children, and mothers should be cautioned about repeating the dosage. Simply drinking the carbonated beverage may allay nausea, and the less concentrated form of the beverage does not present the hazard of the syrup.[68]

This example of a home remedy points out the fact that many such remedies have a sound therapeutic basis and they may offer a real advantage over the use of drugs. However, when used and recommended professionally, all aspects of composition, electrolyte effect, relative advantages and risks, appropriate use, and dosage must be understood as for a drug, and the remedies must be used with sound judgment.

Antiemetics, sedatives, and antidiarrhea preparations are not recommended for use with young children, as these drugs are potentially hazardous either by virtue of their potential toxicity to the child or because of the dangers of compounding the child's problems in maintaining adequate fluid and electrolyte balance. Further, these drugs do not benefit the child in terms of alleviating the underlying pathophysiology of the illness. The family needs to be cautioned not to use medications available on a nonprescription basis. Providing the family with specific instructions regarding dietary management and careful follow-through to monitor the child's progress will enhance their confidence in being able to adequately care for the child without resorting to unnecessary drugs.[68,69]

### Gastrointestinal problems requiring nurse-physician collaboration

**Rumination syndrome.** Rumination is a voluntary regurgitation of ingested food followed by rechewing and reswallowing of portions of the regurgitated food. It is a serious emotional disorder of infancy arising from an inadequate mother-infant relationship and occurs predominantly in infants from poverty-stricken environments. The rumination usually begins between 3 and 6 months of age and may continue for several years. Significant amounts of fluids, electrolytes, and nutrients can be lost, resulting in fluid depletion, electrolyte imbalance, or failure to thrive. The act of ruminating may escape the attention of people in the environment, as the infant tends to ruminate when left alone and when there are no distractions in the environment. Recognition of the possibility of this problem in susceptible infants can lead to indepth assessment that identifies the physiologic state of the infant and the social factors that have contributed to the development of the problem. Intervention consists of correcting fluid, electrolyte, and nutritional problems as rapidly as possible and providing the infant with emotional nurturing and planned stimulation. Negative approaches, such as punishment for ruminating or restraining the infant who uses fingers or objects to stimulate regurgitation, are ineffective.[59,69,214]

**Acute gastroenteritis.** Acute gastroenteritis is most often caused by one of three organisms: enteropathogenic *Escherichia coli*, *Salmonella*, or *Shigella*. *E. coli* causes clinical illness in young infants and children more frequently than in older children or adults. The organism is acquired through contact with hands, linen, or objects that have come in contact with comtaminated feces of another ill individual. The illness is characterized by a sudden onset of explosive watery stools, mild fever, and vomiting in a newborn infant. Young children under the age of 2 years who are affected have a more gradual onset of foul-smelling, slimy, green diarrhea. Fever is minimal, and no vomiting is present. In addition to management of fluid and electrolyte balance, antibiotics to which the organism is sensitive are given. Neomycin is usually effective, and is given in doses of 100 mg/kg/day orally in three divided doses.[57,60,68,159]

Salmonella gastroenteritis is acquired by ingestion of the bacteria from contaminated food or water or by direct contact with contaminated hands or handled objects. Within several hours to three days after contact, the young child exhibits diarrhea, fever, and vomiting. The older child may complain of headache, nausea, and abdominal pain. Diarrhea may be mild to severe and may be watery or contain mucus and in some instances blood. Children under 6 years of age are most frequently affected, and in infants and young children the complications of meningitis and septicemia can occur rapidly.

The symptoms subside within two to four days, and the primary concern is management of fluids and electrolytes. If no complications occur, antibiotic therapy is of little value and may prolong the carrier state of the infant after the infection has run its course.[60,68,159]

*Shigella* organisms are believed to enter the system through the alimentary tract by contact with contaminated people, animals, food, or water. Shigellosis is a serious illness in children under 2 years of age, with a significant mortality rate. The illness is milder in older children. The onset is sudden with abdominal cramping, bloody diarrhea, pus and mucus in the stools, and high fever. The young child may appear lethargic and disoriented, and convulsions can occur. Respiratory symptoms of bronchitis are often present. Often, other members of the family have or recently have had a mild episode of diarrhea. Rapid dehydration is a major threat to the young child, and management of fluids and electrolytes is essential. Ampicillin is usually given intravenously, intramuscularly, or orally in doses of 100 mg/kg/day in four divided doses for five days.[59,60,159]

**Enterobiasis (pinworms).** Pinworm infections are common occurrences worldwide. The infection leads to no serious complications, but the primary manifestation, intense itching of the anus, is bothersome. Often several members of a household are infected, acquiring the worms from ova deposited on clothing, bedding, and hands. The child experiences itching primarily at night and usually scratches the area, depositing ova under the fingernails and transferring them to the mouth, which results in autoinfection. In young girls, vaginitis and pruritis vulvae may also occur. The adult worms reside in the cecum and colon, and gravid females deposit ova in the skinfolds of the anus, especially at night, which causes the itching. The diagnosis is established by a simple tape test. Transparent adhesive tape is applied to the anus and the perianal skin, preferably early in the morning before defecation or washing. The tape is then examined on a glass slide under a microscope to determine the presence of ova. To prevent cross-infection, all members of the household are usually treated. The drug of choice is pyrantel pamoate, given in a single dose of 11 mg/kg,

not to exceed 1 g. Nursing measures include counseling with the family regarding personal hygiene, including clipping of nails and handwashing, and frequent laundering of bed linens and clothing until the infection has been eliminated.[110]

### Infections manifested in the skin (MNPC no. 350.7)
*Pathophysiologic considerations*

The infant and young child's particular susceptibility to skin infection and the immunologic function of the skin and mucous membranes have been discussed in Chapter 9. The infant gradually gains maturity of the skin surface, and the problems of the skin begin to exhibit different characteristics.

The seemingly endless occurrence of skin rashes that many young children suffer may be the result of local or systemic infections or allergies. The infections considered here are those that tend to occur most commonly during infancy or early childhood, and they involve the physiologic characteristics of both the skin and the immunologic competence of the child.

Rashes occurring on the skin of young children are to be fully documented as to the nature of the rash at the time it is observed. Rashes may be described as to color and shading that occur in various areas of the lesion. They may be described as macular (a rash that discolors the skin but is not raised), papular (a raised rash), vesicular (lesions that contain clear fluid), pustular (lesions containing pus), or crusted (lesions that become crusted in the healing stages). Rashes should also be described as to distribution in specific areas of the body and in regard to duration. Exanthemas are rashes that are present on the external skin of the body; enanthemas are those present on mucosal tissues.

### Nursing diagnosis and intervention for local infections

A common skin infection during infancy and early childhood is invasion by either staphylococcal and streptococcal organisms or both, which create the superficial lesions known as impetigo. Nursing criteria for diagnosis of impetigo may include:

1. Documented subjective history of skin le-

sions such as scratches or insect bites. **RATIONALE:** Bacterial entry to the skin is gained through skin lesions in impetigo.

2. Discrete, isolated lesions are observed primarily on exposed surfaces of the body, such as face and extremities.
   **RATIONALE:** Impetigo typically occurs on these surfaces where scratches and minor cuts occur.

3. Early lesions are vesicular, progressing to a pustular and then to a crusting stage.
   **RATIONALE:** Various stages of development of lesions may be objectively observed, confirming the characteristic progression of impetigo lesions.

4. When the crust is removed, a red, inflamed corium is exposed.
   **RATIONALE:** Objective observation of the appearance of the corium suggests the presence of impetigo.

5. Local lymph nodes may be swollen and inflamed.
   **RATIONALE:** Lymph node enlargement may accompany an impetigo infection.

6. Other signs and symptoms of systemic illness are not present.
   **RATIONALE:** Signs and symptoms of systemic illness indicate extensive infection or an accompanying illness, which requires further evaluation.[55,60,162,211]

Impetigo is extremely contagious and is transferred to other areas of the child's body by his own contaminated hands, particularly where superficial scratches cause an opening. Other children also are subject to acquiring the infection by contact with the infected child.

Cultures of the infected lesions may be of interest, but the highly specific clinical description of the infection leaves little doubt as to its type. The lesions leave no scar when healed, indicating that involvement is only in the superficial layers of the skin. However, the serious sequelae of streptococcal infection, particularly acute glomerulitis, are reliably documented in relation to impetigo, and thus vigorous treatment is indicated.

Nursing management of impetigo includes implementing medical antibiotic treatment that will effectively combat the organism cultured from the lesion. When culture evidence is not obtained, an antibiotic is chosen that will effectively combat the possible staphylococcal and streptococcal infection. The drug of choice is penicillin in a dose of 50 to 100 mg/kg/24 hours divided into three to four equal doses. The antibiotic must be administered for a period of ten days if an oral drug is used in order to effectively provide protection against the serious sequelae of the renal system.[60,66]

Local treatment is also indicated. This includes removal of the scabs to expose the red area of involvement, thorough cleansing of the area, and application of topical antibiotic ointment. The scabs must be removed in order for the topical preparation to be effective; this may be accomplished with a minimum of pain and discomfort by soaking the scabs in warm water (a wet pack may be used on the face) and carefully removing the softened scab.

Impetigo arises primarily under conditions where adequate hygiene is neglected, either because of the living conditions of the family or because the children play in areas that expose them to an unusual amount of infected dirt and bacterial growth. For example, a child may play in a yard or field rich with animal wastes and may fail to adequately wash and bathe when returning home. The family may need to examine all possible sources of infection and take measures to prevent the repeated recurrence of the problem.[30,162,163]

**Fungal infections of the skin.** Ringworm is a condition caused by invasion of the superficial layers of the skin by dermatophytes such as *Microsporum canis* and *Trichophyton verrucosum*. The organism grows mainly in the stratum corneum, releasing toxins that result in dermatitis. The appearance of the skin lesion varies. When the infection occurs on the scalp (tinea capitis), thickened, broken-off hairs and erythema and scaling of the scalp are observed. Pustular lesions and a boggy fluctuant mass may be observed. On other areas of the body (tinea corporis), the lesions appear as annular marginated papules with a thin scale and clear center or as an annular confluent dermatitis. The lesions usually fluoresce yellow-green with a Wood's lamp. Topical application of tolnaftate (Tinactin) two to three times daily is usually sufficient to clear the infection. If the

**407**

hair or nail beds are involved, griseofulvin taken orally is required. The dose is 10 to 20 mg/kg/day, continued for six weeks to three months.[162,236]

*Candida albicans* is an organism that invades the oral mucosa and diaper area of infants, causing a condition known as thrush. In the mouth it produces thick white patches with an erythematous base that cannot be removed with a cotton-tipped swab. In the diaper area it produces a bright red diffuse dermatitis. The infant becomes fussy and irritable and refuses to suck. An oral suspension of nystatin (Mycostatin) is given in a dose of 1 ml four times a day for week. Topical application of a cream form of nystatin can be applied to the involved diaper area every three to four hours.[204,236]

### Systemic infections manifested in the skin

Many of the acute exanthematous illnesses that afflict young children are so similar that they may not be distinguishable on the basis of clinical signs and symptoms. Differentiation is important, however, in cases where the nature of the disease has serious implications for others who may be exposed, as when a woman in the first trimester of pregnancy may be exposed to a child with rubella. Although differentiation is often a medical diagnostic problem, a careful nursing interview and history with documentation of the nature of the rash and the systemic signs of illness may provide a sound basis for nursing identification of a particular communicable disease.

The epidemiologic nature of these illnesses often delays exposure and subsequent infection until the child enters day care, nursery school, or school. Infants are prone to develop each of the infections after maternally acquired immunity is lost through contact with a sibling who attends school. Some of the infections are age-limited; they tend to occur only in children within a certain age group. The exact mechanism by which this phenomenon occurs is not clearly understood, but it may be due to the level of active immunity that is acquired, possible universal exposure to the infectious agent during this age period with subclinical occurrences of the illness, or a particular age-dependent interaction that occurs during the susceptible period.

The child's exposure to epidemiologic factors, past history of infectious illness, and immunization history are important in determining the nature of the condition and in ruling out a possible allergic origin. Further, the various acute exanthematous illnesses may be differentiated by three major features of the illness itself: (1) the nature of the prodromal period, or the period just before the appearance of the rash, (2) characteristics of the rash itself, including description of the lesions, distribution, and changes over a period of time, and (3) the presence and nature of accompanying signs of illness or epidemiologic features. In some cases it is not possible to definitively identify specific disease until the full course of the illness has passed. Complete documentation of the full course of an illness is important for knowledge of epidemiologic factors that may be affecting other children. A record of the first two or three children who appear with an illness later documented as exanthema subitum is important in helping other families to know that this particular illness is circulating among young children in the community.[23,49]

The various features of several of the common exanthematous rashes seen during early childhood will be described, including some illnesses that are now preventable through immunization procedures. Fig. 11-16 contrasts some of the features that are described.

**Chickenpox.** Usually there is no prodromal period in young children. Older children and adults may experience a one- or two-day period of fever, headache, malaise, and anorexia before onset of the rash. The rash is specifically characterized by the rapid evolution of the macules to papules, then to vesicles, and finally to crusts. The rash appears most densely on the trunk and sparsely on the face and extremities. Lesions in all stages of development appear in any one anatomic area, including the scalp and the mucous membranes. The child is infectious from several hours prior to the appearance of the first lesion to about the fifth day thereafter. The incubation period is from 12 to 21 days. Transmission appears to be directly from the lesions and by droplet infection.[27,124]

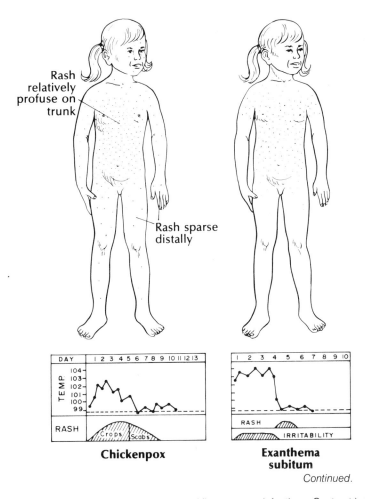

Rash
relatively
profuse on
trunk

Rash sparse
distally

**Chickenpox**

**Exanthema
subitum**

*Continued.*

**Fig. 11-16.** The differences in distribution of rashes of five common infections. Contrast in the accompanying signs and symptoms is indicated. (Adapted from Krugman, S., and Ward, R.: Infectious diseases of children and adults, ed. 5, St. Louis, 1973, The C. V. Mosby Co.)

Complications of chickenpox are uncommon. Secondary bacterial infection of the lesions can occur if the child scratches and adequate measures for maintaining body hygiene are not achieved. Permanent scarring is not common but can be minimized by minimizing scratching and manipulation of the lesions. Itching can be controlled by frequent warm bathing and soaking in water to which baking soda is added. Sedative antihistamines may be considered if the child is extremely uncomfortable and irritable. Antipyretic drugs and other measures to control body temperature are used as indicated. The child should remain isolated from other young children until all of the lesions have dried to the crust stage.[76] Since most children do not feel ill during the major course of the disease, the family is faced with the stress of providing activity and diversion for an active young child who must be relatively isolated. Nursing counsel and guidance in coping with this stress is indicated.

**Enteroviral infections.** Coxsackie virus and enteric cytopathogenic human orphan (ECHO) viruses types 4, 6, and 9 have a very brief, if any, prodromal period; the fever and constitutional symptoms usually coincide with the onset of the rash. ECHO virus type 16 may have a

**409**

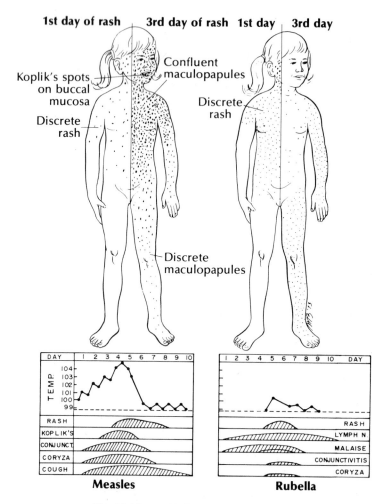

**Fig. 11-16, cont'd.** For legend see p. 409.

three- or four-day prodromal period with moderate fever and irritability. The rash of these infections is maculopapular, discrete, not itchy, and evenly distributed over the entire body. It fades without staining or desquamation. These infections occur most commonly in the summer and fall months. Young children are particularly susceptible to the viruses. The incubation period ranges from 2 to 15 days, and the child is infectious during the time the rash is apparent. Transmission is by respiratory droplets and mechanical spread by various flying insects.[111,124]

Treatment consists of management of the symptoms of fever and irritability. Antipyretic drugs and environmental measures are used to control the fever. The family should be counseled regarding isolating the child until the contagious stage is passed and providing comfort for the young child.

**Erythema infectiosum.** Usually there is no prodromal period; the appearance of the rash is the first sign of illness. The rash begins unaccompanied by other signs of illness and erupts first as a red, flushed-cheek appearance (slapped face appearance) with circumoral pallor, followed by a maculopapular rash over the arms and legs, and finally a gradual fading of the rash in a lacelike appearance. Recurrence of the rash may be precipitated by a variety of skin irritants. Usually the child remains well throughout the course of the infection. Young children

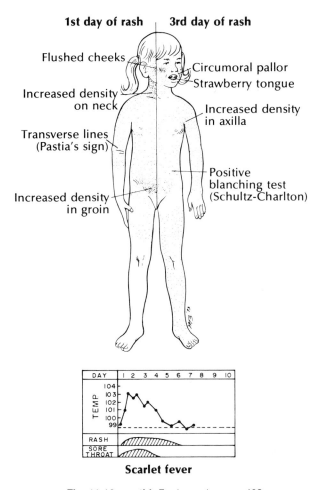

**1st day of rash** | **3rd day of rash**

Flushed cheeks

Circumoral pallor
Strawberry tongue

Increased density
on neck

Increased density
in axilla

Transverse lines
(Pastia's sign)

Positive
blanching test
(Schultz-Charlton)

Increased density
in groin

**Scarlet fever**

**Fig. 11-16, cont'd.** For legend see p. 409.

are primarily affected, and transmission seems to be by droplet infection. The incubation period is estimated to be between 4 and 14 days.[124,125]

**Exanthema subitum (roseola).** There is a three- or four-day prodromal period with a high fever (104° F or higher) and irritability but no other signs of illness. The rash is a typical rose-red maculopapular rash, which usually appears first on the chest and trunk and then spreads to the face and extremities. This lasts from several hours to two days. With the appearance of the rash the fever suddenly subsides, and the child begins to feel well again. Leukopenia may be observed with the appearance of the rash. About 95% of all cases of this illness occur in young children under 30 months of age. The incubation period seems to be about 10 days, but the means of transmission and the period when the disease is definitely contagious are not known. Many subclinical cases of the illness may exist, in which the fever and/or the rash never appear.[124,244]

Intervention is directed primarily to the control of fever during the period prior to onset of the rash. The management approaches described for acute febrile states are implemented, with particular attention to measures to prevent spiking of the temperature and the possibility of febrile convulsion. If the child is under 2 years of age and there is a known incidence of roseola in the community, the family can be

**411**

forewarned that the febrile state may be indicative of this infection and informed of the probable course of the illness.[76]

**Measles (rubeola).** This illness, which is now preventable through immunization, may still be encountered in nonimmunized children. There is a prodromal period of three or four days with fever, conjunctivitis, coryza, and cough. The rash is reddish-brown. It appears first on the face and neck and progresses down to involve the trunk and extremities (see Fig. 11-16). By the third day all parts of the body are involved. The rash on the face, neck, and upper trunk tends to become confluent, whereas the rash on the lower trunk and extremities has a more discrete appearance. By the fifth day the rash begins to fade, with brownish staining and desquamation occurring except on the hands and feet. Children who have received the measles vaccine may, several years later, exhibit an unusual variation of the illness with a mild rash that mimics that of Rocky Mountain spotted fever. Koplik's spots—white desquamated areas on the buccal membranes of the mouth—are the typical diagnostic sign of measles. The child is infectious during the prodromal period and for five or six days after the rash appears. Transmission is from person to person by droplet infection. The incubation period is about ten days. A measles hemagglutination-inhibition test provides an important laboratory diagnosis for children who need to be definitively identified, particularly among those who were previously vaccinated.[101,124,228]

Measles is a severe infection with a high risk of serious complications. The most serious complication is encephalitis, which can result in permanent disability or death. It is believed that the measles virus, which remains latent in the neural cells of infected infants and children, causes a progressive degenerative central nervous system disease years after the initial infection, known as subacute sclerosing panencephalitis. Upper and lower bacterial respiratory tract infections, particularly otitis media and pneumonia, occur in about 15% of all instances of measles infection. Bacterial conjunctivitis is common. Thrombocytopenia and gastrointestinal and cardiac complications occur in some cases.

Good nursing care is essential for the child with measles. The nurse should provide direct assistance to the family in the home to assure their ability to institute specific measures for care of the child. Measures for control of fever and relief of cough, described in earlier sections of this chapter, are essential. Percussion of the chest and saline nose drops are used to provide adequate exchange of gases and prevent serious respiratory infection. Meticulous body hygiene and care of the environment reduces the chances of secondary infection. Of particular concern is care of conjunctiva. Regular cleansing of the conjunctiva with a saline wash helps to prevent secondary infection and provides a soothing effect. The family may need assistance in discovering ways to provide comfort and diversion for the child, such as reading to the child, playing quiet games, or providing music. The child should remain isolated from other children until the rash and cough have subsided, usually a period of seven to ten days after the appearance of symptoms. The nurse should assess the immunization status of all children in the community when an outbreak of measles occurs and take measures to provide for their immunization.[76]

**Rocky Mountain spotted fever.** Fever, chills, headache, joint pains, malaise, and anorexia precede the rash by three or four days. The rash is maculopapular and petechial, with a centrifugal distribution. The palms of the hands and soles of the feet are often involved, and occasionally the face is involved. There is usually a history of a recent tick bite, which is the only mode of transmission. A specific Rocky Mountain spotted fever complement fixation test is available for definitive diagnosis. Nervous system and cardiovascular involvement lead to a wide range of ominous symptoms, and there is about a 20% death rate among affected persons of all ages. Specific antibiotic treatment administered early in the course of the disease is the most important factor in preventing fatality. Recovery is slow and may not be complete for several months.[104,124,243]

**Rubella.** This illness is preventable with immunization protection. In young children the prodromal period may not be clinically present or obvious. The lymphadenopathy is asymptomatic, and if the child has a low-grade fever or feels tired, it is often not clinically obvious. In older children and adults these symptoms are present for one to four days prior to onset of the rash. The rash is pink. It begins to appear on the face and neck and progresses downward to the trunk and extremities, covering the entire body within 48 hours. The lesions are usually discrete, and those that appear first fade first. Within three days the initial lesions are fading, and only the extremities may be involved. The illness is not discomforting to the young child, but may produce fever, lymphadenopathy and joint pains in older children and adults. A positive throat culture for the rubella virus may be obtained as a definitive diagnostic sign. The period of infectiousness is from about one week prior to the rash to about five days after it appears. Transmission is by droplet infection, and the incubation period is from 14 to 21 days.[124,210,227]

Specific intervention consists of symptomatic treatment of any signs of illness that the child exhibits. The primary concern is study of the epidemiology of the illness and identification of any possible contact with pregnant women or susceptible young children in a family where a woman is pregnant. The pregnant woman's previous immunization record is studied, and if indicated her immunity status may be determined. All young children who are susceptible to the infection should be immunized.

**Scarlet fever.** Fever, sore throat, and vomiting begins within 12 hours of onset of the rash. The rash is an erythematous punctiform type of lesion, which balances on pressure. It first appears on the flexural surfaces of the arms, legs, and groin, and rapidly becomes generalized. Desquamation is characteristic and involves the hands and feet. A strawberry appearance of the tongue and exudative or membranous tonsillitis are typically present. Group A beta hemolytic streptococci are cultured from the throat.[124,229] The incubation period from the time of intimate contact with the pathogen is 48 to 72 hours. The incidence is highest in young children and during the cold months.

Antibiotic treatment with 800,000 to 1.2 million units of oral penicillin for ten days is the preferred approach to control of the infection and to prevention of the serious cardiac and renal sequelae that develop from a streptococcal infection. Nursing intervention for the mild discomforts associated with the illness is implemented as needed. Family members and other children with whom the child has been associated should be cultured for the presence of streptococcal organisms in the throat and treated with appropriate antibiotic therapy.[34,60]

### Allergies (MNPC no. 313)
*Pathophysiologic considerations*

The allergic response is initiated by entry into the system of antigens, which are also called allergens because of their ability to stimulate an allergic reaction. The portal of entry is through the respiratory tract, the skin, or the gastrointestinal tract. Fig. 11-17 depicts the basic concepts of the allergic response. When the allergen enters, the antibody-producing cells, or immunoblasts, in the system produce antibodies that may be any one of five classes—IgG, IgM, IgA, IgD, or IgE. Immunoblasts include lymphocytes and plasma cells found in the lining of the respiratory and alimentary tracts, lymph nodes, and circulating blood. The antibodies that are produced affix themselves in some manner to basophils and tissue mast cells, and the individual is sentitized to the allergen. When another encounter with the allergen occurs, several types of allergic reactions may result. Fig. 11-17 illustrates the basic concepts of the atopic allergic reaction. The antigen comes in contact with the antibody that is fixed on the target cell and causes a reaction that activates an enzymatic chain of responses that breaks down the sensitized target cell and releases components such as histamines, slow-reacting substance of anaphylaxis (SRS-A), bradykinin, and eosinophilic chemotactic factor of anaphylaxis (ECF-A). Histamine causes contraction of smooth muscle adjacent to the site of release, as occurs in the bronchi during an asthmatic attack; capillary permeability between the endothelial cells with leakage of intravascular fluids into the tissues, which results in edema; and stimulation of mucus production by mucus glands and cells. SRS-A produces marked prolonged smooth muscle constriction. Bradykinin produces mucus secretion, edema, and smooth

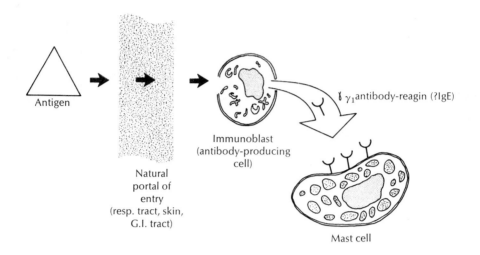

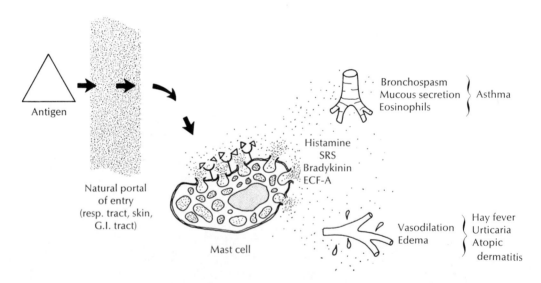

**Fig. 11-17.** Atopic sensitization and reaction.

muscle constriction. ECF-A appears to exert a negative feedback control on the allergic reaction, for the action of ECF-A causes eosinophils to be attracted to the area where the response has occurred, and the eosinophils destroy or inactivate the antigen-antibody complexes. Eosinophils also contain a natural antihistaminic compound that breaks the SRS-A molecule into inactive fragments.[72]

Allergic reactions have been classified as four types, each of which has specific characteristics, but any one or several of the types of reactions can occur simultaneously. These types of responses are as follows:

1. *Type I reaction (anaphylactic-atopic).* This is essentially the reaction illustrated in Fig. 11-15 and described above. When the potent chemicals of histamine, SRS-A, and bradykinins are released, these chemicals affect adjacent tissue cells and cause extreme responses of smooth muscle constriction, leakage of capillary endothelial cells, and stimulation of mucus-producing cells. This reaction produces the symptoms of anaphylaxis. This type of reaction occurs only in individuals who have a genetic predisposition for sensitization to selected antigens.

2. *Type II reaction (cytolytic or cytotoxic).* This type of reaction usually involves antibodies of the IgG or IgM class that activate complement components and result in the breakdown of selected cells. Usually the cell that is lysed, or destroyed, is the target cell itself, or the cell to which the antibody is fixed. An example of this type of reaction is the hemolytic anemia secondary to penicillin-sensitizing red cells. Many kinds of autoimmune reactions are probably of this type, wherein the alteration of the body cell that occurs with the fixing of the antibody causes the body cell to be recognized as foreign, and the body uses the immunologic mechanism to get rid of the "foreign" element.

3. *Type III reaction (Arthus or toxis-complex).* In this type of reaction the antibody is not fixed to a target cell surface, but rather complexes of free antigen and antibody circulate in the blood and tissue fluids. These complexes activate the complement cycle that is chemotactic for leukocytes. Edema, ischemia, and necrosis of the region result. Allergic reactions of the skin are usually of this type.

4. *Type IV reaction (cellular immune or delayed hypersensitivity).* In a type IV reaction, sensitized lymphocytes cause the release of lymphokines, which in turn affect other adjacent cells, causing an inflammatory response. Contact dermatitis is usually this type of response.

The relationship between age and the development of allergic responses has been observed but is not clearly understood. Early in infancy, foods are the most predominant source of allergens that cause the allergic response. The

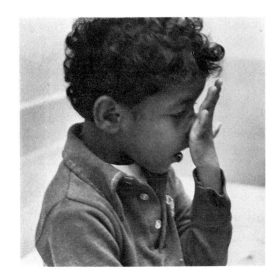

**Fig. 11-18.** The allergic salute.

response during infancy and early childhood is most often in the skin. Contact dermatitis also occurs with frequency during infancy. As the child matures, inhalant allergens become more important and respiratory symptoms of allergic reactions begin to develop with greater frequency. It is recognized that many older children and adults who develop serious forms of allergy have a history of more mild forms of allergy from infancy and early childhood, even though the allergens and the responses to the allergens change over the life span.[72,175]

### Nursing diagnosis and intervention for allergic rhinitis

Allergic rhinitis is a common problem for young children and may occur throughout the year or seasonally. An allergen such as a pollen grain enters the respiratory system and is absorbed. The allergic response illustrated in Fig. 11-17 occurs in the nasal submucosa and causes the release of histamine, SRS-A, and ECF-A. These substances cause increased vascular permeability, itching, secretion of watery mucus, and eosinophil infiltration into the area. The nasal symptoms may be accompanied by itching of the soft palate and the eyes, with excessive tearing and conjunctival injection. The child's voice may sound hoarse, and there may be a hacking cough stimulated by a postnasal drip.

**415**

The child is often a mouth breather and snores during sleep. The symptoms may be worse in the early morning hours, and the child may complain of a sore throat in the morning, which is due to drying which occurs as a result of mouth breathing. A distinctive mannerism of young children with allergic rhinitis is the "allergic salute" in which the child repeatedly rubs the nose in an upward motion with the palm of the hand.

Recommended criteria for nursing diagnosis of allergic rhinitis are:

1. Subjective history and objective observation of persistent coryza, which may be accompanied by any of the following symptoms:
   a. Hacking, nonproductive cough
   b. Hoarseness of the voice
   c. Mouth breathing
   d. Morning sore throat that disappears within an hour or two
   e. Itchiness and excessive tearing of the eyes
   f. Enlargement of the tonsils and adenoids
   g. Allergic salute or facial grimaces accompanied by "sniffling"

   RATIONALE: These signs and symptoms constitute the typical clinical picture of allergic rhinitis.

2. Documented absence of the following signs and symptoms:
   a. Fever
   b. Altered breath sounds
   c. Yellowish or greenish nasal discharge accompanied by redness and inflammation of the mucosa of the nose and throat
   d. Signs of infection of the middle ear
   e. Group A beta-hemolytic streptococcal infection of the throat

   RATIONALE: Presence of these signs and symptoms is indicative of other types of illness requiring further investigation.

3. Documentation of eosinophils in the nasal secretion.

   RATIONALE: Eosinophilia is indicative of the allergic response.

4. The child is over 1 year of age.

   RATIONALE: Symptoms similar to those of allergic rhinitis in infants are indicative of other types of illness, and this type of allergic response during infancy is rare.

Intervention for allergic rhinitis begins with avoiding offending antigens. However, this is often difficult or impossible, as often the offending allergens float freely in the air. If several family members suffer severe symptoms frequently, the family may consider mechanical air filtration for the home, which decreases the amount and frequency to which they are exposed to the allergens. Food allergens may be considered and systematically eliminated from the diet. Antihistamines and/or vasoconstrictors such as ephedrine may be indicated to control symptoms, particularly when the problem is seasonal. Consultation with an allergy specialist may be indicated, particularly if the child exhibits other signs and symptoms of allergy, or if there is a strong family history of serious allergic conditions such as asthma or anaphylactic responses. In the opinion of some allergists, early comprehensive evaluation of an allergic child and hyposensitization or other specific forms of treatment can alter the development of later, more serious allergies.[72,174,175]

### Nursing diagnosis and intervention for allergic dermatitis

Allergic, or atopic, dermatitis is the most common allergic response in children under 2 years of age. Frequently infants who develop early atopic dermatitis develop asthma or other more serious forms of allergic response after the age of 2 years. The most frequent site of the dermatitis is on the cheeks of the face and the diaper area, although the rash may involve all other parts of the body. The typical rash consists of erythematous patches, papules, and/or vesicles. The vesicles rapidly break down and ooze and then crust over, causing a scaly, rough feel and appearance of the skin. The most severe form of the response is called atopic erythroderma, in which the entire body is fiery red and the skin is thickened with scaling and exfoliation. The areas on which the rash appears are itchy, and the infant may appear restless and irritable and may scratch the affected areas.

Recommended criteria for nursing diagnosis of atopic dermatitis are:

1. Documented observation of skin rash that appears as erythematous patches, papules, and vesicles in discrete areas of the body. RATIONALE: This type of rash is typical of allergic dermatitis; extensive involvement of the body skin requires medical evaluation.
2. Documented absence of the following signs and symptoms:
   a. Fever
   b. Central nervous system irritability
   c. Signs of infection of skin lesions
   RATIONALE: These signs and symptoms are indicative of infection or other forms of illness requiring further evaluation.
3. Signs of itchiness, or the child's report of itchiness, including frequent scratching, irritability, restlessness.
   RATIONALE: The itching threshold appears to be lowered in children with allergic dermatitis, and itching stimulates observable behavioral responses.

The most common allergens causing atopic dermatitis are food and materials in the environment that come in contact with the skin. Elimination of specific allergens from contact is basic in treating the condition. The nurse should obtain a detailed food history and explore in detail various materials that might be stimulating the response. Frequently, the environmental allergens during infancy are laundry compounds used on diapers and bedding. Often these articles are laundered separately and harsh detergents and bleaching compounds are used to disinfect. The nurse should identify the compounds used and recommend eliminating these compounds entirely until the condition of the infant's skin is cleared and further study can be made to determine the exact allergen. Laundering with a mild laundry soap, combined with several clear water rinsings, should achieve sufficient cleansing of the diapers and bed clothing.

Foods that are prone to cause allergic dermatitis are eliminated from the infant or child's diet altogether for several days, or until the skin condition clears. All cereals, milk, egg, pork, chocolate, cola, nuts, citrus fruits and juices, and spices are eliminated. Infants who are still on formula are placed on a soy formula. After the condition of the skin has remained clear for several days, each suspected allergen may be reintroduced to determine whether it will in fact stimulate a response. Each suspected allergen is offered to the child one at a time and continued without adding any new suspected allergen for at least three days. If a food stimulates a response, it is immediately withdrawn indefinitely from the diet. A new challenge with the food may be attempted a year or two following the initial identification, as the child's sensitivity to the allergen may change over time.

Care of the skin and control of itching and scratching are important nursing considerations. The child may be given cornstarch or oatmeal baths to relieve itching. Nonallergenic skin lotion may be used to promote skin moisture and prevent excessive drying. A mild topical steroid cream or ointment may be used for a few days after allergen control has been instituted to promote restoring the skin to a healthy state. Cotton mittens on an infant's hands during sleep may help to decrease excessive scratching. The child's fingernails should be kept short and clean. The older child can be taught to gently rub or pat the itchy area rather than scratch.[34,72,174,175]

## Accidental injury (MNPC no. 331)

The tragic occurrence of accidental injury in young children accounts for a great proportion of the morbidity and mortality during this period of life.[235] The common types of accidents will be discussed here, with a brief review of special aspects of nursing care.

**Head injuries.** Injuries to the head occur as a result of severe falls (usually from an unguarded surface), from automobile accidents, or from battering. Specific problems of battering are discussed in a following section; automobile safety for the infant and young child is presented in Chapters 9 and 10. Injuries to the head may affect the scalp, the skull, the nervous system, or any of these in combination. Injuries requiring surgical repair of the scalp or skull require immediate hospitalization, but the major concern is for possible damage to the nervous system, which may not be apparent for several days. Injuries that do not cause damage to the scalp or skull but involve bruising or swelling of the soft tissues beneath the scalp may result in serious damage to the central nervous system. The child may be thoroughly evaluated and observed at home for 24 to 48 hours, with hospitalization delayed until definitive signs of injury to the central nervous system develop. The initial assessment of the child should include:

1. Determination of the nature of the injury and the child's immediate response. If the child cried vigorously or if loss of consciousness was very brief (less than three minutes), hospitalization may not be required.
2. During the period following the immediate reaction, stability of behavior and increasing alertness should have developed. If the level of alertness deteriorates and the child becomes drowsy to the point of being difficult to arouse, hospitalization is indicated.
3. Pulse, respiration, and blood pressure should be within normal range. Transient bradycardia may be noted immediately after a head injury.
4. Vomiting may occur three or four times after the injury. If this persists, hospitalization is indicated.
5. All reflexes and neurologic signs appropriate for the child's age should be present. If these are sluggish or absent, immediate hospitalization is required.
6. The pupils provide a ready means of evaluating the neurologic adequacy and the possibility of intracranial pressure. The parents may be taught to illuminate the eyes and watch for pupil response. If the child is observed at home, the parents should be instructed to awaken him or her at least every three hours during the time that he or she is asleep and determine the pupillary response. If this changes, or if the child is more difficult to arouse than under ordinary circumstances, they should bring the child to the hospital at once.
7. There should be no evidence of spinal fluid otorrhea or rhinorrhea, and no blood should be evident in the ear canal or behind the tympanic membrane. Should these conditions be present, the child must be hospitalized.

If the child is irritable and at times hyperactive or complains of headache, the parents should be cautioned not to use any drug that might mask the symptoms of developing intracranial pressure. Aspirin in doses appropriate for the child's age may be used to relieve headache.[93,112,195,210,223]

**Burns (MNPC no. 350.3).** Burns in young children result from many accidents in the home, and they vary in severity from a small localized surface burn to severe burns covering a great percentage of the body. When young children are burned, there are several factors that determine if they can be cared for at home. These include the following:

1. The burn covers no more than 10% of the child's body surface area (Fig. 11-16).
2. The burn does not involve the face, neck, hands, feet, axilla, groin, or knees.
3. The family is able to care for the child 24 hours a day for several days.
4. The condition of the home is such that infection can be adequately controlled.
5. The burn involves less than the full thickness of the dermis.

Full-thickness injury is indicated by a blanched, ischemic appearance of the area and total absence of feeling immediately over the affected area. Accurate estimate of the thickness of burns is often impossible in the early stages. If the extent of the burn is less than 10% of body area and the home conditions are suitable, it may be desirable to help the family treat the child's burns at home until a more definitive estimate of thickness can be made. Except for very minor burns, injuries involving the face, neck, hands, feet, axilla, groin, or knees require careful evaluation and treatment in order to reduce scarring and maintain full range of motion. If these areas are involved, the child should probably be hospitalized until the full extent of the injury can be ascertained.

In the initial treatment of burns, regardless of the severity or extent, a primary concern is the relief of pain and, in the case of severe burns, the control of fluid and electrolyte losses. The second major concern is for local treatment of the burned area and for control of infection. The ultimate success of burn therapy depends upon infection control, fluid and electrolyte

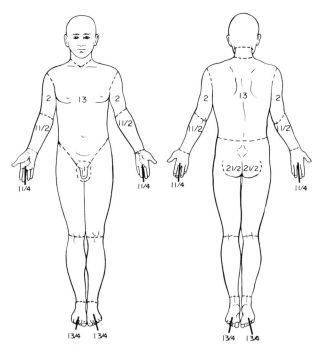

Relative percentages of areas affected by growth

| AREA | Inf. | 1-4 | 5-9 | 10-14 | 15 | Adult | Part. | Full | Total | Donor areas |
|------|------|-----|-----|-------|----|-------|-------|------|-------|-------------|
| HEAD | 19 | 17 | 13 | 11 | 9 | 7 | | | | |
| NECK | 2 | 2 | 2 | 2 | 2 | 2 | | | | |
| ANT. TRUNK | 13 | 13 | 13 | 13 | 13 | 13 | | | | |
| POST. TRUNK | 13 | 13 | 13 | 13 | 13 | 13 | | | | |
| R. BUTTOCK | 2½ | 2½ | 2½ | 2½ | 2½ | 2½ | | | | |
| L. BUTTOCK | 2½ | 2½ | 2½ | 2½ | 2½ | 2½ | | | | |
| GENITALIA | 1 | 1 | 1 | 1 | 1 | 1 | | | | |
| R.U. ARM | 4 | 4 | 4 | 4 | 4 | 4 | | | | |
| L.U. ARM | 4 | 4 | 4 | 4 | 4 | 4 | | | | |
| R.L. ARM | 3 | 3 | 3 | 3 | 3 | 3 | | | | |
| L.L. ARM | 3 | 3 | 3 | 3 | 3 | 3 | | | | |
| R. HAND | 2½ | 2½ | 2½ | 2½ | 2½ | 2½ | | | | |
| L. HAND | 2½ | 2½ | 2½ | 2½ | 2½ | 2½ | | | | |
| R. THIGH | 5½ | 6½ | 8 | 8½ | 9 | 9½ | | | | |
| L. THIGH | 5½ | 6½ | 8 | 8½ | 9 | 9½ | | | | |
| R. LEG | 5 | 5 | 5½ | 6 | 6½ | 7 | | | | |
| L. LEG | 5 | 5 | 5½ | 6 | 6½ | 7 | | | | |
| R. FOOT | 3½ | 3½ | 3½ | 3½ | 3½ | 3½ | | | | |
| L. FOOT | 3½ | 3½ | 3½ | 3½ | 3½ | 3½ | | | | |
| | | | | | | TOTAL | | | | |

**Fig. 11-19.** Burn estimate diagram. (Adapted from Jacoby, F. G.: Nursing care of the patient with burns, St. Louis, 1972, The C. V. Mosby Co.)

control, and optimal comfort for the child, both physically and psychologically.

The local treatment of burns varies greatly both in terms of home first-aid remedies and in relation to professional medical care. Initially, the family should avoid using any of the greasy materials that are recommended for burn treatment. They should be instructed to immerse the burned area in cool water, quickly assess the probable extent of the burn, wrap the burned area in a clean sheet, and take the child to a clinic or a hospital. Small minor burns may be treated at home with continued application of cold water or ice, which eases the pain and reduces the damage caused by high temperature and edema. When the burn has been assessed in a clinic or hospital, the next steps in care include cleansing the burned area thoroughly, assessing the damage, and then instituting the therapy of choice to prevent infection, compensate for fluid and electrolyte losses, control pain, and eventually replace lost skin tissue.

If the extent of the child's burn approaches 10% of the body surface area, and the decision is made to help the family with home care, some consideration may be indicated for compensating for small fluid and electrolyte losses. Encouraging oral intake of fluids and providing some dietary means of solute intake, such as soda crackers or pretzels, may avoid the gradual development of fluid and electrolyte depletion over the first few hours of home care.

Continued use of the affected part of the body, whether it is an entire limb or a single finger, may avoid some of the difficulty resulting from the healing process. Contractions and deformities of the area are difficult to correct and overcome. Minimizing these effects requires persistent, rational intervention from several members of the health care team, particularly physical and occupational therapists, nurses, and physicians.*

**Poisonings.** Even though children under 5 account for only 9% of the total population, about one half of all poisonings occur among this age group.[219] The variety of all toxic agents that a young child may ingest is so great that it would be impractical to list all agents with instructions as to what should be done in the event of ingestion. For this reason regional poison control centers have been established that provide 24-hour 7-day-a-week assistance to parents and health care workers in the event of accidental poison or drug ingestion. In many cases their services extend to any drug problem, including drug interactions, information on appropriate dosage for specific age groups, and other related information and advice that might not be readily available to practitioners through any other source.

When a poisoning does occur, the nurse must be prepared to act quickly and to help the family provide certain important information so that treatment of the child may be accomplished accurately, efficiently, and quickly. Hopefully,

the family is also prepared to meet this emergency.

As soon as the child is discovered after an accidental poisoning he or she should be given an emetic dose of syrup of ipecac: 15 ml for the 1- to 4-year-old child, followed by another 15 ml dose if no vomiting occurs within 20 minutes. Syrup of ipecac in these dosages is ordinarily available over the counter; if not, ipecac should be provided by prescription for all families with young children, and its use carefully understood by all adults who care for children. All vomitus is to be saved for chemical analysis later if this is needed. The only contraindication to administering syrup of ipecac is in the case of ingestion of a caustic substance, such as lye or strong acid. In this case a dose of activated charcoal may be given to the child to provide absorption and neutralization in the stomach and gastrointestinal tract. Subsequently, removal of the products may be accomplished in an emergency setting. When there is a question regarding immediate treatment, the poison control center or physician should be consulted.

As soon as the initial treatment at home is given, the child, the container for the vomitus, and all evidence of the agent that was ingested should be transported to the nearest emergency care facility. Here further measures to remove the poison from the system may be instituted, and specific treatment of any effects of the poison may be utilized. The child may need to be placed under close observation and treatment for several hours or days, depending upon the severity of the poisoning. All signs of the physical status of the child must be evaluated by the health care worker who first contacts the child. Supportive care to maintain gas exchange, to control and prevent peripheral vascular collapse, to maintain fluid and electrolyte balance, and to control central nervous system excitement may be instituted.*

When the immediate crisis of the poisoning episode has subsided, the parents or other adults involved need extra care and attention. Incriminations and lectures on poison prevention are most inappropriate at this time. Equally ludicrous is the approach that conveys the

*References 13, 19, 86, 95, 100, 189, 219, 238.

*References 88, 145, 152, 171, 190, 194, 212, 219.

message, "That's O.K., it happens to everyone." Supportive understanding of their distress and regret over the situation and helping them to experience their feelings can sustain the child's family while they work through the tasks of dealing with their feelings of guilt and shame and of reconstructing a sound, mature approach with the child and accident prevention. A healthy resolution of the situation reveals realistic attempts to provide a safer environment for the children at home but without measures that create an overprotected, unduly compulsive control on the environment and the child's activity. If the child survives and yet suffers permanent damage or handicap, the task for the family is indeed great, and continuing assistance from a number of mental health resources may be required.

## Nutritional inadequacies

Nutritional inadequacies can take the form of *undernutrition*, where children do not receive an adequate supply of an essential nutrient, or *overnutrition*, where they receive more of a certain nutrient than is needed for healthy growth and development. Countries vary in the type of problem that tends to predominate. Where food is plentiful and readily available, overnutrition and problems of obesity present the greater problem; where food is scarce, undernutrition is a predominant concern. For infants and young children in the United States there is, ironically, a combination of these problems. Undernutrition due to unavailability of foods exists in certain areas of the society, and in spite of the availability of foods, there is a widespread incidence of iron deficiency anemia in infants and young children.[142] While this incidence tends to be increased among populations that are generally undernourished, many children who supposedly have an adequate diet available to them are not receiving adequate intakes of iron. The other major problem, overnutrition, results from the ready availability of foods, the popular notion promoted through advertising that to be healthy is to be big, and the idea that fun and enjoyment in life are equated with many culinary delights. While obesity is not condoned as such for older children and adults, it is condoned and considered desirable by many adults for their infants. Thus a fat baby is thought to be a happy, healthy one. The fallacy lies in the belief that a large intake of food provides all the essential nutrients for the infant and that obesity will disappear during early childhood, never to plague him or her again in later life. Recent investigations have demonstrated that these beliefs are fallacious and that, indeed, the reverse may be the case.

**Excessive weight** (**MNPC no. 314**). Excessive body weight during infancy and childhood may result from many factors, and it can involve structural tissue, musculature, or adipose tissue. Children should be considered "overweight" only if they have an excessive amount of adipose tissue; however, there are no reliable means of determining the amount of total body adipose tissue. Plotting body weight in comparison to body height serves as a useful indirect guideline for most children, and the child who exceeds the mean standard body weight by 2 standard deviations is presumed to be overweight. The body weight and body length or height should fall within the same percentile range. A child whose body weight exceeds body length or body height by one 10-percentile range should be considered overweight. Measurement of skin fold thickness is a useful estimate of the amount of adipose tissue.[1]

Recent studies of overweight individuals of all ages suggest that the first critical period for development of a persistent problem of obesity begins during infancy.[122] The number of adipose cells and the size of these cells play important but separate roles in the development of obesity. It appears that once the cell number has increased to an excessive degree, the only way to decrease adipose tissue deposit is to decrease cell size; the number of cells remains the same. There is limited evidence to suggest that if decrease in cell size is possible at all it may occur only during early childhood.[122]

Unfortunately, most infants and children who have a problem with obesity come to the attention of health care workers after the conditions that promote and maintain obesity are well ingrained in the life patterns of the family. Programs for weight reduction and control are extremely difficult to institute, and in most cases they are only temporarily successful if they suc-

**421**

ceed at all. Therefore, the most important aspect of controlling obesity during infancy and early childhood is initial prevention and helping the family to understand basic nutritional needs and food and activity habits that promote adequate but not excessive growth. When the family does come to the health care worker for assistance, or when the health care worker identifies a real weight problem in a young child, the problems of management are immensely complex. Socioeconomic, psychologic, genetic, endocrine, and metabolic factors must be considered in addition to the physical problem of reducing adipose tissue growth while maintaining adequate growth for all other tissues. Simply giving the family lectures on the rationale for weight control and stating the risks of permanent obesity, which include potential cardiovascular problems and diabetes, is of little or no benefit. Any plan for control must fit within the family's own desires, their own life-style patterns, and their available resources.

Psychologic factors related to obesity during infancy and early childhood are complex and not clearly understood. No single psychologic pattern can be identified as clearly related to the development of obesity. In some cases such factors seem to play a relatively small role, in others, eating seems to have become a predominant mechanism for psychologic adjustment. In the feeding of young infants and children the family may not recognize satiety behavior; the mother may feel compelled to provide as much food as possible, which means that the infant is fed far beyond the basic requirements. The child thus learns to ignore satiety signals or develops the habit of eating to satisfy a variety of different needs and feelings.

When a therapeutic or control diet for a young child is indicated, at least on a trial basis, Knittle[122] has recommended the use of 60 calories per kilogram of ideal body weight, with 20% of the calories as protein and the remaining 80% evenly distributed between carbohydrate and fat. Supplements of minerals and vitamins may be provided as needed; iron supplementation is needed for infants or children who do not maintain an adequate hemoglobin level. Weight changes, height gains, behavior patterns, and general health of the young child must be care-

fully monitored, and dietary restriction must be carefully reevaluated at frequent intervals. Presently, there are no means to determine the differential effect of various dietary controls on the deposition of fat and the growth and development of nonfat organs. Thus the many indirect indications that total health is adequately maintained must be carefully monitored. The most ideal program of weight control probably begins in the nursery, and continuing efforts to help a family provide for optimal nutrition includes consideration of preventing excessive weight.[5,122,161,170]

**Iron deficiency (MNPC no. 330.3).** Iron deficiency in the diet of infants and young children begins a series of metabolic events that lead to the development of iron deficiency anemia. The first consequence of prolonged iron deficiency is the depletion of the total body stores of iron. Consequently, there is a gradual decrease in the concentration of serum iron and a concomitant rise in the serum iron-binding protein, transferrin. A transferrin saturation of the serum of 16% or less is typical of iron deficiency. After this deficiency develops, anemia and the characteristic red blood cell hypochromia and microcytosis appear.

It is estimated that from 4% to 8% of infants 12 to 18 months of age in "privileged" American families suffer from iron deficiency anemia, and the percentage rises drastically to about 40% in infants of this age group from economically disadvantaged families. Whether iron deficiency per se is a more extensive problem than is indicated by the incidence of anemia is unknown. In addition the actual adverse effects of iron deficiency or iron deficiency anemia have not been fully elucidated. There is suggestive evidence that iron deficiency, even before the development of the anemic state, results in fatigue, irritability, decreased attentiveness, and decreased ability to concentrate.

When anemia is identified by hemoglobin or hematocrit measurements, the assumption must not be made that the problem is caused by iron deficiency. Although this cause of anemia is predominant among young children, there are other causes, such as occult blood loss, metal poisoning, errors of metabolism, and genetic blood disorders. Each of these requires therapy that is specific and different from that required for iron deficiency, and thus a differential determination should be attempted.

The recommended criteria for nursing diagnosis of iron deficiency anemia are:

1. Mean corpuscular hemoglobin concentration (MCHC) under 32%, calculated as follows:

$$\frac{\text{Hemoglobin (g)}}{\text{Hematocrit (\%)}} \times 100 = \text{MCHC}$$

   RATIONALE: The normal range of MCHC is 32% to 34%; a cell index that falls below this level is indicative of anemia.[83]

2. History of poor dietary intake of iron.

   RATIONALE: Known inadequate intake of iron supports the presumption that anemia is related to iron deficiency.

3. Signs and symptoms that may be present are documented, including:
   a. Pallor
   b. Fatigue
   c. Irritability
   d. Delayed motor development
   e. Poor muscle tone

   RATIONALE: These signs and symptoms may accompany iron deficiency anemia.

4. Red blood cells appear microcytic and hypochromic on microscopic examination.

   RATIONALE: These red cell changes occur with iron deficiency anemia.

5. Documented absence of the following signs and symptoms:
   a. Occult bleeding
   b. Fever and other signs of infection or serious systemic illness
   c. Lead levels in the blood

   RATIONALE: These signs and symptoms are indicative of other possible causes of anemia and need further evaluation.

6. The child's MCHC reaches normal range or moves upward in response to dietary and supplemental iron within three to four weeks.

   RATIONALE: Adequate response to iron intake confirms the etiology of iron deficiency. If a response is not observed, the child should be evaluated for other etiologic factors.

Therapeutic preferences for intervention vary greatly and range from dietary increases of iron intake to vigorous oral or parenteral iron administration. The most predominantly used therapy consists of oral administration of ferrous sulfate, which supplies 5 to 6 mg of iron per kilogram of body weight per day, usually given in three or four divided doses. The anemia should be corrected within three or four weeks, but to replenish iron stores, therapy must be continued for two or three months.*

Teaching and assistance with dietary needs may be indicated for the family; if the child is given therapy but returns to the previously deficient diet, depletion and anemia will eventually recur. This challenge involves the family's life-style, food habits, and socioeconomic condition and often revolves around a basic social dilemma.

## PROBLEMS RELATED TO LEARNING AND THOUGHT, SOCIAL, AND INNER COMPETENCIES
### Behavioral problems
### (MNPC no. 32)

Concern for and willingness to work with the family who is experiencing behavioral problems are relatively lacking in most health care settings. The value assumption that something is wrong with the parent's ability to properly rear their children and control their behavior interferes with the ability to objectively and empathetically understand the real problem and to offer some help for the distressed family. Most children pass through transient stages with behavioral disturbances; a few of these are discussed in Chapter 10. Most of these disturbances involve some aspect of the child-rearing process. The parents' ability to cope adequately with the problem until it runs its natural course varies greatly. The problem may, on the other hand, prove not to be transient, and it may persist because of the parent's inability to adequately help the child through the crisis, their inadvertent perpetuation of the problem, or some other unidentified cause.

---

*References 32, 48, 109, 136, 161, 167, 213, 217, 239.

## Differentiating problem behavior from normal early childhood behavior

Whenever a family expresses concern for any behavioral characteristic of their young child, a problem exists for the family. Intervention for the problem begins by taking the family's concern seriously and listening empathically to their own perceptions of the problem. Complete understanding of their own perceptions is not only therapeutic for the family, it provides real information that makes an accurate assessment of the situation possible. Premature interpretation of the situation interferes with obtaining complete insight, as well as with the therapeutic relationship that might otherwise develop. When a concern is expressed, the initial goal of assessment is to determine if the problem is basically a problem of the child or one of the parents or a problem for both. Problems arising from the parents include emotional, social, or economic pressures that cause the parents to interpret the child's normal behavior as unusual or problematic, a lack of understanding of normal early childhood behavior, and unrealistic expectations for the child's behavior. Primary parental problems are discussed in a following section of this chapter and need to be confronted with compassion while maintaining support and guidance in relation to their perceived problem with the child's behavior. Problems that arise from a real lack of understanding of normal early childhood behavior require counsel and guidance directed to helping the parents reorient their expectations for the child's behavior while meeting their own expressed needs. For example, a family may identify their child as excessively boisterous and active, causing disarray and physical damage to property within the home. The child may indeed have an active, inquisitive, and boisterous personality with normal age-appropriate behavior that results in frequent active movement about the home, such as dragging toys and household objects freely about the house, that results in things being misplaced and broken. The parents, on the other hand, prefer a well-ordered environment with everything in place and a peaceful and restful environment with little activity inside the house. A lack of understanding of normal early childhood behavior and the incompatability between their child's temperament and their own causes concern for the child's behavior, and a desire to solve the problem by changing the child's behavior.

Actual behavior problems in young children may be differentiated from normal early childhood behavior by careful observation and assessment of the child's behavior and of the events in the child's environment. Misbehavior in young children occurs as a result of four basic inner motivations on the part of the child. These include:

1. *Seeking attention.* The child's need for attention may arise out of a real deprivation of sufficient attention directed to the child or from excessive demands for attention. Children vary in the amount of attention they need to satisfy their needs for interpersonal contact. A child who is never satisfied, or very seldom satisfied, with activities that do not require adult attention may be identified as one with excessive demands for attention.

2. *Seeking control.* Since toddlers and preschool children are working through tasks of autonomy and independence, they have a normal need to gain and demonstrate control over others in the environment. The social environment should provide opportunities for the child to obtain the control that is appropriate for this age level, such as choosing activities, toys, snacks, or having others respond to requests for interaction or favors. A young child whose behavior reflects almost constant attempts to gain and maintain control, as with the use of manipulative behavior, may have a real behavior problem.

3. *Seeking retaliation.* Retaliation in the young child is closely related to a desire to maintain control. Retaliation expressed through aggression, deliberate acts of destruction, or consistent resistance to cooperation has a real behavior problem.

4. *Behavior excesses or deficits to cover up a real or imagined disability.* A young child who is actually handicapped or who imagines a handicap will act out in ways to compensate for the disability.

Table 11-3 summarizes the behaviors that are often identified as problem behaviors for young children, the normal expectations related to

**Table 11-3.** Summary of behavior problems during early childhood, normal expectations, and factors that contribute to problem behavior

| Behavior | Normal expectations | Factors contributing to problem behavior | |
|---|---|---|---|
| | | **Child factors** | **Parent/home environment factors** |
| Sleep disorders | Occasional nightmares beginning at about 36 months<br>Ritual bedtime routine, with attempt to delay sleep peaks between 2-3 years<br>Head banging and rocking between 1-4 years providing release of tension<br>Waking between 1-5 AM occurs infrequently after 6 months of age, less than once a week<br>Fearful of darkness between 2-5 years; will settle down with use of rituals, such as having a favorite toy or a night light | Excessive napping during the day<br>Insufficient adult interaction during the day, leading to use of bedtime as opportunity to gain adult attention<br>Unusual fears related to darkness, being left alone; rituals and night light do not suffice<br>Illness<br>Development of nighttime bowel and bladder control | Anxiety for child's safety results in frequent checking on child, disturbing sleep<br>Inability to set and maintain limits on delaying tactics<br>Unrealistic expectations; cannot tolerate bedtime rituals<br>Environment noisy, not conducive to sleep<br>Excessive stimulation before bedtime<br>Frightening TV shows before bedtime<br>Environmental stress, such as new sibling, moving, etc. |
| Temper tantrums | Peak at 2 years of age, decreasing in frequency and intensity until they rarely occur by about 4 years of age<br>Usually occur in response to frustrated desires of a child, such as wanting a toy that cannot be purchased | Used as a manipulative device to gain control of parental behavior<br>Insufficient positive interaction with adults, leading to use of tantrums to gain attention | Inability to set and maintain limits, allowing themselves to be manipulated<br>Insufficient positive approaches to child in response to desired behavior<br>Unrealistic expectations; cannot tolerate any tantrum behavior |
| Toilet training and bedwetting | Child has full physiologic capacity for day control by 3 years, night control by 4 years<br>Daytime and nighttime "accidents" occur throughout early childhood, decreasing in frequency by 4-5 years<br>Regression occurs with environmental or social changes, such as arrival of sibling, moving, divorce | Fears and anxiety in response to negative means of toilet training inhibit ability to gain control<br>Used as an attention-getting device if positive means of gaining attention are lacking<br>Excessive fluid intake before bedtime | Punishment and other negative approaches to toilet training<br>Unrealistic expectations for control; expect normal control prior to physiologic ability or expect the child to be accident-free<br>Inconsistent recognition of child's signals of needing to use the toilet<br>Inadequate provision for child's toileting needs, such as small commode<br>Clothing is too difficult for child to maneuver independently<br>Irregular eating patterns |
| Aggressive or quarrelsome behavior; sibling rivalry | Ability to play cooperatively begins to emerge during 4-5 years<br>Prior to this age, child seldom able to share toys; often wants toys that another child has<br>Predominant use of physical hitting, shoving, to express displeasure; verbal abilities begin to emerge during fifth year | Insufficient positive adult attention leads to deliberate use of aggression to gain adult attention<br>Aggression may arise from actual or perceived adult preference for sibling or playmate | Insufficient positive interaction in response to desired behavior<br>Unrealistic expectations for cooperative and sharing behavior<br>Actual preferential attention given to sibling or playmate |

*Continued.*

**Table 11-3.** Summary of behavior problems during early childhood, normal expectations, and factors that contribute to problem behavior—cont'd

| Behavior | Normal expectations | Factors contributing to problem behavior | |
|---|---|---|---|
| | | Child factors | Parent/home environment factors |
| Inability to separate; excessive shyness | Child can separate easily by 3 years if surroundings are consistent, predictable, positive<br>Continues to protest separation if the environment changes or if confronted by total strangers<br>Shy in new and strange surroundings; relaxed and spontaneous in familiar surroundings | Inadequate establishment of self-concept leading to lack of confidence even in familiar surrounding<br>Uses protest of separation as a manipulative control device<br>Fear of being abandoned | Parental anxiety and guilt over separation<br>Inability to set limits, to leave child after brief, direct explanation<br>Lack of preparation for an anticipated separation, leading to an unpredicted, fearful experience for the child<br>Inconsistent messages and actions, such as telling the child the parent will stay, then sneaking out or not returning at a predicted time |

these behaviors, and the child and parent factors that might contribute to a problem behavior.

### Nursing intervention for behavioral problems

When a behavioral problem exists during early childhood, the family often needs specific counseling and guidance in establishing positive means of communication and discipline with the youngster. The family may need to learn to use clear, brief statements in communicating their desires to the child. Often, the need to provide a signal or a forewarning for the child is not recognized. The parent may ignore the signal that trouble is about to begin or simply fail to warn the child verbally that a situation exists that will lead to a problem. For example, a parent may ignore signs that the child needs to use the toilet or that the child is getting ready to take a toy from another child. The parents may need specific guidance in developing the ability to respond to these signals and to verbally provide warning and guidance for the child, as well as inform the child of the consequences of an undesired action.

One of the most bothersome problems is the establishment of clear expectations and limits and maintaining these limits. The nurse may assist the family to initially determine a selected behavior on which they need to set limits and to plan for enforcing the limits, including role playing the responses that are indicated for each of the child's behaviors that they might anticipate. For example, if the family determines that they need to begin by controlling the child's persistent attempts to delay bedtime, the nurse assists the family to determine the ritual behavior that they will encourage and participate in, including the number of times a particular behavior will be tolerated and the length of time that will be set for the ritual. Their means of warning the child that the deadline is approaching is discussed, such as telling the child "This will be the last story" or "You have two minutes to finish arranging your dolls." Once the deadline has arrived, the parents need to determine how they will enforce and maintain the limits that have been set and how they will respond to the child's attempts to protest. They need to be prepared to encounter tantrum behavior, prolonged crying, or pitiful pleas for one more drink of water. Undesired parental responses, such as bribes offered in advance of bedtime in an attempt to gain the child's cooperation, are also discussed in order to help the parents work through a real determination to maintain the desired course of action.[38,61,63,188,215]

Behavior modification and use of positive reinforcement may be used to bring a specific behavior under control.[94,156] The specific approaches used in planning and implementing such a program of behavior control are presented in Chapter 16, p. 683.

Often parents of young children benefit from a parent group experience. Such groups require skilled professional leadership, because the group experience may create seemingly greater problems than existed before the experience began. Parents with very severe problems and burdens may gain control, or they may begin to use the individuals in the group to meet their own needs at the expense of all other persons' needs. Anxiety and doubt in the parents' own ability to meet the needs of their young children may be fostered by such an unfortunate experience. However, strong, professional leadership for a group can assure the provision of a balanced, freely expressive group that can work together to generate creative, constructive approaches to child-rearing problems. Such a group also provides a means for parents to safely test their own feelings and ideas in regard to various approaches in childrearing. Thus each parent's independence, self-confidence, and realization of the developmental challenges of childhood can be facilitated.

A few families may profit greatly by early, intensive family therapy in a mental health setting by a professional psychotherapist. This may be a frightening and initially unacceptable alternative to many of the families who need such assistance most urgently. Little is to be gained by "prescribing" such an alternative. Rather, the family may require counseling with a respected health care worker in order to reach the independent, self-determined conclusion that this is an acceptable and desirable alternative for their situation. In some cases a parent group experience may help a family come to such a realization.

Unfortunately, many families never receive the kind of help in child-rearing that is desperately needed to facilitate healthy growth and development. Even if help is available, some families are not able to respond. Attempts to find a wider range of assistance for families may yield increased understanding of ways in which young families can be helped to achieve greater success in child-rearing.[22,42,105]

## Social-environmental problems (MNPC no. 332) and parental problems (MNPC no. 363)

The relationship between acute or chronic stress and health is well recognized.[89] The specific effect of social and parental stress on the health of young children has not been studied sufficiently to offer clear understanding, but several inferences and objective observations have led to a description of some major factors that may be involved in a young child's reaction to social stress. It is known that when such stress exists, young children are more prone to physical acute illness and accidents.[89] In addition the young child's limitations in cognitive ability cause cognitive misunderstanding of the problem that exists and emotional misinterpretation. The young child responds to a stress event in an egocentric manner, assuming that he or she caused the event, either by some behavioral misdeed or by fantasy wishes related to the actual event. For example, a young child may experience fantasies of a parent leaving or dying in response to a ordinary parent-child conflict. When the parent later does leave or die, the young child is likely to think that the innocent death wish caused the event to happen. Stress events that threaten an impending loss or result in actual loss are particularly ominous for the infant or young child and create a situation of life-long emotional risk. Such events include divorce or separation of the parents, physical or emotional illness of the parents or other significant family members, and death of a loved one.*

Table 11-4 summarizes the assessment factors that must be considered when an infant or young child experiences a social environmental stress. All children in this age group are emotionally vulnerable. The factors that contribute to minimizing the vulnerability of the child and those that maximize the child's vulnerability are summarized in Table 11-4. Also presented are those resources that can be provided for all young children to minimize the degree of risk and provide long-term protection against the development of serious emotional and physical sequelae.

*References 4, 56, 77, 89, 91, 119, 233, 241.

**Table 11-4.** Assessment and intervention for infants and young children who experience stress of threatened or real loss

| Assessment factor | Minimal risk | Maximum risk | Resources for minimizing risk |
|---|---|---|---|
| Quality of early mother-child attachment | Solid attachment bond formed | Early attachment failure or inadequacy; neglect or abuse | Provide support for existing attachment relationship throughout period of reintegration *or* Provide a new attachment figure, maintaining long-term consistency in the relationship |
| Family relationships | Family relationships predominantly harmonious before stress event | Long-term history of family discord, frequent absence of significant member(s) | Provide support for the reestablishment of satisfying family life after stress event *or* Provide alternate family environment with predominantly harmonious relationships |
| Mental health of parents | Parents mature, well-adjusted, positive outlook, predominantly happy with life before stress event | Previous incidence of parental depression, withdrawal, or other psychiatric illness | Provide intervention for mental health problem Provide a therapeutic relationship for child with an adult who has adequate mental health |
| Information child receives about the stress event | Child is given direct, honest information appropriate to age and in accord with family's religious beliefs | Information withheld from child Inaccurate information conveyed Information distorted to place blame on child | Counsel family regarding the information needs of the child Institute direct therapeutic counseling with young child to uncover child's perceptions of the information received, and support the development of reality-based perceptions |
| Reactions of other family members to stress event | Periods of initial shock, personal disintegration, and reintegration proceed to unfold within the following year | Inadequate initial coping, prolonged period of personal disintegration, failure of signs of reintegration | Long-term therapy for members in personal difficulty Short-term therapeutic support for minimal-risk family members Therapeutic, secure relationship for child with an adult not involved personally in the experience of stress. |

## ACUTE HEALTH PROBLEMS WITH FAR-REACHING EFFECTS

There are several problems affecting the health of the young child that have great implications and far-reaching effects on the life of the child and family. Three such problems are discussed here, with emphasis on health care intervention that must be instituted.

### Child abuse and neglect (MNPC no. 360.6)

The tragic problem of child abuse and neglect is an awesome challenge in the health care of infants and young children. Understanding of the multiple problems involved has led to development of a few definitive guidelines that can be used in identifying cases where abuse is a threat to the child's life and health and in offering more constructive, realistic help to the family than has been typically available in the past.

Parents who abuse their children often arouse strong feelings of disgust and repulsion in health care workers and others in society. The adult's needs and problems are considered insignificant when abuse has been inflicted on a helpless young child. In spite of the fact that these reactions may be justified, they do not facilitate the kind of objective help that these people need. These parents are often frightened, defensive, and angry; they need help and may even want help, but they do not know how to face the reality of the problem.

The foremost challenge is early identification of situations in which a child is likely to be abused or neglected. Observations of the early mother-child relationships may be helpful (see Chapters 5 through 9). It is believed that when a mother and child are not able to establish a satisfactory early relationship, the risk of abuse is greater. However, mothers are not the only adults who might abuse a child; fathers, older siblings, baby-sitters, and day-care workers have also been implicated in specific situations.

Certain personality traits should alert health care workers to the possibility of abuse, particularly when the child is brought to a clinic with symptoms that typically suggest abuse. The adults involved are commonly emotionally immature, self-centered, rejecting, and angry. They are often burdened by multiple problems that they seem unable to handle. They come from every social strata, but their life-style suggests that they are relatively isolated from the usual social group contacts, such as church affiliation, family ties, or social club membership. In the face of stress, they tend to act out in an impulsive way. Very often, adults who batter a child were abused or battered as children. They may not recall such events, but their recollection of their childhood is far from happy and pleasant. When a young, dependent child enters their life, these adults often exhibit signs of turning to the child for their own dependency needs, for nurturing, and human companionship. When the infant or child makes dependency demands and requires nurturing and care, the adult typically strikes out angrily and physically or emotionally abuses the child. Although some abusing adults are chronically depressed, psychotic, or criminally inclined, more commonly these problems do not contribute to the abuse tendency.[82,218]

Growing awareness of sexual abuse of young children has led to increased identification of this form of child abuse. The actual incidence is not known, for there remains an awesome aura of fear, shame, and guilt on the part of adults who might be aware of the problem, and young children are unable or too frightened to inform someone who might intervene on their behalf. Sexual abuse is most often inflicted by the child's father, another close family member, or older child or adult who is well known to the child. In many instances the child's mother or another adult is aware that sexual molestation has occurred or that the adult involved has been involved in sexual molestation of other children or adolescents. The signs of sexual abuse are very similar to those of other forms of abuse and neglect and should always be considered as a possible form of abuse whenever abuse of any sort is suspected. Specific signs of sexual abuse include evidence of oral, anal, or genital penetration with or without trauma, presence of semen in the mouth and throat, anus, or vagina, and evidence of venereal disease in the child.[29,81,98,208]

The variety of problems that an abused child might exhibit includes single or multiple physical injuries, failure to develop, or behavior disturbance. Because physical injuries are common under normal circumstances in children of this age, it may be difficult to determine whether the child has been battered. The child may have a head injury or fractures of the arms and legs or ribs. A useful clue in differentiating an accidental fracture from one that is imposed by battering is radiologic evidence of multiple fractures in other areas of the body that are in different stages of healing. The child may have been treated for another fracture at another health care facility or may have suffered a minor fracture without receiving medical attention. Bruises, intestinal injuries, and burns are also seen. Less obvious but equally important results of abuse include poor skin hygiene, undernutrition, failure to thrive, undue irritability, and excessive appetite with undergrowth. The child often exhibits developmental retardation.[31,70,127]

When a child with these problems is identified and an adult member of the family appears to exhibit traits commonly associated with abuse, the family should be brought into some sort of intensive evaluation and appropriate therapy program should be started with the intention and hope of preventing further hazard to the child's health and well-being. Therapy centers that are investigating ways to help families experiencing this sort of stress have been instituted, and initial evidence indicates significant success.[74,116,157,166,173]

When adults in the family are not available for interview regarding a child's condition, when they delay in instituting follow-through care or treatment, or when the report of the "accident" is bizarre or inconsistent, suspicion of a problem is warranted. The many legal implications regarding the identification of a battering adult and the decisions required to ensure the child's safety vary among states and counties. In general, some legal recourse to protect the child's welfare is provided, and the provisions of the area should be understood.*

**Lead poisoning (MNPC no. 331.1).** The tragic incidence of lead poisoning, a totally preventable social problem, claims the lives of about 200 children in the United States annually. A total of about 12,000 children are treated for lead poisoning each year. Other cases of poisoning probably go unrecognized and untreated and these children may suffer permanent effects of lead ingestion.

Lead poisoning occurs as the result of the young child ingesting nonfood substances. This practice of pica in the young child is a natural outgrowth of the normal exploratory tendency to mouth objects and substances in the environment, but continued practice of pica is not a normal developmental trait. Most children experiment temporarily, but they are either discouraged by adults and older children or by the disagreeable taste of the nonfood substances. Whether pica develops as a result of malnutrition or hunger is not definitely understood; emotional factors of understimulation or loneliness may also be related.

Lead poisoning occurs predominantly in children from 1 to 3 years of age who live in deteriorating, overcrowded, slum housing. The main sources of lead are paint and plaster that chip off the wall. The child's mother is not usually aware of the potential problem, and although she often is not impressively attentive to the child's needs and may be under great social and economic stress herself, she is seldom neglectful or prone to inflict deliberate harm.

The child's symptoms vary from mild gastrointestinal signs mimicking infectious illness to severe central nervous system reactions and convulsions, coma, and death. The action of lead in the system is systemic, affecting primarily metabolic processes of the cells. It inhibits certain enzymatic reactions that are essential in the transport of substances across cell membranes. The predominant effects are on the renal, blood, and nervous systems. Renal effects are usually reversible, but chronic disorders later in life may be associated with early lead intoxication. The effects on the blood are usually first noticed as a gross anemia, but effects on hematopoiesis are grave, although most often reversible. The effects on the central nervous system are the most significant, because these effects are probably irreversible. Even in the absence of acute lead poisoning symptoms, children with elevated lead levels have been demonstrated to exhibit certain learning disabilities later in life.[54]

The child may be thought to have an acute gastrointestinal illness (vomiting, diarrhea, abdominal cramping), iron deficiency anemia (low hematocrit, fatigue, irritability), or behavioral problems that the parents describe as laziness, inability to get along with playmates, clumsiness, or loss of recently acquired developmental skills. When a child from a suspicious environment is seen to exhibit such symptoms, a determination of the blood lead level should be made, and intervention should be aimed toward immediately removing the source of lead.

The Surgeon General of the United States Public Health Service has recommended that a blood lead concentration of more than 40 $\mu$g/100 ml of whole blood be designated as evidence of undue absorption of lead.[144] At this level a child will usually not exhibit obvious symptoms of lead poisoning but should be followed closely, the environment should be evaluated for sources of lead, and the parents and older siblings should be cautioned to discourage pica behavior in this child. When blood lead concentrations exceed 80 $\mu$g/100 ml of whole blood, the child should be actively treated, because the grave and imminent danger to permanent health is very real.

Treatment for lead poisoning includes immediate withdrawal of the source of lead ingestion, eliminating the lead that remains in the system with chelating agents that facilitate rapid urinary excretion, and careful treatment of the child's blood and nervous system symptoms.*

---

*References 11, 15, 37, 41, 44, 85, 115, 117, 128, 151, 160, 186, 203, 286.

*References 2, 36, 40, 51, 54, 58, 113, 121, 131, 144, 153, 177, 193.

### Sudden infant death syndrome (SIDS)

Sudden, unexpected death in apparently well infants occurs in approximately 15,000 infants annually in the United States. Incidence is highest between 1 and 8 months of age. The fact that the infant is well and exhibits no sign of illness other than a mild cold in some instances accentuates the grave alarm and disbelief experienced by the family whose infant is suddenly found dead in the crib. The usual course of events includes a mild cold that involves only rhinorrhea, which is present within two weeks of death. The infant is placed in bed for the night and may be noted to be sleeping peacefully before the parents retire; the next morning the infant is found dead. No sign of distress, crying, or coughing alerts the family to the crisis that occurs.

There have been multiple theories proposed to explain the cause for sudden infant death. Autopsy findings have been remarkably similar, including pulmonary congestion and edema, intrathoracic petachiae, and minor pharyngeal edema, but none of these findings offer an etiologic explanation. Investigation is continually pursued in an effort to find some clues to explain the occurrence and offer means of identifying susceptible infants so that prevention can be initiated. No answers have been found. The evidence available to date substantiates the fact that death does not occur from suffocation, which is often the primary concern of the parents. The infant may be found face down or covered by a blanket, but suffocation did not cause death. Young infants are not affected, seasonal variation in occurrence is consistent, and pathologic findings among infants who are found face down do not differ from infants found in other positions. In about 10% of the cases of SIDS, a congenital or definitive diagnosis can be made. Accurate, thorough autopsy findings are essential in helping the family understand their infant's death and in gathering further evidence that may lead to eventual understanding of this mysterious syndrome.

The grief and reaction of the parents are the significant concerns for all health care workers. Often the child had been examined in a well-baby visit within a week or two of death. The family is eager to know if there were any clues that might have predicted the infant's untimely death. Guilt and despair lead them to blame themselves, one another, the physician, or any other person involved at the time. Frustration over not being able to identify a cause or any action they might have taken to prevent the death is initially intolerable, but as the parents begin to realize that this is indeed true, these facts may be used to help them realize that no one is to blame. Several counseling encounters with a qualified health care worker who understands the problems typically experienced by such families may be needed. Parent groups have been organized in many communities, and the National Foundation for Sudden Infant Death can supply literature and recent information on research findings.

When another infant is born in the family following a sudden infant death, the new infant is invariably affected. In spite of counseling and support for the family and their own desire to overcome the effects of the tragic experience, the new child is vulnerable to unexpected, spontaneous protective efforts and concerns. These reactions occur particularly when the infant has a mild upper respiratory infection or when conditions similar to those present at the time of the prior infant's death are noticed. Empathetic understanding of the mother's concerns can help her during a difficult period.*

## INTEGRATING CARE DURING ACUTE ILLNESS WITH COMPREHENSIVE HEALTH CARE
### Implementing the goals of health care

When reflecting over the general goals of comprehensive health care presented in Chapter 2, we are reminded of the significant opportunity available during an episode of acute illness to promote the child and family's motivation to seek health and to promote their use of their own resources to attain, maintain, or regain optimal health and function. The value that the family puts on "health" determines the meaning, for them, of each encounter with acute illness. As children grow and learn to adopt the notion that the family holds of health and health care practices, they begin to incorporate standards for their own health practices

*References 12, 14, 45, 46, 73, 139, 146, 158, 172, 220, 225.

that will probably influence them for the rest of their lives.

If children are adequately evaluated in relation to all aspects of functioning during times when they are not ill, working with them and the family during times of minor illness becomes well integrated into the total health care needs of the child and the family. On the other hand, many children come to the health care setting only when illness strikes. Health assessment and teaching during this encounter become vitally important, and an effort should be made to follow the child for any specific concerns that are identified.

During this brief encounter, however, the central goal of helping the family use their own resources in relation to their health care needs is often overlooked. Brief, hurried instructions are given to the parents (the child is usually excluded regardless of age), and the family is dismissed to go home. They have little or no notion of their central role in caring for the child's physical and emotional comfort during the illness, and there is little consideration for the health and well-being of the rest of the family, including the mother who is often tired and discouraged with the care of the sick child. Instead, in the health care encounter, the family should gain a realistic picture of the child's illness. They should know the signs of complications that warrant further medical or nursing attention. They should be realistically reassured in their capacity to take care of the situation and to apply these understandings to other situations in the future. The effort and time spent in helping a family in this manner may be great initially but is well compensated as the family gains better understanding. The goal is primarily to give realistic assistance with the task of learning more about health care and incorporating this into the family's own resource for self-care.[33] All aspects of health are considered, as are all factors that influence this particular family and child.

## The effect of acute illness on competency development

Physical illness during infancy and early childhood often causes the child to experience a brief, transient regression to earlier forms of behavior and capability. Recently acquired developmental skills may be temporarily lost. The child may return to the bottle or begin to wet the bed at night. Speech and language capacities may return to a level typical of an earlier period. Dependence upon mother and father returns to an earlier, more infantile level. The way in which parents respond to these changes can be significant for children; they either have the security of being cared for when something is wrong or they feel rejected when they are less than well. Children may be encouraged and helped to grow through the experience of an acute illness. They can learn about life and health, how to cope with the discomfort and frustration of not feeling well, and how people live and work together to help one another in times of need.[33]

Although children's physical competency may be temporarily affected by the illness, their ultimate growth and development may be enhanced in all areas of competency, or their ability in one or more areas may be permanently impaired. If they are treated with disgust and annoyance during illness, they learn to regard themselves as not worthy of continued love and care. If severe complications develop physically, they may be left with permanent effects in regard to learning and thought. Illness, even a very minor encounter, can be an instrument for further growth, or it can adversely inhibit the child's ultimate growth potential.

## STUDY QUESTIONS

1. Identify a nursing care problem that you may have encountered in the past (e.g., decreased peripheral circulation, headache, grief, fatigue). Describe how you would assess the exact nature of the problem, and establish criteria upon which to formulate a nursing diagnosis. Specify what nursing intervention would be indicated, and the specific aspects of the situation that would need to be considered in planning care. Also indicate the definitive role of medical or other health care professionals who would necessarily be involved in certain aspects of care.
2. Choose for comparison two drugs that might be used in the treatment of a single childhood problem, such as aspirin and acetaminophen or penicillin and erythromycin. Investigate the use of each drug thoroughly, including pharmacologic information and recent research findings. Indicate each consideration that must be understood in making a choice between the drugs and the

rationale for choosing one drug or the other in any given situation.

3. Describe ways in which a family with very limited resources and no running water in the home might be helped to find better ways to achieve adequate skin hygiene for children who suffer from repeated skin infections such as impetigo. Explore ways in your community that such a family might be helped.

4. Determine the location of the nearest poison control center or some other resource for obtaining help when a child has suffered from accidental poisoning. Investigate the range of services offered by this facility, and determine each step that is involved in the use of the facility, beginning with the initial call, the advice that is given to the family, the cost involved in using the facility, and what kind of care is available for the severely poisoned child.

5. Determine what action, if any, has been taken in your community to control the hazards of lead poisoning. Investigate the screening procedures that are available for determining blood lead levels, and ascertain the cost to the family. What standard value is recommended by the laboratory in interpreting the dangerous level of lead in the blood?

6. Visit a local drug store and identify all preparations that are available to treat one of the common problems mentioned in this chapter. Study the label of each preparation thoroughly, and identify the action of each compound. Choose one or two of these drugs for more indepth investigation. Determine what research has been conducted on the drug; correspond with the company that manufactures the drug and determine in detail their recommendations for use. Determine what side effects the drug may have, the possible interactions with other drugs, and what precautions the company recommends in its use. Determine how much of this information is accurately available on the label, and how the drug might be inadvertently misused by a parent.

7. Determine what measures are being taken by various groups in your community to help battered children and their families. What legal protections are offered to the child, to the parents, and to community agents who might be involved in identifying a case of child abuse. Determine how local practitioners in your area seek to protect children through early identification and how help for the child and family is instituted once identification is confirmed.

8. Choose a home remedy for one of the common childhood problems discussed in this chapter. Investigate all aspects of its composition, physiologic basis for use, and possible hazards. Describe what your recommendations for use would be.

## REFERENCES

1. Adebonojo, F. O.: Primary exogenous obesity; a conceptual classification, Clin. Pediatr. 13:715, Sept., 1974.

2. Adebonojo, F. O., and Strahs, S.: Reducing the lead burden of urban ghetto children, Clin. Pediatr. 13:310, April, 1974.

3. Aiai, M.: Pyrogenic infections of the central nervous system. In Cooke, R. E., editor: The biologic basis of pediatric practice, New York, 1968, McGraw-Hill Book Co., p. 1299.

4. Anthony, E. J.: Children at risk from divorce; a review. In Anthony, E. J., and Koupernik, C., editors: The child in his family; children at psychiatric risk, New York, 1974, John Wiley and Sons, p. 461.

5. Asher, P.: Fat babies and fat children; the prognosis of obesity in the very young, Arch. Dis. Child. 41:672, 1966.

6. Asnes, R. S., and Grebin, B.: Pharmacotherapeutics; a rational approach, Pediatr. Clin. North Am. 21:81, Feb., 1974.

7. Aspinall, M. J.: Nursing diagnosis—the weak link, Nurs. Outlook 24:433, July, 1976.

8. Avery, M. E.: Disorders of the lung. In Cooke, R. E., editor: The biologic basis of pediatric practice, New York, 1968, McGraw-Hill Book Co., p. 295.

9. Barich, D. P.: Steam vaporizers—therapy or tragedy? Pediatrics 49:131, 1972.

10. Bass, J. W., and others: Adverse effects of orally administered ampicillin, J. Pediatr. 83:106, July, 1973.

11. Bates, T.: Child abuse. In Green, M., and Haggerty, R. J., editors: Ambulatory pediatrics, II, Philadelphia, 1977, W. B. Saunders Co., p. 231.

12. Beckwith, J. B.: The sudden infant death syndrome; a new theory, Pediatrics 55:583, May, 1975.

13. Bellack, J. P.: Helping a child cope with the stress of injury, Am. J. Nurs. 74:1491, Aug., 1974.

14. Bergman, A. B.: Sudden infant death, Nurs. Outlook 20:775, Dec., 1972.

15. Besharov, D. J.: Building a community response to child abuse and maltreatment, Children Today 4:2, Sept.-Oct., 1975.

16. Blair, J., and Fitzgerald, J. F.: Treatment of nonspecific diarrhea in infants, Clin. Pediatr. 13:333, April, 1974.

17. Bleyer, W. A.: Surveillance of pediatric adverse drug reactions, Pediatrics 55:308, March, 1975.

18. Bluestone, C. D., and Shurin, P. A.: Middle ear disease in children; pathogenesis, diagnosis, and management, Pediatr. Clin. North Am. 21:379, May, 1974.

19. Boericke, P. H.: Emergency! II. First aid for wounds, severe bleeding, and shock, Nursing '75 5:40, March, 1975.

20. Breese, B. B., and others: The treatment of beta hemolytic streptococcal pharyngitis, Clin. Pediatr. 16:460, May, 1977.

21. Brem, J., and others: Salicylism, hyperventilation, and the central nervous system, J. Pediatr. 83:264, Aug., 1973.

22. Browder, J. A.: Needs and techniques for counseling parents of young children, Clin. Pediatr. 9:599, Sept., 1970.

23. Brown, M. S.: What you should know about communicable diseases, III. Nursing '75 5:55, Nov., 1975.

24. Brown, M. S.: Over-the-counter gastrointestinal drugs. III. Antidiarrheal drugs, Nurse Practitioner 2:23, Sept.-Oct., 1976.

25. Brown, M. S., and Alexander, M. M.: Physical examination; examining the nose, Nursing '74 **4**:35, July, 1974.

26. Brown, M. S., and Collar, M.: Over-the-counter drugs for upper respiratory symptoms, Nurse Practitioner **2**:18, Jan.-Feb., 1977.

27. Brunell, P. A.: Chickenpox. In Top, F. H., and Wehrle, P. F., editors: Communicable and infectious disease, ed. 8, St. Louis, 1976, The C. V. Mosby Co., p. 165.

28. Buchanan, N., and Rabinowitz, L.: Infantile salicylism—a reappraisal, J. Pediatr. **84**:391, March, 1974.

29. Burgess, A. W., and Homstrom, L. L.: Sexual trauma of children and adolescents; pressure, sex, and secrecy, Nurs. Clin. North Am. **10**:551, Sept., 1975.

30. Burnett, J. W.: Infections of the skin. In Rudolf, A. M., editor: Pediatrics, ed. 16, New York, 1977, Appleton-Century-Crofts, p. 876.

31. Caffey, J.: The whiplash shaken infant syndrome; manual shaking by the extremities with whiplash-induced intracranial and intraocular bleedings, linked with residual permanent brain damage and mental retardation, Pediatrics **54**:396, Oct., 1974.

32. Cantwell, R. J.: Iron deficiency anemia of infants, Clin. Pediatr. **11**:443, Aug., 1972.

33. Carey, W. B., and Sibinga, M. S.: Avoiding pediatric pathogenesis in the management of acute minor illness, Pediatrics **49**:553, April, 1972.

34. Carver, D. H., and Hodes, H. L.: Bacterial and viral infections. In Rudolph, A. M., editor: Pediatrics, ed. 16, New York, 1977, Appleton-Century-Crofts, p. 389.

35. Chadzik, G. M., and Yaffe, S. J.: Drug interaction; an important consideration for rational pediatric therapy, Pediatr. Clin. North Am. **19**:131, Feb., 1972.

36. Challop, R., McCabe, E., and Reece, R.: Breaking the childhood lead poisoning cycle—a program for community casefinding and self-help, Am. J. Public Health **62**:655-57, May, 1972.

37. Chamberlain, N.: The nurse and the abusive parent, Nursing '74 **4**:72, Oct., 1974.

38. Chamberlin, R. W.: Management of preschool behavior problems, Pediatr. Clin. North Am. **21**:33, Feb., 1974.

39. Chandra, R. K.: Immunocompetence in undernutrition, J. Pediatrics **81**:1194-1200, Dec., 1972.

40. Chisolm, J. J.: Screening for lead poisoning in children, Pediatrics **51**:280-283, Feb., 1973.

41. Clark, A. L.: Recognizing discord between mother and infant and changing it to harmony, Mat. Child Nurs. **1**:100, March-April, 1976.

42. Combs, A. W., Avila, D. L., and Purkey, W. W.: Helping relationships; basic concepts for the helping professions, Boston, 1971, Allyn and Bacon.

43. Committee on Drugs: Inaccuracies in administering liquid medication, Pediatrics **56**:327, Aug., 1975.

44. Committee on Infant and Preschool Children: Maltreatment of children; the battered child syndrome, Pediatrics **50**:160, July, 1972.

45. Committee on Infant and Preschool Child: The sudden infant death syndrome, Pediatrics **50**:964, Dec., 1972.

46. Committee on Infant and Preschool Child: Home monitoring for sudden infant death, Pediatrics **55**:144, Jan., 1975.

47. Committee on Infectious Diseases: Ampicillin-resistant strains of hemophilus influenzae type B, Pediatrics **55**:145, Jan., 1975.

48. Committee on Nutrition: Iron fortified formulas, Pediatrics **47**:785, May, 1971.

49. Communicable Childhood Disease—USA—1974: Clin. Pediatr. **15**:488, May, 1976.

50. Copeland, L.: Chronic diarrhea in infancy, Am. J. Nurs. **77**:461, March, 1977.

51. Croft, H., and Frenkel, S.: Children and lead poisoning, Am. J. Nurs. **75**:102, Jan., 1975.

52. Cunningham, A. S.: Homemade electrolyte solutions, J. Pediatr. **81**:417, Aug., 1972.

53. Davidson, M., and Silverberg, M.: Acute and chronic diarrhea. In Shirkey, H. C., editor: Pediatric therapy, ed. 5, St. Louis, 1975, The C. V. Mosby Co., p. 631.

54. de la Burde, B., and Choate, M. S.: Does asymptomatic lead exposure in children have latent sequelae? J. Pediatr. **8**:1088-1091, Dec., 1972.

55. Dillon, H. C., Jr., and Derrick, C. W., Jr.: Beta hemolytic streptococcal infections. In Shirkey, H. C., editor: Pediatric therapy, ed. 5, St. Louis, 1975, The C. V. Mosby Co., p. 422.

56. Dower, J. C.: Assessment and care of the child. In Rudolph, A. M., editor: Pediatrics, ed. 16, New York, 1977, Appleton-Century-Crofts, p. 17.

57. Drachman, R. H.: Acute infectious gastroenteritis, Pediatr. Clin. North Am. **21**:711, Aug., 1974.

58. Eidsvole, G., Mustalish, A., and Novick, L. F.: The New York City Department of Health; lessons in a lead poisoning control program, Am. J. Public Health **64**:956, Oct., 1974.

59. Einhorn, A. H.: Rumination syndrome. In Rudolf, A. M., editor: Pediatrics, ed. 16, New York, 1977, Appleton-Century-Crofts, p. 987.

60. Eller, J. J.: Infections; bacterial and spirochetal. In Kempe, C. H., Silver, H. K., and O'Brien, D., editors: Current pediatric diagnosis and treatment, ed. 4, Los Altos, Calif., 1976, Lange Medical Publications, p. 710.

61. Elliott, R. N.: Influencing the behavior of children in emotional conflict, Nurse Practitioner **2**:18, Sept.-Oct., 1977.

62. Ellis, E. F.: Asthma. In Green, M., and Haggerty, R. J., editors: Ambulatory pediatrics, II, Philadelphia, 1977, W. B. Saunders Co., p. 325.

63. Erickson, M. L.: Assessment and management of developmental changes in children, St. Louis, 1976, The C. V. Mosby Co.

64. Feinstein, A. R.: Clinical judgment, Baltimore, 1967, The Williams & Wilkins Co.

65. Fernald, B. W., Collier, A. M., and Clyde, W. A., Jr.: Respiratory infections due to mycoplasma pneumoniae in infants and children, Pediatrics **55**:327, March, 1975.

66. Ferrieri, P., Dajani, A. S., and Wannamaker, L. W.: Benzathine penicillin in the prophylaxis of strepto-

coccal skin infections; a pilot study, J. Pediatr. 83:572-577, Oct., 1973.

67. Fischer, C. C., Doxiadis, S. A., and Ziai, M.: Fever. In Ziai, M., editor: Pediatrics, ed. 2, Boston, 1975, Little, Brown and Co., p. 805.

68. Fitzgerald, J. F.: Diarrhea. In Green, M., and Haggerty, R. J., editors: Ambulatory pediatrics, II, Philadelphia, 1977, W. B. Saunders Co., p. 113.

69. Fitzgerald, J. F.: Vomiting. In Green, M., and Haggerty, R. J., editors: Ambulatory pediatrics, II, Philadelphia, 1977, W. B. Saunders Co., p. 110.

70. Fleisher, D., Ament, M. E.: Diarrhea, red diapers, and child abuse—clinical alertness needed for recognition; clinical skill needed for success in management, Clin. Pediatr. 16:820, Sept., 1977.

71. Fogelson, M. H., and Shelburne, S. A.: Management of febrile convulsions, Clin. Pediatr. 10:27, Jan., 1971.

72. Frick, O. L.: Allergy. In Rudolf, A. M., editor: Pediatrics, ed. 16, New York, 1977, Appleton-Century-Crofts, p. 329.

73. Friedman, S. B.: Psychological aspects of sudden and unexpected death in infants and children, Pediatr. Clin. North Am. 21:103, Feb., 1974.

74. Friedman, S. B., and Morse, C. W.: Child abuse; a five-year follow-up of early case finding in the emergency department, Pediatrics 54:404, Oct., 1974.

75. Frothingham, T. E.: Fever. In Green, M., and Haggerty, R. J., editors: Ambulatory pediatrics, II, Philadelphia, 1977, W. B. Saunders Co., p. 32.

76. Fulginiti, V. A.: Infections; viral and rikettsial. In Kempe, C. H., Silver, H. K., and O'Brien, D., editors: Current pediatric diagnosis and treatment, ed. 4, Los Altos, Calif., 1976, Lange Medical Publications, p. 680.

77. Furman, R. A.: A child's capacity for mourning. In Anthony, E. J., and Koupernick, C., editors: The child in his family; the impact of disease and death, New York, 1973, John Wiley and Sons, p. 225.

78. Gardner, H. G., and others: The evaluation of racemic epinephrine in the treatment of infectious croup, Pediatrics 52:52, July, 1973.

79. Gardner, P.: Antimicrobial drug therapy in pediatric practice, Pediatr. Clin. North Am. 21:617, Aug., 1974.

80. Gebbie, K. M., and Lavin, M. A.: Classification of nursing diagnoses; proceedings of the first national conference, St. Louis, 1975, The C. V. Mosby Co.

81. Geiser, R. L., and Norberta, Sr. M.: Sexual disturbance in young children, Mat. Child Nurs. 1:186, May-June, 1976.

82. Gelles, R. J.: Child abuse as psychopathology; a sociological critique and reformulation, Am. J. Orthopsychiatry 43:611, July, 1973.

83. Githens, J. H., and Hathaway, W.: Hematologic disorders. In Kempe, C. H., Silver, H. K., and O'Brien, D., editors: Current pediatric diagnosis and treatment, ed. 4, Los Altos, Calif., 1976, Lange Medical Publications, p. 358.

84. Goulding, R.: Acetaminophen poisoning, Pediatrics 52:883, Dec., 1973.

85. Green, M.: The pediatric disturbances of parenting. In Green, M., and Haggerty, R. J., editors: Ambulatory Pediatrics, II, Philadelphia, 1977, W. B. Saunders Co., p. 426.

86. Grosfeld, J. L., and Ballantine, T. V. N.: The skin; lacerations, abrasions, and burns. In Green, M., and Haggerty, R. J., editors: Ambulatory pediatrics, II, Philadelphia, 1977, W. B. Saunders Co., p. 238.

87. Gwaltney, J. M., Jr., and Hendley, J. O.: Acute respiratory infections. In Top, F. H., and Wehrle, P. F., editors: Communicable and infectious diseases, ed. 8, St. Louis, 1976, The C. V. Mosby Co., p. 91.

88. Haggerty, R. J.: Accidental poisoning. In Green, M., and Haggerty, R. J., editors: Ambulatory pediatrics, II, Philadelphia, 1977, W. B. Saunders Co., p. 260.

89. Haggerty, R. J.: Family crises and intervention. In Green, M., and Haggerty, R. J., editors: Ambulatory pediatrics, II, Philadelphia, 1977, W. B. Saunders Co., p. 221.

90. Haggerty, R. J., and Roghmann, K. J.: Noncompliance and self medication; two neglected aspects of pediatric pharmacology, Pediatr. Clin. North Am. 19:101, Feb., 1972.

91. Haka-Ikse, K.: Child development as an index of maternal mental illness, Pediatrics 55:310, March, 1975.

92. Halpern, L. M., and Bonica, J. J.: Analgesics. In Modell, W., editor: Drugs of choice 1978-1979, St. Louis, 1978, The C. V. Mosby Co., p. 205.

93. Hammill, J. F.: Trauma to the nervous system. In Barnett, H. L., editor: Pediatrics, ed. 16, New York, 1977, Appleton-Century-Crofts, p. 1827.

94. Harper, R. G.: Behavior modification in pediatric practice; a description of operant conditioning and positive and negative reinforcements, Clin. Pediatr. 14:962, Oct., 1975.

95. Hartford, C. E.: The early treatment of burns, Nurs. Clin. North Am. 8:447, Sept., 1973.

96. Hawkins, D. B., and Clark, R. W.: Orbital involvement in acute sinusitis, Clin. Pediatr. 16:464, May, 1977.

97. Henderson, B.: Nursing diagnosis; a concept analysis, unpublished paper, Houston, 1977, Texas Woman's University.

98. Herman, J., and Hirschman, L.: Incest between fathers and daughters, Sciences 17:4, Nov., 1977.

99. Hicks, J. N.: Upper respiratory tract (otorhinolaryngologic disorders). In Shirkey, H. C., editor: Pediatric therapy, ed. 5, St. Louis, 1975, The C. V. Mosby Co., p. 669.

100. Hill, L. L.: Burns in children. In Cooke, R. E., editor: The biologic basis of pediatric practice, New York, 1968, McGraw-Hill Book Co., p. 1608.

101. Hinman, A. R.: Resurgence of measles in New York, Am. J. Public Health 62:498-503, April, 1972.

102. Hirschhorn, N., and others: Ad libitum oral glucose therapy for acute diarrhea in Apache children, J. Pediatr. 83:562, Oct., 1973.

103. Honig, P. J., Paquariello, P. S., and Stool, S. E.: Influenzae pneumonia in infants and children, J. Pediatr. 83:215, Aug., 1973.

**435**

104. Hovenden, H. G.: Rocky Mountain spotted fever, Am. J. Nurs. **76**:419, March, 1976.

105. Howell, S. E.: Psychiatric aspects of habilitation, Pediatr. Clin. North Am. **20**:203, Feb., 1973.

106. Howie, B., and Ploussard, H. H.: Treatment of serious otitis media with ventilatory tubes, Clin. Pediatr. **13**:919, Nov., 1974.

107. Islur, J., Anglin, C. S., and Middleton, P. J.: The whooping cough syndrome; a continuing pediatric problem. Observation on epidemiology, bacteriology and clinical responses to therapy, Clin. Pediatr. **14**:171, Feb., 1975.

108. Janeway, C. A.: Recurrent infections. In Green, M., and Haggerty, R. J., editors: Ambulatory pediatrics, II, Philadelphia, 1977, W. B. Saunders Co., p. 73.

109. Jelliffe, D. B., and Jelliffe, E. F. P.: The at-risk concept as related to young child nutrition programs, Clin. Pediatr. **12**:65, Feb., 1973.

110. John, T. J., and Heyneman, D.: Infections; parasitic. In Kempe, C. H., Silver, H. K., and O'Brien, D.: Current pediatric diagnosis and treatment, ed. 4, Los Altos, Calif., 1976, Lange Medical Publications, p. 760.

111. Johnson, K. M.: Enteroviruses: Coxsackie and echo virus infections. In Top, F. H., and Wehrle, P. F., editors: Communicable and infectious diseases, ed. 8, St. Louis, 1976, The C. V. Mosby Co., p. 252.

112. Johnson, M. R.: Emergency management of head and spinal injuries, Nurs. Clin. North Am. **8**:389, 1973.

113. Joselow, M. M., and Bogden, J. D.: Lead content of printed media (warning: spitballs may be hazardous to your health), Am. J. Public Health **64**:238, March, 1974.

114. Judy, W. V.: Body temperature regulation. In Selkurt, E. E., editor: Physiology, ed. 4, Boston, 1976, Little, Brown and Co., p. 677.

115. Kauffman, C., and Neill, K.: Care of the hospitalized abused and his family; nursing implications, Mat. Child Nurs. **1**:117, March-April, 1976.

116. Kempe, C. H.: Family intervention, Pediatrics **56**:693, Nov., 1975.

117. Kempe, C. H., and Helfer, R.: Helping the battered child and his family, Philadelphia, 1972, J. B. Lippincott Co.

118. Kempe, C. H., Silver, H. K., and O'Brien, D. O.: Current pediatric diagnosis and treatment, ed. 4, Los Altos, Calif., 1976, Lange Medical Publications.

119. Keniston, K., and the Carnegie Council on Children: All our children; the American family under pressure, New York, 1977, Harcourt, Brace, Jovanovich.

120. Keynan, A., and Winter, S. R.: Respiratory infections in nursery school children, Clin. Pediatr. **16**:128, Feb., 1977.

121. Klein, R.: The pediatrician and the prevention of lead poisoning in children, Pediatr. Clin. North Am. **21**:277, May, 1974.

122. Knittle, J. L.: Obesity in childhood; a problem in adipose tissue cellular development, J. Pediatr. **81**:1048-1059, Dec., 1972.

123. Kogutt, M. S., and Swischuk, L. E.: Diagnosis of sinusitis in infants and children, Pediatrics **52**:121, July, 1973.

124. Krugman, S., Ward, R., and Katz, S. L.: Infectious diseases of children, ed. 6, St. Louis, 1977, The C. V. Mosby Co.

125. Kuberski, T. T., and Rosen, L.: Erythema infectiosum. In Top, F. H., and Wehrle, P. F., editors: Communicable and infectious diseases, ed. 8, St. Louis, 1976, The C. V. Mosby Co., p. 279.

126. Lampert, R. P., Robinson, D. S., and Soyka, L. F.: A critical look at oral decongestants, Pediatrics **55**:550, April, 1975.

127. Lauer, B., Broeck, E. T., and Grossman, M.: Battered child syndrome; review of 130 patients with controls, Pediatrics **54**:67, July, 1974.

128. Leake, H. C., III, and Coleman, R. O.: Preparing for and testifying in a child abuse hearing, Clin. Pediatr. **16**:1057, Nov., 1977.

129. Lecks, H. I.: Explosive asthma in the infant and young child under two years; clinical features; anatomic and physiologic peculiarities, Clin. Pediatr. **15**:135, Feb., 1976.

130. Lee, C. A., Stroot, V. R., and Schaper, C. A.: When acid-base problems hang in the balance, Nursing '75 **5**:32, Aug., 1975.

131. Lin-Fu, J. S.: Preventing lead poisoning in children, Child. Today **2**:2, Jan., 1973.

132. Linneman, C. C., and others. Febrile illness in early infancy associated with ECHO virus infection, J. Pediatr. **84**:49, Jan., 1974.

133. Linneman, C. C., and others: Pertussis; persistent problems, J. Pediatr. **85**:589, Oct., 1974.

134. Lipow, H. W.: Respiratory tract infections. In Green, M., and Haggerty, R. J., editors: Ambulatory pediatrics, II, Philadelphia, 1977, W. B. Saunders Co., p. 36.

135. Lohr, J. A., and Hendley, J. O.: Prolonged fever of unknown origin; a record of experiences with 54 childhood patients. Clin. Pediatr. **16**:768, Sept., 1977.

136. Lovric, V. A., Beal, P. J., and Lammi, A. T.: Iron-deficiency anemia, J. Pediatr. **86**:194, Feb., 1975.

137. Lucius, N. J.: The nursing management of the child with acute otitis media, unpublished master's thesis, University of Utah, 1972.

138. Maloney, S.: A health care protocol for otitis media. In Brandt, P. A., and others, editors: Current practice in pediatric nursing, II, St. Louis, 1978, The C. V. Mosby Co., p. 185.

139. Mandell, F., and Wolfe, L. C.: Sudden infant death syndrome and subsequent pregnancy, Pediatrics **56**:724, Nov., 1975.

140. Manning, P., Avery, M. E., and Ross, A.: Purulent otitis media; differences between populations in different environments, Pediatrics **53**:135, Feb., 1974.

141. Marks, M. B.: Differential diagnosis of wheezing in children, Clin. Pediatr. **13**:225, March, 1974.

142. Mauer, A. M.: Malnutrition—still a common problem for children in the United States, Clin. Pediatr. **14**:23, Jan., 1975.

143. McCarthy, P. L., and Dolan, T. F.: The serious im-

plications of high fever in infants during their first
three months, Clin. Pediatr. **15**:794, Sept., 1976.

144. Medical aspects of childhood lead poisoning: Statement approved by the surgeon general, U.S. Public
Health Service, Pediatrics **48**:464, Sept., 1971.

145. Mennear, J. H.: The poisoning emergency, Am. J.
Nurs. **77**:842, May, 1977.

146. Merritt, T. A., Bauer, W. I., and Hasselmeyer, E. G.:
Sudden infant death syndrome; the role of the emergency room physician, Clin. Pediatr. **14**:1095, Dec.,
1975.

147. Metcoff, J.: Regulation of the body fluids. In Cooke,
R. E., editor: The biologic basis of pediatrics, New
York, 1968, McGraw-Hill Book Co., p. 95.

148. Mikal, S.: Homeostasis in man, Boston, 1967, Little,
Brown and Co.

149. Milko, D. A., Marshak, G., and Striker, T. W.: Naso-
tracheal intubation in the treatment of acute epiglottitis, Pediatrics **53**:674, May, 1974.

150. Millichap, J. G.: Paroxysmal disorders of the central
nervous system. In Cooke, R. E., editor: The biologic
basis of pediatric practice, New York, 1968, McGraw-
Hill Book Co.

151. Mitchell, B.: Working with abusive parents; a case-
worker's view, Am. J. Nurs. **73**:480, March, 1973.

152. Mofenson, H. C., and Greenshear, J.: Keeping up
with changing trends in childhood poisonings, Clin.
Pediatr. **14**:621, July, 1975.

153. Mooty, J., Ferrand, C. F., and Harris, P.: Relationship of diet to lead poisoning in children, Pediatrics
**55**:636, May, 1975.

154. Mundinger, M. O., and Jauron, G. D.: Developing a
nursing diagnosis, Nurs. Outlook **23**:94, Feb., 1975.

155. Murray, J. D., and others: Acute bacterial meningitis
in childhood; an outline of management, Clin. Pediatr.
**11**:455, Aug., 1972.

156. Murray, M. E.: Behavioral management in pediatrics, applications of operant learning theory to problem behaviors of children, Clin. Pediatr. **15**:465, May,
1976.

157. Nagi, S. Z.: Child abuse and neglect programs; a national overview, Children Today **4**:13, May-June,
1975.

158. Nakushian, J. M.: Restoring parents' equilibrium after
sudden infant death, Am. J. Nurs. **76**:1600, Oct.,
1976.

159. Neter, E.: Salmonella, Shigella, and Enteropathogenic E. Coli infections. In Rudolph, A. M., editor: Pediatrics, ed. 16, New York, 1977, Appleton-Century-
Crofts, p. 486.

160. Newberger, E. H., and others: Reducing the literal
and human cost of child abuse; impact of a new hospital management system, Pediatrics **51**:840, May,
1973.

161. Nitowsky, H. M.: Nutrition. In Cooke, R. E., editor:
The biologic basis of pediatric practice, New York,
1968, McGraw-Hill Book Co., p. 891.

162. Noojin, R. O.: Pediatric dermatology. In Shirkey,
H. C., editor: Pediatric therapy, ed. 5, St. Louis,
1975, The C. V. Mosby Co., p. 863.

163. Norins, A. L.: Pediatric dermatology. In Green, M.,
and Haggerty, R. J., editors: Ambulatory pediatrics,
II, Philadelphia, 1977, W. B. Saunders Co., p. 81.

164. Nursing problem classification for children and youth:
Department of Health, Education and Welfare, Ma-
ternal and Child Health Services, Research grant
MC-R-270058, Minneapolis, Feb., 1976, Minnesota
Systems Research, Inc.

165. O'Grady, R., and Dolan, T.: Whooping cough in infants, Am. J. Nurs. **76**:114, Jan., 1976.

166. Olson, R. J.: Index of suspicion; screening for child
abusers, Am. J. Nurs. **76**:108, Jan., 1976.

167. Oski, F. A.: Designation of anemia on a functional
basis, J. Pediatr. **83**:353, Aug., 1973.

168. Ouellete, E.: The child who convulses with fever,
Pediatr. Clin. North Am. **21**:467, May, 1974.

169. Paradise, J. L.: Why T & A remains moot, Pediatrics
**49**:648-651, May, 1972.

170. Parra, A., and others: Correlative studies in obese
children and adolescents concerning body composition
and plasma insulin and growth hormone levels, Pediatr. Res. **5**:605, Nov., 1971.

171. Parthion poisoning alert: Clin. Pediatr. **12**:511, Sept.,
1973.

172. Patterson, K., and Pomeroy, M. R.: Nursing care begins after death when the disease is; sudden infant
death syndrome, Nursing '74 **4**:85, May, 1974.

173. Pavenstedt, E.: An intervention program for infants
from high risk homes, Am. J. Public Health **63**:393,
May, 1973.

174. Pearlman, D. S.: Allergic disorders. In Kempe, C. H.,
Silver, H. K., and O'Brien, D., editors: Current pediatric diagnosis and treatment, ed. 4, Los Altos, Calif.
1976, Lange Medical Publications, p. 862.

175. Pearlman, D. S., and Szentivanyi, A.: Excessive reac-
tivity of defense mechanisms—allergy. In Cooke, R.
E., editor: The biologic basis of pediatric practice,
New York, 1968, McGraw-Hill Book Co., p. 536.

176. Pinney, M. S.: Postural drainage in infants, Nursing
'72 **2**:45, Oct., 1972.

177. Piomelli, S., and others: The FEP (free erythrocyte
porphyrins) test; a screening micromethod for lead
poisoning, Pediatrics **51**:254-259, Feb., 1973.

178. Pizzo, P. A., Lovejoy, F. H., Jr., and Smith, D. H.:
Prolonged fever in children, Pediatrics **55**:468, April,
1975.

179. Plotkin, S. A.: Antibiotics—1975, Clin. Pediatr. **14**:
816, Sept., 1975.

180. Plotkin, S. A., and Arbeter, A. M.: New antibiotics
and old diseases, Clin. Pediatr. **16**:472, May, 1977.

181. Proctor, D. F.: The air passages. In Cooke, R. E.,
editor: The biologic basis of pediatric practice, New
York, 1968, McGraw-Hill Book Co., p. 273.

182. Quinn-Bogard, A. L., and Potsic, W. P.: Stridor in the
first year of life; the clinical evaluation of the persistence of intermittent noisy breather, Clin. Pediatr.
**16**:913, Oct., 1977.

183. Randolph, M. F., and others: Streptococcal pharyngitis; Posttreatment carrier prevalence and clinical relapse in children treated with clindamycin palmitate or

phenoxymethyl penicillin, Clin. Pediatr. 14:119, Feb., 1975.

184. Rapkin, R. H.: Tracheostomy in epiglottitis, Pediatrics 52:426, Sept., 1973.

185. Rapkin, R. H.: Bacteriologic and clinical findings in acute pneumonia of childhood, Clin. Pediatr. 14:130, Feb., 1975.

186. Rausen, A. R.: Symposium on child abuse, Pediatrics, (suppl.) vol. 51, April, 1973.

187. Rees, T. S.: Tympanometry as an aid in the diagnosis of middle ear disease, Clin. Pediatr. 15:368, April, 1976.

188. Reinhart, J. B., and Pisula, D.: Phobic symptoms in a toddler; early intervention can forestall serious developments, Clin. Pediatr. 16:1100, Dec., 1977.

189. Rinear, C. E., and Rinear, E.: Emergency! III. Care for aspiration, burns, and poisoning, Nursing '75 5: 40, April, 1975.

190. Robertson, W. O., Robertson, K. A., and Peters, J. W.: Poison control; retrieving stored information, J. Pediatr. 83:461, Sept., 1973.

191. Robinson, L. A., Roger, K. E., and Fischer, R. G.: Nursing considerations in the use of non-prescription analgesic-antipyretics; aspirin and acetaminophen, Pediatr. Nurs. 3:18, July/Aug., 1977.

192. Romlinson, W. A.: Parents' knowledge of respiratory disease, Pediatrics 56:1009, Dec., 1975.

193. Rosen, J. F., Zrate-Salvador, C., and Trinidad, E. E.: Plasma lead levels in normal and lead-intoxicated children, J. Pediatr. 84:45, Jan., 1974.

194. Rosenstein, G., and others: Warning; the use of Lomotil in children, Pediatrics 12:132, Jan., 1973.

195. Rosman, N. P.: Increased intracranial pressure in childhood, Pediatr. Clin. North Am. 21:483, May, 1974.

196. Rowe, D. S.: Acute suppurative otitis media, Pediatrics 56:285, Aug., 1975.

197. Roy, C., Silverman, A., and DuBois, R. S.: Gastrointestinal tract. In Kempe, C. H., Silver, H. K., and O'Brien, D., editors: Current pediatric diagnosis and treatment, ed. 4, Los Altos, Calif., 1976, Lange Medical Publications, p. 414.

198. Rumack, B. H., and Matthew, H.: Acetaminophen poisoning and toxicity, Pediatrics 55:871, June, 1975.

199. Rumach, B. H., and Temple, A. R.: Lomotil poisoning, Pediatrics 53:495, April, 1974.

200. St. Geme, J. W.: Progress in virology; pathways in the progression of respiratory tract invasions, Clin. Pediatr. 15:164, Feb., 1976.

201. St. Geme, J. W., Coh, W. L., and Meyer, D. L.: Otitis media; bacteriology and antibiotics, Pediatrics 49:785, May, 1972.

202. Samter, M.: Bronchial asthma; new definition for an old disease, Clin. Pediatr. 13:406, May, 1974.

203. Savino, A. B., and Sanders, R. W.: Working with abusive parents; group therapy and home visits, Am. J. Nurs. 73:482, March, 1973.

204. Schmitt, B. D.: Ear, nose and throat. In Kempe, C. H., Silver, H. K., and O'Brien, D.: editors: Current pediatric diagnosis and treatment, ed. 4, Los

Altos, Calif., 1976, Lange Medical Publications, p. 240.

205. Sell, S. H. W., and others: Long-term sequelae in hemophilus influenzae meningitis, Pediatrics 49:206, Feb., 1972.

206. Sell, S. H. W., and others: Psychological sequelae to bacterial meningitis; two controlled studies, Pediatrics 49:212, Feb., 1972.

207. Seto, D. S. Y., and Heller, R. M.: Acute respiratory infections, Pediatr. Clin. North Am. 21:683, Aug., 1974.

208. Sgroi, S. M.: Sexual molestation of children; the last frontier in child abuse, Children Today 4:18, May-June, 1975.

209. Sharer, J. E.: Reviewing acid-base balance, Am. J. Nurs. 75:980, June, 1975.

210. Shillito, J., Jr.: Head injuries. In Green, M., and Haggerty, R. J., editors: Ambulatory pediatrics, II, Philadelphia, 1977, W. B. Saunders Co., p. 247.

211. Shinefield, H. R.: Infections of skin and soft tissue. In Shirkey, H. C., editor: Pediatric therapy, ed. 5, St. Louis, 1975, The C. V. Mosby Co., p. 517.

212. Shulman, B. H., and Reddy, G. D.: "Purse" poisons, Pediatrics 51:126, Jan., 1973.

213. Shumway, C. N.: Iron deficiency in children, Pediatr. Clin. North Am. 19:855, Nov., 1972.

214. Silverberg, M., and Davidson, M.: Vomiting. In Shirkey, H. C., editor: Pediatric therapy, ed. 5, St. Louis, 1975, The C. V. Mosby Co., p. 41.

215. Simonds, J. F.: Enuresis, Clin. Pediatr. 16:79, Jan., 1977.

216. Soyka, L. F., and others: The misuse of antibiotics for treatment of upper respiratory tract infections in children, Pediatrics 55:552, April, 1975.

217. Starfield, B., and Scheff, D.: Effectiveness of pediatric care; the relationship between processes and outcome, Pediatrics 49:547-552, April, 1972.

218. Steele, B. F., and Pollock, C. B.: A psychiatric study of parents who abuse infants and small children. In Helfer, R. E., and Kempe, C. H., editors: The battered child, Chicago, 1974, The University of Chicago Press.

219. Stein, J. M.: Burns in childhood. In Rudolf, A. M., editor: Pediatrics, ed. 16, New York, 1977, Appleton-Century-Crofts, p. 770.

220. Steinschneider, A.: Prolonged apnea and the sudden infant death syndrome; clinical and laboratory observations, Pediatrics 50:646, Oct., 1972.

221. Strauss, M. B., editor: Familiar medical quotation, Boston, 1968, Little, Brown and Co., p. 410.

222. Sutton, E., and Soyka, L. F.: How safe is acetaminophen?; some practical cautions with this widely used agent, Clin. Pediatr. 12:692, Dec., 1973.

223. Swift, N.: Head injury! Essentials of excellent nursing, Nursing '74 4:26, Sept., 1974.

224. Swigart, E., and Stool, S. E.: Hearing sensitivity and physical characteristics of the eardrum observed during otoscopic examination, Clin. Pediatr. 16:556, June, 1976.

225. Tonkin, S.: Sudden infant death syndrome, Pediatrics 55:650, May, 1975.

226. Tooley, W. H., and Lipow, H. W.: Respiratory function and pulmonary disease in older infants and children. In Rudolf, A. M., editor: Pediatrics, ed. 16, New York, 1977, Appleton-Century-Crofts, p. 1544.

227. Top, F. H., Sr.: Rubella. In Top, F. H., and Wehrle, P. F., editors: Communicable and infectious diseases, ed. 8, St. Louis, 1976, The C. V. Mosby Co., p. 589.

228. Top, F. H., Sr., and Wehrle, P. F.: Measles. In Top, F. H., and Wehrle, P. F., editors: Communicable and infectious diseases, ed. 8, St. Louis, 1976, The C. V. Mosby Co., p. 425.

229. Wannamaker, L. W., Rammelkamp, C. H., and Top, F. H., Sr.: Streptococcal infections. In Top, F. H., and Wehrle, P. F., editors: Communicable and infectious diseases, ed. 8, St. Louis, 1976, The C. V. Mosby Co., p. 655.

230. Washington, J. A.: The steam vaporizer, Pediatrics 50:168, July, 1972.

231. Weed, L. L.: Medical records, medical education and patient care, Cleveland, 1970, Press of Case Western Reserve University.

232. Wehrle, P. F.: Meningitis. In Top, F. H., and Wehrle, P. F., editors: Communicable and infectious diseases, ed. 8, St. Louis, 1976, The C. V. Mosby Co., p. 436.

233. Wessel, M. A.: Helping a child cope with the death of a loved one. In Green, M., and Haggerty, R. J., editors: Ambulatory pediatrics, II, Philadelphia, 1977, W. B. Saunders Co., p. 226.

234. West, S., and others: A review of antihistamines and the common cold, Pediatrics 56:100, July, 1975.

235. Westaby, J. R.: A bookshelf on injury control and emergency health services, Am. J. Public Health 64:394, April, 1974.

236. Weston, W. L., Philport, J. A., and Philport, O. S.: Skin. In Kempe, C. H., Silver, H. K., and O'Brien, D., editors: Current pediatric diagnosis and treatment, ed. 4, Los Altos, Calif., 1976, Lange Medical Publications, p. 192.

237. Wichlacz, C. R., Randall, D. H., Nelson, J. H., and Kempe, C. H.: The characteristics and management of child abuse in the U.S. Army—Europe, Clin. Pediatr. 14:545, June, 1975.

238. Wiley, L., editor: Shock. II. Different kinds, different problems, Nursing '74, 4:43, May, 1974.

239. Wilson, J. F., Lahey, M. E., and Helner, D. C.: Studies on iron metabolism. V. Further observation on cow's milk-induced gastrointestinal bleeding in infants with iron-deficiency anemia, J. Pediatr. 84:335, March, 1974.

240. Wilson, J. T.: Compliance with instructions in the evaluation of therapeutic efficacy; a common but frequently unrecognized major variable, Clin. Pediatr. 12:333, June, 1973.

241. Winograd, M.: Pathological mourning. In Anthony, E. J., and Koupernik, C., editors: The child and his family; the impact of disease and death, New York, 1973, John Wiley and Sons, p. 233.

242. Winter, S. T.: The age factor in acute diarrhea during childhood, Clin. Pediatr. 13:17, Jan., 1974.

243. Wisseman, C. L., Jr.: Rickettsial diseases. In Top, F. H., and Wehrle, P. F., editors: Communicable and infectious diseases, ed. 8, St. Louis, 1976, The C. V. Mosby Co., p. 567.

244. Wright, H. T., Jr.: Exanthem subitum. In Top, F. H., and Wehrle, P. F., editors: Communicable and infectious disease, ed. 8, St. Louis, 1976, The C. V. Mosby Co., p. 283.

# Shana—PROBLEM-ORIENTED RECORD
# Stacy—PLAY ASSESSMENT

Cheryl Boyd Hundley

## HEALTH STATUS LIST

| Onset | Date | No. | Active | Date | Inactive/resolved |
|---|---|---|---|---|---|
| | 9/30/77 | 1 | Incomplete data base | | |
| ? | 9/30/77 | 2 | Unable to use descriptive words | | |
| 9/8/77 | 9/30/77 | 3 | Developed "cold" after playing in weeds | 9/30/77 | No. 3 |
| ? | 9/30/77 | 4 | Nutrition | | |
| ? | 9/30/77 | 5 | Laceration of L foot | 9/30/77 | No. 5 |
| 3/2/77 | 9/30/77 | 6 | New baby in the family | | |
| 6/9/74 | 9/30/77 | 7 | Mother had "high B/P" during labor with Shana | | |

Client _____ **Shana S.** _____ Sex ___ F ___ Age _3 yr. 3 mo._ B.D. _____ 6/9/74 _____

Date _9/30/77_ Race _____ Black _____

**Information sources:** Shana
Mother

**Reason health care worker sought client**

Shana was sought as a client for a primary mode nursing assessment for learning and for health intervention.

**Reason for seeking health care (mother and child's comments)**

Shana accompanied her mother and her baby sister Tina to the clinic.

**What events led up to the situation?**

Came to the clinic for follow-up exam for recent "cold."

**When did this situation occur?**

A cold developed after playing in the weeds.

**Describe the situation and/or how you are feeling. What made you decide to seek health care?**

Shana replied she "felt good" about getting "to play" with us for a while.

**What do you and your family do when something like this happens?**

Mother brings children to clinic before they "get real sick."

**How is this affecting you and your family at the present time?**

Mother has to take off work to bring children to clinic. Can leave children with grandmother when sick. **441**

## MOTHER PROFILE
HEALTH HISTORY
### Present health status
"Good." No major illnesses or surgeries. Two children: Shana and Tina.

### Previous medical-surgical events
In the brief interview could not recall anything.

PRENATAL HISTORY WITH THIS CHILD (SHANA)
### Medical supervision
Yes

### Nutrition, diet
Could not recall restrictions. Weight gain about 25 pounds.

### Illness, infections, complications
None until onset of labor. Then blood pressure "went up."

### Treatments, procedures
None recalled.

### Anesthesia
Remembered only "a shot in the hip."

### Course of labor and delivery
"Real high blood pressure" started during labor. Shana was delivered vaginally.

### Availability in home
Works six days a week as a maid in a hotel.

### Number of people in the home
Has an uncle who lives with them; Shana calls him "a brother." Unable to explore this further due to time factor as mother had to leave clinic.

### Employment/work environment
Leaves at 8 AM. Gets home 5:30 PM. Frequently has to work extra.

### Date of last menstrual period
No information obtained.

## FATHER PROFILE
There is no father in this home. Mother is unmarried.

### Present health status
Not applicable.

### Previous medical-surgical events
Not applicable.

### Number of people she supports
She supports herself and her two children. Income is supplemented by government assistance. There is no child support from father of the children.

### Availability in home/work habits
Not applicable.

### Employment/work environment
Not applicable.

**Range of income**

Mother makes $2.50 per hour. $66 weekly in assistance.

**Insurance**

None.

LIFE CHANGE EVENTS

Death (family, close friend) _____ New baby Tina—less than 1 year old

Divorce _____ Marital separation _____ Return to school _____

Injury, illness _____ Job loss _____

Change of residence "Recently" Retirement _____

**Pedigree** (include chronic, inherited conditions, allergies, causes of death, illness in siblings)

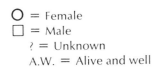

○ = Female
□ = Male
? = Unknown
A.W. = Alive and well

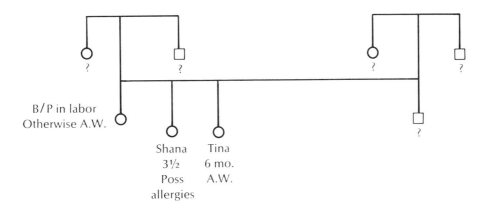

B/P in labor
Otherwise A.W.

Shana  Tina
3½  6 mo.
Poss  A.W.
allergies

**Does your family see itself as a healthy family or as a sick family?**

Everyone "feels good" most of time except for "little things."

**CHILD PROFILE**
HEALTH HISTORY
**Neonatal status (risk, Apgar, congenital abnormalities)**

No congenital abnormalities seen in physical examination. Records for risk and Apgar not available.

**Postnatal course**

"Normal baby."

**Previous illnesses (dates)**

Recently (2-3 weeks ago) "ran through a bunch of weeds and got a cold." Medicine from UMC physician "dried it up."

**Medications**

Medication for "cold" in last 2-3 weeks. Not taking any medication now.

**Accidents and injuries (dates)**

Scar on L heel, inner aspect about 2 by 4 cm; healed, nontender, no inflammation. "I stepped on a piece of glass when the dog bit me."

**Nutrition history (example of 24-hour intake)**

Time not sufficient to do 24-hr intake. Obtain more data on next visit.

BREAKFAST          LUNCH          SUPPER          SNACKS

Mother related briefly that Shana eats meats, fruits, and vegetables "good." Presently she refuses to drink milk and she dislikes cheese. Mother expressed "worry" about this.

**Formula: type/amt.**

On prepared formula until she was 8 months. Formula stopped as she was "getting heavy."

**Compare weight/height/age ratio**

3½ yrs., weight = 35 lbs. (60%); height = 42 in. (90%)

**Identify developmental milestones (DDST)**

Unable to do DDST and identification of milestones at this time.

**Sleep patterns/disturbances**

None.

**Allergies**

Possibly allergies to pollens, the mother thinks.

**Immunizations**

"Up-to-date" according to mother. No objective data to confirm.

PSYCHOLOGIC PROFILE (data here to be obtained during interactions, inquiry, observation, DDST)

### Cognition

CONCRETE OPERATIONS: PRECONCEPTUAL
THOUGHT (2-4 YEARS)

_____ Believes everyone views world as he does

Yes Play is chief activity; assigns elements of reality to toys, objects

Yes Centering: can identify only one quality of an object

_____ Imitates parental model

_____ Events judged by outward appearance

_____ Unable to perform a completed process in reverse (reversibility)

### Ego

AUTONOMY VS. SHAME AND DOUBT
(12 MOS-3 YEARS)

Yes Sense of will: "I want" "me" "mine"

Yes Collects, hoards

_____ Interacts more with father

_____ Seeks reassurance from parental model after new self-exploration

Yes Plays with a world of small manageable toys

Yes Unable to stay in a designated place

INITIATIVE VS. GUILT (3-6 YEARS)

_____ Cares for own body, toys, pets

Yes Observes differences between men and women

_____ Interacts more with parents and peers

_____ Intrusive behavior, questioning, noisy

_____ Rivalry with older siblings; solitary play or group play with peers; plays out feelings

_____ Identifies with parent of the same sex

### Comments

Play was her central activity throughout the exam. She named the doll Shana (element of reality). She identified parts of the face on the doll figure. Only able to center on naming the parts of the dolls' faces and was unable to focus on whether a doll was "big" or "little" (centering).

Used the words "me" and "mine" at intervals during handling of toys. Segregated dolls into boys and girls, man and momma. Had to periodically move about the room. Played continually with the small toys provided. Hoarded and grouped the toys at regular intervals. Just moving into the initiative vs. guilt phase.

**School progress**                                                Case

Not applicable to Shana.

**Perception of self**
**Describe yourself to me**

I'm a little girl.

**Tell me things you like about yourself; dislike**

Unable to explore this, due to no response.

**Let's pretend you could change something about yourself. Would you change anything?**

Unable to explore this.

**Describe how you feel about what's happening to you now.**

"Liked to play" with me. (She was relaxed, confident.)

SOCIAL COMPETENCY PROFILE
**Personal-social (DDST)**

Unable to test specifically.

**Father/mother–child interaction**

Eye contact _Good_
Touching _Eagerly took mother's hand_
Tone of voice of parent _Soft, gentle_
Child-parent activities _No information_
Ease of separation _Separated for the examination without tears_

**Position of child in family**

First child

**Describe life-style**

Obtain in home visit
Is more than one language spoken in the home? _No_

ENVIRONMENTAL PROFILE
**Pollutants**
**Population density** } Check with city/county health department.
**Infestations**
**Fire hazards** } Obtain in home visit.
**Medications/poisons**
**Crime**

Check city statistics.

**Availability of transportation**

Mother has her own car.

PHYSICAL PROFILE
**Measurements**

Head circumference _50 cm_   Chest circumference _48 cm_   Ht _42 in._   Wt _35 lbs._

**Neuromuscular system**

Development history, H/A, weakness, numbness in extremities, convulsions.
Mother reports no history of convulsions, weakness or numbness, headaches or incoordination.

**Present neurological status**

Nervous system intact, functioning without any gross abnormalities.

**445**

### Social affect

Relaxed, eager, inner controls during this new situation.

### Developmental status

Appropriate for age (see cognition and ego).

### Speech development

During exam she did not know what "up" or "down" meant. Could not identify salt and sugar with any words.

### Memory

Not tested.

### Posture, muscle tone

No kyphosis, muscle flaccidity.

### Reflexes

2+, negative Babinski
Moro NA
Plantar, palmar NA
Sucking, rooting NA
Babinski Neg.
Tonic neck NA

### Cranial nerves

Intact. See below in exam.

### Cerebellar function

Romberg negative. Walked heel to toe in straight line.

### Fine motor function

Not tested specifically.

### Parietal lobe function

Identified key and rubberband with eyes closed.

### Proprioception

Inconclusive as she was unable to relate to "up" and "down" words by pointing finger in big toe test.

### Tactile capacity

Could feel sharp, dull sensations on arms and thighs.

### Skin (condition, description, hydration)

Pliable, supple, hydrated skin without rashes, scars (except on L heel).

### Head (circumference, fontanel measurement, palpation, transillumination)

Negative to palpation. Fontanels closed. Transillumination not performed. Symmetry bilaterally equal.

### Face (expression, placement of ears, palpebral fissures, percussion of sinuses, skin)

Ears aligned with outer canthus of eyes. Eyes alert, relaxed face. Structures symmetrically placed. Face symmetry equal.

### Hair, scalp (hairline, hygiene)

Hair and scalp clean; well-groomed hair, texture coarse but pliant. Hairline not receded or lowered.

### Eyes (acuity, peripheral fields, color, EOMs, retina, conjunctiva, strabismus)

EOMs intact. PERRLA. Red reflex present bilaterally. Conjunctiva pink. Vision not tested. Could not identify any colors. All colors were identified as black. PE negative for strabismus. DEST normal— CNII intact.

### Nose (patency, discharge, smell)

Nose patent. Unable to detect discharge. Mucosa pink, lubricated. No erythema. Identifies smells—CNI intact.

### Mouth and throat (teeth, gums, pharynx, tongue, palates, throat culture, swallowing)

No caries. Mouth and tongue clean; no gingivitis. Throat not reddened. No deviations of palate structure. Uvula midline to "ahh." CNXII intact, CNIX intact.

### Ears (structure, hearing, bilaterally symmetrical in location and size)

External ears nontender. R tympanum pearly gray with cone of light at 4-5 o'clock position. L tympanum not visualized due to wax occluding the canal. Bony landmarks visualized on R tympanum. No scars on tympanum. Heard watch tick about 2 inches from ears. Negative Weber and Rhinne. CNVIII intact.

### Neck (palpation, motion)

Negative for adenopathy. ROM not tested. Good shoulder shrug against resistance (CNXI).

### Chest (nodes, nipples)

Bilaterally symmetrical and nipples at the same level. Palpation negative for edema, nodes, or masses. Tactile fremitus negative.

### Heart (size, position, PMI, sounds)

PMI is L of MCL at the 4th ICS. Boundaries of the heart not percussed. No extra sounds heard by auscultation. Rate 108/minute apically, regular rhythm. Pulses equal bilaterally (unable to palpate popliteals). $S_1$ loudest at PMI $S_2$ loudest at pulmonic. No murmur.

### Lungs (movement, sounds)

Negative for adventitious sounds. Chest clear to percussion. Exclusion equal bilaterally.

### Abdomen (size, contour, bowel sounds, umbilicus, femorals)

Negative for palpation. Bowel sounds present (25-26/min). Liver edge palpated with some difficulty. Spleen not palpable. Femorals equal bilaterally. Umbilicus dry and clean.

### Back and spine (structure)

Negative for scoliosis, kyphosis, pilonidal dimple.

### Extremities (palmar creases, ROM, hip abduction)

Full passive ROM in arms and legs. No clicks felt during ROM. Active ROM revealed equal strengths bilaterally. Symmetry and length of extremities equal. Scar on L inner aspect of heel from stepping on glass 2 × 4 cm; healed and nontender to pressure.

### Urinary tract (characteristics of voiding, urinalysis)

Mother reports no problems.

### Genitalia (structure, secondary sexual characteristics)

Not examined.

### Anus (structure, function)

Not examined.

## INITIAL PLAN

9/30/77    **No. 1    Incomplete data base**

Plan: Obtain complete data base by 10/7

Obj. 1   Shana and family will plan to meet 10/7 with clinical specialist for completion of data base.

9/30/77    **No. 2    Unable to use descriptive words**

**S**   Unable to use up, down, sweet, salty as descriptions during exam upon request. Did not identify any color but "black."

**O**   No testing for color blindness. DDST not administered to validate subjective responses as correct. No objective data to evaluate language skills.

**A**   At 3 years and 3 months she should have a beginning usage of common descriptors, prepositions, and color recognition (3 out of 4) according to the DDST.

**P**   Obj. 1   Shana should develop language skills appropriate to her age.

9/30/77    **No. 3    Developed "cold" after playing in weeds**

**S**   Mother stated Shana 2-3 weeks ago had a "cold" after playing in the weeds, which only resolved after taking prescribed medication.

**O**   No nasal discharge. Nasal mucosa not examined. Throat not reddened. Chest clear to auscultation. Conjunctivae pink and moist. No tearing.

**A**   "Colds" of a recurrent or seasonal nature are sensitivity responses to environmental allergens. Such recurrent respiratory responses are childhood precursors to adult onset of C.O.P.D. many times. Desensitization can prevent or reduce this hazard.

**P**   Obj. 1   Shana should demonstrate no chronic inflammatory response of a respiratory nature.

9/30/77    **No. 4    Nutrition**

**S**   Mother stated Shana recently refuses milk in any form. Dislikes cheeses.

**O**   Musculoskeletal development appropriate for age. Tongue is pink, clean. Shana is energetic.

**A**   Milk and milk products are essential in well-balanced nutrition for growth of bones, teeth, for enzymatic and cellular activities, and for supplemental sources of vitamins A and D.

**P**   Obj. 1   Shana should demonstrate intake of milk and/or milk products three times a day.

9/30/77    **No. 5    Laceration of L heel**

**S**   "Cut my foot when the dog bit me when I was outside."

**O**   Scar (granulated in) about 2 by 4 cm on inner aspect of L heel. Healed, nontender to pressure.

**A**   Cuts, burns, falls resulting in injury are a leading cause of injury and death in children under 5, and they occur generally at home. Many of these home injuries are preventable with knowledge of how to remove or reduce environmental hazards that can precipitate accidents.

**P**  Obj. 1  Shana should be able to live in an environment safe from prevent-  Case
able or reduceable hazards.

9/30/77  **No. 6  New baby in the family**

**S**  Mother said Tina was Shana's new sister and that Shana was her first child.

**O**  Mother accompanied by Tina who looked about 6-7 months old.

**A**  Entry of a new infant into a family structure introduces stress into the family system in which adaptation must be made by all persons within the system. Shana is at an age developmentally where she is learning new motor and language skills and is needing to interact more with parents and peers. She developmentally can only know that everyone views the world as she does. Therefore, it is important to determine how the baby has affected her own thoughts and how she is viewing the change. Since the mother's time is divided between two children, Shana can no longer be the only recipient of her mother's attention.

**P**  Obj. 1  Shana should be able to identify feelings about new sister.

9/30/77  **No. 7  Mother had "high B/P" during labor with Shana**

**S**  Developed "high B/P" during labor with Shana.

**O**  None

**A**  High blood pressure in pregnancy and abrupt onset in labor and delivery is associated with toxemia. While toxemia is not present with every pregnancy, it potentially can occur with each subsequent one. Toxemia is a killer and damager of mothers and unborn infants. Hypertension of a secondary and of an essential type is a major health problem. Health management is necessary to prevent the complications of early stroke, arteriosclerotic vascular disease, and kidney damage.

**P**  Obj. 1  Ms. S. should be able to seek health guidance for evaluation of presence or absence of hypertension.

## NURSING ORDERS

| | | PERSONNEL |
|---|---|---|

9/30/77  **No. 1  Incomplete data base**

    Obj. 1  Compile a complete data base.

        A. Make a home visit and complete a thorough     C.S.
evaluation of Shana. 10/7

           1. Interview of mother

           2. Physical exam of Shana

        B. Perform a family assessment. 10/7     C.S.

9/30/77  **No. 2  Unable to use descriptive words**

    Obj. 1  Develop language skills appropriate to her age.

        A. Administer D.D.S.T. to evaluate rudimentary     C.S.
language skills. 10/7

        B. Administer Ishihara test for color perception to     C.S.
determine an organic basis for inability to iden-
tify colors. 10/7

        C. In a home setting, attempt to evaluate the qual-     C.S.
ity and quantity of time mother spends with
Shana. 10/7

        D. Determine if Shana watches educational TV     C.S.
(i.e., Sesame Street) and the type of games and
toys she plays with. 10/7

        E. Referral to resource to assist in speeding lan-     C.S.
guage development.

9/30/77  **No. 3  Developed "cold" after playing in weeds**

    Obj. 1  Demonstrates no chronic inflammatory response of
a respiratory nature.

        A. Complete a careful history of respiratory condi-     C.S.
tions from mother and health records. 10/7

        B. Evaluate home and play environments for al-     C.S.
lergens, air temperatures (heating and air conditioning, humidification). 10/7

        C. Refer Shana for allergy testing with a positive     C.S.
history of URI's or "hay fever" symptoms.

        D. Health teaching on how to prevent URI's, and     C.S.
the long-term hazards of URI's to mother.

9/30/77  **No. 4  Nutrition**

    Obj. 1  Demonstrate intake of milk and/or milk products
three times a day.

        A. Perform an in-depth nutrition history; observe a     C.S.
mealtime if possible. 10/7

        B. Explore mother's knowledge of the basic four,     C.S.
particularly the milk products group. 10/7

        C. Suggest alternatives to milk, and cheese, i.e.,     C.S.
yogurt, cereal with milk, ice cream. 10/7

        D. Determine financially how much of the family's     C.S.
income can be spent on food; explore quantity
and quality of grocery purchases. 10/7

9/30/77 **No. 5 Laceration of L heel**                              Case

  Obj. 1 To live in an environment safe from preventable hazards.
- A. Obtain history of cuts, falls, burns for the family. 10/7 — C.S.
- B. Teach mother about safety measures to prevent accidents by reducing hazards, i.e., pans on stove with handles in, wearing shoes when outside, safety locks for cabinet doors, cleaning solutions on top shelves. 10/7 — C.S.
- C. Home visit to identify safety hazards in the home and in play areas. 10/14 — C.S.

9/30/77 **No. 6 New baby in family**

  Obj. 1 Identify feelings about new sister.
- A. Talk with Shana about new baby; design a play session with a doll (new baby) and observe and record behaviors. 10/14 — C.S.
- B. Observe interactions of mother, Shana, and the new baby. 10/7 — C.S.
- C. Obtain information from mother about how Shana was prepared for baby. 10/7 — C.S.
- D. Explore with the mother how she is coping with the change within the family. Explain adaptations that should occur after a new child comes into the family. — C.S.

9/30/77 **No. 7 Mother had "high B/P" during labor with Shana**

  Obj. 1 Seek health guidance for evaluation of possible hypertension.
- A. Obtain a blood pressure reading and review health records for hypertensive episodes. 10/14 — C.S.
- B. Obtain maternity and family histories. 10/14 — C.S.
- C. Teach the hazards of hypertension, the need for consistent health follow-up and the need for immediate obstetrical management in the event of pregnancy. 10/14 — C.S.

## HEALTH STATUS LIST—Stacy

| Onset | Date | No. | Active | Date | Inactive/resolved |
|---|---|---|---|---|---|
| | 12/5/77 | 1 | Incomplete data base | | |
| | 12/5/77 | 2 | Cognitively ready for symbolic thought | | |
| | 12/5/77 | 3 | Advanced developmentally in language skills | | |
| | 12/5/77 | 4 | Child health maintenance | | |
| | | 4A | Normal growth parameters | | |
| | | 4B | Incomplete immunization schedule | | |

# PLAY ASSESSMENT TOOL

Client __Stacy Lane M.__   Sex __F__   Age __23 mos.__   B.D. __12/30/75__
Date __12/5/77__   Race __Caucasian__   Phone __801-3092__
Mother __Margaret   12008 Sunnyvale__   Father __Thomas B. M.   12008 Sunnyvale__

**Information sources:** Preschool records.

## MOTHER PROFILE
**Marital status**
Married.

**Employment (hours, place, days off)**
Works M-F Campbell Inc., phone 802-1067.

**Educational level**
High school graduate.

## FATHER PROFILE
**Marital status**
Married.

**Employment**
City Police Department.

**Educational level**
College education.

**Life change events (state dates and whether it involves mother and/or father if parents are divorced)**

**History of illnesses (chronic, inherited, allergy)**
Parents in good health without any chronic conditions.

**Siblings**
None.

## CHILD PROFILE
HEALTH HISTORY
**Present health status**
Good except for "runny nose."

**Prior accidents, injuries, illnesses (dates)**
Parents report none on school record.

**Nutritional status**
Active, alert, healthy skin. Slightly overweight by observation.

**Weight/height/age ratio**
No data available or obtained.

**Developmental milestones appropriate to age**
Uses four to six word sentences, uses plurals, gives first and last names. Holds small glass with one hand. Follows simple verbal directions. Correctly names objects in a book (cat, bird, bunny). Engages in parallel play but is starting some interactive play. Names and points to body parts on herself, pictures, or dolls accurately. Recognizes colors verbally: black, red, yellow. Assists in tasks at school, i.e., putting up toys and handing out place mats. Indicates verbally without prompting that her parents are "at work." Appears advanced developmentally in language.

## Sleep patterns, disturbance

Bedtime 9 PM; arises 7 AM.

## Allergies/medications

None.

## Immunizations

| | DPT | | POLIO | TUBERCULOSIS | MMR |
|---|---|---|---|---|---|
| #1 | 2/25/76 | #1 | 2/25/76 | None | None |
| #2 | 3/24/76 | #2 | 4/29/76 | | |
| #3 | 4/29/76 | #3 | 6/30/76 | | |

## Nursery school information

Hours at school: Arrives 7:45 AM; leaves 5:30 PM.
Number of days: M-F.
Special precautions/instructions: None.

SOCIAL PROFILE

Interactions with parent; with teachers; with other children. Interacts congenially with adults and peers. Seems relaxed and self-assured.

## Eye contact

Good during verbal interchanges.

## Touching

Asks to be held. Will sit in lap for 5-10 minutes contentedly.

## Position in the family (birth order)

First child.

## Languages spoken in the home

English. No information about other languages.

## Life-style

Resides at a home (single dwelling) address.

## Additional data

Pediatrician: Malcolm Smith. Last exam 7/1/77.

PLAY EXPERIENCE

Time allowed: no limit.
Time used: approx. 10 minutes.

**Limits** (responsibility of the child, use of materials, behavioral guidelines)

Child must demonstrate interest in the object to be hidden. The child must retrieve the hidden object.

## Theory or concept to be tested

Piaget's concept of object permanence, specifically the visual pursuit and search for hidden objects. (Test sequence was adapted from The Uzgiris-Hunt Infant Assessment Tool of Ordinal Scales of Psychological Development.)

**Setting** (materials, environment, controlled variables)

Three screens were used and were of a texture and opacity that would not reveal the outline of the hidden object. The child was seated on a rug so that there was working area surrounding and the hands could be free to manipulate objects.

## PLAY ASSESSMENT TOOL—cont'd

### Purpose of the assessment

To test the ability of the child to visually pursue a hidden object with variations in the type of hiding requiring alteration of search behavior to obtain the object. Successful completion of the visual pursuit of hidden objects gives empirical evidence of the ability of the child to differentiate between himself or herself and the object and the different spatial contexts of the object. This is necessary cognitive development for symbolic thought.

**Special considerations** (language level, use of touch, developmental level, maturational level, cultural background)

The child should be near the end of the sensory-motor period to complete the visual pursuit.

### Description and assessment of the experience

12/5/77 Earlier in the morning, I approached Stacy and told her we were going to play "some games" later on. Thinking that noises and other children would distract her, I performed the play exercise while the other children were outside. I seated her on the rug and placed three cloth screens between us. From my sack, I selected a yarn bee and a small white wind-up bunny. She immediately showed interest in the bunny and that was used as the object to be hidden.

In the first hiding the bunny was hidden under the three screens. Stacy immediately tore off the screens and retrieved the bunny. Secondly, the bunny was placed in a box and hidden under one screen. After inspecting the empty box, she retrieved the bunny again. Then a second screen was placed to her other side. When the bunny was placed in the box and deposited under the second screen, she again retrieved the object from under the screen where the box disappeared.

Then she became distracted and wanted to play with just the bunny. I unsuccessfully tried to interest her in another object.

Using the third screen and placing the bunny in the box the object was deposited randomly under a screen and again after direct search she retrieved the object.

The bunny was placed and hidden in my hand. Then I put my hand under the first, the second, and the third screen (where the object was deposited). My hand paused momentarily between the screens. Stacy immediately searched under the last screen from which my empty hand had emerged.

Then the positions of the screens were changed. The object was hidden under the first screen but my hand went under screen two and three and then I showed Stacy my empty hand. On the second try in this event, Stacy searched in reverse order (starting with screen 3) to find the bunny under screen one. She successfully completed the displacements in the visual pursuit exercise. This indicates that she can discriminate between objects and self and the spaces an object can occupy. This gives evidence that cognitively she is capable of symbolic thought and will be assimilating intellectually by imaginative (symbolic) play. She is capable of using concrete objects to represent a mental image of what she is thinking, for example, using a block as a telephone.

### Additional data

Stacy correctly identified the object as a bunny. She quickly and dextrously wound up the rabbit. She acknowledged that this was "a game." She was very curious about other items in my paper bag.

### Suggestions for future planning and intervention

In a repeat performance I would not allow her to bring a toy or object she was previously interested in as the doll she brought was a distraction for her when she became the least bit tired of the hiding exercise. In choosing a setting, I would make sure there were no interruptions, as one of the teachers passing through the room distracted her. Becoming more efficient in the hiding series would improve the quality of the response, as a child's attention span at this age is short, and they are easily distracted. Since Stacy demonstrates advanced cognitive behaviors, particularly in language, it would be interesting to devise an experience to see how far along she is in the preconceptual phase of cognitive development.

## INITIAL PLAN

12/5/77 **No. 1 Incomplete data base**

**S** Unable to interview the parents.

**O** Information was obtained from the school record and from observations of Stacy before and during the play exercise.

**A** Need to talk with parents for accurate and complete data.

**P** Obj. 1 If possible, talk with parents to obtain a complete data base.

12/5/77 **No. 2 Cognitively ready for symbolic thought**

**S** Plays with block using it as a telephone. States mother and father are "at work."

**O** Successfully completed the visual pursuit of hidden objects following a visible and invisible displacement in the described play experience.

**A** Data indicates that the child can distinguish an object as separate from herself, that it exists even though it is not always visible, and that it can occupy different spaces. This level of thinking is a foundation for symbolic play in which there is imaginative as well as imitative characteristics. This type of thinking is characteristic of the preconceptual thought between the ages of 2 and 4. This is a foundation for cognition in which play eventually will develop into intellectual activity.

**P** Obj. 1 Stacy will be able to participate in make-believe games and use symbols in the thought process

12/5/77 **No. 3 Advanced developmentally in language skills**

**S** Uses four to six word sentences, plurals, first and last name. Recognizes colors by naming: black, red, yellow. Identifies objects in books—cat, bird, bunny.

**O** No test data to validate responses. Diction and enunciation are distinct.

**A** Color recognition, giving of first and last name, use of plurals do not usually begin until later in the second year. At 23 months, there is usually a combination of two different words to form a beginning sentence. Testing will provide a base on which to accurately assess Stacy's language ability. Since she appears advanced, it is necessary to give her stimulation appropriate to her developmental, rather than chronological, age level. According to Piaget, certain cognitive functions within each developmental period must be fostered at that time or the cognitive task if delayed will not develop as well in a later stage as optimum time has passed.

**P** Obj. 1 Stacy should be able to demonstrate language skills advanced beyond chronological parameters.

12/5/77 **No. 4 Child health maintenance.**

4,A Normal growth parameters.

**S** None.

**O** No measurements, but she appears to weigh more than she should.

**INITIAL PLAN—cont'd**

12/5/77    **No. 4   Child health maintenance—cont'd**

**A**    Two-year-olds should approximately quadruple their birth weight. Comparing weight, height, and head circumference measurements allows comparisons with norms and previous measurements for nursing intervention in presence of a deviation or sudden change. If obesity develops as a childhood problem, it creates alterations in the body image that threatens a positive self-concept.

**P**    Obj. 1   Stacy should demonstrate normal parameters of height, weight, and head circumference

4,B   Incomplete immunization schedule

**S**    None.

**O**    School record does not show any immunizations since 6/30/76, 18 months ago.

**A**    DPT and TOPV are given at 2, 4, and 6 months. The tuberculin skin test and the MMR are given at 15 months. At 18 months another DPT and TOPV are given. These are necessary to protect the child from preventable diseases, many of which inflict permanent damage on children.

**P**    Obj. 1   Stacy should demonstrate up-to-date immunizations.

## NURSING ORDERS

12/5/77   **No. 1**   **Incomplete data base**          **PERSONNEL**

Stacy should:
Obj. 1   To obtain data for a complete data base

    A. Try to talk briefly with parents when they bring     C.S.
       Stacy to school.

    B. Visit with parents over the phone.     C.S.

12/5/77   **No. 2**   **Cognitively ready for symbolic thought**

Stacy should:
Obj. 1   Participate in make-believe activities.

    A. Discuss the data from play experience with   Teachers
       teacher and parents. Provide make believe ac-   Parents
       tivities:     C.S.

        1. Songs—"I'm a Little Teapot."

        2. Let's pretend games.

        3. Mr. Rogers' Neighborhood—educational
           TV which has make-believe activities.

    B. Encourage Stacy to elaborate any make-be-   Teachers
       lieve activity by introducing the remainder of the   Parents
       scheme of the activity. For example, if pretend-   C.S.
       ing a block is a phone, engage her in a phone
       conversation and follow through with hanging
       up, dialing, etc.

    C. Share this information (A and B) with parents   C.S.
       and teach them the reason and the means to
       stimulate her.

    D. Teach parents that children need:   C.S.

        1. Privacy for play

        2. Special place for play

        3. Nondescript play items like blocks, simple
           wheeled vehicles of hand size, natural mate-
           rials (clay, sand, water) for creative play

12/5/77   **No. 3**   **Advanced developmentally in language skills**

Stacy should:
Obj. 1   Demonstrate language skills beyond chronological
      age

    A. Administer DDST to screen for language pa-   C.S.
       rameters

    B. Ishihara color test to validate color recognition.   C.S.

    C. After DDST, give Peabody Picture Vocabulary   C.S.
       Test.

    D. Share this information with parents and teach-   C.S.
       ers.

    E. Talk with parents about how they perceive   C.S.
       Stacy developmentally and refer for intelligence
       testing for planning appropriate stimulation pro-
       grams.

## NURSING ORDERS—cont'd

12/5/77  **No. 4   Child health maintenance**

4,A   Normal growth parameters
Stacy should:
Obj. 1   Demonstrate normal parameters of height, weight,
and head circumference.

    A. Measure and compare and record height,    C.S.
weight, and head circumference with norms.

    B. Obtain measurements at birth and at Dr.'s visits    C.S.
from physician's records (or from mother if she
has a record) and compare with new measurements.

    C. Talk with parents and teachers to perform a nu-    C.S.
tritional assessment if weight above norm for    Parent
her age, or if increased proportionately from    Teacher
previous measurements.

    D. Share all information with parents.    C.S.

    E. If dietary therapy is necessary consult and refer    C.S.
problem to child nutritionist and her pediatri-
cian.

4,B   Incomplete immunization schedule.
Stacy should:
Obj. 1   Demonstrate up-to-date immunizations.

    A. Call physician's office to ascertain if Stacy has    C.S.
been immunized since 6/76 without being re-
corded at school.

    B. Ask parents to bring her record so school can    C.S.
update if necessary.

    C. Teach parents hazards and potential conse-    C.S.
quences of out-of-date immunization of their
child.

    D. Assist them in making provisions for updating    C.S.
these, if necessary.

**REFERENCES**
**Stacy**

Caplan, F., and Caplan, T.: The Power of play, New York, 1974, Anchor Press/Doubleday.
Moustakas, C.: Children in play therapy, Jason Aronson, Inc.
Shaefer, C., editor: The therapeutic use of child's play, Jason Aronson, Inc.
Uzgiris, I. C., and Hunt, J. McV.: Assessment in infancy, Urbana, 1976, University of Illinois Press.
Vaughn-Wroebel, B. C., and Henderson, B.: The problem-oriented system in nursing, St. Louis, 1976,
The C. V. Mosby Co.

# Later childhood

As children enter the traditional school environment offered in Western societies, they begin to experience new influences, which make a significant impact on development. New people, new surroundings, and new events provide for physical, learning and thought, social and inner development. Because children are mastering challenging learning and thought competencies that enhance development in each of the other competencies, they often center attention on the ability to use newly acquired skills in everyday life. They are intense in attempts to gain increasingly adultlike competencies and to master the developmental skills that increasing physical capacities allow.

In this unit attention is focused upon the development and health care of children during these later childhood years. The purposes of Chapter 12, "Later Childhood: The Age of Widening Experience," are (1) to present the scientific bases for development that have been demonstrated or hypothesized in biologic and behavioral sciences and (2) to discuss both the means of assessment of competency development and the child's health maintenance needs.

Chapter 13, "Common Health Problems of Later Childhood," covers (1) the basis for nursing diagnosis of minor health problems that tend to occur during these years of development, (2) nursing management that is needed to assist the child and family in attaining and maintaining the goals of health, and (3) the concerns and goals shared in common by health care workers and persons in education and the means by which these professions can mutually achieve better health for children.

# Later childhood: the age of widening experience

For most people the years of later childhood are the healthiest time of life. Children at this age reach a level of physiologic maturity that enables the system to effectively fight off most infection. Their capacity to recover from injury or infection is rapid and relatively complete, and their energy level is great. They reach a level of motor coordination and mastery that enables them to accomplish many tasks of adulthood, opening a wide world of possibilities for participation and learning.

## HEALTH MAINTENANCE DURING LATER CHILDHOOD

Since children from 6 to 12 years are usually healthy and free from illness, they are seldom the subject of specific consideration in discussions of health care. Their physical health risks are not as great as those of the infant and younger child, and the physical changes typical of earlier childhood and of adolescence are not present during these middle years. In addition, those concerned with mental health have in the past regarded this time of life as relatively calm and stable, when risks for development of emotional disturbance are minimal and when children are generally in a state of equilibrium. While these assumptions and characteristics may be justifiable for some children, they do not apply to all children in this age period. Indeed, all children of this age group encounter important physical and emotional developmental events, and their health care needs are important. By the end of later childhood, children should have reached total independence in providing for their own personal hygiene, in being capable of choosing and eating nutritious foods, in recognizing signs of illness, in preventing accidents and injuries, and in being able to cope with emotional stresses of everyday living, including knowing how to find help when they are troubled.

Health maintenance is aimed toward implementing the basic goal of health care in direct relationship to the child as an individual. The aim is to promote the child's motivation to seek health and to use various resources to attain, maintain, or regain optimal health and function. Children are still an integral part of the family, and responsible adults must be included in the implementation of this goal. However, they now begin to learn to act in relation to their own needs independently. They gradually begin to assume more responsibility for themselves and for others around them. Adults and children beyond the family circle become significant and may participate in certain aspects of health care and maintenance, helping them to learn

**461**

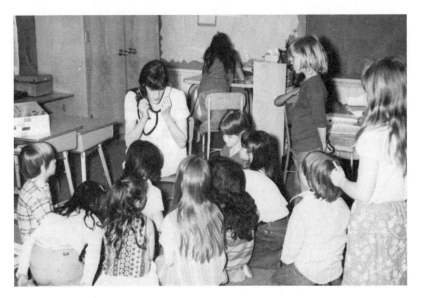

**Fig. 12-1.** The school system provides health education programs.

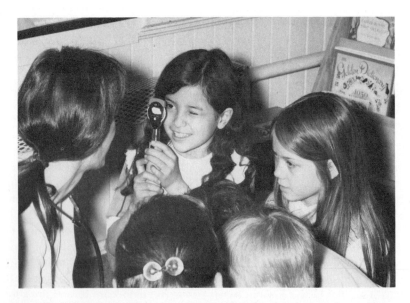

**Fig. 12-2.** School-age children are eager to actively participate in real experiences.

to assume a more central role in their own care.

## THE SCHOOL AND HEALTH CARE

As an integral part of the total community, the school system has specific responsibilities in health care and planning to provide a healthful school environment, an adequate school health service, and a comprehensive health education program.[14] School systems vary greatly in the extent to which they fulfill these roles, and the extent to which they agree that these are real functions of the school. Most schools take specific steps to assure a level of safety and cleanliness in the environment, but an individual school may represent either extreme in providing a healthy physical and emotional environment. School health service in the United States and other countries also varies greatly. In some areas nurses, physicians, and other health care workers are integrally involved in the school health program, which includes health care and maintenance as well as education. In other areas the school health program considers educational aspects only. Health education programs range from an occasional mention of body care and the changes of puberty to a full program integrating physical and mental health principles into all aspects of the educational experience.[1,12,14,36,62]

While the ideal role of the school in providing health care remains a matter of debate, the fact remains that the school does influence and participate in children's health and well-being. As they begin to spend an increasingly greater percentage of their waking hours in and around the school, this environment begins to exert an influence on their lives that may, at times, outweigh the current influence of the home. The attitudes that the school conveys in regard to health and well-being begin to influence children's attitudes, and they contribute to the shaping and formulation of the concept of health. If health concepts are avoided and disliked by those in and around the school, children learn that these concerns are not to be taken seriously or incorporated into their areas of interest. If they are taught that mental health is a matter for concern and that people can bring about changes in their environment that con-

tribute to better mental health, they begin to incorporate these ideas into their own values and thought systems. If the school treats puberty and sexual roles with great delicacy and embarrassment, children begin to learn that these are not acceptable, wholesome topics to pursue with knowledgeable adults. Thus the school has a central role in determining the environment in which children grow and develop during these years.

## SCIENTIFIC BASES FOR DEVELOPMENT DURING LATER CHILDHOOD
### Developmental physiology
#### Neurologic development

The neurologic system of the middle-age child continues to grow and develop in function at a gradual rate. The brain has achieved most of its ultimate size by the age of 6 years, and by the onset of puberty it has almost reached adult proportions. The development of the sulci of the cortex proceeds as intellectual function expands, and myelination probably reaches completion. Full voluntary control of gross and fine motor function is achieved; the gains in size and strength of small, fine motor musculature account for the increasing capacity in this regard. The child's memory capacity begins to approach a maximal level. The ability to conceptualize and form mental structures grows significantly. These capacities are discussed in more detail in the following section on learning.

Little is known about the role of stimulation of the nervous system during later childhood. Understimulation during later childhood is often a continuation of similar circumstances that existed during earlier childhood, and specific effects during the later years have not been subject to investigation. Limited observations of temporary sensory deprivation, as when a child is isolated during hospitalization, suggest that the effects are similar to those for an adult. The effects, while significant to the child, are not permanent in the sense of damage to the central nervous system, and they may be overcome.

When children entering the school system are discovered to have certain specific neurologic handicaps that interfere with academic achievement, specific skilled intervention may help the child overcome a portion of the handi-cap. Such problems, which are termed learning disabilities by educators, include visual, lan-guage, and auditory handicaps. Explanations of the ways in which these changes are mediated neurologically are speculative. The child may be able to make alternate neurologic associations, or myelination may occur later than normal for these children. This evidence suggests that some neurologic plasticity exists in later child-hood.

Full capacity to imitate sounds linguistically develops during the later childhood years. The capacity to learn foreign languages is probably at an optimal level of potential; the child pos-sesses the full articulation capacity and full au-ditory-mental-speech-visual association capac-ities. The motor development of the muscula-ture of the mouth and throat is not permanently established; thus function is not limited. The child's ability to listen and to make associations with the incoming auditory stimuli is fully ma-ture by 7 years of age.

Visual capacity should reach optimal function by the sixth or seventh year. The child's periph-eral vision should be fully developed, and the ability to discriminate fine differences in shad-ing of colors s fully developed. Acuity should be at maximum level of development, or at least 20/30 in each eye as measured by the Snellen chart. The child who is myopic at the onset of later childhood will probably never achieve ade-quate visual acuity and should have correction for the problem at the earliest possible time. Since such a child has probably never experi-enced maximal acuity, he or she does not realize that the visual images are not adequate. The de-light and surprise when the world is first seen in full focus are long remembered.

The child is able to coordinate eye move-ments, to see a single image, and to associate incoming visual stimuli with past and present mental images and functions. Further develop-ment of full potential through use and practice is one of the many tasks of later childhood.[30,50,75]

### Metabolic and homeostatic mechanisms

The tissues of the gastrointestinal and res-piratory systems achieve adultlike maturity dur-ing later childhood. Differences in lung capacity are a function of size during this period of life, but difference in lung function is negligible. Primary teeth are lost and the permanent teeth begin to erupt.

Endocrine control of homeostasis and the ability to respond to stress increase gradually. By puberty all endocrine functions except those regulating reproduction approach adult capac-ity. The renal and circulatory functions that are regulated by endocrine control mature in pro-portion to endocrine maturity. Immunologic functions of the body approach adult capacity, and as the structures that are exposed to infec-tions enlarge and gain maturity in composition, danger from infection decreases significantly. Complications arising from minor infections are seldom encountered as the ability of the body to localize infection becomes effective.[30,69,75]

### Structural tissues

The skin, which is one of the maturing struc-tures related to defenses from infection, gains structural maturity and begins to approach adult appearance and texture. Sebum production re-mains minimal throughout childhood, as does eccrine sweat production. The ability of these glands to respond to temperature and emotional stimuli increases slightly. The skin provides better protection from insensible water loss. As the renal system acquires the ability to conserve water and the circulatory system is able to alter blood flow, the child's ability to maintain tem-perature and fluid and electrolyte balances in-creases.

The most dramatic physiologic events during later childhood occur in the musculoskeletal systems. While growth is not as rapid as during infancy or adolescence, a significant proportion of growth occurs during these years. The growth of this period is relatively gradual and constant, although individual children tend to demon-strate "spurts" of growth alternated with periods when growth is minimal. The deposition of adi-pose tissue begins to accelerate during the years of later childhood, and thus the child gains in girth as well as height and weight. There may be some observed differences between girls and boys in the relative gains of muscle or adipose tissue mass, but during this period such differ-ences are probably more closely related to greater use of muscle tissue among boys than girls. Some active girls gain muscle mass and relatively little adipose tissue, whereas some less active boys gain adipose tissue and relatively little muscle mass. These activity habits arise partly from the child's temperament and the family's life-style, and while these traits tend to persist into later life, identification with appropriate sex roles does not seem to be related to differences in growth in later childhood.

The fact that the child is constantly building new bony tissue during the entire period of childhood accounts for the rapid repair of any fractures that occur during childhood. The ongoing ability to provide the needed tructural elements nor growth also enhances the provision of these same materials for repair.[30,50,69,74,75]

## Cognitive development
### Piaget's theory of cognitive development

The theory of Jean Piaget offers insight into the cognitive development of the middle-age child. Piaget refers to the span from age 7 to 11 years as the *concrete operations subperiod*. This and the previous subperiod (preoperational) comprise the entire *concrete operations period*. A review of the discussion in Chapter 10 may be helpful, since the preoperational subperiod will be contrasted to the concrete operations subperiod.

During the preoperations subperiod, perceptions were the dominant mental activity of the child. Gradually, at about the age of 7 years, the child begins to move into a period when perceptions are dominated by intellectual operations, which are the dominant mental activity of the concrete operations period. These operations (the ability to order and relate experience to an organized whole) begin to occur within a framework of relationships that make possible mobility of thinking. Rather than being bound to irreversibility as before, the child begins to be able to reverse mental operations and return to the starting point. Rather than being bound by egocentrism, the child begins to be able to take into account another person's point of view. Instead of centering on one dimensional property of a situation, the child is able to focus on several properties in sequence and to quickly move from one to another.

The operations of this period are termed concrete, because the child's mental operations still depend upon the ability to concretely perceive what has happened. The child cannot perform a mental experiment without dependence upon perception. The basic ability from which concrete operations develops is the ability to mentally form ordering structures, which Piaget terms groupings (or nestings) and lattices. *Groupings* are systems that fit together because of some relationship between the smaller parts and their all-inclusive whole. For a group to be formed, several principles from mathematical logic are applied. The details of these principles are important in studying experimental and theoretical details of Piaget's work but will not be described here.

*Lattices* refers to a special form of grouping in which the focus is upon the connection between two or more objects and the objects that are connected. This allows the child to form a classification hierarchy system, in which there is understanding, for example, that all people are vertebrates, but not all vertebrates are people. Altogether there are nine types of groupings that appear in the concrete operations period, each of which involves a specific logical operation. The appearance of each type of thinking may be described, and it appears sequentially in order. The exact time of appearance is variable, but Piaget found a certain consistency in the developing abilities of children.

By examining some of the typical experiments that Piaget and others have conducted to describe the thinking of the preoperational and concrete operational subperiods, the reader can begin to understand how the child's behavior reflects cognitive capacity. One of the abilities that appears at about the age of 7 years is conservation of number. To demonstrate this thought process, the child is presented a line of vases and a cluster of flowers and then is asked to arrange the flowers, one flower for every vase, as many vases as flowers. The child in the preoperational subperiod arranges all of the flowers in a line that equals in length the line of vases and is surprised to discover that if he places one flower *in* every vase, there are flowers left over. The child centers on the length of the row of the two objects and is not able to change to the concept of numbers. If the flowers are taken out of the vases and placed in a cluster on the table and the child asked if now there are more flowers or more vases, he or she will respond that there are more vases. There is still centering on the length of the row of vases as opposed to the flowers, and the child cannot reverse the operation even when the equal number of flowers is observed to be removed from the vases.

When the concrete operations subperiod begins to emerge, the child is able to arrange the flowers correctly in the beginning and is not fooled when they are placed in a cluster. The child is now able to reverse the operation, and is no longer centering on one aspect of the problem. The interesting point that should be remembered as these experiments are described is that children are not taught these concepts and operations deliberately. They emerge; they are constructed by the environment and by experience, but they are not taught. Most adults are not even aware of their operational mental capacity, which they use easily and without analysis.

Conservation of quantity (substance, amount of space occupied by an object) also emerges at about 7 or 8 years of age. Conservation of weight emerges at about 9 years of age, whereas conservation of volume emerges close to the end of the concrete operational period.

Part-to-part and part-to-whole relationships are examined by investigating the child's ability to perceive the composition of classes of objects. A typical experiment involves presenting the child with three boxes, one of which contains 20 wooden beads. Eighteen of the beads are brown and two are white. All of the beads are visible in the bottom of the box. The brown beads are removed from the box and placed in another box. The child is asked if there will be any beads left when all the brown ones are gone. He or she responds that there will be two white beads left. The experimenter then refers to the white beads as wooden ones, asking if any beads will be left in the box when the wooden beads are placed in the other empty box. The young child replies that there will not be. The child is then asked which would make the longer necklace, the wooden beads or the brown ones. The pre-

operational subperiod child will respond, "the brown ones," centering on the property of color. The concrete operations child, on the other hand, will respond that the wooden beads will make the longest necklace, for this category includes all of the brown plus the white beads. The child is able to perceive the properties of both material and color, and the associations between them, reversing from color to material and back to color again.

Egocentricity changes are illustrated in an experiment in which the child is placed at a square table with three molded mountains of varying height on it. There are three empty chairs at each side of the table. A doll is placed in each of the three chairs sequentially, and each time the child is asked what the doll sees when looking at the mountains from that side of the table. The child may be given cardboard cut-outs of the mountains to arrange as he or she imagines the doll would see them or the child may draw the doll's image. From one side of the table the big mountain would be near the doll, with smaller mountains behind it; from another side the big mountain would be to one side with both smaller mountains on the other side. Before the concrete operations subperiod, the child cannot conceive of what the doll's view might be. The problem is often not sufficient to engage the child's interest. However, after about age 7 years the child begins to show some interest in the problem and is able to erratically represent the doll's point of view. Toward the latter part of the period, the child begins to accurately represent the doll's view from all sides of the table.

This trait of egocentrism is also observable in children's conversations with one another. The preoperational child, in talking with another child of about the same age, will engage in collective monologues. Each child pursues his or her own private conversation regardless of what the other child says. When concrete operations develop, the child begins to be able to take into account the other child's point of view and to incorporate the partner's conversation into his or her own. Thus more meaningful intercommunication begins to emerge, and the children carry on a dialogue, responding directly to what the other has just said. These traits do not emerge suddenly and completely; they tend to flow into one another, with the new skill being demonstrated in behavior only occasionally at first and then emerging with increasing frequency as the child's mental capacity and experience grow.[54-56,59]

## Learning capacity

The theoretical ideas related to learning that were discussed in Chapters 9 and 10 continue to apply to the later childhood years. The principles of positive and negative reinforcement, conditioning, and punishment have received some specific investigation in relation to learning processes, and these principles may continue to function in certain areas of learning. The effects of practice, which has been an established mode of teaching and learning for many decades, have also been studied. The role of motivation has received extensive investigation, but the problems in defining and identifying the motivational phenomena have limited definitive study.[37] Insight, intuition, understanding, problem-solving, creativity, conceptual constructs, attitudes, moral development, acquisition and retention phenomena, and many other principles have received limited attention from theorists and investigators. What has been learned about learning continues to be limited, but some advances have been made. There have been severe limitations in transferring newly acquired understandings and theoretical propositions into teaching practice. To more fully refine theoretical ideas and inspect their effects in the real world of learning in children, this transfer must be accomplished.

### Bruner's theory of education

Jerome Bruner[11] has discussed several ideas regarding the nature of learning and the role of the environment. This discussion does not fully describe Bruner's propositions and ideas about learning and education but will consider a few of the predominant themes upon which his work is based.

For Bruner, growth of the mind and the ability to learn are a function of the culture in which the child lives and grows. The limits of growth depend on how the culture assists the individual to use his or her intellectual potential. The culture provides this growth-provoking stimulation by providing amplification systems to which human beings, equipped with appropriate skills, can link themselves. For example, there are amplification systems for action, such as hammers, wheels, and motors; there are prescribed programs, or appropriate behavior patterns, into which such actions are to be directed. There are amplifiers of the senses, including the culturally prescribed ways of noticing, seeing, and feeling, which render meaning to sensory experiences of the world. Some sensory data are noticed and attended to; others are ignored. Finally, there are amplifiers of thought processes and ways of thinking that employ the languages of symbolic speech, mathematics, and logic through which the individual processes incoming data and is able to use it to direct his action and behavior. All cultures, primitive and modern, provide for the acquisition of the amplifiers of the particular culture. The modern society has chosen the setting of the school to accomplish this function after about the age of 6 years and has further assigned the school with the specific function of converting knowledge and skill into more symbolic, abstract, and verbal forms.

For Bruner, knowledge exists within children's minds and thought before they are able to put what they know into words. Knowledge is acquired intuitively at the outset or at the time that an individual first approaches a new body of knowledge. Imitation and modeling is one important means of acquisition during this period of the learning process. Once intuitive knowledge is acquired, the child must proceed to the stages of making this knowledge part of the self, of being able to verbalize and put the knowledge into language form, and of transferring it to other similar problems and situations. Balanced learning, then, is what enables the child to proceed intuitively when necessary and to then use full analytic powers when this is appropriate.

Bruner has described certain traits of human learning that place very real constraints on formal attempts to educate children. These may be briefly summarized as the necessary strategies that the human uses to maximize limited capacities to learn. The human mind is significantly limited in function, and in order to compensate for its own limitations, these strategies are developed and used to overcome, or compensate for, the limitations of neural functioning:

1. The mind is selective. It attends to some things and not to others. Those things that are given attention are often the things that the culture has prescribed should be attended to.

2. The mind is economical for the sake of speed and strain reduction. The learner utilizes minimal cues and does not linger with information in reaching decisions about the phenomena under consideration.

3. The learner is sensitive to steady properties. The minimal cues that are selected are invariant features, for the learner, of things that are attended to. In this way structures that predict the outcome of things happening in the environment begin to emerge.

4. The mind is connective. The features that are steady for the individual are put together as working models, forming an idea of the way in which things happen, as causes and effects.

5. Deviance causes alarm and attention. When something happens that does not fit the way in which prior learning has indicated it should happen, some degree of alarm is experienced. How a child deals with this alarm is part of the learning process.

6. People extrapolate meanings beyond the information with which they are confronted by very natural, innate processes of inference. The accuracy of these extrapolations, or the meanings attached to experiences, in part determines the success of the learning experience.

Thus for Bruner, it is the processing of information that yields the significance of the learning experience and not the receipt of information. How the child uses each of these strategies and the meaning outcomes that they create are the measure of successful learning.[11]

In Western technological societies, when children enter school they encounter certain social demands that may be different and new. These demands are most closely related to their abilities to learn, reason, and understand.

### Factors that influence learning performance

**Sensory capacity.** The capacity of the child's sense organs is a vital factor in the ability to learn. From these sensory experiences, including vision, hearing, tasting, smelling, kinesthetic moving, and touching, the child has received perceptions throughout the growing years. The vital importance of these experiences in infancy and early childhood has been discussed. By the time of later childhood the child has begun to use these perceptions to form increasingly complex concepts and understandings of the world. Since no two children have exactly the same sensory acuity, sensitivity, or discrimination, all children build perceptions and conceptions of the world around them that are slightly different.

**Health.** The relationship between the child's state of health or well-being and capacity to learn is poorly understood. It is presumed that a serious state of illness or some physical malfunctioning is detrimental to the ability to concentrate and use mental capacity. But the child who suffers repeated acute minor upper respiratory infections, who is undernourished, or whose endurance and stamina are less than optimal is often ignored in relation to the influences of these conditions on the learning process. Limited evidence supports the suggestion that these factors may indeed be important for the child of school age. Most children who attend school are presumed to be well, but on closer assessment they may be suffering from any of several underlying, not easily recognized, health problems, which may be vitally important in relation to academic achievement.[12]

**Intelligence.** The level of intelligence with which the child is endowed, plus the environmental factors that influence the development of intelligence, also determines the effectiveness of a child's learning. Intelligence has not been comprehensively defined, because of the great difficulty in identifying exactly which capacities are involved in general mental abilities. Several contrasting statements that have been suggested as definitions of intelligence illustrate the problem.[17]

. . . tendency to take and maintain a definite direction; the capacity to make adaptations for the purpose of attaining a desired end; and the power of auto-criticism (Binet)

. . . the ability to do abstract thinking (Terman)

. . . the power of good responses from the point of view of truth or fact (Thorndike)

. . . the property of so recombining our behavior patterns as to act better in novel situations (Wells)

Intelligence test scores tend to differ because of the fact that each test, or each form of the same test, measures slightly different samples of abilities such as those indicated in the various definitions. Further, the nature of the tests tends to reflect the author's philosophy of the nature of intelligence. For example, the Stanford-Binet test places a heavy emphasis on abstract thinking. The Weschler series emphasizes aggregate, or global, knowledge. The Peabody Picture vocabulary test emphasizes verbal skills.

The younger the child, the less well developed these skills are, and the more difficult they are to measure. As language ability and mental functioning increases during later childhood, the more reliable and valid is the measurement of intellectual capacity.[17]

**The nature of environmental experiences.** Environmental opportunities for learning and the nature of these experiences greatly influence children's learning skills. Previous chapters have presented discussions of how these factors affect children during infancy and early childhood, and these early factors continue to influence learning abilities in later childhood. If young children have been encouraged to use their natural potential for scholastic learning, they come to the school setting well prepared to continue the learning patterns established earlier.

All children learn whether or not they are encouraged specifically to learn. However, the content and process of their learning may be entirely different from what is required in the school setting. Unfortunately, little is understood about learning that does not involve scholastic achievement or specific behavior change. The term "cultural deprivation" is particularly limited in describing the disadvantage that many children have in dealing with scholastic achievement. All children have a valuable culture that helps them learn those things that are important to their way of life. The learning patterns established and encouraged may be totally different from those required by the school or by standard intelligence tests, but may demand, in reality, a very skilled level of functioning in ways essential for the child's life.[12,76]

If children's learning experiences have primarily involved physical survival, they may be poorly equipped to deal with the abstractions and mental forms of operating that are required for scholastic learning. Their intelligence levels may be identified as adequate, inadequate, or gifted, but ways of learning and directing their own behaviors are not established in relation to the scholastic abilities valued by schools. For example, their symbols may be primarily cues in the environment, such as signals of rain; behavioral, nonverbal cues that one's motives are suspected; cues indicating an opportune moment to get away with something; or indications that a stranger is "one of us" or "one of them." Geometric symbols may be seldom, if ever, encountered with any attached meaning. Verbalization skills may not be necessary or important in relation to the kinds of symbols they learn to deal with. In addition the structures that they form mentally to predict the world about them and to perform mental tasks may differ from those needed for scholastic performance. When children must continue to function in real life with the cultural capacities developed earlier, but at the same time must perform in the ways of the scholastic world, increasingly difficult problems emerge unless the specific phenomena that are operating can be identified and the learning environment adapted to meet their particular needs.[27]

Most children of modern technological societies encounter a significant exposure to the mass media. A great many children from all social and economic environments encounter daily the influences of television, radio, or printed material. These media have been used in recent years in the United States to attempt to influence the experiential background of young children in preparing them with some of the skills required in the academic setting. Television programs designed especially for children in the preschool and early school years have proliferated to provide a means of widening the experiences of children in relation to meanings of geometric symbols, verbalizations, number concepts, and abstract reasoning abilities. The effect of such attempts is not yet fully determined.[33]

**The child's personality and emotions.** It is widely recognized that emotional and personality factors play a significant role in the learning performance of children. The extent to which they are able to adapt to novel situations, to solve problems, and to grow and develop in their capacity to acquire and use new knowledge and skills is enhanced by good mental health and adequate personality development. These abilities are hampered by poor mental health and personality problems. Even temporary disturbances such as disruption of family life, fear of a teacher or another child, or worry about an impending disaster or problem may be implicated in a change from the child's past ability to learn.[26,31,33,34]

## Social development

### Significance of peer groups

Probably the most predominant feature of the later childhood years is the change in socialization focus that occurs for children in modern, technological society. Whereas influences of the family predominated in forming children's social responses and interactions earlier in life, the world of school and their peers becomes a predominant influence on social behavior. This change is neither sudden nor complete. Children who attend a day-care or preschool setting during early childhood begin to experience this shift away from the family at a younger age. All children continue to be significantly influenced by their family, the culture of the family, and many other environmental factors. However, at about the age of 7 years, there is a relative shift in children's focus of attention and desires for socialization. They shift away from the influences of the immediate family and its culture to those of the school, teachers, and peers. It now is the peer group who begins to influence life-style, habits, and speech patterns, and who formulates standards of behavior and performance. The standards of the peer group become vitally important, and all efforts are made to conform. It becomes more important to be accepted by the peer group than by anyone else. Children begin to face the fact that their own goals, desires, and aspirations might be very different from those held by the peer group or the school, and they must find some way to cope and to perform according to the new standards if they are to succeed. Their success or failure

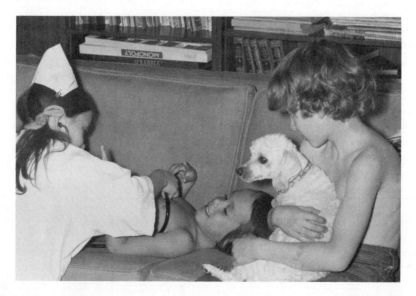

**Fig. 12-3.** Through identification and play, the school-age child relates to significant adults within and outside the family circle.

may be judged more harshly among peers than they were previously among the family group. While the devastation of failure with the group may be more severe than any they have experienced before, the feelings of success that come when they achieve group approval is a powerful and gratifying experience. The degree to which a child is able to fit in socially, to make the adjustment, to learn to cope, and to receive satisfaction from the group is a powerful determinant of healthy socialization.

As children are able to observe increasingly broader ranges of behavior, attitudes, and values, they begin to examine and to try out for themselves those attributes that they see as desirable. Through identification, they begin to relate to significant adults within and outside the family circle. Identification serves to provide children a means by which they can strengthen, direct, and control their own behavior in such a manner that it matches that of adults or children whom they view as admirable. Children usually perceive some similarity between themselves and the models they choose. A child often chooses a model of the same sex who has similar physical or behavioral traits. This mechanism of socialization during the first year or two of later childhood is the child's strongest link with the family. During these years, children may or may not maintain a strong identification with the parent of the same sex, but they also tend to adopt other adult models with whom they can identify.[37]

In relation to practicing increasing complex social skills, middle-age children tend to become preoccupied with the rules of the game, with rightness and wrongness of behavior, with responsibility, and with justice and fairness in all aspects of interaction. They seek to follow, as intently as they can, the exact code by which they feel things should be done. At the same time, they begin to try out judgments and ways of behaving that may be unacceptable to the family group but that are sanctioned or desired by their peers. For example, modes of dress become those that the peer group chooses and finds attractive. They begin to develop, with their best friends, a small world that only the group can share, a world that is secret and well guarded from intrusion by other children or

adults. The group's standards of loyalty and behavior in relation to the group members, to outsiders, and to adults are clearly delineated. Violation of the standards by any individual member results in severe group criticism and possible exclusion.

### Moral development

The moral development of children during later childhood has received substantial attention in the study of social and personality development during these years, since this appears to be one of the most dominant aspects of socialization that occurs during this period of life. Six aspects of development have been identified by Kohlberg[39] as clearly developing during the grammar school years in Western societies.

First, the child enters the school-age period judging behaviors in relation to real outcomes, or physical consequences. If a child of this age is asked whether it is worse to break five cups while helping mother set the table or to break one cup while stealing a cookie, most young children would think it is worse to break five cups. As middle childhood progresses the act begins to be judged in terms of the intention of the offender, and thus the stealing incident is considered the worse of the two acts.

Second, younger children view behaviors as totally right or totally wrong. Later they begin to be able to weigh several aspects of the situation and to use judgment in regard to the relative rightness or wrongness of the act.

Third, early in the middle years children will state that an act is wrong because it will bring punishment or displeasure from an adult. Later, they develop the insight that an act is wrong because it breaks a rule, offends another person's rights, or does harm to another.

Fourth, the fact of reciprocity is used in terms of what will happen to the child when he or she offends or is offended. In other words, children are able to calculate that they would hit back when hit, and that they would be hit if they were to hit someone else. By the age of 10 or 11 years, children are able to place themselves in the position of the other person and to begin to exercise the "Golden Rule" of doing unto others as you would have done unto you.

Fifth, younger children usually recommend

**471**

severe punishment for the misdeeds of others. Later, they begin to recommend a milder form of punishment and then an approach that would lead to the reform of the offender.

Finally, young children tend to view accidents or misfortunes as being punishments for wrong-doing. Later, such naturally occurring misfortune is not confused with punishment.[39,53,77]

## Personality development

Through each of the developmental processes of physiologic growth, cognitive development, learning capacity and social development, children are engaged in an important process of self-discovery, of building and creating their own personalities, and of becoming exposed to a wider range of possibilities for their own behavior, attitudes, and values. While a significant foundation for personality was developed during infancy and early childhood, the years of later childhood offer a valuable time during which children may begin to participate more actively in the assumption of specific traits and the choosing of values and attitudes. Although they tend to adopt those traits from which they continually receive family, school, or peer group reinforcement, they are often placed in a position of making a choice between conflicting values and traits. They begin to formulate their own sexual role through identification with the parent of the same sex. They encounter adult teachers, club leaders, adult friends, or peers who also present models of appropriate roles associated with their sexual identification, and they ultimately adopt a unique combination of these roles as appropriate for themselves.

Children's esteem for themselves is directed, to a large extent, by the degree to which they experience esteem from peers. They must have some contact with other children their own age who value them and who see them as worthy and desirable in order to experience such feelings for themselves.

### Erikson's theory of personality

The theoretical framework of Erik H. Erikson[15,22,23] offers one way in which to view this aspect of development during the school-age years. The major task to be accomplished, according to Erikson, is full mastery of whatever the child is doing. The child's concerns tend to be directed toward social tasks, so that the major arena in which this mastery is accomplished is in relation to age mates. Erikson calls this a sense of industry. The primary hazard of this period of life, on the other hand, is the development of a sense of inferiority. Fear of being seen as inferior as a person is supported by the very fact that he or she remains a child, and many limited capacities limit total performance. Yet the child can experience mastery through interaction with peers, and it is out of these dynamics that the intense devotion and preoccupation with the peer group grow. As the child wields mastery of the tools of the culture in relationship to those of the peer group, a sense of worth and of understanding of the self is developed. The original Freudian theory termed these years "latent"; for Erikson, these years are vital and important. The child is intense, interested, involved, and is concentrating on developing knowledge and skills. Interests appear to be directed away from children of the opposite sex, but at the same time there is a desire for knowledge about the biologic aspects of sexual function.[15,22,23]

As society has begun to narrow the dichotomy of appropriate sex roles and no longer encourages vast differences between man and woman concerning interests, behavior, appearance, or personality traits, the lack of interest in children of the opposite sex during this phase of development as described by Erikson may begin to change. In some cases, there is less discrimination in choosing children of the same sex for playmates, and interaction between boys and girls tends to continue throughout later childhood into adolescence.

### Lewin's field theory

The theory of Kurt Lewin[37,38,41] is of special value in attempting to understand personality development of the child during the middle years. This theory of personality holds application for any person at any point in life but is discussed here because it emphasizes the role of the complex environment in the development of personality and behavior.

For Lewin, personality is a function of the

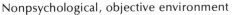

Nonpsychological, objective environment

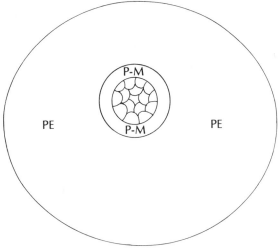

Nonpsychological, objective environment

**Fig. 12-4.** Person (represented by the circle) plus the psychologic environment (PE) comprise the life space. The person is comprised of regions, including the perceptual-motor area, which mediates between the person and the environment and the cells of the inner-personal region.

field that exists at the time the behavior occurs. The person exists within a psychologic environment. Both the person and the psychologic environment comprise the life space. The life space may be thought of as containing all of the possible facts or the whole of psychologic reality. In Fig. 12-4 the person is represented as a circle existing within the psychologic environment; together they comprise the total life space of the individual. The person is further differentiated by an outer circle, which is called the "perceptual-motor area." This area mediates between the inner-personal region and the environment, either in relation to influences of the environment on the person or in relation to influences of the person on the environment. The inner-personal region is further differentiated by peripheral cells and central cells. These cells, or areas of functioning, develop progressively and begin to differentiate as the individual grows and matures. The specific cells of personality function may be thought of as individual units, which are either rigid, fixed, and inflexible or flexible, in a state of change, and open or closed to the environment. Some aspects of the personality remain fairly well pro-

tected both from external influences and from communication with other areas of the personality. Other personality traits are subject to influence from any source. Areas that are represented as being close to one another are believed to possess a quality of communication. Those that are remote tend not to communicate with other remote areas. The boundaries surrounding areas of functioning may be represented as firm or weak, rendering them more or less prone to change or influence.

The environment, likewise, may be represented as composed of many different areas and facts. These areas, like those of the person, are subject to change and influence by the many dynamic properties of the total life space. Lewin did not deal extensively with the factors that lie outside of the life space in the objective, nonpsychologic environment, but these are supposed to influence the life space also. The number of regions or cells in any area of the life space is determined by the number of separate psychologic facts that exist at any one given moment for the individual. For many young children the environment may contain only one or two regions, such as mother and father or the home. Later this expands to include other regions, such as the school and peers. In Fig. 12-5 the person is represented as existing within the regionalized environment, and at a particular point in time the person is within one particular region. The person moves about from moment to moment among the various regions of the environment. (Remember that Lewin is referring to the psychologic environment, so that a child may be physically in school, but psychologically on the playground.) In understanding the person, it is necessary to map out the relationship of each of the regions of the life space as accurately as possible, including representing them in accurate approximation to one another and determining the characteristics that render them subject to change and influence. For Lewin, only those facts that currently exist in some concrete form can have real bearing upon the personality at a given time. Thus factors from earlier childhood are important only as they can be identified as exerting a real influence on the child's life space at one particular point in time.

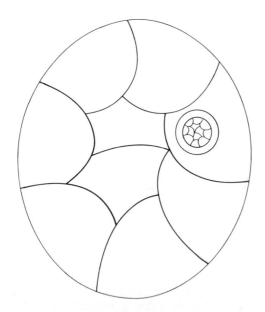

**Fig. 12-5.** The psychologic environment of the person is regionalized into areas that represent all of the facts influencing behavior at any given time. The person moves about from one region to another. The region within which the person is operating at a given moment is the region of greatest influence.

For Lewin, changes in the structure of the life space are accomplished as a result of several dynamic processes. These are need, psychic energy, tension, force or vector, and valence. In locomotion or in restructuring the person uses one or more of these processes to accomplish tension reduction and need satisfaction, or a state of equilibrium. Thus a child might discover something that was not known before, which alters the way of valuing a certain trait, and the valence (the positive or negative perception of the trait) changes. The child may, in another instance, have a desire (need) for candy and must obtain money from mother. The child moves from the playground to the mother to obtain the money, motivated by the tension or vector of the intention to obtain the candy.

In summary, Lewin's theory offers a useful way to conceptualize personality development during the years of later childhood. The psychologic environment becomes increasingly complex, and the person develops increasingly complex structure as the total life space changes, interacts, and the person performs the dynamic processes of locomotion and restructuring. Each region in the life space is important in determining the child's behavior at any given time, and understanding the features of each of the influencing regions is essential to understanding the individual child. Increasing age, by virtue of widening experiences, contributes to the complexity and diversity of the regions of the person and the psychologic environment, and to the complexity of the dynamic processes used by the person. However, one cannot account for behavior in terms of the age of the child; one must explore the total life space in terms of the field which determines the behavior.[41]

## NURSING ASSESSMENT OF PHYSICAL COMPETENCY

Regardless of the setting, the nurse performs a complete assessment of the school-age child in order to establish the data base from which to identify health care needs and problems. Those aspects of the assessment that relate to physical competency are considered initially, along with specific related health maintenance needs during later childhood.

## Past development and health maintenance

The past history of the child's development and health care may be determined either from the health care record or through a detailed interview. Features of pregnancy, labor and delivery, family medical history, developmental milestones, medical or surgical problems, and pattern of health maintenance in the past should be explored and documented. The child's immunization history is important, and it is recommended that booster immunizations for polio and for diphtheria, tetanus and pertussis be given at the time of entry to the school system (see Chapters 9 and 10).[38]

## Growth and vital signs

Growth in body weight and height are plotted on a sequential growth chart to determine consistent growth patterns within the established percentile range for the individual child. The heart rate, respiratory rate, and blood pressure are obtained and compared with developmental norms (see Appendix). Obesity and hypertension are increasingly recognized as potential hazards for the school-age child, and related factors of nutrition, eating patterns, and patterns of daith activity are assessed to assure adequate health practices that prevent such problems from developing.[3,7,60]

## Neuromuscular system

Functioning of the neuromuscular system is one of the most useful tools in evaluating adequacy of development during the later childhood years. The gradual changes in ability that occur over these years are difficult or impossible to fully demonstrate in isolated health assessment encounters, but the functioning of all school-age children should reflect a level of ability that approximates adult capacity in kind, but with a degree of expected immaturity in strength, quality, and fine coordination.

The function of the cranial nerves is deter-

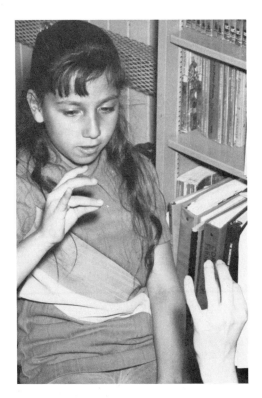

**Fig. 12-6.** The school-age child can tap each finger with the opposing thumb in rapid, coordinated succession.

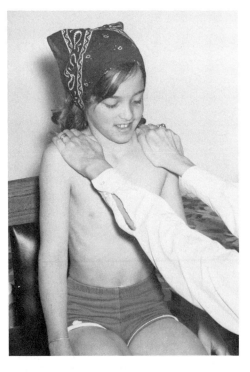

**Fig. 12-7.** The strength of muscle function in the shoulders is equal on both sides.

Later childhood

mined as described in Chapter 10. Even though these nerves reach maturity during the early childhood years, their function should be estimated periodically throughout childhood. By the seventh or eighth year children should develop full capacity to perform all gross and fine motor tasks with an adultlike level of coordination. They should be able to walk heel to toe, balance on one foot with eyes closed, touch the tip of the nose with each index finger with eyes closed, tap each finger with the opposing thumb in rapid, coordinated succession, and follow specific instructions accurately. The eye reflexes should be intact, as well as all other reflexes that do not fade, such as the knee jerk, the biceps, and triceps reflexes.

The child's muscular strength should be equal on both sides, with some predominance detected on the side of predominant function, or handedness. The areas of particular concern are the hands, arms, neck, shoulders, and legs. Incoordination or lack of strength on one side of the body is a definite deviation requiring further evaluation.

Children's handedness should be well established by the time that they enter school. They should be able to write letters of the alphabet early during the sixth year and indicate visual associations of the meaning of the figures written or drawn. They should be able to draw a figure of a person that is recognized as such, with at least six distinct body parts. By the end of later childhood most children can use shading and line effects to achieve a desired tone or mood in their drawing.

During the interview the child should indicate that he or she is not troubled by dizziness, headaches, blurred vision, ringing in the ears, or any other sign indicating a problem of functioning in the central nervous system.[2,38,48]

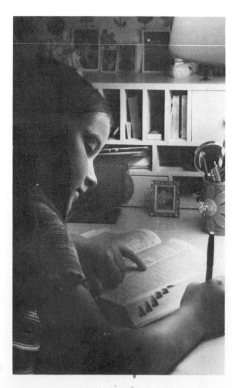

**Fig. 12-8.** Handedness is well established by the beginning of the school years. The child gains capacity to write legibly and to make increasingly complex visual associations with written and drawn figures.

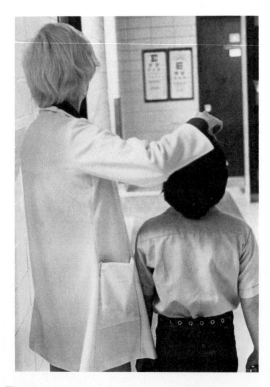

**Fig. 12-9.** Snellen screening for visual acuity is often a routine screening procedure conducted by the school system.

## Sensory capacity

This assessment is one of the most crucial of all determinations in regular health maintenance during later childhood, because sensory function is vitally important for adequate performance in the school setting. Snellen screening or some other screening procedure for visual acuity should be conducted as accurately as possible, with faithful adherence to recommendations for standardization.[13] Estimating the visual coordination of eye movements, equality of pupil reaction to light, peripheral vision, accommodation, and convergence is an essential component of assessment of visual capacity. (Techniques for assessment are found in Chapter 10.) Ability to recognize colors is ideally evaluated using a color-blindness test. The nurse may ask the child to read in order to observe for indications of impaired visual function, such as squinting or holding the book close to the face, or signs of impaired visual-mental-speech associations.

The child's hearing capacity is most accurately determined using audiometric procedures. However, this ability may be estimated by using a tuning fork, or by using any of several methods for estimating capacity in different ranges (see Chapter 10, p. 339).

The child's ability to feel and differentiate small objects may be estimated by placing objects in the hands behind the back. Being able to differentiate between various coins indicates fine touch discrimination and provides evidence of adequate introduction to the world of coin exchange used in society. The child may be given a cotton ball, rubber band, button, safety pin, plumber's washer ring, paper clip and other small items to identify by tactile feel alone, indicating a breadth of experience as well as tactile sense. The sense of touch may be tested

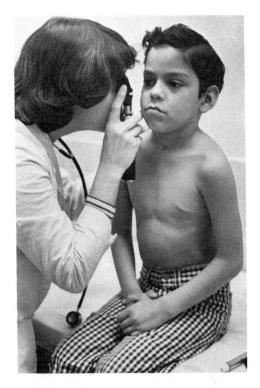

**Fig. 12-10.** The eyes are inspected for pupil reaction, adequacy of muscle coordination, peripheral vision, accommodation, convergence, and adequacy of eye grounds.

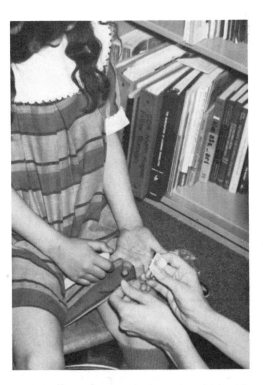

**Fig. 12-11.** The microhematocrit can be obtained in a school setting as a screening procedure.

over the entire body, and the sense of cold and warmth may be evaluated by having the child report the location and nature of the sensation when it is felt, keeping the eyes closed.

An estimate of kinesthetic motion may be determined by moving parts of the body with the eyes closed, and having the child report the direction of movement. This estimate confuses that of pressure sensations, and for finer discriminations the child should be placed in a rocking, rotating chair with the eyes covered and asked to report the direction of movement that is felt when the chair is moved about.

Smell is estimated by the child's report of familiar odors presented with the eyes covered. Taste is likewise determined by having the child differentiate between salt and sugar or other contrasting tastes.[4,38]

## Circulatory and blood systems

The adequacy of circulation to each extremity is determined by observing for pulse, warmth, and color in peripheral areas of the extremity. Heart sounds are auscultated, locating the point of maximal impulse, the apex beat, and estimating heart size. The apex beat gradually shifts from the fourth interspace to the left of the midclavicular line to a location at the fifth interspace at the midclavicular line by about the age of 7 years. Percussion of the heart further confirms adequate heart size and placement, indicating achievement of adultlike placement. (See Chapter 10 for description of the technique of scratch percussion.) In thin, hyperactive or excited children, a visible cardiac impulse may be detected, but such an impulse should be discretely located rather than diffuse in appearance. On auscultation the heart sounds should be sharp and clear, with a normal rhythm. Any unusual rhythm, splitting of sounds, or murmurs should receive further evaluation to distinguish such sounds as normal or abnormal.[4] The child's hemoglobin or hematocrit level is determined periodically and should be expected to reach the age-appropriate values indicated in the Appendix, p. 879. Appropriate blood pressure and heart rate values are also determined.[4,10] Respiratory and circulatory responses to exercise may be estimated by comparing at-rest values with values obtained

after the child has run in place for a full minute.

In talking with the child it is desirable to obtain some estimate of daily exercise and rest patterns. The child should be able to relate some active, outdoor sport or game that he or she enjoys regularly, either in summer or winter. The amount of time spent playing out-of-doors is not as important as the fact that the child deliberately seeks and enjoys regular activity that involves large muscle use, with substantial stimulation of muscular, circulatory, and respiratory systems.

## Respiratory system

The child's breath sounds are auscultated to determine the nature of the sounds in each quadrant of the chest. The adequacy of aeration of all lobes should be estimated under normal breathing conditions as well as during a sigh, or a prolonged, deep breath.

The child's ears, nose, and throat are inspected for signs of infection. Throat cultures to detect pathogenic group A, beta hemolytic streptococci are important screening measures in programs for prevention of rheumatic fever.[24,73]

## Gastrointestinal system

The child's mouth and teeth are inspected for adequate hygiene, dental repair, and evidence of adequate function. The foods that the child likes to eat and that are actually eaten for regular meals and snacks are determined by interviewing the child and the adult who prepares the meals. Adequacy of nutrition is primarily determined by factors indicating the total nutritional cycle, including intake, absorption, and utilization of dietary components. Such signs include adequate growth, healthy appearance and texture of the skin and mucous membranes, adequately formed and growing skeletal tissue, and adequate hemoglobin level. The child should not experience discomfort related to gastrointestinal functions either before or after meals and should indicate that bowel elimination function is adequate.[4,38,63]

## Genitourinary system

Renal function is estimated by determining the adequacy of a urine sample. Tenderness of

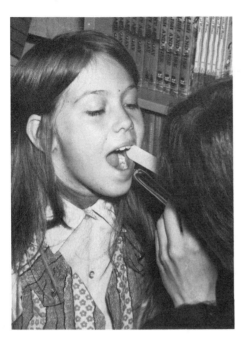

**Fig. 12-12.** The child's mouth and teeth are inspected for adequate hygiene, dental repair, and evidence of adequate function.

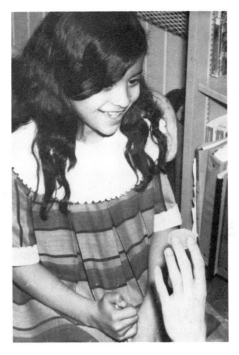

**Fig. 12-13.** The child is asked to obtain a urine specimen for screening of renal function.

the kidney region in the back or increased size of the kidneys detected by deep palpation should be ruled out.

The genitalia of both boys and girls should be observed under appropriate circumstances, particularly if talking with the child or parents leads to any question about a health problem involving the genitalia. Boys beginning to engage in competitive sports may experience periodic trouble with skin irritations or infections of the genitalia. A boy with undescended testicles that have not spontaneously descended by the age of 8 or 9 years needs to be evaluated to determine the desirability of surgical intervention.

Girls may also develop irritations and infections around the labia and in the vagina; occasionally a young girl will not realize that a condition of itchiness, discharge, or odor is not normal or expected, and so she does not mention such discomforts even when asked specifically. Visually observing for these problems, particularly when general body hygiene seems to be inadequate, can lead to discovering these health problems.[4,38,47]

## Skeletal system

The child's skeletal system is evaluated thoroughly in regard to adequacy of alignment of all structures and range of motion of all joints. Any joint swelling, pain, or tenderness to pressure indicates a need for medical evaluation. The child, particularly a girl, who is approaching puberty should be evaluated specifically for adequacy of growth and development of the spinal column. Without clothing from the waist up, the child is asked to bend over and touch her toes. The configuration of the entire spinal column is observed and palpated, noting particularly that the level of curvature of the shoulders is equal on both sides.[70,71]

The child's posture is observed in lying, sitting, standing, and walking positions. When the child is in a supine position, the lower costal margin of the ribs flare slightly, but the circumference of the chest is not increased, nor is there an increased anteroposterior diameter. The lower rib flaring should disappear early during adolescence. In a sitting position the child's spine should be relaxed but straight, the shoulders

**479**

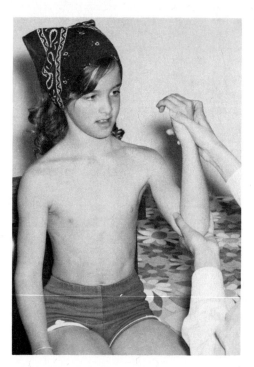

**Fig. 12-14.** The function of all joints is evaluated for adequacy of range, tenderness, and swelling.

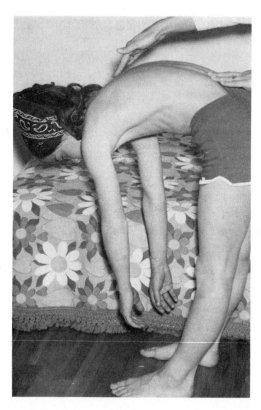

**Fig. 12-15.** The curvature and function of the spine are noted, particularly for a girl who is in the later childhood years. The level of curvature of the shoulders is equal when she bends over to touch her toes.

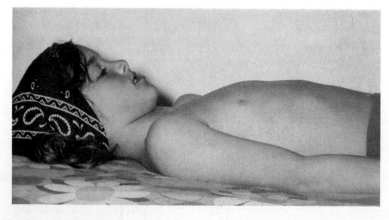

**Fig. 12-16.** When the child is in a supine position, the lower costal margin of the ribs flares slightly. This lower flare should disappear during puberty.

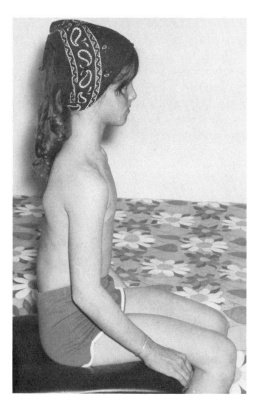

**Fig. 12-17.** In a sitting position, the child's spine should be relaxed but straight, with shoulders and hips horizontally equal.

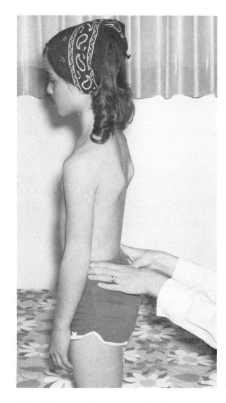

**Fig. 12-18.** While standing, the child's hips are horizontally equal.

and hips horizontally equal. While standing, the hips should be horizontally equal, legs straight and the feet directed forward at a 90-degree angle. The arms should fall in straight alignment along the trunk, with the palms of the hands facing the thighs with a slight posterior rotation. While walking, the child should demonstrate an even gait, with the feet maintaining straight alignment and arms swinging slightly and comfortably at the side.[4,10,13]

## Skin

The child's skin is inspected for signs of adequate hygiene and hydration, as well as signs of injuries or infection. The skin of the scalp

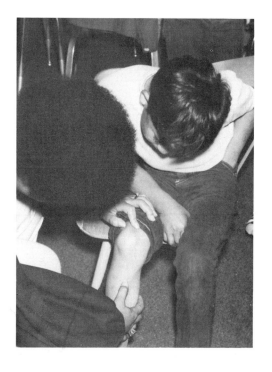

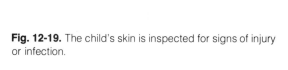

**Fig. 12-19.** The child's skin is inspected for signs of injury or infection.

should also be inspected, and the child may be asked how he or she takes care of the skin. Dryness and itching, particularly in cold, dry climates, may present a problem to the child and assistance may be needed in reducing the discomfort.[4]

### Signs of onset of puberty

The first signs of the onset of puberty usually occur physically several weeks or months before the child may be said to have entered adolescence (see Chapter 14). Secondary sexual characteristics including genital, underarm, and facial hair begin to appear. The boy's scrotum enlarges, followed by relative enlargement of the penis. The girl begins to have enlargement of the areola and nipples, followed by gradual growth of breast tissue.[4] A significant growth spurt, documented on the sequential growth graph, usually heralds the onset of puberty.

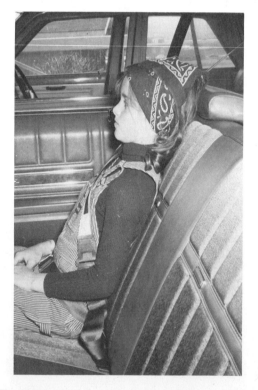

**Fig. 12-20.** Safety factors that the child should incorporate include adequate use of car safety belts. For the child over 4 feet tall, the shoulder belt should be used with the lap belt.

### Assessment of environmental conditions

The conditions of the child's environment should be determined, either by observation, report from the child and family, or by community statistics. The pollution problems of the environment should be determined, including food, air, water, and garbage conditions. Safety factors of the child's total environment should be explored, particularly in relation to traffic hazards in the home and school communities. The child's knowledge of pedestrian, bicycle, and automobile safety rules should be determined.

### Nutrition and eating behavior

Detailed assessment of nutritional status and eating behavior includes many of the details of assessment described above. Particular attention is given to the child's snacks and preferred foods, for there is more autonomy and responsibility assumed by the child in choosing and obtaining foods. The child's own understanding of the basic nutritional requirements, and the degree to which this understanding is used in selecting foods for meals and snacks should be determined. A detailed summary of the complete nutritional assessment is presented in Table 12-1.

### NURSING ASSESSMENT OF LEARNING AND THOUGHT COMPETENCY

During the course of the physical assessment, the nurse observes many cues that indicate learning and thought competencies. Determination of specific age-appropriate ability requires psychologic evaluation, but developmental lags may be detected through the estimates of general capacity obtained by the nurse. Areas of physical performance that specifically indicate learning and thought competency are those requiring neurologic functioning. The neurologic assessment, particularly in regard to the child's ability to perform tasks requiring gross or fine motor coordination, are often correlated with learning and thought capacity. The child should be able to follow directions accurately and without hesitation. All sensory capacities should function adequately.

When a concern arises regarding learning and thought competency, further evidence may be

**Table 12-1.** Levels of nutritional assessment for children (ages 6 to 12 years)*

| Level of approach† | History | | Clinical evaluation | Laboratory evaluation |
| | Dietary | Medical and socioeconomic | | |
|---|---|---|---|---|
| Minimal | 1. Source of iron<br>2. Vitamin supplement<br>3. Milk intake (type and amount)<br>4. Probe about snack foods; determine whether salt intake is excessive | 1. Birth weight<br>2. Length of gestation<br>3. Serious or chronic illness<br>4. Ask about medications taken; drug abuse | 1. Body weight and length<br>2. Gross defects | 1. Hematocrit<br>2. Hemoglobin<br>3. Urine protein and sugar |
| Midlevel | 1. Semiquantitative<br>  a. Iron-cereal, meat, egg yolks, supplement<br>  b. Energy nutrients<br>  c. Micronutrients—calcium, niacin, riboflavin, vitamin C<br>  d. Protein<br>2. Food intolerances<br>3. Baby foods—processed commercially; home cooked | 1. Family history: Diabetes Tuberculosis<br>2. Maternal Height Prenatal care<br>3. Infant Immunizations Tuberculin test | 1. Head circumference<br>2. Skin color, pallor, turgor<br>3. Subcutaneous tissue paucity, excess<br>4. Blood pressure | 1. RBC morphology<br>2. Serum iron<br>3. Total iron binding capacity<br>4. Sickle cell testing |
| In-depth level | 1. Quantitative 24-hour recall<br>2. Dietary history | 1. Prenatal details<br>2. Complications of delivery<br>3. Regular health supervision | 1. Cranial bossing<br>2. Epyphyseal enlargement<br>3. Costochondral beading<br>4. Ecchymoses<br>5. Changes in tongue, skin, eyes | Same as above, plus vitamin and appropriate enzyme assays; protein and amino acids; hydroxyproline, etc., should be available; BUN |

*Adapted from: Christakis, G., editor: Nutritional assessment in health programs, Am. J. Public Health, (suppl.) **63**:46, Nov., 1973.
†It is understood that what is included at a minimal level would also be included or represented at successively more sophisticated levels of approach. However, it may be entirely appropriate to use a minimal level of approach to clinical evaluations and a maximal approach to laboratory evaluations.

elicited by determining the child's orientation in time and space, by estimating memory capacity, by giving fairly complex instructions to follow, and by asking the child to read aloud age-appropriate material or to write a sentence that the nurse dictates. The child should be able to recall the day, month, and year by about 8 years of age, and the ability to tell time appears at about the same age. Children should know their home address by the time they enter first grade and should be able to describe how they travel from school to home and back again. They should be able to remember past events and to repeat more than four digits that have some meaning, such as the address or telephone number. They may be asked to perform several tasks in succession and be given the instructions all at once to determine the ability to remember and follow complex instructions. The child may, for example, be asked to walk to the other side of the room, turn right, tap the head three times, turn right again, and return. While these games and exercises do not yield specific or definitive information, they provide observation of a variety of types of performance involving learning and thinking capacity and thus give evidence that may help to differentiate between general developmental lag and inability to function in just one or two areas.[4,71]

During the transition period from early childhood to the school-age years, the child's language ability should be screened to determine accomplishment of adultlike language competency. Scholastic ability depends to a great extent on the child's receptive and expressive ability with the language of the school, and teaching and testing of vocabulary strength is a major focus during the early years of school. If the language of the child's family differs from that of the school, particular attention needs to be given to the range of exposure and experience that the child has had with the language used in the school. If the child has some ability with using the school's language, the equivalent developmental ability with that language may be estimated using the guidelines presented in the table entitled "Landmarks of Speech, Language, and Hearing Development," which is found in the Appendix. If on entering school the child appears to have a well-developed receptive ability and the major lag appears in expressive ability, the child is likely to be able to acquire sufficient expressive ability rapidly when experiences in use of the language increase. However, if receptive ability for the language of the school is lacking, the child needs special learning provisions, either to acquire the language of the school or to learn in a setting that uses the language of the home.

Temporary regression in the use of language may occur during the early school-age period in response to adjustment to the school experience or in response to unusual stressors. If such a period of regression is observed, attention needs to be directed to the child's underlying problem.

The Peabody Picture Vocabulary Test is a useful screening tool for verbal intelligence ability of middle-class English-speaking children.[21] The ability of the child to print or write words at a comprehension level appropriate to the grade level should be screened. The child's writing style should be observed; writing style does not approach adultlike maturity until the end of later childhood, but the child's writing should reflect the child's handedness, there should be no reversal of letter forms by the age of 7 or 8 years, and the relative size of letters should be uniform. Firm fine motor control should be evident by the eighth or ninth year of

age, in that the letter strokes are firm, even, and flow with ease. The child should be able to recognize and correct spelling and grammar errors by the eighth or ninth year of age.

## NURSING ASSESSMENT OF SOCIAL COMPETENCY

Because adequate social functioning is of vital importance to the child's total health during later childhood, it is important to determine the adequacy of adjustments and interactions with other children and adults. When the teacher expresses a concern for a child's social competency, the nurse may wish to explore this aspect of development thoroughly. This may be accomplished by interviewing the child, talking with the family, siblings, and friends, and observing the child's behavior in social situations. The specific feelings expressed by the child, such as loneliness, feelings of being liked or disliked by other children, excessive anger and aggression, or hostility toward conforming to behavioral norms, are important indications of social competency.

The maturity of the child's moral judgment may be estimated by discussing various fictitious situations involving moral acts. For example, the nurse may present a situation involving the problem of fair play and sharing as follows:

Five children run a race. Two of the children tie for first place, and the other three are so close behind that nobody can tell who came in second or third. There are three candy bars for the children who came in first, second, and third. How would you give out the prizes?

The nurse then discusses the child's responses to explore the child's concept of fairness. If the child suggests, for example, that they should run the race over, the nurse might ask how Susan, who won the race the first time, would feel if she did not even place in the second race. Because such concepts are dependent upon the child's cultural heritage and expectations, there are no "right" or "wrong" answers, but the child is likely to encounter social problems in school if his or her concept of fairness is incongruent with that of the predominant social culture of the school. In the predominant social culture of the United States, a child entering school would be expected to respond to the above situation with an inflexible set of rules and justice, which can be described and explained by the child. The child may insist that the first race was "no good" since there was not a winner that the only solution is to run the race over so that real winners can be determined and these children be given their prizes in return for their accomplishment. At a later period of early childhood the child's responses would be more flexible, and the relative feelings of each character in the story would be taken into account, with an attempt made to impart justice for all of the children in the race. For example, the child of 10 or 12 years might come to the conclusion that the children who tied for first place should be given a candy bar each, and the other three children should split the third candy bar equally.[19]

Assessment of peer group relationships can be estimated by asking the child questions regarding who he or she would choose for companionship or friends in relation to specific activities and exploring why these friends are chosen. For example, the child might be asked who he or she would choose to sit next to in class, to share a secret with, or to borrow money from or loan money to. At the time the child enters school, friends are likely to be chosen based on specific acts or behaviors that the child identifies as pleasant or good. A single transgression perceived by the child can quickly change the child's feeling of friendship association, but in turn friendship can be readily reestablished by acts of good will between the children. By about the age of 9 or 10 years, the child begins to sense the constant traits of trustworthiness in other children and identify as the basis for friendship those traits that are indications of a more consistent trustworthiness. Toward the end of later childhood, friends are selected because of a feeling of mutual understanding and willingness to assist with one another's innermost struggles.[19]

The child's attitudes toward authority, including their conceptualization of who holds authority, why that person has the right to hold authority, and the reasons for a child obeying that authority are assessed. A story dilemma involving an authority choice is given to the child, and the child's reactions to the story are elicited. For example, the child might be told a story involving a child whose mother has made a rule that the child must put all the toys away before going out to play, but one day the child's best friend wants to go out to play, and the child tells mother that he or she will pick up the toys later. The nurse then explores the child's impressions of what should be done and why.

In the predominant American culture, when children enter school, authority is legitimized by attributes in the authority figure that enable the person to enforce the commands, such as physical or social power. Obedience is motivated more out of respect for that power than out of a desire to avoid undesired outcomes, although the desire to avoid undesired outcomes (which predominates during earlier childhood) is still a factor in the child's thinking. At about 7 or 8 years of age, the child begins to base obedience on a sense of reciprocating favorable acts that the authority figure has demonstrated in the past. The authority figure's legitimate right of authority is appreciated because of that person's demonstrated ability to act out of generosity or kindness. Toward the end of later childhood, the child begins to integrate situational factors in deciding a situational dilemma. The right of the authority figure to exert authority is partially derived from the situation itself and might change if the situation changes. For example, a teacher might have the right to exert authority in the classroom but not necessarily on the playground, where a peer such as the captain of the ball team would be viewed as having greater authority. Obedience is viewed as a cooperative effort that results in benefit to all concerned.[19]

Social influences may occur which direct a child to begin to experiment with deviant social behaviors, including behaviors that are socially appropriate for adults but not children. Experimentations with drugs, alcohol, smoking, or sexual function are particularly disturbing for the adults responsible for the child's behavior in the home or the school. These problems will be discussed in detail in Chapters 13 and 14, but they can and do occur during later childhood,[61] and the nurse should be alert to cues that suggest their occurrence.

The child's behavior early in the school-age years reflects a continuing adult dependency mixed with a gradual shift toward peer dependency. Young children will use verbal and physical means to establish attachment and dependency with adults and peers. They may, for example, show a need to sit on the teacher's lap or to hug and wrestle with their friends. Gradually during later childhood this trait begins to disappear in most Western cultures, and the child shifts to visual and verbal means of establishing and maintaining social attachments. Likewise, acts of physical aggression and hostility occur with greater frequency among children in the younger school grades. As age and maturity increase, there is a shift to the use of verbal and other nonphysical means of expressing hostility.[19,40]

The *Vineland Social Maturity Scale* is designed to assess the child's performance and ability in progressing toward independence. The scale estimates ability in self-help skills, self-direction, locomotion, occupation, communication, and social relations. The data is obtained by direct observation of the child's behavior and by interview of the child or parent.[20]

## NURSING ASSESSMENT OF INNER COMPETENCY

As during all other ages, the interrelationships between inner competency and each of the other competencies are real and significant. Children during the school years discover further dimensions of the self and continue to understand and realize the inner nature of their existence through experiences with physical, learning and thought, and social competencies. Paradoxically, they are significantly impaired in the ability to develop capacity with each of the competencies unless their sense of inner satisfaction and realization is healthy and strong. If they have developed this sense during infancy and early childhood, they can progress through the later childhood years relatively unhampered in the industrious pursuit of mastery and realization of full potential for each area of competency. A child may be limited in intellectual capacity or by physical handicaps, but his or her own full potential is the goal toward which a child reaches. The child who has developed and continues to experience adequate inner competency is self-confident, happy, energetic, and able to cope with stress. Such a child relates satisfying experiences with friends and adults but is also realistic in discussing things that are not satisfying, relationships that are not enjoyed, or activities to which he or she must conform but does not like. The child can discuss with relative ease encounters with conflict, fear, worry, insecurity, loneliness, or doubt and is able to relate how he or she has dealt with these feelings in the past or how one might deal with them in other situations.[60-63]

One approach in assessment of inner competency for the school-age child is asking the child to draw a self-portrait. When the drawing is completed, the nurse asks the child to discuss features of the drawing and feelings that the drawing might suggest. The child of school age can respond to direct questions about inner perceptions of the self with great candor. For example, the self-concept may be estimated by asking the child questions such as "Are you smart?" "What do your friends think of you?" "Are you good at playing games?" "What makes you worry?". The child's self-portrait reveals the developing body image and should be roughly accurate in presenting certain observable details, such as curly hair. If a child is having difficulty incorporating certain physical features into the body image, this conflict may be revealed in the drawing. For example, after abdominal surgery a child may draw a self-portrait from the waist up, with the upper torso of the body filling the entire sheet of paper. The child may be given a blank outline of a human body and asked to draw on it certain inner structures of the body, such as the heart, lungs, and stomach, to estimate the extent and accuracy of concepts that have developed with regard to inner organ structure and function. The child's sexual identity is also explored using the self-portrait and interview. The school-age child has acquired many behaviors and concepts that have been culturally conveyed as appropriate for his or her sex. Questions such as "In what way are you like your mother (and father)?" or "What are girls (or boys) supposed to do?" reveals the child's conceptualization of specific sex-role behavior and the way in which

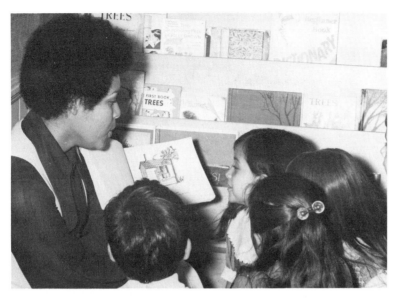

**Fig. 12-21.** The child's teacher is often able to offer specific information related to a particular problem the child is experiencing.

the child has identified with each of the parents.[5,8,31,49,58]

## HEALTH MAINTENANCE, PROMOTION, AND PREVENTION OF ILLNESS

Increasingly the school has been viewed as an important setting for the provision of health maintenance, promotion, and prevention of illness, for the school-age child is at a critical period of life when responsibility for health care is gradually transferred from the family to the individual child. The following sections present a comprehensive discussion of the health concerns that exist for the child of school age, with particular attention on the school as a health care setting. Regardless of the setting in which the nurse encounters the school-age child, however, these health care concerns need to be addressed on the child's behalf.

### The school and the nurse

Comprehensive school health services require an interdisciplinary, coordinated effort between health care professional workers and educators. The nurse, either as a private practitioner, a member of the community health care team, or a health care provider within the school itself, is often in a position to plan and direct comprehensive health care services for school-age children. These services should include planning for the delivery of direct health maintenance and restoration for the school-age child, providing nursing services for school-age children, coordinating referral services from other health care providers, planning and implementing actions to assure a healthy physical and emotional milieu for the school, planning and participating in the health education curriculum, and providing screening and health care for health problems that interfere with the learning process. While the underlying philosophy of school health programs usually assigns primary responsibility for the health of the individual child to the family, the provision of the full range of comprehensive services outlined above is considered essential in assuring optimal learning potential for all children and enhances the family's ability to identify and respond to their own health care needs.*

The role and responsibility of the nurse is dependent upon many factors inherent in the particular situation but may involve any of the com-

---

*References 9, 14, 16, 18, 25, 34, 42, 43, 45, 46, 62, 68.    **487**

prehensive dimensions of health programs. The central focus of the nurse is the direct delivery of nursing care for school-age children, but each dimension of the comprehensive health care program should be considered and drawn upon in providing nursing care. The following sections describe each of these dimensions in further detail.

## Health education for assumption of health care

Recognition of the school-age child's growing ability to serve as his or her own agent in health care provides the major thrust for health education programs in schools. The child needs adequate knowledge of all dimensions of health in order to make responsible choices that serve to protect his or her health status and to seek health care services when they are needed. The total health education program should involve all persons implementing the curriculum, for these concepts need to be integrated into every facet of the educational program as well as planned as a separate curriculum experience for every grade level. In addition the nurse is often involved in health teaching for individual children and families in relation to particular areas of concern that arise from the child's cur-

rent health status. Another important dimension is that of evaluation of the health education program, an effort that requires careful planning and follow-through.[68]

### Nutrition education

One of the predominant areas of health care that the school-age child begins to assume as a personal responsibility is that of selecting foods for snacks and meals. During the early grades the child should be introduced to the concepts of the basic four food groups and the importance of selecting foods in each group daily. In addition the hazards of foods that cause dental caries need specific attention, as this is one of the primary health problems of school-age children. During the later grades children need to learn more detail regarding each of the essential nutrients and their relationship to adequate growth and health. For example, the child needs to be introduced to the concepts of essential proteins, vitamins, minerals (especially iron), carbohydrates and fats, and the appropriate amounts of intake needed for optimal growth and health.

In addition to the learning concepts needed for each child, the school health team should give careful attention to the planning and evalu-

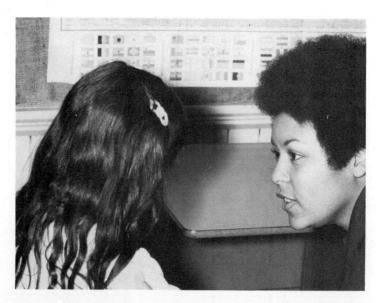

**Fig. 12-22.** It is vital to establish understanding of the child's point of view of a situation and to help her participate in the solution of a problem.

ation of snack foods and meals available for consumption by children at the school. Snack food machines should contain a selection of high-protein, noncariogenic foods. Foods containing empty calories, particularly cariogenic foods, need to be eliminated. Snack foods and meals should be evaluated for their appeal for the group of children in the school, and the pattern of selection planned to enhance wise food choices among the children. This dimension of the health program promotes acquisition of food preferences among children, which helps to shape their tendency to select nutritious foods when confronted with a variety that includes less desirable selections.

### Body hygiene

Another area of self-care that is assumed early during the school years is that of providing for body hygiene. Typically, the school-age child has little interest in bathing and grooming, but attention should be given to assisting the child to acquire an understanding of the importance of adequate skin care in preventing bacterial and fungal infections. Often this aspect of health care is integrated with the physical fitness and sports program by teaching the child to bathe following rigorous physical activity. Specific discussion of the areas of the body that need particular and regular attention, such as bathing the genitalia, care of the feet, tooth brushing, and shampooing the hair, should be planned as a part of the health education program. In addition, children need guidance in learning how to care for minor skin injuries and to promote optimal healing.

### Exercise and physical fitness

Providing a planned, age-appropriate program of physical fitness in the school not only enhances the child's level of physical fitness during the school-age years but also provides the opportunity for the child to develop the habit of regular physical exercise. Fitness exercises should be planned to appeal to the children of each age group, and specific instruction given regarding the physical benefits that are derived from each type of physical exercise. Learning programs that deal with body mechanics, coordination and efficiency of movement,

adaptation of activity levels with physical capacity, the nature of fatigue, the importance of sleep and rest and relaxation, and prevention of injuries related to physical activity are incorporated into the health education curriculum.

The school health care team is often involved in assessing a school-age child for activity levels of tolerance, particularly if the child has suffered a major illness or injury. Physical fitness guidelines have been developed, but it has not yet been possible to accurately predict the upper levels of tolerance for an individual child. Medical evaluation by an experienced person who is familiar with the school's physical fitness program should be obtained for any child who has a health problem. The nurse should screen all children for exercise tolerance by obtaining vital signs before and after a standard exercise task, such as running in place for one minute. The pulse and respiratory rate should not rise more than 20/min and should return to the preexercise level within one to three minutes. The child needs to be aware of signs of undue fatigue, and the physical fitness supervision should respond to a child's expression of fatigue rather than force a child to reach beyond levels of tolerance.

### Concepts of prevention of illness and accidents

Accidents during later childhood often arise from the child's lack of judgment and inability to predict a potentially dangerous hazard and in knowing how to take adequate precautions. The potential sources of burns from chemicals, electrical appliances, and fire need to be included in the health education program. In a community where swimming is a popular activity, the sources of swimming accidents, such as diving into shallow water or attempting a distance beyond the level of tolerance and ability, need to be discussed. If a child swims regularly and frequently, life-saving instruction should be given during the upper grades. Bicycle and pedestrian safety concepts need to be presented during the early grades and reinforced throughout the school-age years.

Concepts of prevention of illness may be integrated into the science curriculum, including the processes of communicable disease transfer,

**489**

immunization, and other means of controlling the environment to minimize transfer of infection. Concepts of host defenses against communicable diseases and the role of physical fitness, rest, and nutrition in building optimal defenses should be included for the older school-age child.

Prevention of dental caries and gingivitis should be taught to the school-age child. This includes teaching, demonstration, and return demonstration of use of the toothbrush and dental floss and teaching concepts of regular dental evaluation of the mouth and teeth and concepts of nutrition for prevention of dental caries.[57]

### Protection of sensory capacity

During later childhood the importance of preserving optimal sensory capacity, particularly sight and hearing, should be brought to the child's attention. The child needs to understand that these abilities have now reached their full potential and that specific measures need to be taken to preserve optimal ability. Appropriate measures in caring for the eyes, optimal settings for reading, and the importance of resting the eyes periodically during prolonged reading need to be taught. Classroom situations need to be periodically evaluated to assure that such measures are provided in the classroom itself. The dangers of imposing hearing loss through exposure to prolonged or repeated loud sounds, particularly music, needs to be brought to the child's attention.

### Human sexuality

Planning a human sexuality curriculum for school-age children has produced much debate among parents and educators in local communities. The extent of the formal curriculum needs to be reviewed and evaluated for adequacy in meeting the needs of the school-age child, and most important, in the effect that the content and presentation have on attitude development among school-age children. When the school curriculum is limited in the range of content provided in the school, the sources from which children obtain information should be identified and evaluated for accuracy and attitude formation. In many schools, study of the life cycle provides the focus for children in the lower

grades, and the study of reproduction, with particular attention to preparation for the changes of puberty, is included in the upper grades.

Beyond the specific curriculum, the school provides a major influence in the development of human sexuality for the school-age child. Sex-role typing in children's textbooks has received considerable attention, and efforts have been made by publishers to remove this bias from their books. Learning units designed to introduce children to jobs and careers have been increasingly planned for removal of sex-role typing of jobs and careers. Learning experiences that help the child to develop mature social relations and communication skills provide an important basis for developing concepts of human sexuality. The presence of role models in the school itself, such as men teachers in the classroom, women in roles of authority, and involvement of fathers in parent-teacher activities, has an effect on formation of attitudes toward human sexuality. Provision of physical fitness and sports activities for girls equivalent to that offered boys is another dimension in responding to changing attitudes toward sex-role typing.

Preparation for the changes of puberty is a health care concern that can no longer be neglected by the schools, using the rationale that the family must assume this responsibility. In some communities, there is a particularly strong feeling that specific content instruction should not be included in the school curriculum, but even in these settings the school health team must be sensitive to this need in relation to changing physical and emotional and social dynamics that emerge for the later school-age child. For example, when a girl in a fourth-grade class has a sudden growth spurt, breast development, and begins menstruating, the individual and social impact of this on the entire group of children cannot be ignored, and families are not in a position to respond adequately to the learning and mental health needs of each child within the group. The school health team and the teachers need to assess the attitudes of the group of children, assist them in maintaining sound social relationships, and facilitate the children's understanding of the changes of puberty, and the development of healthy attitudes toward these changes. Many schools include in the curriculum content a study of life cycle changes, with attention on the ranges of normal during puberty, in an effort to prepare children for the acceptable fact that some children experience these changes early, while others experience the changes later. Boys and girls should be included together in most discussions related to these units of learning in order to facilitate learning to understand and appreciate the phenomena for both sexes and to develop open communication and acceptance between boys and girls.

Children's questions should be answered openly and with an attitude of matter-of-fact acceptance. In schools where human sexuality is a planned part of the curriculum, open discussion of masturbation should be planned, with the aim of dispelling many of the misunderstandings and myths that children acquire related to masturbation. The focus of all such discussion should be on the ways in which sexual feelings and stimulation are valuable dimensions of human living and how these can be used for healthy relationships between people.[6,65]

## Prevention of drug abuse

Prevention of drug abuse begins with early discussions with school-age children in which they can obtain information about drugs, including alcohol, tobacco and caffeine, ask questions, and express their feelings about people's use of drugs. The establishment of open dialogue between school-age children, their teachers, and the health care team is essential in providing openess and trust so that young children can seek sound answers to their questions and discuss their concerns. Of particular concern is the use of alcohol and tobacco among young school-age children. They need to discuss the underlying reasons why people may use drugs to cope with stress and fear, discuss healthy alternatives that can be used for coping, and experience the use of such alternative methods in the school setting. The use of alcohol and tobacco as a way of feeling "grown up" needs to be discussed, and the children encouraged to discuss and think about behavior that is more completely indicative of being "grown up."

Sources of availability of drugs should be explored, including the availability of alcohol and tobacco in the home, as well as sources of illegal drugs on the street. Children need to discuss their encounters with available drugs and explore the choices with which they are confronted when such drugs are available and the reasons for making each of the choices.[44]

## Prevention of illness and accidents

A specific program for the prevention of illness and accidents in and around the school should be planned by the school health care team. The school environment needs to be periodically evaluated for sources of health hazards. Pedestrian and automobile traffic patterns should be assessed for safety and altered when a definite safety hazard exists. Worn out and broken playground equipment should be removed and replaced. Adequate ice and snow removal should be available in winter months. Procedures for physical maintenance of the school building should include consideration of safety provisions, such as standards for the maintenance of toilet facilities and prompt repair of broken fixtures, stairways, and desks. Fire prevention is usually mandatory by law and includes regular fire drills to acquaint teachers and students of procedures to be used in the event of fire. All classrooms, libraries, and hallways should be equipped with adequate lighting. Techniques used in the preparation of food should receive regular critical review.

The aesthetic environment of the school should be assessed for its impact on mental status. A bleak environment in the school will have a much different effect than a colorful and stimulating environment. On the other hand, areas that need to be used for concentrated attention should provide minimal distracting stimuli and a choice of wall color that is conducive to quiet and calm, such as light blue or brown.

All children in school should be assessed in terms of their immunization status, and immunizations provided for any child who has not received adequate protection. In the event of a communicable illness epidemic, appropriate measures should be taken to protect the health of all persons in the environment. If a mass immunization program is available, as for a particular strain of influenza, the children and teachers need to be informed of the availability of the immunization and the benefits and risks of receiving the vaccine.[51] Special attention is given to detecting early signs of illness in a child or teacher and providing for that individual to be isolated from the other children. Screening of children on return to school may be needed to assure that they have recovered sufficiently to attend classes.

Detection and treatment of streptococcal throat infections are important aspects of prevention of rheumatic heart disease and other serious sequelae to this common infection. Many communities have instituted prevention programs in which all school-age children are screened for streptococcal organisms in the throat during periods of peak incidence during the year. A throat culture for streptococcal infection should be obtained on any child complaining of a sore throat and is often available free of charge from the state health department. If a culture reveals the presence of the organism, treatment with appropriate antibiotic therapy can be instituted. The school nurse often provides evaluation and follow-through to assure that the child receives full treatment with antibiotics to ensure the effectiveness of treatment in prevention of serious sequelae.[35,73]

## Management of minor illness and accidents at school

Policies regarding the management of minor illnesses and accidents at school vary widely from state to state, community to community, and school to school. The nurse should be aware of all state and local laws and policies that affect the scope of nursing activity in the school and consider the legal implications of all such activities. While the legitimate scope of nursing practice has been expanded in many areas, the legal risks of nursing practice have become increasingly complex. Each of the dimensions of assuring personal and legal protection, discussed in Chapter 2, should be reviewed and current practice in schools planned to assure maximum provision of services to children while providing protection for the nurse.

When a child is determined to have common symptoms of illness such as fever, vomiting or diarrhea, the child should remain isolated from the classroom and provided a place to rest until the end of the school day or until someone can come to take the child home. If it is possible to administer an antipyretic drug, this may be done for the child who has a fever. Other means of reducing body fever, such as cold packs to the head, may be used to make the child more comfortable. The nurse should institute measures to assure adequate fluid intake and periodically reevaluate the child's condition while he or she remains at school.

Minor injuries to the skin should be carefully assessed to determine the exact extent of the injury and to evaluate whether medical repair might be needed. Cuts on the face and hands, even though of minimal severity, may require stitching to minimize scarring in these areas. The wound should be thoroughly cleaned and bandaged if needed to protect from further injury or infection.[28]

During later childhood, usually at about 9 years of age, children begin to complain of various physical aches and pains that have no apparent organic cause. Headaches, abdominal pains, and pains in the limbs (growing pains) are the most frequent complaints. The symptom is usually transient but may tend to recur for a particular child. The school health care team needs to develop a standard protocol for the management of such complaints, including an adequate history, interview and physical assessment to rule out serious organic problems, and an acceptable approach in managing the child's symptoms, including reassurance for the child, the use of drugs, and adequate reevaluation to determine resolution of the symptom. The child's parents need to be informed that such intervention was needed, so that they are aware of the child's symptoms in the event the condition develops further at home.[28,29,47]

## Detection and prevention of learning problems

Screening of vision and hearing problems at regular intervals is necessary to detect children who may be at a disadvantage in the classroom because of inadequate sensory capacity. The teacher and the school health care team must work closely together in evaluating a child whose performance in school does not seem to be meeting the child's potential, for often a health problem is involved.

When a general lag is suspected, nursing intervention includes further exploration of the problem and collaboration with appropriate health care team members to delineate the nature and extent of the difficulty. The child's family may have specific concerns that support the nurse's findings. On the other hand, they may be unaware of any problem, and conditions of the home may indicate a lack of stimulation or little opportunity to develop scholastic and academic skills and concepts. In such a case, it may be important to determine the areas of function within the child's own culture and environment that might indicate adequate learning and thought competency.

The child's teacher may be able to offer more specific information, and consultation with psychologic or education resources may be helpful in finding an appropriate plan of intervention for the child.

## Promoting healthy social relationships

As in other areas of health care, prevention of problems is the most effective way in which to help a child grow and develop socially. However, in spite of all efforts to provide for optimal social interactions, reinforcement from the group, and assistance with group interactions and coping with group stress, social problems continue to constitute a major concern for many children during this period of life. Children may experience difficulty in making the initial transition away from the family and in establishing dependency and satisfaction from the group of peers. They may make the initial adjustment but then continue to interact with friends and with adults in a relatively immature fashion, failing to form increasing mature social judgments and ways of interacting. When problems such as these arise, the child's entire life space must be explored, and all persons involved must be encouraged to help the child achieve more satisfying social relationships. The nurse's role in such an undertaking may be central or peripheral for any given child, but as appropriate each adult and health care worker who is involved with the child should seek to work together to understand the child's problem and to find ways

in which he or she might be helped. It is vital to establish knowledge of the problem from the child's point of view and to clearly understand his or her perception of the problem itself and how the problem might be resolved. To the extent that the child is actively involved in understanding the dilemma and in finding ways to resolve it, success and real inner satisfaction for the child will be enhanced.

Helping a child to achieve and maintain mental health is a complex task that is far beyond the scope of any single health care worker, the family, or the school alone. Each individual who becomes a part of the child's life contributes to ongoing formulation of mental health at any given time.

Ways in which people can achieve inner security, happiness, and satisfaction need to be understood by children. They need to know that no human being has yet discovered a ready-made formula and that inner knowledge and peace are things that each person seeks and finds in their own way. There are certain things that most people find conducive to inner and emotional health, including ways to cope with frustration and disappointment, ways to alleviate anxiety, and ways to achieve peace and approval from and with other people. One of the most important concepts for children to develop during these years is that it is right and good to ask for help when they are troubled. Knowing where and how to get help from someone is a great advantage in continuing to attain and maintain increasingly strong inner competency. At times children might need to turn to their best friend; at other times they need help from an adult. They need to learn how to discriminate when to seek help and who might be the best person to turn to.

**STUDY QUESTIONS**

1. Observe a group of children about 6 years of age and a group about 10 or 11 years of age. Contrast the behaviors of each group that you see. Identify the ways in which they communicate with one another, express attachment or dependency, or hostility. Contrast the interests and games in which they engage.
2. Plan and implement a nursing assessment of a child in this age period. Describe the approach that you plan to use, ways of interacting on the child's level, of promoting comfort, and of establishing rapport. Document the

health care needs that you ascertain as being met by the family, those the child is able to provide, those the school provides, and those that need nursing intervention.

3. Describe in your own words how the theories of Piaget, Erikson, and Lewin can be applied to nursing practice. Discuss your ideas with those of your classmates, and draw comparisons with other theories with which you might be familiar.

4. Plan an interview with a teacher in an elementary school setting. Determine what health problems he or she feels are important in this particular classroom and what resources are available in the school to help with health care and education problems. How is the environment of the school planned and supervised to promote the physical and emotional health of the children and teachers.

5. Describe the health education curriculum of an elementary school. Evaluate the adequacy of this curriculum in relation to the goals of health care and your own philosophy and beliefs about maintaining health.

6. Observe the area surrounding a school during the time that the children are leaving the building for the day. What provisions have been made to ensure traffic and pedestrian safety in the area. What behavioral traits of the children do you notice that might influence the child's safety at this particular time.

## REFERENCES

1. Anderson, C. L., and Creswell, W. H., Jr.: School health practice, ed. 6, St. Louis, 1976, The C. V. Mosby Co.
2. Angle, C. R.: Locomotor skills and school accidents, Pediatrics **56**:819, Nov., 1975.
3. Bailey, E. N.: Screening in pediatric practice, Pediatr. Clin. North Am. **21**:123, Feb., 1974.
4. Barness, L. A.: Manual of pediatric physical diagnosis, ed. 4, Chicago, 1972, Year Book Medical Publishers, Inc.
5. Beardslee, C.: Acquisition of appropriate sex-role behavior; a review of the literature, Mat. Child Nurs. J. **3**:139, Summer, 1974.
6. Bell, A. I.: Psychologic implications of scrotal sac and testes for the male child, Clin. Pediatr. **13**:838, Oct., 1974.
7. Botwin, E. D.: Should children be screened for hypertension, Mat. Child Nurs. J. **1**:152, May/June, 1976.
8. Brodie, B.: Views of healthy children toward illness, Am. J. Public Health **64**:1156, Dec., 1974.
9. Brown, G. W.: School; Child advocate or adversary? Clin. Pediatr. **16**:439, May, 1977.
10. Brown, K., and others: Prevalence of anemia among preadolescent and young adolescent urban black Americans, J. Pediatr. **81**:714-718, Oct., 1972.
11. Bruner, J. S.: The relevance of education, New York, 1971, W. W. Norton and Co., Inc.
12. Chinn, P. L.: A relationship between health and school problems; a nursing assessment, J. School Health **43**: 85, Feb., 1973.
13. Chinn, P. L., and Leitch, C. J.: Child health maintenance; a guide to clinical assessment, ed. 2, St. Louis, 1977, The C. V. Mosby Co.
14. Committees on pediatric manpower and committee on school health: Concepts of school health programs, American Academy of Pediatrics, Pediatrics **55**:140, Jan., 1975.
15. Coppersmith, S.: The antecedents of self-esteem, San Francisco, 1967, W. H. Freeman and Co.
16. Creighton, H., and Squaires, G. M.: School nurses; legal aspects of their work, Nurs. Clin. North Am. **9**: 467, Sept., 1974.
17. Cronbach, L. J.: Essentials of psychological testing, ed. 3, New York, 1970, Harper & Row, Publishers, pp. 200-202.
18. Cronin, G., and Young, W. M.: Posen/Robbins; a model school health care project, Nurse Practitioner **2**:22, Sept.-Oct., 1977.
19. Damon, W.: The social world of the child, San Francisco, 1977, Jossey-Bass Publishers.
20. Doll, E. A.: Vineland social maturity scales, Circle Pines, Minn., 1965, American Guidance Service, Inc.
21. Dunn, L. M.: Peabody picture vocabulary test, Minneapolis, 1965, American Guidance Service, Inc.
22. Erikson, E. H.: Childhood and society, ed. 2, New York, 1963, W. W. Norton & Co., Inc.
23. Erikson, E. H.: Identity, youth and crisis, New York, 1968, W. W. Norton & Co., Inc.
24. Feeney, R.: Preventing rheumatic fever in school children, Am. J. Nurs. **73**:265, Feb., 1973.
25. Fine, L. L., and Bellaire, J.: The school nurse—an obsolete professional revisited, Pediatr. Nurs. **1**:25, Jan.-Feb., 1975.
26. Glasser, W.: Schools without failure, New York, 1969, Harper & Row, Publishers.
27. Gordon, E. W.: Programs of compensatory education. In Deutsch, M., Katz, I., and Jensen, A. R., editors: Social class, race, and psychological development, New York, 1968, Holt, Rinehart & Winston, Inc., p. 381.
28. Green, M. I.: A sign of relief; the first-aid handbook for childhood emergencies, Washington, D.C., 1977, Capitol Publications, Inc.
29. Grunberg, E.: Standing orders for the school health room, Nurs. '75 **5**:62, Feb., 1975.
30. Guyton, A. C.: Textbook of medical physiology, ed. 5, Philadelphia, 1976, W. B. Saunders Co.
31. Harns, D. B.: Children's drawings as measures of intellectual maturity, New York, 1963, Harcourt, Brace & World.
32. Hunt, J. McV.: Environment, development and scholastic achievement. In Deutsch, M., Katz, I., and Jensen, A. R., editors: Social class, race, and psychological development, New York, 1968, Holt, Rinehart & Winston, Inc., p. 293.
33. Hurlock, E. B.: Child development, ed. 5, New York, 1972, McGraw-Hill Book Co.
34. Igoe, J. B., and Silver, H. K.: Improving health care in the school setting, Nurse Practitioner **2**:7, Sept.-Oct., 1977.
35. Jackson, H.: Prevention of rheumatic fever; A compara-

tive study of clindamycin palmitate and ampicillin in the treatment of group A beta hemolytic streptococcal pharyngitis, Clin. Pediatr. 12:501, Aug., 1973.

36. Jenne, F. H.: Variations in nursing service characteristics and teachers' health observation practices, J. School Health 40:248, 1970.

37. Kagan, J.: Understanding children: Behavior, motives and thought, New York, 1971, Harcourt, Brace, Jovanovich, Inc.

38. Kempe, C. H., Silver, H. K., and O'Brien, D., editors: Current pediatric diagnosis and treatment, ed. 4, Los Altos, Calif., 1976, Lange Medical Publications.

39. Kohlberg, L.: Development of moral character and moral idiology. In Hoffman, M. L., and Hoffman, L. W., editors: Review of child development research, vol. 1, New York, 1964, Russell Sage Foundation, p. 383.

40. Leighton, D. C.: Measuring stress levels in school children as a program-monitoring device, Am. J. Public Health 62:799-806, June, 1972.

41. Lewin, K.: Field theory in social science; selected theoretical papers, edited by D. Cartwright, New York, 1951, Harper & Row, Publishers.

42. Lewis, M. A.: Child-initiated care, Am. J. Nurs. 74:652, April, 1974.

43. McAtee, P. A.: Nurse practitioner in our public schools? An assessment of their expanded role as compared with school nurses, Clin. Pediatr. 13:360, April, 1974.

44. Montana, E.: Project DDD; dialogues on drug dependence, Clin. Pediatr. 12:355, June, 1973.

45. Nader, P. R.: The school health service; making primary care effective, Pediatr. Clin. North Am. 21:57, Feb., 1974.

46. Oda, D. S.: Increasing role effectiveness of school nurses, Am. J. Public Health 64:591, June, 1974.

47. Oster, J.: Clinical phenomena noted by a school physician dealing with healthy children, Clin. Pediatr. 15:748, Aug., 1976.

48. Page-El, E., and Grossman, H. J.: Neurologic appraisal in learning disorders, Pediatr. Clin. North Am. 20:599, Aug., 1973.

49. Paluszny, M.: Sexual identity and role in children; how do these develop? Clin. Pediatr. 13:154, Feb., 1974.

50. Penfield, W.: The uncommitted cortex, the child's changing brain. In Bernard, H. W., and Huckins, W. C., editors: Exploring human development; interdisciplinary readings, Boston, 1972, Allyn & Bacon, Inc., p. 189.

51. Phillips, C. F., and others: Killed subunit influenza vaccine in children, Pediatrics 52:416, Sept., 1973.

52. Philips, L.: Youth, permissiveness, and child development, Pediatrics 49:1-4, Jan., 1972.

53. Piaget, J.: The moral judgment of the child, New York, 1932, Harcourt, Brace.

54. Piaget, J.: The language and the thought of the child, New York, 1965, The World Publishing Co.

55. Piaget, J.: The theory of stages in cognitive development, New York, 1969, McGraw-Hill Book Co.

56. Piaget, J., and Inhelder, B.: The psychology of the child, New York, 1969, Basic Books, Inc., Publishers.

57. Polson, A. M.: Gingival and periodontal problems in children, Pediatrics 54:190, Aug., 1974.

58. Porter, C. S.: Grade school children's perceptions of their internal body parts, Nurs. Res. 23:384, Sept.-Oct., 1974.

59. Pulaski, M. A.: Understanding Piaget—an introduction to children's cognitive development, New York, 1971, Harper & Row, Publishers.

60. Rance, C. P., Argus, G. S., Balfe, J. W., and Kooh, S. W.: Persistent systemic hypertension in infants and children, Pediatr. Clin. North Am. 21:801, Nov., 1974.

61. Ray, O. S.: Drugs, society and human behavior, St. Louis, 1972, The C. V. Mosby Co.

62. Recommendations on Educational Preparation and Definitions of the Expanded Role and Functions of the School Nurse Practitioner; a Joint Statement of the American Nurses' Association and the American School Health Association. J. School Health 43:594, Nov., 1973.

63. Ripa, L. W.: The role of the pediatrician in dental caries detection and prevention, Pediatrics 54:176, Aug., 1974.

64. Roberts, S. O.: Some mental and emotional health needs of Negro children and youth. In Wilcox, R. C., editor: The psychological consequences of being a black American, New York, 1971, John Wiley & Sons, Inc., p. 332.

65. Rybicki, L. L.: Preparing parents to teach their children about human sexuality, Mat. Child Nurs. 1:182, May-June, 1976.

66. Schmitt, B. D., Jordan, K., and Hamburg, F. L.: The role of the pediatrician in helping children develop a sense of responsibility, Clin. Pediatr. 11:509-513, Sept., 1972.

67. Schmitt, B. D., Jordan, K., and Hamburg, F. L.: How to help your child be responsible for his schoolwork, Clin. Pediatr. 11:514-515, Sept., 1972.

68. Schour, M., and Clemens, R. L.: Fate of recommendations for children with school-related problems following interdisciplinary evaluation, J. Pediatr. 84:903, June, 1974.

69. Selkurt, E. E., editor: Physiology, ed. 4, Boston, 1976, Little, Brown and Co.

70. Sells, C. J., and May, E. A.: Scoliosis screening in public schools, Am. J. Nurs. 74:60, Jan., 1974.

71. Shifrin, L. Z.: Scoliosis—current concepts, early recognition and aggressive treatment, Clin. Pediatr. 11:594, Oct., 1972.

72. Stamler, C., and Palmer, J. O.: Dependency and repetitive visits to the nurse's office in elementary school children, Nurs. Res. 20:254, May-June, 1971.

73. Wang, R. M.: Streptococcal sore throat, Am. J. Nurs. 77:1797, Nov., 1977.

74. Wara, D. W., and Ammann, A. J.: Immunologic disorders of childhood. In Rudolf, A. M., editor: Pediatrics, ed. 16. New York, 1977, Appleton-Century-Crofts, p. 299.

75. Whipple, D. V.: Dynamics of development; Euthenic pediatrics, New York, 1966, McGraw-Hill Book Co.

Later childhood

76. Whiteman, M., and Deutsch, M.: Social disadvantage as related to intellective and language development. In Deutsch, M., Katz, I., and Jensen, A. R., editors: Social class, race, and psychological development, New York, 1968, Holt, Rinehart & Winston, Inc., p. 86.

77. Whiteman, P. H., and Kosier, K. P.: Development of children's moralistic judgments; age, sex, I.Q. and certain personal-experiential variables. In Noll, V. H., and Noll, R. P., editors: Readings in education psychology, ed. 2, New York, 1968, Macmillan Publishing Co., Inc., p. 29.

# CHAPTER 13

# Health problems of later childhood

Although the years of later childhood are ordinarily characterized by health and well-being, there are typical health problems that all children encounter periodically. Many of these problems are preventable, and many are subject to nursing intervention. The extent to which they interfere with the children's abilities to function and to learn is not known, and children are relatively inarticulate in conveying the nature of their physical or emotional stress. They remain in need of advocates who can help to determine the level of their need and who can help to guide and teach them in approaches to regain and maintain health.

Included in this chapter is a discussion of a few altered health states that involve chronic or long-term underlying pathology but are manifested in intermittent acute episodes. Such conditions as seizures, asthma, and other allergic responses produce acute episodes of illness, while most of the time the child is well and fully able to function. The goal of intervention is to control the manifestation of their health problem and assist them in developing as healthy, well-rounded individuals. To the degree that this is possible, the child will avoid developing a self-image of "chronic" illness.

## NURSING DIAGNOSIS AND CARE OF THE SCHOOL-AGE CHILD WITH ACUTE HEALTH PROBLEMS

The principles of nursing diagnosis and problem identification were presented in Chapter 11, p. 372. These principles should be reviewed, as they apply to the approach used in this chapter for nursing management of acute problems in school-age children.

### Challenge of the school-age child

The school-age child is beginning to assume increasing responsibility for health maintenance and care and as maturity increases is less dependent upon adult family members to recognize signs of altered health states or to communicate health care needs. Children gain ability to speak on their own behalf and begin to provide subjective information regarding their physical and emotional health that may be unique to the individual and different from perceptions of adult family members. If children have the benefit of a comprehensive school health program, as described in Chapter 12, their ability to recognize and interpret their own health needs is enhanced, but nursing care of the individual child focuses on helping the child develop in this regard.

Through the school and other community agencies, the school-age child often has access to health care services independent of the family. Full family involvement is desired and legally required; however, the nurse's role in serving as an advocate for the child demands appropriate confidentiality and respect for the child's own individuality and privacy. During the later years of the school-age period, children are likely to encounter health problems similar to those

**497**

described for the adolescent and may desire assurance of some privacy from full family involvement. The legal considerations of providing health care for children and adolescents are presented in Chapter 14, p. 569. In most instances, school-age children will not meet legal requirements for receiving health services without parental consent, and their own needs, the situation of the family, and the local legal requirements must be carefully weighed in providing for the child's care. The nurse can plan with the child the manner in which parental involvement will be sought and maintained, with the goal of promoting family health and strengthening mutual understanding between the child and the family.

School-age children can provide a major portion of information required by interview, even in the presence of adult family members. The adult family member should be relied on to provide a history of family health problems and the history of the child's early development, but the child should provide information regarding a present alteration in health. Adult corroboration of the child's report of changes is helpful in estimating the accuracy of the child's perceptions and report. The adult's willingness and encouragement of the child's ability to provide his or her own information is indicative of the nature of family interactions and of the atmosphere in the family for promoting increasing independence for the child.

### Tools for nursing management during later childhood

The measures for comfort and symptomatic relief described in Chapter 11, p. 375, are used for many acute health problems during later childhood. Older children may need prolonged rest following the acute stage of an illness, and their ability to tolerate prolonged rest is enhanced by their increased attention span and independent ability to provide for diversion in the form of reading, maintaining interest in television programs, or involvement in quiet games and hobbies. As an example, special exercise that might be needed following an injury can be pursued by children independent of adult involvement, but they continue to need adult support and encouragement.

Fluid and electrolyte maintenance during acute illness does not present the delicate problem that existed earlier in life, because homeostatic mechanisms for compensation begin to approach adultlike maturity during later childhood. However, protecting the child from unnecessary fluid and electrolyte imbalance remains a major consideration, and the younger the child, the more supportive assistance is needed in this regard.

Drugs are used with continuing caution during later childhood, with the preferred means of calculating dosages being the estimation of body surface area (see p. 904). With increased maturity of the gastrointestinal system, liver function, and renal function, the danger of inadvertent drug intoxication is reduced. However, the child and family should be carefully guided in the conservative use of drugs and cautioned against prolonged use of over-the-counter preparations beyond the time required for symptomatic relief.

Play remains an important tool for nursing intervention during later childhood. Children continue to be able to communicate more effectively through the medium of play than in a direct manner, although direct communication is increasingly observed during later childhood years. Play is particularly useful when a subject of concern is emotionally laden for the child. For example, if a child's illness or injury is suspected to result from abuse or neglect, the child will be able to communicate much more about his or her plight through play than to reveal objective details through direct interview. Techniques of mutual story-telling, puppets, role-playing with a doll family, and drawing, as described in Chapter 16, are useful in such a situation.

During later childhood, children may be given more complete advance information in preparation for a painful procedure. Depending upon the child's temperament, warning of a painful procedure may be given well in advance of the procedure, and the interim time used to help the child consciously work through feelings of fear and anxiety and gain awareness of the ability to master the difficult situation independently. Gaining the child's understanding and voluntary cooperation is increasingly impor-

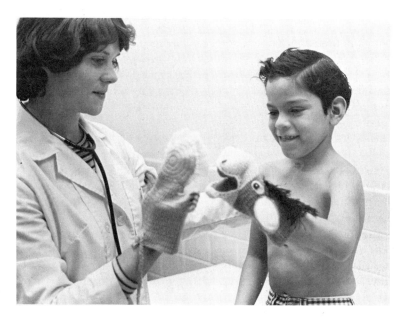

**Fig. 13-1.** During the school-age period, children are often able to communicate more effectively through puppets and other mediums of play than through direct verbal communication.

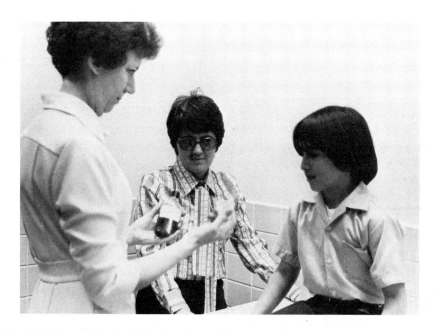

**Fig. 13-2.** The child is directly involved in teaching concerning the use of prescribed drugs.

tant as the child grows in physical strength and size, for with these increasing abilities, passive restraint becomes increasingly impossible. Further, the child gains a positive sense of mastery when he or she is able to demonstrate an independent ability to cope with the reality of fear and pain.

Teaching and counseling are directed to complete involvement and understanding of the child as an individual, while the focus of teaching and counseling with the family is aimed toward providing a supportive, augmentary role for the child's own understanding and ability. For example, rather than direct teaching of drug use to the adult family members, during later childhood the child is most directly involved in drug use teaching in order to encourage assumption of individual responsibility for therapeutic drug use. The child should understand the required dosage, the frequency of administering the drug, the means of administration, and the duration of time that the drug is to be used. The family is included in the learning experience in order to provide assistance and support for the child. The child and family both need to be aware of undesirable side effects of any drugs used, of any potential problems of drug incompatibility, and how to recognize and manage these signs and symptoms.

### Evaluation of care

As during other periods of childhood, complete evaluation of care is needed to assure attainment of an optimal health state following an acute illness and to use an episode of acute illness to teach the child and family increased ability in self-care and health maintenance. The nurse assesses and documents complete recovery from the illness and provides evidence of plans that are made to maintain optimal health based on the health care goals established by the child and the family.

### NURSING PROBLEMS RELATED TO PHYSICAL COMPETENCY
### Acute respiratory health problems

Many of the problems involving the respiratory tract that were discussed in Chapter 11 continue to occur with significant frequency during later childhood. The older child has an

increased capacity to localize infection, and the larger, more mature structures of the respiratory tract are not as prone to communication of infection from one area of the system to another. In addition the child's susceptibility to developing complications is greatly reduced as a result of greater immunologic resistance, ability to localize infection, and maturity and increase in size of the structures. During later childhood the anatomy of the ear begins to approach adultlike proportions, and the incidence of acute otitis media begins to decline. The incidence of common colds approaches that typical of adulthood. There is a decline in frequency compared to early childhood, but colds continue to occur as often as three or four times a year.

Acute febrile states occur with less frequency during later childhood and are more frequently associated with other signs of illness, particularly illness involving the respiratory, gastrointestinal, or renal systems. Fever does not threaten to rise as sharply as during early childhood.

Nursing management of fever and symptomatic relief and treatment of specific problems remains the same for the older child as that described for the infancy and early childhood periods. The prevention of all complications remains a vital aspect of comprehensive nursing care, but the dangers of febrile convulsions and fluid and electrolyte imbalances are relatively lessened in later childhood.

#### Nursing diagnosis and management of viral and streptococcal throat infections (MNPC no. 350.5)

For health care during later childhood, a local health care team may choose to identify the diagnosis and management of children with streptococcal throat infections as within the legitimate scope of nursing practice, making provisions for adequate medical collaboration in respect to the administration of antibiotic treatment. Where feasible, such an approach provides increased effectiveness of a streptococcal prevention and control program, for comprehensive care can be implemented that provides adequate follow-through, health teaching for the child and family, and identification of other children or adults who may also be infected.

Streptococcal infections continue to constitute a major health problem among school-age children in the United States.[90] Although these infections are not limited to children of this age group, the highest incidence is between 6 and 12 years of age. Likewise the incidence of rheumatic cardiac and renal sequelae is highest for this age group. The incidence of the disease is highest in areas where the weather is temperate and during the cold winter months. The mode of transmission is primarily by direct contact with an infected person, but indirect transmission can occur. The kind of disease that the child develops as a result of contact with pathogenic group A beta hemolytic streptococci (BHS) depends upon the interaction among a group of significant factors. These include the immunologic state of the child, the mode of transmission of the disease, and properties of the particular type of streptococcus encountered. Because serious sequelae can occur in response to streptococcal infection, prevention and control of the spread of this infection are major health concerns for children of later childhood years.[52,58,84]

The primary forms of streptococcal infections are tonsillitis, pharyngitis, scarlet fever, and skin eruptions such as impetigo. Streptococcal tonsillitis or pharyngitis is essentially scarlet fever without the skin rash. The child's tonsils are enlarged, reddened, and covered with patches of exudate. The pharynx is edematous and beefy red in appearance. Although a classic picture of group A BHS infection may be readily diagnosed by skilled clinical observation of the condition of the throat, pathologic infections can exist without causing the classic observable symptoms in the throat. Therefore, the only reliable means of determining the presence of group A BHS infection is by culture.[47,52,79,84,90]

The onset of streptococcal infection is sudden and may be accompanied by fever, abdominal pain and vomiting, headaches, and chills. When scarlet fever is manifested, the typical skin rash appears within 12 to 48 hours after onset of throat and constitutional symptoms (see Chapter 11, p. 413).

The single criteria that is used for nursing diagnosis of group A, beta hemolytic streptococcal infection of the throat is:

1. Positive identification of group A, beta hemolytic streptococci by direct culture of the pharynx.

   RATIONALE: Differentiation of this bacterial infection from viral organisms causing similar clinical signs and symptoms can only be obtained by accurate throat culture.

Nursing intervention is indicated in any instance when a positive culture is obtained. The following criteria should be documented in the child's record to provide evidence of the manifestations of illness exhibited by the child and to support any conclusion drawn regarding the extent of the child's illness and whether other problems coexist with the throat infection:

1. Appearance of the pharynx, including degree of induration and swelling of the tissues, amount and color of exudate, if present
2. Nature of breath sounds
3. Condition of the nasal passages, mucous membranes of the eyes, mucous membranes of the mouth
4. Appearance of the tympanic membranes
5. Location and size of enlarged lymph nodes, report of subjective tenderness of nodes
6. Current body weight, with estimate of any weight loss that has occurred since the onset of symptoms
7. Current body temperature
8. Presence and characteristics of vomiting and/or diarrhea or abdominal pain
9. Subjective report of lethargy
10. Duration of signs and symptoms

As many as 20% of all children who have positive evidence of the streptococci organism in the throat will have few or no signs or symptoms of illness.[90] Therefore, once a child has been identified as harboring the infection, cultures should be taken from all other children and adults with whom the child has been in contact to determine the possible presence of an infection, regardless of their having or not having specific symptoms of illness.

Table 13-1 summarizes the signs and symptoms that are characteristic of acute streptococcal infections and those of viral infections. Relatively few children exhibit all the symptoms

**Table 13-1.** Characteristic signs and symptoms of viral and streptococcal throat infections*

| Assessment dimension | Typical viral infection | Severe streptococcal infection |
| --- | --- | --- |
| *Nature of onset of symptoms* | Gradual | Sudden |
| *Systemic symptoms* | | |
| Lethargy | Mild to moderate | Moderate to severe |
| Abdominal pain | Rare | Common |
| Vomiting | Rare | Common |
| Headache | Rare | Common |
| Fever | Moderately elevated, below 103° F | Elevated to 105° F |
| *Respiratory tract and mouth* | | |
| Cough | Common | Rare |
| Hoarseness | Common | Rare |
| Nasal congestion | Common | Rare |
| Conjunctivitis | Common | Rare |
| Sore throat | Common | Common and severe |
| Tonsillar erythema | Minimal to moderate | Moderate to extensive |
| Tonsillar exudate | None to small | Small to extensive |
| Petechial mottling of soft palate | Rare | Common |
| *Anterior cervical nodes* | | |
| Enlarged | Minimal to moderate | Moderate to extensive |
| Tender on palpation | Minimal to moderate | Moderate to severe |

*Adapted from Lipow, H. W.: Respiratory tract infections. In Green, M., and Haggerty, R. J., editors: Ambulatory pediatrics, II, Philadelphia, 1977, W. B. Saunders Co., p. 44.

listed in this table. If they do, the infection is considered severe, and antibiotic treatment may be started before results of the throat culture are received. Once started, the antibiotic therapy should continue for the full course of ten days, even if the throat culture results are negative.[61]

Nursing diagnosis depends upon accurate, positive throat culture results. Routine throat cultures are obtained by vigorous swabbing of each tonsil and then the pharynx, with three or four rotary motions. The swab is then transferred to an appropriate medium and processed by standard laboratory methods. The results of such cultures are readily available to most health care facilities within 24 to 48 hours, and adequate antibiotic treatment may be instituted. When a child has a severe infection that is readily recognized by severe clinical symptoms, the culture may be obtained for confirmation and differential diagnostic purposes, but antibiotic treatment is begun immediately to relieve the child's severe distress. When antibiotic therapy is instituted within seven days of the onset of the infection, deleterious sequelae are prevented.

Investigations related to the choice of antibi-

otics have consistently confirmed penicillin as the superior drug in treatment of the streptococcal infection and in prevention of cardiac and renal sequelae. The recommended doses for school-age children are:

5-10 years of age: penicillin G or V, 200,00 units orally every six hours for ten days, or one dose of 600,00 units of bicillin intramuscularly

10-15 years of age: penicillin G or V, 400,000 units orally every six hours for ten days, or one dose of 1:200,000 units of bicillin intramuscularly

Children who are allergic to penicillin are given erythromycin, 250 mg, every six hours orally for ten days.[58,61,90]

Supportive treatment of symptoms is instituted to provide comfort and prevent complications. Antipyretics may be used to control fever, and dietary management is used for control of vomiting and diarrhea. The patient should be encouraged to consume fluids to provide adequate maintenance of fluids and electrolytes. If the infection is of viral origin, symptomatic treatment alone is used.

Several other important aspects in the control and prevention of group A BHS infection and its sequelae include early detection of children who have the disease, isolation from schoolmates and siblings until the diagnosis is confirmed and treatment has been instituted, and throat cultures have been taken from schoolmates or siblings who have been in close contact with the infected child since the illness began. Early treatment of asymptomatic children who have pathologic culture findings contributes significantly to control and prevention programs.[61,84]

### Respiratory allergies (MNPC no. 313)

**Allergic rhinitis.** Although detailed allergy diagnosis and management of the more severe forms of allergy require careful and skilled specialist attention (see Chapter 18), those forms that mimic the common cold can be effectively controlled with skilled nursing intervention. The allergic reaction is chronic, and symptoms may appear sporadically in response to exposure to seasonal allergens, such as pollens, or to exposure to household allergens, such as pets or household dust. The child exhibits frequent or nearly continuous symptoms like the common cold, with rhinitis and watering of the eyes predominating. Criteria for nursing diagnosis and management of the common cold and for allergic rhinitis are presented in Chapter 11, pp. 388 and 415. These criteria and the approaches to management are appropriate for school-age children as well as younger children.

Knowledge of the underlying mechanisms of allergic disorders is essential to obtain an adequate and detailed data base from which to determine the possible allergenic agents (see Chapter 11). When all possible allergens are explored in the child's environment, management begins with an attempt to remove suspicious allergens from contact with the child. If there is relief from the symptoms in response to the change in the environment, the allergen that caused the child's reactions can be definitely identified. This seemingly simple identifying procedure is the ideal treatment, because the child's symptoms are completely and immediately relieved. However, it is seldom possible to eliminate a specific allergen from the child's environment, as when pollens are the offending substance. If symptoms occur only in the spring of the year, some environmental allergen present only at this time of the year is probably responsible for the child's allergic reaction but isolating the specific agent is not possible by environmental elimination.

The second line of approach in management of mild allergic rhinitis is administering symptomatic treatment, usually in the form of antihistamines. If these drugs control the discomfort of the symptoms and symptoms return on withdrawal of the drug, the problem is probably allergic in origin. The antihistamines most commonly used for children include diphenhydramine hydrochloride (Benadryl), tripelennamine hydrochloride (Pyribenzamine), chlorpheniramine maleate (Chlor-trimeton), and brompheniramine maleate (Dimetane). Combinations of antihistamines and nasal decongestants, such as triprolidine hydrochloride and pseudoephedrine hydrochloride (Actifed), may be more effective for some children. Antihistamines often cause drowsiness, which may interfere with their usefulness for some children; one agent may be less prone than another to produce such an effect for an individual child. Decreasing the dosage of the drug may be indicated in the event of drowsiness, and a lesser dosage may be sufficiently effective in controlling the allergic symptoms. The use of nose drops and sprays is discouraged because of their limited usefulness in relieving symptoms, the rebound complication, the interference with the normal ciliary action of the mucosa, and drying and irritation of the mucosa.[7,77]

When the child's problem does not meet the criteria for nursing diagnosis and management of an allergy, the child's problem should receive thorough medical evaluation. An allergy specialist is most completely equipped to determine the origin of a specific problem and to manage any specific treatment, such as hyposensitization. Nursing management may be indicated in relation to allergic treatment, and particular nursing expertise in the management of allergic problems in childhood may be developed through specialized study and experience.

**Asthma.** Asthma is a chronic allergic condition that causes mild-to-severe acute episodic illness, with the child remaining well between attacks. Although this is basically a chronic illness, asthma is considered in this chapter because the acute episodic illness produced by

**503**

asthma accounts for a large percentage of all absences from school associated with chronic illness. The primary feature of asthma is the hyperreactivity of the lung in response to a wide variety of physical and emotional stimuli, causing large and small airway obstruction that is reversible, either spontaneously or in response to treatment. During the school-age period, asthma is twice as common in boys as in girls; after puberty the incidence is equal for boys and girls. Most children who exhibit asthma during the school-age period have a history of frequent upper respiratory infections during early childhood, which may or may not have been identified as asthmatic in nature (see Chapter 11).[28,29,76]

Early in an asthmatic attack, smooth muscle spasm is a primary factor, particularly if the onset of the attack is sudden. As the attack progresses, mucous membrane edema and increased mucous secretions are predominant in producing airway obstruction. Status asthmaticus, which is a severe, sudden attack causing marked airway obstruction from mucus plugs, can result in death from asphyxiation. The onset of asthmatic attacks and severity of the attacks varies significantly from child to child, and the etiologic factors include irritants of the environment such as sulfur dioxide, tobacco smoke, noxious odors, cold air and rapid temperature or humidity changes in the air, environmental allergens such as pollens, house dust, animal hair, and foods, and viruses. The respiratory syncytial and parainfluenza viruses have been particularly associated with provoking asthmatic attacks. Emotional factors, which were once thought to have etiologic significance, are now believed to contribute to the symptomatic course of the illness and precipitate onset and severity of symptoms but not to cause them. The asthmatic attack is a frightening and anxiety-producing experience for the child and family, creating a vicious cycle of illness onset, fear, worsening of the symptoms, and increased fear and anxiety.[17,28,70,86]

The onset of symptoms of an attack may be sudden or insidious and may last for several hours or several days. Episodes associated with identifiable allergens tend to be sudden in onset, and the attack subsides rapidly with removal of the allergen. If the attack is associated with a respiratory infection, the onset tends to be more gradual and lasts for a prolonged period of time. Initially, the child exhibits pallid cyanosis, dry mucous membranes, restlessness, apprehension, fatigue, or drowsiness. A distressing cough, with increasing prolongation of expiration and wheezing, develops. The child becomes dyspneic, with varying degrees of respiratory distress. Breath sounds diminish as the severity of the attack progresses, indicating air trapping in the lungs. Prolonged expiration, high-pitched rhonchi, and wheezes throughout the chest are observed. Diagnosis of asthma rests upon observation of these signs and symptoms, eosinophilia of sputum and blood, and restoration of normal (or near normal) pulmonary function in response to an injection of epinephrine, 1:1000, 0.3 ml, subcutaneously, or inhalation of isoproterenol, 1:200 dilution.

A severe asthma attack is an emergency, and the child should be given epinephrine as quickly as possible. The epinephrine dose may be repeated at 20-minute intervals three times to ease the severity of the attack. The child should be hospitalized following such an attack and given respiratory support, monitoring of acid-base and fluid balance and blood gases, and careful management of imbalances that have occurred[15,106,107] (see Chapter 16).

Children who have mild and moderate attacks usually do not require hospitalization, and in some instances the family may learn to institute early intervention on their own, preventing the need to rely on health care resources. Intervention is directed to five major areas:[22]

1. Institution of symptomatic intervention early in the attack
2. Administration of bronchodilators to reduce airway obstruction and promote exchange of gases
3. Administration of expectorants to promote clearing of the airway of secretions that form in the lungs
4. Maintenance of hydration to reduce problems arising from fluid and acid-base imbalance created by the respiratory distress and to promote liquefaction of mucus
5. Intervention for any coexisting bacterial infection

Early symptomatic intervention is achieved by injection of epinephrine as described above or by use of inhalation of epinephrine 1:100. Nebulized epinephrine depends upon the vapors reaching the lower portion of the lung, and the child must be able to inhale the medication as it is nebulized. Overuse of nebulized epinephrine is a hazard, and its prolonged use is not encouraged.

Ephedrine sulfate is a useful bronchodilator with a duration of action of about five hours. It is useful early in an attack to prevent a mild episode from progressing to a more serious attack. The recommended dose is ⅛ to ⅜ gr, usually combined with phenobarbital to minimize the side effects of ephedrine, such as palpitation, nervousness, and tremors. Isoproterenol hydrochloride, 5 to 10 mg, is less effective than ephedrine but does not have the undesirable side effects. It is administered sublingually for older children.

The xanthines, such as aminophylline or theophylline, are valuable bronchodilators. Rectal administration yields a more satisfactory blood level than does oral administration, although oral administration may be desirable and effective when used in combination with other bronchodilators. Suppositories of aminophylline (250 mg) are used for children over 6 years of age, with the dose repeated two to three times a day.

Reduction of the viscosity of respiratory secretions and clearing the airway are achieved by maintenance of adequate hydration and with the use of drugs. Iodides are the most frequently used drugs for this purpose. Saturated solution of potassium iodide (1 gr/drop) at a dose of 1 gr per year of age (up to 15 gr) three times a day may be used with relative safety. Side effects that may occur are gastrointestinal irritation, rhinorrhea, parotitis, and acnelike skin rash. If a child is sensitive to iodides, ammonium chloride is used in doses of 1½ to 5 gr every three to four hours.

Antihistamines are not used for children with asthma as they offer little benefit and exert a drying effect on bronchial mucus that aids the production of mucus plugs and interferes with clearing of the airway. The child and family should be warned against use of over-the-counter drugs containing antihistamines.

Steroids may be used for symptomatic management of persistent, intractible asthma. Cromolyn sodium, which appears to act on the mast cell to inhibit the release of chemical mediators (see Fig. 11-17, p. 414) has been demonstrated to be a valuable drug in controlling episodic attacks of asthma.*

Nursing management includes teaching and assisting the family in learning to use the drugs that are medically prescribed for the child, including learning the particular hazards and potential side effects of use of the drugs. In addition the nurse can provide valuable support and counseling in helping the child and family identify specific environmental and situational circumstances that precipitate asthmatic attacks and learn ways of avoiding or reducing these circumstances. In addition to the potential hazards of long-term sequelae of emphysema and atelectasis and other physical sequelae of repeated asthma attacks, the child and family are at risk for developing a psychologic invalidism. There are many factors that contribute to such a problem, but it often arises from an overcautious avoidance of ordinary experiences and activities in an attempt to avoid the fearsome attacks. Assisting the family to identify specific allergens and other precipitating factors helps them cope with these problems specifically and avoid developing unnecessary caution regarding possible precipitating factors. If physical exercise has been demonstrated to be a precipitating factor, for example, the family and the school teachers can be assisted in developing a program of physical exercise and education that will promote the child's involvement but not unduly stimulate undesirable attacks. The child, family, and school can be assisted in learning to use prophylactic bronchodilators before exercise and to have available appropriate medication to abort an impending asthmatic attack. Such an approach provides the child with as normal and healthy a life-style as possible, within the limits needed for control of asthmatic attacks.[24,39,59,94,96]

The child and family also need to gain understanding of the nature of the health problem and to be reassured that the long-term outlook

---

*References 9, 14, 22, 55, 57, 76, 102, 109.

for the child is very good. Many school-age children who suffer from asthma completely "outgrow" the problem by the end of adolescence, and with adequate early intervention for repeated attacks, the long-term consequences can be avoided.[39,59]

## Gastrointestinal problems (MNPC no. 350.4)

The incidence and type of gastrointestinal problems during the school-age period change from that of early childhood to a more adult-like problem, reflecting the maturity of the gastrointestinal tissues and of the immunologic responses. Minor acute gastrointestinal infections occur as a result of local viral epidemics, but the dangers of complication from delicate fluid and electrolyte imbalance in the presence of such infections is greatly decreased over that of early childhood. As at any older age, the child and family need to understand how to protect themselves from excessive fluid loss during such illness and how to appropriately cope with the symptoms. Symptomatic intervention is primarily dietary, restricting intake to clear liquids for at least 24 hours. Over-the-counter drugs for control of vomiting and diarrhea should not be used during later childhood; if symptoms become severe or cause intolerable discomfort, the family needs to consult the health care service for medical evaluation of the possibility of serious bacterial infection or other gastrointestinal disorder before using the drugs.[34]

### Encopresis (MNPC no. 351.3)

Encopresis is a problem that occurs primarily in young school-age boys and is characterized by involuntary passage of formed stool into the clothing. It is most commonly associated with emotional problems related to school adjustment or an unhappy home environment. It can be associated with spinal cord lesions or anorectal stenosis. The young child may experience abdominal discomfort and is usually unable to verbalize information about the problem. The abdomen is usually mildly distended and has a "doughy" feel on palpation. Large amounts of fecal material are palpated, and bowel sounds may be normal or decreased in frequency. Stool is observed on the underclothing and around the anus. The anus has poor sphincter tension, and the anal canal is noticeably shortened. The symptoms arise from the child's withholding of stool until large amounts collect in the lower colon and involuntary passage occurs. Medical treatment for neurologic or stenotic lesions of the anus is required. When the problem is caused by emotional problems, the nurse must obtain a complete family and school assessment in order to evaluate the nature of the child's distress. Inadequate toilet facilities in the school for young boys that do not provide individual private stalls for defecation may contribute to a problem of encopresis. The child's family and teachers need to be involved in helping to identify the possible difficulties that the child is experiencing and in planning a positive approach to help the child overcome the problem. Intervention is also directed to clearing impactions, overcoming the withholding patterns, and establishing regular bowel habits. Hypertonic phosphate solution enemas (3 ml/kg body weight) are used every 12 hours initially to clear the impaction. Thirty to 75 ml of light unflavored mineral oil are given to the child twice a day to stimulate evacuation of the bowel. This is given between meals so that the oil does not interfere with fat-soluble vitamin absorption from foods. The child and family are instructed to have the child maintain regular meal patterns, particularly in the morning and in the evening, and to sit on the toilet for five to ten minutes after the morning and evening meals. The child's diet is evaluated for the presence of adequate fluids and residue in the form of bran, whole grain cereals, and fresh fruits and vegetables, which the child should be encouraged to eat.

The mineral oil is continued and slowly tapered over a period of six months, during which the child should establish a regular bowel habit. If soiling reoccurs, a new impaction has probably occurred and the bowel must be cleared with enemas and the mineral oil dosage must be reestablished.[35]

## Problems of the skin and skeletal systems

Injuries involving the skin and skeletal systems during later childhood are related to the child's changing activity and behavior patterns. Children become increasingly mobile, active, and daring and are exposed to greater dangers in the course of expanding experiences. Encounters with traffic hazards change and increase as children become cyclists or pedestrians. Participation in active contact or competitive sports leads to injuries. Children's willingness and daring to try increasingly difficult physical feats in running, jumping, climbing, and diving lead to injuries. While this trend in activity patterns exposes children to increasing hazards, it is to be encouraged and supported. Protecting children should be accomplished by helping them to judge imminent dangers and to protect themselves from known hazards rather than by limiting their activity. Their interest and participation in active sports, attempts at physical mastery, and increased mobility are indicative of health and well-being both physically and emotionally; these activities are necessary and important for growth and development.

Insect bites and communicable skin problems also create health problems for the child during later childhood. Communicable problems affecting the skin include impetigo and the childhood communicable illnesses that are manifested by a skin rash (see Chapter 11). Animal bites and insect bites and stings become more frequent as the child's activities extend beyond the indoors.

### Skeletal system injury (MNPC no. 350.3)

Bone, muscle, and joint injuries occurring during later childhood require the attention of a specialist in skeletal trauma care. However, initial care of the child and assessment of the condition of all systems are critical parts of total care of the child and can influence the eventual outcome.

When a child receives an injury affecting the skeletal system, the nature of the injury may be assessed by determining the presence and extent of dislocation or distortion of the injured area, accompanying skin lesions, and evidence of bruising. Measures should be taken to prevent bleeding, promote comfort, and to protect the injured area from further insult during efforts to move or reposition the child.

If there is no evidence of distortion of the injured area, the extent of the injury may be further assessed by determining the child's ability to actively move the injured part. For example, if a child's finger is injured in catching a ball, dislocation of the joint or fracture of a bony part may be ruled out by observing the ability to move the finger. If movement is present, the extent of injury is likely to be contusion of the muscle and the soft tissues. When normal range of motion is not possible or when there is any other evidence of a possible fracture, x-ray films of the injury should be obtained to determine the nature and extent of the injury.

Dislocations of joints, muscle injuries, and ligamentous injuries may be treated immediately after the injury by application of ice packs to the injured area. The extent of the injury is quickly assessed, and a decision is made in regard to the subsequent course of management and treatment. The immediate application of ice to the injured area prevents excessive swelling of injured tissues and provides some relief of pain or discomfort. Experience in assessing the nature of skeletal injuries leads to development of the ability to manage certain types of minor injuries, such as dislocation of a finger joint. If there is no evidence of hemarthrosis (bleeding into the joint and surrounding tissue) or ligamentous tearing, the dislocation may be adequately and quickly reduced by pulling on the injured finger. Should the finger joint fail to snap into alignment, open reduction may be required.*

### Skin injuries (MNPC no. 350.3)

When a minor injury to the skin occurs, a decision regarding the extent of the injury and the treatment of choice must be made. The initial impression of the extent of the injury based on the amount of bleeding may be misleading; many injuries involve areas of generous vascularization and result in copious bleeding from a relatively minor laceration. When the bleeding is controlled, the injury can be inspected to determine its extent and to locate any foreign material that may be lodged in the area. The na-

---

*References 32, 41, 45, 75, 83, 99, 101, 103.

ture and cause of the injury must be identified and related hazards of possible infection determined. The wound is cleansed thoroughly and irrigated with water, or water and soap, to remove any foreign material and infectious organisms. Protection against tetanus infection should be considered in the event of any injury to the skin, particularly if the injury occurred in an outdoor area such as a field, yard, or street. If the child has not received active immunization within the past year, a booster dose of tetanus toxoid should be given within 24 hours of the injury.

Lacerations on the face or scalp should be repaired surgically to prevent disfiguration. Even a very small superficial wound may cause permanent scarring over bony prominences, and the more skillful the repair, the fewer the scars. Superficial cuts that occur where cosmetic results are inconsequential for the child may be repaired by closure with adhesive "butterfly" strips or skin clips. When the wound occurs over a moving joint, immobilization of the joint is required until healing is complete.

Signs of infection of the laceration site must be understood by the child and family. Pain, swelling, redness, drainage, and failure to heal indicate that infection may have begun in the wound. Prevention of infection and promotion of rapid healing are accomplished by exposing the injury to air, keeping the area dry, and protecting it from contamination, dirt, or reinjury.[46]

### Septic joint disease

Signs and symptoms of joint disease in children require prompt medical attention and intervention in order to obtain adequate treatment and maintain adequate growth and function of the skeletal system. A frequent complaint of school-age children is joint pain, and it is most often associated with "growing pains" of unknown origin, discussed in a later section of this chapter, p. 519. Various forms of arthritis and osteochondrosis can account for joint pain and may be accompanied by swelling of the joints, limp, limitation of range of motion, and signs of systemic illness. Septic joint disease, or transient synovitis, is the most common cause of joint pain requiring specific medical intervention. It affects boys more often than girls and is characterized by a sudden onset of mild or severe pain in the hip or knee, sometimes accompanied by palpable swelling and limitation of motion. The child usually has fever but may be afebrile. The child often has a recent history of trauma to the joint, recent streptococcal or viral infection, or allergy. Orthopedic intervention is required to provide a specific diagnosis, which rests on isolating an infectious organism in the joint. Hospitalization, with drainage of fluid from the joint, traction, and antibiotic therapy, is required. The illness usually lasts from a few days to three weeks or more.[11,45,68,71,88]

### Bites and stings (MNPC no. 350.3)

Puncture wounds or lacerations from animal bites are treated the same as other injuries to the skin, with additional concern about the possibility of rabies. Although the incidence of human rabies is relatively rare, the disease continues to persist to a significant degree among animals, particularly foxes, skunks, raccoons, and bats. Domestic dogs and cats are susceptible to the disease and should be protected with antirabies vaccine as a means of protecting children who may be bitten. Every effort should be made to capture the animal after the bite and to keep it under observation for signs of rabies for at least ten days.

Snakebites occur most frequently among school-age children during the summer months when camping and hiking are popular. Health care workers likely to be serving such children should be thoroughly familiar with emergency use of antivenom, since this is the only effective and desirable treatment when a poisonous snake bite occurs. Immobilization of the bite area may be helpful in preventing rapid spread of venom to the system. In addition, an incision into the fang area to the muscle fascia, followed by suction by bulb or mouth, may be helpful in removing a significant amount of toxin from the area before it disperses to the systemic circulation.

Insect bites occur with increasing frequency as children play in fields during warm months of the year. Mosquitoes, fleas, and chiggers cause bothersome itchy bites involving some degree

**Table 13-2.** Classification of stinging-insect sensitivity*

| Grade | Signs and symptoms |
| --- | --- |
| I. Slight general reaction | Generalized urticaria, itching, malaise, and anxiety |
| II. General reaction | Any of the above plus two or more of the following: generalized edema, constriction in chest, wheezing, abdominal pain, nausea and vomiting, and dizziness |
| III. Severe general reaction | Any of the above plus two or more of the following: dysphagia, hoarseness or thickened speech, confusion, and feeling of impending disaster |
| IV. Shock reaction | Any of the above plus two or more of the following: fall in blood pressure, collapse, incontinence, and unconsciousness |

*From Mueller, H. L., Schmid, W. H., and Rubinsztain, R.: Stinging-insect hypersensitivity; a 20-year study of immunologic treatment, Pediatrics **55:**531, April, 1975.

of local erythema; excessive scratching that leads to breaks in the skin and resulting infection are the major associated hazard. Bees, wasps, hornets, ants, and spiders can inflict more serious stings and may cause histiminic, hemolytic, and neurotoxic effects. Immediate treatment of complications from an insect sting includes administration of an antihistamine, epinephrine, or a bronchodilator. Children who have had a severe reaction to an insect sting should be taught to take every possible precaution against further exposure to similar insect bites, and first aid treatment should be readily available when they are likely to be exposed.[16]

Table 13-2 presents a classification of stinging-insect sensitivity. When a child develops such an allergic sensitivity to insects bites and stings, grade III and IV reactions are relatively rare but are likely to occur later in adult life when exposed to the same or a similar bite or sting. Therefore, attention must be given to providing long-term protection for the child in the form of immunologic treatment for stinging-insect hypersensitivity. Desensitization is accomplished by administration of immunizing infections with aqueous whole-body insect extracts over a period of three years or more. The

child and family should always have available in their home and car emergency aqueous epinephrine, 1:1000, and know how to administer the injection immediately after a sting or insect bite, for serious reactions usually occur within minutes of the sting once a child is known to have an allergic sensitivity.[69,73]

## Urinary tract problems (MNPC no. 350.8)
### Signs of urinary tract disorders

Continued adequacy of urinary tract function depends upon intact structure and function involved in glomerular filtration, tubular reabsorption, tubular secretion, and movement of urine through the emptying system. The child who is born with obvious malformations is readily identified in the newborn period, but a significant number of children gradually develop symptoms of inadequate renal function during later childhood. The underlying nature of the problem may be chronic or acute. The alarming frequency of chronic progressive renal disease in adults that can be associated with previously undetected urinary tract malfunction has led to increased awareness of the potentially serious nature of all identified urinary tract disorders in children. The child who begins to exhibit persistent symptoms regardless of their actual severity must be thoroughly evaluated urologically in order to detect or prevent permanent renal disease. There remains wide divergence of opinion and practice in regard to when and how a child should be subjected to a complete urologic evaluation. Research evidence is continually accumulating to clarify the many issues involved, including prediction of permanent residual effects of a disorder, precision in diagnosis, effective intervention, and significance of diagnostic findings.[23,92,93,98]

Signs of urinary tract disorders that may occur during later childhood include the following:[5,65,91,93,108]

1. *Abdominal masses.* If an abdominal mass is discovered, the child should have a complete diagnostic medical evaluation. Tumors or kidney enlargement due to vascular changes may be identified as the cause of the enlargement and require immediate and vigorous intervention.

2. *Disturbances of urination.* The child who

509

suffers from straining, dribbling, daytime or nighttime enuresis, or infrequent urination may be suffering from urinary tract disorder. These problems may have been present throughout the early childhood period, but they are occasionally considered by the child and family as typical of normal developmental urinary function, or they are not recognized as being significantly different from normal urinary patterns. As later childhood begins, the symptoms may or may not be recognized as extraordinary. A careful history in regard to past and present urinary function in children at this age is essential in determining the adequacy of the urinary system.

3. *Abdominal or back pain.* Complaints of pain in these areas are frequent among children of later childhood years and are exceedingly difficult to evaluate. Psychogenic, orthopedic, infectious, gastrointestinal, and metabolic disorders as well as abnormal renal function may be implicated. The child who repeatedly complains of abdominal discomfort should be screened for the signs of urinary tract infection as one possible source of the pain.

4. *Abnormal urinalysis findings.* When a urine sample is found to contain more than 10 to 15 white blood cells per high power field or if bacteria or protein is identified, the child should be further evaluated. In some instances, analysis and culture of a more recent, adequately collected sterile specimen will rule out infection or malformation in the system, but if this step identifies further indication of a problem, complete urologic investigation must be considered.

5. *Hypertension.* When a child is found to have persistent hypertension, one of the primary associated causes to consider is malformation or disease of the kidney. Thorough urologic evaluation is required.

6. *Unexplained fever and malaise.* Often a child will exhibit only nonspecific and vague symptoms, including low-grade fever and general malaise. These signs in the absence of other physical findings often lead to the impression of a psychogenic problem or of an acute minor viral illness. Obtaining a sterile urine specimen for analysis and possible culture and determining the child's blood pressure may be helpful in detecting urinary tract infection.

*Team intervention*

Health care related to urinary tract infections in childhood involves a coordinated team approach, which is essential for adequate treatment and prevention of potential serious sequelae. The diagnostic procedures may be long, involved, and difficult for the child and the family to understand, and continuing efforts are needed by all team members to continually reinterpret procedures and assure the family's understanding of the problems. Subsequent treatment may likewise entail a long, continuing course in spite of the disappearance of the child's overt symptoms. Support, encouragement, and continuing involvement of appropriate health care workers are essential in order to integrate the child and the family into the management plan and thus achieve their full understanding, cooperation, and participation.[56]

**Infection.** When infection is identified, thorough investigation of the urinary tract to discover the source of the child's problem begins with detailed urinalysis, intravenous pyelography, and micturition cystourethrography. These procedures usually enable the specialist to identify all normal structures of the upper and lower tract and most abnormalities, except in the presence of severe renal impairment. A trial of treatment is often undertaken to observe the response of the child and in an effort to eradicate the infection before it causes permanent damage to the system. In some cases, surgical correction of a defect is required. If the initial studies fail to reveal the source of infection or if the child continues to suffer from infection after a thorough course of chemotherapy, further investigation using cystourethroscopy, retrograde pyelography, ureteric collections for culture, angiography, or surgical exploration may be indicated.

Treatment includes correction of the structural abnormality combined with a thorough course of chemotherapy. When no structural cause for the infection is identified, chemotherapy is used alone. Infections involving the upper tract require more prolonged chemotherapy, but the principles of treatment are the same. An organism-sensitive antibiotic that tends to affect the tissues, such as ampicillin, and a high-concentration urinary agent such as nitrofurantoin or nalidixic acid are used. The antibiotic is required for about two weeks and the urinary agent should be used for four weeks at full dosage, then reduced to half-dosage for three months. Analysis and culturing of the urine monthly during the treatment period and for several months thereafter provide evidence of the response to treatment. Increased fluid intake to promote frequent emptying of the bladder and attention to personal hygiene of the vulvular area for girls are often important aspects of care.[2,25,95]

**Enuresis.** Night enuresis occurring without evidence of urinary tract infection is a most disturbing problem for the child and for the family. The problem is poorly understood, and there does not appear to be a consistent relationship with the symptom and any of several possible etiologic factors. Many associated problems, such as psychologic disturbance or behavioral disorders, urologic lesions, or allergies have not been demonstrated to have a real causative relationship, and management of the problem remains primarily symptomatic. A variety of devices and approaches has been promoted as effective in the treatment of bedwetting, and often the family tries several approaches before the problem is somehow resolved.

The technique of conditioning a child to awaken when beginning to urinate while sleeping by a bell that sounds in response to wetness of the sheet has been demonstrated to be effective in about one third to two thirds of children in experimental trials. Drugs, diet therapy, and fluid restriction before bedtime have received some trials, but the results are inconclusive. Bladder training, including gradual increase of bladder capacity in the daytime by forcing fluids and deliberate retention of urine, plus practicing bladder control by having the child stop and start the stream, has provided an effective and lasting treatment for at least one third of the children in the experimental trials reported. When an initial approach does not seem to be effective for a particular child, more detailed evaluation of the total health of the child and the environment may be indicated.[38,63,66,92]

## Neurologic and sensory organ problems
### Head injury (MNPC no. 350.3)

When a head injury occurs during later childhood, immediate assessment of the extent of the injury to the scalp, skull, and brain must be performed and a judgment made regarding the need for hospitalization or immediate medical attention or the safety of observation of the child at home. The child is able to report subjective symptoms reliably during later childhood, but the signs of intracranial injury are essentially the same as those observed for the younger child. Criteria for immediate hospitalization and medical evaluation are:[89]

1. Severe concussion or increasing intracranial pressure
   a. Unconsciousness immediately after the injury that continues for longer than five minutes
   b. Progressive loss of consciousness after the injury
   c. Ominous vital signs, including persistent bradycardia, systolic hypertension, and widening of the pulse pressure, irregular respirations, or fever
   d. Vomiting more than two or three times after the injury
   e. Subjective report of severe or worsening headache
   f. Disoriented behavior
2. Signs of focal brain damage that might be indicative of a local clot formation
   a. Focal neurologic deficit, such as hemiparesis, aphasia, facial asymmetry, unilateral Babinski sign
   b. Dilatation and nonreactivity of one pupil
   c. Focal or generalized convulsions
3. Signs of intracranial hemorrhage
   a. Hemorrhages in the fundus of the eye
   b. Meningismus without neck injury
   c. Extreme or rapidly developing pallor
   d. Hemorrhages from the nose or ears; signs of blood behind the tympanic membrane
4. Evidence of fracture of the skull
5. Scalp laceration requiring surgical repair
6. Associated spinal cord injury
7. Criteria for home observation not clearly met (see below)

If none of the above conditions are noted on the initial assessment, further assessment and observation are made to determine if the child meets criteria for observation at home. These criteria are as follows:

1. There is no loss of consciousness following the injury, or loss of consciousness persists for less than five minutes.
2. The state of alertness is stable and improves.
3. Pulse and respiration rates are normal, blood pressure is normal, and temperature is not elevated.
4. If vomiting occurs, there are no more than three episodes that occur immediately after the injury (within the first 30 minutes).
5. Neurologic assessment is normal.
6. Pupils react equally to light.
7. There is no evidence of injury to the skull or scalp.
8. There is no evidence of spinal fluid otorrhea or rhinorrhea.
9. There is no evidence of intracranial bleeding, such as blood behind the tympanic membranes or bleeding from external canals.
10. The family is able to observe the child at home constantly for the next 24 to 48 hours.
11. The family is sufficiently reliable to understand and interpret signs of complications.

The family is given detailed instructions regarding the danger signs for which to observe. These should be available in writing, along with written instructions as to who to contact and what to do if any of these signs develop. In addition the nurse may want to have the parents demonstrate their ability to elicit reactivity of the pupils and testing for equal muscle strength in the extremities in order to determine their ability to make these observations reliably and to promote their own confidence in caring for the child at home.

The danger signs for which the family needs to be alert are:[89]

1. Drowsiness and failure to respond when aroused. The family should awaken the child at regular intervals throughout the first night and should have no more difficulty awakening the child than they would ordinarily experience.
2. Vomiting. Any incidence of vomiting after the child has arrived at home is an ominous sign.
3. Weakness on one side. This can be tested by the family by having the child squeeze their hands simultaneously and having the child resist the adult's effort to bend his or her knees.
4. Unequal reactivity of the pupils to light.
5. Complaints of double vision.
6. Difficulty or change in speech.
7. Worsening headache.
8. Focal or generalized convulsions.

### Convulsive disorders (MNPC no. 315)

Convulsive disorders arise from a chronic problem of multiple etiology characterized by paroxysmal and excessive neuronal discharge that results in a wide variety of signs and symptoms. The term "epilepsy" is no longer used to label children with this disorder because of the negative social stigma associated with it and the association that is made between epilepsy, mental retardation, and stigmatized heredity. Most children with a convulsive disorder have normal intelligence and are able to lead healthy lives; furthermore their convulsive episodes can be controlled or greatly decreased with adequate drug management. While most children with convulsive disorders exhibit signs and symptoms during the preschool period, many are not detected until later childhood, because a previous seizure was not observed, was ignored, or not reported by the family. When the child enters school, even mild seizures become apparent, or the child encounters a related learning or social problem that leads to diagnostic identification of the underlying neurologic problem. Fifty percent of all children who exhibit a febrile convulsion during early childhood develop a convulsive disorder during later childhood; the fact that the early seizure was associated with a fever during early childhood obscures the identification of a chronic neurologic problem.

Evidence of genetic inheritance of a lowered convulsive threshold has been demonstrated for a few conditions, and familial abnormal electroencephalograms are occasionally detected. However, for most children with convulsive disorders, hereditary factors are not evident and are not considered to be a primary etiologic factor. Brain injury during the prenatal, perinatal, or postnatal periods is the most commonly identified etiologic factor. Often the exact nature of the injury is not defined but is presumed from a history of prenatal, perinatal, or postnatal events that often yield cerebral insult, hypoxia, edema, or hemorrhage.[42,48]

Table 13-3 presents a classification of convulsive disorders based on the origin of the abnormal neuronal discharge and the type of seizure exhibited. Information related to the drugs used to control the seizures is presented in Table 13-4.

Generalized convulsions are characterized by an episode of stiffening accompanied by extension of the head and rolling up of the eyes. After this tonic posturing, a period of clonus follows within minutes, and with continued clonus the child may develop apnea, cyanosis, salivation, and chewing movements. When the seizure ceases, the child is drowsy and may go to sleep. The EEG pattern may be normal or it may be slow for the age of the child. The EEG may be used to identify the exact location of origin of the abnormal discharge if an abnormality is demonstrated on the pattern. Children whose convulsions of this type begin after the preschool period do not often have associated mental retardation, behavioral, learning, or motor problems.

Petit mal seizures occur almost exclusively in children between the ages of 5 and 12 years. They are characterized by staring or blinking episodes that last for 5 to 30 seconds, which may be accompanied by slight movement of the mouth or hands. The child does not lose con-

**Table 13-3.** Classifications of convulsive disorders*

| Type of seizure (approximate percentage) | Anatomic region and spread | EEG pattern | Recommended drugs | Associated problems |
|---|---|---|---|---|
| Generalized grand mal Major motor—15% | Cortex Centrencephalon† Spinal cord | Bilateral; spikes or slow waves | Barbiturates Dilantin Mysoline | Social, learning problems |
| Petit mal Absence; lapse—5% | Centrencephalon Cortex | Bilateral; 3/sec spike wave | Zarontin Valium Diamox Barbiturates | Rare |
| Myoclonic Salaam; akinetic—10% | Centrencephalon Spinal cord | Polyspike and waves; hypsarrhythmia | Steroids Valium Gemonil Ketogenic diet | Mental retardation; choreoathetosis; spasticity |
| Focal motor Jacksonian march; adversive; tonic postural; focal sensory—25% | Frontal lobe Parietal lobe | Focal spikes, slow waves, or spike waves | Dilantin Mebaral Valium | Behavior, motor disorders |
| Psychomotor Temporal lobe limbic—35% | Temporal lobe Amygdala Hippocampus | Temporal spike or slow waves | Dilantin Mysoline Zarontin Celontin Barbiturates | Behavior, learning, language disorders |
| Convulsive equivalent Abdominal, visceral epilepsy—10% | Diencephalon (?) Temporal lobes | 14/6 per sec positive spikes, or temporal lobe spikes | Dilantin Mebaral Valium Librium | Behavior, learning disorders |

*From: Jabbour, J. T., Duenas, D. A., and Gilmartin, R. C., Diseases of the nervous system. In Hughes, J. G., editor, Synopsis of Pediatrics, 4th edition, St. Louis, 1975, The C. V. Mosby Company, p. 825.
†The term *centrencephalon* refers to the subcortical nuclear masses that have bilateral connections to the cortex, brain stem, and spinal cord. The thalamus, basal ganglia, and reticular activating system are thought to be the primary areas of electrical response.

**Table 13-4.** Drug dosage and toxicity of anticonvulsants*

| Drug | Indications | Dosage (mg/kg/24 hr) | Side effects | Preparations |
|---|---|---|---|---|
| Barbiturates | | | | |
| Phenobarbital | All seizures | 4-6 | Drowsy; hyperactive; rash; ataxia | 15, 30, 60, 100 mg tablets (white); elixir, 20 mg/5 ml (red) |
| Mephobarbital (Mebaral) | All seizures | 8-10 | Drowsy, ataxia, irritable | 32, 50, 100, 200 mg tablets (white) |
| Metharbital (Gemonil) | Massive spasms; myoclonus | 15 | Drowsy; ataxia | 100 mg tablets (white) |
| Primidone (Mysoline) | All seizures; psychomotor, except petit mal | 10-20 | Drowsy; ataxia; vomiting; anemia | 50, 250 mg tablets; 250 mg/4 ml suspension (white) |
| Hydantoins | | | | |
| Diphenylhydantoin (Dilantin) | All seizures, except petit mal | 5-9 | Gum hyperplasia; rash; nystagmus; ataxia; lethargy; leukopenia; thrombocytopenia | 30, 100 mg capsules; 50 mg Infatabs; 100 mg/4 ml suspension (orange); 30 mg/4 ml suspension (red); 250 mg injection (clear) |
| Other | | | | |
| Diazepam (Valium) | Myoclonic seizures; generalized status epilepticus; petit mal | Neonates, 0.5-1; infancy, 1-2; childhood, 2 | Lethargy; ataxia | 2 mg tablets (white); 5 mg tablets (yellow); 10 mg tablets (blue); 2 ml/10 ml ampules, IM, IV |
| Acetozolamide (Diamox) | Myoclonus; petit mal; generalized | 15-30 | Lethargy; rash; dehydration; acidosis; agranulocytosis; thrombocytopenia | 250 mg tablets (white) |
| ACTH | Infantile spasms; myoclonus (massive) | 5-50 units/ 24 hr | | |
| Succinimides | | | | |
| Methsuximide (Celontin) | Petit mal; psychomotor; myoclonus | 15-30 | Skin rash; nausea; vomiting; ataxia | 150, 300 mg capsules (yellow orange) |
| Phensuximide (Milontin) | Petit mal; psychomotor | 20-40 | Skin rash; nausea; vomiting; ataxia | 500 mg capsules (white pink) |
| Ethosuximide (Zarontin) | Petit mal; psychomotor | 20-50 | Vomiting; rash; ataxia; lethargy | 250 mg capsules (orange) |

*From Jabbour, J. T., Duenas, D. A., and Gilmartin, R. C.: Diseases of the nervous system. In Hughes, J. G., editor: Synopsis of pediatrics, ed. 4, St. Louis, 1975, The C. V. Mosby Co., p. 834.

sciousness but does have a sudden arrest in activity and does not remember having the seizure. The seizures may occur infrequently, or often throughout the day, and may be mistaken by the teacher for daydreaming. A typical EEG pattern of a 3 cycle/second spike-and-wave pattern appears during sleeping states and sometimes during waking states. Many children have a spontaneous remission of the problem within two years of onset, although generalized convulsions may develop during puberty that can be successfully controlled and are unlikely to persist. Associated disorders of learning or behavior are rare.

Akinetic or myoclonic convulsions are characterized by a momentary loss of trunk and limb muscle tone or sudden myoclonic jerks, causing the child to fall, stumble, or appear clumsy. The child does not experience loss of consciousness or any altered state of conciousness following the seizure. The seizures tend to occur with a frequency ranging from a few to hundreds of episodes a day. Children with myoclonic convulsions frequently have associated disorders, including cerebral lipidosis or other metabolic problems. The EEG pattern is either normal or is characterized by polyspike or multiple spike-and-wave patterns appearing on a slow background.

There are several clinical patterns of focal motor convulsions, which arise from circumscribed areas of the cerebral cortex. These seizures begin on one side of the body only but may spread during the course of the seizure and result in a generalized convulsion. The Jacksonian march is a clonic convulsion that begins on one side of the body characterized by twitching of the mouth or eyes spreading to the face, arm, trunk, or leg muscles. After the seizure there may be a transient limb weakness, known as Todd's paralysis, which may last several minutes or hours. There is no drowsiness or loss of conciousness during this postseizure phase if the seizure is confined to one side of the body. Another type of focal motor convulsion, the tonic postural convulsion, is characterized by a tonic extension of the limbs on the side of the body toward which the head is turned. Focal sensory convulsions involve paresthesias, numbness, tingling, prickling or pain sensations that begin in the face and may spread to other parts of the body. Hypertonia or peculiar posturing may also occur, and the child may report visual sensations such as flashing colored lights or formed images or objects. The location of the origin of these seizures can be determined by the location of EEG patterns of spikes and/or slow waves.

Psychomotor convulsions, or temporal lobe convulsions, consist of a wide variety of bizarre, unpredictable combinations of motor, sensory, autonomic, and psychic signs and symptoms. There may be an arrest of activity similar to that observed with the petit mal seizure. Oropharyngeal signs of lip smacking, chewing, drooling, swallowing, and nausea or abdominal pain are common, followed by a generalized stiffening of the body and a period of sleep. The primary feature of many psychomotor seizures is a period of behavioral confusion, with purposeless movement such as walking, kicking, running, incoherent speech, inappropriate laughter and smiling, followed by confusion and sleep. In some instances the seizure is primarily psychic,

with auditory, visual or olfactory hallucinations, illusions, or feelings of apprehension and fear. Visual hallucinations may involve objects or people that change in shape, size, and color; auditory hallucinations may involve familiar voices. The child does not lose conciousness during the attack, although after the seizure the child may not be able to remember the sensations and usually is drowsy or sleepy. An abnormal EEG pattern is localized most often in the temporal region but may be observed in the frontal or occipital lobe.

The convulsive equivalent, also termed abdominal-visceral-diencephalic, or autonomic, seizure, is characterized by headache, abdominal pain, nausea, vomiting, pallor, cyanosis, or rubor. Behavioral, learning, and emotional problems occur frequently with this type of disorder, and fever, generalized weakness, and chest and leg aches have been associated. Generalized, psychomotor, or focal convulsions may also occur in children who exhibit this type of seizure.[42,48]

The selection of an appropriate drug is of primary importance and may require several trials until the ideal drug for the individual child has been determined. Usually a single drug that has been demonstrated to be effective for the type of seizure diagnosed is started at a relatively low dose, and the dosage is gradually increased until full tolerance is reached, as determined by the ability of the drug to control the seizure, the appearance of side effects or toxic reactions, and the effectiveness of the drug in combination with other drugs. When a child has several different types of seizures, three or four drugs may be required to adequately control the seizure episodes.[42,48]

Teaching and counseling is the primary focus of nursing care for the child and the family. Often the success of control of seizures and establishing a normal life pattern is dependent upon the extent to which the family is able to understand the nature of the child's problem and work through feelings and ambivalence in order to establish a healthy attitude toward the child's problem. The following areas of teaching and counseling are of vital importance:

*Understanding the nature of the convulsive disorder.* The nurse assists the family in understanding their child's problem by interpreting the diagnostic results, answering questions, and helping them work through misconceptions, fears, and feelings of guilt. Many families will still feel the social stigma associated with convulsive disorders, particularly if the child's problem was first recognized in school or in other public settings. They need to work through feelings of shame and embarrassment and establish healthy ways of acknowledging the child's problem. The child particularly needs counseling in resolving feelings of shame, incompetence and guilt and in establishing satisfying social relationships with peers. If other children in school have witnessed a seizure, the nurse and teachers may plan for learning experiences and group discussions that can help all the children in the group understand the nature of the problem, and establish positive social interactions.

*Establishing a realistic outlook for the future.* Often the family fears that the seizures will recur and that the child might die as a result of a severe attack. They need to understand that death rarely occurs during a seizure and that the outlook for the child is very good, with 80% of all children with convulsive disorders achieving control or significant decrease in seizure activity. If the child has normal intelligence and few associated problems, the outlook for control is extremely good. They need to understand the nature of societal implications for the child as an adult, which vary with the type of disorder. With severe forms of the disorder, adult limitations in choice of career or jobs may exist; in less extensive forms, adult limitations will not exist.

*Learning to respond to the child when a seizure occurs.* The family needs to learn how to prevent the child from injury and support him or her during and following a seizure.

*Understanding the drugs used, the trials that may be required, and the expected side effects of drugs.* Both the family and the child need to understand the nature of the drugs used and the reasons for altering the drugs in successive trials until satisfactory control is achieved. They need to be aware of predictable side effects and of signs of drug intolerance that should be observed if they occur. Their understanding should be observed in the form of actual ability

to administer the drugs as prescribed, to maintain the drug program consistently over a prolonged period of time, and to reliably describe any undesirable side effects.

*Achieving sound emotional development for the child and the family.* The child should be encouraged to engage in full participation in school and community activities, and the interactions with peers and family members should not be altered or remain altered as a result of the convulsive disorder. Various forms of counseling and support of parenting ability may be needed, depending upon the personal and social resources of the family. The family assessment can provide the basis for helping the family identify their own goals and meaningful resources for support.

### Headaches (MNPC no. 319)

Headaches are a common symptom during later childhood but only occur in about 5% to 10% of children with systemic illness as compared to about 50% of adults. Most commonly, headache is associated with a minor and transient health problem, such as viral infection, infection of the sinuses, allergic problems, or transient emotional tension. If such a related factor exists and the headache does not persist, it can be presumed to have been associated with these factors. Headaches associated with allergic problems will dissipate when the other symptoms of the allergy are controlled by removal of the antigen or the use of antihistamines.

Rarely, a headache signals a serious condition that needs complete medical evaluation and treatment. Table 13-5 summarizes the major types of headaches that occur during later childhood and contrasts the associated symptoms and character of these types of headache. If a headache is associated with a serious illness, it will not dissipate, and other signs and symptoms of the problem will be present or emerge within a brief period of time.[40,43,48,67]

### Eye injuries and infections

The most common type of eye injury that occurs during later childhood is a foreign body in the eye. Most often, the foreign body rests under the margin of the upper lid, and can be removed readily by pulling the upper lid forward

**Table 13-5.** Headache in childhood*

| Disorder or disease | Location and character | Other symptoms | Diagnostic studies | Treatment |
|---|---|---|---|---|
| Convulsive equivalent | Frontotemporal region; dull ache | Abdominal discomfort, nausea, pallor | EEG, positive spikes or temporal lobe spikes | Dilantin |
| Tension headache | "Band" about head; constant, dull ache | Insomnia, anxiety | EEG, CSF studies | Librium, Mellaril, psychotherapy |
| Migraine headache | Unilateral frontotemporal region; throbbing | Nausea, vomiting, sees bright colors, followed by sleep | Family history | Cafergot, Gynergan, barbiturates |
| Meningitis, encephalitis | Generalized headache; dull ache | Nausea, vomiting, fever, nuchal rigidity, convulsions | CSF studies, EEG | Acetylsalicylic acid (aspirin), Darvon |
| Sinusitis allergy, systemic infections | Frontal region about the eyes; dull ache | Fever, fatigue | Sinus radiographs, CBC | Antihistamine, decongestant, ASA |
| Brain tumor | Frontal or occipital regions; dull ache | Personality and behavior changes, ataxia, convulsions | Air studies, cerebral angiogram | Surgery and/or radiation |
| Eye problems (astigmatism, refractive errors, squint) | Frontal or occipital regions; dull ache | Astigmatism, squint, refractive errors | Ophthalmologic evaluation | Glasses, eye exercises, surgery |

*From Jabbour, J. T., Duenas, D. A., and Gilmartin, R. C.: Diseases of the nervous system. In Hughes, J. G., editor: Synopsis of pediatrics, ed. 4, St. Louis, 1975, The C. V. Mosby Co., p. 841.

and downward while the child blinks. This maneuver causes an increase in tearing and removal of the foreign body without the danger of injury to the eye with manual removal of the foreign body. If this maneuver is not successful, further inspection of the eye, including the appearance of the cornea and the upper and lower conjunctiva is required to determine the presence of a foreign body or signs of other problems such as trauma to the cornea or infection of the conjunctiva. If a foreign body cannot be located, the child should receive immediate medical attention to determine the source of the discomfort and appropriate intervention.

Ecchymosis of the eyelids occurs during later childhood as a result of a blow to the eye, usually in physical contact sports or physical attack. If there is no evidence of blood in the anterior chamber, lacerations, or skeletal injury, the injury may be treated with cold compresses to reduce further hemorrhage and edema. If the injury is extensive or any of the above signs are present, the child should receive immediate medical attention.

Blepharitis, or granulation of the eyelids, is caused by either seborrhea or by a staphylococcal infection. The eyelid margins are itchy and burning, and there is redness and crusting of the lids. The crust is oily in the seborrheic type, and seborrhea of the scalp may also be present. With a staphylococcal infection, the scales are dry and small ulcerative lesions of the skin are present. Conjunctivitis is a more common form of infection and can be caused by bacterial, viral, or fungal infections. Symptoms may include redness, purulent discharge, pain, and necrosis. These infections require specific identification of the invading organism, appropriate antibiotic treatment, and/or symptomatic treatment for discomfort.[30]

## Cardiovascular and hematologic problems

### Epistaxis

School-age children are prone to nosebleeds that occur spontaneously, as a result of trauma, or in association with an upper respiratory infection. If a child suffers frequent repeated nosebleeds, medical evaluation is indicated to determine the possibility of a coagulation disorder or abnormality of the nasal mucosa. Nosebleeds are usually controlled by direct pressure applied for ten minutes from the lateral side of the nose against the nasal septum. The child should remain in a quiet, reclining position while pressure is applied and for a period of time after the

517

bleeding has ceased. The child should be cautioned against picking at the scab that forms in the nose and instructed to not attempt to clear the nose with forceful blowing. After the nasal mucosa has stabilized and the blood clot has formed with sufficient healing of the traumatized tissue, the airway will be restored with gentle blowing to clear loose scab particles.[6,53]

### Hypertension

Hypertension in children is now recognized as a real health problem that can have long-lasting effects on the health of the child in future years. Evidence regarding the pathophysiology and the predictive significance of hypertension during later childhood is insufficient to draw definite conclusions, but the literature reflects the general opinion that children who exhibit borderline high or high blood pressure during childhood are at increased risk for later cardiovascular disease in adulthood. Intervention during childhood is generally accepted to be indicated in an attempt to lower the risk for these children.

Hypertension that is symptomatic of an underlying health problem is usually accompanied by other signs and symptoms of illness, although hypertension may be the first symptom that is recognized. Primary hypertension, or increased blood pressure for which there is no apparent cause, may be related to excessive weight, increased salt intake, or hereditary factors reflected in a family history of high blood pressure or premature cardiovascular disease. The most common underlying problem that occurs with hypertension is a variety of renal disorders, including pyelonephritis, glomerulonephritis, renal tumor, and abnormalities of the renal system. The most common cardiovascular disorder associated with hypertension is coarctation of the aorta. Other factors that may be associated include lead poisoning, mercury poisoning, increased intracranial pressure, excessive ingestion of licorice, and acute bacterial endocarditis.

Table 13-6 presents the upper limits of normal, which can be used as a guideline in identification of a child with hypertension. If a child approaches the upper limit of normal, blood pressure should be assessed repeatedly, using appropriate blood pressure equipment and

**Table 13-6.** Criteria of upper limits of normal for blood pressure measurement in children*

| Sex | Age in years | Upper limit of normal (mm Hg) | |
| --- | --- | --- | --- |
| | | Systolic | Diastolic |
| Girls and boys | 0-3 | 110 | 65 |
| Girls and boys | 3-7 | 120 | 70 |
| Girls and boys | 7-10 | 130 | 75 |
| Boy | 10-15 | 140 | 80 |
| Girls | 10-13 | 140 | 80 |
| Girls | 13-15 | 140 | 85 |

*Adapted from Lieberman, E.: Essential hypertension in children and youth; a pediatric perspective, J. Pediatr. **85:**1, July, 1974.

technique (see p. 338), to determine if the child exceeds the limits of normal. If the child's blood pressure is excessive, in-depth assessment should be pursued to identify any other signs or symptoms of illness. Of particular importance is the study of the renal system. If the child is known to be taking any compound that might contribute to a hypertensive state, these should be altered or discontinued. Such compounds include licorice, sympathomimetics, and corticosteroids. If the child is overweight, a weight reduction or control program should be instituted (see Chapter 14). The child's diet needs to be assessed for excessive intake of salt and measures taken to restrict salt intake. Salt intake in most American diets exceeds the minimum daily requirement for salt, but the child's salt intake should be at least no more than the minimum daily requirement. Salt intake of 2 g of sodium chloride per day, which is essentially a no-salt-added diet, is recommended.[44,60,62,74,85]

### Rheumatic fever

Rheumatic fever remains an important acute problem for children between 5 and 15 years of age, even though the incidence and severity of the disease has been greatly reduced with the use of antibiotics and conscientious detection and treatment of group A, beta hemolytic streptococcal infections. Total eradication of rheumatic fever is possible with intensive detection and control of this strain of streptococci, but in reality large segments of the population do not have access to an intensive control program, and the incidence of rheumatic fever remains just below 1 per 1000 among school-age children in the United States.[74] While there appears to be a hereditary disposition to develop rheumatic fever, the sole environmental trigger for the disease is the group A beta-hemolytic streptococcal infection. Evidence supports the theory that rheumatic fever develops from an autoimmune response of the host to the antigens. The child's system produces antibodies against the antigens of the strep infection, and these same antibodies are somehow capable of attacking similar antigens in the child's system, specifically in the heart in the instance of rheumatic fever.

Medical diagnosis of rheumatic fever is traditionally based on Jones Criteria (revised). These criteria and a description of the related signs and symptoms are presented here to emphasize the importance of recognition of these signs and symptoms in the nursing assessment as worthy of further medical evaluation. Supporting evidence of a preceding streptococcal infection in the form of an increased ASO titer or previous positive throat culture is required, plus two major or one major and two minor criteria are required for a presumptive diagnosis of rheumatic fever. The major and minor criteria are as follows:

1. Major manifestations
   a. Active carditis, as demonstrated by either a significant new heart murmur associated with mitral insufficiency or aortic insufficiency, a pericardial friction rub or evidence of pericardial effusion, or evidence of congestive heart failure
   b. Polyarthritis involving two or more joints simultaneously or in a migratory fashion, associated with signs of inflammation such as heat, redness, swelling, pain, and tenderness
   c. Subcutaneous nodules that are movable under the skin, and observed most commonly over the joints, scalp, and spinal column
   d. Erythema marginatum, consisting of a macular erythematous rash with a circinate border that appears primarily on the trunk and extremities
   e. Sydenham's chorea, characterized by involuntary movements, muscle weakness, and emotional instability

2. Minor manifestations
   a. Fever, usually low grade, sometimes reaching 103° to 104° F
   b. Polyarthralgia consisting of pain in two or more joints without signs of inflammation associated with the major criteria of polyarthritis
   c. Electrocardiogram evidence of prolongation of the P-R interval
   d. Acute phase reactants, including an accelerated sedimentation rate and C-reactive protein; leukocytosis usually present
   e. History of acute rheumatic fever; presence of inactive rheumatic heart disease

3. Essential manifestation—evidence of prior group A, beta-hemolytic streptococcal infection

Treatment of the child during the acute stage of illness requires adequate anti-infection therapy, antiinflammatory therapy with aspirin and/or corticosteroids, therapy for congestive heart failure, and management of appropriate bedrest and exercise. After the acute episode the primary concern of therapy is prevention of a subsequent streptococcal infection, for the child who has once exhibited rheumatic fever will be at a greatly increased risk for developing rheumatic fever again after a streptococcal infection. The preferred prophylactic approach is 250,000 units of oral Penicillin G taken twice daily. Monthly injections of benzathine penicillin G, 1.2 million units, may be used instead of the oral route of administration.[3,51,74]

## Nonspecific problems of physical competency
### Somatic complaints (MNPC no. 324)

A common problem encountered in working with school-age children is recurrent complaints of abdominal pain, headaches, or joint pain ("growing pains"). When no organic base can be identified, these pains are presumed to be psychogenic; however evidence of serious psychologic disturbance is often lacking. Adjustment problems or anxiety may be identified. Abdominal pain and headaches are more frequently associated with a clear emotional upset than are limb pains, which are reported by most school-age children at some time during this period of development. Limb pains are not associated with peak periods of growth, even though the term "growing pains" implies such an association. Children who report recurrent somatic pain may be responding to pain sensations in a manner that is characteristic of the family, or there may be a familial lowered pain threshold. Widespread controversy exists regarding the appropriate intervention that is indicated for a child with recurrent somatic pain, and each individual child's circumstances and the personality of the health care worker must be taken into account. Counseling is indicated if a specific emotional crisis or stress is known to exist. Assistance may be obtained in helping the child with an adjustment problem in school or at home from teachers and parents. The nurse may work with the teachers and the parents to help the child engage in diversionary activities and relaxation exercises. Caution should be taken against overattending the child's symptom of pain in favor of providing positive reinforcement for positive actions and behaviors of the child. Drug intervention is not indicated for this type of pain, as the pain does not interfere with the child's ability to function and positive nonpharmocologic means of coping can be an important learning experience for the child.[8,27,78,80]

### Tension-fatigue syndrome

This allergic disorder is poorly understood and infrequently recognized as an allergic problem, but the symptoms are frequently encountered among school-age children. Determination of the allergic nature of the problem requires careful and skillful management. When symptoms simulating this complex syndrome are recognized, other types of illness such as infection, metabolic disorders, anemia, and neurologic disturbance must be considered. However, by using a skilled approach to seek and eliminate an allergen or by treating the child with trial antihistamines, early identification of the source of the problem may be achieved.

Opinion varies regarding the exact physiologic mechanism involved in the creation of the syndrome, but evidence seems to suggest that there is a direct allergic reaction of the central nervous system in response to food allergens or, occasionally, respiratory allergens. Seven common signs and symptoms of the syndrome have been identified, and most children exhibit at least three or four of these.[105] They are:
1. Respiratory tract allergy, such as seasonal allergic rhinitis or asthma
2. Abdominal discomfort
3. Headache
4. Nervous tension, irritability
5. Facial pallor and dark circles under eyes
6. Tiredness, easy fatigability
7. Musculoskeletal discomfort

Foods suspected as being allergens, such as milk, wheat, corn, or chocolate, are removed from the diet for a trial of 5 to 14 days. If symptoms disappear, as they will if the causative allergen has been removed, definitive diagnosis is achieved by challenging with each food substance separately for a period of several days at a time. When symptoms recur, the diagnosis of definitive tension-fatigue syndrome may be made. It is imperative that complete withdrawal of the food be accomplished, and the "hidden" forms of a product such as milk must be understood by the mother and child to accomplish this. When milk is withdrawn, a source of calcium must be provided either in the form of a soybean product or a commercial calcium substitute such as Neo-Calglucon syrup. Many nondairy milk substitutes contain proteins closely related to whole milk, and may not provide suitable nutritive values. Thus these agents should not be used during an allergy trial. For reasons not completely understood, the allergy tends to be somewhat alleviated during summer months, and children often reach a point where they can tolerate small amounts of the offending food in the diet. As the child and family begin to understand the nature of the problem, they often become adept in controlling the symptoms through food trials and challenges.[76,105]

## HEALTH PROBLEMS RELATED TO LEARNING AND THOUGHT, SOCIAL, AND INNER COMPETENCIES

Of the many variations of problems that may be identified as health problems related to learning and behavior, three will be discussed here. The interrelationships among these three problems will be evident. Since most of the problems that relate to learning and behavior in the child are incompletely understood, intervention and management are currently based on subjective preference or impressions gained through observational experience. There is little or no conclusive scientific evidence available to guide and direct sound clinical practice. Some of the predominant issues involved with these and similar problems are discussed here, but the reader is referred to literature specific to a given problem for more detailed study of advances being accomplished in each field of concern.

## Care of the child on behavior-modifying drugs

Recently, from 4% to 10% of all children in later childhood have been identified as having specific learning disabilities. These children are receiving increasing attention from educators who are seeking to provide better ways to help them achieve in the learning situation. These children have near-average, average, or above-average intelligence, and yet they are not able to achieve academic success because of some deficit in behavioral, perceptual, language, reading, or motor function (see Chapter 19). Many of these children exhibit a characteristic hyperactivity, or hyperkinesis. As an adjunct to the primary intervention implemented by the educator in the school setting, the child may be placed on drug therapy in an attempt to alter the behavior patterns and to promote the establishment of mental functions that appear to enhance learning ability. When such a situation evolves, the health care team and those involved in the educational program become an essential unit in working to promote both the education and health care goals.

Since the problem is primarily one that involves learning, the specialized educator is the most appropriate person to assume direct leadership in planning and coordinating the total plan of intervention for the child, but health care workers become integrally involved as the evaluation of organic injury or defects is attempted, when the child encounters a health crisis, or as drugs are used in intervention.[20]

Not all children benefit from the use of drugs, and decisions regarding initiating or continuing usage require careful consideration of the total life space of the child.

The drugs of choice in behavior control during later childhood are the stimulant drugs, such as dextroamphetamine (Dexedrine) and methyl phenidate (Ritalin). The action of these drugs for children in this particular age group is opposite that experienced by older individuals; they become relatively subdued and calmed. Their attention span is lengthened, and distractibility is lessened. This paradoxical effect of stimulant drugs in this age group is not understood, but several theories have been advanced to explain the action. One such theory proposes that the behavior exhibited by the child with the hyperkinesis syndrome results from the fact that there is a low level of central nervous system arousal or activation possible because of disordered functioning of the reticular activation system. This means that the normal cortex of the child does not receive adequate stimulation from arousal mechanisms that allow it to use its full inhibitory and regulating capacities. The cerebral-stimulating drugs mediate the function of the arousal systems, allowing full regulation by the cortex to occur. This hypothesis does not offer an explanation for the facts that this drug effect is observed only in children and that some children respond favorably while others do not. Nevertheless, the low incidence of side effects and the relative success with many children has led to widespread use of such drugs in behavior control for over 30 years in the United States. Only in recent years have the effects of the drugs begun to be studied in well-controlled clinical trials.[29-31]

One of the most frequently voiced concerns related to the use of these drugs is the fear that they will be abused by these children during adolescence or adulthood or that the drug will be abused by another family member. This concern is justified primarily in relationship to the availability of the drug for other family members; children who are on the drug for behavior control do not tend to become abusers later in life. This may be due to the fact that these children do not experience the pleasurable effects that lead to abuse.[9,26,31,54,82]

To reach a decision regarding the desirability of using and continuing drug therapy for a particular child, several complex factors must be considered. The cooperation of the child, the family, and the school is required in providing accurate and reliable information. First, the child's family life and state of equilibrium within the family must be known. Drug therapy is not suitable for children who experience disorganization and excessive distress in the home. It is often difficult to distinguish the etiology of the behavior problem as an organic functional disorder or as one having emotional basis. Children who benefit from drug therapy experience behavior disorders or hyperactivity clearly related to learning, concentration, or other tasks requiring attention focus, mental activity, and control; this occurs both in the home and in the school setting. Most children who have this syndrome appear to achieve some relief from their distress during the summer months when they can actively work off their energy and activity drives. Such relationships do not usually occur when the child's behavior is in response to an unhappy home life.

Second, the child must be known to be adequately nourished. Malnourishment or disturbances that interfere with the child's ability to sustain an adequate level of glucose in his or her system may result in behavior patterns similar to those of the hyperkinetic child. Correcting the nutritional deficiency, even through the relatively simple approach of supplying an adequate breakfast before school, may distinguish the hungry child from one who has a real disability.

Third, the classroom environment must be known. If the child is in a class setting that is overcrowded, poorly equipped, or if the teacher is overwhelmed by the conditions of the class, the child's behavior may be a response to these factors. Drug therapy is obviously not indicated in such a situation.[26]

When a child begins drug therapy, several important factors need to be considered in order to achieve success and to accurately evaluate the child and the response to the drug. The entire family, including the child and the teachers involved in the school situation, need to be thoroughly familiar with the drug to be used, its name, hazards, side effects, potential for abuse, and particular effects on children of this age group. Teachers and parents are often concerned about the abuse potential of the drug, and they need to understand the relative safety in this regard for the child who is being treated. Failure to inform them fully of the exact nature of the drug creates a dangerous situation with enhanced potential for inadvertent abuse or misuse.

The family and school workers need to understand the procedure to be used in establishing the ideal dosage level for this child over the first few weeks of administration, and they must be aware of their individual roles in helping to achieve success with drug therapy. Knowing the difference between serious side effects and certain transient initial effects helps families, children, and teachers to tolerate the initial adjustment period and to anticipate the positive changes that are expected to occur with the use of the drug.

Dosage of the drugs varies considerably, as does the approach used in establishing the desirable dosage for individual children. Methylphenidate doses range from 5 to 60 mg per day in one or two doses; dextroamphetamine doses range from 5 to 40 mg per day in one or two doses. Each child's response to these drugs is entirely individual; one child may do well on one drug and not on the other, while another child will experience exactly the opposite response. Side effects include anorexia, insomnia, increase in activity rather than decrease, irritability, headaches, depression, excessive crying, and gastrointestinal discomfort. Heart rate and blood pressure may increase slightly, but this is not known to be associated with a harmful effect. In rare instances urticaria, facial tics, hallucinations, and dyskinesias develop. Tolerance to the drug may develop, and thus the withdrawal of the drug over summers and holidays is recommended.*

## Repeated absence from school (MNPC no. 332.0)

Because most schools rank health problems as the major acceptable reason for missing school,

---

*References 14, 26, 36, 81, 100, 104.

absentee rates are often used to determine the supposed health status of children in a given school situation. Closer examination of the reasons for repeated absence from school suggests that factors other than health problems are more important. Although illness may be the actual reason for daily absence, observation of general absence patterns among all school-age children reveals that these patterns differ according to socioeconomic level, ethnic group, sex, attitudes toward health care, and distance of the home from the school.[13,50,72]

The exact effect of each factor thought to influence school attendance is not known. The child's socioeconomic level appears to be the most predominant factor relating to repeated school absence. A child may be kept at home for illness alone or sent to school when exhibiting signs of illness known to the parents. Some families are not aware, it seems, that certain symptoms of illness are deserving of having the child remain at home.[18,50,72]

It appears that factors leading to absence from school constitute a complex group of interacting variables that are not completely understood. These factors deserve study and exploration in order to determine what type of health care would be most effective for different groups of school-age children. Comprehensive health care for school-age children is assumed to lower absenteeism by providing a means to prevent health problems and by providing for immediate attention and early treatment of existing problems. However, it is clear that this is not the only factor involved in preventing absence; providing comprehensive health care may not always result in significant lowering of absenteeism.[10,18,50,72]

## Nonspecific psychogenic problems (MNPC no. 323)

During the later childhood years complaints of nonspecific symptoms such as those comprising the tension-fatigue syndrome are frequent. Because of the multiplicity of possible causes of such symptoms, a premature assumption is often made regarding the possible etiology. Such problems are often treated nonspecifically based on insufficient criteria, or they are dismissed as being emotionally based somatic complaints, as discussed earlier in this chapter. The child who exhibits physical symptoms that are emotionally based is providing an important signal of distress, and such problems should not be overlooked. Relief of the underlying distress may be difficult or impossible, but some way may be found to help the child cope with the problem. Because of the relative frequency of somatic complaints that are mild enough to ignore but interfere occasionally with the child's attendance at school, with performance in school, or with social relationships, it is important to understand guidelines that may be useful in making an accurate assessment of a possible serious emotional base for the distress. Further, when an emotional problem is present, it is essential that a sound judgment be made regarding the need for psychiatric evaluation and management. Transient emotional problems or developmental disturbances that occur periodically and are normal for a particular child should not be mistaken for a serious emotional disorder. Serious problems, on the other hand, should not be dismissed as a developmental trait, thereby delaying needed psychiatric intervention.

One of the first tasks in evaluating the possible psychogenic origin of a health problem is determining the nature of the child's environment, both from the child's perspective and from an objective point of view. Common sources of emotional stress among school-age children include psychologic illness in a close family member, family disorganization, parental preoccupation with illness, absence of a parent, school problems, unsatisfying parent-child relationships, and difficulty in handling aggressive, hostile, or sexual feelings. Symptoms that are commonly encountered include abdominal pain, cough, headaches, joint aches, skin abrasions and rashes, and self-inflicted injuries. Usually a symptom exists alone, and a pathophysiologic basis for the disorder cannot be identified. The functional symptom, such as cough, is observable and real, but underlying signs of infection or other illness cannot be identified.

Several basic psychologic phenomena may be operating in the production of a psychogenic illness, such as conversion reaction, malingering, hypochondriasis, self-destructive behavior, psychosomatic illness, and hysterical personality disorder. In many cases these problems are serious and chronic; in others they may represent an extreme reaction to emotional stress that may be transient. A few of these problems are considered briefly in order to illustrate the features that distinguish a transient problem from a more serious one requiring psychiatric intervention. More detailed discussion is found in Chapter 20.

A *conversion reaction* occurs when the child cannot repress an inner conflict that is too painful to acknowledge and feel, and it is displaced to a neutral part of the body where somatic symptoms are manifested. The symptoms are usually sudden, bizarre, and dramatic in onset. They follow no anatomic, neurologic, or structural pattern, but they always disappear during sleep. The child exhibits little concern over the problem, and usually a parent, teacher, or friend brings the problem to someone's attention. Definitive diagnosis requires psychiatric evaluation, and treatment may lead to alleviation of the somatic symptoms.

*Malingering* is a conscious pretense of illness or disability and can often be related to instances when the child has a secondary objective, such as remaining at home on a particular school day. The child is adamant in complaining about the symptoms, and yet the complaints may vary upon repeated questioning. The child who has a mild response to transient stress is easily distracted from the malingering complaint and the duration of the problem is relatively brief. Adjustments in the environment that might be contributing to undue stress often relieve the malingering pattern. Severe forms of the problem do occur, however, and require psychiatric evaluation.

*Hypochondriasis* is closely related to malingering, but is typified by a preoccupation and worry about possible signs and symptoms of illness that may or may not exist. Rather than complain that a particular symptom is present in order to achieve a secondary gain, the child expresses repeated worry and fear that something really might be wrong. Like malingering, hypochondriasis can occur in response to temporary stress, and counseling with the objective of

helping the child to identify both the source of stress and the steps that will alleviate it may bring relief.

*Self-destructive behavior* is a serious problem requiring definitive psychiatric evaluation and care. Likewise, *psychosomatic illness* requires psychiatric care and may be differentiated from other forms of psychogenic symptoms by the fact that underlying organic illness may be identified. Increased emotional stress can lead to the development of a psychosomatic illness, but removal of the stress seldom alleviates the organic illness. Since these forms of emotionally related problems present a serious threat to the health of the child, early recognition and treatment are essential.[19,33,37,64,87]

## THE SCHOOL AND THE HEALTH CARE TEAM

As has been illustrated in previous discussions, the health care team and those working with the child in school must achieve a close alliance. Regardless of the system from which the nurse works, the child's school setting and significant people within the school must be considered in the management of health problems during this period of life. Thus an expanded team is formed, with important contributions from each member being essential to the success of health care. The teacher has a particular advantage in being able to observe the child's behavior for long, continuous periods of time. Many teachers are also equipped with professional skills of observation and may be able to participate in health care intervention that requires some understanding and skill.

### The role of the teacher in health care

The role of the teacher in relation to health is often poorly defined or not considered at all. Certain aspects of health education may be incorporated into the curriculum, and there may be a teacher policy regarding illness or treatment of injuries. With minimal effort the teacher can be a most valuable agent in the detection of health problems, in observing behavior indicating response to treatment, and in contributing to a definitive identification of a nonspecific health problem.

A teacher may make an observation but not

associate it with a possible health problem. For example, a child may be noticed who is underweight, but health intervention for the problem is not considered appropriate unless health care workers are available and have interpreted their role in relation to health care. Interpreting to teachers the kinds of problems that are significant as signs of possible health problems can facilitate early identification of those children who are in need of health care. Once a referral has been made, the teacher may be involved in the plan of care, at least to the extent that he or she is aware of what has been planned and implemented and knows how this process is expected to affect the child in school. The teacher can often contribute observations of changes (either expected or not expected), which lend relevant and valuable information in ongoing health care for the child.

## Health care related to educational goals

Just as teachers and other working in the educational system are a valuable addition to the health care team during the school-age period, so does the health care worker provide valuable assistance and contribution to the educational system. This reciprocity was illustrated in the discussion of the management of the child on behavior-modifying drugs. Collaborative efforts directed toward the facilitation of the child's achievement in learning are essential for success. Each health problem that is encountered during later childhood may be conceptualized as involving just such an interaction and intimate association. Increased success in health care and education depends upon the ability of both systems to join forces toward the realization of mutual goals.[10,12,18,49]

## STUDY QUESTIONS

1. Investigate the provisions for culturing for group A beta hemolytic streptococcal infections in your community. What is the cost to the family and how long does it take to obtain the results of the culture? Is there an organized program directed toward the prevention of rheumatic heart disease in your community? Describe such a program either in your own community or in another community that is described in the literature.
2. What seasonal allergies commonly afflict individuals in your area? Identify the pollens, grasses, and weeds that tend to cause allergic reactions, presenting either a specimen or a drawing of the plant.
3. Demonstrate and discuss nursing management of a specific skin or skeletal injury. If possible, obtain samples of equipment, drugs, or supplies needed in order to adequately care for the injury you choose, and delineate the cost of obtaining and maintaining such supplies in an appropriate health care facility.
4. Review carefully the history of an older child or adult who has a chronic urinary tract disorder. Determine the evolution of the problem for this particular individual, including the age at which signs of the problem first appeared. Describe the onset of symptoms and, if possible, the diagnosis and treatment that was instituted initially and at each subsequent phase of the problem.
5. Visit a family or school where you can observe a child who is on behavior-modifying drugs. Determine the drug used and the manner in which the dosage for this child was ascertained. If possible, determine the child's own perception of the problem and the nature of the drug he or she is taking. Describe the behavior you observe, contrasting it with that of other children.
6. Review the absence records of a school or a class for a selected period of time. Seek to ascertain the reason for absence and what follow-through, if any, would be indicated by the health care team or by the school. If such follow-through is available in the situation, describe this service, its purpose, and the outcome for the child.
7. Select one of the health problems discussed in this chapter for further, in-depth study. Explore recent research dealing with issues involved in diagnosis and treatment, and compare the various points of view which you discover. Identify and formulate criteria for nursing care related to the comprehensive health care plan.

## REFERENCES

1. Adams, J.: Clinical neuropsychology and the study of learning disorders, Pediatr. Clin. North Am. **20:**587, Aug., 1973.
2. Amar, A. D., and Chabra, K.: The practical management of urinary tract infections in children, Clin. Pediatr. **13:**533, June, 1974.
3. Ammann, A. J., and Wara, D. W.: Collagen vascular diseases (rheumatic diseases). In Rudolf, A. M., editor, Pediatrics, ed. 16, New York, 1977, Appleton-Century-Crofts, p. 373.
4. Arnold, L. E.: The art of medicating hyperkinetic children; a number of practical suggestions, Clin. Pediatr. **12:**35, Jan., 1973.
5. Askin, J.: The excretory system; developmental disorders. In Cooke, R. E., editor: The biologic basis of pediatric practice, New York, 1968, McGraw-Hill Book Co., p. 1012.
6. Baehner, R. L.: Bleeding. In Green, M., and Haggerty, R. J., editors: Ambulatory pediatrics, II, Philadelphia, 1977, W. B. Saunders Co., p. 192.
7. Bailit, I. W., and Mueller, H. L.: Allergic disorders. In Shirkey, H. C., editor: Pediatric therapy, ed. 5,

St. Louis, 1975, The C. V. Mosby Co., p. 889.

8. Bain, H. W.: Chronic vague abdominal pain in children, Pediatr. Clin. North Am. 21:991, Nov., 1974.

9. Baldessarini, R. J.: Symposium; behavior modification by drugs. I. Pharmacology of the amphetamines, Pediatrics 49:694, May, 1972.

10. Basco, D., and others: Epidemiologic analysis in school populations as a basis for change in school-nursing practice—report of the second phase of a longitudinal study, Am. J. Public Health 62:491, April, 1972.

11. Baum, J., and Pless, I. B.: Juvenile rheumatoid arthritis. In Green, M., and Haggerty, R. J., editors: Ambulatory pediatrics, II, Philadelphia, 1977, W. B. Saunders Co., p. 139.

12. Beal, P. B.: The school nurse role—a changing concept—use of system analysis in program planning, J. School Health 40:189, 1970.

13. Berger, H. G.: Somatic pain and school avoidance, Clin. Pediatr. 13:819, Oct., 1974.

14. Bergner, R. K., and Bergner, A.: Rational asthma therapy for the outpatient, J.A.M.A. 235:266, Jan. 19, 1976.

15. Bierman, C. W., and Pierson, W. E.: The pharmacologic management of status asthmaticus in children, Pediatrics 54:245, Aug., 1974.

16. Carithers, H. A.: Bites and stings. In Green, M., and Haggerty, R. J., editors: Ambulatory pediatrics, II, Philadelphia, 1977, W. B. Saunders Co., p. 256.

17. Chai, H.: Intermediary mechanisms in asthma, Clin. Pediatr. 13:409, May, 1974.

18. Chinn, P. L.: A relationship between health and school problems; a nursing assessment, J. School Health 43:85, Feb., 1973.

19. Chused, J. F., Sibler, T. J., and Kodish, I.: Differential diagnosis of a functional symptom (persistent cough), Clin. Proc. Child. Hosp. 27:107, April, 1971.

20. Clemmens, R. L., and Kenny, T. J.: Clinical correlates of learning disabilities, minimal brain dysfunction and hyperactivity, Clin. Pediatr. 11:311, June, 1972.

21. Conners, C. K.: Symposium; behavior modification by drugs. III. Psychological effects of stimulant drugs in children with minimal brain dysfunction, Pediatrics 49:702, May, 1972.

22. Crawford, L. V.: Allergic diseases. In Hughes, J. G., editor: Synopsis of pediatrics, ed. 4, St. Louis, 1975, The C. V. Mosby Co., p. 667.

23. Demaria, W. J. A., Krueger, R. P., and Anderson, E. E.: Urinary tract abnormalities in the nephrotic syndrome; seven cases demonstrating such an association, Clin. Pediatr. 11:530, Sept., 1972.

24. Dewey, J.: 18 ways to live with asthma, Nursing '75 5:48, April, 1975.

25. Dolan, T. F., and Meyers, A.: A survey of office management of urinary tract infections in childhood, Pediatrics 52:21, July, 1973.

26. Eisenberg, L.: Symposium; behavior modification by drugs. III. The clinical use of stimulant drugs in children, Pediatrics 49:709, May, 1972.

27. Elliott, R. N.: Influencing the behavior of children in emotional conflict, Nurse Practitioner 2:18, Sept.-Oct., 1977.

28. Ellis, E. F.: Allergic disorders. In Vaughan, V. C., III, and McKay, R. J., editors: Nelson's Textbook of pediatrics, ed. 10, Philadelphia, 1975, W. B. Saunders Co., p. 492.

29. Ellis, E. F.: Asthma. In Green, M., and Haggerty, R. J., editors: Ambulatory pediatrics, II, Philadelphia, 1977, W. B. Saunders Co., p. 325.

30. Ellis, P. P.: Eye. In Kempe, C. H., Silver, H. K., and O'Brien, D., editors: Current pediatric diagnosis and treatment, ed. 4, Los Altos, Calif., 1976, Lange Medical Publications, p. 213.

31. Erenberg, G.: Drug therapy in minimal brain dysfunction; a commentary, J. Pediatr. 81:359-365, Aug., 1972.

32. Felman, A. H.: Bicycle spoke fractures, J. Pediatr. 82:302, Feb., 1973.

33. Ferry, P. C.: Diagnosis and office management of headaches in children, Clin. Pediatr. 11:195, April, 1972.

34. Fitzgerald, J. F.: Diarrhea. In Green, M., and Haggerty, R. J., editors: Ambulatory pediatrics, II, Philadelphia, 1977, W. B. Saunders Co., p. 113.

35. Fitzgerald, J. F.: Encopresis. In Green, M., and Haggerty, R. J., editors: Ambulatory pediatrics, II, Philadelphia, 1977, W. B. Saunders, p. 121.

36. Freeman, R. D.: The drug treatment of learning disorders; Continuing confusion, J. Pediatr. 81:112-115, July, 1972.

37. Friedman, R.: Some characteristics of children with psychogenic pain, Clin. Pediatr. 11:331, June, 1972.

38. Galdston, R., and Perlmutter, A. D.: The urinary manifestations of anxiety in child, Pediatrics 52:818, Dec., 1973.

39. Ghory, J. E.: The ABCs of educating the patient with chronic bronchial asthma; how we do it, Clin. Pediatr. 16:879, Oct., 1977.

40. Golden, G. S., and French, J. H.: Basilar artery migraine in young children, Pediatrics 56:722, Nov., 1975.

41. Goode, R. L., and Spooner, T. R.: Management of nasal fractures in children, Clin. Pediatr. 11:526-529, Sept., 1972.

42. Green, J. B.: Seizures. In Green, M., and Haggerty, R. J., editors: Ambulatory pediatrics, II, Philadelphia, 1977, W. B. Saunders Co., p. 306.

43. Green, M.: Headaches. In Green, M., and Haggerty, R. J., editors: Ambulatory pediatrics, II, Philadelphia, 1977, W. B. Saunders Co., p. 153.

44. Greenfield, D., Grant, R., and Leiberman, E.: Children can have high blood pressure, too, Am. J. Nurs. 76:770, May, 1976.

45. Griffin, P. P.: Musculoskeletal trauma. In Green, M., and Haggerty, R. J., editors: Ambulatory pediatrics, II, Philadelphia, 1977, W. B. Saunders Co., p. 253.

46. Grosfeld, J. L., and Ballantine, T. V. N.: The skin; lacerations, abrasions, and burns. In Green, M., and Haggerty, R. J., editors: Ambulatory pediatrics, II,

Philadelphia, 1977, W. B. Saunders Co., p. 238.

47. Hable, K. A., Washington, J. A., and Hermann, E. C., Jr.: Bacterial and viral throat flora, Clin. Pediatr. **10:**199, 1971.

48. Jabbour, J. T., Duenas, D. A., and Gilmartin, R. C..: Diseases of the nervous system. In Hughes, J. G., editor: Synopsis of pediatrics, ed. 4, St. Louis, 1975, The C. V. Mosby Co., p. 811.

49. Jacobsen, R. F., and Siegel, E.: Comprehensive health planning in the space age; the role of the school health program, J. School Health **41:**156, 1971.

50. Kaplan, R. S., Lave, L. B., and Leinhart, S.: The efficacy of a comprehensive health care project; an empirical analysis, Am. J. Public Health **62:**924, July, 1972.

51. Kaplan, S.: Diseases of cardiovascular system. In Shirkey, H. C., editor: Pediatric therapy, ed. 5, St. Louis, 1975, The C. V. Mosby Co., p. 698.

52. Katz, H. P.: Accuracy of a home throat culture program; a study of parent participation in health care, Pediatrics **53:**687, May, 1974.

53. Landeen, J. M.: Ear, nose, and throat emergencies. In Stephenson, H. E., Jr., editor: Immediate care of the acutely ill and injured, St. Louis, 1974, The C. V. Mosby Co., p. 202.

54. Laufer, M. W.: Long-term management and some follow-up findings on the use of drugs with minimal cerebral syndromes, J. Learn. Disabil. **4:**518, 1971.

55. Lecks, H. I.: Appraisals of cromolyn sodium and corticosteroids in the treatment of the asthmatic child, Clin. Pediatr. **16:**861, Oct., 1977.

56. Levin, S.: The excretory system; infection. In Cooke, R. E., editor: The biologic basis of pediatric practice, New York, 1968, McGraw-Hill Book Co., p. 1023.

57. Levison, H., Collins-Williams, C., Bryan, A. C., Reilly, B. J., and Orange, R. P.: Asthma; current concepts, Pediatr. Clin. North Am. **21:**951, Nov., 1974.

58. Levy, J. S., and Lovejoy, G. S.: Management of pharyngitis by pediatric nurse practitioners, Clin. Pediatr. **15:**415, May, 1976.

59. Lewiston, N. J., and Bergman, A. S.: A self-help group for parents of asthmatic children, Clin. Pediatr. **16:**888, Oct., 1977.

60. Lieberman, E.: Essential hypertension in children and youth; a pediatric perspective, J. Pediatr. **85:**1, July, 1974.

61. Lipow, H. W.: Respiratory tract infections. In Green, M., and Haggerty, R. J., editors: Ambulatory pediatrics, II, Philadelphia, 1977, W. B. Saunders Co., p. 36.

62. Londe, S., and Goldring, D.: Hypertension in children, Am. Heart J. **84:**1, Jan., 1972.

63. Marshall, S., Marshall, H. H., and Lyon, R. P.: Enuresis; an analysis of various therapeutic approaches, Pediatrics **52:**813, Dec., 1973.

64. McClelland, C. Q., and others: The practitioner's role in behavioral pediatrics, J. Pediatr. **82:**325, Feb., 1973.

65. McCrory, W. W.: The excretory system; anatomic and physiologic considerations. In Cooke, R. E., editor: The biologic basis of pediatric practice, New York, 1968, McGraw-Hill Book Co., p. 989.

66. McKendry, J. B. J., and Stewart, D. A.: Enuresis, Pediatr. Clin. North Am. **21:**1019, Nov., 1974.

67. Menkes, M. M.: Personality characteristics and family roles of children with migraine, Pediatrics **53:**560, April, 1974.

68. Miles, J. S., and Solomons, C. C.: Orthopedics. In Kempe, C. H., Silver, H. K., and O'Brien, D., editors: Current pediatric diagnosis and treatment, ed. 4, Los Altos, Calif., 1976, Lange Medical Publications, p. 500.

69. Miller, W. V.: Injuries resulting from animal contact and their initial care. In Stephenson, H. E., Jr., editor: Immediate care of the acutely ill and injured, St. Louis, 1974, The C. V. Mosby Co., p. 113.

60. Minor, T. E., and others: Greater frequency of viral respiratory infections in asthmatic children as compared with their nonasthmatic siblings, J. Pediatr. **85:**472, Oct., 1974.

71. Molteni, R. A.: The differential diagnosis of benign and septic joint disease in children, Clin. Pediatr. **17:**19, Jan., 1978.

72. Moore, G. T., and Frank, K.: Comprehensive health services for children; an exploratory study of benefit, Pediatrics **51:**17, Jan., 1973.

73. Mueller, H. L., Schmid, W. H., and Rubinsztain, R.: Stinging-insect hypersensitivity, Pediatrics **55:**530, April, 1975.

74. Nora, J. J., and Wolfe, R. R.: Cardiovascular diseases. In Kempe, C. H., Silver, H. K., and O'Brien, D., editors: Current pediatric diagnosis and treatment, ed. 4, Los Altos, Calif., 1976, Lange Medical Publications, p. 301.

75. Oh, W. H., Craig, C., and Banks, H. H.: Epiphyseal injuries, Pediatr. Clin. North Am. **21:**407, May, 1974.

76. Pearlman, D. S.: Allergic disorders. In Kempe, C. H., Silver, H. K., and O'Brien, D., editors: Current pediatric diagnosis and treatment, ed. 4, Los Altos, Calif., 1976, Lange Medical Publications, p. 862.

77. Pearlman, D. S., and Szentivanyi, A.: Excessive reactivity of defense mechanisms—allergy. In Cooke, R. E., editor: The biologic basis of pediatric practice, New York, 1968, McGraw-Hill Book Co., p. 536.

78. Pearson, L. B.: A protocol for the chief complaint of headache, Nurse Practitioner **2:**12, Sept.-Oct., 1976.

79. Peebles, T. C.: Identification and treatment of group A beta hemolytic streptococcal infections, Pediatr. Clin. North Am. **18:**145, 1971.

80. Poznanski, E. O.: Children's reactions to pain; a psychiatrist's perspective, Clin. Pediatr. **15:**1114, Dec., 1976.

81. Quinn, P. O., and Rapoport, J. L.: Minor physical anomalies and neurologic status in hyperactive boys, Pediatrics **53:**742, May, 1974.

82. Report on the Conference on the Use of Stimulant Drugs in the Treatment of Behaviorally Disturbed Young School Children: Washington, D.C., 1971, Office of Child Development.

83. Rotman, C. B., and Schmalz, E.: Illnesses and in-

juries in a summer camp, Am. J. Nurs. **77:**821, May, 1977.

84. Rowe, R. T., and Stone, R. T.: Streptococcal pharyngitis in children; difficulties in diagnosis on clinical grounds alone, Clin. Pediatr. **16:**933, Oct., 1977.

85. Salt intake and eating patterns of infants and children in relation to blood pressure; Report of the Committee on Nutrition, American Academy of Pediatrics: Pediatrics **53:**115, Jan., 1974.

86. Samter, M.: Bronchial asthma; new definition for an old disease, Clin. Pediatr. **13:**406, May, 1974.

87. Schmitt, B. D.: School phobia—the great imitator; a pediatrician's viewpoint, Pediatrics **48:**433-441, Sept., 1971.

88. Shands, A. R., Jr., MacEwen, G. D., and Cowell, H. R.: Pediatric orthopaedics. In Shirkey, H. C., editor: Pediatric therapy, ed. 5, St. Louis, 1975, The C. V. Mosby Co., p. 1150.

89. Shillito, J., Jr.: Head injuries. In Green, M., and Haggerty, R. J., editors: Ambulatory pediatrics, II, Philadelphia, 1977, W. B. Saunders Co., p. 247.

90. Sieber, O. F., Jr., and Fulginiti, V. A.: Streptococcal infections. In Vaughn, V. C., III, and McKay, R. J., editors: Nelson's Textbook of pediatrics, ed. 10, Philadelphia, 1975, W. B. Saunders Co., p. 569.

91. Slosky, D. A., and Todd, J. K.: Diagnosis of urinary tract infection; the interpretation of colony counts, Clin. Pediatr. **16:**698, Aug., 1977.

92. Starfield, B.: Enuresis; its pathogenesis and management, Clin. Pediatr. **11:**343, June, 1972.

93. Stephens, F. D.: Urologic aspects of recurrent urinary tract infection in children, J. Pediatr. **80:**725-737, May, 1972.

94. Symposium on exercise and asthma: Pediatrics **56:** (suppl.)843, Nov., 1975.

95. Todd, J., and others: A nonculture method for home follow-up of urinary tract infections in childhood, J. Pediatr. **85:**514, Oct., 1974.

96. Verman, S., and Hede, J. S.: Physical education programs and exercise-induced asthma; individualized gym programs allow asthmatic youngsters to participate with great benefit, Clin. Pediatr. **15:**697, Aug., 1976.

97. Waite, D. E.: Pediatric fractures of jaw and facial bones, Pediatrics **51:**551, March, 1973.

98. Walker, D., and Richard, G. A.: A critical evaluation of urethral obstruction in female children, Pediatrics **51:**272, Feb., 1973.

99. Wappel, F. A.: Athletic emergencies. In Stephenson, H. E., Jr., editor: Immediate care of the acutely ill and injured, St. Louis, 1974, The C. V. Mosby Co., p. 118.

100. Warren, S. A.: Adult expectations and learning disorders, Pediatr. Clin. North Am. **20:**705, Aug., 1973.

101. Webb, K. J.: Early assessment of orthopedic injuries, Am. J. Nurs. **74:**1048, June, 1974.

102. Weinberger, M. M., and Bronsky, E. A.: Evaluation of oral bronchodilator therapy in asthmatic dhilren, J. Pediatr. **84:**421, March, 1974.

103. Whitehead, D. J.: Emergency care in orthopedic injuries, Nurs. Clin. North Am. **8:**435, Sept., 1973.

104. Winsberg, B. G., and others: Dextroamphetamine and methylphenicate in the treatment of hyperactive children, Pediatrics **53:**236, Feb., 1974.

105. Wolf, S. I.: Tension-fatigue syndrome, Clin. Proc. Child. Hosp. **27:**25, Feb., 1974.

106. Wood, D. W.: Childhood status asthmaticus revisited; a synopsis of a program for management of childhood patients, Clin. Pediatr. **12:**555, Sept., 1973.

107. Wood, D. W., and Lecks, H. I.: Deaths due to childhood asthma; are they preventable? Clin. Pediatr. **15:**677, Aug., 1976.

108. Woodard, J. R.: The prognostic significance of fever in childhood urinary infections, Clin. Pediatr. **15:**1051, Nov., 1976.

109. Zepp, E. A., Thomas, J. A., and Knotts, G. R.: Some pharmacologic aspects of the antihistamines, Clin. Pediatr. **14:**1119, Dec., 1975.

# Brad R.—AGE 9

Cheryl Boyd Hundley

## HEALTH STATUS LIST

| Onset | Date | No. | Active | Date | Inactive/resolved |
|-------|------|-----|--------|------|-------------------|
| | | 1 | Incomplete data base | | |
| | | 2 | Child health maintenance | | |
| | | 2,A | Physical competency | | |
| | | 2,B | Learning and thought competency | | |
| | | 2,C | Inner competency | | |
| | | 2,D | Social competency | | |
| | | 3 | Need for knowledge and anticipatory guidance in managing late childhood and preadolescence | | |
| | | 3,A | Developmental tasks for forthcoming year | | |
| | | 3,B | Education in preparation for puberty | | |

Client **Brad R.**   Sex <u>M</u>   Age <u>9</u>
Date <u>5/22/78</u>   Race <u>Caucasian</u>

**Information sources:** Brad
Mother

**Reason health care worker sought client**
**Reason for seeking health care (mother and child's comments)**
Brad needs an exam before going to camp this summer. Mother would also like son to be more aware of taking care of his body.

**What events led up to the situation?**
Preparations for summer camp and health teaching concerning personal hygiene.

**When did this situation occur?**
Brad has been going to camp for last two summers and always has a physical at this time. Brad states mother always gets up in the morning to see that he has taken a bath, brushed his teeth, or washed hair.

**Describe the situation and/or how you are feeling. What made you decide to seek health care?**
Brad stated he "loved camp" and wants to be ready to go. This is "really why I'm here."

**What do you and your family do when something like this happens?**
Try to prepare in advance the camp experience. Mother has tried to talk with Brad about the need to "take care of his body" but her attempts "haven't been too successful."

**529**

### How is this affecting you and your family at the present time?

Mother believes camp is a good experience for son, as it allows for more contact with peers and other adults. Is a little frustrated with Brad's level of hygiene.

### MOTHER PROFILE

Sandra S, age 36. She and Brad constitute the family, live at 404 S. 26th Street. Is divorced and is a hairdresser by trade.

HEALTH STATUS
### Present health status

Mother states she is "healthy" without any acute or chronic problems except for a "cold" at this time.

### Previous medical-surgical events

Hysterectomy in 1970. Has two other children by a prior marriage. The two L & D's were uncomplicated. Children live with father (first husband) in California.

PRENATAL HISTORY WITH THIS CHILD (BRAD)

Pregnancy during second marriage. Brad was result of her third pregnancy. (Was divorced from Brads father six months after his birth.)

### Medical supervision

Regular visits to obstetrician during pregnancy. At this time gives herself prescribed estrogen injections. Visits gynecologist yearly.

### Nutrition, diet

"Tried to eat well." Weight gain about 25 pounds, she thinks.

### Illness, infections, and complications

None during the pregnancy.

### Treatments, procedures

Remembers none.

### Anesthesia

Had no anesthesia until right before delivery when she was "knocked out with gas."

### Course of labor and delivery

Membranes ruptured. Labor started and stopped several times during the 24-hour period after ROM.

### Availability in home

Brad and mother have only a few hours in the evening together. States Brad "gets upset with me because I have to work so much." Brad stays after school until 6 or 7 PM at the baby-sitter's. Spends Saturday there, too. Baby-sitter is 55 and cares for three other children, all preschoolers. Baby-sitter's grown son (25) and husband spend time with Brad. Baby-sitter encourages Brad to use manners if opening doors for guests, etc., and he helps some with minor chores around house. Has stayed here since first grade.

### Number of people in the home

Brad and mother.

### Employment/work environment

Works anywhere from 8 to 14 hours per day six days a week in a beauty shop. Is a hairdresser.

### Date of last menstrual period

Before hysterectomy in 1974.

### FATHER PROFILE

Father lives several hundred miles away and never sees child as he does not send child support money.

**Present health status**

Brad's mother believes father to be in good health.

**Previous medical-surgical events**

Information not available.

**Number of people he supports**

Himself and second family. Does not contribute to Brad's support.

**Availability in home/work habits**

Works for railroad.

**Employment/work environment**

Information not known.

**Range of income**

Not sure how much but thinks his salary is good. Mother's income $12,000 per year.

**Insurance**

Income protection, life insurance. No hospitalization. Carries car insurance.

LIFE CHANGE EVENTS (dates)

Death (family, close friend) <u>Father 1970</u>   New baby <u>No</u>
Divorce <u>1970 of Brad's parents</u>   Marital separation ____   Return to school <u>No</u>
Injury, illness <u>No</u>   Job loss <u>No</u>
Change of residence <u>No</u>   Retirement <u>No</u>

**Pedigree** (include chronic, inherited conditions, allergies, causes of death, illness in siblings)

◯  = Female
▢  = Male
 ? = Unknown
A.W. = Alive and well

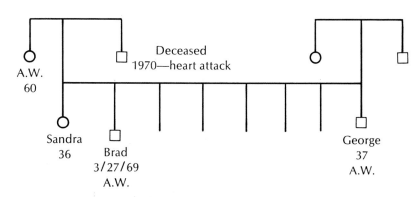

**Does your family see itself as a healthy family or as a sick family?**

Believes they are "healthy as horses."

**CHILD PROFILE**
HEALTH HISTORY
**Neonatal status (risk, Apgar, congenital abnormalities)**

No problems. No congenital abnormalities.

Later childhood

## Postnatal course

A "healthy baby."

## Previous illnesses (dates)

Brad relates he was "real sick" with flu a year ago. No chronic sore throats or ear infections. Measles and mumps—mother can't remember when.

## Medications

Takes vitamins occasionally.

## Accidents and injuries (dates)

Brad has never had stitches for any cuts. Mother cannot recall any accidents or injuries.

## Identify developmental milestones (DDST)

Not applicable.

## Sleep patterns/disturbances

Bedtime 10 PM. Arises at 7 AM. Sleeps all night.

## Allergies

None to environmental allergens. None known to medications.

## Immunizations

Brad remembers a booster at kindergarten. Mother believes they are up-to-date. Does not have a record.

## Nutrition history (example of 24-hour intake)

Brad proudly related he fixes his own breakfast. Has school lunches. Mother and child have supper together.

| BREAKFAST | LUNCH | SUPPER | SNACKS |
|---|---|---|---|
| Cereal/milk or oatmeal/milk, juice | "Some meat, vegetable, milk, dessert, bread" | Pork chop, mixed vegetables, choc. chip cookies, milk | Fruit, leftovers, cookies, milk, sometimes candy |

## Food groups

Meats (2) 2    Veg. (4) 2    Fruit 2    Breads/cereals (4) 2    Milk products (3) 4

## Formula (type/amt.)

Not applicable.

## Compare weight/height/age ratio*

9 years, weight = 65 lbs. (62%); height = 54 in. (50%)

*Chart percentiles from Children's Medical Center, Boston-Anthropometric Chart.

PSYCHOLOGIC PROFILE (Data here to be obtained during interactions, inquiry, observation, DDST)     Case

| Cognition | Ego |
|---|---|
| **Concrete operations: Operational thought (8-11 years)** | **Industry vs. Inferiority (6-13 years)** |

| Cognition | | Ego | |
|---|---|---|---|
| Yes | Operational thought: mentally orders and relates the experience to an organized whole | No | Concentrates on communication with peers |
| Yes | Sees events from different perspectives | Yes | Activities segregated by sex |
| Yes | Able to return to starting point of an operation (reversibility) | No | Competitive activities |
| Yes | Deduction from simple experiences | Yes | Participates eagerly in learning activities |
| | | Yes | Play: relives real-life situation |
| | | Yes | Identifies with an adult other than a parent |

**Comments**

Related step-by-step how to make clay from his art class. Related how to bake pottery step by step. Uses "I think of course you may think different"—able to see other points of view.

Described a game at school where boys and girls were playing like a marriage ceremony. Identifies with one of mother's men friends. Likes school and speaks enthusiastically about learning activities in art and science. Brad not observed in situation with communication with peers or in competitive activities.

**SCHOOL PROGRESS:**
**What would you like to tell me about school?**
"I have 24 to 43 friends—all the kids in my grade."

**What do you like or dislike most about school?**
Dislikes math but very much likes school plays, lunch, recess, art, and science class.

**Talk with parent or teacher about memory**
Mother states Brad's recall is accurate. In interview had difficulty with time recall.

**Tell me, What kind of a student do you think you are?**
"Medium" student. (Grades reflect average and above average work.)

**PERCEPTION OF SELF**
**Self-evaluation**
(Describe yourself to me.)
"I have blue eyes, a silver coat, a Star Wars watch, dirty pants, and I need new shoes."

**Tell me things you like about yourself; dislike**
I'm glad to be alive and I like that. Stated he "hated to be alive" when he was upset or disappointed.

**Let's pretend you could change something about yourself. Would you change anything?**
Would like to change when "I get mad at my Mom."

**Describe how you feel about what's happening to you now.**
Described how he is eagerly awaiting camp as he is going to "learn to ride a horse."

SOCIAL PROFILE
**Personal-social (DDST)**
Not applicable.

**Father/mother–child interaction**
Appears to be a warm relationship. Mother expresses praise and how she loves him. "Couldn't do without him."
Eye contact Good

Later childhood    Touching <u>None seen</u>

Tone of voice of parent <u>Soft and affectionate when speaking of Brad</u>

Child-parent activities <u>Brad states they go to the fair and occasionally go to the park. States "there's</u> not enough time" to do too many things together.

Ease of separation <u>Apart from mother most of the day. Seems to be accepting of this.</u>

### Position of child in family

Third child by birth. The only child in the present family unit.

### Describe life-style

Live in an apartment. Brad states they buy what they can "depending on how much money Mom and I have." Spends much time at babysitter's home.

Is there more than one language spoken in the home? <u>No</u>

ENVIRONMENTAL PROFILE

### Pollutants

Check with city.

### Population density

Check with city.

### Infestations

None obvious.

### Fire hazards

Will check during home visit.

### Medications/poisons

No information about this.

### Crime

Check city statistics.

### Availability of transportation

Mother has car and takes Brad to school. He can walk one block from school to the babysitter's house.

REVIEW OF SYSTEMS

### General

Energetic, smiles a lot, inquisitive. Seems in good health. Jeans and shoes are dusty.

### Hair and scalp (dandruff, lice, cradle cap, itching, and hair loss)

No history of above. Only likes to wash hair once every three weeks.

### Skin (infections, scaling, burns, allergies)

Takes a bath "once, maybe twice a week." Mother does not recall any impetigo or scaling or burns of skin. No allergic skin reactions known to occur.

### Hematopoietic (anemias, bleeding, bruising)

Does not bruise easily, have nose bleeds. No bleeding from urinary tract or blood with stools. Has never had anemia.

### Eyes (infections, blurred vision, squinting, color blindness)

Does not wear glasses. Eye testing at school negative for astigmatism, myopia, hyperopia. Correctly identifies colors. No past eye infections mother can remember.

### Ears (infection, discharge, eardrum perforation, foreign objects, wax removals, decreased hearing)

No history of ear infections, decreased hearing, or discharges of purulent nature.

**Nose, throat, sinuses (runny nose, colds, decreased smell, foreign body, broken nose, tonsil-litis)**

Has occasional runny nose and sore throat. Has never had broken nose or septal deviation.

**Mouth and dentition (dental caries, gingivitis malocclusion, cleft lip and/or palate)**

Two years ago had all of lower deciduous molars filled and one upper molar on R. Was not born with any cleft structures. Mother believes occlusion is normal.

**Respiratory (bronchitis, pneumonia, whooping cough, histoplasmosis, tuberculosis, cough)**

Negative history for the above except for cough associated with infrequent URI.

**Cardiovascular (heart murmurs, cyanosis)**

No history of above.

**Gastrointestinal (nausea/vomiting, diarrhea, constipation, jaundice, pain, colic, gas, hernias, anorexia)**

Occasionally may have diarrhea when ill with "flu." Otherwise negative history for the above.

**Genitourinary (frequency, urgency, burning, toilet training, bedwetting, odor, stream)**

No history of bedwetting, urgency, burning, and frequency. Toilet trained completely by age 3.

**Reproductive (irritations/rashes, deviations, secondary sexual characteristics)**

No history of deviations in reproductive structures. Onset of puberty is not evident according to mother.

**Neuromuscular (convulsions, headache, imbalance, incoordination, muscle weakness, numbness, tremors, tics)**

Brad states he has headaches once a year. Mother denies any occurrence of the above.

**Psychologic (thumb sucking, fears, masturbation)**

Did not suck thumb after 12 months of age. Mother does not know of any fears.

PHYSICAL PROFILE
**Measurements**

Head circumference 22 in.   Chest circumference 25 in.   Ht. 54 in.   Wt. 65 lbs.

**Vital signs**

B/P 140/60   H.R. 80/min (apical)   R.R. 22/min   Temp. 98.4° F

**NEUROMUSCULAR SYSTEM**
**Present neurological status**

Posture erect, coordinated movements of limbs. Muscle masses firm. Walk is straight. Feet are mildly arched.

**Social affect**

Smiles most of the time, has good eye contact in conversation. Cooperative attitude is one of enthusiasm. Feelings congruent to spoken words.

**Speech development**

Is able to express thoughts. Articulation of words precise.

**Reflexes**

Biceps 3+   Triceps 3+   Brachioradialis 3+  } Equal response
Patellar 3+   Achilles 3+                        } bilaterally
Babinski Negative   Eye Corneal reflex not tested

Later childhood

## Cranial nerves

I (olfactory): Intact. Identified smell of alcohol.

II (optic): Intact. Snellen 20/20. Peripheral vision at 90 degrees bilaterally. Can distinguish colors.

III, IV, and VI (oculomotor, trochlear, and abducens): EOM's present without deviations. III, IV, and VI intact.

V (trigeminal): Intact. Detects light touch in maxillary and mandibular areas. Good blinking reflex. Jaw bite coordinated and equal.

VII (facial): Intact. Mimics eye squint, grimace, frown with equality of lines an contours during movements. Discriminated salt and sugar tastes.

VIII (acoustic): Intact. Can hear watch tick at shoulder line bilaterally. Negative Weber and Rinne test.

IX, X (glossopharyngeal and vagus): Intact. Salivates. Gag reflex present. Tongue in midline coordinates swallowing.

XI (accessory): Intact. Equal strengh of shoulder lift and head turn bilaterally.

XII (hypoglossal): Intact. Moves tongue from side to side. Can apply pressure to cheek with tongue.

## Cerebellar function (Rhomberg, walk heel-toe, run in place, touch tip of nose, copy hand movements, pincer grasp, draw and copy geometric shapes)

Negative Rhomberg. Coordinated movements in heel-to-toe, running in place. Accurately copied geometric shapes. Able to touch tip of nose and copy hand movements.

## Parietal lobe (object identification)

Identified key, safety pin, rubber band by touch.

## Proprioception (positional sense of toe)

Correctly identified position of big toe.

## Tactile capacity (cold, two-point discrimination, pin prick)

Can discriminate hot and cold. Has two-point discrimination of pin prick.

## Skin (scars, lesions, turgor, bruises, moles)

Skin is hydrated and without scars, lesions, or moles. Feet dirty. Light hair on legs and arms.

## Head (circumference, fontanel measurement, palpation, transillumination)

Circumference 54 cm. Palpation negative for masses. Bilaterally symmetrical shape and placement of structures.

## Face (expression, palpebral fissures, placement of ears, percussion of sinuses, symmetry)

Pleasant facial expression. Ears in line with outer canthus of eyes. No tenderness over sinuses. Facial structures bilaterally symmetrical.

## Hair, scalp (hairline, hygiene, distribution)

Hair needing washing. Thick hair with normal hair line. No scaling of scalp.

## Eyes (amblyopia, strabismus, nystagmus, discharge, red reflex)

Negative for strabismus, amblyopia. Red reflex present. PERRLA. Good convergence.

## Nose (patency, discharge, smell)

Nares patent. Watery mucus drainage without an odor coming from nose. Nose in midline of face.

## Mouth and throat (teeth, gums, pharynx, tongue, palates, swallowing, tonsils)

Mixed dentition—12 teeth upper and lower. All of lower molars filled. Upper and lower molars encircled with plaque. No caries seen. Palate arched. Tonsils present without inflammation or exudates. Gums not inflamed.

## Ears (landmarks, structure, hearing)

Ear structure pliant. Ears close to head. Hearing intact (see C.N. VIII) Wax occluded L ear completely. R tympanum partially visualized but unable to see (due to wax) landmarks. Tympanum pearly gray. Periphery of tympanium reddened at 9 o'clock.

### Neck (nodes, masses, bruits, ROM)

Neck negative for nodes, masses, bruits. Full ROM. No openings for residual brachial clefts.

### Chest (symmetry, excursion, nodes, nipples)

Chest equal in symmetry and excursion and placement of nipples. No nodes or masses palpable on chest wall. No findings after tactile fremitus. No swelling or discharge at nipples.

### Lungs (breath sounds, fremitus, percussion, duration of inspiration, expiration, rate)

Slight flaring of lower costal margin. Clavicles level. Inspiration to expiration 1:2. Ausculation negative for adventitious sounds. Vocal fremitus revealed negative findings, as did percussion. Rate is 22 per minute.

### Heart (size, position, PMI, sounds)

PMI at 4th ICS 1-2 cm to right of nipple. $S_1$ loudest at apex, $S_2$ loudest at pulmonic with splitting upon inspiration. No murmurs heard or thrills palpated. Head borders not percussed. Apical rate 80 and regular. Pulses present and equal. Conjunctiva pink. Extremities warm. No peripheral cyanosis. No clubbing of fingers.

### Abdomen (size, contour, bowel sounds, umbilicus, liver, spleen, femorals)

Nô respiratory movements. Musculature firm and contour slightly concave. Liver, spleen not palpable. Umbilicus clean. Bowel sounds present and heard about every 10 seconds. No hernias palpable. Femorals equal.

### Back and spine (structure, symmetry, column curvature)

Column is midline, scapulas bilaterally symmetrical. No defects palpated in column or openings seen or felt in sacral area.

### Extremities (palmar creases, ROM, hip abduction)

Palmar creases of normal configuration. Full active and passive ROM in extremities. Equal and strong hand grasp. Negative Ortalani's sign. Warm and perfused extremities. No scars or bruises or lesions.

### Urinary (position of meatus, charae of voiding, appearance of urine)

Urine is yellow, clear. Meatus normally placed.

### Genitalia (structure, secondary sexual characteristics)

Normal male anatomy with descended testes. No axillary or pubic hair. Not in stage I of puberty.

### Anus (structure, function)

Patent. Regular bowel movements daily.

**INITIAL PLAN**

5/22/78   **No. 1   Incomplete data base**

    **S**   Mother desires that son care for his body.

    **O**   Brad needs some teaching about personal hygiene as revealed by interview and exam. Data reveals Brad physically fit for camp.

    **A**   Family assessment to further identify the stressors in their lives and to identify mother's expectations for herself and Brad in the future.

    **P**   Obj. 1   The family should be able to continue interaction with clinical specialist for further need identification.

5/22/78   **No. 2   Child health maintenance**

    2,A   Physical competency

    **S**   Mother states Brad is "healthy as a horse" and was "healthy baby with no problems." Brad claims he's never ill and is hungry a lot. Mother believes immunizations are up-to-date but has no record. Brad remembers "a booster shot" at kindergarten. Brad related a 24-hour intake of food and proudly related he fixes own breakfast. Gets about eight or nine hours' sleep a night. Goes to doctor yearly (only because of camp physical) and hasn't been to dentist in two years. Mother nor child can recall any serious illnesses and/or accidents. Does not have allergies of any kind. Brad relates that he bathes once a week, washes hair every three weeks, maybe brushes teeth in the morning, and almost never washes his ears. Mother states Brad needs to care for his own body. Mother does not always arise to fix breakfast or to check Brad's hygiene (according to Brad).

    **O**   PE revealed plaque on teeth with caries or gingivitis. Feet were dirty, ears not clean, and hair needed washing. Clothes were dusty, shoes too small. No physical abnormalities or conditions revealed after physical assessment. The quick nutrition history indicates basically good nutrition with need to increase vegetables and cereal intake. Postures sitting and standing are straight and gait is coordinated. Weighs 65 pounds (62nd percentile for age). Height 54 inches (50th percentile for age). Head circumference 22 inches (50th percentile for age). Chest circumference 25 inches (50th percentile for age). Cranial nerves and reflexes are intact. No sensory deficits. Cardiovascular and respiratory exams reveal negative findings. No data to confirm adequacy of immunizations. Has fillings in sixth year molars. Is physically preadolescent.

    **A**   At this age health maintenance is directed toward implementing the basic goal of promoting his own motivation to seek health. The most dramatic physiologic events are in the musculoskeletal system with increased muscle mass for boys. Sensory capacity is most crucial of all the determinations as sensory function is vitally important to the school setting. Hygiene should be understood by the school-age child, and he should be able to care for his personal hygiene needs and to have firmly established daily hygiene habits. He should demonstrate increasing neuromuscular skills for games and work. Should eat approximately an adult meal. Dentition is mixed. Lymphoid tissues reach height of development and increases the vulnerability of mucous membranes, increasing the possibility of congestion and inflammation due to excessive tissue growth. His fillings are in first sixth year molars, which is keystone for the permanent dental arch. Lordosis is gone and posture should be straight. Because of refined eye-hand coordination the 9-year-old is skillful in physical activities. Basic

**538**

four should include at least 1900 calories per day. Immunizations for rubella and mumps should be given if they have not been already.

**P** Obj. 1 Brad should demonstrate adequate nutrition appropriate to his age.

Obj. 2 Brad should demonstrate up-to-date immunizations.

Obj. 3 Brad should demonstrate ability to perform daily hygiene procedures.

2,B Learning and thought competency

**S** Brad sees himself as a "medium" student. Related directions on how to make clay and fire pottery.

**O** Grade card confirms that he is an average student with above average grades in art and science. These subjects he enthusiastically discussed. "I think, of course, you may think different" indicated cognitively he can accommodate different perspectives from his own. Can mentally order and relate an experience to an organized whole. Follow a direction correctly during exam. Peabody Picture Vocabulary indicates age-appropriate language usage skills. Speech is articulate with adequate vocabulary to express his meanings. Is able to carry on discussion.

**A** The child of 9 is cognitively in stage of concrete operations. He is not altogether egocentric and can take into account another point of view. Can focus on several properties in sequence within a given situation. Concrete operations means he can only know what he can perceive through his senses. Needs to formulate a concept of health at this age that can be mediated by attitudes of adults in his personal life, school teachers, and health care person with whom he has contact. Successful learning is demonstrated by how he processes information for outcomes for successful living.

**P** Obj. 1 Brad should demonstrate cognitive skills necessary for foundation of formal operational stage (logical deduction and hypothesis testing for reasoning)

Obj. 2 Brad should demonstrate concept of health as applied to his own body needs.

2,C Social competency

**S** Talks of all kids in class being friends. Mother and Brad relate that they have little time together. There is no father in the home. Brad spends many hours at the babysitter's, and there is no one his age there. Does not attend church or belong to any groups. Goes to camp every summer. Few child-parent activities. Plays with boys and girls at school.

**O** Mother speaks warmly of Brad. Brad matter-of-factly relates he does not see much of his mother. He did not relate that he had a "chum" or close friend. Only child in the family unit.

**A** Developmental tasks of the school-age child include decreasing dependence upon family and gaining some satisfaction from peers and other adults, learning basic adult concepts and knowledge, and being able to reason and engage in tasks of everyday living. About 9 or 10 the child moves from interaction with peer group to a special friend of the same sex or age. From sharing with a "chum" ideas and feelings the child learns more about himself or herself, as well as other people. The child learns

**539**

**INITIAL PLAN—cont'd**

5/22/78 **No. 2  Child health maintenance—cont'd**

competition, compromise, and collaboration in order to get along with others. Should this not be learned, socialization will be inhibited. Through identification begins to relate to significant adults in and out of the family circle. Identification serves to provide the child a means by which to strengthen, direct, and control behavior in such a manner that it matches an adult or a child whom he or she admires.

**P**     Obj. 1   Brad should demonstrate social interactions necessary for age-appropriate social competency.

2,D   Inner competency

**S**     "Glad to be alive" was Brad's remark as to things he liked about self. Would like to change himself when he "get mad" at mother. The only bodily physical feature he described was "blue eyes." Self-image was projected with features of clothing, i.e., "dirty pants, silver coat and Star Wars watch." Has "43 friends" or all the kids in class for friends. Relates he belongs to no special groups. Plays mostly with boys, sometimes with girls. Related he and boys and girls were playing like they were at a wedding. Only enthusiastic about science and art and play times at school. "Likes" one of his mother's male friends. Never sees father who makes no initiative to visit child.

**O**     Brad's mother expresses concern over his hygiene yet takes no mentioned steps to help him with these areas. Brad seems rather unconcerned with hygiene—may be an attention-getting device since there is little mother-child interaction. Doesn't like himself when "he's mad" at mother—very somber and quiet for a while after this statement. Never mentioned father or any adult specifically that he admires or interacts with. Did not describe himself by physical characteristics but by things worn on his person. Slightly self-conscious about removing shirt and slacks. Not enthusiastic about learning except for science and art. No talk of specific friends.

**A**     Is in industry vs. inferiority stage of affective development. Industry results with successful resolution of the maturational crisis, which is characterized by a child feeling he can learn and solve problems, by wanting to participate in the real world, by seeking recognition for efforts, and by concentrating on a task. The child should feel pride in doing something well and should exhibit diligence, self-control, cooperation, and compromise. Inferiority may develop in the child as he feels inadequate, unable to learn or do tasks, unable to compete, compromise, or cooperate. This can cause the child (and later the adult) to lack perserverance, be meek and isolated or, conversely, aggressive, bossy, and overcompetitive. Parents can contribute to a sense of industry by not having unrealistic expectations of the child. The child's self-esteem is directed by the extent to which he experiences esteem from his peers. Perceptions of the child by the parent, teachers, and adults are very important to the child. By this age he should care for his own body. May be critical of his own and other's behavior. The child with adequate inner competency is happy, energetic, confident, and able to cope with stress.

**P**     Obj. 1   Brad should demonstrate positive self-concept.

5/22/78    **No. 3   Need for knowledge and anticipatory guidance in managing late childhood and preadolescence.**    

3,A   Developmental tasks for forthcoming year

**S**   Mother wants nurse to impress upon Brad the need to care for his body. Few mother-child interactions. Spends much time with baby-sitter.

**O**   No comments about preparing child for future events. No mention of what she wishes Brad to attain.

**A**   Knowing the hazards of each developmental period is essential to providing a safe home environment. By age 6 will be in stage of Industry vs. Inferiority affectively until age 13. By 11 he should enter the formal operation phase (Piaget). Industry vs. inferiority stage is referred to from the Freudian view as latency. In this time children are concerned with learning and peer group activities, and it is a relatively peaceful period for the parent. Children of preadolescence are beginning to experience some inner turmoil directly before and at the onset of puberty. A parent who wishes to cling to the peace of latency may force the child to not share his questions and fears about changes he perceives to be near and/or is experiencing. His behavior may be one of politeness without consideration, mechanical performance of tasks without personal involvement, and conversation without content, all reflecting an effort to mark the diffusion being experienced. Mastery of the developmental tasks in the affective realm are necessary for establishing identity of the adolescent. Inability to master cognitive concepts of the concrete operations phase may impair the potential for adultlike intellectual skills.

**P**   Obj. 1   The mother should demonstrate application of developmental tasks of rearing of son.

3,B   Education in preparation for puberty

**S**   None.

**O**   At 9 Brad may soon start to have body changes and the development of secondary sexual characteristics.

**A**   The prepubescent male demonstrates increases in height and weight, vasomotor instability, increased perspiration, and active sebaceous glands. Sebaceous materials may produce blemishes or acne. Uncontrollable blushing is a manifestation of vasomotor instability. Physical changes include increase in size of testes, changes in scrotum color, temporary enlargement of breasts, appearance of lightly pigmented hair at base of penis, and increase in length and width of penis. A boy's fears about his changing body may be ignored. Mothers may be embarrassed to talk about them. Parents must assist the child as he adjusts to his new body image and they must also alter their image of the child. The child needs to understand the changing requirements of hygiene as puberty begins. Preparation for puberty is vitally important throughout the later childhood years. Needs education about his body, general sex education and what is happening as to changes in his opposite-sex peer.

**P**   Obj. 1   The mother should be able to identify body changes of the preadolescent.
      Obj. 2   The mother will be able to prepare Brad for puberty.

**NURSING ORDERS**

5/22/78 **No. 1 Incomplete data base** PERSONNEL

Obj. 1 The family should be able to continue interaction with clinical specialist for further need identification.
  A. Make appointment for home visit to obtain family assessment. (5/28) C.S.*
  B. Give mother phone number should she need clinical specialist (done). C.S.

5/22/78 **No. 2 Child health maintenance**

2,A Physical competency

Obj. 1 Brad should demonstrate adequate nutrition appropriate to his age.
  A. Do an in-depth nutritional assessment next visit. (5/28) C.S.
  B. Elicit from mother and Brad their knowledge of the basic four and essential vitamins and minerals. (5/28) C.S.
  C. Supply them with learning aids about basic four. (5/28) C.S.
  D. Correlate good nutritional status with preventive health care as with teeth and bone formation and increasing blood components. (5/28) C.S.
  E. Inquire if summer camp has any resources or groups teaching children about nutritional needs. (5/28) C.S.

Obj. 2 Up-to-date immunizations
  A. Call Brad's physician to obtain record of immunizations. (5/23) C.S.
  B. Give this information to the mother and teach her the importance of record keeping. (5/28) C.S.
  C. Refer Brad to clinic for rubella and measles immunization if he is deficient. (5/30) C.S.
  D. Provide mother with a record booklet so she can maintain record of immunizations. (5/28) C.S.

Obj. 3 Ability to perform daily hygiene procedures
  A. Elicit from mother how much commitment as to time and input she is willing to demonstrate. (5/28) C.S.
  B. Elicit from Brad his knowledge of what constitutes adequate daily hygiene. (5/28) C.S.
  C. With Brad and mother outline on a week calendar hygiene measures. Have Brad mark off on calendar as he completes tasks daily with mother verifying task performance. (6/1) C.S.
  D. Institute a reward system (praise, mother-son outing) with Brad and mother jointly deciding what reward should be after a week of fulfilling contract. (6/1) C.S.

*Clinical Specialist.

|  |  | PERSONNEL |
|---|---|---|
| E. | Demonstrate tooth care—brushing and flossing to Brad. (5/28) | C.S. |
| F. | Provide teaching aids about how bacteria work on skin and excretory products to produce odors. (5/28) | C.S. |
| G. | Check health science museum to see if they have a health hygiene program. (5/23) | C.S. |

2,B  Learning and thought competency

Obj. 1  Cognitive skills necessary for foundation for formal operational stage.

|  |  | |
|---|---|---|
| A. | Talk with mother and teacher about Brad's learning performance in school. (5/23) | C.S. |
| B. | Elicit from Brad projects or activities he would like to do. (5/28) | C.S. |
| C. | Collaborate with mother and teacher and design play experiences for Brad that will allow for perfection of cognitive tasks involving classification, seriation, conservation, and reversibility. (6/7) | C.S. |
| D. | Investigate the type of learning experiences he will be having at camp this summer. (6/7) | C.S. |
| E. | Educate mother to the fact that Brad's self-confidence and self-esteem will be increased with increasing competency in school achievement and activities for play that allow for learning. (5/28) | C.S. |

Obj. 2  Brad should demonstrate concept of health as applied to his own body.

|  |  | |
|---|---|---|
| A. | Talk with teacher and school nurse as to experiences provided for health learning. (5/23) | C.S. |
| B. | Plan a session for Brad and teach him how parts of his body work and how he can maintain them. (6/7) | C.S. |
| C. | Elicit from him his knowledge of how he expects his body to change as he "grows up." (5/28) | C.S. |
| D. | Continue ongoing teaching and intervention about hygiene and nutrition. | Mother<br>Teachers<br>C.S. |
| E. | Provide Brad with a book to explain the changes that will take place in his body soon. (5/28) | C.S. |
| F. | Discuss with Brad how he can use the information from the book as applied to his own body. (6/7) | Brad<br>C.S. |

**NURSING ORDERS—cont'd**

5/22/78    **No. 2   Child health maintenance—cont'd**        PERSONNEL

     2,C   Social competency

         Obj. 1   Brad should demonstrate social interactions necessary for age-appropriate social competency.

| | |
|---|---|
| A. Encourage mother to plan suppertime as one where companionship and conversation allow for Brad to relate his activities and school experiences each night. (5/28) | Mother C.S. |
| B. Encourage mother to take Brad on shopping trips so he can learn about spending money, choosing his own clothes, and see new places. (6/7) | Mother C.S. |
| C. Inquire about community resources that might have activities for Brad that are close to the baby-sitter's house (Big Brother programs, YMCA groups, scouts, church groups). (5/23) | C.S. |
| D. Explore with mother and teacher Brad's social interactions with peers and any close friends his age. (5/23) | C.S. |
| E. Encourage mother to periodically accompany Brad on an outing of his choosing. (5/28) | C.S. |
| F. Teach mother the developmental needs and implications for achieving successful social interactions. | C.S. |

     2,D   Inner competency

         Obj. 1   Brad should demonstrate a positive self-concept

| | |
|---|---|
| A. Teach mother that a great deal of Brad's self-esteem is determined by how much his friends value him. (5/28) | C.S. |
| B. Ascertain if her expectations behaviorally for son at this time are age-appropriate. (6/7) | C.S. |
| C. Ask mother to consider exploring with Brad tasks and jobs for which he would like responsibility. (5/28) | C.S. |
| D. Encourage mother to consider for Brad a group activity with peers that is service-oriented. (6/7) | C.S. |
| E. Explore further with Brad how he perceives himself and his strengths and weaknesses. (6/7) | C.S. |
| F. Teach Brad that being clean and well groomed will provide a sense of well-being and pride. (5/28) | C.S. |
| G. Further explore Brad's coping mechanisms. (6/7) | C.S. |
| H. Talk with teacher about peer relationships. (5/23) | C.S. |

5/22/78    **No. 3   Need for knowledge and anticipatory guidance in managing later childhood and preadolescence**

     3,A   Developmental tasks for forthcoming year

         Obj. 1   The mother should demonstrate application of developmental tasks in rearing of son.

| | PERSONNEL | Case |
|---|---|---|

A. Ascertain the mother's and baby-sitter's knowledge of Brad's present and future developmental needs. — C.S.

B. Elicit from mother what she perceives as important events within the next year. (6/7) — C.S.

C. Teach her those cognitive and affective tasks that she and baby-sitter can promote. (6/7) — C.S.

D. Provide basic reading about developmental needs and discuss it with her and baby-sitter on a return visit. (5/28) — Mother, Baby-sitter, C.S.

E. Investigate his materials and space for activities and play — C.S.
   1. Home
   2. Baby-sitter's home (6/7)

F. Explore how she plans to cope with Brad as an adolescent. (6/7) — C.S.

3,B   Education in preparation for puberty

Obj. 1   The mother should be able to identify body changes of the preadolescent.

A. Ascertain mother's knowledge of body changes associated with puberty. (6/7) — C.S.

B. Inquire as to how she presently has planned for preparing Brad for this period. (6/7) — C.S.

C. During a home visit teach her (using booklets, pictures) about body changes and approaches to the child. (6/14) — Mother, C.S.

D. Teach mother that masturbation is a normal activity for the release of sexual tension. (6/7) — C.S.

Obj. 2   The mother will be able to prepare Brad for puberty.

A. Give mother names and authors of books that she can provide for Brad about puberty and sexual interactions. (5/28) — C.S.

B. Have mother role play a situation in which she could teach Brad about forthcoming physical events. (6/14) — C.S.

C. Serve as a role model for the mother if necessary. (6/14) — C.S.

D. Teach her to question Brad about what he already knows and to clarify his new knowledge for accuracy and for questions. (6/14) — C.S.

## REFERENCES

Kostenberg, J.: The effects on parents of the child's transition into and out of latency. *Parenthood: Its Psychology and Psychopathology,* In Anthony, E. J., and Benedeck, T., Boston: Little, Brown and Company. 1970, pp. 289-307.

Murray, R., and Zentner, J.: Nursing assessment and health promotion throughout the life span. Englewood Cliffs, N.J., 1975, Prentice-Hall, Inc.

Vaughn-Wrobel, B. C., and Henderson, B.: Problem oriented record in nursing practice, St. Louis, 1976, The C. V. Mosby Co.

# Adolescence

Adolescence has become both a mystery and a challenge in modern technological societies. The child becomes a young adult and is suspended for several long years between childhood and adulthood. The young person's confusion and ambivalence are confounded by the confusion and ambivalence of society toward the individual who is experiencing this change, and adolescent behavior reflects the multitude of interacting problems.

For several years during this period of development, young people appear like neither children nor adults; they behave like neither age group. They are simply adolescents, and they experience the great ambivalence imposed upon them by the type of transition required in society. The transition for some young people and families is exceedingly difficult; for others it is relatively smooth.

Because young adolescents are neither children nor adults, their own peer group becomes of paramount importance. They can only be understood by others who are experiencing the same transition, and they experience their whole world in relationship to their peer group. In fact, they seem unable to relate to the world as individuals and must achieve satisfying, intense peer group relationships in order to accomplish the transition required. They invest themselves in those who will share the future with them and somewhat painfully break the ties that they must leave behind.

The purposes of Chapter 14, "Adolescence: The Age of Transition," are (1) to present the scientific bases for development during adolescence that have been demonstrated or hypothesized through the biologic and behavioral sciences, (2) to discuss the means of nursing assessment and identification of development in each competency, and (3) to discuss the management of health maintenance needs that occur during this period of life.

Adolescence     In Chapter 15, "Health Problems of Adolescence," the purposes
are (1) to consider the basis for nursing diagnosis of health problems
that tend to occur during adolescence, (2) to discuss the management
needed for each of the problems considered, and (3) to discuss the
special health care needs of socially alienated youth in our world today.

# Adolescence: the age of transition

The period of adolescence, like other developmental stages, is impossible to define in exact chronological terms. While it is often thought of as beginning with the onset of puberty and ending with the achievement of a certain level of maturity, these landmarks are difficult to identify, and they do not seem adequate in describing the many complex factors that comprise adolescence in Western cultures. Adolescence may most appropriately be conceptualized as the period of life during which emancipation from the primary family unit is the central task of the individual. The term "puberty" will be used to denote the period of time that involves the development and maturation of the reproductive, endocrine, and structural systems. Adolescence, on the other hand, refers to the period of life characterized by the psychologic, emotional, and social changes that result in emancipation from one's family unit and the formation of a sense of personal identity. Adolescence usually begins just before, or concurrent with, the changes of puberty, but it lasts for an extended period of time after puberty has been completed.

During later childhood, children become capable of performing in a relatively individual, autonomous, and independent manner. A few limitations in relation to size, strength, sexual immaturity, and economic dependence influence total capacity. As these developmental accomplishments begin to emerge or become possible during adolescence, children begin to desire increasing independence from the ties that identified them as children, and they seek entry into the adult world. In cultures and societies where immediate or rapid entry into adult living is possible, adolescence as a stage of behavioral development does not occur. Entry into adult living and responsibility has been increasingly delayed in technological, Western cultures, and adolescence has become an important and difficult stage of development unlike any that precedes or follows.[28]

There is ample evidence indicating that the complex problems and tasks of this period of life are not caused by the physical and sexual changes that occur at puberty. There has been speculation that behavioral turmoil of adolescence is related to a period of physiologic instability created by the massive changes that are taking place in the system. However, studies have failed to demonstrate physiologic instability. There is a change in many of the functions of the body, but the transition appears to be relatively gradual, with little fluctuation for one individual from day to day.[83] These changes may become a significant factor involved in the problems for a given adolescent, but the changes do not cause the upheaval, the behavior changes, or the struggles that are observed and felt.[30,40,47,60]

Social attitudes toward adolescence and the cultural definition of the role of the individual during this period of life have created the multiple circumstances that cause this stage of development to be what it is in Western societies.[59,75] We shall seek to explore each of the major factors that influence the individual, and discuss the meaning of these factors in relation to health maintenance.

## SCIENTIFIC BASES FOR DEVELOPMENT DURING ADOLESCENCE

The study of adolescence has led to both confusion and understanding. Where confusion predominates, we shall attempt to consider several points of view and encourage further exploration of the problem. Where understanding seems to have emerged, we will consider evidence that provides this confidence.

### Developmental physiology

The significant surge in growth and development that occurs during the early adolescent years and the variety of physiologic and behavioral changes, including the attainment of sexual function, provide visible evidence of the child's transition into adult physical capacity.

#### Changes related to the reproductive and neuroendocrine systems

At the point of life when physical changes begin to occur that lead to the development of reproductive function, the levels of estrogen and testosterone production gradually increase. These hormones are thought to be involved in the stimulation of accompanying growth acceleration, but the exact nature of this involvement is not clear. They do not appear to be necessary for growth to occur, but they are essential for the development of secondary sex characteristics, such as the typical broadening of the shoulders and increased muscle mass for boys and widening of the hips for girls. The differential distribution of adipose tissue in girls and boys is also a significant part of the changes that occur at this point.

It has become clear in recent years that the onset of puberty is controlled by neural regulatory function. This phenomenon is viewed as resulting from a series of maturational events that follow a complex sequential schedule involving several brain areas. The hypothalamus, which is sensitive to the circulating levels of gonadotropin hormones, is involved in the feedback mechanisms controlling their release. However, this area is also subject to influence from the higher centers of the central nervous system. The limbic system, which forms a rim around the brain stem, has been studied with particular attention to the phenomena of the onset of puberty. It appears that a particular structure within the limbic system, the amygdala, exerts an inhibitory effect on the production of the gonadotropins throughout childhood. While these hormones remain at a very low level in the prepubertal periods, the structures involved in their production and release appear mature and capable of releasing a substantial amount of hormonal material. The amygdala, through some mechanisms not completely understood, appears to inhibit the release of these hormones until puberty. At this point the amygdala appears to change in activity and function. The main pathways of relay between the amygdala and the hypothalamus become functional, and the threshold for the mature feedback pattern of hormonal production begins (see Chapter 4). Low levels of estrogen and testosterone during maturity stimulate the function of the pituitary and production of FSH and LH. It is thought that this function does not occur in response to low estrogen and testosterone levels during the prepubertal period, either because of a higher threshold of hypothalamus sensitivity to circulating hormonal levels or because an inhibitory compound prevents FSH and LH production until puberty.[52,83] One of the problems that remains controversial is that of the initial phenomenon that occurs at the onset of puberty. Whether increased hormonal production is a primary or a secondary event in the beginning of reproductive function remains obscure.

In addition to the effects and changes occurring in sex hormones, other endocrine functions are known to contribute to the changes of puberty. Again, the exact mechanisms are not known, and the role of each of these functions is not clearly understood. They appear to affect either general, nonspecific growth and development or to act directly on brain maturation. Adrenocorticotropin hormone (ACTH), growth hormone, and thyroid appear to directly affect brain maturation and are known to affect the onset of reproductive function.

The effects of the estrogens, progesterone, and testosterones during puberty are externally observed in the appearance of secondary sex characteristics. The changes that occur in reproductive structures, as well as changes in distribution of body hair and adipose tissue occur in a defined sequence. As with all areas of development, the rate and time of occurrence are highly variable. Girls ordinarily begin the changes of puberty between the ages of 10 and 14 years; boys between the ages of 12 and 16 years. A world-wide trend in recent years toward earlier onset of puberty, as well as persistent geographic differences in the age of onset, is part of a complex phenomenon that has stimulated a great deal of study. The effects of relative exposure to daylight, altitude, season of birth, genetic inheritance, and differences in nutrition are a few of the factors that have been investigated in relation to the age of onset of puberty. The

issue remains complex, and evidence supporting one point of view is not consistent enough to draw definitive conclusions.[34,72,80,83]

The stages of development of secondary sexual characteristics are summarized in Table 14-1. These changes occur for girls over a period of time ranging from 1.5 to 8 years and for boys over a time period ranging from 1.8 to 4.7 years.[52,57,58] Delay in initiation of the first stage of puberty beyond the seventeenth or eighteenth years is unusual and requires thorough investigation.

The beginning of reproductive capacity is heralded by the onset of menstruation for girls and the beginning of seminal emissions for boys. Menstruation is initially irregular and may not be accompanied by ovulation for several months. It first occurs about two years after the first appearance of secondary sex characteristics and after the peak height velocity. A critical weight of 48 kg has been associated with menarche.[18,33] Seminal emissions occur spontaneously and independently of sexual stimulation and may take place at periodic intervals of approximately two weeks. Mature spermatozoa

**Table 14-1.** Developmental stages of secondary sex characteristics*

| Stage | Male genital development | Pubic hair development | Female breast development | Other changes |
|---|---|---|---|---|
| 1 | Prepuberty | Prepuberty; hair over the pubic area similar to that on the abdomen | Prepuberty; increased pigmentation of the papilla only | |
| 2 | Initial enlargement of the scrotum and testes; reddening and texture changes of the scrotum | Sparse growth of long, straight, downy hair at the base of the penis or along the labia | Enlargement of areolar diameter; small area of elevation around the papillae | Usual time of peak height velocity for girls |
| 3 | Initial enlargement of the penis; further growth of testes and scrotum | Hair becomes darker, more coarse and curly; spreads sparsely over the entire pubic area | Further elevation and enlargement of breasts and areolas, with no separation of the contours | Usual point of onset of menstruation. Facial hair begins to grow and voice deepens for boys |
| 4 | Further enlargement of the penis and testes and scrotum; growth in breadth and development of the glans | Further spread of hair distribution not extending to the thighs | Areolas and papillae project from the breast to form a secondary mound | Usual time of peak height velocity for boys; axillary hair begins to grow |
| 5 | Adult in size and contour | Adult in amount and type | Adult, with projection of the papillae only; recession of the areolas into the general breast contour | |

*As defined by Tanner, J. M.: Growth at adolescence, ed. 2, Oxford, 1962, Blackwell Scientific Publications, Ltd.

may not be produced for several months.

Sexual desire in young adolescents is under the domination of the cortex. There are significant differences in the early development of sexual desire for girls and boys, which interact with cultural and family expectations for sexual performance to produce the particular behavior that is usual for boys or girls in a given society. Physiologically, girls who have reached reproductive maturity experience a pleasing sensation, which is generalized in reaction, to mild sexual stimulation arising from cognitive processes. The feeling is not usually localized to the genital area, although engorgement of the vulva and erection of the clitoris occur. Physical stimulation such as kissing or petting produce further generalized and localized sensations, but the desire for coitus is not necessarily present. As the girl matures sexually, the desire for coitus increases, but the fulfillment of female physical sexuality involves a long development sequence including coitus, achievement of pregnancy, lactation, and final involution at the menopause.

The adolescent boy, by contrast, experiences a localized sensation centered about his genitalia. Arousal in response to cognitive stimulation creates some response, and physical contact stimulates the production of spermatozoa and the abundant flow of secretions from the accessory glands. These secretions build up pressure and tension that excite the ejaculatory reflex, and the boy is stimulated to seek relief by ejaculation; thus the desire for coitus is stronger than that felt by the young adolescent girl. Physical sexuality for boys is primarily centered upon the fulfillment of the sex act, although developmental changes in desires and behavior occur throughout life. The resulting differences in sexual interests, concerns, and behavior are attributable at least in part to this basic physiologic difference.[80,84]

### Structural tissues

Several physiologic changes that occur related to the reproductive changes have been mentioned. Growth in skeletal size, muscle mass, adipose tissue, and skin is particularly significant during the adolescent period. The fact that differential growth in these systems occurs

between girls and boys indicates that the sex hormones may play a significant role in stimulating and regulating this growth; however, evidence supporting this effect is controversial.[80,83] The genetic inheritance that renders an individual male or female probably carries influences other than hormonal that regulate and control the differential development during puberty.

Skeletal growth differences between boys and girls are illustrated by the typical increased length in legs and arms for boys in relation to trunk size. This relatively greater length is thought to arise from the prolonged prepubertal growth period of boys, along with accelerated limb growth relative to trunk growth during these years. In addition, boys develop greater shoulder width, a difference that occurs primarily during the pubertal growth spurt. Ossification of the skeletal system is not completed for boys until late adolescence or early adulthood. Ossification for girls is more advanced throughout childhood and is completed at an earlier period during adolescence. Estrogen influences ossification and early unity of the epiphyses with the shafts of long bones, leading to the shorter stature of these structures in girls.[33,37,83]

Muscle growth occurs during late adolescence for boys, but no appreciable change in muscle size occurs for girls beyond what is proportionate to growth in other supportive tissue. The presence of androgens seems to be directly related to the increased muscle mass. Adipose tissue distribution, on the other hand, occurs predominantly for girls. Particular deposition over the thighs, buttocks, and breasts results in the contour that is characteristic of the mature female figure.[37,62,69,83]

Changes in the skin are particularly significant during the adolescent years. At puberty there is a rapid acceleration in growth and maturation of skin and all of its structures. The hair distribution of the body changes, with some characteristics common to both boys and girls. Axillary and pubic hair grows as described in Table 14-1. Boys experience a generalized increase in body hair, particularly facial hair. Boys' body hair tends to become more coarse and dense in distribution, depending partially upon genetic endowment. Androgens appear to affect the distribution of body hair, stimulating increases in all areas of the body except the scalp. Baldness occurs as an interaction between a genetic factor and the presence of testosterone.[84]

The sebaceous glands become extremely active during puberty. These glands, located primarily on the face, scalp, and genitals, increase in size and production. Acne results from an abnormal amount of sebum and keratin (a byproduct of the epidermis) within a dilated sebaceous gland.[84] Some degree of acne is expected and within normal limits during adolescence; problems in relation to this condition are discussed in Chapter 15.

The eccrine sweat glands become fully functional during puberty, with boys developing a greater functional capacity than girls. The response of these glands to emotional stimulation is particularly increased. Sweating in response to psychic or thermal stimuli differs in body location. Emotional stimuli produce sweat on the palms and soles and axillae. Thermal conditions produce sweat on the forehead, neck, trunk, extremities, and finally the axillae.[84]

Apocrine sweat glands, which remain nonfunctional throughout the prepuberty years, begin to secrete during puberty. These glands develop in relation to hair follicles and occur in the axillae, genital and anal areas, external auditory canals, around the umbilicus, and around the areola of the breasts. Apocrine sweat is produced continuously and stored, and is released onto the skin in response to emotional stimuli only. The secretion is odorless when it reaches the surface of the skin but contains fats that are acted upon by skin bacteria and produce characteristic odors.[84]

### Cardiovascular system

Cardiovascular function undergoes significant changes during adolescence. For girls, this change is specifically associated with menarche and occurs somewhat earlier than the same change in boys. For both boys and girls the increase in size and strength of the heart and the increase in blood volume account for the functional changes. The systolic pressure increases significantly because of a greater basal stroke volume (the amount of blood pumped out of each ventricle with each beat). The pulse pressure increases, and the pulse rate per minute decreases. Pulse rate may show a transient increase during the period of peak rate of height growth. The differential changes that occur for boys and girls produce the characteristic adult differences in pulse rate, blood pressure, and body temperature. Girls establish a pulse rate that is about 10% higher than boys, a lower systolic pressure, and a higher basal body temperature. These characteristic differences have been attributed to differences in size and strength of the heart and/or differences arising from the genetic or sexual endowment.[83]

### Formed elements of the blood

Hematopoietic function is affected by the changes of adolescence and is known to be dependent upon the sex hormones. Androgens are known to stimulate the process of erythropoiesis, either by direct stimulation of erythropoietin or by potentiating the action of erythropoietin. For girls, erythropoiesis depends upon a proper ratio of estrogen and progesterone, but the effects of each of these hormones are not understood. It is speculated that estrogens block the action of erythropoietin through some unknown mechanism and that progesterone antagonizes this depressant effect. The observed outcome of these hormonal effects includes a gradual rise in hemoglobin and red blood cells for both boys and girls at puberty, with the increase continuing for boys throughout adolescence and resulting in an average higher red blood cell volume (measured clinically as the hematocrit). The hemoglobin level likewise becomes higher for boys than for girls.

There is some suggestion that total muscle mass is related to some of these differences, since it is observed that blood volume is increased in persons with larger proportionate amounts of muscle regardless of sex. However, red cell volume per body weight is consistently increased in men when the muscle/fat ratio is equivalent as far as can be determined with the methods presently available to study these parameters. The sedimentation rate, or the amount of time required for erythrocytes to sink in a mass in a volume of drawn blood, reaches

**553**

adult values at puberty and is higher for girls than for boys.[83]

White blood cells also change with the onset of adolescence. Adult values are reached early in adolescence, with characteristic differences between boys and girls developing at this time of change. Each type of white blood cells gradually decreases in number, and platelets increase. Girls reach an average greater number of platelets than do boys.

### Respiratory system

Since respiratory function is under neural and chemical regulation, changes at adolescence are primarily related to increased maturation of the specific nervous structures involved in regulatory control. Sex differences that develop at adolescence are related to differences in structural size and volume. Boys gain relatively greater shoulder width and chest size, resulting in a greater respiratory volume (amount of air inspired per minute), greater vital capacity (maximal expiration following maximal inspiration), greater maximum breathing capacity (volume breathed during a 15-second period when breathing as fast and deeply as possible), and increased inspiratory and expiratory flow rate (rate of air flow at 40 respirations per minute). These functions increase for both boys and girls to a greater extent at puberty than at any other point in life since infancy, with the function in boys becoming greater than that for girls.

The composition of inspired and expired air also begins to manifest sex differences at puberty. These differences are probably related to size and structural increases for boys, since the differences become insignificant when adjustments are made for body size regardless of sex. Percentage of oxygen decreases and carbon dioxide increases in expired air for both boys and girls, but to a greater extent for boys.

### Fluids and electrolytes

The changes that occur in fluids and electrolytes during adolescence reflect the changes in body composition in terms of proportionate bone, muscle, and adipose tissues. Thus the differences between boys and girls are related to the relative differences in body composition. The percentage of body water gradually declines during childhood until adult levels are reached during adolescence. Boys and girls remain essentially similar in percentages until the changes in body composition occur, and then boys reach fluid composition of about 60% of total body weight (reflecting a relatively greater percentage of muscle tissue), and girls reach an average of about 50% of total body weight in water (reflecting the relatively larger percent of body fat). Renal capacity in response to fluid and electrolyte stress becomes fully mature as the endocrine systems mature.

Extracellular fluid volume and total exchangeable sodium and chloride are relatively high at birth and decline throughout childhood. The adult levels are reached early in adolescence, representing about 20% of total body weight (see Table 8-2). Intracellular fluid and total body potassium, on the other hand, rise gradually over the childhood years, with a brief decline between the eighth and twelfth years, and then once again rise with the onset of adolescence. This pattern of change reflects the growth rate of muscle tissue during the childhood and adolescent years; muscle tissue contains a high percentage of water, and maturation demands increasing levels of potassium for increased function. Thus boys have about a 15% greater potassium concentration over the normal level for girls.

### Metabolic rate and response to exercise

The adolescent reaches full adult capacity in relation to chemical and energy transformations as body size, structure, and function reach maturity. The basal metabolic rate in a resting state slowly declines throughout life, with boys having a consistently higher metabolic rate than girls. The sex difference is thought to be a function of androgenic steroids throughout life rather than the difference in muscle mass and strength. Given equivalent muscle mass, boys continue to exhibit higher metabolic rates and higher oxygen consumption levels. At adolescence there appears to be a transient arrest in decline or rise in basal metabolic function, which is thought to result from the rapid growth and physiologic changes.

Physical stress and exercise responses change significantly during adolescence as adult capacity is reached. For the first time the child has the ability to adapt to strain or stress equal to or in excess of that of the adult. This capacity is primarily a function of change in size and strength, but it also depends upon the increased capacity of specific structures involved in a given task. For example, the child can begin to run with increasing speed and stamina because of the increase in muscle size and strength, particularly in the legs. This ability is also due to increased capacity of the lungs and accompanying structures, which serve to restore oxygen to the tissues after intensive exertion and to facilitate recovery of normal function once the exercise is over. Heart rate, respiratory rate, reflexive shunting of blood from resting to working muscles, blood pressure, and electrolyte and fluid responses are a few of the many varied and complex reactions reaching full capacity in responding to exercise. The rate of recovery after exercise has been used as a parameter to measure physical fitness, but standardized measures of this function that give a meaningful index of fitness are difficult to obtain.

Adolescence and young adulthood are periods of life when physical capacity is at its height of development; thereafter, the ability to sustain strain and stress and to recover following exercise gradually decreases. Exercise is known to improve the general status of health, endurance, and appearance during these years of maximal function, but the effects on the quality of health and longevity of life during later years is not known.[37,59,83]

### Central nervous system

Neural regulation of endocrine function has been discussed. Further changes in neural function occur that affect all systems and the ability to function at full adult capacity. Myelination is considered to have developed in all areas by the age of about 2 years but apparently continues throughout adolescence and into the middle adult years in some structures of the central nervous system, particularly in the reticular formation and the greater cerebral commissures.[83,88] There is some suggestion that the sex hormones stimulate myelination processes during adolescence.[83] The precise difference in function that is possible with advanced development of the myelination process is not clear. Once the sheath is sufficiently formed to allow for intact, rapid nerve conduction, there are presently no means of measuring differences in quality of function that occur as myelination develops. Increased fine motor control functions and intellectual capacity that develop as a result of practice and learning may be related to further development of the myelin sheath.

Brain tissue appears to reach qualitative maturity at about the time that sexual maturity is achieved.[83] Regulatory and functional changes of the brain at puberty are known to exist but have been impossible to study in detail. Because the neurologic changes of the first six years are rapid and easily demonstrated in the child's motor, language, sensory, thought, and social performance, this early period has been studied much more thoroughly than other developmental stages. The functional changes that occur between later childhood, adolescence, and adulthood are exceedingly difficult to quantify and measure. They occur very gradually, and many are subtle to the extent that they are not recognized. For example, the young school-age child's ability to execute the fine motor task of handwriting is very different from that of the adult and differences in adolescent and adult performance may be detected, but the basic ability is present throughout this period. Identifying, quantifying, and measuring the changes in this ability have not been pursued in relation to neural function. It is speculated that this change reflects maturation of the central nervous system, but it is not known whether measuring and studying such capacities in these periods of life would be helpful in interpreting the quality of performance, capability, or living.

## Behavioral and personality development
### Piaget's theory of cognitive development

To consider the changes that take place in the cognitive abilities of the child, we return to the theory of Jean Piaget, which was considered in Chapters 9, 10, and 12. It should be remembered that Piaget's theoretical stages are typified by the ability that most recently emerges. Children who have entered the formal operations period begin to use more mature thought patterns, but they will not always do so. By the age of 15 years, children of adequate intellectual ability will have begun to demonstrate the ability to think in the ways that Piaget describes, but they may continue to use concrete operations to a significant degree.

In addition, we are considering a theory of cognitive development that is one scientist's proposition about reality. It provides one of several ways of representing reality and has been used to organize and develop investigations that are intended to provide further understanding of the children and their thought patterns. While some of the ideas may seem valid to the reader, it should be remembered that many possibilities yet exist and that these relatively new ideas remain to be fully tested.

The early part of adolescence, ages 11 through 15 years, is the period when Piaget's formal operations begin. Thought processes develop into mature, adultlike patterns, with specific traits that allow for adult accomplishments in thinking. Piaget believes that development evolves as a result of the maturation of the cerebral structures. The main feature of this period of thought is the fact that children can enter into the world of possibilities beyond the world of reality. They are able to think beyond the present and to consider things that do not exist but that might be. This type of thinking involves real logic and an organized, consistent approach to thinking. The term "formal" is used by Piaget to represent the fact that children at this stage of cognitive development center upon the "form" of thought, objects, and experiences rather than upon the exact content. Children in the period of concrete operations respond to things about them with a number of structures for organizing and ordering but always in relation to what is reality for them—what is readily available to perception. Adolescents, by contrast, respond in a way that indicates a far greater range of possibilities for thinking, for problem-solving, and for decision-making.

The young person develops a concept of relativity in approaching problems by means of two accomplishments. These are the application of hypotheses, or propositional statements, and the use of implications. In applying these newly formed abilities, adolescents make reality secondary to possibility. Thus, in a sense, they combine certain traits of cognition from earlier periods of life. They are capable of the fantastic flights from reality that are typical of the preoperational period and yet order their ideational material in a manner similar to organizational patterns used for sensory reality in the operational periods. Reality is recognized but becomes only a subset of many other possibilities. As these patterns of thought emerge, adolescents are observed to be extremely idealistic, to constantly challenge the way things are, and to consider the way things could be or ought to be. They may totally discard what is. During this early part of the formal operations period, young people return to a kind of egocentrism in thinking. Their propositions and flights from reality allow them to see themselves as omnipotent and to bring reality in line with their own thinking. While this trait may be irritating to others, it is a necessary stage into formal operational thinking. Once this has been mastered, young people can move on into more fully mature thought patterns that make use of the propositional, organized approach but that take into account more fully the social and cosmic universe to which they are applied.

In solving a problem, young people in the formal operations period can try out a variety of solutions in their minds without having to actually manipulate materials. They can operate solely through symbolism. They can even hold several relevant variables constant while they systematically manipulate one and hypothesize about the outcome under each condition. This approach is the classic method of experimental science, but young people rarely realize that they are using it with such sophistication.

A typical experiment that contrasts concrete operational thought and formal operational thought illustrates the refinement in thinking that emerges in problem-solving. The child is presented with a bucket of water and several different objects that are small enough to fit into the bucket. He or she is then asked to classify the objects according to whether or not they will float and to explain the basis of classification. After the initial explanation, the child is encouraged to experiment with the materials and to explain the cases that do not follow his or her predictions and is further encouraged to look for a law that will tie all floating objects together.

The child who is in the preoperational period applies arbitrary predictions and explanations for each separate object without becoming concerned when the predictions do not apply. The concrete operational child makes arbitrary predictions, based on common properties, such as size or weight, but becomes troubled when predictions do not hold true. The child then begins to look for ways in which he or she can classify objects that will provide adequate predictions for the remaining objects. For example, the child notices that certain large objects (block of wood) float and certain small objects (nail) sink. The child then begins to determine that size is not relevant and turns to another category, such as weight. Some sort of classification system is created that predicts that some objects will float, some will sink, and some are not predictable. The child's eagerness to solve the problem leads to additional confusion, and he or she is unable to follow a solution to a successful end because of the limitations in escaping from the absolute, real qualities that are observable by the senses.

During the formal operational period, on the other hand, young people can reach an accurate conclusion. It may be stated in very unsophisticated terms, but the ideas that they propose are systematically applied to each of the objects until they find one that consistently predicts the ability of all objects to float. They may identify the fact that wood floats because it has air spaces between the spaces of wood. Steel objects are more solid, without any air spaces. They may then be able to conclude that weight and volume are interacting variables that determine the ability of an object to float. They may not fully solve the problem and arrive at the notions of density or specific gravity, but they provide reasonable hypotheses for solving the problems, test them, discard those that are not valid, and try new ones. If contradictions occur, they are able to recognize them and proceed to untangle the confusion or discard those aspects of their thinking that lead to confusion.[63]

When presented with an argument, young people in the formal operations period are able to respond to the form of the argument and disregard the content. For example, consider the following sentence: "I am very glad that I do not like spinach, for if I liked it, I would always be eating it and I hate eating unpleasant things." The formal operations person is capable of responding to the logical inconsistency of the statement while ignoring the content. The concrete operations child, on the other hand, responds to the content of the statement.[63,64,65]

This cognitive capacity is very significant for the emergence of mature moral values and attitudes. Piaget has contributed a great deal to understanding morality development in children (see Chapter 12). Young people begin to develop a new type of morality through their newly acquired social and ideational position in thinking. Objects become relative in terms of appropriate usage. Properties of objects become relevant according to the demands of the situation. The value of objects is seen as being entirely explained by human value systems. Young people become engrossed in weighing, classifying, reevaluating, organizing, and examining different social points of view without actually committing themselves to any one of them. This cognitive experimentation may be thought of as resembling the imitation aspect of development that was typical of the preoperational child. The mental thought processes are used to imitate, in a sense, another person's attitude or behavior without the intention of adopting it and without the necessity of actually acting out the behavior. This also allows the person to deal with intangible experiences, such as religion, philosophy, lawmaking, and theory-building.

Thus young people are able to develop a more mature notion of morality. They can reason beyond the cause and effect of a situation and can take into account many aspects of a situation to determine their rightness or wrongness. When presented with a problem involving two children who disagree over taking turns with a single toy, the concrete operational child would only be able to think in terms of realistic cause-and-effect aspects of the situation, such as who had the toy first. Although the formal operations young person might finally solve the problem in this manner, he or she is capable of considering many aspects of the situation from each child's point of view and of reaching a decision based on the larger context. This is termed judgment by implication. One important aspect of implication becomes the issue of intentionality. This is illustrated in the definition of lying that emerges during the formal operations period. Rather than judging a statement as a falsehood based on some code of true and false, the young person begins to define anything that is intentionally false as a lie because of its intentional aspect. Thus a statement that does not represent the truth may result from misinformation, no information, or intentional falsehood. Only the latter is considered a lie.

Justice becomes a greatly expanded concept during this period of development. The young person begins to define justice in terms of equality for all. Wrong-doing is not simply a matter to be punished, but rather it is an event to be examined and explored from the point of view of all concerned. Punishment of a group in order to punish unknown offenders, an acceptable approach earlier in childhood, now becomes viewed as injustice to the innocent of the group.

For Piaget, the period of formal operations results in a final accomplishment of equilibrium because of four major cognitive processes that develop. These are:

1. The social world is conceptualized as an organic unit that has its laws and regulations and its division of roles and social functions.
2. Egocentricity is "dissolved" by a sense of "moral solidarity," which is consciously cultivated by the young person.
3. Development throughout the remainder of life becomes dependent upon an exchange of ideas by social intercommunication in place of simple mutual imitation.
4. A sense of equality supersedes submission to adult authority.[64]

### Social development concept of Coleman

While social and inner development are intimately interdependent, there are aspects of each that present special concerns, and thus we will discuss them as separate entities. The reader should remember that in reality no aspect of competency development is separable from the others, and the theories that we consider will emphasize this point.

Social development in Western societies has emerged as a special consideration in terms of the adolescent individual. It has long been recognized that this is a period of final preparation

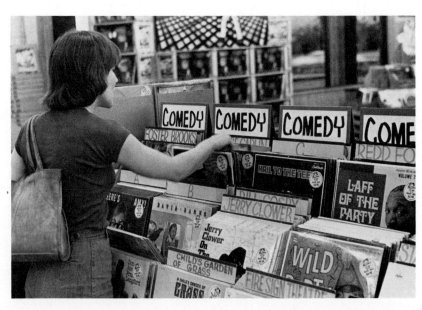

**Fig. 14-1.** The adolescent has become a very important economic consumer.

for the assumption of adult roles, but the increasing importance of the social experience of the adolescent has drawn a considerable amount of attention.[13,32] Coleman[13] has identified five factors in American culture that have led to the development of an "adolescent society." These factors affect the major social developmental tasks of adolescents, and are as follows:

1. A mutual lack of communication and understanding between adolescents and their parents has developed, because of the extremely rapid changes in society that have left gaps in skills, knowledge, and values of the two generations.

2. Adolescents no longer receive vocational training from the family or parents. They must begin this endeavor on their own, leaving no personal relationship to the way of life of the family.

3. Adolescents are no longer essential in providing income for the family. The family is thus not obligated to teach young people many of the skills that are essential for maintaining economic independence.

4. Adolescents have become very important economic consumers. Without being expected to provide a source of income, they are seen commercially as an important market for such commodities as entertainment, clothing, cosmetics, food, and automobiles.

5. The school includes a much wider range and variety of adolescents than ever before, because of compulsory school attendance. Thus the range of opportunities for social interaction are greatly enhanced.

### Lewin's Field Theory

The theory of Kurt Lewin discussed in Chapter 12 is useful in understanding the influence of social factors upon the adolescent. These factors may be thought of as regions of the life space during adolescence. They tend to exert a strong influence on the behavior of the adolescent, and they interact with internal developmental processes to produce the observed behavior. For example, we shall consider in following sections adolescents' inner needs to become independent and autonomous from the family. The extent to which mutual communica-

tion and understanding between adolescents and families are possible influences the way in which adolescents will be able to accomplish this inner need.

Lewin[54] considered adolescence in particular in relation to his theoretical proposition and identified three factors in a young person's life space that create adolescent behavior typical of Western societies. These factors are:

1. Expansion of the psychologic field, with a new degree of freedom of movement within the life space. Young people are able to come and go with fewer restrictions. They acquire machinery to enhance mobility and form associations in increased numbers of areas.

2. A "marginal person" status in relationship to childhood and adult groups, in that they do not appropriately belong to either group and experience conflicts between the attitudes, values, ideologies, and styles of living of each group. Adolescents are caught between the two groups. In one situation they apply codes of

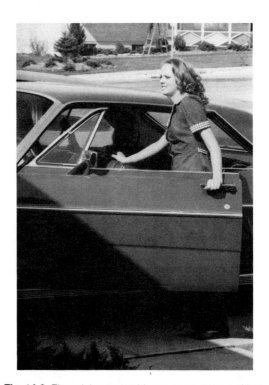

**Fig. 14-2.** The adolescent achieves a new degree of freedom of movement within his or her life space.

justice, logic, or problem-solving traits of the child. In another instance they adopt those of the adult. Likewise, they are treated in ambivalent ways by those around them.

3. Biologically determined changes in the life space as a result of the body changes. Young people appear physically neither as adults nor children. They experience rapid body changes requiring the creation of a new body image several times throughout adolescence.

For Lewin the type of adolescent behavior that emerges is directly dependent upon the strengths of these forces of the life space.[54]

### Adler's social-psychologic theory

The influence of adolescent peer group and subculture is incompletely understood, since this cultural development is a relatively new phenomenon. However, some aspects have been clarified even though there has not yet developed a unified frame of conceptual or theoretical propositions that provide adequate predictions of adolescent behavior and development. The social-psychologic theory of Alfred Adler provides some ideas about personality that appear to have special relevance to the study of adolescence, although this was not the original intention for the theory.[62]

One of the central concepts developed by Adler is that of fictional finalism, or subjective expectations for the future held by an individual. It is these future-oriented notions that motivate people and shape present behavior. These are not part of a predestined or teleologic design, but rather are the inner strivings and hopes that an individual creates for himself or herself. Past experience may influence the person's formulation of goals, but it is no longer important in understanding the basis for behavior. This particular function of the personality, when considered in relation to Piaget's proposition of cognitive capacity of the adolescent, becomes very important for the individual at this stage in life.

Another concept of Adler's theory is that of striving for superiority. This is thought of as a striving for completion or for self-actualization; it is not to be confused with seeking a competitive sort of social position. Each person achieves this completion in a slightly different way. For

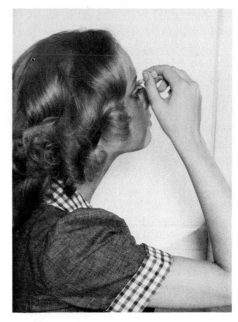

**Fig. 14-3.** Adolescents must reconstruct their body images and adjust to biologic changes.

Adler, the individual who is not healthy strives toward esteem in the eyes of others, power, and self-aggrandizement in seeking personal completion. The healthy individual, on the other hand, seeks completion through goals that are primarily social in character.

The concept of inferiority feelings and compensation further clarifies Adler's notion of striving for superiority. Individual experience feelings of inferiority as they strive for completeness, because they recognize that they have not reached the goal of completeness. These feelings of incompleteness represent a need to overcome inferiority and a desire to reach completion and provide an impetus for action. When these factors are in balance, people have a healthy capacity to adapt and adjust in reaching the goals that they have determined for themselves. When feelings of inferiority are excessive, they suffer from disability that prevents healthy striving.

When these factors of the individual are considered in relation to Adler's concept of social interest, the particular application of his ideas to the social development of the adolescent begins to emerge. Social interest is the true and inevitable compensation for all the individual natural weaknesses of human beings. It involves such dynamic processes as cooperation, interpersonal and social relations, identification with the group, and empathy. Individuals are never able to completely reach the fictional goals that they project for the future, but through the group they are able in some manner to fulfill many of them. People are embedded in a social framework that influences and shapes their lives from the beginning. By learning to work toward a common goal, individuals may compensate for many of their own weaknesses that prevent them from perfect goal attainment. Adler believes that people are innately social in nature. They will strive for social goals that transcend their own, because the satisfaction of social goals is more completely realized and rewarded. This social capacity, while innate, must be nurtured and guided throughout development in order for it to be used by the individual to its fullest capacity. Thus one of Adler's central professional involvements was in the establishment of child guidance clinics, improving education of children, and helping parents to develop child-rearing practices that are indicated by his theoretical propositions.[2]

The concept of life-style is a distinctive and pervasive aspect of Adler's theoretical statements. This is perhaps one of the most influential and far-reaching ideas that Adler proposed. It is the system principle by which the individual functions. It is the single unique feature of a person's life that distinguishes his or her life from those of others. The people behave, the way they strive toward completion, the goals that they identify for the future, and their attitudes and feelings are all determined by their life-styles. For Adler this feature of the personality is formed very early in life, by about the age of 4 or 5 years. From that point onward, everything the individual learns, feels, perceives, or does reflects the individual style of life. All things that do not fit the life-style the person ignores and discards.

The creative self is a concept that Adler proposed to explain how the individual's life-style comes into existence. For Adler, the self is the prime mover, creatively dictating all else that happens. People construct their own personality out of their own heredity and experience. During the early part of life, this prime mover is responsible for the creation of the life-style. Thereafter, the self operates within the context of the life-style to further develop the personality from the added experiences of life. Heredity gives the individual abilities, environment gives the impressions. How the individual simultaneously interprets and experiences these factors is a function of the creative self.[5,39]

Although Adler focused upon early childhood experiences in the unfolding of the person, his ideas provide useful insights in relation to the adolescent. Young people have previously established personality traits and life-styles and now possess many adult capabilities. Yet they are not independent and autonomous and must fit into the social world. As they begin to formulate goals for the future that include the peer group rather than the primary family, they must make a significant transition. If, indeed, the idea of social interest exists as an innate quality of human motivation, the adolescent's need for recognition, achievement, and accomplishment through the group may be viewed as a significant factor in development of this dimension. Through the creative self, adolescents learn to identify personally meaningful goals for the future that are relevant in relation to other people and that achieve benefit for the greater good of the group. Individuals must succeed in relation to the group in order to achieve compensation for their individual weaknesses. The dynamics that lead to the two major departures from achievement of this socialization process of adolescence—alienation or delinquency—may be viewed and studied in terms of some inadequacy or imbalance in the factors that Adler describes.

Adolescent success as a group member may or may not follow peer group success as a school-age child. Several factors have been investigated, apart from any specific theoretical formulation, that seem to be related to the level of group success achieved. Physical maturation and the timing of this event is important for boys. An individual who matures after about age 15 is often considered to be less than adequate by adults and by other adolescents, and the

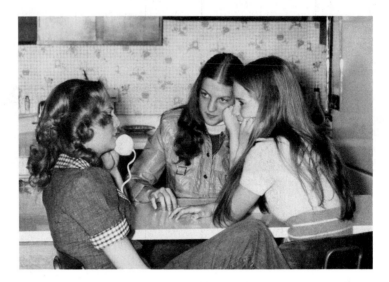

**Fig. 14-4.** Belonging to a clique is the primary means in Western culture for adolescents to make the transition from primary allegiance to the family to a colleague in a peer group.

boy's self-esteem and ability to relate to the group are seriously jeopardized. Such boys are not capable of conveying a good impression on others. They tend to be dependent, less self-controlled, and less responsible than boys who mature at an average age. These effects appear to last into the adult years. Girls, on the other hand, tend to be less influenced by the timing of maturation, with early maturation being a greater handicap than late maturation. The girl who matures early tends to be larger, and she exhibits different interests from those of her peers, especially in relationship to the boys who mature later than girls of the same age.[46]

Belonging to a clique, or specific group that is organized informally, is the primary means in Western societies for adolescents to make the transition from primary allegiance as a child in the family group to a colleague in the peer group. There develops within the group a sense of commonality that follows no set rules or regulations but that demands loyalty and group solidarity. This type of group membership requires that the individual lay aside personal goals and gain in order to achieve what is desired for the group as a whole. Identification with the group is proclaimed through conformity to standards of clothing, behavior, language, and values. This feature of the adolescent subculture persists in spite of the strong inclination in family and social structures toward greater levels of individuation (see Chapter 3). However, the adolescent group is a vehicle for movement out and away from the family unit and, as such, it provides a means of achieving the goals of individuation.

It should be noted that Adler's concept of social interest is a seeming paradox to his concepts of the creative self and the unique individual life-style. For Adler the innate social interest of human beings provides balance and meaning for the individual creative self. He does not advocate a self-centered, hedonistic approach to life, but rather he proposes that the individual who is healthy strives toward socially relevant and meaningful goals, thus achieving a balance between development of the self and development of society. Adolescents appear to be seeking to find the healthy balance. At some points they seem to be totally dedicated to the fulfillment of group goals with no thought of individual uniqueness or future goals. At another point they appear to be totally dedicated to fulfillment of personal goals that have little or no relationship to the group.

## Peer group identity and family alienation

To understand the problems that occur when young people alienate themselves from family and society, we need to explore certain aspects of normal alienation and departure from accepted norms of social behavior that occur during this stage of life in Western societies. This alienation is disturbing to families, to adult members of the community, and to young people themselves. Faced with the need to become autonomous, to achieve sexual function and identity, and to become economically self-sufficient and productive, adolescents must turn away from the family unit. This creates a great deal of anxiety and apprehension, which they do not fully comprehend, but which leads them to perform the acts of leaving the family unit with distorted, ambivalent, and confused behavior. They are not able, at this point in development, to achieve identity as an individual without some degree of alienation and denial of the primary family unit.

Family standards must be rejected to some extent in order to adopt the standards of the peer group. Many adolescents in modern societies discard these standards by rejecting the value, rightness, or desirability of the family expectations. It is not possible to fail in relation to standards that are wrong in the first place. For example, if young people can view their familys' standards of dress as an unworthy or wrong standard, then they are not really failing or violating anything when they do not conform to it.

Another mechanism that may be used to achieve separation from the family unit has arisen from the intellectual class, which has grown in Western societies along with the youth culture. While few youths are intellectual, the development of the two cultures has been significantly related. Many young people reach a higher level of education at an earlier age than did their parents and thus have exceeded their parents' skill, knowledge, and capacity to perform.[60] Because this has often been a desired goal of the parents for their child, a situation arises where the older, more mature adults stand in awe and respect of their young offspring, and an interesting interaction between parents and children evolves. Children often

adopt the approach of the typical "intellectual," viewing as worthy only the most vital aspects of life (as defined by the individual). Simultaneously, they adopt an attitude of derogation toward those who act in more mundane or more routine capacities. Young people adopt an attitude of superiority, which may be fostered by the parents. Because neither the parent nor the young person understands the dynamics of the situation, rejection and lack of communication build until a level of adult maturity and equilibrium is approached by the young person, when rejection of the family does not constitute a threat to individual autonomy.

Another significant problem that has evolved in more recent years concerns the more well-educated parents who hold highly respected social positions. These parents cannot be outstripped in education or in social status, and in fact their offspring may not be able to meet many of their standards for education and achievement. In a society that still places high value upon achievement and status as measured by education and material goods, young people are placed in a position of increasing pressure and conflict. The outcome of this conflict is often alienation (see Chapter 15) and, indeed, an increase in this pattern of adolescent and young adult behavior bears out the fact that social problems in our societies today are great.[59,73,78]

The problems faced by minority group adolescents in the larger society of America are different from those of the Anglo, middle-class teenagers, but many of the outcomes are similar. The social conflicts that arise in the individual's quest for social identity, in achievement of self-completion within society, and in dealing with the pressures of modern living that may exceed their capacity to respond lead to the development of significant social problems for young minority group people.[14,68]

## Erikson's theory of identity

We return once again to the theory of Erik Erikson[25,26] in considering the development of the inner self during adolescence. Erikson has focused upon the problems of development during this period of life more intensely than most personality theorists, and his ideas provide a framework to examine and understand many of the traits of the years of youth. Some of the ideas are similar to those of other theorists, but examining them in the light of Erikson's framework gives additional insight.

The central task of adolescence is the establishment of identity, with the primary risk being identity confusion. Erikson conceptualizes the youth culture that has developed in technological societies as an attempt to establish identity formation. It may appear that the youth creating the culture are involved in a final, rather than a transient or initial, identity formation, but dedication to the adolescent culture provides a means of moving into and through the identity crisis of the period. Through the group, individuals find support and help with the many inner problems of developing a new body image, finding sexual identity, establishing intimacy with the opposite sex, and dealing with the many conflicting possibilities and choices of the present and the future. Erikson views the adolescent clique as a means of testing one's ability to remain constant and loyal in the midst of inevitable conflicts of values.

The adolescent identity crisis involves a restaging of each of the previous stages of development. The stage of infancy, with the development of trust in oneself and others, is again encountered as the adolescent looks intently for people and ideals to have faith in for which one might prove oneself trustworthy. Because young people fear a foolish, strong commitment, they often express their need for faith in insistent and cynical mistrust.

The stage of developing autonomy is reestablished in young people's search for avenues to express their right to will freely. At the same time, they must avoid the hazard of behaving in a manner that would expose them to self-doubt or to ridicule from their friends. They intensify their search for an occupational role through which they can express themselves in an autonomous, freely chosen direction. The accomplishment of this task and the avoidance of shame lead to a rather interesting paradox. Adolescents would rather behave shamelessly in the eyes of their parents than be forced into behavior that would bring ridicule from their peers.

The third stage of life, when a sense of initiative develops, also is reenacted as young people seek identity. Their unlimited imagination over what they might become is tempered only by a sense of guilt over the excessiveness of their ambition. Thus they aspires to great accomplishment at one point, and then loudly denounce themselves for exceeding the possible.

The school-age period of developing a sense of industry is carried into the adolescent period as young people begin to make a choice in occupation. The typical confusion and hesitation in making this choice arise from a fear of entering a career that will not afford them the chance to excel.

The extent to which the earlier tasks were successfully completed or resolved influences adolescents' success in finding an identity. Young people who have primarily experienced success are often very resourceful during adolescence in finding ways of making up a gap that might have been left in earlier stages of development. Erikson believes that when young people feel that society is depriving them of all the

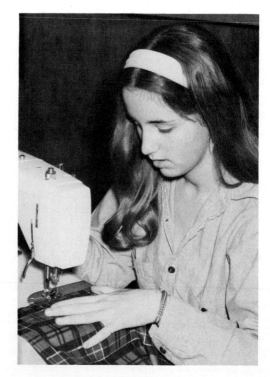

**Fig. 14-5.** Adolescents continue to develop their sense of industry, incorporating increased abilities for creativity.

forms of expression that permit them to integrate the various steps of their previous development, they resist violently and feel forced to defend their development of identity. When the threat of identity confusion is exceedingly great, delinquent or borderline psychotic episodes occur. Such a threat is enhanced by conditions such as a strong previous doubt of one's ethnic and sexual identity, role confusion in the society and family, or longstanding hopelessness in regard to the plight of individuals and society.

Erikson views industrial democracy as posing special problems for the youth of society by insisting on self-made identities that are characterized by strength, tolerance, readiness to take advantages of opportunity, and readiness to adjust to change. Democracy must present its young people with certain ideologies that can be shared by young people of many different backgrounds and subcultures and yet maintain the ideal of freedom of self-realization and freedom of choice. Erikson views these ideologies as a psychologic necessity and as an institution that is the guardian of identity. It is through these ideologies that young people are able to become the creators of the coming society, to effect evolutionary change, and to bind what is relevant from the past with what is relevant in the future.

The pursuit for something to be devoted to and the search for a meaningful ideology often create a puzzling combination of shifting devotion and sudden extremes in action. Erikson views this behavior as an attempt to try out various extremes and to search for some stable principle that might last through the testing of extremes. Individuals seldom have great insight into the dynamics of their behavior, but the testing eventually serves to allow them to settle on a chosen course. These extremes, particularly in a time of ideological confusion and widespread marginality of identity, may include rebellious, deviant, and self-destructive tendencies. Much of Erikson's work has been devoted to finding interpretations of youth behavior cast in relation to the entire life-history of the individual and to thus differentiate behavior that is truly pathologic during adolescence from that which is normal and useful in completing the ages of man.[25,26]

## Carl Rogers' concept of the phenomenal self

The theory of Carl Rogers[70,71] provides another useful framework from which to view the adolescent and the interaction between the inner strivings of the person and the conditions of the environment that promote the achievement of self-identity and healthy development.[62] Rogers' theoretical propositions have stimulated much research, some of which has provided favorable support for his ideas and some of which has not. However, the ideas have provided one the most significant contributions to personality development in the field of humanistic psychology, and they are important because of the positive, personal, and uniquely human approach that is proposed.

Rogers describes several salient human characteristics, which might also be considered his basic assumptions about people. First, people are seen as unique organisms with a specific evolutionary ancestry and development. People are basically social beings, with a tendency to enter into secure, close, communicative relationships. When such a tendency is not exhibited, the person is not healthy, and some means of therapy may be necessary to restore the innate ability of the person to respond to a meaningful human relationship. As a unique organism, persons also exhibit the tendency toward psychologic and physiologic development, differentiation, and maturation. They tend to be self-enhancing and self-preserving, but under favorable circumstances their behaviors tend also to be toward the enhancement of the species.

Human nature is directional. People follow a predictable, directional pathway in the forward thrust toward wholeness and growth. When external conditions are conducive to growth, both psychologic and physiologic, and when the alternatives of movement are known to them, they always choose a direction of growth rather than of regression.

The human tendency toward directional movement may be further described as being toward self-actualization. People move inherently toward the full realization and development of all of their potentialities in ways that tend to maintain or enhance the self and the species. This process of self-actualization involves meeting the basic physiologic needs for food, air, water, and shelter as well as the needs for total organismic experience and fulfillment. Rogers differentiates between the organism and the self. The organism is the locus of experience. The total organismic experience constitutes the total phenomenal field. Portions of the phenomenal field that are symbolized are available to conscious awareness. Those that are not symbolized remain unavailable to awareness, or unconscious.

The self is that portion of the phenomenal field that becomes differentiated as "me." For Rogers, this is the total perception, or gestalt, of all the characteristics of the individual along with all the characteristics of relationships to others and to various aspects of life and the values that are attached to these perceptions. The self is available to awareness, but it may not be totally in awareness. It is a fluid and changing process.

People's experience includes their higher mental functions but is by no means limited to these functions. When people are functioning optimally, they exhibit a certain trust of all areas of reaction, not limiting these to the intellect. Thus people are wiser than their intellect. Rogers describes this phenomenon as the capacity to sense an ongoing process and to respond to inner feelings and processes that may not be totally available to awareness.

Human potentiality for awareness is a significant aspect of their unique existence. The more fully they are able to be aware of their total organismic experience, the more satisfactory is their level of functioning and growth. At the same time, they may use the symbolization and awareness process to deceive themselves and thus behave in an unhealthy fashion. When a situation or event is perceived as potentially threatening to the self, it may be distorted in awareness. People simply cannot see, with accuracy, those experiences, feelings, or reactions that are at variance with their picture of themselves. This results in the development of neurosis, which Rogers describes as the divergence between the meaning of an experience for the organism and the meaning that the conscious mind and self attach to the experience. Rogers

calls this divergence incongruence. When the two experiences are in accord with one another, the person experiences congruence. One of Roger's primary concerns is the discovery of how the self and the organism can achieve greater levels of congruence.

Humans possess a basic need and hunger for a relationship in which they can be totally themselves. In spite of the fact that most cultures are organized on the basis of roles and role status and behavior is largely determined by cultural expectations, people seek relationships that express their full potentiality apart from their societal roles. This relationship was described by Martin Buber as the "I-Thou" relationship and is necessary, as Roger agrees, for continued healthy development throughout life. Such a relationship has no concern for time, practicalities, status, role, or consequences. It is simply the total experiencing of the other person and being experienced by another.

One of the most controversial features of Rogerian theory is his proposition that humans have the capacity for sound choice. To the extent that individuals achieve congruence and learn to rely on their total organismic experience, they will always make a sound choice based on the principle of growth and self-fulfillment, including the principle of species fulfillment. Rogers concedes that this tendency depends upon having available a wide and complex range of accurate data, and that the choices made may not be totally infallible. However, when people are functioning on the level of organismic experience, they are able to make the adjustments in their behavior that would quickly redirect them toward growth. The defects in this process that most humans experience result from including information that does not belong in the present situation or excluding relevant information. When, for example, memories and previous learning are used in the present decision-making process as if they were a real part of the present situation, erroneous decisions result. Past experience is relevant to the present situation only to the extent that it is a real part of the present. One example of this might be the change that takes place in the child's definition of lying that we discussed earlier. Children initially respond to lying based on what their parents and others have told them is absolutely right or wrong. As they mature, they are able to weigh many aspects of the situation and reach a more mature judgment in such a moral issue. If, however, they persist in responding to the memory and previous learning that all statements that are not true are morally wrong, they will not respond adequately to their total organismic experience of the situation and may reach an erroneous conclusion.

People are also conceptualized by Rogers as living subjectively. This means that they cannot successfully objectify themselves. Objectification, or the process of intellectualizing one's personal living, leads to erroneous choices, because of the tendency to respond only to those things that are symbolized and that are thus part of the intellect. In spite of efforts to do this, people cannot succeed, and the very effort leads to a condition of incongruence. People who are developing their full potential live subjectively; they think and feel and experience life as a total human person, not as an object in whom these events occur.

Finally, Rogers sees people as being trustworthy to the extent that they are fully functioning. When they are basically congruent, moving in self-selected directions and choosing responsibility, their actions, behavior, and choices can be trusted. When individuals are given even an imperfect opportunity to grow toward self-fulfillment, they tend to grow and move toward self-actualization and to leave behind the negative human traits of brutality, cruelty, deceit, defensiveness, and abnormality.

We have referred several times to conditions that promote growth. Rogers has defined these from his experiences in developing a specific counseling approach known as client-centered therapy. However, the traits of a growth-producing relationship extend to any form of counseling or therapy and include any human relationship, such as the parent-child, teacher-child, or friend-friend relationship. These conditions are:

1. Two persons must be in psychologic contact.
2. One of the persons is in a state of relative incongruence.
3. The other person is relatively congruent, or integrated, in the relationship.
4. The congruent person experiences unconditional positive regard for the other person.
5. The congruent person also experiences empathic understanding for the other person's internal frame of reference or phenomenal field.
6. The incongruent person is able to sense the unconditional positive regard and the empathic understanding of the other person.

Two new concepts, unconditional positive regard and empathic understanding, have been introduced in relation to the necessary conditions for growth and change. Rogers conceptualizes unconditional positive regard as being a warm acceptance of the other person's phenomenal field as it exists for the other person. There are no conditions of acceptance and no selective evaluative attitudes toward the person. The individual is sensed as being totally acceptable. Moral value judgments, which might be associated with certain aspects of the person, are not considered. All aspects of the person, the unhealthy as well as the healthy, the bad and the good, the immature and the mature, are accepted. The person is valued and cared for because of the self, with the right to possess whatever traits exist for the separate individual. Thus the value and moral judgments of the congruent person are not transferred to the incongruent person, because they are irrelevant and meaningless in relation to that individual. If such values are relevant, they must be the person's own experiences and feelings and not those of another. In a therapeutic relationship of any kind, there is a mixture of conditional and unconditional positive regard, and negative regard. Rogers clarifies this fact by stating that there is a relatively frequent incidence of feelings of unconditional positive regard, with a relative infrequency of conditional positive regard and negative regard.

Empathic understanding is a concept that is closely related to positive regard. The person's feelings, emotions, reactions, impressions, and confusions are sensed as if they were one's own but without losing the "as if" quality of the experience. This leads to a complete understanding of the other person's world, making it possible to enter into the process of symbolizing the other person's world accurately when the other person may not be able to do so.[39,70,71]

The applications of Rogers' ideas for the adolescent are primarily related to the young person's striving for identity and growth.* Rogerian theory does not deal with the life span from a specific developmental point of view, but from Rogers' discussion of the basic assumptions of human beings, it is clear that there is a progressive directional movement throughout the life span toward ultimate fulfillment. The adolescent may be close to achieving a level of development that can center on self-fulfillment, and yet there are certain aspects of development that are particularly involved in this period of life.

First, adolescents are in the process of formulating and differentiating essential aspects of the self apart from the total phenomenal field. Their changing body size and structure, changing roles, and changing societal expectations for behavior lead to a great deal of confusion as they try to sort out the self. If the conditions for growth are present, Rogers' theory would suggest that growth toward self-identification should proceed with a minimum of confusion and distortion. The young person would be able to move forward, forming an accurate perception of the self.

The conditions for growth may be provided for adolescents from a number of sources. The two most important sources would be the individual's family and peer group. If one of the important social groups does not provide the necessary ingredients of unconditional positive regard and empathic understanding, at least to a relative degree, young people are likely to exhibit disturbance in behavior and be in need of a therapeutic relationship to help them achieve their growth potential.

The source or sources that provide the growth-promoting conditions externally probably exert a significant influence during the adolescent years in helping young people bring phenomenal experiences into accurate aware-

ness. The more this capacity develops, the more completely are individuals able to fully experience themselves and identify that which is the self. Without intellectualizing or treating the self objectively, young people need to verify the accuracy of their perceptions about themselves and to detect their distortions. This is similar to the act of looking into a mirror, or seeing yourself as others see you. As individuals move toward more complete fulfillment, they reach the point where verification of experiences comes increasingly from within. However, in the earlier stages of growth and during the therapeutic experience, clarification of distortions and verification of accurate perceptions help individuals grow and develop.

The peer group is probably the most significant agent for this function in adolescence because the group may either significantly promote distorted awareness functions or facilitate the development of accurate perceptions. As individuals receive an ever increasing range of input from many different sources, they begin to develop either a trust or mistrust of their own inner feelings. For example, as teenagers seek to form a new body image when the massive changes of puberty occur, they waver between feeling unattractive and ugly and feeling attractive and physically acceptable. They go through a significant period of testing the reality of the situation and trying to discover how other people view their physical appearance.[23] If their awareness of their appearance remains distorted and confused, they will receive distorted and confused verification from the peer group. If they begin to formulate a predominantly healthy body image and have this awareness verified from peers and other significant people, they learn to trust their own inner feelings.

As adolescents grow toward a more complete identification of self and fulfillment of their total potential, their behavior becomes increasingly trustworthy and they are able to make their own decisions in the direction of growth and for the good of society. While we may point to many instances where this may appear to be an overly optimistic viewpoint of the adolescent individual, there are many instances in which this concept is demonstrated. Rogers proposes that when this growth potential is not realized, the

*These applications of Rogerian theory are the author's own.

individual is suffering from a lack of external growth conditions or a relatively great degree of incongruence. Therapy is directed toward facilitating the development of congruence through growth-promoting conditions.

## LEGAL ISSUES IN HEALTH CARE FOR ADOLESCENTS

During the 1960s and early 1970s in the United States, a significant trend emerged in the formation and application of laws that recognize adolescents as individuals with growing maturity, capability, and responsibility for their own health care. Further, courts of law have recognized the very real need for adequate health care for young people who avoid such care if they are required to reveal the nature of their problem to parents or must obtain their consent. The normal developmental conflict that emerges during adolescence and young people's desire to assume responsibility for their own affairs produce in many instances in which parental knowledge and involvement is not desired and adequate health care is sacrificed in order to maintain autonomy. When given the opportunity to obtain health care under circumstances in which adolescents can consent to health care without the involvement of parents, many adolescents will seek out and accept adequate care. In many such instances a relationship is then possible between health care workers and teenagers that makes it possible for teenagers to eventually involve their parents with the assistance and guidance of health care workers.

The legal trend has been to view adolescents who are away from home with or without parental consent and who are making the majority of daily decisions and managing their own financial affairs (regardless of the source of income) as sufficiently emancipated to grant consent for health care on their own behalf. Further, there has been a trend to support a mature minor rule that permits unemancipated minors to grant consent on their own behalf if they have sufficient intelligence and understanding of the nature and consequences of the health services and if those health services can be defended as beneficial. Several states have enacted comprehensive laws that give certain defined groups of adolescents, such as those described above, the right to consent to all health care services. A few states have enacted specific laws that grant the right to consent for minors who seek health care for specific problems. Most states have enacted such a law for treatment of venereal disease so that an adolescent can seek diagnosis and treatment with total confidentiality. A few states have also enacted laws that protect the confidential rights of adolescents seeking family planning services or prenatal health care. Professional health care groups have urged communities to recognize the need for permitting teenagers to obtain health care services on their own consent.[4,42] The nurse needs to be aware of the local laws governing teenagers' access to health care on their own consent and facilitate informing teenagers in the community of their legal rights and responsibilities in this regard.

## NURSING ASSESSMENT OF PHYSICAL COMPETENCY

Health maintenance related to all areas of development is optimal when this is an ongoing process extending throughout the childhood period. Increased mobility in modern society makes this ideal unlikely, but the family may be able to provide previous health care information that will demonstrate the child's unique pattern of growth and development, as well as identify any specific health problems. When the child is known to the nurse, the assessment during the adolescent period is facilitated, since the approach to the young person is more comfortable and the individuality of this person is known. The assessment should include all aspects that are described in detail for earlier stages of development as long as they are appropriate, but this section will consider primarily those aspects peculiar to the adolescent. For example, full evaluation of the skeletal system includes observation of range of motion and symmetry of growth and development, size, and relative shape of the structures. In addition, adolescent aspects of growth and change discussed here are of particular concern.

Factors that promote maintenance of physical competency during adolescence include the condition and function of physical systems, as well as environmental factors that uniquely af-

**569**

fect physical health and competency during this period of life.

## Assessment of physiologic systems

Each of the systems of the body is assessed during adolescence in much the same manner as during later childhood. Young people who are being examined by a health care worker of the opposite sex may be reluctant to undress or to discuss function related to the genitourinary system. Skill in approaching teenagers in a matter of fact, open manner often helps to allay their apprehensions and to facilitate their cooperation. When invasion of the teenager's modesty and privacy is not essential to the assessment, it may be wise to postpone these aspects until a later encounter.

The reproductive and endocrine changes that occur during the early puberty stages should be documented. Secondary sexual characteristics may be identified, and the child's stage of development may be classified according to Tanner's description of stages as presented in Table 14-1. Development of each of the areas usually proceeds simultaneously and in sequence, so that a girl would be expected to be in stage 2 of breast and hair development at the time that she is experiencing a peak velocity of height growth, but variations in timing can occur.[41,51,55]

The development of female genitalia should be observed by abdominal palpation, requiring internal as well as external palpation. The size and location of the uterus and ovaries can be estimated, and the cervix and vaginal mucosa are visualized. Increases in vaginal and cervical secretions normally occur at puberty and should be distinguished from discharges representing an infection or other abnormal condition. The external appearance and structure of the labia majora, labia minora, clitoris, vaginal vestibule, and urinary meatus are observed. There should be no signs of infection or injury, and no masses should be evident upon palpation. The distribution of pubic hair should be observed for the typical female pattern of growth, in a downward sweeping curvature over the mons pubis.[9]

The adolescent girl's breasts are gently palpated to determine the absence of masses. Each quadrant of each breast is palpated from the outer circumference toward the nipple, with the opposite hand providing support for the breast as it is palpated. Assymmetry of breast size is common during early adolescence, for often one breast will develop slightly in advance of the other. As the nurse assesses the breasts, frank discussion should be attempted in order to teach the girl self-examination of the breast and to counsel her in regard to any concerns that she has related to development of her breasts.

The genitalia of the boy are inspected and palpated to determine adequacy of structure. The penis and testes will appear like that of a child until the onset of puberty, at which time there is significant growth in the size of these structures. Both testes should be observed to have descended into the scrotal sac. The urinary meatus should be centered at the tip of the penile shaft. If the boy is not circumcised, the foreskin should be retracted and the tissues observed for integrity and hygiene of the skin. The femoral and inguinal areas are palpated to determine the absence of hernias or abnormal masses.[3,12]

Hygiene and care of the external genitalia may be estimated and may give an indication of the young person's understanding and attitudes toward changes of genital functioning during this period. Adolescents who are ordinarily very meticulous about care of their bodies, especially hair and skin, may neglect the pubic area because of feelings of modesty, lack of understanding, or fear of touching this area of their body.

Changes in structural growth and development are assessed by measurements of height and weight, as well as observations of changes in body proportions and symmetry. The head continues to grow slightly in diameter during adolescence. It should be measured and determined to be growing in proportion to the previous percentile rank. Development of increased muscle size and strength in both boys and girls may be observed, and the levels and type of physical activity may be assessed. Optimal capacity is reached by the end of puberty, with the potential for performance being greater than at any other period of life. Adultlike capacity may be estimated by comparing performance, strength, and quality of small and large muscles with that of another adult or the nurse.

Experience in testing strength—for example, by testing the young person's ability to "Indian hand wrestle"—can be developed with rough general guidelines for the individual nurse in terms of the amount of effort required to compete with a teenager in such a muscle strength task.

The skin is an area of particular concern during adolescence. All teenagers demonstrate some change in the condition of the skin during the years of reproductive and endocrine development. The teenager's own approaches for treating acne should be determined, including methods of hygiene used for all areas of the body. The beginning of function of the apocrine sweat glands is suggested by changes in body odors and hygiene needs.

Evaluation of the cardiovascular system is conducted through measurement of the pulse rate and blood pressure and auscultation, palpation, and percussion of the heart and peripheral vessels. Particular attention is given to expected changes in each of these parameters and to the response of the system to exercise. Interpretation of the response to exercise is inexact at this time, but the child should be expected to return to a preexercise state of cardiovascular function within five to ten minutes, depending upon the severity of exercise. If the teenager is asked to run in place for one minute, the pulse rate and blood pressure should rise and then return to a preexercise state within about five minutes. A boy or girl who is in an athletic training program will have a slower than usual resting pulse rate, and the recovery period may be more efficient than that observed for an individual not undergoing athletic training.[74] Cardiovascular function is probably at an optimal level of functioning during adolescence and young adulthood.

The blood is evaluated with standard laboratory measurements of hematocrit, hemoglobin, and white blood cell evaluation and screening for sickle cell disease. Renal function should also be determined by evaluation of the urine. Increases in the red blood cell and hemoglobin content should be observed, with boys being expected to have a higher level than girls (see Appendix, p. 879). Renal function reaches full capacity as endocrine maturation is achieved,

including the full adult level of response to stress.[7,21,27]

The respiratory system is assessed by auscultation, percussion, palpation, and inspection. The individual reaches full adult capacity, and lung function may be studied in detail with special equipment for determining volume, capacity, and gas content of inspired and expired air. The diameter and configuration of the chest increase significantly for boys, and some increase occurs for girls. The slight flaring at the lower edge of the costal margin, which is observed in a supine position during childhood, begins to disappear as the teenager attains adult proportions. The structure of the middle ear should also reach adult proportions.

Neurologic function is estimated by (1) observation of muscle function and strength; (2) evaluation of sensory capacity in vision, hearing, touch, taste, and kinesthetic movement; (3) evaluation of the primitive reflexes; and (4) evaluation of the function of each of the cranial nerves as outlined in Chapter 10. The adolescent's capacity in each of these areas should be optimal, with the exception of vision. Visual capacity is expected to remain optimal throughout adolescence and young adulthood, but variations in acuity occur, which need correction in order to obtain optimal visual capacity (see Chapters 9 and 10). Changes in visual function during adolescence are most likely to be in the direction of deterioration, and they usually occur during the period of peak growth velocity.

The gastrointestinal system is evaluated as described for the earlier stages of life. The development and care of the mouth and teeth are particularly important during early adolescence, since during this period dental caries are particularly prone to develop with the physiologic changes of the body and the dietary habits of young people. The adequacy of the child's bite, with optimal alignment of the mandible and maxilla and function of the joint are assessed. If orthodontic intervention is indicated and possible, this should be instituted no later than the early adolescent period.

Patterns of eating, sleeping, and elimination may be determined by asking the teenager to relate typical daily occurrences. Nutrition and diet during these years are of particular con-

**Table 14-2.** Levels of nutritional assessment for adolescents

| Levels of approach | History | | Clinical evaluation | Laboratory evaluation |
|---|---|---|---|---|
| | **Dietary** | **Medical and socioeconomic** | | |
| Minimal level | 1. Frequency of use of food groups<br>2. Habits-patterns<br>3. Snacks<br>4. Socioeconomic status | 1. Previous diseases and allergies<br>2. Abbreviated system review<br>3. Family history | 1. Height<br>2. Weight | 1. Urine, protein, and sugar<br>2. Hemoglobin |
| Midlevel | 1. Above<br>2. Qualitative estimate<br>3. 24-hour recall | 1. Above in more detail | 1. Above<br>2. Arm circumference<br>3. Skinfold thickness<br>4. External appearance | 1. Above<br>2. Blood taken by vein for albumin (serum), serum iron and TIBC; vitamins A and beta carotene; RBC indices; blood urea nitrogen (BUN); cholesterol; zinc |
| In-depth level | 1. Above<br>2. Quantitative estimate by recall (3-7 days) | 1. Above | 1. Above<br>2. Per ICNND Manual bone density | 1. Above<br>2. *Blood tests:* folate and vitamin C; alkaline phosphatase; RBC transketolase; RBC glutathione; lipids<br>3. *Urine:* creatinine; nitrogen; zinc; thiamine; riboflavin; loading tests (xanthurenic acid/FIGLU)<br>4. *Hair root:* DNA; protein; zinc; other metals |

From Christakis, G., editor: Nutritional assessment in health programs, Am. J. Public Health (suppl.). **63:**55, Nov., 1973.

cern, and teenage fads in this regard should be integrated into a pattern of adequate nutrition as much as possible. Sleep habits are often erratic and unsatisfactory, even to teenagers themselves.

**Environmental conditions**

Several aspects of the environment should be evaluated. Safety factors of the school, home, community, and work settings should be determined, with particular attention to the increased mobility of the teenager. The use of cars and motorcycles increases during this period, with all associated hazards.

Availability and use of drugs, tobacco, and alcohol present a significant physical health problem to the adolescent. These problems also involve social and emotional development and are discussed in this and the following chapter in relation to social competency. When a young person decides to use any of these agents, the difference between moderate use as defined by adult standards and misuse or abuse must be determined. For example, a young person may choose to smoke and to limit consumption so that it does not interfere with the desires of the school or family. On the other hand, smoking may be used to deliberately interfere with social relationships in the home or school, in which case a different kind of problem exists. When young people choose to begin adult habits of social consumption of alcohol or tobacco or to experiment with certain kinds of drugs, their understanding of the physical health risks must be determined, and health teaching or guidance should take into account this prior understanding. They can be given sound, accurate information, but their right and privilege to choose their own course of behavior remain.[23,38,70,77,87]

Exposure to environmental hazards and pollution may change for adolescents as they enter the world of work. There may be special hazards peculiar to the kind of job and the sort of materials used. Working in and around an automotive garage may involve gas inhalant, fire, or electrical hazards. Factories may expose young people to certain kinds of chemical poisonings, such as lead or mercury. The risks for individuals should not be overemphasized, but they should be known to young people and their own understanding of the measures that are necessary for protection should be determined.

## Assessment of nutrition and eating behavior

Many adolescents assume total responsibility for selection and provision of their own meals during adolescence. Further, most adolescents select their own snacks, often without adult guidance. Food fads of all types are often used as one expression of rebellion against traditional life-styles of older adults. In particular, vegetarian diets, diets emphasizing natural, organic, and other kinds of health foods, and the Zen macrobiotic diet are being adopted by many groups of adolescents. Special diets for weight control are also used extensively by teenagers, and often those chosen are the latest fad among adults or peers. Another kind of eating pattern that might emerge is a relative disregard for the selection of foods and eating patterns that respond to hunger with the most easily accessible, often least expensive, snacks in the form of chips, candy, carbonated drinks, and other forms of empty calories.[31]

In approaching the nutritional assessment, the nurse seeks to establish an accurate accounting of the actual foods eaten and the influence of fads, economic factors, and emotional factors. If the teenager is aware that his or her eating habits are not acceptable to parents and other adults, there may be a reticence to reveal the actual eating pattern. If the teenager understands that the nurse is sympathetic to whatever is the underlying motivation in selecting an unusual eating style and will assist in evaluating that pattern for essential nutrients, willingness to openly discuss food habits may be enhanced.

Weight control and control of skin problems are the most frequent concerns of teenagers regarding selection of foods. These concerns should be discussed, and their own knowledge and understanding assessed in order to plan for nutrition guidance and counseling. Table 14-2 summarizes the levels of nutritional assessment for adolescents.

## NURSING ASSESSMENT OF LEARNING AND THOUGHT COMPETENCY

Nursing evaluation of learning and thought competency during adolescence is limited, and definitive assessment must be conducted by a qualified psychologist. However, many indications of learning and thought capacity may be detected throughout the health care encounter with a young person, and specific approaches to obtain evidence are similar to those described for the school-age child (Chapter 12).

In observing an adolescent's learning and thought capacity, the nurse may detect the emerging thinking patterns described by Piaget. When the nurse and young people enter into a problem-solving task together, teenagers may be given an opportunity to express their thoughts, to consider several aspects of a problem, to generate a logical and consistent argument in favor of one or more alternatives, and to systematically discard hypotheses that they determine will not work. They should be able to make these kinds of mental associations and reach conclusions without having to physically try them out. However, if their problem-solving ability is not sophisticated, this is not indicative of a developmental lag; it should be remembered that this is a newly acquired skill. Several observations over an extended period of time or observations from other people in different situations may be required to identify a real developmental lag.

The Peabody Picture Vocabulary Test may be used for middle-class, English-speaking teenagers as an estimate of verbal intelligence ability.[22] Scores on academic achievement tests may be available to the nurse to determine how the teenager's academic performance has been evaluated. These scores should indicate an academic level of performance that is congruent with that of the earlier school years. The teenager may be asked to read aloud a passage of adult-level reading material to determine maturity in reading ability and then asked questions regarding comprehension of the content of the passage. Teenagers should be able to read such a passage without hesitations or stumbling and should be able to indicate accurate comprehension of the content.

The nurse may give the teenager a series of instructions to follow as a further estimate of level of comprehension of language. For example, the teenager may be asked to read the instructions for folding a paper bird and then make a bird using the instructions.

Acquisition of social concepts is another indicator of learning and thought competency. The adolescent's sense of justice, described in the following section, indicates acquisition of complex thinking ability. Familiarity and ability to use money, knowledge of checking and charge accounts, the ability to compare relative economic value of products in stores, and the ability to use library resources can be used to estimate the degree to which the teenager has acquired adultlike abilities in these areas. The nurse may also explore the teenager's ability to identify a long-range goal for future attainment and the means by which the teenager plans to reach that goal. The means should be consistent with an accurate assessment of the teenager's ability and congruent with a realistic expectation for reaching the goal. For example, a teenager may identify a goal of purchasing a car in the future but identify an unrealistic time span for earning sufficient money for the purchase given the actual price of cars and earning capacity of the teenager.

## NURSING ASSESSMENT OF SOCIAL COMPETENCY

Social behavior during adolescence is the major dimension that sets teenagers apart from all other groups in society. There is a constantly changing adolescent code of what is acceptable and what is not, which is defined by each generation of peers in an effort to establish a unique identity for the group and for the individuals within the group. Manner of dress, speech, style of music, and preferred activities are altered in response to that which is considered

"new" or at least not popular among older adults. Adult society as a whole responds initially with contempt, dislike, or disinterest to the latest adolescent fads but often gradually begins to migrate toward the adolescent style, stimulating yet another change in the prevailing adolescent value system. Social behavioral excesses or deficits occur for most teenagers at some point during adolescence, which provides for the teenager the opportunity to try reaching beyond various societally imposed limitations. These transient experimentations may be innocent and serve a useful purpose for the teenager but often cause family and school stress and can result in some form of harm. Experimentation with drugs, sex, law infractions, tobacco, and alcohol, for example, may represent a transient and innocent phase of experimentation or may be indicative of more serious, long-range disturbance. Differentiating between a serious problem and a transient one may extend beyond the expertise of the nurse.[35,66] However, several guidelines are helpful in making an initial judgment until further evidence is available.

Friendships during adolescence are formed on the basis of perceived personality traits of trustworthiness and because of a perceived understanding and sympathy with inner conflicts and problems.[20] One or two close friends are likely to be established fairly early during adolescence and continue to hold lasting value throughout the teenage years. There may be periodic disagreements and breaks in the friendship tie, but the friendship may be restored. Romantic friendships tend to be transient in nature, lasting from a few days to one or more years. The nurse should obtain from the teenager a description of the current group of best friends, an indication of why the teenager considers these people best friends, and a description of how they work out problems among themselves. The teenager may also be willing to describe the nature of romantic friendships and discuss problems encountered in that type of friendship. The adolescent's perceptions of friendships that have "broken up" and the circumstances of the break are useful in revealing how he or she copes with interpersonal stress and the level of insight that is used in retrospect.

Whether the young person is having to resort to socially unacceptable and personally damaging behavior in order to obtain vitally important social contact should be assessed. If teenagers have not been able to identify with a particular age group clique, they are invariably in some difficulty and may display behavior that is designed to attract attention and to enlist friendship. They may have turned to friendship with a person outside of their own age group, such as a much younger child or an adult. Although these patterns of behavior may not constitute gross and permanent abnormality in all instances, in American society they are likely to indicate a serious problem and should be evaluated; some sort of therapy should be instituted as appropriate.

Young people who have become members of a small peer group may or may not have done so with complete success. The group with whom they finally identify may not be the desired group, either from the point of view of the young people or from the point of view of their family. When teenagers are not liked by those whom they seek as companions, they experience a significant loss of self-esteem and may turn to a group of peers with whom they can identify and find some level of esteem and success, even though they inwardly do not prefer this group. Without forming moral judgments or prejudicial implications, the nature of the relationships within teenage groups, their inner feelings of satisfaction with the group, the kinds of activities that the group prefers, and the responses of the group to others outside of their own informal organization can be explored. Parents or teachers may object to a teenager's group because of attitudes that the group encourages, activities of the group, or the ethnic or social background of group members.

## Relationship with parents

Another major area of social competency is teenagers' relationships with their parents. When a behavior problem has occurred that suggests serious difficulty, the parents' attitudes toward their adolescent child may need to be explored in order to view the problem from several perspectives. Parents who recognize teenage behavior traits as a normal manifestation of

adolescence, who recognize and encourage efforts toward emancipation from the family unit, and who respond appropriately to the ambivalent needs expressed in the independent-dependent struggle of their teenager are likely to have minimal difficulty with the ongoing adjustments during adolescence. Such a family is not immune, however, to experiencing instances when teenage behavior is distressing, anger provoking, or embarrassing.

The family assessment, including an interview of the parents alone, is useful in gaining insight of the parent-teenager relationship. Parents may view their adolescent in a manner that does not facilitate healthy growth and development, and recognition of these patterns of response to adolescent offspring is important in assessing the teenager's social competency. Anthony[6] has identified several adolescent stereotypes that may be adopted by parents who respond to their children as the embodiment of negative ideas rather than as real people. When a stereotypic reaction is identified, the family and the teenager are probably in some difficulty.

One such reaction is the representation of the adolescent as a dangerous and endangered object. Teenagers are seen as suddenly able to devastate the family who has cared for them all these years, and thus excessive restrictions are suddenly placed on their behavior and mobility that did not apply earlier in life. Just as teenagers are reaching a point of being able to assume increasing responsibility, they are further restricted. At the same time young people are viewed as being in need of excessive protection from harm that might come to them from the outside. Girls particularly are suddenly viewed as not able to defend themselves or to protect themselves from the evils of the world. Such a parent resists efforts to have their teenagers exposed to knowledge about certain subjects, such as sex and drugs, and adamantly refuses to allow the child to be exposed to dangers of the cruel world.

The transition of the individual from a child not capable of generating sexual interest and activity to a person fully endowed with sexual capacity may produce a significant reaction from one or both parents. The child toward whom the parent could express love and affection may now become a stimulating and forbidden object, and varying degrees of strain between teenagers and parents occur. Sexual experimentation at this point may be related to disturbed relationships in the home, but such an assumption must not be made until ample, accurate evidence is available. Psychiatric evaluation may be necessary in order to determine these aspects of a situation.

The stereotypic response to adolescents as maladjusted individuals is viewed by Anthony as the fulfillment of a parental expectation that has been expressed throughout the child's growing years. Teenagers know that their parents expect adolescence to be a state of acute disequilibrium and disturbance and they proceed to fulfill the prophecy. Further, to the extent that they are treated as maladjusted individuals and not as worthy individual persons, their behavior continues to develop in the direction of disequilibrium. Adolescents themselves express the opinion that this sort of behavior is invariable, that they have a right to excessive mood swings, and that they are caught in the midst of impending insanity. When attention is drawn to such behavior, both teenagers and families are further convinced that adolescents are primarily maladjusted and their fear that this disturbance will become a lasting condition may paralyze realistic responses to efforts to assist with a relatively transient problem.

Parents who are able to view their adolescents as basically healthy individuals are able to flexibly swing with the youngster's mood swings and to respond to their ambivalent, confused expressions of dependence and independence. Parents who see their adolescent as basically disturbed are always suspicious when behavior appears relatively sane and normal. This parent expresses the conviction that at any minute now things will change for the worse.

Parents who have a relatively healthy attitude toward their own adolescence are likely to respond to their teenagers on a person-to-person basis. The parent is able to express remembrance of his or her own conflicts and problems during adolescence, along with a sense of satisfaction in having consciously worked through and resolved the conflicts.

Socially healthy adolescents achieve a relative balance between conforming to the authority of parents and conforming to the authority of the peer group. The adolescent should be able to identify clearly those parental wishes and desires that are respected and adhered to and the reasons for conforming. Likewise, they can identify those areas in which the peer group exerts sufficient demand or respect that their behavior conforms to those standards. Where conflict exists, they usually will discuss the conflict openly or indicate a friend or confidant with whom they would discuss the conflict. Teenagers are also aware of points of disagreement between themselves and their parents and can describe the ways in which they handle the disagreements at home. In some instances, they are able to understand their parents' point of view but can discuss their reasons for holding an opposing point of view.

### Moral development

During adolescence, young people acquire an intense sense of ideals or a system of values evolved from that which they project could be, not necessarily what is. They sometimes align their beliefs with a particular religion or intellectual school of thought or some other formal system that provides a basis for the formulation of the ideals. The teenager uses these ideals in weighing the situational dimensions of decisions of right or wrong, best or worst, important or not important. The ideal system may change drastically several times during adolescence, and this changing process provides the young person with different ranges of experience upon which to later base lasting choices. When presented with a right or wrong dilemma as a part of the nursing assessment, the ideals of the teenager will emerge as the various dimensions of the situation are explored and as various alternatives are presented and mentally tested.

## NURSING ASSESSMENT OF INNER COMPETENCY

Inner competency is central to all aspects of adolescence. It is both a product and producer of behavior.[15] In considering physical, learning and thought, and social competencies we have referred repeatedly to aspects of inner competency development that affect each area of development. Each of the theories that we have considered also illustrate the central nature of the development of the self during adolescence. This task remains universal for all people as they enter the social arena of adulthood, but the prolonged nature of this entry in Western societies has created unique developmental tasks for many adolescents in today's world.

## Evaluation of competencies for indications of inner development

Nursing assessment of the individual's inner competency during adolescence is achieved partially through evaluation of each of the other major competencies; as during all other stages, this remains an area of indirect observation. Teenagers who have a healthy self-concept perform appropriately physically, keep their physical appearance acceptable and appropriate according to the standards of their peers, their learning and thought performance is adequate, and their social behavior is appropriate as defined in the discussion of social competence. In assessing adolescent social behavior, we emphasized the need to make a judgment concerning the meaning of the behavior for teenagers' themselves, that is, whether behavior represents a serious inner or social difficulty, or whether it is a transient experimentation needed in order to define and discover one's own self. The assumption that is made in making such a judgment is that a single behavioral experiment during adolescence may represent a wide range of social inadequacies, serious inner distress, or the normal quest in seeking an inner identity. When a judgment is made that the adolescent is involved in the normal identity-seeking task, an estimate may be made of the adequacy of development by estimating each of the major components of inner competency. This estimate may require a great deal of advanced experience and skill, and validation of one's impressions with a particular adolescent may be necessary from a professional specialist in psychology or psychiatry. Teachers, parents, peers, siblings, or the adolescents themselves may be able to provide some validation for the impressions of the health care worker.

Once a relationship of mutual acceptance and rapport has developed with young people, they are often very open and eager to talk about their inner development. The quality of the self-concept may be estimated by what teenagers say about themselves, how they see themselves as being perceived by others, and how they feel about their own performance, worth, and acceptability. The extent to which they achieve a balance between inner direction and direction derived from peers and society is one estimate of the way in which their self-concept functions. The development of future-oriented goals and the striving for self-fulfillment and satisfaction from activities in this regard are also important indices of function.[59] Here it is important to discard all notions of competitiveness with peers, siblings, or social standards; individual teenagers should be evaluated only in relation to what is reasonable and appropriate for them. Individuals who are limited in talent, academic potential, or economic resources have as great a potential for development of a healthy inner self

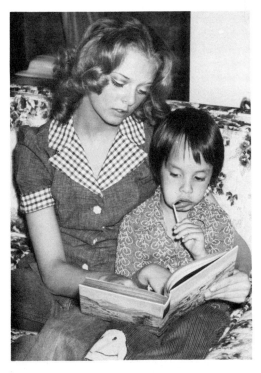

**Fig. 14-6.** Adequacy of inner development is indicated by the young person's ability to assume responsibility and satisfying relationships with others.

as any other person, and their strivings for self-fulfillment and satisfaction should be encouraged in relationship to what is appropriate for them.

Teenagers' attitudes toward themselves, as well as behavior and social relationships that reflect inner competency, may be assessed in regard to the continuums that apply to the structure of the self-concept[59] including:

1. Rigidity—flexibility
2. Inaccuracy—accuracy (as compared with other significant peoples' perceptions of the individual)
3. Simplicity—complexity
4. Narrowness—breadth

### Interview related to inner competency

The nursing interview for assessment of inner competency during adolescence can be struc-

tured to explore the functions of inner competency described in Chapter 2. Table 14-3 presents each of these functions and related interview questions to elicit the teenager's perception and a summary of expected adolescent responses.

In approaching the nursing interview, which will involve significant self-disclosure on the part of the teenager, the nurse must fully inform him or her of the purposes for the interview and discuss the relationships that will be defined between the teenager, the nurse, the parents, and the school. The child health nurse or school nurse is an advocate for the adolescent. Confidentiality of information shared by the teenager should be totally respected and adhered to; however the nurse needs to initially discuss with the adolescent that together they will identify and plan for the areas of health care

**Table 14-3.** Interview for nursing assessment of adolescent inner competency

| Area of function | Interview questions | Optimal responses |
|---|---|---|
| I. Self-evaluation | 1. How would you describe yourself? 2. What do you like best/worst about yourself? 3. If you could change something about your body right now, what would it be? 4. How are you like your mother/father? 5. What do your friends think of you? | Teenagers can take into account many factors in responding; teenagers should be able to explore and reflect on various dimensions and how they interact. The responses should be accurate to the observed behavior, relatively positive and favorable, flexible in describing different dimensions of the self suited to different situations. |
| II. Prediction of success or failure | 1. Tell me about your plans after high school. 2. What can you do best? How do you think you might use this in the future? 3. What is the most difficult thing that you have to do? | Plans for the future should begin to take shape at about 15 to 16 years; expectations should be realistic, taking into account each factor affecting their plans, such as financial, family preferences, peer influences, ability of the self. Responses should focus on goals and means that assure realistic success. |
| III. Obtaining personal survival, acceptance, comfort, enhancement, competence, and actualization | 1. What is the biggest problem you have ever had with a friend, and how did you work it out? 2. In what ways do you agree/disagree with your parents? 3. How do you spend your spare time? 4. What do you like best/least about school? | Teenagers can identify an interpersonal problem and resolution of the problem. The resolution should indicate taking the other person's point of view into account and some degree of compromise. There are areas of agreement and disagreement with parents and school; these should not pose a threat to the teenager. Spare time is valued for pleasant, desired, and positive activity. |
| IV. Instigation of behavior mediated by one's own desires and values or by the society's desires and values | 1. Who influences you the most and why? 2. Have you ever made a decision completely on your own? What was it? What happened? 3. What would you do differently if you were completely on your own? Why? | The primary influence should come from peers or adults outside of the family, although dimensions of family influence should be acknowledged and viewed as relatively positive. Decisions should be motivated from inner desires predominantly. There is a sense of wanting complete independence, but the transient state of dependence on the family is viewed as necessary and not unduly constricting. |

that need to involve their parents or the school. In assuring advocacy and confidentiality for the adolescent, the nurse can identify those instances when the parents might be interviewed alone, such as during the initial family assessment, and share with the adolescent the basic purpose and content of such an interview. After the initial period of assessment, all encounters with the parents should either be planned by the nurse and the adolescent together to meet the needs of the adolescent or the adolescent should be present and involved as a participant on his or her own behalf.

The interview should be conducted in a relaxed atmosphere, and the effectiveness of the interviewer will be determined by the warmth, compassion, and respect for the teenager as a competent individual. Teenagers are often eager for an understanding adult advocate outside of the family and will respond with behavioral indications of willingness to accept the nurse as such a personal advocate if he or she senses trustworthiness and sincere respect from the nurse. The nature of the nurse-teenager relationship needs to be periodically discussed and any concerns acknowledged openly. If a teenager begins to use the relationship with the nurse to compete with the family, to reject or manipulate the family, or as a source of identification with preferred values outside of the family, these dynamics need to be openly discussed. The nurse needs to acknowledge and respect the teenager's developmental thrust of breaking family ties and establishing identity outside of the family and assist him or her in thinking through the specific dimensions of family life that the teenager might wish to reject and the preferred identities from other sources.[40,89]

## HEALTH MAINTENANCE, PROMOTION, AND PREVENTION OF ILLNESS

Many health care needs of the adolescent have been implied in the discussion of assessment, particularly needs for health teaching and guidance. The assessment defines and directs appropriate intervention for the individual young person. For example, in evaluating the dietary and nutrition habits, some patterns will be relatively adequate, requiring little intervention; others will require a great deal of health care, teaching, and guidance.

## School health programs and adolescent clinics

The school health program and special adolescent clinics have designed programs to meet the special developmental and health care needs of adolescents. Each of the components of a comprehensive health program for schools, described in Chapter 12, are integrated into the health program of the middle and upper, or high schools, with curriculum designs appropriate to the health care concerns of adolescents.[10] The health care workers who participate in these programs need to have a thorough understanding of the developmental traits of adolescents, be skilled in interpersonal approaches that are essential in working with adolescents, understand their particular health care needs, and have a thorough knowledge of the protocols for management developed by the adolescent health care team.

The Minnesota Nursing Problem Classification system for children and youth has provided two major diagnostic categories for anticipated guidance for adolescents. These are the "need for knowledge and guidance in adolescence (14-17 years)," classification group no. 308, and "need for knowledge and guidance in late adolescence (18-21 years)," classification group no. 309 (see Appendix, p. 887). The following sections present a detailed description of management approaches for health maintenance, promotion, and prevention of illness that is needed to achieve these health maintenance and guidance needs during adolescence.

## Nutrition and eating behavior

The nutrition assessment described previously in this chapter is used as a basis for health promotion. Many adolescents, regardless of their actual weight and body size, are preoccupied with weight control as a dimension of their preoccupation with their own developing self and body image. The exact concern that the teenager expresses with regard to weight control should be analyzed to determine the extent to which the young person understands basic nutrition principles and the relationship between activity and weight control. In some instances the adolescent's concern may really center on fashion and grooming, and the young person would be more realistic to center attention on studying the effect of various fashions and grooming approaches that will highlight the physical appearance they wish to achieve. Another area of concern might be the adolescent's attempt to lose or control weight in an attempt to alter a basic body build that is not to their liking. For example, a teenager with large bone structure and stocky build might think that losing weight will result in attaining a slim and more delicate figure. This misconception needs to be acknowledged, but the focus should be on assisting the teenager to begin to value his or her own body build for the advantages that it offers and to find ways in which to use these advantages. The nurse and teenager might discuss well-known persons of similar body build, such as television stars, and discuss ways in which their body build contributes to their image as a star. This adolescent might also need assistance in selecting fashions and grooming styles that complement his or her body build but realize that these are not measures to achieve a different body image.

When an adolescent is overweight, several approaches are needed to assist the adolescent in achieving adequate weight control. Fender[29] has described a group approach in working with obese teenage girls. This approach was designed to assist young girls to learn about appropriate means of increasing caloric output through physical activity and to enhance the teenage girls' self-esteem through positive group interaction. Many adolescent girls who are overweight do not actually consume excessive amounts of calories, but they are relatively inactive and their self-concept is low. The group experience provided girls the opportunity to share their feelings and concerns, to obtain therapeutic correction of misconceptions about weight control and nutrition, build self-confidence and a more accurate, realistic self-image, and develop skills in participating in group physical activity as well as learn means of integrating physical activity into their daily lives. Specific dietary management was not used with this group, based on evidence that indicates

adolescents are not able to follow through with a selective diet and that often they are not consuming excessive amounts of calories. Nutrition guidance in terms of knowing the relative food values of different foods, including relative calorie content, and in selecting a well-balanced eating pattern that integrates moderate amounts of favorite foods was included. The major emphasis on increasing physical activity and acquiring a positive self-identity was based on evidence indicating that these factors are more frequently associated with the life-style patterns that lead to establishing and maintaining obesity during adolescence.[29]

When an adolescent has adopted a particular food fad, such as health foods, a macrobiotic diet, or a vegetarian diet, nutrition guidance is needed to correct any nutrition deficit that might exist while maintaining respect for the adolescent's determination to adhere to the particular food preferences. The macrobiotic diet usually does not provide sufficient nutritive intake, and counseling may need to be focused on the particular psychologic or spiritual basis for the adolescent's selection of this particular diet. The hazards of the diet should be discussed but not in a manner which conveys disapproval or rejection of the adolescent's right to exert individualism and self-direction. The health food diets and vegetarian diets can provide adequate nutrition provided the young person has a sufficient understanding of the basic nutrition requirements and the food sources that are important in meeting these requirements, within the limits of the diet preferences.[11,31]

Adolescent girls continue to be prone to iron deficiency anemia. The teenager's nutrition may appear adequate as determined by the diet history, but the hemoglobin level may not approach normal adult values. The girl's economic resources, home eating patterns, school food service, between-meal eating habits, and social influences are all considered in attempting to attain a lasting adequate hemoglobin level. Dietary increase of iron intake is often the most economical method, but this may not be possible if the girl's family eating patterns and the school food service are not adequate, or if she tends to depend upon between-meal snacks for a significant percentage of her calorie intake.

Supplementary iron tablets may be used for a time, but the girl's understanding of the problem and her desire to cooperate are significant factors in whether she actually consumes the tablets daily. Changes in gastrointestinal and eliminative function in response to the supplemental iron may further discourage her intake of the tablets. Thus adequate health care in relation to such a problem involves many different aspects of the total life of the individual, and health maintenance involves a wide range of concerns.

## Sexual competence

The adolescent needs to have a great deal of support and help during the changes of puberty and the onset of reproductive function. Intellectual knowledge of the function of male and female reproduction and sexual functions should be obtained during later childhood, but assuming such knowledge may leave a great gap of understanding between the health care worker and the teenager. In a tactful and unobtrusive manner the teenager's knowledge of sexual functioning for both sexes should be estimated, and offers of further explanation and clarification may be made as appropriate. Teenagers may have questions and concerns that they are afraid to ask, and experience in working with young adolescents helps the nurse to develop an acceptable manner of approaching the concerns of young people.

Most adolescents are able to discuss their concerns only when their parent is not present, but the presence of a friend may enhance the discussion. Girls tend to be concerned about adequacy of development of their breasts, menstrual problems, and social relationships with boys. Sexual feelings are diffuse, not centered on genital function, and tend to be very romanticized. Questions and concerns about pregnancy, both in relation to initiation through coitus and the conduct of pregnancy through labor and delivery, begin to emerge as adolescence progresses. Concerns about homosexual feelings or experiences and masturbation occur among girls but are usually not freely disclosed.

Boys, on the other hand, are primarily concerned about the development of their genital organs and secondary signs of masculinity and specific aspects of coitus. Because their sexual arousal is centered in the genital area and leads directly to desire for relief of tension through orgasm, boys experience a relatively early concern for this particular function. In relation to this they are curious and concerned about the female body and its function, but questions and concerns about pregnancy and the initiation of pregnancy are not prominent. The urge to masturbate may be quite significant for the boy, and his feelings about the acceptability of this practice may be a very important concern. Misunderstandings in relation to masturbation may be gross at this point in life. Desire for social contact with girls is a prominent concern, but it is not romanticized as for girls, and permanent mate-seeking is not as prominent an urge for boys.

Intellectual understanding before or during puberty may not alleviate the emotional concerns and problems encountered during adolescence in relation to sexual functioning. These matters are crowded into individuals' thinking, living, and behaving, and they become central to all that they do at certain points of adolescent development. These are not easily discussed, and often young people must approach the subject themselves before successful health guidance can be attempted. This is one instance where printed material is almost always received and read carefully, for young people find the subject irresistible and eagerly seek all information that they can possibly find. Materials that are directed to their level of interest and that include a discussion of all the physical and emotional concerns that they might be experiencing are particularly helpful. Young people may be given the opportunity to discuss what they are given to read when they are ready, but they may indicate their desire and readiness to talk in a very subtle manner. Skill in approaching and working with the adolescents cannot be overemphasized in developing the ability to recognize and respond to their unique concerns.

It may be helpful to ask to see any reading material that teenagers themselves have found. They may feel embarrassed to share this with a health care worker either because of the source of the material or because the material is considered undesirable by their society. However,

**581**

it is helpful to identify some of young people's misunderstandings and inaccurate perceptions related to sexual functioning by knowing the type of literature they are finding on their own.

### Masturbation

Masturbation is a particularly difficult topic to pursue in our society. Many people still consider masturbation as evil and leading to a variety of ill effects, such as blindness, severe acne, baldness, convulsions, impotency, and insanity. Many children have been threatened with physical calamity if masturbation occurs or persists, and the child is burdened with worry and guilt over the desire and urge to masturbate. More subtle attitudes that masturbation is "not nice," that it should be discouraged, that youngsters will outgrow the habit, or that they should be encouraged to find better things to do encourage the same sort of worry, guilt, and emotional conflict.[49,84]

The adolescent boy needs to understand that masturbation is a normal activity for the release of sexual tension. There is no more danger that a teenage boy will carry this activity to excess than that he might indulge in any other pursuit to an excessive degree. The individual who is healthy and normal will engage in a wide diversity of activity related to a single function and will not pursue one aspect of functioning to the exclusion of all others. Masturbation becomes a problem when it is engaged in exclusively, when the individual is excessively preoccupied with this activity, or when he uses it in socially perverse ways. Other kinds of human activity such as eating, talking, or sleeping are similar in relation to misuse and overindulgence, yet masturbation has been subject to particularly inappropriate attitudes over many centuries, which persist to influence young people today. The boy who feels free to masturbate as a normal activity from time to time in response to sexual tension is developing a normal, healthy attitude. He understands how his body functions, has a healthy attitude toward all aspects of his sexuality, accepts his body as a part of a healthy concept of himself, and feels good about growing into adulthood.[84]

Because of the physiology of the girl's sexual feelings, masturbation does not arise as a pre-dominant concern or problem. However, female masturbation can and does occur as a normal activity and may be pursued during the time that the girl is seeking to explore and know her own anatomy, which is largely hidden from view. This activity is also completely normal. Masturbation for the female is not usually carried to the point of orgasm, and girls often seek a wide variety of means of releasing sexual tension, which are not completely understood.[50,84]

### Contraception

Another important aspect of health care in relation to newly acquired reproductive capacity is information and counseling regarding family planning, or contraception.* Adolescents should become thoroughly acquainted with the available methods. Professional health care workers must put aside moral judgments in counseling with individual teenagers and in recognizing a very real health need that young people may have in this regard. Both boys and girls should understand each of the methods of contraception, and they should know where to obtain help and advice when they need it. The community and the family of an individual teenager may have reservations or strong objections to the availability of such information, and the impact of these preferences should be fully understood and respected. However, the individual teenager has the right and privilege to obtain information and to make an autonomous choice in the matter as long as he or she understands the consequences of the choice and is willing to assume responsibility for it. Teenagers can be encouraged to know and understand the teachings of their culture, family, and religion in regard to family planning, and to make their own choice based on each aspect of the situation. While they are limited in regard to legal rights and responsibilities by being identified as minors in American society, they retain personal rights that must be advocated if health care needs are to be adequately met.†

The rhythm method of contraception involves determining the time of ovulation during the female cycle and abstinence from coitus during

---

*References 1, 16, 67, 76, 79, 86.
†References 4, 8, 19, 42, 43, 45, 85.

the normal life span of sperm before ovulation and for the life span of the ovum after ovulation. Ordinarily, ovulation occurs 14 days before the last day of a uterine cycle (see Chapter 4), but variation in timing of ovulation from cycle to cycle and from individual to individual makes exact prediction of this event difficult. To use the rhythm method with some assurance, the woman's cycle must be fairly regular from month to month.

An estimate of the usual time of ovulation is made by identifying the longest and the shortest cycles that occur over a period of time and then estimating the range of time when fertilization is possible. The days of abstinence from coitus for all future cycles is then estimated until either a shorter or a longer cycle is experienced, and then the days of abstinence are reestimated. The first day of abstinence is calculated by subtracting 18 from the length of the shortest cycle. The figure 18 is derived by adding two days of sperm life and two days for possible variation of the time of ovulation to 14, the theoretical day of ovulation counting backward. The last day of abstinence is determined by subtracting 11 from the longest cycle. The figure 11 is derived from subtracting two days for possible variation in time of ovulation and one day for the life span of the ovum from the 14-day theoretical ovulation time. This gives the widest theoretical range during which fertilization might occur. Thus if a woman records her shortest cycle as being 23 days, and her longest as being 28, she must abstain from coitus from the 5th through the 17th day of all future cycles.

Reliability of the rhythm method may be increased for some women by using body temperature to estimate the time of ovulation. Ovulation is presumed to occur when basal awakening body temperature is the lowest, and the time of fertilizability of the ovum is considered to be past when the temperature has elevated at least 0.5° F and continues this elevation for at least 72 hours. Thus abstinence may begin as estimated by the 18-11 method, but the time of engaging in sexual relations again may be determined by the basal body temperature.

The rhythm method is reported to have a failure rate of 14% to 40% in people using it for a year, as defined by the number of pregnancies that occur while this method of contraception is being used. Since the risk of becoming pregnant when no control method is used is 80%, the rhythm method of control has some value, but the pregnancy risk must be understood. When the basal body temperature is combined with the rhythm method, the failure rate is significantly lowered.[44]

The diaphragm is a small rubber dome molded onto a circular rim, which is fitted over the cervical os in order to occlude the entry of sperm into the uterus. It is used in combination with a spermicidal cream or jelly and thus provides both a mechanical and chemical barrier. The device must be obtained from a health care agency and is not available in drug stores, since it must be fitted to the size of the woman's cervix. Use of the diaphragm requires some amount of manipulation, which is troublesome and inconvenient, and the failure rate is about 12%. However, the diaphragm has become increasingly popular because of the relative safety of this method over all others in relation to the woman's own health. The risk of pregnancy can be significantly reduced by using a chemical contraceptive, such as cream or jelly or foam, in conjunction with using the diaphragm.

The male condom is also used to provide a mechanical barrier to the entry of sperm into the uterus. This method of contraception is probably attempted by most young teenage boys, and the peer-group sources of sex information usually include some description of the use of condoms. They are not considered popular for most adults because of the decrease in sensation for the man and inability of the woman to feel ejaculation, but they are undoubtedly popular because of their availability. Condoms are recommended as a protection against venereal disease, but because only a portion of skin area is covered by the sheath, protection is limited. The sheaths are made of rubber or plastic material and are usually supplied in a rolled form ready to be unrolled onto the erect penis. A small portion of the sheath is left at the end as a receptacle for the seminal fluid. The failure rate with proper usage is about 18%.[44]

Chemical contraceptives are also readily available in drugstores without prescription. They come in the form of creams, jellies, and foams, and their use is relatively simple and inexpensive. However, they must be applied just prior to coitus, and they involve some decrease in sensation and some inconvenience. The failure rate is high, averaging about 30%, and thus they are usually recommended in combination with another method of control.

The female oral contraceptive pill first became available in the United States in 1960, but because of reports of hazards and potential complications, its popularity as a form of contraceptive control has decreased. The exact action of each form of the pill varies, but the basic principle is the prevention of ovulation by chemically altering the usual endocrine cycle. Most forms of the pill contain estrogen, which raises the circulating level of this hormone early in the menstrual cycle. Since high levels of estrogen prevent the release of FSH by the pituitary, ovarian follicles are not stimulated to mature, and ovulation is prevented. When progesterone is added to the estrogen preparation, the endometrium of the uterus is stimulated to develop as during a normal cycle, and withdrawal of the pill causes a menstrual period to occur that simulates the normal ovulatory cycle (see Chapter 4).

The pill has certain bothersome side effects for many women, including weight gain, nausea, and breast tenderness that simulate a pregnant state. Other side effects include headaches, regression of gum tissue around the teeth, eye complications, and blood pressure increase. Serious side effects that have been substantiated are the risks of thromboembolic disease, heart disease, hypertension, and cancer. Thus the pill is never recommended for a woman who has had prior blood clotting problems or who has a strong family history of these problems. The risk of serious illness or death from the use of the pill is less than that expected from normal pregnancy and childbirth, and the pill is still considered to be safe, convenient, and reliable form of contraception. The woman who uses the pill enhances safety of use by having regular evaluations of her progress and condition supervised by a health care professional, and most physicians and dispensing agents require that the woman seek annual health care before prescription for the drug is renewed.

Use of the pill requires that the woman take 20 pills on consecutive days beginning with the fifth day of each cycle. If a pill is forgotten, it is taken as soon as the error is discovered. If the time span exceeds 12 hours after the usual time of taking the pill, another form of contraception should be used for the remainder of the cycle. Women who find remembering to take the pill daily difficult or impossible should use another form of contraception. The failure rate of the pill when it is used correctly is about 0.6%. Most instances of failure result from forgetting to take the pill regularly.[17]

The intrauterine device (IUD) is a small plastic or metal device that is placed in the uterus and remains indefinitely. It prevents pregnancy by interfering with implantation of the fertilized ovum. The exact mechanism by which this interference occurs is not known, but it appears that the device may affect the timing of when the fertilized egg reaches the endometrium, or it may interfere with implantation by causing the accumulation of cytotoxic compounds within the uterus. The most common side effects of the IUD are increased menstrual flow and associated pain, particularly in the early months after insertion. Serious risks include perforation of the uterine wall during insertion and transmission of infection into the uterus and abdominal cavity. These risks may be significantly decreased with appropriate insertion techniques.

Risk of pregnancy with the IUD has been decreased in recent years with improved devices to as low at 1.1% to 3%. Spontaneous expulsion of the device may occur, and a string is left on most devices that hangs below the level of the cervix so that the woman may determine the IUD's continued placement.[56]

### Abortion

When contraception fails or is not used and an unwanted pregnancy occurs, the problems for the adolescent girl are complex. These will be discussed in detail in Chapter 15. Termination of pregnancy by means of abortion is mentioned here because of the growing use of this approach as a method of birth control in the United States. This has been the chief means of population control in the world for many centuries, and the illegal use of this procedure has created health problems for many years in the United States. Information in regard to legal abortion is still relatively difficult for young people to obtain in most American cities, and social and legal aspects of the question remain extremely controversial. Abortion is condemned on philosophical, religious, social, and political grounds that require individual evaluation and personal judgments. Fears of physical or psychologic harm are common, even though there is no scientific evidence of untoward effects when a sound, acceptable method is used.

Abortion is most safe and efficiently accomplished before the end of the twelfth week of pregnancy. Local anesthesia may be used, and the abortion is accomplished either with dilatation and curettage (D and C) or with vacuum or suction aspiration of the uterine lining. The procedure may be done without hospitalization. If abortion is required after the end of the first trimester, hospitalization is required and the surgical and medical procedures are conducted under very close supervision.

### Venereal disease prevention

An important consideration related to sexual function is that of venereal disease. Because the everyday information passed among friends during adolescence often includes discussion and descriptions of these diseases, most young people have some prior impression of the problem. Like other matters of sex, venereal disease is a very sensitive subject to approach, but it is most desirable to provide some access to the subject from a health care source. One of the most important aspects of venereal disease control is detection of infected persons, and the fact that infection is shameful and embarrassing to most people in our society interferes with an effective detection program. Young people should be given information regarding prevention of infection and sources of assistance when a need arises.[24,44]

Although the term venereal disease can apply to any disease that is transmitted by sexual intercourse, the term is usually limited to five infections. The formidable aura and social stigma that accompanies such a label are not appropriate to many of the minor disorders that might be appropriately labeled as such. The five infec-

tions that traditionally receive this label are syphilis, gonorrhea, chancroid, granuloma inguinale, and lymphogranuloma venereum. Specific manifestations of the diseases and treatments are discussed in Chapter 15. Young people need to be aware of the potential hazards of these infections and the means of prevention, detection, and diagnosis. Prevention of the diseases is primarily through avoidance of sexual contact with an infected person; however, a partner's state of infection is often not recognizable. Use of condoms or thorough washing with soap and water may help to inhibit transfer of disease. Local health departments in the United States usually provide services to those who wish to determine the possibility of having contracted a venereal disease, and immediate treatment is available if infection is detected.[24,44]

### Breast self-examination

Adolescents need to be taught the technique and importance of breast self-examination. Girls should form the habit of regular examination of the breasts following each menstrual period. This can be taught during the physical assessment, but films and group discussions are helpful in reinforcing the importance and acceptability of this self-care responsibility. The girl should observe the contour of the breasts in the mirror, looking for visible masses or depressions or excessive drooping of a breast. The girl makes this visual observation with arms lowered and with arms raised. Each breast and axilla are then palpated thoroughly to detect any palpable mass, depression, or tenderness. Detailed instructions on breast self-examination are shown in Fig. 14-7. Young women also need to know what to do if they detect any unusual signs and discuss current methods of treating breast cancer in women.

## Skin care

Care of the skin during adolescence is another major health concern.[61] The many remedies and cosmetic preparations available to the young person are irresistible once the problem of acne begins. Because even relatively mild cases of acne can cause permanent physical and emotional scars, every effort should be

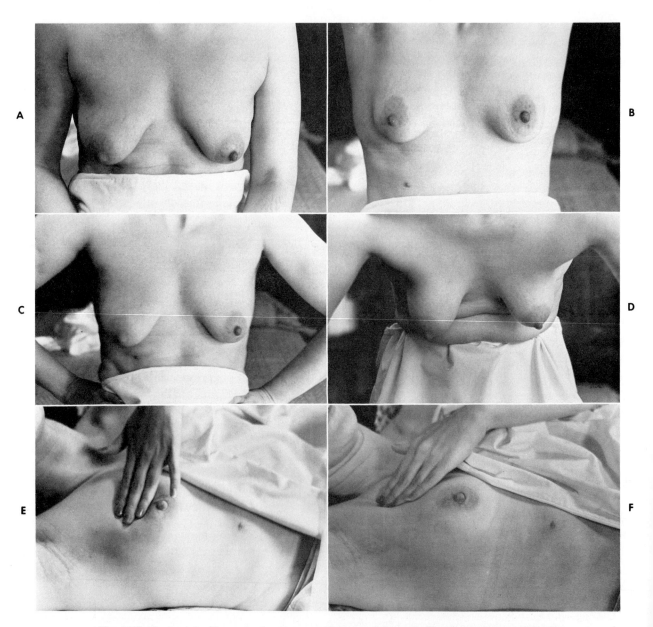

**Fig. 14-7.** The breast self-examination is accomplished as follows: **A,** Standing before a mirror, the woman should visually inspect the breasts for the usual contour and the appearance of visible excessive drooping, masses, or depressions. **B,** The same observations are made with the arms raised over the head. **C,** The arms are then placed on the hips with pressure applied to the hips, and the breasts are observed for any unusual changes in contour. **D,** The breasts are observed for contour and symmetry as the woman leans forward. **E,** Lying on the bed with a pillow under the shoulder, the woman palpates the breast near the areola, **F,** toward the neck and shoulder.

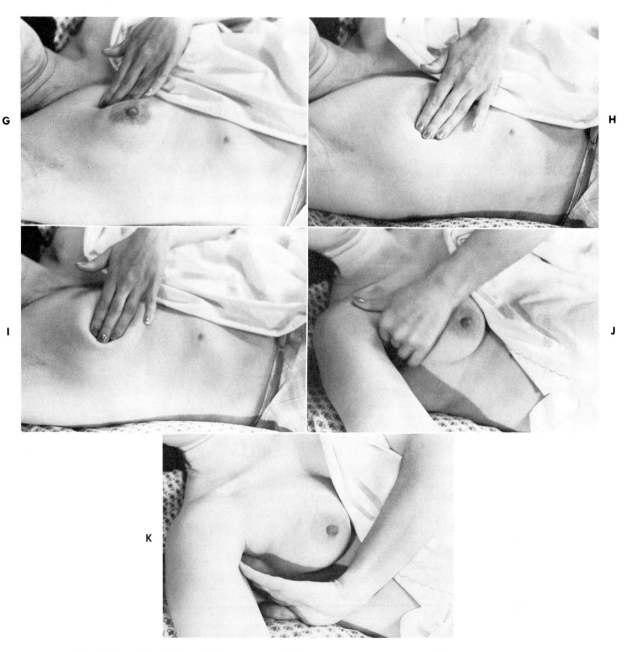

**Fig. 14-7 cont'd. G,** Toward the sternum and, **H,** around toward the axilla. **I,** The area beneath the areola and nipple is palpated. The axilla is palpated over the rib cage **(J)** and over the arm **(K).**

made to help the young person with the problem. When the approaches described below are not effective in controlling the problem, dermatologic assistance must be sought.

First, the young person must keep the skin immaculately clean, washing affected areas three or four times daily. Prevention of bacterial growth on the skin and in the sebaceous glands is essential in preventing infection, increased scarring, and worsening of the condition. In addition, washing helps to keep accumulated dirt and secretions of the sebaceous glands at a minimum, preventing some of the buildup that occurs in the gland and on the skin surface. Application of alcohol may have some beneficial effect as long as the skin does not become too dry.

Removal of the pustules and papules that form should not be attempted by the adolescent but may be accomplished by a nurse or parent with a comedo remover, which expresses the blackhead or pus with gentle suction, causing minimal damage to the skin. Squeezing the lesion may result in further irritation of the gland and permanent injury to the skin.

Skin abrasives may be used to remove dirt and sebum, but they should be used cautiously and infrequently to avoid excessive dryness of the skin. Topical medications such as steroids may help to temporarily alleviate an extensive problem. Peeling agents such as Fostril, Seba-Nil, and ProBlem alcohol are useful in inhibiting bacterial growth, drying the skin, and moderating the production of sebum.

Makeup should be carefully selected. Many cosmetic preparations do not carry appropriate indications of their contents, and they may contain agents that actually irritate and encourage acne. Most preparations that are applied extensively over the face prevent maximal exposure to air and light and cause the accumulation of dirt particles on the skin. Any cosmetic that has a grease or fat base should be avoided.

Ultraviolet light is known to have a beneficial effect in the treatment of acne. Exposure to the sun in the summertime often results in a marked improvement of the condition. Exposure to an artificial sun lamp for five or six minutes on each side of the face several times a week may be beneficial when sunlight exposure is not possible. The light should be at least 15 inches away from the face, and the length of exposure should be only 15 to 30 seconds at first until the reaction of the skin is determined and burns are not a problem.

The effect of diet on acne remains a highly controversial issue. Whether or not certain foods promote the severity of the condition for a given individual can be determined only by food trial and challenges similar to that employed for the identification of food allergens. All suspected foods, such as chocolate, nuts, carbonated beverages, fried and fatty foods, or fish, can be withdrawn for a trial period of two weeks. At the end of two weeks, each food is reintroduced into the diet, one at a time, for a two-week period, to see if the condition of the skin is affected. If the food causes an adverse reaction, the food should be withheld until the period of acne has resolved during later adolescence or early adulthood. Girls should be cautioned not to challenge with a food during the ten days before a menstrual period, as the condition of the skin may respond to the endocrine changes at this time of the cycle.

One of the benefits of approaching dietary control in this manner is the fact that the teenagers themselves participate in a reasonable plan of problem identification and solution. Rather than arbitrarily and severely limiting the diet for a prolonged period of time, teenagers are able to see any reaction of the skin to specific foods and then know what they must do with the diet if the skin is to remain relatively clear.

Social effects and success of adolescents in dealing with skin problems are vitally important. The family should understand that constant reminding and nagging about the problem are irritating and distressing to young people, who are already unhappy over their appearance. Understanding and support may be best expressed by relative silence except when the teenager expresses a desire to discuss the problem. The responsibility for management of the problem should be clearly assigned to young people themselves; carrying through the necessary measures is then clearly their own responsibility.

## Exercise, rest, and body hygiene

The adolescent's need for regular exercise and rest are similar to those during other periods of life, but the pattern for many teenagers tends toward excesses or deficiencies in one area or another. Erratic mood swings during adolescence often contribute to this imbalance, and a certain degree of imbalance is expected. However, important features of the life-style that will continue throughout adulthood are being formed during this period of life, and it is important to assess the predominant tendency of the adolescent and assess understanding of the importance of adequate daily activity and rest. If a relatively sedentary style seems to predominate, the adolescent should be encouraged to discover a satisfying type of activity that will be pursued each day and that will provide for stimulating the cardiovascular and respiratory systems. Means of integrating activity into the daily life pattern, such as using stairs instead of elevators, walking when possible rather than riding, or pursuing participation in a noncompetitive sport, such as jogging, swimming, or hiking, should be discussed.

When an adolescent appears to get insufficient sleep at night, the factors contributing to the predominant pattern should be explored. If the teenager is working long hours to earn a living or save for future goals, discussion should center on the relative value of the work-related goals and the possible detrimental health effects. If the adolescent expresses a desire and need for relief, alternate financial planning or some form of financial assistance may be needed. If the sleep deficiency is related to an apparent emotional turmoil that interferes with sleep, the underlying emotional problem needs to be addressed in a therapeutic manner.

Participation in sports and physical fitness programs requires regular assessment to determine continued fitness for the type of sports activity and tolerance for the level of stress. Continued intact function of the cardiovascular and neurologic systems is essential. The teenager's nutritional adequacy needs to be assessed thoroughly, and the eating patterns followed in meeting nutritional requirements should be determined. The relationship between the use of drugs, including alcohol and tobacco, and performance in athletic competition, should be assessed.

Regular body hygiene becomes a central concern for most adolescents as their attention turns to developing an adult self-image. Particular assistance is needed in care of the hair, use of deodorants as apocrine sweat glands mature, care of the genitalia, and care of the skin. Skin care was discussed in detail in the previous section. Hair care and grooming needs should be discussed, with attention to informed selection of products for hair care from among the many marketed products.

## Prevention of drug misuse and abuse

Detailed discussion of drug misuse and abuse is found in Chapter 15. The health education program should continue measures to inform teenagers of the hazards of drug misuse and abuse as described in Chapter 12. Particular attention should be directed to the misuse of the socially sanctioned alcohol and tobacco products available to teenagers. The effects of health education on use of tobacco and alcohol have not been confirmed to be effective; in fact the incidence of smoking among school-age children and teenagers has grown during recent years.[48] However, teenagers and children report that drug education has influenced their decisions regarding use of drugs, alcohol, and tobacco, and the related health hazards are perceived accurately by those groups that have been surveyed. The young person tends to view the adverse health effects as having an effect far in the future and to indicate an intention to worry about that later. The attitudes of parents and teachers appear to be very important; these factors need to be assessed and the health care team in the high school should plan a program that they project will be of value and then evaluate the actual effectiveness of their efforts.[48,53,81,82]

## Prevention of illness and accidents

Principles of prevention of illness, including adequate immunizations and environmental protection, were discussed in Chapter 12 and should be applied in the high school setting. Accident prevention remains the major threat to life and health for adolescents, with automobile accidents being the primary type of accident suffered during adolescence. Often, such accidents are associated with misuse of alcohol or other drugs. Driver education is mandatory in many states in order for teenagers to obtain driver's licenses and/or insurance coverage. These programs often include detailed discussion of the hazards of mixing drug use with driving.

### Maintaining adequate school performance

As during later childhood, adolescents need to experience some degree of success in their academic life. Young adolescents are particularly vulnerable to slumps in relation to school achievement, because they are involved in dealing with massive changes of their physical body, new social accomplishments, a new school situation, and the need to begin to establish new peer relationships. Their uncertainty regarding their ability in each of these areas and wavering in terms of their own identity are significant, whether these are causes of poor school performance, results of poor school performance, or parallel events with no cause-effect relationship. Teenagers who are able to excel in school performance during this period of adjustment may find themselves in a particularly uncomfortable relationship with peers who envy their academic success. Thus failure to achieve in school may result from the overwhelming need to experience group approval.

Further, teenagers often experience conflicting messages about what is considered adequate achievement in school. The teachers in a junior or middle school may define achievement in slightly different ways than what the child experienced in an elementary or primary school. Parents may begin to express increased concern as teenagers approach the stage when grades are important for potential college entry. Friends and peers, on the other hand, may express rebellion, disgust, or rejection of the academic standards of teachers and parents in an attempt to break away from the family unit. Because each of these dynamics is intimately associated with emotional and physical health, the nurse who is in contact with adolescents may become involved in helping teenagers

whose initial identified problem is inadequate performance in school.

Helping teachers and parents understand some of the aspects of an individual adolescent or of adolescents in general may be a desirable approach. Teachers and parents can contribute significantly to the nurse's understanding of the total situation of teenagers, and together they may be able to more accurately differentiate a serious problem from one that is within the range of normal adolescent behavior.

### Counseling and guidance related to adolescent behavior

Assessment of social and inner competency form the primary basis for decisions related to counseling and guidance when adolescent "acting out" behavior occurs. The health care team is often involved when a teenager engages in some form of behavioral experimentation that brings an extreme reaction from parents or teachers, or when the behavior initiates some kind of health crisis for the teenager. Distinguishing between a normal phase of behavioral experimentation and a serious problem is often difficult, but the comprehensive assessment described previously in this chapter provides a basis for making such a distinction.

If, for example, a young person is found to be experimenting with drugs, and the situation at home, at school, and with age peers is determined to be satisfactory, then the behavior may be viewed as a normal, transient behavioral experiment. Counseling and guidance may be indicated for the parents, the teenager, or both in relation to drug usage, but the incident should not be overattended. On the other hand, if the teenager's social relationships are determined to be inadequate in all areas of life, he or she probably is in serious difficulty and needs psychiatric referral. Should one or two areas of social contact seem adequate and the others are identified as having a real or potential inadequacy, a judgment must be made to either wait and obtain further information, have another professional person obtain more complete assessment of the total situation, or refer the child for immediate psychiatric evaluation and treatment based on the evidence available and the severity of the problem.

To achieve some level of success in working with an adolescent and his or her family in the face of social and behavioral experimentation, some level of confidence and confidentiality must be attained. One single person may not be able to accomplish this because he or she may not be able to relate to both the teenager and the parents. Thus cooperation and coordination among several persons are essential when adolescent problems arise. Helping the family to recognize a single behavioral event as a transient, normal occurrence may be a difficult or impossible task and may require a team effort. If more than one person assesses the teenager's social situation from different perspectives and each arrives at a similar conclusion regarding the problem, efforts toward helping the family place the problem in perspective may be enhanced. Whatever counseling, guidance, or therapy is indicated requires the full understanding and support of the parents and the teenager in order to achieve some degree of success. Consider, for example, an instance where a teacher, social worker, and nurse decide mutually that a teenage boy's involvement in destruction of property should be viewed as a normal behavior experiment, and that, beyond his responsibility for restoring the damaged property, the incident should be forgotten. If the parents in their distress and embarrassment are prone to make a much larger issue of the incident and are not included in the deliberation of factors that led to the professional decision, the decision simply remains on paper. Implementation is thwarted by the well-intended attempt of the parents to appropriately intervene. As a result, conflict with the school may arise, and the child's behavior becomes a matter of undue focus, which in the professional plan was specifically to be avoided.

### Counseling related to identity crisis

The normal adolescent identity crisis brings about the need for frequent validation and feedback for adolescents of their worth and desirability. The peer group is most important in this respect, but a health care professional person is in a unique position to provide such therapeutic assistance. The nurse can find many opportunities to discuss the teenager's strengths, to discuss realistic expectations for daily living, and to assure teenagers that many of the feelings and experiences of this period of development are acceptable, normal, and indeed very valuable in establishing adult abilities and lifestyle.

Physical health care, including the teaching, guidance, and nursing care related to sexual function and skin conditions described earlier, holds a great potential for helping adolescents establish their own identity and deal with their inner concerns. As the health care worker is able to contribute to certain aspects of care related to learning and thought and social competencies, promotion of the young person's inner development is always an intimate concern. Youngsters who are developing normally through the transient crises of self-identity are in great need of an adult advocate and a mature counselor other than a parent with whom they can share their problems, trials, and searching. They may need a single encounter with a person whom they identify as being able to give them advice or information, and as the interaction progresses they may be able to unload a specific inner concern. Additional contact may be indicated and is appropriate when their concerns are primarily assessed to be in the realm of normal adolescent development. When a serious problem or unusual difficulty in development is identified, the young person should receive counseling and therapy with an experienced, qualified therapist, and referral to such a team member is indicated.[3,59,68]

### Preparation for adult family living

Many high school health programs include a specific curriculum on preparation for marriage and family living or preparation for parenthood. This kind of learning responsibility has been increasingly assumed by schools because of the evidence that modern nuclear isolated families are not able to provide for the range of experiences needed to assume adult responsibility for family living and parenthood. Many teenagers today have little or no responsible contact with younger children and therefore have developed no concept of the responsibilities involved in child-rearing. They are relatively protected from a wide range of interpersonal dynamics in-

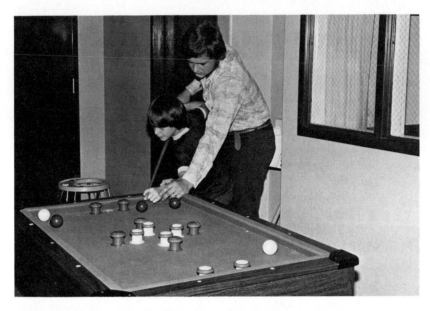

**Fig. 14-8.** Preparation for adult family living includes learning to assume responsibility for younger children and to pursue a satisfying range of leisure activities.

volved in family living as the range of family members living in one household has decreased. Many teenagers have experienced and witnessed breakdown in interpersonal relationships in the home, leaving few role models of satisfying, long-term interpersonal relationships. Their expectations for their own intimate family relationships as adults are often romanticized and center on the pleasures of intimate sexual relationships and sharing of intimate leisure time. The realities of meeting financial obligations, working through interpersonal differences, establishing a mutually satisfying daily life-style, and setting mutually agreeable realistic family goals are seldom considered seriously by teenagers. These concerns need to be addressed in planned learning experiences and group discussions. Experiences that encourage trial assumption of responsibility for earning money and planning for financial responsibility, child care, resolving interpersonal conflict, and conducting the daily affairs of household management need to be provided for all teenagers. Specific discussion needs to be directed to planning for marriage or other forms of intimate adult relationships and for assumption of parenthood. Teenagers need to consider if these goals are consistent with their real desires or if their expectations are derived from societal expectations of what people should do. Their reasons for seeking these life experiences, delaying them until a later period of adulthood, or rejecting them should be explored and discussed.

This formative period of life is critical in the opportunity to make decisions that affect the health of each individual, and the health of generations to come. Health care workers and teachers need to provide sincere and sympathetic attention to the needs of each teenager and assist in helping this generation of young people establish a sound basis for future family living.[36]

## STUDY QUESTIONS

1. Determine the availability in your community of special services for adolescents. Is there a specific clinic, either private or public, designed to meet the needs of adolescents? Determine the availability of family planning information and information related to sexual function. What resources are available to help the teenage unwed mother?

2. Describe the health education program of a local junior

high school (grades serving the child during puberty). What aspects of health are included in the educational program, and how comprehensive is the program? What facilities are available in the school to help individual young people with specific health problems?

3. Investigate the legal implications of providing family planning information for young people in your community. Discuss the rationale given by civic, religious, or political groups who strongly support or oppose this practice.

4. Survey the cosmetic, medicinal, and family planning products locally available to adolescents in your community. Describe the contents of treatments for acne and cosmetics that are popularly used. Discuss the relative cost of comparable products, the advertising appeal, and the hazards of use. Describe the advertising claims of comparable contraceptive products and the relative availability and cost of each.

5. Choose one of the theorists discussed in this chapter and study the propositions of the theory in more complete detail. Identify a counselor, educator, or therapist who subscribes to the theorist's ideas, and describe how the theory is applied in practice.

6. Choose a book or article describing a particular counseling approach that is appropriate for teenagers and study the contents in detail. If possible, try to apply the ideas in an encounter with an adolescent in a health care setting, and describe the experience. If possible, tape-record your interview and critique its contents, and repeat the experience several times to improve your ability to relate to young people as a professional health care worker. Some of the books that might be used are:

Combs, W. W., Avila, D. L., and Purkey, W. W.: Helping relationships; basic concepts for the helping professions, Boston, 1971, Allyn & Bacon, Inc.

Glasser, W.: Reality therapy; a new approach to psychiatry, New York, 1965, Harper & Row, Publishers.

Gordon, T.: Parent effectiveness training, New York, 1970, Peter H. Wyden, Inc.

## REFERENCES

1. Abernethy, V.: Illegitimate conception among teenagers, Am. J. Public Health 64:662, July, 1974.
2. Adler, A.: Social interest, New York, 1939, C. P. Putnam's Sons.
3. Alexander, M. M., and Brown, M. S.: Physical examination. XIV. Examining male genitalia, Nursing '76, 6:39, Feb., 1976.
4. A model act providing for consent of minors for health services. Report of the Committee on Youth of the American Academy of Pediatrics: Pediatrics 51:293, Feb., 1973.
5. Ansbacker, H. L., and Rowena, R., editors: Superiority and social interest by Alfred Adler, Evanston, Ill., 1964, Northwestern University Press.
6. Anthony, E. J.: The reactions of parents to adolescents and to their behavior. In Anthony, E. J., and Benedek, T., editors: Parenthood; its psychology and psychopathology, Boston, 1970, Little, Brown and Co., p. 307.
7. Bailey, E. N.: Screening in pediatric practice, Pediatr. Clin. North Am. 21:123, Feb., 1974.
8. Blake, J.: The teenage birth control dilemma and public opinion, Science 180:708, May 18, 1973.
9. Brown, M. S., and Alexander, M. M.: Physical examination. XV. Examining female genitalia, Nursing '76, 6:39, March, 1976.
10. Bruce, N. M., and Dawson, A. E.: The school—its relationship to health services. In Kalafatich, A. J.: Approaches to the care of adolescence, New York, 1975, Appleton-Century-Crofts, p. 49.
11. Caghan, S. B.: The adolescent and nutrition, Am. J. Nurs. 75:1728, Oct., 1975.
12. Chard, M.: An approach to examining the adolescent male, Matern. Child Nurs. 1:41, Jan.-Feb., 1976.
13. Coleman, J. S.: The adolescent society, Glencoe, Ill., 1961, The Free Press.
14. Coles, R.: Children of the American ghetto, Harper's 235:16, Sept., 1967.
15. Combs, A. W., Avila, D. L., and Purkey, W. W.: Helping relationships; basic concepts for the helping professions, Boston, 1971, Allyn & Bacon, Inc.
16. Counseling opportunities in human reproduction. Report of the Committee on Youth, American Academy of Pediatrics: Pediatrics 50:492, Sept., 1972.
17. Cowarts, M.: Oral contraceptives; how best to explain their effects to patients, Nursing '76 6:44, June, 1976.
18. Crawford, J. D., and Osler, D. C.: Body composition at menarche; the Frisch-Revelle hypothesis revisited, Pediatrics 56:449, Sept., 1975.
19. Cutright, P.: Illegitimacy; the prospect for change, Am. J. Public Health 63:765, Sept., 1973.
20. Damon, W.: The social world of the child, San Francisco, 1977, Jossey-Bass Publishers.
21. Daniel, W. A.: Hematocrit; maturity relationship in adolescence, Pediatrics 52:388, Sept., 1973.
22. Dunn, L. M.: Peabody Picture Vocabulary Test, Minneapolis, Minn., 1965, American Guidance Service, Inc.
23. Dempsey, M. O.: The development of body image in the adolescent, Nurs. Clin. North Am. 7:609, Dec., 1972.
24. Eberly, F. W.: Venereal disease in the adolescent. In Kalafatich, A. J., editor: Approaches to the care of adolescents, New York, 1975, Appleton-Century-Crofts, p. 109.
25. Erikson, E. H.: A memorandum on identity and Negro youth, J. Social Issues 20:29, Oct., 1964.
26. Erikson, E. H.: Identity; youth and crisis, New York, 1968, W. W. Norton & Co., Inc.
27. Faigel, H. C.: Hematocrits in suburban adolescents; a search for anemia, Clin. Pediatr. 12:494, Aug., 1973.
28. Faigel, H. C.: A developmental approach to adolescence, Pediatr. Clin. North Am. 21:353, May, 1974.
29. Fender, J.: Obesity in teenage girls. In Kalafatich, A. J., editor: Approaches to the care of adolescents, New York, 1975, Appleton-Century-Crofts, p. 79.
30. Fine, L. L.: What's a normal adolescent? A guide for

the assessment of adolescent behavior, Clin. Pediatr. **12:**1, Jan., 1973.

31. Frankle, R. T., and Heussenstamm, F. K.: Food zealotry and youth; new dilemmas for professionals, Am. J. Public Health **64:**11, Jan., 1974.

32. Friedenberg, E. A.: Coming of age in America; growth and acquiescence, New York, 1965, Random House, Inc.

33. Frisch, R. E., and Revelle, R.: Height and weight at menarche and a hypothesis of menarche, Arch. Dis. Child **46:**695, 1971.

34. Frisch, R. E.: Weight at menarche; similarity for well-nourished and undernourished girls at differing ages and evidence for historical constance, Pediatrics **50:** 445-450, Sept., 1972.

35. Giuffra, M. J.: Demystifying adolescent behavior, Am. J. Nurs. **75:**1724, Oct., 1975.

36. Grady, B. H.: A family living course for young adolescents, Children Today **2:**18, July-Aug., 1973.

37. Guyton, A. C.: Textbook of medical physiology, ed. 5, Philadelphia, 1976, W. B. Saunders Co.

38. Haggerty, R. J.: Adolescence. In Green, M., and Haggerty, R. J., editors: Ambulatory Pediatrics, II, Philadelphia, 1977, W. B. Saunders Co., p. 415.

39. Hall, C. S., and Lindzey, G.: Theories of personality, ed. 2, New York, 1970, John Wiley & Sons, Inc.

40. Hall, G. S.: Adolescence; its psychology and its relations to physiology, anthropology, sociology, sex, crime, religion, and education, New York, 1904, D. Appleton and Co.

41. Hammar, S. L.: The approach to the adolescent patient, Pediatr. Clin. North Am. **20:**779, Nov., 1973.

42. Hofman, A. D., and Pilpel, H. F.: The legal rights of minors, Pediatr. Clin. North Am. **20:**989, Nov., 1973.

43. Hoyman, H. S.: Sex education and our core values, J. School Health **44:**62, Feb., 1974.

44. Hubbard, C. W.: Family planning education; parenthood and social disease control, St. Louis, 1973, The C. V. Mosby Co.

45. Inman, M.: What teen-agers want in sex education, Am. J. Nurs. **74:**1866, Oct., 1974.

46. Jones, M. C., and Bayley, N.: Physical maturing among boys as related to behavior. In Meyer, W. J., editor: Readings in the psychology of childhood and adolescence, Waltham, Mass., 1967, Blaisdell Publishing Co., p. 64.

47. Kalafatich, A. J.: Adolescence—a separate stage of life. In Kalafatich, A. J., editor: Approaches to the care of adolescents, New York, 1975, Appleton-Century-Crofts, p. 1.

48. Kelson, S. R., Pullella, J. L., and Otterland, A.: The growing epidemic; a survey of smoking habits and attitudes toward smoking among students in grades 7 through 12 in Toledo and Lucas County Public Schools—1964-1971, Am. J. Public Health **65:**923, Sept., 1975.

49. Kinsey, A. C.: Sexual behavior in the human male, Philadelphia, 1948, W. B. Saunders Co.

50. Kinsey, A. C.: Sexual behavior in the human female, Philadelphia, 1953, W. B. Saunders Co.

51. Kogut, M. D.: Growth and development in adolescence, Pediatr. Clin. North Am. **20:**789, Nov., 1973.

52. Kulin, H. E., and Reiter, E. O.: Gonadotropins during childhood and adolescence; a review, Pediatrics **51:** 260, Feb., 1973.

53. Levy, R. M., and Brown, A. R.: Untoward effects of drug education, Am. J. Public Health **63:**1071, Dec., 1973.

54. Lewin, K.: Field theory and experiment in social psychology; concepts and methods, Am. J. Sociol. **44:**868, 1939.

55. Maloni, J. A.: Seven adolescents' experience of menstruation, Matern. Child Nurs. J. **3:**49, Spring, 1974.

56. Manisoff, M. T.: Intrauterine devices, Am. J. Nurs. **73:**1188, July, 1973.

57. Marshall, W. A., and Tanner, J. M.: Variations in the pattern of pubertal changes in girls, Arch. Dis. Child **44:**291, 1969.

58. Marshall, W. A., and Tanner, J. M.: Variations in the pattern of pubertal changes in boys, Arch. Dis. Child **45:**13, 1970.

59. McCandless, B. R.: Adolescents; behavior and development, New York, 1970, Holt, Rinehart & Winston.

60. Mead, M.: Culture and commitment; a study of the generation gap, Garden City, N.Y., 1970, Natural History Press/Doubleday & Company Inc.

61. Norins, A. L.: Pediatric dermatology. In Green, M., and Haggerty, R. J., editors: Ambulatory pediatrics, II, Philadelphia, 1977, W. B. Saunders Co., p. 81.

62. Perrone, P. A., Ryan, T. A., and Zeran, R. R.: Guidance and the emerging adolescent, Scranton, Pa., 1970, International Textbook Co.

63. Phillips, J. L., Jr.: The origins of intellect; Piaget's theory, San Francisco, 1969, W. H. Freeman and Co.

64. Piaget, L.: The moral judgment of the child, New York, 1932, Harcourt, Brace and World.

65. Pulaski, M. A. S.: Understanding Piaget, New York, 1971, Harper & Row, Publishers.

66. Rajokovich, M. J.: High schools need nurse counselors, too. In Fagin, C. M., editor: Readings in child and adolescent psychiatric nursing, St. Louis, 1974, The C. V. Mosby Co.

67. Rauh, J. L., Hornson, L. B., and Burket, R. L.: The reproductive adolescent, Pediatr. Clin. North Am. **20:** 1005, Nov., 1973.

68. Roberts, S. O.: Some mental and emotional health needs of Negro children and youth. In Wilcox, R., editor: The psychological consequences of being a black American; a sourcebook of research by black psychologists, New York, 1971, John Wiley & Sons, Inc., p. 332.

69. Roche, A. R., and Davila, G. H.: Late adolescent growth in stature, Pediatrics **50:**874, Dec., 1972.

70. Rogers, C. R.: A theory of therapy as developed in the client-centered framework. In Ard, B. N., Jr., editor: Counseling and psychotherapy; classics on theories and issues, Ben Lomand, Calif., 1966, Science Behavior Books, Inc., p. 43.

71. Rogers, C. R.: A humanistic conception of man. In Bernard, H. W., editor: Readings in adolescent devel-

opment, Scranton, Pa., 1969, International Textbook Co., p. 41.

72. Root, A. W.: Endocrinology of puberty. I. Normal sexual maturation, J. Pediatr. **83:**1, July, 1973.

73. Ross, D. C., and Ross, D. C., Jr.: Youthful alienation and social mobility; a re-evaluation of the whole social mobility ethos is urgently needed, Clin. Pediatr. **12:** 22, Jan., 1973.

74. Shaffer, T. E.: The adolescent athlete, Pediatr. Clin. North Am. **20:**837, Nov., 1973.

75. Shenker, I. R., and others. A curriculum guide for adolescent medicine by the Committee on Education, Society for Adolescent Medicine, Clin. Pediatr. **16:** 516, June, 1977.

76. Siegel, E., and Morris, N. M.: Family planning; its health rationale, Am. J. Obstet. Gynecol. **118:**995, April 1, 1974.

77. Statement of marajuana; Report of the Committee on Youth, American Academy of Pediatrics: Pediatrics **49:** 461-462, March, 1972.

78. Stone, L. J., and Church, J.: Childhood and adolescence; a psychology of the growing person, ed. 3, New York, 1975, Random House.

79. Sundstrom, C.: A bookshelf on family planning, Am. J. Public Health **64:**666, July, 1974.

80. Tanner, J. M.: Growth of adolescence, ed. 2, Oxford, 1962, Blackwell Scientific Publications.

81. Tennant, F. S., Weaver, S. C., and Lewis, C. E.: Outcomes of drug education; four case studies, Pediatrics **52:**246, Aug., 1973.

82. Tennant, F. S., Jr., and others: Effectiveness of drug education classes, Am. J. Public Health **64:**422, May, 1974.

83. Timiras, P. S.: Developmental physiology and aging, New York, 1972, Macmillan Publishing Co., Inc.

84. Whipple, D. V.: Dynamics of development; euthenic pediatrics, New York, 1966, McGraw-Hill Book Co.

85. Wolfish, M. G.: A clinic for the ambulatory adolescent; essentials, scope, and patterns of operation, Clin. Pediatr. **12:**13, Jan., 1973.

86. Wolfish, M. G.: Adolescent sexuality; counseling, contraception, pregnancy, Clin. Pediat. **12:**244, April, 1973.

87. Yacenda, J. A.: Smoking behavior and young people; the need for new directions, Clin. Pediatr. **12:**13A, Jan., 1973.

88. Yakolev, P. I., and Lecours, A. R.: The myelogenetic cycles of regional maturation of the brain. In Minkowski, A., editor: Regional development of the brain in early life, Oxford, 1967, Blackwell Scientific Publications, Ltd.

89. Zelter, L. K., and others: The adolescent clinic—a model and profile, Clin. Pediatr. **16:**426, May, 1977.

# CHAPTER 15

# Health problems of adolescence

Adolescence is a relatively healthy period of life, with automobile accidents comprising the leading cause of death during this period. There are many health problems that require a preventive approach, and a great deal of attention to health education is necessary in order to avoid more serious encounters with illness and emotional or social disturbance. These health maintenance aspects of care were the focus of the discussion in Chapter 14. Such problems as acne, issues related to sexual function, and drug use are confronted by all normal teenagers in technological societies today. When problems such as these lead to illness, unwanted pregnancy, drug misuse, or emotional disturbance, the young person is in need of specific health care. Working with adolescent health problems requires a very special commitment and a sincere empathy for young people and their problems, along with the ability to offer mature counsel in a manner that is appealing and acceptable to the individual. Even though many health care workers in the community and special agencies know and understand some aspects of adolescent problems, special concentration on problems of this age group may be desirable in gaining the skill and understanding that facilitate an effective relationship.

The approach for nursing diagnosis and nursing problem statements, described in Chapter 11, p. 372, is used here in defining adolescent health problems. This section should be reviewed in preparation for study of the health problems presented in this chapter.

Health care for adolescents experiencing many of the health problems discussed in this chapter includes the issue of legal consent for health care by the young person without obtaining the consent of parents. As was discussed in Chapter 14, p. 569, there has been a major trend toward redefining the legal rights of minors in confidential consent for their own health care, especially when the young person might otherwise avoid health care if consent of parents is required. When adolescents wish to have their health problem treated without parental knowledge or consent, the health care team must document evidence of meeting the local legal requirements for proceeding with care for the young person and discuss each of the ramifications of such care with the young person. Assurance of confidentiality can be given if all legal requirements can be documented, and this confidentiality must be maintained until such time that the young person consents to informing the parents of the problem. Health care workers should counsel the young person, without coercion, of the desirability and need to establish open communication with parents and if possible help the young person to use the health care crisis as a means of establishing improved family relationships. The following guidelines are offered by the American Academy of Pediatrics as factors that define a situation when health care for adolescents on their own consent is justified:[21]

1. The young person is known to make most of his or her own decisions about the conduct of daily affairs.
2. There is substantial independence in coming and going from home, and the young person is able to move about the community easily and independently.
3. Even though the young person may be supported by parents, the day-to-day management of money is accomplished by the young person and some of the total money needed for personal expenses is earned by the young person.
4. He or she has initiated and sought health care, is not accompanied by parents, is able to state the nature of the health problem, and seems able and motivated to follow through with the required health care.
5. The young person appears to understand the risks and the benefits of the health care needed.
6. The young person expresses an inability to communicate with his or her parents about health problems and concerns.

## MANAGEMENT OF ADOLESCENTS WITH SPECIFIC PROBLEMS

Many of the health problems discussed in Chapters 11 and 13 also occur during adolescence. Respiratory infections, gastrointestinal disturbances, urinary tract infections, repeated absenteeism from school, nutrition and weight problems, and accidents during adolescence are similar in manifestation and management to that of earlier age groups. Adolescents who experience a short-term acute illness may be reluctant to be subjected to the temporary isolation or rest that may be required, since they feel that social activities and obligations are far more important. Young people have reached a stage in life when they are responsible for selecting a significant portion of their nutrition, for caring for their personal body needs, and for taking care of special health problems when they arise. The measures required in response to an acute infection or minor illness should be understood and practiced independently by adolescents, with some supervision and assistance from a more experienced member of the family or a health care worker. The problems that are discussed in this chapter are those that are likely to be encountered for the first time during the adolescent years and, therefore, often require specific resources of the health care system.

### Drug misuse

Drug misuse includes all encounters and trials with drugs that occur outside the realm of prescribed or acceptably safe medical or social standards for use. The term "misuse" is used to imply all injudicious uses of drugs, including the indiscriminate use of antibiotics or vitamins or the use of a drug when another form of therapy might be preferred. Increased drug use and misuse is an integral part of our developing cultures. To eliminate many of these practices would be to demand major changes in beliefs and attitudes and desires that many would not support.[79,84] Even as readers progress through this discussion, they may recognize many forms of their own drug use and misuse. The purpose of this discussion is to neither condemn nor condone various forms of drug use or misuse but to provide information and concepts that are helpful in making judicious judgments regarding drug use.

Intense controversy may exist regarding what is safe or acceptable use of a given agent, and the individual's personal judgment may be influenced by religious, moral, cultural, or peer group preferences. Confusion and uncertainty in available scientific evidence add to the difficulty in determining what is acceptable use of certain drugs. There are five categories of commercially available psychoactive drugs in the United States today. These are (1) prescription drugs, (2) over-the-counter drugs, (3) mood- and consciousness-alerting chemicals, known as social drugs, (4) chemicals sold for nondrug purposes, and (5) drugs and chemicals that are not sold legally and therefore are referred to as illegal drugs.

The patterns of drug use in the United States have shifted away from the misuse of opiates during the 1970s, but there has been an increasing misuse of hallucinogens, amphetamines, sedatives, and social drugs. Factors that contribute to misuse of drugs are not related to socioeconomic status but rather appear to be related to a satisfying inner personal experience or to meeting some felt need. Adolescents may engage in drug misuse to prove their courage by indulging in risk taking, as a means of acting out rebellion and hostility toward authority, to facilitate sexual desires and performance, to elevate themselves from loneliness or despair, or to attempt to find meaning in life.*

There is a basic assumption in American society that all drug use by young people is dangerous and results in serious health sequelae. Concomitantly, there is a failure to recognize the uses and abuses of drugs among responsible adults. This societal attitude and paradox are based on fear of unknown results of many forms of adolescent rebellion and behavior and the fact that results remain unknown for many of the substances prone to transient experimentation or moderate use. Health care workers should understand the known effects of various substances, the dangers involved in use, and the differences between drug experimentation, rational use of a substance, and abuse (see Chapter 14). Cultural and moral values inevitably influence the judgments that are made by the individual; however, the primary responsibility is to convey reliable information about the properties of the drugs themselves and to help the young person understand the related value issues that affect him or her through his or her own culture.[79]

Psychoactive drugs of all types primarily affect the functional transmission of neuronal information at the synapse. The production, release, action, or breakdown of neurotransmitters is affected in such a way as to either excite or dull the impulse in the axon. Thus, intraneural activity is secondarily affected by the change in the synapse brought about by drug action. Drug effects are highly individual. Psychoactive drugs, particularly, exhibit a highly personalized effect, and the behavioral dimensions that tend to be altered are those that are highly complex, abstract, and newly acquired. A well-learned habit is usually not changed significantly by most drugs in most individuals.[84]

### Prescription drugs

The prescription drugs available today that have an effect on the nervous system and are prone to misuse may be classified as narcotic and nonnarcotic drugs. The narcotic drugs have been known and used for many centuries, while most of the nonnarcotic nervous system agents are relatively new as agents for human consumption.

Nonnarcotic drugs have been produced in response to the need for more humane treatment of people suffering varying levels of emotional disturbance. These antipsychosis, antianxiety, antidepression, and antimania compounds are sold only by prescription, and the illnesses that they are designed to treat are often very difficult to diagnose. Diagnosis is based on behavioral, feeling, and thinking changes, which are not directly available for objective observation and scrutiny; thus the prescription of these agents is often made on the basis of the individual's subjective report of recent feeling changes. Drugs are often used to try to achieve some alleviation of the subjective symptoms. Just as diagnosis is inexact and difficult, so is the evaluation of the effect of the drugs, especially when the individual's symptoms are relatively mild and transient. The use of the drug may or may not be fully warranted. These factors have led to widespread availability of prescription mind-altering drugs, because the stresses and problems of modern living have created a great demand for relief from symptoms that simulate or suggest the presence of some degree of nervous or emotional disturbance.

Phenothiazines (Thorazine, Vesprin, Compazine, Stelazine, Trilafon, Dartal, Mellaril) have been used since the early 1950s in the treatment of schizophrenia. Although these drugs are generally thought of as tranquilizers, their action is highly specific and they do not affect certain tension and anxiety symptoms that are ordinarily favorably affected by tranquilizers. The symptoms that are alleviated are emotional withdrawal, hallucinations, delusions and other disturbed thinking, paranoid projection, belligerence, and hostility. The main action is depression of the hypothalamus and the

*References 1, 40, 51, 64, 72, 88, 95.

reticular activating system. Effects that block adrenergic, cholinergic, and histaminic activities of the body account for the side effects commonly associated with the drugs; these include dry mouth, nasal congestion, muscle spasms, and constipation. The drugs are not addicting, and they are not effective suicidal drugs, since death occurs only rarely with extremely high doses. The phenothiazines potentiate and prolong the action of sedatives, narcotics, and anesthetic drugs.[38,75,84]

Mood disorders are seemingly more common than disorders in thinking, and drugs that affect mood are more commonly available to the general population. Depression, mania, and neurosis are the most common mood disorders seen today, and the severity of the problems is highly variable. People with acute depression and mania are most often identified and seen for treatment; people with moderate or mild forms of neurosis may seek treatment, but it is relatively casual and often involves simply the prescription of one of the minor tranquilizers. Chlordiazepoxide (Librium) and diazepam (Valium) are the two most common drugs prescribed. Meprobamate (Miltown, Equanil) and the barbiturates are also used for tranquilizing and treating the symptoms of anxiety. The primary action of Librium and Valium seems to be on the limbic system, with few side effects experienced by most people with therapeutic doses. Like barbiturates, the antianxiety drugs are addicting, and tolerance to the drugs can occur. Abrupt withdrawal from the drugs can be dangerous, producing acute withdrawal symptoms.[38,75,84]

Drugs that alter the arousal and activity level, known as stimulants and depressants ("uppers" and "downers"), are widely available. These drugs are most commonly prescribed for middle-aged and older adults and thus are prone to misuse by people in this age group particularly. Overweight and fatigued, excitable, and anxious housewives and businessmen are particularly prone to have and use stimulants and depressants. The availability of these drugs for experimentation by teenagers in the home of the legitimate user presents a special concern, but chronic misuse is relatively rare among young people.

The action of these agents is primarily on the reticular activating system of the brain. The primary stimulant that is prone to misuse are the amphetamines. These drugs are discussed in Chapter 13 in relation to use for behavior modification of hyperkinetic children. In addition, they are used therapeutically for weight control by adults and as a bronchodilator when inhaled. As weight control drugs, the amphetamines decrease appetite until tolerance is experienced. However, because of the relative lack of lasting weight control with the use of amphetamines and the dangers of misuse, there appears to be little justification for the use of the drug for this purpose. Tolerance, which develops after four to six weeks, causes the appetite reduction effect to disappear, and the individual's basic pattern of overeating returns. The experience of euphoria, increased levels of attention and arousal, and the ability to perform in the face of fatigue may be the basis for continuing use of the drug after it has been used for weight control.

These drugs are often used for the stimulant effects by people who desire or need to perform beyond the fatigue level for a period of time. Students, truck drivers, and military personnel, in particular, have used these drugs to delay the need for sleep and to fight the effects of fatigue.[16,84]

Amphetamines (Benzedrine, Methedrine, Dexedrine) are known by young people under a wide variety of names, which change from time to time in order to maintain a certain level of secrecy and privacy in labeling within the youth culture. "Speed" is the most common colloquial term and the effects of the drug are described as "turning on." The user experiences some level of arousal and hypersensitivity, depending on the dosage used and the reaction to the drug. In low or moderate oral doses the effect begins to occur about two to three hours after ingestion and seems most commonly to prevent the decrement in performance that would occur as a result of fatigue or boredom. Whether the drug enhances the rested person's performance is a matter of debate, particularly in relation to athletic performance.

In high doses, amphetamines taken orally cause a person to feel euphoric, alert, talkative, and sensitive to environmental stimuli. Feelings of hyperactivity, nervousness, and jitteriness may also accompany high doses of amphetamines, and to combat this the user may take a barbiturate simultaneously. High doses taken intravenously produce a "flash," which is described as a sudden awakening feeling, or a full-body orgasm. The user then experiences a prolonged euphoric, hyperactive, hypersensitive period. The person has decreased desire to eat, but when the effects of the drug wear off he or she becomes depressed and hungry. When combined with heroin (speed balls), there is a "flash" and a prolonged drowsy, drifting feeling of more moderate euphoria. Some disturbing behavior changes and symptoms may occur for some individuals, including paranoid psychosis, suspicious and hostile feelings that lead to violence, the feeling of something crawling under the skin and the resulting scratching and cutting to rid the skin of the "bugs," and compulsive and repetitive behavior.

Amphetamines may be misused in a variety of ways, leading to a variety of problems and differing implications for solution. The drug does not appear to be addicting, and sudden withdrawal does not appear to be life threatening. When the person who has been on high doses over a prolonged period of time withdraws, the resulting depression, hunger, and fatigue symptoms disappear in about a week, and continued need for the drug does not seem to occur beyond the possible desire for another drug experience. The young person who uses the drug in moderate doses regularly for "weight control" and the youth who is "shooting" speed intravenously on a regular basis are both misusing the drug, but the problems and the end results are drastically different.

The depressant drugs commonly misused that are available in the United States by prescription include the barbiturates and several nonbarbiturates such as chloral hydrate, paraldehyde, and bromides. Chloral hydrate and paraldehyde are much like alcohol in their effects. Chloral hydrate combined with alcohol, known as a "Mickey Finn," has been known for several decades to cause dramatic effects such as transient unconsciousness. Chloral hydrate and paraldehyde are both relatively safe depressant drugs; they cause little respiratory and cardiovascular depression while effectively inducing sleep. Paraldehyde is not in widespread use because of the noxious taste and odor. The bromides are not widely used because of serious toxic effects with prolonged usage, but they bear mention because of their continued use in over-the-counter sleeping preparations. "Bromism" consists of dermatitis, constipation, motor disturbance, delirium, and psychosis.

The barbiturates are the most commonly misused prescription depressant available. These drugs are classified as long-acting (phenobarbital, barbital), intermediate acting (amobarbital), and short-acting (phenobarbital, secobarbital), depending on the length of time that is typically required for the drug to be metabolized in the liver. Tolerance probably develops because the drugs enhance the microsomal enzyme activity of the liver, causing increasingly more rapid reactivation of the drug. Addiction does occur, particularly in the face of prolonged high dosages. Therapeutic uses for the barbiturates are for treatment of anxiety, insomnia, epilepsy, and the induction of anesthesia. Very small doses of phenobarbital are sometimes used temporarily for the infant colic syndrome. The effects of the barbiturates are very similar to those of alcohol, including the initial euphoria, loss of inhibition, and behavioral stimulation. Subsequently depression of the peripheral sensory and motor pathways develops, leading to sleep and dulling of consciousness. In normal therapeutic uses the barbiturates have few toxic effects. However, they interact seriously with other drugs. Death has been reported repeatedly as a result of respiratory failure when a therapeutic sleeping dose of barbiturate was used following alcohol consumption.[84]

Barbiturate intoxication is similar to that of alcohol; increasing problems develop with increasingly high doses, and withdrawal from addiction is a life-threatening problem. Upon withdrawal from the drug, the user experiences an initial improvement of his or her condition over that of the intoxicated state and then begins to have increasing anxiety, insomnia, tremulousness, weakness, difficulty maintaining cardiovascular function, anorexia, nausea, and vomiting. Convulsions begin to develop by the second or third day following withdrawal, and a psychosis then develops with confusion, disorientation, and visual and auditory hallucinations. Withdrawal may cause death, but once the critical period has passed, the individual lapses into a deep sleep and begins to improve.

Barbiturates are highly effective suicide agents; once the lethal dose has been ingested, the individual lapses into a deep coma within a few minutes. This form of suicide accounts for about one fifth of all suicides in the United States annually.

Narcotic drugs have a long and interesting history, and their powers have long been known. They have always been associated with legitimate therapeutic use and with misuse, although it has only been in relatively recent times that misuse has been labeled a criminal offense. This labeling has come as a result of the indirect harm that comes to individuals and society from the misuse of the drugs. The actual taking of the drug and addiction to it are health problems, as are the accompanying problems of malnutrition, personal neglect, preoccupation with drug-taking, and infection.[63,84] The effects on society, including disruption of interpersonal relationships, economic cost, and crimes against people and property that arise from preoccupation with drug-taking, are social problems that many recent societies have legislated against. However, legislation has been relatively ineffective in controlling the problems of narcotic misuse, and there is growing controversy over the legal approaches that have been developed in the United States.

The narcotic drugs, which include the opiates and synthetics that have similar activity, are the most effective analgesics known today. They are particularly effective against visceral and skeletal pain, and mediate both intense, acute pain and dull, aching pain. The physiologic mechanism by which these drugs mediate pain is still unknown. Morphine, codeine, and heroin are isolated or derived from opium; methadone and meperidine (Demerol) are the most commonly used synthetic agents that mimic the action of the opiates. Morphine remains the classic standard against which all other narcotic agents are judged. In addition to the analgesic property for

which the narcotics are used therapeutically, they produce a euphoric sensation, which is the basis for much of the misuse of the drugs, and a physiologic dependency exceeding that of most other drugs. Tolerance to the analgesic and euphoric effects develops, so that increasingly larger doses of the drug are needed to obtain the desired effects.

The narcotic drugs do not seem to directly affect either the sensation of the pain stimulus or the threshold for pain. Instead, they appear to alter the individual's response to the pain. This action is thought to result from direct action of the cortical arousal system, resulting in a change in awareness and perception of the pain, and on the limbic system of the brain where emotional responses are mediated. The respiratory centers are affected, leading to the primary side effect of the drugs, although some narcotic agents exert a stronger effect on this function than do others. Death caused by narcotic overdose is a result of this depression of the respiratory centers. Constriction of the pupils of the eyes results from any dose of narcotic agents, and tolerance to this effect is minimal, so that this sign has become an important physical symptom of narcotic intoxication. Other less common but significant side effects are nausea and vomiting, decrease in body temperature, body fluid retention, and depression of the pituitary gland. The gastrointestinal tract is affected by a decrease in peristaltic contraction and slowing of passage of food through the tract. A significant amount of water is absorbed through the tract, and constipation develops. Tolerance to this side effect develops very gradually, if at all.

The term "addiction" refers to the fact that physiologic symptoms occur with the withdrawal of the drug after regular use and are relieved by taking another dose of the drug. This differs from dependency, which implies a desire to continue the use of a drug with minimal or no withdrawal effects occurring after regular use. Addiction occurs when the person recognizes the physical withdrawal symptoms for what they are and relieves the discomfort by taking another dose of the drug. When the symptoms are not recognized as related to the drug or are attributed to some other cause, the drug is not likely to be taken again and addiction does not develop. An individual becomes addicted either out of the desire to experience the pleasure and euphoria or from the need to avoid the discomfort and pain that results from withdrawal and return to the world of nondrug use.

The effects of narcotics experienced with regular use are highly variable and depend more on traits of the individual using the drug and the setting in which it is used than upon factors inherent in the drug itself. The "drug culture," which promotes the use of narcotics and makes them available to users on an illegal basis, also defines expectations for behavior, patterns of addiction, and drug use just as any other culture prescribes acceptable behavior. While people are using an optimal maintenance dose of a narcotic, they are physically able to function well in a job, to pursue their ordinary interests and hobbies, and maintain suitable interpersonal relationships. This has been demonstrated by those professional medical and health care workers who have ready access to "legitimate" narcotics and who carefully maintain an adjusted drug dose and continue to work successfully for many years. The dosage ultimately exceeds the level at which successful performance can be maintained, or discovery of drug use is made by colleagues and the habit is terminated in some manner. Contrary to popular belief, addiction occurs over a period of time of drug use, and some intentional effort is required to develop a real addiction.[60,84] Likewise, the withdrawal syndrome is highly variable among people, and becomes excruciatingly painful and life threatening only after a long period of regular use of high doses of the drug.[84]

The kind of treatment program that should be sought for young people who have experimented with or become addicted to narcotic drugs depends upon many factors related to the nature and level of drug use, the individual traits of the users, and the community and social climate in which they developed the misuse pattern. Several effective programs have begun in the United States and other countries, including psychosocial rehabilitation programs and pharmacologic maintenance programs (methadone maintenance), but the needs and demands for therapy far exceed the ability of society to provide treatment programs. Prevention of narcotic misuse remains the most desirable and necessary step in controlling the social and health problems related to narcotic misuse, but few effective prevention programs have been developed thus far.*

### Over-the-counter drugs

Over-the-counter (OTC) drugs are of particular concern because of the widespread availability of a vast array of agents that can be misused. Governmental controls have been instituted in recent decades to remove some dangerous drugs from over-the-counter availability, but a host of agents remain, and any drug is a potentially dangerous agent. Home treatment of minor ailments that tend to spontaneously resolve is a common and integral part of health care today. Throughout our discussions we have emphasized the desirability of helping families understand minor health problems and to become reliable and independent regarding their own health care. This ideal component of understanding symptomatology and using rational care measures, including appropriate OTC drugs, is often overlooked by professional health care workers, and the family is most often left to their own devices about adequate self-care. Labeling of agents available in drug stores has improved, but there is no immediate resource available to the family for judging the relative adequacy of the available agents or for integrating the drug into a sound plan of total care in the home, which includes therapeutic use of food, fluids, warmth, cold, laws of physics, rest, humidity, and so forth (see Chapters 2 and 11). Drug safety in regard to the young infant and toddler has been discussed, and realization of the toxic effects of all drugs on the young child can usually be understood and comprehended by most parents and older children. However, the potential dangers of drugs in the home for young people and adults, particularly in times of stress, is often not adequately appreciated by most families, as the casual approach to home remedies and frequent use of common drugs testify.

One of the greatest problems related to the

---

*References 16, 50, 54, 59, 66, 67, 84.

availability of OTC drugs is the advertising to which everyone is subjected. Several attempts have been made in the United States to control both the claims and the implications conveyed in advertising campaigns. However, the fact remains that there is widespread exposure to the message that pills are available to cure a host of common ailments and complaints, and that one can solve all problems and can achieve happiness, love, contentment, status, and security by ingesting drugs (including tobacco and alcohol). A significant portion of advertising in the United States in recent years has been directed away from claims about the symptom-relieving property of a drug; rather claims are made concerning the attainment of happiness and comfort, and solution of obscure life problems through the use of a particular agent. For example, a typical advertisement might claim that when you have a cold, you may take a certain agent to relieve the discomfort, but most importantly your family will love you more and you will no longer have the social problems that arise from being grouchy. Thus we have thoroughly indoctrinated young people, particularly since the advent of television, with the fact that pill popping is the way to live. While this factor is only one of many that have led to the increased misuse of drugs in our society, it has contributed to the fact that people today turn to drugs rather than to some other means for relief from the stresses of living.

Aspirin is probably the most widely used OTC drug available today. This truly miraculous drug has few side effects when taken in therapeutic doses, and it contains highly effective analgesic, antipyretic, and anti-inflammatory properties (see Chapter 11). However, when taken in overdoses, severe toxic effects occur at all ages, and intentional or accidental overdoses are a common hazard among individuals of all age groups. Among adolescents, aspirin is commonly used in supposed suicide attempts. Death from an overdose of aspirin is much more likely for the young toddler, because a severe metabolic acidosis is likely to develop in the young child in response to the initial respiratory alkalosis resulting from hyperventilation. The teenager's more mature system is better able to achieve electrolyte balance in response to the

hyperventilation, which is the hallmark of salicylism. Vomiting, hyperpyrexia, and sweating lead to dehydration, which compounds the dangers of electrolyte imbalance. As the severity of poisoning progresses, delirium, hallucinations, convulsions, coma, and acute pulmonary edema occur. Withdrawal of the drug from the system brings dramatic relief of the symptoms, but supportive fluid and electrolyte therapy may be needed until all of the salicylate that has already reached the circulatory system is excreted.[3,75,84]

Cold and cough remedies are among the most commonly used OTC drugs. They are considered here particularly because they contain agents that are prone to abuse by young people. These are the sympathomimetics and anticholinergic compounds. Phenylephrine and amphetamine are sympathomimetic agents found in inhalers, nasal drops, and sprays that are used to shrink mucous membranes of the nose and decrease nasal congestion. Antihistamines, scopolamine, and belladonna alkaloids exert an anticholinergic effect. Cough suppressants containing codeine or dextromethorphan act by depressing the central nervous system, but in most cases these agents are used at such a low level that it is not possible to obtain the desired misuse effects without suffering from an overdose of the cough remedy. The relatively high alcoholic content of many of these preparations in combination with the psychoactive agents leads to experimentation in attempting to achieve a "high."[75,84,91]

### Social drugs

Mood- and consciousness-altering chemicals known as "social drugs" may be difficult to conceptualize as drugs because of their widespread use as social and mild therapeutic agents. The principal active chemicals contained in the many available compounds are ethyl alcohol, nicotine, and caffeine. Products made from fermentation and distillation processes, from tobacco, and from the cocoa nut have been used for centuries in societies all over the world, and the acceptability of such compounds has varied from culture to culture and from generation to generation.

Ethyl alcohol is a depressant with action primarily on the reticular activating system of the brain. It is absorbed directly into the bloodstream from the stomach and the small intestine with no digestive processes necessary and is metabolized in the liver. The liver is limited in the rate at which alcohol can be metabolized, and as intake exceeds the rate of oxidation, the alcohol circulates in the blood and body fluids until full metabolism is possible. Alcohol provides a ready source of energy but cannot be stored in any form in the body. Because alcohol is readily available for energy demands at the time of consumption, other foods and energy sources are not utilized but are stored, resulting in the weight gain that may accompany a high alcoholic intake. There is some evidence that heavy, habitual alcohol drinkers have an increased rate of oxidation and metabolism of alcohol, and therefore they can drink more volume without attaining a circulating level that the moderate or light drinker would experience. Behavioral tolerance to alcohol develops with heavy and habitual usage, as does tolerance to the undesirable aftereffects of hangover symptoms. Alcohol blood levels of 0.35% produce a surgical anesthesia, and alcohol was used for this purpose in the past. However, because this level is very close to the lethal dose, alcohol is not a safe or desirable agent for anesthesia.

The exact mechanism of the action of alcohol is not clearly understood, but it appears that the primary effect is on the neuronal membranes themselves and not the synapse, as with most other psychoactive drugs. As the reticular system is the first area of the brain to be affected, the initial effect is a general good feeling, with decreased ability to integrate complex and abstract material and loss of the ordinary inhibitions. Because of inhibitory loss, alcohol is mistakenly believed to be a stimulant, but in actuality the changes observed in behavior are the result of the depression of inhibitions. Thus the exact behavioral effect that is experienced with alcohol is highly individualized and depends upon the person's past experiences and the particular behavioral inhibitions that have been learned throughout life. As the circulating blood level of alcohol increases, the individual experiences more direct effects on the cerebral functions of the brain, with loss of motor and sensory capacities, depression of awareness, and finally

coma and death. Death probably results from depression of the respiratory control mechanism of the medulla.

Alcohol today is used therapeutically only informally as a sedative and a minor tranquilizer. Moderate intake and social use are reported by a significant number of people—about 80% of urban adults and about half of rural adults in America.[84] The problems of misuse of alcohol and eventual addiction to this drug have been only partially studied, and understanding of these problems is clearly limited. Personality and cultural factors seem to be the most pervasive determinants of alcohol misuse, but there are few indices that can be used to predict the eventual use pattern of a young person who begins to experiment with alcohol. Most young people who come from homes where alcohol is used in moderation become users themselves, but there is no evidence to indicate that such young people are more likely to become abusers than are those from homes maintaining abstinence. Alcohol is one of the most important drugs of abuse in America today, and the social cost of problems resulting from the use of alcohol is incalculable. Efforts to control the use of alcohol through legal means have been relatively ineffective, and there appears to be no simple approach to alcohol abuse problems. The high prevalence of use in societies for centuries has not led to the development of ways to avoid the pitfalls of misuse; neither has such prolonged use aided in the understanding of the problems that lead to misuse. Young people can and should be exposed to factual information about the use of alcohol and about the dangers involved in trying to perform certain skills, particularly driving, while alcohol is affecting their higher mental processes. Knowledge alone does not ensure the sound judgment of human beings, and the added insights that lead to sound judgment and moderation are difficult or impossible to define.[84,86]

Inhalation of nicotine through tobacco smoke is also a well-established social habit throughout the world. Nicotine has no therapeutic uses, and it has not been studied as extensively as either alcohol or caffeine. However, since the deleterious effects of this drug on health and longevity have been realized, an increasing interest in the physiologic effects of nicotine and tobacco smoking has developed. While it is clear that cigarette smoking is related to the development of serious disease, the nature of this relationship is not clearly understood, and much speculation has developed around conflicting reports of research evidence. Like many of the "social drugs," nicotine has multiple effects upon the body, and it appears that some people smoke for one effect while others smoke for another. Some research evidence indicates that nicotine is a stimulant at a certain optimal dosage level, and that smoking is continued for this stimulant effect, with the individual selecting the dosage that produces this effect. Other indications are that it is a depressant following a brief period of stimulation, and that smoking is continued for the mild tranquilizing effect achieved.

Nicotine is one of the most toxic drugs known, having an extremely rapid lethal effect at a relatively low dosage. The lethal dose is about 60 mg for humans, the amount contained in two to three filter cigarettes. When cigarette smoke is inhaled, only about 10% of the nicotine is delivered to the lungs of the smoker, and about 90% of that is absorbed. It is gradually deactivated by the liver and excreted by the kidney. While in the active form, it exerts a blockage of cholinergic synapses and stimulates the release of adrenaline from the adrenal glands and other sympathetic sites. It blocks selected sensory receptors such as the chemical receptors found in some large arteries and the thermal and pain receptors in the skin and tongue. The nicotine delivered while smoking one cigarette can inhibit hunger contractions of the stomach for up to one hour.[84]

In addition to the effects of nicotine, carbon monoxide from the smoke is delivered to the lungs and blood, which combines with the hemoglobin molecule and causes a significant decrease in the oxygen-carrying capacity of the blood. This factor is at least partially responsible for the increase in heart rate, increased metabolic rate, increased oxygen consumption, and shortness of breath on exertion. In spite of its hazards, cigarette smoking produces some effects that people obviously want, and ways to approach the health problems resulting from cigarette smoking are as elusive as for the problem of alcohol consumption. The United States government and several other countries have begun to control the advertising of cigarettes, as well as requiring a specific label that warns of the health hazards that occur with use. These measures are designed to discourage the beginning of use of tobacco by young people. Dependency and addiction may develop before the young person has reached a point when adequate judgment can be made considering the serious health consequences. Whether these control measures have had an appreciable effect on the use of tobacco by young people remains uncertain (see Chapter 14).[44,61]

The pharmacologically active agents contained in certain drinks popular in America and other countries are a group of stimulants known as xanthines. These are primarily caffeine, theophylline, and theobromine. Caffeine is responsible for the action of coffee, cola, and tea; theophylline is found in tea, and theobromine is in the fruit of the chocolate tree. Caffeine has the most potent effect on the central nervous system. It is not significantly toxic to humans, but it does create dependency and mild withdrawal symptoms of headache. Tolerance to the effects of the drug develops, and it may take more than two months of abstinence to return to an originally sensitive state. A dose of about 150 to 250 mg of caffeine (about 2 cups of coffee) causes stimulation of the cortex and some increase in heart rate, blood pressure, and metabolic rate occurs. The renal excretion of urine and salivary gland secretion is stimulated, and sleep may be disturbed. There are varying effects on the blood vessels and vascular muscles, with dilation occurring in some areas of the body and constriction occurring in others, primarily the brain. There is some evidence that caffeine increases blood levels of lipids and glucose, and this is thought to be related to the fact that caffeine users develop a higher incidence of angina and myocardial infarction than do nonusers. However, users seem to have a better chance of surviving a myocardial infarction than do nonusers, and the evidence in this regard remains controversial.[84]

Theophylline is the most potent xanthine affecting the cardiovascular system. Theobromine exerts almost no effect on either the central nervous system or the cardiovascular system, requiring much higher doses for an effect to occur. While there are adverse side effects of the xanthines, they appear to be far removed from the use of the drugs, and the exact mechanism of action is poorly understood. As mild stimulants they are relatively safe, the dosage is easily adjusted, and the drinks in which they occur, such as chocolate and tea, remain socially popular.[84]

### Nondrug chemicals

Many chemicals that are sold for nondrug purposes actually exert a drug effect, and produced in a slightly different form may in fact be intended for drug use. Aromatic hydrocarbons are the substances most prone to misuse by preadolescent children. These are readily available in most households in many forms, including model airplane glue, spot removers, innertube repair cement, aerosol deodorants, furniture polish, hair spray, paint thinner, nail polish remover, and gasoline. Inhaling or sniffing these substances produces a euphoric sensation and excited, cheerful behavior. Tolerance to these substances develops as with other dependency-producing agents, and increasingly large doses are required to produce the desired effects. Children and young people may use a plastic bag as a container to hold and concentrate the sniffed substance, leading to suffocation, which can cause death. In addition, freezing of the larynx and lung tissue by various spray products has caused instantaneously lethal effects. The common vapors found in these products include toluene, benzene, trichloroethane, trichlorofluoromethane, and cyrofluorane. Labels are required to identify the substance contained, as well as a warning regarding the dangerous effects of inhalation of the substance.[16,91]

Various easily obtained products derived from plants are also misused by young people and children. Morning glory seeds (Heavenly Blues, Pearly Gates) produce an effect similar to LSD when ingested in large quantities, including perceptual distortions, confusion, giddiness, euphoria, hallucinations, and sometimes an intense anxiety reaction. Catnip smoked and inhaled produces a sensation similar to that of marijuana, but a larger dose is required to achieve the effect. A teaspoonful of nutmeg produces euphoria, hallucinations, excitement, and delirium.[91]

### Illegal drugs

The hallucinogenic chemicals that are available today have a complex and interesting history. Peyote, which has been used in religious and ritualistic ceremonies for centuries by the American Indian, continues to be used as an integral part of the religious and ritual ceremonies of many groups of American Indians. It is believed to possess magic powers and to be useful in curing illness. Peyote, which is derived from the cactus Lophophora williamsii, contains over 30 psychoactive alkaloids. The earliest to be identified is mescaline, which is known to be responsible for vivid visual perceptions. The hallucinogenic drugs that have come into use in technological societies have also been associated with seeking mystical, religious, or mind-expanding experiences. Scientific experimentation has been attempted in order to explore possible therapeutic uses, particularly in the treatment of emotional disorders. The effects are not understood, but are thought to be mediated by action on the neurotransmitted serotonin. The synthetic chemical lysergic acid diethylamide (LSD) has received particular attention, since it was one of the first widely publicized hallucinogenic drugs during the 1960s. Because of fears of chromosomal damage and "bad trips" from impure forms of the drugs, its use has declined, and mescaline and peyote have become the most frequently used hallucinogenic drugs.

The exact pharmacologic action of LSD is not clearly understood, but of the many possible explanations, interaction with the neurotransmitter serotonin seems to be the predominant theory. It is a powerful sympathomimetic, and thus the first effects to appear after ingestion are dilation of the pupils, elevation of temperature and blood pressure, and an increase in salivation. It is metabolized in the liver relatively rapidly and excreted by the kidneys in an inactive form. Tolerance develops within two or three days of repeated use, but recovery from the tolerance is equally rapid, with weekly doses producing the same effect from week to week. The drug does not act directly on sensory pathways themselves, except perhaps in the visual system, but it does increase the effect of sensory input, causing the experience of vivid sensory experiences.

Either alone or in combination with other drugs, particularly the amphetamines, LSD can cause the experiences known as "bad trips." There is an increasing awareness of the massive sympathomimetic effects of LSD and/or the stimulant drugs, which lead to panic and intense anxiety. After the initial autonomic symptoms, there is a gradual increase in mood alterations, abnormal body sensations, decrease in sensory impression, abnormal color perception, space and time disorders, and visual hallucinations. During the second hour, major personality disruptions occur for some users, usually centering about an intense depersonalization. Sensory experiences seem to be outside of the body, or a feeling of having no body at all develops. Distortions of the body are common, as is loss of self-awareness and control of behavior. During this phase of reaction the person on a "good trip" experiences feelings of expansiveness and feels grandiose, hypomanic, and/or creative. The "bad trip" is characterized by feelings of constriction, with limitations in movement, and feelings of paranoia and persecution. As the drug begins to be metabolized and the circulating level decreases, the person slowly begins to regain normal sensory capacities and control of behavior. Difficulty in returning to the nondrug reality may occur, particularly for individuals who have a tenuous hold on reality in the first place. "Flashbacks" can occur, meaning that there is a recurrence of the symptoms several months after use of the drug.

The way in which the individual interprets the hallucinogenic drug experience depends on past experiences and the way in which he or she normally experiences the world. Persons who have emotional problems, difficulty relating socially, or a weak self-concept tend to have bad experiences with the drugs. Many people, on the other hand, tend to view the drug experiences as being magnificent, mind expanding, a great stimulus to creativity, personally revealing, and deeply spiritual. Memory of the drug experience is vivid for most people, so regardless of the interpretation, it may have a significant impact on the individual's reaction to nondrug reality.

Perhaps the most controversial of all psychoactive agents available for use today is that derived from the *Cannabis sativa* plant. The flowering tops of the plant have the greatest concentration of resin, which contains the psychoactive agent and is prepared and marketed under the names of hash, hashish, or cannabis. The leafy and fibrous lower parts of the plant contain lesser concentrations of resin and are prepared as marijuana. Opinion and scientific evidence are widely divergent; there are few clear understandings and many misconceptions about the drug. There have been widely variant reports through recorded history of the various therapeutic uses of *Cannabis* and it has been used recently in therapeutic trials for treatment of glaucoma and other illnesses. The drug is highly variable in strength of action, depending upon the part of the plant used and the geographic location of cultivation. *Cannabis* is insoluble in water and therefore not easily prepared for injectable use. The onset of effect is usually prolonged, and with oral use can be as long as one to two hours.

The immediate effects of inhalation of marijuana are dose related. At typical social levels of intake there is an increase in pulse rate, reddening of the eyes, and dryness of the mouth and throat. In increased doses there are some gastrointestinal effects, including slowing of movement of food through the tract and relaxation of the smooth muscles. Increases in appetite are also experienced. Effects on the lung are not completely demonstrated, but evidence thus far indicates that the smoking of marijuana may not be as damaging as smoking tobacco containing nicotine. The behavioral and physiologic effects of marijuana are difficult to isolate and distinguish, because they are highly individualized and subject to learning and conditioning by the social environment in which use occurs. It appears to have properties similar to stimulant, sedative, analgesic, and psychotomimetic drugs. Some claim that the marijuana "high" is similar to that experienced with alcohol, without the effects of a hangover after intake. Others claim that the experience is quite different and more pleasurable than that of alcohol. Dependency on the drug does not develop, and there are no withdrawal symptoms when regular use of the drug is terminated. For these reasons proponents of the legalization of marijuana claim that it is far safer than alcohol and tobacco. Those who oppose legalization claim that the evidence is not complete enough to say that it is less harmful than alcohol or nicotine and that is has become a means of entering into the world of severe drug misuse. There are convincing arguments and evidence in either direction, and the use of marijuana continues to be widespread in the United States. There is a relative lack of evidence relating marijuana use to harmful physiologic or psychologic effects, but moderate social use does impair the individual's immediate performance capacity and thus leads to dangers similar to those of intoxication from alcohol. There is no basis for the belief that marijuana use leads directly to the use of the opiates or hallucinogens; the social and emotional climates in which marijuana use occurs are far more important factors in determining whether marijuana use will lead to the use of other more harmful drugs.*

### Health care and crisis intervention

The identification of drug misuse or abuse remains somewhat speculative and based on highly individualized information related to the drug being used, the factors that may contribute to the misuse or abuse for the individual, and social factors that contribute to the behavior. Further investigation is needed to establish criteria that might be used in relation to formulating a problem statement. The Minnesota Nursing Problem Classification provides several different categories for a problem of drug misuse or abuse. Drug misuse is classified under the general category of need for knowledge and guidance for each age group: no. 306.6 (5 to 9 years); no. 307.6 (10 to 13 years); no. 308.6 (14 to 17 years); and no. 309.6 (18 to 21 years). The classifications for abuse and crisis include no. 363.2 (parental drug and/or alcohol abuse); no. 322.2 (alcohol abuse/addiction); no. 322.3 (drug abuse /addiction); and no. 351.3 (drug crisis).

---

*References 3, 16, 28, 32, 44, 50, 54, 57, 61, 62, 67, 84, 86, 91.

In Chapters 12 and 14 we considered primarily the problems of differentiating between transient drug experimentation during adolescence and factors indicating the beginning of habitual use and misuse. Prevention of habitual use or misuse is a significant concern in health care and primarily involves rational transfer of real information upon which a personal judgment can be made. Because some form of drug use is inevitable for most individuals in modern society, it is important to convey and to practice rational and conservative approaches toward use and to recognize all forms of misuse of all types of drugs. Although all drugs are potentially dangerous and subject to misuse, some drugs and pharmacologically active substances are safer than others when used in moderation and with sound judgment. For example, the xanthines are relatively harmless, as is alcohol in moderate usage. However, even when used moderately, environmental and social factors may identify a misuse situation, as is the case when the relatively harmless drug marijuana is used as a deliberate social introduction into the "hard" drug culture. Because of the dangers resulting from loss of motor control with alcohol intoxication, this agent has far greater social and physical implications than those related to the direct effect of the drug on the body.[79,84]

While legal and illegal labels on drug use are defined clearly, though not always optimally, the concepts of drug use and misuse are much less clearly defined. There appears to be a continuum between the two extremes, and definition of a particular situation depends upon many complex factors. It appears that there is no drug that is not misused in some way by a certain percentage of those using it. Drugs appear to offer one alternative to many of the unmet needs of individuals in a society and thus are a major outlet and expression of these needs. Therefore, one of the first approaches in health care related to drug misuse is to help the individual identify the personal factors that led to the use or misuse of the agent. Professional health care workers are in a particularly significant position to provide information and guidance regarding the judicious use of drugs. Unfortunately, professional injudicious use of drugs is all too common and represents a conflicting message with the primary goal of achieving maximal health. If a potentially harmful drug is to be used therapeutically, it is essential that the young person understand the hazards of use and the potential for misuse. Most young people will take appropriate measures to control their use of a given agent when they understand the problems involved. When such personal efforts are not taken, a problem of misuse develops and specific psychosocial or medical therapy must be considered.*

To many young people who use or misuse drugs, alienation and the related search for identity apart from the established society are very real factors. Traditional health care systems and the professional people who work in them are considered to be a significant part of the society from which the youth is seeking alienation. The expected response from the health care worker is condemnation, moralization, and punishment. Some effort is needed to establish a meaningful relationship and to soften the image of the health care worker as being judgmental and moralistic. Indeed, the health care worker cannot condone many of the drug practices of alienated youth, but the problems of the young person must be understood, and an empathic, nonjudgmental, confidential approach must be used in helping the young person find a solution to those problems for which he or she seeks help. Scare tactics are seldom if ever effective, because the young person has access to many facts that discount predictions of severe sequelae to drug use. Concern for all aspects of the young person's life, including needs for self-identity, social needs, and physical health maintenance, must be included when helping an individual reach a rational decision regarding the use of drugs and related problems.

When a young person comes to a health care setting or is found in the community suffering from a drug crisis, a "bad trip," or an emotional crisis arising from drug use, immediate and energetic approaches are indicated. The specific crisis therapy that is indicated depends upon the drug ingested; thus the first crucial factor is

to identify, if possible, which agent was taken. Often there is no reliable source of information, and the patient's signs and symptoms are the only clues. The toxic effects of some of the common drugs have been discussed above; specific assistance from a local poison control center may be needed to identify probable agents causing the symptoms that are observed. Table 15-1 summarizes the adverse reactions that are observed when a drug crisis occurs.

Principles of care that apply to all poisonings are applied in most misuse crises. As much of the drug as possible must be removed from the system, and the individual's physiologic and homeostatic mechanisms must be supported by all therapeutic means indicated. Exchange of gases must be maintained, fluid and electrolyte balance must be preserved, and cardiovascular function supported. When behavior changes lead to self-inflicted injury, protection is necessary. In the case of withdrawal reaction from a narcotic drug, a variety of therapeutic approaches is advocated. Some health care centers support the person through the withdrawal without using the drug to alleviate the withdrawal symptoms; other centers use some form of the drug or an equivalent drug to relieve the withdrawal temporarily and to give the individual a chance to voluntarily enter into some kind of treatment program.

Specific antidotes may block or reverse the severe effects of toxic doses of some of the misused drugs. For example, chlorpromazine blocks or reverses the effects of LSD; naloxone is an effective narcotic antagonist.[54,84] However, because the full effects of many of the drugs are not fully understood, the addition of yet another pharmacologically active agent to the system further complicates the homeostatic mechanisms of the body. In addition, the exact drug that is involved may not be known, and it may be impossible to use a drug antidote.

Of great importance for the person involved in a physical or emotional crisis is physical and emotional support through the crisis experience. The value of this kind of support is recognized by those who have experimented with LSD in research efforts to understand the action of this drug. When drug intake is made experimentally for scientific purposes, there is always

*References 16, 54, 56, 74, 79, 84.

**Table 15-1.** Symptoms of commonly misused drugs and poisons*

| Agent | Symptoms | Agent | Symptoms |
|---|---|---|---|
| Ampheta-mine | CNS stimulation with restlessness, apprehension, irritability, delirium, hallucinations, tremors, and convulsions, followed by profound depression<br>Gastrointestinal distress<br>Dilated pupils, dry mouth | Ethyl alcohol —cont'd | Gastrointestinal manifestations—one or more of the following:<br>Anorexia<br>Intermittent vomiting<br>Abdominal pain<br>Constipation |
| Antihista-mines | CNS depression (children may be stimulated)<br>Atropinelike symptoms, dryness in mouth, fixed dilated pupils, flushing<br>Gastrointestinal distress | | CNS manifestations—one or more of the following:<br>Irritability<br>Drowsiness<br>Persistent vomiting<br>Incoordination |
| Aspirin | Gastrointestinal distress<br>Hyperventilation<br>Hyperpyrexia<br>Hypoprothrombinemia<br>Metabolic acidosis<br>Hypoglycemia | | Convulsions<br>Coma<br>Weakness or paralysis<br>Hypertension<br>Papilledema and/or optic atrophy<br>Paralysis of one or more cranial nerves |
| Barbiturates | Respiratory center depression with slow, shallow breathing; cyanosis often present<br>Circulatory depression and shock due to depression of the vasomotor center, as well as direct action on smooth muscle in blood vessel wall<br>Water loss from skin and lungs; decrease in urine output; electrolytes variable | | Elevated cerebrospinal fluid protein content<br>Cerebrospinal fluid plocytosis<br>Elevated cerebrospinal fluid pressure<br>Hematologic manifestations—one or more of the following:<br>Hypochromic microcytic anemia<br>Significant degree of basophilic stippling of red blood cells |
| Chloral hydrate | CNS depression<br>Cardiovascular depression<br>Gastrointestinal distress<br>Banana odor and blanching of lips<br>"Knockout drops" are mixture of chloral and alcohol, producing potent depressant effect<br>Caustic effects with exophagitis (stricture) and gastritis | | 75%-100% red fluorescence in erythrocytes examined under ultraviolet light<br>Radiologic density at metaphyses of long bones |
| | | Marijuana | Exhilaration, euphoria, talkative, conjunctivitis, dryness of mouth<br>Later quiet, drowsy, sleepy |
| Codeine | CNS depression with muscular twitching and convulsions<br>Weakness, disturbed vision, miosis, dyspnea<br>Respiratory depression, collapse, coma | | Chronic effects are tremors, anorexia, pallor, weakness, mental deterioration, with reduction of will power and concentration<br>Users have odor of burnt rope on person or clothing |
| Ethyl alcohol | CNS depression<br>Blood levels of 0.05%-0.15%—slight muscular incoordination and visual impairment and slowing of reaction time<br>Blood levels of 0.15%-0.3%—slurring of speech, definite visual impairment, muscular incoordination, sensory loss<br>Blood levels of 0.3%-0.5%—marked muscular incoordination, sensory loss, blurred or double vision, approaching stupor<br>At 5% concentration—coma, slowed and labored respiration, decreased reflexes, and sensory loss; death can occur | Meproba-mate | CNS depression<br>Respiratory and cardiovascular collapse<br>Stupor, coma, hypotension, miosis, loss of reflexes |
| | | Morphine | Profound CNS depression from above downward and stimulation from below upward<br>Stupor, coma, miosis, slow and shallow respiration, cyanosis, tremors, convulsions<br>Severe retching and nausea |

*Adapted from Arena, J. M.: Poisoning and its treatment, Table 16-2. In Shirkey, H. C., editor: Pediatric therapy, ed. 5, St. Louis, 1975, The C. V. Mosby Co.

**Table 15-1.** Symptoms of commonly misused drugs and poisons—cont'd

| Agent | Symptoms | Agent | Symptoms |
|---|---|---|---|
| Nicotine | CNS stimulation followed by depression; clonic convulsions, followed by collapse and respiratory failure<br>Gastrointestinal distress, severe<br>Caustic effects on mouth, throat, esophagus, stomach | Parathion (phosphate ester insecticides) —cont'd | Muscarine effects<br>Miosis<br>Sweating, salivation, tearing<br>Pulmonary edema<br>Bradycardia and hypertension<br>Abdominal cramps, vomiting, diarrhea |
| Parathion (phosphate ester insecticides) | Nicotinic effects<br>Incoordination<br>Fasciculation<br>Paralysis | | Effects<br>Apathy<br>Convulsions<br>Coma |

another person present who is not using the drug and who supports the experimenting individual through the experience. When a physical crisis is not involved, young people may be relatively far removed from the drug experience, as when they have been discovered to have illegal drugs in their possession. Sincere concern for individuals and their problems and an appreciation of their total life space are essential for effective helping relationships in the crisis.*

### Rape (MNPC no. 351.7)

Rape and the problems resulting from it have been increasingly acknowledged by the public and have become the object of investigation and social action during the 1970s. Yet the traditional misconceptions and prejudices surrounding rape persist in the minds of men and women, and rape victims are often unable or unwilling to report their plight. When they do, they are often treated with suspicion, disrespect, and rejection, and their real needs are misconstrued, ignored, and denied. Traditionally, the emphasis in definitions of rape has been on the role of the victim of the assault rather than on the person rendering the assault, and investigations by police, legal authorities, and health care workers have focused on an investigation of the victim's role in the crime, a policy that does not exist for any other type of criminal act. Most reports of investigation of rape incidents label the incident as "alleged rape" or "suspected rape,"

further implying the focus of the victim's role in defining whether a crime was committed and indicating a basic distrust of the report of the crime. When a prepubertal child has been assaulted, the crime is likely to be labeled sexual abuse, and the criminal act may be taken more seriously, but the child's primary caretaker often becomes the target of suspicion, and distrust related to his or her failure to protect the child against the crime or in some way contributing to the incident is evident.[12,15,48,96]

Rape exists in epidemic proportions in the United States, a fact that is readily clear even if the statistics of reported rape alone are examined. In 1974, reported rapes had increased over 200% over reported rapes in 1960. It is estimated that only one in ten rape crimes is reported to the law enforcement officials or the health care system. These estimates are based on the traditional view and definition of rape, which focuses on the role of the victim in the crime; if the victim's experience of sexual trauma were used in labeling and reporting such crimes, the statistics would mount considerably.[96]

For the purposes of this discussion, rape is defined as any physical encounter between an attacker and a victim involving the use of sex, strength, and power against the will of the victim and violating the victim's right to preserve physical and emotional integrity. The victim is usually a girl or woman but can be a boy or man. The attacker is usually a man, but instances in which a woman performs acts of sexual assault are increasingly recognized.

---

*References 2, 19, 54, 67, 84, 98.

## Nursing diagnosis

Counseling programs and rape crisis centers have been developed in many communities in an attempt to correct the complex problems of inadequate response and care for the rape victim. Their efforts and careful study of the problems involved have led to a new understanding of the rape crime and of the needs of victims of rape. Holmstrom and Burgess[48] have developed three categories of diagnosis of rape, which are based on the victim's perception of the distress experienced and which reflect a more comprehensive conceptualization of what constitutes a rape experience than has been traditionally acknowledged. These diagnostic categories are as follows:

1. *Rape trauma syndrome.* The rape trauma syndrome develops as the result of forced, violent sexual penetration against the victim's will and without the victim's consent or from an attempted attack of this nature. There is an acute phase of disorganization in the victim's life-style and a long-term phase of life-style reorganization. Each of these phases may last months or years. During the acute phase the victim experiences physical symptoms of gastrointestinal irritability, muscular tension, sleep-pattern disturbance, genitourinary discomfort, and a wide range of emotional responses. The long-term phase involves changes in life-style such as change in residence, seeking support from family members, friends, and professional helpers, and learning to cope with repetitive nightmares and phobias. There are two types of expression of the rape trauma syndrome that may be observed: the compounded reaction and the silent reaction. The compounded reaction involves the experience of the rape trauma syndrome as described above, compounded by the reactivation of symptoms of previous conditions such as physical or psychiatric illness. The silent reaction is one in which the victim does not reveal either the fact of rape or the symptoms of the rape trauma syndrome to anyone. The physical and emotional symptoms are present, but the victim is unable or unwilling to report them to anyone. Signs of this type of reaction should alert the nurse to consider a diagnosis of rape trauma syndrome. The signs include increasing anxiety during an interview, including such behavior as withdrawal and long silences, a report of abrupt changes in relationships with men, significant changes in sexual behavior and attitudes, sudden onset of phobic reactions, or increase in nightmares.

2. *Accessory-to-sex reaction.* This reaction occurs when the victim is incapable of giving consent to sexual activity because of the stage of personality or cognitive development but is coerced into cooperation and thus contributes to the offense in a secondary manner. The victims are most often children or adolescents, but this type of rape can occur at any age. The offender coerces the victim and gains access in one of three ways: (1) by pressuring the victim to accept material goods such as candy or money in return for cooperating, (2) by pressuring a socially deprived victim to accept human contact, and (3) by convincing the victim that sexual activity is appropriate and enjoyable. The reaction of the victim involves gradual social and psychologic withdrawal, especially when the offense is repeated with the same offender over an extended period of time and the victim is sworn to secrecy. How and when the offense is revealed is an important diagnostic factor.

3. *Sex-stress situation.* Sex-stress occurs when both parties have consented to the sexual activity initially, but the sex situation produces trauma and anxiety for one of the participants. This occurs when the offender demands sexual perversion as perceived by the victim or is violent or sadistic. Sex-stress can be created when other people in authority, such as parents, law enforcement officers, or health care workers, become aware of the sexual activity, thus creating a situation of sex-stress. The reaction of the victim may involve physical and emotional symptoms similar to that of the rape trauma syndrome and often involves feelings of guilt and shame arising from the fact that initial consent for the sexual activity was given. This may be expressed in terms of "I should have known better," or "It was my fault."[48]

### Counseling the rape victim

The initial interview and long-term counseling and support are essential in helping the rape victim reconstruct a healthy life-style. An open-ended protocol for the initial interview of the rape victim is presented on p. 614. This interview approach facilitates accurate understanding of the crisis request of the victim and promotes the development of a long-term plan for support based on the client's perceived needs. Burgess and Holmstrom[15] identify five categories of crisis request that account for the expressed needs of rape victims as identified in the initial interview just after reporting the rape. These are:

1. *Need for medical intervention: "I need a physician."* The victim is seeking reassurance of her physical condition and often wants some intervention to alleviate fears of pregnancy and venereal disease that might have resulted from the rape. She views the health care services as offering traditional medical intervention for physical lacerations, abrasions, bruises, and other injuries, and the primary concern is establishing an opinion of the degree of physical injury.

2. *Need for police intervention: "I need a policeman."* This is often the primary expressed need of the victim who has been physically beaten as well as raped and includes the expression of the need for protection and for assistance in retaliation against the assailant. The victim has a strong desire to ensure that justice is met, and a friend or a family member who is accompanying the victim may join in this intent.

3. *Need for psychologic intervention: "I need to talk to someone."* Victims in this group usually request medical and police assistance but also see the health care system as a resource for counseling and support and a means of ventilating feelings about the experience and obtaining information. They express feelings of shock and talk spontaneously about their feelings.

4. *Uncertain: "I'm not sure I want anything."* Victims with this reaction usually seek medical or police assistance because of the advice of a friend or family member and are not sure if anyone can really help them or of their own feelings toward the experience. They may be relieved to be in a health care setting, angry and resentful toward the fact of being there, or may feel indifferent. They are usually ambivalent about what to do as a result of the rape experience and are willing to go along with the advice of other people.

5. *Control: "I need control."* These victims arrive at the health care setting in an incoherent state, often high on alcohol or drugs or in a psychotic state. Contrary to popular belief, this type of reaction is relatively rare, but it occurs with such drama that the distress of the victim cannot easily escape the attention of police officers, family members, or friends. This type of victim is usually accompanied by someone when they arrive in the health care setting, and the victim is usually unable to verbalize her needs or provide an account of what has happened until after she has been assisted in gaining control.[15]

The response to the primary request at the time of the initial interview is crucial in the adjustment that the victim makes to the rape trauma experienced. If the health care worker responds appropriately to the victim's initial request, the victim is able to progress; if the response is inappropriate, the victim is likely to regress or not make progress toward reintegration of life-style. As the weeks and months pass after the initial experience, there is usually a change in the expressed needs of the rape victim. These long-term needs and related counseling needs are described by Burgess and Holmstrom[15] as follows:

1. *Confirmation of concern: "It's nice to know you are available."* Many of the victims who exhibit this response in the long-term adjustment period are children and young adolescents who are relatively inarticulate in expressing their emotions and feelings. Often their parents express a need for ventilation or clarification (see below), and the young person may rely on these family members for support. Often the initial response was a request for medical intervention (initial crisis response no. 1 above) without the expressed need for emotional support or counseling.

This type of response requires active participation on the part of the helper. The contacts that are made with the victim involve active questioning about the daily activities of the person, such as getting back to school or work, and reestablishing satisfying social contacts with friends. Positive feedback for positive features of adjustment provides confirmation of the person's feelings and perceptions and reinforce-

## Initial interview guide of the rape victim*

### Introductory phase

SETTING: Concern for privacy (the right of the victim to retain emotional and physical privacy).

INTRODUCTION: Purpose of interview and who the counselor is (the right of the victim to understand what is being done).

COMMUNICATION: Request of the victim and request of the counselor (the right of the victim to influence care and to be carefully listened to).

### Working phase

THE ASSAULT

1. Circumstances: When and where was the victim approached? Why was she there? Where did the rape itself occur?
2. Assailant: Who did it? Was he of the same race? Was he known to the victim? A stranger? Number of assailants?
3. Conversation: What kind of conversation occurred prior to the rape between victim and assailant? Did he try to help her or con her? Did he threaten her? Did he make humiliating comments? Did he talk during the rape? Did he offer to pay her? What did she say to the assailant?
4. Sexual details: What type of sex did the assailant demand (e.g., vaginal, oral, or anal intercourse)? What type did he actually obtain from her? What other degrading acts, such as urinating on her, did he perform? How did she react to what she was forced to do?
5. Physical and verbal threats: Did the assailant have a weapon? Did he threaten the victim physically or verbally? What kind of violence, such as slapping or striking, did he inflict?
6. Struggle: Did the woman struggle? How does she feel about this?
7. Alcohol and drug use by assailant or victim: Does she think the assailant was under the influence of drugs or alcohol? Had she been using drugs or alcohol? How does she feel about this?
8. Emotional reaction: How did the victim feel emotionally at the time? How does she feel emotionally now? What is the most painful part to think about?
9. Sexual reaction: What does the sexual assault actually mean to the victim? Is this her first sexual experience? Or what has been her normal sexual style? What are her feelings about sex? Has she been attacked or raped before?

AFTER THE ATTACK

1. Seeking help: Where did she go for help? Was there any delay to clean up or to change clothes before seeking help? Who did she talk with or helped her decide what to do? Did *she* decide to seek help or was the decision made for her?
2. Encounter with the police: Did the victim report the rape to the police? What is her reaction to this experience? Did the police encourage or discourage her from taking it to court? How did she feel she was treated by the police?
3. Encounter with the hospital: After the victim arrived at the hospital, how did she feel about being there? Was she seeking medical attention? Did the gynecological examination upset her? What concerned her most as a result of the rape, such as possible pregnancy, venereal disease, or feelings about the rape?
4. Pressing charges: Is the victim to cooperate with the police and to testify in court? How does she feel about this?

SOCIAL NETWORK

Family and friends: Who is the victim's family? Which people are important to her? Who will she tell in her family? What friends are there at work or school and which friends will she tell? Does she have a counselor or a therapist?

Insuring safety for the victim: The victim should not be released alone from the hospital, unless it is her request. Try to insure that she has safe transportation to her destination.

Assessing crisis reaction and possible difficulties: Has the victim prior psychiatric or social difficulties which should be noted? What previous physical difficulties has she had? Has she been hospitalized or under the care of a doctor?

### Concluding phase

FOLLOW-UP:

What type of follow-up, such as telephone or home counseling or office visits, will be possible for the victim? (The right of the victim for continuity of care.)

RECORDING THE INTERVIEW:

The right of the victim to have an objective record written of the incident, including all signs and symptoms of trauma.

---

*From Burgess, A. W., and Holmstrom, L. L.: Crisis and counseling requests of rape victims, Nurs. Res. **23**:198, May-June, 1974, p. 198.

ment for healthy patterns of adjustment. Even though the victim may be unable to express her desire for such confirmation, her response is indicative of feeling reassured that someone cares and understands and is available for assistance.

2. *Ventilation: "It helps to get this off my chest."* This type of response involves an openness and eagerness to talk at length about the rape experience and about feelings that are experienced as the long-term adjustment period progresses. The victim is dependent upon the opportunity to talk to someone about the experience at regular intervals and feels relieved after talking. After a period of time the victim begins to feel in control of her feelings and reactions and constructs a means of continuing her life-style without the aid of counseling. Victims whose initial response is for medical or psychologic assistance in the initial period may be prone to need long-term support for ventilation of feelings.

Active listening is the preferred counseling approach for a person who needs to ventilate. The helper gives positive feedback for healthy means of working through the feelings that are being expressed and helps to correct misconceptions and feelings of damaged self-esteem. The predominant role of the listener is to ask the victim to clarify her thoughts and feelings and reflect back what has been said in order to assist in ventilation of feelings.

3. *Clarification: "I want to think this through."* This type of response is similar to the need for ventilation, but the victim is asking in addition for active assistance in reconstructing the crisis and her response to it. There are direct questions related to facts needed and requests for feedback as to whether her efforts are reasonable and healthy. The victim is able to express her feelings openly and to acknowledge her distress and uses the counselor's comments and assistance in an active manner. The counselor's response should be one of active listening combined with direct response to questions and requests for clarification, following the verbal lead of the victim. This type of response is likely to come from persons whose initial response to the crisis was to ask for psychologic support.

4. *Wants nothing: "I don't need counseling services."* In the initial interview persons who respond to the crisis by stating that they are fine and do not need long-term counseling are likely to either refuse to give an address or telephone number where they can be reached or they make themselves unavailable for follow-through counseling. This type of response indicates that either the victim does not view the health care workers as an appropriate source of support and counseling, that their efforts to give support were unacceptable in the initial encounter, that the individual prefers to receive support from another nonprofessional source, or perceives no need for long-term counseling.

5. *Advice: "What should I do?"* The victim who makes this response usually has isolated a specific problem with regard to the rape crisis and seeks specific guidance from a professional helper. Examples of the problems identified include making a decision whether to press charges against the assailant and whether to tell friends and family members about the incident and learning how to obtain protection and security and to deal with rejection by family members and friends who know about the incident. The counselor needs to provide specific alternatives that are available to the victim and help the victim consider the consequences of each alternative in arriving at a solution for herself. If the alternative that is selected is one that is difficult for the victim to implement, support and assistance may be needed as she works through the stress of putting her decision into action.[15]

## Venereal disease (MNPC no. 350.6)

Prevention and education related to venereal diseases were discussed in Chapter 14. Here we will consider the specific signs of two venereal infections, treatment approaches, and epidemiologic measures.

### Syphilis

Syphilis is caused by the bacterial organism *Treponema pallidum.* It is an extremely fragile organism, which requires specific conditions in order to live and reproduce. The primary requirement is a living human host; the organism is not acquired naturally by animals, and it is not successfully grown under laboratory conditions. Light, cold, moderate heat, lack of moisture, the presence of air, weak antiseptics, and exposure to soap and water effectively and rapidly destroy the organisms. Therefore, the only possibility for becoming infected remains direct skin contact with active, exposed syphilitic lesions.

As with most other infections, the individual reaction and manifestation of the disease differ greatly from person to person. Definitive diagnosis depends upon identification of the spirochete organism by microscopic darkfield examination of exudate from the lesions or special diagnostic tests of blood or spinal fluid. There are a few typical signs and symptoms of the infection, which may serve as clues to the presence of the disease. The incubation period from the time of the initial infection to the first appearance of symptoms varies from ten days to ten weeks. During this period the individual cannot infect others. The appearance of the first lesion, or chancre, that is characteristic of syphilis marks the beginning of the primary stage of the illness. There may be one or more chancres, and they are usually found in the anogenital area. Occasionally they are also present in or around the mouth, trunk, or fingers. The sore appears at the site or sites of germ entry. The appearance of the chancre is highly variable but often resembles an ulcerated area surrounded by a firm, raised border. The ulcerated portion and its exudate are highly infectious. The lesions may be as large as 2 cm in diameter. They may appear reddened but are usually painless. They disappear spontaneously without treatment of any kind after four to six weeks and seldom leave a scar. Because the lesions are usually painless and disappear spontaneously, the individual often assumes that the problem was of no consequence. Further, in some cases, chancres do not appear at all, they are small enough to escape notice, or they occur only internally. Thus signs of illness may escape notice altogether. Within a few days of infection, however, blood testing for syphilis is usually positive, and this remains the most conclusive and definitive diagnostic and screening tool for detection of infected persons.

The time of onset of the secondary stage of syphilis is also highly variable, beginning as early as during the primary stage to several months or years following the disappearance of the primary chancre. The symptoms of secondary syphilis arise from the fact that the organism lives and multiplies in the blood vascular system, and secondary lesions occur throughout the body at sites that are peculiarly susceptible for the infected individual. There is often a skin rash, but this may be generalized, localized, profuse, or sparse. A localized outbreak may appear only on the palms of the hands and soles of the feet, which is an alerting signal to the nature of the disease, since syphilis is one of the few diseases that can cause a rash in these areas. The rash is highly variable in character and may resemble chickenpox, measles, smallpox, or scarlet fever. Genital and mucous membrane lesions may also be present, along with swollen and painful lymph nodes, low-grade fever, headache, bone and joint pain, sore throat, hair loss, eye inflammation, jaundice from liver involvement, albumin in the urine, or syphilitic meningitis. It should be remembered that the illness in this stage may be relatively minor and mild or quite severe and disturbing. The individual is highly contagious during the period of time that the secondary rash and mucous membrane lesions appear. The lesions, like those of the primary stage, disappear spontaneously without treatment within two to six weeks, and there is no scarring or tissue damage.

During the months and years following the first outbreak of secondary signs, there may be several more outbreaks of similar nature. Once the rashes and lesions of the secondary stage have ceased, the infection is rarely transmissible again, with the exception of the pregnant mother, whose infected blood transfers direct infection to the fetus. During the latent period, when the secondary symptoms of the illness have ceased, the only means of identifying the infection is through blood testing. The latent period may last for many years, or it may follow the secondary stage immediately. Late symptomatic syphilis is characterized by specific organ degeneration caused by invasion of the organisms. For some people destruction is extremely slow, and the organs affected do not endanger life or cause significant debilitation. The skin may again be infected, but the resulting lesions are not infectious, and massive tissue damage occurs. During late syphilis antibiotic treatment is effective against the organisms, but the effects of organ damage are irreversible. The cardiovascular and neurologic systems are usually affected in the very late stages of the disease, if at all, and damage to these essential structures is life threatening. During any stage of syphilis, antibiotic treatment must be maintained at high levels for a minimum of ten days. Blood tests for the presence of active infection may remain positive throughout the person's life, making detection of a new infection extremely difficult.[49]

When a teenage girl becomes pregnant, she is screened for the possibility of active syphilis infection, as are all pregnant women, because congenitally acquired syphilis can cause a number of destructive effects. In most states there is a requirement that all pregnant women be screened for the infection at the onset of pregnancy. However, infection that occurs during the course of pregnancy can also affect the fetus, and congenital syphilis can pass unnoticed unless the mother's blood is tested at the time of delivery. There may be no signs of the disease in either the infant or the mother. The first signs of syphilis to appear for the infant are those of secondary syphilis, since there is no point of skin contact but only direct infection of the bloodstream. The skin rash may appear to a variable degree; mild or severe lesions of the mucous membranes may cause continuous discharges, which from the nose may resemble a common cold. Positive blood testing is again the only definitive diagnostic sign available. After the initial symptoms appear, which may be as late as the early childhood period, the child experiences a latent period that may last as late as adolescence or young adulthood.

### Gonorrhea

This infection is caused by the bacterial agent *Neisseria gonorrheae*. The organism is found in human reproductive organs and may or may not give rise to disease symptoms. It can invade the uterus, fallopian tubes, ovaries, urethra, and peritoneal membrane, but not the mature vaginal mucosa. The male genitourinary tract may be invaded. Occasionally, other specific tissues

of the body, such as the mouth, throat, rectum, and conjunctiva, are affected. Because of this tissue specificity, the symptoms for men and women differ. Definitive diagnosis rests on laboratory culture of the specific organism. Microscopic observation of a stained smear taken from the pus-containing discharge from the male urethra or the female cervical os reveals a gram-negative diplococci. The organism can be cultured in a laboratory medium, but there is currently no blood test specific for gonorrhea; this makes diagnosis difficult when a discharge specimen cannot be obtained. Unlike the syphilis organism, gonococci can survive away from the human host for several hours and can infect an individual from contaminated clothing or other objects.

The infection has an incubation period of three to nine days but, unlike syphilis, the infected individual is contagious during this time and remains infectious throughout the untreated course of the disease. The infection is usually self-limiting, but the effects that can occur during the course of infection are serious and sometimes life-threatening, especially for women. The early symptoms of infection may never be evident to a woman, and she may harbor the infection for many years without realizing that she is infected. Discovery of the problem may come when a sexual partner becomes infected. If there are any early symptoms, the woman may have a mild cervicitis and vaginal discharge. If the organism travels beyond the cervix, this occurs during the first, second, or third menstrual period following infection. The invasion may cause severe, acute inflammation of the fallopian tubes, uterus, and ovaries, and the entire peritoneal cavity. This infection may lead to a surgical crisis, necessitating removal of the reproductive organs; or it can become a chronic, lingering type of infection that produces no noticeable symptoms for several years. During chronic infection invasion of the blood is possible, with subsequent septicemia, gonococcal arthritis, heart disease, or any one of several other debilitating conditions. Permanent damage to the affected tissues can occur, unless antibiotic treatment is instituted before permanent damage has begun. A fetus can be infected during any stage of pregnancy. When infection of the newborn occurs during delivery, infection of the newborn's conjunctiva is the most common manifestation leading to serious damage and blindness. For this reason most states require routine prophylactic treatment of the eyes of all newborns.

When a man is infected, there are typical early symptoms of the infection that usually lead him to seek some sort of treatment. There is a sudden onset of thin, watery, white discharge from the urethra after the incubation period. Within a day the discharge becomes yellowish and thick, because of the body's attempts to suppress the infection. There is usually an uncomfortable stinging or burning during urination. Occasionally an infected man does not experience symptoms that lead him to seek treatment, and the infection may invade the prostate.

In addition to the hazards to the newborn infant from the infected mother, infected young people and adults can infect children of all ages by contact of their own contaminated hands with the eyes, genitalia, or mouth. In preadolescent girls the vagina is susceptible to invasion by the gonococcal organism, leading to gonococcal vulvovaginitis.[65]

### Health care and epidemiology

Treatment for gonorrhea requires specific antibiotic therapy. The dosage and the type of antibiotic used depend upon the complications that are present at the time of treatment. Aqueous procaine penicillin G is the drug of choice for most instances of gonorrhea. Syphilis, on the other hand, must be treated with procaine penicillin in oil and aluminum monostearate. Unfortunately, gonococcal organisms can develop resistance to the antibiotics used in treatment, and therefore every effort is needed to treat the infection specifically and judiciously. Alternative antibiotics may be used in treatment when the organism seems to be resistant or when the individual cannot take penicillin.

One of the most important aspects of control of venereal disease is the identification of sexual contacts during the periods of contagion.[10,68] Because the highest rate of infection occurs between the ages of 15 and 29 years, particular attention is directed to adolescent and young

adult groups in the community for both education and treatment. The incidence of these infections has increased worldwide in recent years in spite of efforts on the part of the World Health Organization and individual countries to control their spread. One of the problems that has been a significant deterrent to adequate detection and treatment of the illness is the requirement that minors under the age of 21 years of age must obtain parental consent before treatment can be instituted. Fear of informing the parents causes many young people to avoid seeking appropriate health counseling and diagnosis or to avoid pursuing the appropriate treatment. Thus, there has been an effort to adjust the legal requirements that would allow a minor to obtain medical treatment for venereal disease on his or her own request.*

## Teenage pregnancy (MNPC no. 354 and no. 355)

Some of the effects of teenage pregnancy on the welfare of the fetus and infant were discussed in Chapter 5. We now turn our discussion to the problems that affect primarily the young people involved when pregnancy occurs during adolescence.

### Etiologic factors

Teenage pregnancy often arises from developmental and behavioral characteristics of adolescence. The young people may or may not perceive or desire the possibility of pregnancy occurring as a result of sexual experimentation, and their immaturity of judgment interferes with their taking this possibility into account. Nakashima[77] has identified several behavioral factors that cause sexual experimentation and pregnancy in the teenage years, including a love of risk-taking, feelings of omnipotence, impulsive action, lack of judgment, a desire for peer approval, and curiosity. A depressed adolescent may be sexually acting out for self-destruction, and young people who are victims of neglect or rejection often use sex to gain emotional and physical closeness. Younger adolescents present the greatest problem, for they may use sex as a means of expressing these and other adolescent

*References 5, 11, 13, 20, 49, 70, 71, 78, 83.

behavioral traits and may unexpectedly become pregnant or frightened because of a late or missed menstrual period and may seek contraception or abortion or further act out as a means of masking their underlying distress.[77]

### Emotional and social problems

As noted in Chapter 5 the physiologically optimal age at which a young woman bears children is about 18 years.[9] However, the social and emotional stresses that often accompany teenage pregnancy in current societies seem to outweigh any physiologic advantage to the young mother; the outcome for the fetus is generally not as favorable, and the stresses for the mother are great. It should be remembered that not all teenage pregnancies are unwanted; many are planned and deliberate, and social stigma attached to pregnancy out of wedlock has begun to change in recent years. Marriage may occur in the traditional sense, or another form of deliberate commitment may exist between young people who have initiated pregnancy. Adolescent boys are often intimately involved in the problems and events surrounding the gestational period of a child they have fathered, and social and cultural pressures can be as great for the young father as for the young mother.

When a pregnancy occurs during the adolescent years, there are several problems that affect the health and well-being of the young mother whether she is married, unmarried, living with parents, or on her own. When the child's father is involved, these factors influence him also. First, there is often an economic crisis, which results in a decreased standard of living from that of the family of origin. The young mother finds herself needing health care, and there are expenses that she had not planned on. In addition, plans for the future, such as a job or an education, must be altered. A young adolescent who is beginning a family is unskilled, inexperienced, and in an unfavorable position to earn a wage substantial enough to adequately support more than one person. In addition, because the limited income must now be directed toward support of a young child, plans for completing one's educational goals are seriously jeopardized. The young person, whether the mother or the father, must cope with the reality of either bringing a child into the world and providing a home or seeking other alternatives.

Compounding the economic problem is the emotional and personal crisis created by the pregnancy. The planned, deliberate pregnancy during adolescence involves a certain emotional advantage, but emotional and experiential immaturity remain disadvantages to the young person as the realities of pregnancy, economic stresses, and family responsibilities begin to unfold. If the pregnancy is not deliberately or consciously planned, the young person faces an unexpected task in development and search for identity. While sexual and reproductive capacity may be fulfilled to some extent, these aspects of identity and their interrelationship with other aspects of identity become seriously challenged and precarious at this point of crisis. If the girl's cultural heritage identifies any young person who becomes pregnant as bad, sinful, or unworthy, then any previous efforts to establish herself as a good, righteous, and worthy individual in her own estimate and in the estimate of others are in serious jeopardy. If the culture is less punitive, then the person may be less threatened by the advent of an unplanned pregnancy but may face a reorientation task of another sort. A young girl may have begun to fashion herself as a career-seeking woman whose eventual marriage and family responsibilities would fit into the framework of her career. With the advent of an unplanned pregnancy, she now must face the necessity of either readjusting her personal goals and concepts of what she is to become, or of finding alternatives that preserve what she has built for herself thus far.

The emotional response of the adolescent who is pregnant reflects the developmental tasks and behavioral characteristics of this period of development and presents a special challenge for health care workers who are involved with her during pregnancy. There is an enormous concern about body image, which is congruent with the normal adolescent narcissism and self-absorption. The body changes of pregnancy are not compatible with the socially accepted body image for young women, and a significant conflict and preoccupation with this problem often exist. Many adolescents are openly hostile to restrictions that are imposed, such as dietary alterations and restrictions, changes in required exercise and physical activity, and social restrictions. Often the adolescent begins pregnancy with an unrealistic optimism that the fact of pregnancy will not change or affect her life-style or life goals, and when she is faced with the reality of the problems that emerge, she is disillusioned and angry or depressed. Adolescent perceptions of appropriate maternal behavior and child care are based in fantasy and often appear more like an expectation of "playing house" than the reality of mothering. An adolescent may proceed through pregnancy with very little difficulty and even enjoy the extra attention that she receives during pregnancy, but when faced with the reality of infant care, she begins to express typical behavioral responses to stress, such as open hostility and depression.[77]

### Health care, counseling, and education

Although the alternatives available to the adolescent pregnant mother are currently broader than at any time in the past, the decisions that must be made are of great importance to the young girl, the young boy involved, and the child who may be born. Counseling and guidance are essential for most young people if they are to make satisfying adjustments and decisions, and many young people rely heavily on several forms of informal counseling and guidance from peers, respected adult friends, and, under some circumstances, parents. Because the fact of pregnancy is usually confirmed in a health care setting, professional health care workers need specific skills in helping the young girl find appropriate counseling resources that can help with the problems that are likely to occur. The young girl who delays or avoids appropriate health care because of lack of knowledge, socioeconomic disadvantages, or fear is in a particularly difficult position.

The basic initial choice available to the young pregnant teenager today is to either maintain the pregnancy through term or to take steps to terminate the pregnancy. Some teenage girls never consider terminating the pregnancy and center on the choices available to them at the time the pregnancy ends. Others immediately consider the termination of pregnancy and may try to induce abortion on their own, find an illegal source for obtaining such a service, or seek a legitimate abortion. Since Colorado, in 1967, significantly amended its abortion law, many states have followed in providing safe, legal means of obtaining abortion services, and federal programs have been developed to assure the availability of safe and legal abortion services for persons who meet specified guidelines.[58,82] If a young woman does not consider abortion, this alternative probably should not be advocated, although in some situations the professional judgment may be made that this is a sound and desirable consideration. Regardless of the intellectual and emotional capacity of the young woman, the decision must be her own to the greatest extent possible.[4]

Abortion counseling is an essential aspect of care for any teenager who considers this alternative. Whether abortion is conducted or not, she needs to have sound and mature guidance in considering possible action. The counselor should approach the encounter in a nonjudgmental and supportive manner, regardless of the circumstances of the pregnancy or the personal attitudes of the counselor. Such counseling may not be possible for health care workers who hold strong beliefs and values against the practice of abortion, and this personal preference should be expressed and such counseling needs referred to those who can freely and willingly guide the young person to her own decision.[4,14,89]

The experience should be an educational one for the young girl and for the young father who may be involved. Because of the growing acceptance and desirability of obtaining abortion services, the emotional factors for some young people may be minimal, while for others they may be mammoth. In addition to learning about the medical and surgical procedures required, about health care maintenance before and after the procedure, and about prevention of future unwanted pregnancies, young people should have support and help in learning more about themselves and the culture in which they live. They should explore the cultural attitudes and values by which they have been reared, and the implications that may exist if they violate some of these by turning to abortion. Ways of coping with such conflict can be acknowledged and understanding of one's self gained.[4,27,55,90]

Finally, the health care worker who assists a young person in reaching a decision regarding abortion must be alert to factors that indicate a need for continued counseling and therapy following the termination of pregnancy either through abortion or through delivery. Such factors include:

1. A history of some form of emotional disturbance in the past, including regular drug abuse, previous postpartal psychotic reaction, multiple previous unplanned pregnancies, suicidal attempts, depression, impulsive behavior, or poor self-concept
2. A history of a culture and family environment that strongly opposes abortion
3. History or question of mental retardation
4. Evidence that the girl is being coerced into making a decision to either have an abortion or not to have one
5. Evidence that the girl is suffering from marked inability to make a decision, as if she is paralyzed by the stress of the problems, or the opposite extreme where she appears to have no ambivalence whatsoever, her decision is clearly and certainly made with no need to consider the other possibilities involved
6. Evidence that the girl is having an unusually difficult development of her concept of sexuality and of her role as a woman*

The next decision point comes when the teenage girl has decided to continue the pregnancy throughout the normal gestation period. The alternatives then available are to either claim the infant as her own and attempt to provide a home (either as a single parent or in some form of a family arrangement) or to renounce her parenthood of the infant and pursue her own personal goals for the future. In addition, she may attempt to combine these alternatives and to provide for the child as well as pursue her personal goals. Because the latter alternative is being increasingly attempted by young mothers

*References 4, 18, 24, 36, 76, 97.

today, special services to assist them through the economic, educational, social, and emotional difficulties have been instituted in the interest of the welfare of the young mother and of her infant. The effectiveness of such services remains to be evaluated, and the changing social climate in which we live will surely affect the success with which young women can realistically achieve their goals.[26,33,69,73,93]

## Infectious mononucleosis
### Pathophysiologic considerations

Infectious mononucleosis (glandular fever, "kissing disease") is a viral infection that typically occurs during the late adolescent years. There is evidence that it occurs in younger children, but apparently the infection is not as severe, and accurate diagnosis is either overlooked or not possible with present tools for identifying the problem. The causative virus appears to be the Epstein-Barr virus, and specific antibodies seem to be developed as protection against the infection. There is controversy over whether this illness exists as a single entity; several related illnesses may be identified clinically as "infectious mononucleosis."

The symptoms of illness may be mild or severe and include enlarged lymph nodes, fever, pharyngitis, malaise, facial or periorbital edema, anorexia, headache, chills, and liver and spleen enlargement. A skin rash occurs in about 10% of all confirmed cases, and occasionally the person experiences arthralgia and diarrhea, mimicking the "flu." There appears to be about a 40-day incubation period, and transmission is by droplet infection. There is currently no evidence supporting the former theory that the infection is spread by kissing, although close contact does seem to be required, since the infection is not notably contagious. Thus epidemics seem to develop most frequently in college dormitories or military barracks.[8,17,23,30,53]

There are relatively few complications of the illness, but it can become a prolonged illness for some adolescents. This may be related to lack of needed bed rest. Medical diagnostic criteria for the illness include:

1. Clinical manifestations of the illness.
2. Lymphocytosis with atypical lymphocytes present, with the total percentage of lym-

phocytes in the differential reaching 50% or more.

3. Heterophil antibody titer of 1:112 or higher. This test rests upon the presence of high titer agglutinins against sheep cells in the serum of persons with infectious mononucleosis. Since the Epstein-Barr virus seems to be the causative agent, the Epstein-Barr virus antibody titer is the most significant diagnostic tool, but measurement of this antibody titer is not generally feasible at the present time.

4. Possible evidence of liver involvement. It appears that infiltration in all the visceral organs occurs in a majority of those affected by the infection, but liver dysfunction seems to be present in at least 90% of all infections. This problem is usually of little significance but can lead to complications of jaundice, prolonged malaise, anorexia, and disability related to lack of stamina.

### Supportive care

Care is primarily directed toward relieving discomfort and providing adequate rest until the body has had a chance to effectively fight off the infection. Bed rest is usually required for a period of a week or more, or until the subjective clinical symptoms of the illness have subsided. The symptoms appear to recur or to be prolonged when adequate rest is neglected. Aspirin may be needed to control fever and to relieve the discomforts of sore throat and arthralgia. Occasionally a beta hemolytic streptococcal infection is present simultaneously, requiring specific antibiotic treatment. When symptoms are severe or when complications develop, such as anemia, neurologic involvement, or severe hepatic involvement, corticosteroids may be indicated.[30,53]

A comprehensive approach to care during infectious mononucleosis demands the inclusion of the teenager and the family, particularly in relation to the therapeutic need for rest. Facilitating the intake of food when the young person has no appetite and helping him or her to endure a long period of relative confinement may present a challenge to the most innovative of families. Objective nursing diagnosis related to the various clinical symptoms that may occur and identification of the severity of involvement for a particular teenager can be important steps in helping the teenager and the family understand and treat the problem. For example, assessment may indicate a significant level of fatigue, with almost no endurance for ordinary household and personal care skills at the onset of the illness. Maximal bed rest is indicated at this stage. As the condition improves, the fatigue may lessen, but endurance continues to be severely limited. Even though the desire to pursue normal activities is present, bed rest continues to be indicated for a certain portion of the day, and adequate guidance and nursing care may assist the young person in achieving this particular requirement of care.

## Dysmenorrhea
### Physiologic considerations

Problems in establishing normal menstrual cycles are not unusual during early adolescence. Discomfort associated with the onset of menstrual flow may begin after ovulatory cycles begin and includes discomfort in the lower abdomen from cramping, backache, headache, pain in the thighs, anorexia, nausea and vomiting, diarrhea, constipation, or fainting. The exact mechanism by which these symptoms occur in the absence of an apparent organic disorder is obscure but is thought to be a function of irregular, large uterine contractions of varying amplitude that occur in response to the rising levels of progesterone. Older adolescents and mature women may continue to experience some degree of discomfort in the early days of the period, but this usually does not cause a disruption in normal daily activities. The young girl who experiences such severe discomfort that school attendance and other activities are interrupted may be experiencing some emotional difficulty in adjusting to the onset of menstrual function, or there may be other problems of development, with the physical problems associated with menstruation becoming a focus of attention. However, the physical symptoms often occur without evidence of psychologic difficulty.

### Health care

There should be an effort to help a young girl express her fears and concerns about the symptoms she experiences and to understand some of the physical and emotional factors that can occur. There are often misunderstandings arising from cultural attitudes and beliefs toward menstruation, including beliefs about the causes of discomfort, such as unacceptable behavior or thoughts, exercise, bathing, exposure to heat or cold, or foods. Misunderstandings should be clarified but within the context that cultural beliefs and pressures will continue to operate for the young girl. Health care and measures for relief must be adjusted to fit the girl's cultural pattern.

Relief from the cramping and pain may be accomplished with moderate doses of an analgesic compound. Occasionally an antispasmodic drugs, such as Isoxsuprine, may be helpful in reducing the cramping. There are a multitude of over-the-counter agents sold specifically for the relief of menstrual discomfort. The value of these agents remains questionable, and many contain compounds that are unrelated to the relief of pain. These agents are also prone to misuse. The young girl may misuse a drug simply out of a desperate attempt to obtain relief by taking the drug too often or doubling the single recommended dose.

When an acceptable dosage of an acceptable analgesia is not effective in controlling the discomfort, medical management may be indicated. Low doses of estrogen may be given for several months to produce anovulatory cycles, after which the discomfort of menstruation may be somewhat lessened.[22]

Protocols for management may be developed within a given health care setting with criteria of nursing, medical, and psychologic referral and management carefully delineated.

## Nutrition and body size problems

Although we have discussed the problems of nutrition and body size related to other age groups, these problems during adolescence need special attention. Deviations from the ideal body size produce significant psychosocial problems for the teenager, even if the deviation is a relatively transient one. The adolescent's food intake often does not provide a totally balanced diet, and the degree to which this affects performance and body size varies among individual young people.

### Deviations in stature and sexual development

Excessive height growth for girls or unusually delayed height growth for boys presents special problems throughout adolescence. Because boys tend to experience the peak velocity of height growth somewhat later than girls of the same age, there is a period when most boys and girls are particularly sensitive to their body height. Their body sizes are exactly the opposite of the cultural ideal of tall, large men and small, petite women. When unusual advances or delays in growth occur and are accompanied by unusual delays or advances in the development of secondary sexual characteristics, there may be an endocrine disorder influencing the growth pattern, and complete medical evaluation is indicated.* When an advance or delay is within the limits of normalcy but deviates enough to cause a significant psychosocial disturbance for the young person, several aspects of the total situation must be considered in determining which health care team member can give the youngster the needed support and care during the adjustment period. If there is evidence that medical evaluation is not essential for several months and might be desirably delayed, counseling and psychologic support may be indicated until medical evaluation becomes more clearly indicated.

Gynecomastia is enlargement of one or both breasts in boys during puberty. The underlying physiology is not known, but it is speculated that testicular or adrenal androgens may be converted to estrogens, which stimulate breast enlargement. Rarely, gynecomastia is associated with serious problems such as Klinefelter's syndrome, liver disease, severe malnutrition, obesity, feminizing endocrinopathies, or carcinoma of the testes. The physiologic form of gynecomastia occurs frequently, however, and is a benign condition that usually reverses within six months. It creates considerable anxiety for

---

*References 7, 22, 34, 35, 45, 52, 85.

young boys and can result in serious emotional disturbance. If breast enlargement is severe and the young boy is at risk for serious emotional disturbance, surgical intervention may be considered.[22]

### Excessive weight (MNPC no. 314)

Excessive weight rarely appears as an initial problem during adolescence. More commonly there has been a history of excessive weight during the earlier developmental periods. However, there often is an urgent desire to do something about the weight problem with the onset of adolescence. This desire leads to a variety of independent measures taken by a large number of teenagers in efforts to reduce weight, with a varying degree of success. The approach taken is usually a drastic interruption of ordinary food intake alternated with periods of resumption of usual eating patterns. The results of such programs are often disappointing. Teenagers with some means of financial income often become prey to the many commercial programs for weight reduction, with varying degrees of success (see Chapter 15).

When the young person with a weight problem seeks assistance from a health care worker, every attempt should be made to assist the individual in successfully achieving a weight reduction goal and to maintain a reasonable weight activity, and eating pattern throughout adult life. Motivation may be optimal during this period. Assessment includes a thorough understanding of the approaches attempted by the young person in the past, because this information gives an idea not only of the individual's past eating patterns but also of the level of dietary and nutritional understanding the young person possesses. Histories of weight and height and blood pressure patterns of other members of the family may be helpful in establishing a realistic goal for this individual. Family attitudes toward food and exercise are particularly relevant in helping the young person establish a realistic weight reduction program. The exact nature of the weight reduction program may vary considerably, but the essential components are a reasonable intake of calories combined with a reasonable level of regular exercise. The program need not involve extra expense to the young person or the family; indeed, it may result in a savings. The entire family may become involved, and in many instances this is the only way to achieve successful weight control. The family members may not have the weight reduction needs of the young person, but cooperation is necessary in establishing understanding, encouragement, and support of the young person's efforts to control weight.*

### Iron deficiency anemia

The adolescent stage of development, particularly for girls, is a period of risk for development of iron deficiency anemia. The increased metabolic needs that are stimulated by rapid growth, combined with a tendency to neglect adequate nutritional requirements, account for the prevalence of iron deficiency during adolescence. Iron deficiency in adolescent girls may be associated with menstruation, particularly if the flow is excessive or prolonged. The criteria for nursing diagnosis and the approach to treatment are the same as that described in Chapter 11, p. 423.[6,37,94]

## Sports injuries

Sports activities are extremely important during adolescence in that they provide a means for social and personality development that is not afforded by any other type of activity. In addition to valuable exercise, sports provide experience in competition, team effort, handling conflict in a mature and socially acceptable fashion, and development of self-esteem. However, young people are particularly prone to injury resulting from sports activities due to the fact that their coordination skills are not fully developed, their judgment is often immature and inadequate, the epiphyses are not yet closed, and the extremities are poorly protected by stabilizing musculature. Further, school athletic programs are often underserved by health care workers who can provide consultation in prevention of sports-related injuries and immediate attention to young people who suffer an injury. It is estimated that approximately 600,000 injuries a year occur in high school football alone in the United States, and with growing programs for

---

*References 22, 25, 29, 41, 45, 46.

other athletic sports and athletic programs for girls, this figure is probably an underestimate.[80,81]

### Head injuries

Injuries to the head and brain are of special importance, because of the possibility of long-term neurologic damage or death. Immediate evaluation is required in order to establish appropriate intervention, and the guidelines presented in Chapter 13, p. 511, should be used for evaluation and judgment regarding an adolescent who has received a head injury. The nurse may also provide a service for high school teachers and sports directors to assure their knowledge of assessment of head injury and appropriate actions to be taken in order to assure rapid and appropriate intervention for the young person immediately after the injury.

### Spine and spinal cord injuries

Spine and spinal cord injuries are often serious in nature and result in long-term disability or death. Cervical spine injuries are the most common and are related to hyperflexion, hyperextension, or flexion compression of the vertebral column. It is extremely important to obtain information as to how the injury occurred, for this will provide a judgment as to which type of spinal lesion might exist. Flexion and hyperextension injuries are more likely than others to result in cord damage. Spinal shock follows cord injury below the level of the injury and occurs as a result of edema or ischemia of several cord segments. There is temporary loss of motor, sensory, and reflex function in those parts of the body innervated by the cord distal to the lesion. Upper cervical cord injury results in respiratory impairment due to damage of the intercostal and diaphragmatic neurons. In lower cervical cord injury the diaphragm remains functionally intact, but the intercostal muscles are paralyzed, resulting in impaired respiration.

The young person must be immediately immobilized after a known or suspected cord injury. He or she is placed on a flat board or surface, and sand bags are used to stabilize the head. If respiratory support or assistance is needed, this must be provided immediately. The reflexes of the extremities should be noted, and if the person is alert, sensory perception of pin pricks, heat, and cold should be estimated, and the ability to move the extremities should be determined. The young person should be transported immediately to an acute care setting, where further assessment and treatment can be given. Recovery from even a minor injury may require several weeks of bed rest with traction and physical therapy. The young person's ability to continue to participate in sports is usually altered, and full evaluation of the risks of further injury, in light of the risks of the particular sport, needs to be evaluated in order to make a wise judgment in this regard.[80]

### Skeletal injuries

Ankle injuries, particularly sprains, are common. There is usually swelling and tenderness at the site of the damage, and limited ability to invert the foot. Sprains are due to incomplete rupture of the lateral ligament of the ankle and are treated by wrapping the ankle in an elastic bandage, elevating the foot, and applying ice packs for 24 hours. After this period of time, heat may be applied to facilitate circulation, and the young person should maintain bed rest and refrain from bearing weight on the ankle. A fracture of the lateral or medical malleoli can be detected by x-ray examination. Closed reduction of a displaced fracture may be possible, but open reduction is usually required to achieve perfect restoration. The extremity is immobilized in a below-knee walking cast for four to six weeks, and active range-of-motion exercises are prescribed to reduce edema and prevent joint stiffness and muscle wasting.

Foot injuries include puncture wounds, lacerations, and torn or pulled muscles and fractures. Puncture wounds and lacerations are thoroughly cleaned, soaked in Betadine solution, and irrigated with sterile water and saline solution. Butterfly or suture closure may be needed. Tetanus immunization and antibiotic treatment may be indicated. Strains and sprains of the ligaments are treated as ankle aprains, described above. Fractures require x-ray examination and immobilization. Fractures of the toes are immobilized by splinting the injured toe to the next toe, except for the large toe, which may require plaster casting.

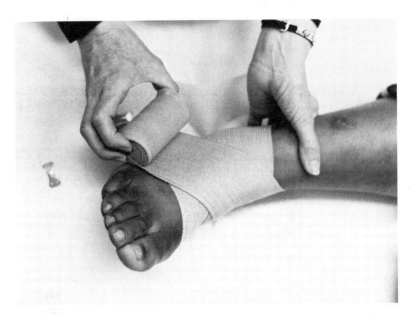

**Fig. 15-1.** An elastic bandage is applied by wrapping the foot and heel loosely toward the toes, then proceeding from the toe over the ankle with firm pressure.

Adolescents are prone to knee injuries because of the undeveloped strength of the ligaments and lack of strength and coordination of the musculature surrounding the joint. Injuries tend to occur when the foot is locked to the ground or otherwise immobilized, and a lateral force causes the femur to adduct while the tibia rotates externally, with a medial hinging action between the femur and the tibia. Knee injuries involve derangement of the joint, ligament injury, and cartilage tears. These injuries must be thoroughly evaluated and treated appropriately with the first few days after the injury in order to assure adequate recovery and full function of the knee. Repeated knee injuries are more likely following insufficient correction of even a minor injury. Mild knee injuries are treated with compression, ice packs, immobilization by splinting or casting, elevation of the extremity, and aspiration of blood and excessive fluid that accumulates in the joint. Surgery is required for more serious injury involving tears of the ligaments or cartilage.

Fractures of the tibia, fibula, and femur must be identified by x ray and are treated with appropriate surgical reduction, immobilization by casting, and intensive physical therapy to maintain adequate function of the extremity. Stress fractures of the tibia are characterized by mild, gnawing pain of insidious onset in the lower portion of the leg, which disappears with rest but which recurs with activity. Changes may not be evident on x-ray film for weeks or months after the injury. Treatment consists of rest and application of compression bandages until after the fracture has healed.

Contusions of the quadriceps, known as charley horse, result in pain, swelling, and spasms of the thigh muscles. These injuries are treated by application of a firm pressure bandage from the toes to the groin, elevation of the leg, and application of ice packs for 24 hours. After this period of time, heat is applied to facilitate circulation. Exercise and activity are gradually increased after the symptoms subside, which usually occurs within 10 to 14 days.

Tenosynovitis results from muscle injury of the calf and is characterized by pain, tenderness, and palpable crepitus of the muscle. Local injections of hydrocortisone or prednisolone and rest are required until the symptoms subside.

Sprains and fractures of the arms, wrists, elbows, and hands are treated similarly to injuries

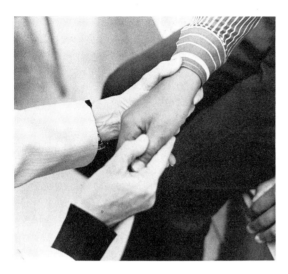

**Fig. 15-2.** A mild finger dislocation should be reduced immediately by pulling firmly on the finger or thumb as shown here.

described for equivalent structures of the legs. Injuries of these structures can result in permanent disability if prompt assessment and treatment are not obtained. Injuries to the wrist and hands are the most common. X-ray evaluation should be obtained to determine the extent of injury of these structures. Dislocated fingers should be reduced promptly, which is often possible by closed reduction. A mild finger injury can be reduced immediately by pulling firmly on the finger, which will result in reduction of the injured joint and immediate alleviation of pain. More serious dislocations and fractures may require open reduction and immobilization with Kirschner wires to maintain the injured parts in the reduced position and in a position of maximal function. Intensive physical therapy is required to maintain and achieve optimal function of the hand.[80]

## HEALTH AND SOCIALLY ISOLATED YOUTH

Socially isolated youth in recent years have established communities characterized by countercultural values and life-styles. The community may be found within the ghetto of a large city or in a geographically isolated area. Some older adults may be members of the group, but a large proportion of the members are young people. They may be permanently committed to the community, or they may be transient members experimenting with alternative life-styles. Because of many problems of economic support, transience, communal living, and discrimination from many segments of society, including the traditional health care system, the health problems of these young people are significant.

Several factors of living conditions chosen by isolated youth contribute to susceptibility and exposure to disease, nutritional inadequacies, and accidents. Sleeping accommodations are often inadequate and patterns of sleep irregular. Food may be scarce. Facilities for maintaining adequate body hygiene may be lacking, particularly in a communal living situation. Drug use may be present. These factors contribute to a high incidence of communicable disease, venereal disease, hepatitis, drug overdoses, skin problems, and psychologic crises. A health problem may be neglected or self-treated for a prolonged period because of reluctance to approach a traditional health care facility where the services are geared to middle-class American culture and where understanding for the self-imposed health problems of these young people is often lacking.

In an effort to provide some means of acceptable health care to these young people and to encourage the incorporation of health maintenance into the particular life-style and value system chosen by the individual, special types of health care facilities have been established in selected areas. Persons providing the health care have often integrated themselves into the isolated community in order to gain a personal understanding of the values and problems of the young people. Often the professional services are provided on a voluntary basis, and the cost of operating the facility is low. Financial support may be derived from donations and contributions from the community and from those who receive health care. The success of such programs remains to be fully evaluated, but they represent a significant effort toward the incorporation of sound health care goals into the life-style of a particular segment of today's society.*

---

*References 31, 39, 42, 43, 47, 87, 92.

## STUDY QUESTIONS

1. Choose a common symptom of illness for which an adolescent might attempt self-medication, such as menstrual cramps, flu, cold, headache. Investigate the drugs and agents available in local drug stores, and discuss the potential agents found for abuse. Identify those agents in which the ingredients are appropriate and instructions on the package provide clear, adequate guidance for safe usage.

2. Identify agencies and programs in your community that are designed to serve adolescents with health problems, particularly social alienation, drug abuse, venereal disease, or pregnancy. Describe the kind of program offered, ways in which individuals can establish contact and receive services, and the cost to the individual.

3. What are your state laws related to giving medical or health care to young people under 21 years of age? Discuss the effect of these laws on the kind of health care that can be offered to young people who have particular problems.

4. Choose one of the health problems related to adolescence. Identify related nursing diagnosis, developing criteria for diagnosis and a protocol for management or nursing care plan. Substantiate your criteria and protocol with underlying physiologic and psychologic principles.

5. Discuss the everyday types of drug misuse that occur in most households, including your own. Compare these problems with the drug abuse of the "drug culture." Articulate as clearly as you can your own attitudes and beliefs regarding each type of drug misuse, and how you would subjectively react to another person's drug misuse in each of these categories. How would these attitudes enhance or distract from your ability to work with a person as a health care worker? Exchange reactions and impressions with your colleagues in an effort to explore more fully how your attitudes affect an interaction situation.

## REFERENCES

1. Alcohol consumption; An adolescent problem: Pediatrics 55:557, April, 1975.
2. Alonzi, J., and Faigel, H. C.: A structured, therapeutic approach to drug abuse, Pediatrics 50:754, Nov., 1972.
3. Arena, J. M.: Poisoning and its treatment. In Shirkey, H. C., editor: Pediatric therapy, ed. 5, St. Louis, 1975, The C. V. Mosby Co., p. 101.
4. Asher, J. D.: Abortion counseling, Am. J. Public Health 62:686-688, May, 1972.
5. Atwater, J. B.: Adapting the venereal disease clinic to today's problem, Am. J. Public Health 64:433, May, 1974.
6. Baehner, R. L.: Anemia. In Green, M., and Haggerty, R. J., editors: Ambulatory pediatrics, II, Philadelphia, 1977, W. B. Saunders Co., p. 184.
7. Bailey, J. D.: Management of the teenager with retardation of physical growth or sexual maturation, Pediatr. Clin. North Am. 21:1029, Nov., 1974.
8. Barnes, A., Jr.: Infectious mononucleosis, Cont. Educat. Family Physician 2:34, Dec., 1974.
9. Birch, H. G., and Gussow, J. D.: Disadvantaged children; health, nutrition and school failure, New York, 1970, Harcourt, Brace and World, Inc.
10. Blount, J. H.: A new approach for gonorrhea epidemiology, Am. J. Public Health 62:710-712, May, 1972.
11. Brown, M. S.: Syphilis and gonorrhea; an update for nurses in ambulatory settings, Nursing '76 6:71, Jan., 1976.
12. Brownmiller, S.: Against our will: Men, women and rape, New York, 1975, Simon and Schuster.
13. Buchta, R. M.: It is important to search for mixed vaginal infections in sexually active young women with endocervical gonorrhea, Clin. Pediatr. 16:1001, Nov., 1977.
14. Bullough, V., and Bullough, B.: Pregnancy, contraceptives, and abortion, Health Values 1:166, July-Aug., 1977.
15. Burgess, A. W., and Holmstrom, L. L.: Crisis and counseling requests of rape victims, Nurs. Res. 23:196, May-June, 1974.
16. The Child Study Association of America: You, your child and drugs, New York, 1971, The Child Study Press.
17. Chretien, J. H., and Esswein, J. G.: How frequent is bacterial superinfection of the pharynx in infectious mononucleosis? Clin. Pediatr. 15:424, May, 1976.
18. Clancy, B.: The nurse and the abortion patient, Nurs. Clin. North Am. 8:469, Sept., 1973.
19. Combs, A. W., Avila, D. L., and Purkey, W. W.: Helping relationships; basic concepts for the helping professions, Boston, 1971, Allyn & Bacon, Inc.
20. Committee on Youth, American Academy of Pediatrics: A model act providing for consent of minors for health services, Pediatrics 51:293, Feb., 1973.
21. Committee on Youth, American Academy of Pediatrics: The implications of minor's consent legislation for adolescent health care; a commentary, Pediatrics 54:481, Oct., 1974.
22. Cooper, H. E., Jr., and Nakashima, I.: Adolescence. In Kempe, C. H., Silver, H. K., and O'Brien, D., editors: Current pediatric diagnosis and treatment, ed. 4, Los Altos, Calif., 1976, Lange Medical Publications, p. 175.
23. Copperman, S. M.: "Alive in Wonderland" syndrome as a presenting symptom of infectious mononucleosis in children, Clin. Pediatr. 16:143, Feb., 1977.
24. Danon, A. H.: Organizing an abortion service, Nurs. Outlook 21:460, July, 1973.
25. deCastro, F. J., and others: Hypertension in adolescents, Clin. Pediatr. 15:24, Jan., 1976.
26. DeLissovoy, V.: Child care by adolescent parents, Children Today 2:22, July-Aug., 1973.
27. Donovan, C., Greenspun, R., and Mittleman, F.: The decision-making process and the outcome of therapeutic abortion, Am. J. Psychiatry 131:1332-1337, Dec., 1974.
28. Effect of marihuana on man: Pediatrics 56:134, July, 1975.
29. Fender, J.: Obesity in teenage girls. In Kalafatich, A. J., editor: Approaches to the care of adolescents,

New York, 1975, Appleton-Century-Crofts, p. 79.

30. Fernback, D. J., and Starling, K. A.: Infectious mononucleosis, Pediatr. Clin. North Am. 19:957, Nov., 1972.

31. Fielding, J. E., and Nelson, S. H.: Health care for the economically disadvantaged adolescent, Pediatr. Clin. North Am. 20:975, Nov., 1973.

32. Fisher, G., and Strantz, I.: An ecosystems approach to the study of dangerous drug use and abuse with special reference to the marijuana issue, Am. J. Public Health 62:1407, Oct., 1972.

33. Foltz, A., Klerman, L. V., and Jekel, J. F.: Pregnancy and special education: Who stays in school? Am. J. Public Health 62:1612, Dec., 1972.

34. Frasier, S. D.: A review of growth hormone stimulation tests in children, Pediatrics 53:929, June, 1974.

35. Gallagher, J. R.: Adolescents and their disorders. In Cooke, R. E., editor: The biologic basis of pediatric practice, New York, 1968, McGraw-Hill Book Co., p. 1970.

36. Gedan, S.: Abortion counseling with adolescents, Am. J. Nurs. 74:1856, Oct., 1974.

37. Githens, J. H., and Hathaway, W.: Hematologic disorders. In Kempe, C. H., Silver, H. K., and O'Brien, D., editors: Current pediatric diagnosis and treatment, ed. 4, Los Altos, Calif., 1976, Lange Medical Publications, p. 358.

38. Goodman, L. S., and Gilman, A., editors: The pharmacological basis of therapeutics, ed. 5, New York, 1975, Macmillan Publishing Co., Inc.

39. Gordon, J. S.: The kids and the cults, Children Today 6:24, July-Aug., 1977.

40. Greene, M. H., and Dupont, R. L., editors: The epidemiology of drug abuse, Am. J. Public Health vol. 64(suppl.), Dec., 1974.

41. Gross, I., Wheeler, M., and Hess, K.: The treatment of obesity in adolescents using behavioral self-control; an evaluation, Clin. Pediatr. 15:920, Oct., 1976.

42. Guthrie, A. D., and Howell, M. C.: Mobile medical care for alienated youths, J. Pediatr. 81:1025, Nov., 1972.

43. Harding, E. H., Harrington, C., and Manor, G. J.: The Berkeley Free Clinic, Nurs. Outlook 21:40, Jan., 1973.

44. Harlin, V. K.: The influence of obvious anonymity of the response of school children to questionnaire about smoking, Am. J. Public Health 62:566, April, 1972.

45. Heald, F. P.: Anatomy, physiology, and pharmacology. In Cooke, R. E., editor: The biologic basis of pediatric practice, New York, 1968, McGraw-Hill Book Co., p. 1649.

46. Heald, F. P., and Kahn, M. A.: Teenage obesity, Pediatr. Clin. North Am. 20:807, Nov., 1973.

47. Hofman, A. D.: Health care of innter-city adolescents, Clin. Pediatr. 13:570, July, 1974.

48. Holmstrom, L. L., and Burgess,, A. W.: Assessing trauma in the rape victim, Am. J. Nurs. 75:1288, Aug., 1975.

49. Hubbard, C. W.: Family planning education; parenthood and social disease control, St. Louis, 1972, The C. V. Mosby Co.

50. Hughes, P. H., and others: The natural history of a heroin epidemic, Am. J. Public Health 62:995, July, 1972.

51. Kandel, D., Single, E., and Kessler, R. C.: The epidemiology of drug use among New York State high school students; distribution, trends, and change in rates of use, Am. J. Public Health 66:43, Jan., 1976.

52. Kaplan, J. G., and others: Constitutional delay of growth and development; effects of treatment with androgens, J. Pediatr. 82:38, Jan., 1973.

53. Karzon, D. T.: The exanthems. II. Chickenpox varicella and herpes zoster, herpes simplex, infectious mononucleosis, erythema infectiosum. In Cooke, R. E., editor: The biologic basis of pediatric practice, New York, 1968, McGraw-Hill Book Co., p. 639.

54. Kaufman, D. M., Hegyi, T., and Duberstein, J. L.: Heroin intoxication in adolescents, Pediatrics 50:746, Nov., 1972.

55. Kelly, M.: Birthright; alternative to abortion, Am. J. Nurs. 75:76, Jan., 1975.

56. Kepler, M. O.: The abuse of drug abuse; some implications for medicine and religion, Clin. Pediatr. 11:386, July, 1972.

57. Klerman, G. L.: The therapeutic future of mind-altering drugs, J. School Health 43:116, Feb., 1973.

58. Knowles, J. H.: The health system and the Supreme Court decision; an affirmative response, Family Planning Perspectives 5(2):113, 1973.

59. Kolton, M.: The humanistic treatment philosophy of innovative drug programs, J. Humanistic Psychol. 13:47, Fall, 1973.

60. Kramer, J. P.: The adolescent addict; the progression of youth throughout the drug culture, Clin. Pediatr. 11:382, July, 1972.

61. Lanese, R. R., and others: Smoking behavior in a teenage population; a multivariate conceptual approach, Am. J. Public Health 62:807-813, June, 1972.

62. Lieberman, C. M., and Lieberman, B. W.: Marihuana—a medical review, N. Engl. J. Med. 284:88, 1971.

63. Litt, I. F., and others: Liver disease in the drug-using adolescent, J. Pediatr. 81:238-242, Aug., 1972.

64. Litt, I. F., and Cohen, M. I.: End of an epidemic? J. Pediatr. 86:293, Feb., 1975.

65. Litt, I. F., Edgberg, S. C., and Finberg, L.: Gonorrhea in children and adolescents, J. Pediatr. 85:595, Nov., 1974.

66. MacKenzie, R. G.: A practical approach to the drug-using adolescent and young adult, Pediatr. Clin. North Am. 20:1035, Nov., 1973.

67. Maidlow, S. T., and Berman, H.: The economics of heroin treatment, Am. J. Public Health 62:1397, Oct., 1972.

68. Marino, A. F., Pariser, H., and Wise, H.: Gonorrhea epidemiology—is it worthwhile? Am. J. Public Health 62:713, May, 1972.

69. McAnarney, E. R.: Adolescent pregnancy—a pediatric concern? Clin. Pediatr. 14:19, Jan., 1975.

70. McCormack, W. M., and others: Evaluation of two methods of following women who have been treated

because of exposure to gonorrhea, Am. J. Public Health **64:**714, July, 1974.

71. McGrath, P., and Laliberte, E. B.: Level of basic venereal disease knowledge among junior and senior high school nurses in Massachusetts; a survey, Nurs. Res. **23:**31, Jan-Feb., 1974.

72. McKee, M. R.: Drug abuse knowledge and attitudes in "middle America," Am. J. Public Health **65:**584, June, 1975.

73. Mercer, R.: Becoming a mother at sixteen, Mat. Child Nurs. **1:**44, Jan.-Feb., 1976.

74. Minkowski, W. L., Weiss, R. C., and Heidbreder, G. A.: A view of the drug problem; a rational approach to youthful drug use and abuse, Clin. Pediatr. **11:**376, July, 1972.

75. Modell, W., editor: Drugs of choice, 1976-1977, St. Louis, 1976, The C. V. Mosby Co.

76. Nadelson, C.: Abortion counseling; Focus on adolescent pregnancy, Pediatrics **54:**765, Dec., 1974.

77. Nakashima, I. I.: Teenage pregnancy—its causes, costs and consequences, Nurse Pract. **2:**10, Sept.-Oct., 1977.

78. Noona, A. S., and Adams, J. B.: Gonorrhea screening in an urban hospital family planning program, Am. J. Public Health **64:**700, July, 1974.

79. Noshpitz, J. D.: Drugs and adolescents, Clin. Proc. Child. Hosp. **27:**138, April, 1971.

80. O'Broyle, C. M.: Sports injuries in adolescents; emergency care, Am. J. Nurs. **75:**1732, Oct., 1975.

81. Ostaszewski, T. M., and Marshall, J. L.: Prevention and treatment of sports injuries, Am. J. Nurs. **75:**1737, Oct., 1975.

82. Paul, E. W., Pilpel, H. F., and Wechsler, N. F.: Pregnancy, teenagers and the law, Family Planning Perspectives **6**(3):142-147, 1974.

83. Quirk, B., and Huxall, L.: VD, the equal opportunity disease, J. Obstet. Gynecol. Neonatal Nurs. **4:**13, Jan.-Feb., 1975.

84. Ray, O. S.: Drugs, society, and human behavior, ed. 2, St. Louis, 1978, The C. V. Mosby Co.

85. Root, A. W.: Endocrinology of puberty. II. Aberra-

tions of sexual maturation, J. Pediatr. **83:**187, Aug., 1973.

86. Rubin, E., and Lieber, C. S.: Alcoholism, alcohol, and drugs, Science **172:**1097, 1971.

87. Schatz, B. E., and Ebrahimi, F.: Free clinic patient characteristics, Am. J. Public Health **62:**1354, Oct., 1972.

88. Stephenson, J. N.: Drug abuse in adolescence. In Kalafatich, A. J., editor: Approaches to the care of adolescents, New York, 1975, Appleton-Century-Crofts, p. 131.

89. Teenage pregnancy and the problem of abortion. Report of the committee on Youth, American Academy of Pediatrics: Pediatrics **49:**303, Feb., 1972.

90. Thiebaux, H. J.: Self-prescribed contraceptive education by the unwillingly pregnant, Am. J. Public Health **62:**689, May, 1972.

91. Thomas, J. A., Mawhinney, M. G., and Knotts, G. R.: Substances with potential for abuse for elementary and secondary school pupils; an informational reminder, Clin. Pediatr. **12:**17A, Jan., 1973.

92. Turner, I. R.: Free health centers; a new concept? Am. J. Public Health **62:**1348, Oct., 1972.

93. Wallace, H. M., and others: The maternity home; present services and future roles, Am. J. Public Health **64:** 568, June, 1974.

94. Webb, T. E., and Oski, F. A.: Iron deficiency anemia and scholastic achievement in young adolescence, J. Pediatr. **82:**827, May, 1973.

95. Weitman, M., Scheble, R. O., and Johnson, K. G.: Survey of adolescent drug use, Am. J. Public Health **64:** 417, May, 1974.

96. Welch, M. S.: Rape and the trauma of inadequate care, Prism **3:**17, Sept., 1975.

97. Williams, S. J., and McIntosh, E. N.: Requirements for abortion services, Am. J. Public Health, **64:**716, July, 1974.

98. Yancy, W. S., Nader, P. R., and Burnham, K. L.: Drug use and attitudes of high school students, Pediatrics **50:**739, Nov., 1972.

# Donna R.—ADOLESCENT

Cheryl Boyd Hundley

## HEALTH STATUS LIST

| Onset | Date | No. | Active | Date | Inactive/resolved |
|-------|------|-----|--------|------|-------------------|
| | | | Incomplete data base | | |
| 2/8/60 | 6/1/78 | 2 | | 2/8/60 | Apneic at birth |
| 2/8/60 | 6/1/78 | 3 | | 5/60 | Colic |
| 1965 | 6/1/78 | 4 | | 1965 | Tonsillectomy and removal of melanoma |
| 1967-1968 | 6/1/78 | 5 | | | Childhood diseases |
| | | | | | 1967—Mumps |
| | | | | | 1968—Chickenpox |
| 1970 | 6/1/78 | 6 | | 1970 | Pneumonia (staphylococcal) |
| 3/78 | 6/1/78 | 7 | Dysmenorrhea | | |
| 2/8/60 | 6/1/78 | 8 | Child health maintenance | | |
| | | 8,A | Physical competency | | |
| | | 8,B | Learning and thought competency | | |
| | | 8,C | Social competency | | |
| | | 8,D | Inner competency | | |

Client **Donna R.**  Sex F  Age 18  B.D. 2/8/60
Date 6/1/78  Race Caucasian

**Information sources:** Donna
　　　　　　　　　　Mother

### Reason health care worker sought client

Upon request nurse made home visit to interview Donna and mother and to assess for the need for intervention concerning menstrual cramps.

### Reason for seeking health care (mother and child's comments)

"Menstrual cramps" are worse lately. Has come home from school with them, according to mother and daughter.

### What events led up to the situation?

Periods started at age 12½, but cramps have progressed from mild discomfort to painful. Amount of bleeding has not increased; no new premenstrual signs.

### When did this situation occur?

Started about 3 months ago. Pains feel like spasms in lower abdomen at times. Worse the first two days. Flow is not heavier; no clots are passed according to Donna.

## Describe the situation and/or how you are feeling. What made you decide to seek health care?

Has a part-time job and is busy with school activities, and this is causing her to periodically be absent from school and work. Going to college in the fall and would like to see if anything can be done for her cramps.

## What do you and your family do when something like this happens?

Takes aspirin, uses a heat pad to the abdomen, and sits or lies down as much as possible. Recently these measures have not been giving relief.

## How is this affecting you and your family at the present time?

Mother is concerned at this much discomfort. Has disrupted school and work schedules. Doesn't want cramps to interfere with summer job she'll be starting soon.

## MOTHER PROFILE
HEALTH HISTORY

Carol, age 36. Full-time instructor at the local university.

### Present health status

No health problems at this time, except a "stuffy nose."

### Previous medical-surgical events

Kidney surgery at 4 years. Didn't know much about reason for surgery as mother died when she was 7, and father didn't know about details of her condition. Past surgeries include appendectomy, D and C, and a tubal ligation in 1975. Is gravida ii, para ii. No history of recurrent renal problems as to flow obstruction or infections.

PRENATAL HISTORY WITH THIS CHILD (DONNA)

Was ill most of the time with first severe morning sickness and vomiting and nausea all during pregnancy and for a few weeks afterward.

### Medical supervision

Good obstetrical care, since they were military personnel.

### Nutrition, diet

Ate anything she desired as she vomited most everything she ate. Gained eight pounds. Discovered with second pregnancy that in leaving off the iron preparation, she no longer had nausea and vomiting.

### Illness, infections, complications

Nausea and vomiting nine months and six weeks postpartum. Had a "full blown" urinary tract infection for six weeks postpartum.

### Treatments, procedures

Can remember none.

### Anesthesia

IV Demerol, which caused her to be nauseous and vomit as she is allergic to it. Saddle block.

### Course of labor and delivery

In labor 36 hours. Obstetrician ruptured membranes after 26 hours of labor. Husband with her most of this time.

### Availability in home

Works full-time. Usually home in the evenings and weekends. Donna helps with or prepares supper sometimes.

### Number of people in the home

Three: Carol (mother), Donna (daughter), Terry (son).

**Employment/work environment**

Instructor at local university. Works 8 to 10 hours daily, five days per week. Has to drive 20 miles to work.

**Date of last menstrual period**

Tubal ligation, 1975.

**FATHER PROFILE**

Donna's parents were divorced 3/12/70. Father lives several hundred miles away. She sees him on weekends. Speaks of him fondly, will live with father to attend the university there.

**Present health status**

Healthy according to Donna and Mother.

**Previous medical-surgical events**

They can remember none.

**Number of people he supports**

Her stepmother, Donna, and Terry.

**Availability in home/work habits**

Not known.

**Employment/work environment**

Retired military and is now a self-employed businessman.

**Range of income**

Mother earned $24,000 last year. Father contributes 25% toward support of children.

**Insurance**

Mother—hospitalization, health care, and life insurance. Father—not known.

LIFE CHANGE EVENTS (DATES)

Death (family, close friend) <u>Maternal grandfather 1970</u>  New baby _____

Divorce <u>Mother-stepfather (Feb. 1978)</u>  Marital separation _____  Return to school _____

Injury, illness _____  Job loss _____

Change of residence _____  Retirement _____

**Pedigree (include chronic, inherited conditions, allergies, causes of death, illness in siblings):**

O = Female
□ = Male
? = Unknown
A.W. = Alive and well

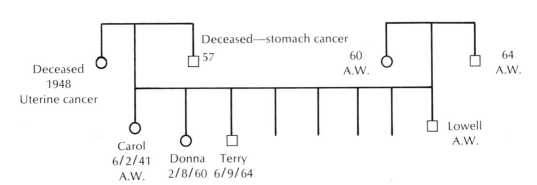

**633**

**Does your family see itself as a healthy family or as a sick family?**

Donna believes they are a "very healthy" family.

**Compare weight/height/age ratio**

Weight = 110 lbs.; height = 64 in.

**Identify developmental milestones (DDST)**

Not applicable.

**Sleep patterns/disturbances**

Needs ten hours of sleep but often only gets eight. Gets tired because of eye strain. Wears "contacts."

**Allergies**

None.

**Immunizations**

Last booster, age 14. Rubella vaccination at that time.

PSYCHOLOGIC PROFILE (data here to be obtained during interactions, inquiry, observation, DDST)

| Cognition | Ego |
|---|---|
| **FORMAL OPERATIONAL PHASE (11-15)** | **IDENTITY VS. IDENTITY DIFFUSION (13-18)** |
| __Yes__ Uses systematic ways for problem solving (relativity) | __Yes__ Secondary sexual characteristics |
| __Yes__ Uses implications from logical deduction for reasoning | __Yes__ Self-image and how others see him is congruent |
| _____ Reasons with propositions | __Yes__ Making long-range plans for occupation in rudimentary form |
| __Yes__ Thinks beyond his own world and beliefs | __Yes__ Seeks contacts with members of the opposite sex |
| | Not discussed "Being against" some societal establishments |
| | Not discussed Expresses some basic philosophy and faith |
| | __Yes__ Experiments with various roles; enjoys music, literature, company of others |
| | __Yes__ Peers are center of social interests |

**Comments**

Good academic performance, accepted into university for pre-medical curriculum. Grades in school reflect competency in concept of relativity and use of implication.

Dates, no steady relationship with a boy now. Has fully developed secondary sexual characteristics. Has long-range occupational plans for medicine. Is active in National Honor Society, biology club, math club, and attends school sport activities. Enjoys reading and "likes people at school." Most activities involve peers. Need more contact to explore ideologies and philosophies. No expression of anti-societal views during visit. Is in late phase of identity formation.

**SCHOOL PROGRESS**

**What would you like to tell me about school?**

"I really enjoy school." Rarely ever misses. Enjoys her clubs and activities.

**What do you like or dislike most about school?**

Likes the people at school, especially "the guys." Dislikes about school being hassled about being absent by school personnel.

**Talk with parent or teacher about memory**

Confirms that it is good.

**Tell me, What kind of a student do you think you are?**

"A good student." Mother confirms that she is an "A" student.

PERCEPTION OF SELF
**Self-evaluation**

(Describe yourself to me.)
Believes she likes how she looks, feels "good about me." Upset because her long hair was trimmed "too short."

**Tell me things you like about yourself; dislike**

No specific response to this just—I like myself except I wish I had "more up front." She then laughed jokingly.

**Let's pretend you could change something about yourself. Would you change anything?**

Would like larger breasts.

**Describe how you feel about what's happening to you now**

She's excited about going to college and preparing for a career in medicine. Wants very much to rid herself of the distraction of painful menstrual cramps so it won't interfere with studies or activities.

SOCIAL PROFILE
**Personal-social (DDST)**

Not applicable.

**Father/mother–child interaction**

Warm interchanges, some joking together. Relaxed communications.
Eye contact  Good.
Touching  Yes. Mother put arm around Donna's shoulders.
Tone of voice of parent  Soft, teasing sometimes.
Child-parent activities  They like to shop together on weekends.
Ease of separation  Easy. Donna is looking forward to college and leaving home.

**Position of child in family.**

First-born child.

**Describe life-style**

Comfortable suburban home. Kids help run household. Donna has her own car. Open communications.
Is there more than one language spoken in the home?  No

ENVIRONMENTAL PROFILE
**Pollutants**

Check statistics of city.

**Population density**

Check city figures.

**Infestations**

None seen.

**Fire hazards**

None seen.

**Medications/poisons**

No information.

**635**

Adolescence

## Crime
Check city statistics.

## Availability of transportation
Mother has car. Donna has a car.

REVIEW OF SYSTEMS
## General
Slender, attractive with brown eyes and hair. Dressed in jeans and a T-shirt. "Never sick." Busy with activities.

## Hair and scalp (dandruff, lice, cradle cap, itching, hair loss)
Denies any of the above.

## Skin (infections, scaling, burns, allergies)
None of the above. Melanoma removed from L breast at age of 5.

## Hematopoietic (anemias, bleeding, bruising)
Will bruise with a hard blow. No history of anemia, nose bleeds, or bleeding from bladder or bowel.

## Eyes (infections, blurred vision, squinting, color blindness)
Got glasses in seventh grade. She is nearsighted. Doesn't know the correction. Got contacts three years ago. Never had any of the above.

## Ears (infection, discharge, eardrum perforation, foreign objects, wax removals, decreased hearing)
Some ear infections when very small. Negative history for remainder of items.

## Nose, throat, sinuses (runny nose, colds, decreased smell, foreign body, broken nose, tonsillitis)
Tonsillectomy age 5. Occasional runny nose. Otherwise negative history.

## Mouth and dentition (dental caries, gingivitis, malocclusion, cleft lip and/or palate)
Hasn't gone to dentist for two years. Never had braces. Has had a few teeth filled.

## Respiratory (bronchitis, pneumonia, whooping cough, histoplasmosis, tuberculosis, cough)
Pneumonia at age 10. Negative history otherwise. Does not smoke.

## Cardiovascular (heart murmurs, cyanosis)
Negative history.

## Gastrointestinal (nausea/vomiting, diarrhea, constipation, jaundice, pain, colic, gas, hernias, anorexia)
Negative for any of the above.

## Genitourinary (frequency, urgency, burning, toilet training, bedwetting, odor, stream)
Toilet trained at age 2 years, 6 months. Otherwise negative history.

## Reproductive (irritations, rashes, deviations, secondary sexual characteristics)
LMP  5/15/78
Menarche age 12½ years. Periods are every 30 days. Cramps recently. Obvious secondary sexual characteristics.

## Neuromuscular (convulsions, headache, imbalance, incoordination, muscle weakness, numbness, tremors, tics)
Occasional headache that she believes to be caused by wearing contacts too long.

## Psychologic (thumb sucking, fears, masturbation)
Sucked three fingers as a baby.

PHYSICAL PROFILE

**Measurements**

Head _Omitted_   Chest _Omitted_
Ht. _5'4"_   Wt. _110_

**Vital signs**

B/P _110/70_   H.R. _78/reg._
Resp. _20/min_   Temp. _98.4° F_

**Neuromuscular system**

Well-muscled arms and legs. Walk is aligned straight with relaxed swinging of arms. Posture is erect sitting and standing.

**Present neurological status**

Neuromuscular system is intact; has reached almost full development.

**Social affect**

Relaxed, smiling, likes to relate incidents, funny situations. Communicates with words accompanied by congruent feeling tones. Good eye contact with interviewer.

**Speech development**

Articulate speech with wide vocabulary.

**Reflexes**

Biceps _3+_
Triceps _3+_
Brachioradialis _3+_   } Response equal bilaterally
Patellar _3+_
Achilles _3+_
Babinski _Negative_
Eye _Active blink_

**Cranial nerves**

I (olfactory): Intact. Identified smell of rubbing alcohol.
II (optic): Snellen 20/20 with contacts. Peripheral vision at 90 degrees. Can distinguish colors.
III, IV, and VI (oculomotor, trochlear, abducens): Intact EOM's intact. Good convergence and blink.
V (trigeminal): Intact. Can feel light touch in maxillary and mandibular areas bilaterally. Equality of bite.
VII (facial): Intact. Lines and contours of the face symmetrical. Able to mimic squint, frown. Tasted salt and sugar on tongue.
VIII (acoustic): Intact. Negative Rinne and Weber tests. Heard watch tick 4 inches from ears.
IX, X (glossopharyngeal, vagus): Intact. Salivates. Articulates speech sounds. Gag reflex present. Tongue in midline. Swallow is coordinated. Uvula midline.
XI (accessory): Intact. Equal strength in shoulder and neck.
XII (hypoglossal): Intact. Can move tongue from side to side. Can apply pressure to cheek with tongue with equal strength.

**Cerebellar function (Rhomberg, walk heel-toe, run in place, touch tip of nose, copy hand movements, pincer grasp, draw and copy geometric shapes)**

Negative Rhomberg. Able to walk heel-toe, run in place, touch top of nose with eyes closed.

**Parietal lobe function (object identification)**

Identified tactually a key, safety pin, and rubber band.

**Proprioception (positional sense of toe)**

Accurate sense of up and down positions of big toe with eyes closed.

Adolescence

**Tactile capacity (cold, two-point discrimination, pin prick)**

Recognizes hot, cold, pressure and pin prick on inner and outer aspects of arms and thighs.

**Skin (scars, lesions, turgor, bruises, moles)**

No lesions, bruises, or moles seen. Surgical scar size of nickel below left breast. Skin reflects turgor and hydration.

**Head (circumference, fontanel measurement, palpation, transillumination)**

Negative results from palpation. Head circumference inadvertently omitted.

**Face (expression, palpebral fissures, placement of ears, percussion of sinuses, symmetry)**

A few blemishes on face. Equal symmetry and placement of features. Sinuses nontender.

**Hair, scalp (hairline, hygiene, distribution)**

Long straight clean hair, medium thickness, and normal hair line.

**Eyes (amblyopia, strabismus, drainage, deviation red reflex and structures)**

Conjunctivae pink, not inflamed and moist. No exudates. Negative, i.e. for strabismus, ambylopia, PERRLA (see cranial nerves). Red reflex present.

**Nose (patency, discharge, smell)**

Patent nares, no discharge. Able to smell alcohol (see cranial nerves)

**Mouth and throat (teeth, gums, pharynx, tongue, palates, swallowing, tonsils)**

Two fillings in lower back molars on right. Complete permanent dentition. Teeth aligned. No malocclusion. Pharynx not reddened. Teeth clean. No gingivitis.

**Ears (landmarks, structure, hearing)**

Pliant, firm pinnae. Canals clean. Tympanums pearly gray. Bony landmarks on identified. Cone of light at 5 o'clock on right, at 7 o'clock on left.

**Neck (nodes, masses, bruits, ROM)**

Full range of motion. No palpable masses or bruits. No lymphadenopathy.

**Chest (symmetry, excursion, nodes, nipples)**

Equal bilateral symmetry, excursion and placement of nipples. No flaring of lower costal margin. Breasts equal in size—no masses palpable. Donna knows how to examine her breasts, verified with self-demonstration. Chest wall had no palpable masses. No lymph adenopathy.

**Lungs (breath sounds, fremitus, percussion, duration of inspiration, expiration, rate)**

Clear to percussion, auscultation, vocal fremitus. Inspiration to expiration 1:2. Rate 20 per minute.

**Heart (size, position, PMI, sounds)**

Rate = 78 and regular. Borders not percussed. PMI at 5th ICS at MCL. $S_1$ loudest at the mitral area. $S_2$ loudest at pulmonic area in sitting and lying positions. No murmurs heard. No palpable thrills. No clubbing of fingers or facing of nares at rest. Extremities perfused.

**Abdomen (size, contour, bowel sounds, umbilicus, liver, spleen, femorals)**

Concave contour. Bowel sounds present. Negative findings for masses or tenderness with light and deep palpation. Liver edge felt. Femorals equal in character and rate.

**Back and spine (structure, symmetry, column curvature)**

Straight, in midline. No structural deviations palpable. Posture erect in sitting position. Scapulas bilaterally symmetrical with no flaring. No openings visualized or palpable in sacral area.

**Extremities (palmar creases, ROM, hip abduction)**

Light color hair on arms, legs shaved. Full active and passive ROM without joint crepitus. No hip clicks. Extremities warm and perfused. No peripheral cyanosis.

**Urinary (position of meatus, charae of voiding, appearance of urine)**

Yellow clear urine. Position of meatus above vaginal outlet.

**Genitalia (structure, secondary sexual characteristics)**

Deferred until seen in clinic setting for pelvic examination. Has never had pelvic examination or Pap smear.

**Anus (structure, function)**

Patent. Daily bowel movement.

**INITIAL PLAN**

### No. 1   Incomplete data base

**S**   Mother and daughter concerned with daughter's recent development of menstrual cramps of increased severity.

**O**   Home visit did not allow for complete physical exam, which would include pelvic examination.

**A**   Need further data to have more in-depth assessment of physical and psychosocial aspects. Factors possibly related to onset of dysmenorrhea of increasing severity.

**P**   Obj. 1   The client should plan for visit to clinic for further interaction and pelvic examination by clinical specialist.

6/1/78   **No. 7   Dysmenorrhea**

**S**   Started periods at 12½ years of age. Periods occur about every 30 days. LMP 5/15/78. In past three months cramps have progressed from uncomfortable to painful. Has come home from school because of pain, mother states. Has a part-time job and has been busy with school activities, and menstrual cramps have interfered with these. Going to college in the fall, working this summer, and desires to get relief from monthly pain. Regular comfort measures are ineffective. Pain is worse during first one or two days of menstrual flow. No increase in flow, no passage of clots. Does not believe she has any new premenstrual signs.

**O**   None. Need pelvic exam for base-line objective data. Not presently menstruating.

**A**   Dysmenorrhea is a term used to describe painful menstruation. It is generally accepted that strong or abnormal uterine contractions are major cause of discomfort. There may be no apparent organic disorder, but it is thought the large uterine contractions occur in response to rising levels of progesterone. Menstruation following an ovulatory cycle is more commonly associated with uterine cramps. Claim that cramps will subside after childbirth is not a pertinent promise to an unmarried teenager and there are no valid studies to confirm this. Onset of dysmennorhea after several years of minimal discomfort with cramps is referred to as secondary dysmenorrhea. Diseases or alterations of the uterus or reproductive structures are possibilities with secondary dysmenorrhea. A careful pelvic examination often provides necessary clues. Patients with secondary dysmenorrhea should be treated with the intent of removing the etiologic factor.

   As in all instances involving pain consider the individual's attitude toward the pain, attitude and interrelationship with peers and families. Symptomatology ranges from mild cramps to an intense suffering with severe cramps and symptoms, suggesting vaginal irritation such as diarrhea, bladder tenesmus, vomiting, and fainting.

**P**   Obj. 1   Donna should demonstrate relief from dysmenorrhea.

6/1/78   **No. 8   Child health maintenance**

8,A   Physical competency

**S**   Donna believes herself to be healthy with no chronic or acute health problems at this time. History reveals Donna was apneic at birth and resuscitated without any other neonatal complications. Colic in first three months of life. Tonsillectomy and removal of melanoma mole at the age of 5, mumps when 7, chicken pox when 8, and pneumonia at age of 10. Menarche at age 12½. No dental visit in two years. Does not smoke. Concerned about breast size.

**O** Ht. is 5 feet 4 inches; wt. is 110 pounds. B/P 110/70, H.R. 78 and regular. Respiratory rate 20 per minute. Temperature 98.4° F. Physical examination negative for abnormalities. Neurological exam reveals sensory and motor systems intact. Sleeps 8 to 10 hours daily. Nutrition needs supplementation with more vegetables and fruits. Nickel size scar below L nipple. Active and alert. Wears contacts. No dental caries. Well-muscled arms and legs. Posture erect. Tonsils absent. Hygiene is good. Fully developed secondary sexual characteristics. Nontender abdomen, without palpable nodes or masses. Few blemishes on the face. Omitted inadvertently head and chest measurement.

**A** Adolescence is conceptualized as the period of life during which empancipation from the primary family unit is the major task of the individual. Adolescence is the final growth cycle to yield optimal development and to resist the degradation of matter and energy. Maturation of systems is designed for maintenance of steady physical states. The newly formed shape of youth stabilizes with maturity. Adolescent stress emerges from internal drives and impulses toward maturation, accentuated by demands of the environment. Studies show that the adolescent females are one of the most poorly fed groups in the U.S. Their diets are frequently low in iron, calcium, and vitamins A and C. Physical health hazards for adolescents are motor vehicle accidents, acne, pregnancy, venereal diseases, and drug abuse. Knowledge of sexual function and contraception and the above-mentioned health hazards should be considered as essential knowledge to the health maintenance of the adolescent. It is important not to assume an understanding of health maintenance because of the seeming sophistication of the adolescent. Immunizations remain an important ingredient of health protection. Also girls have a tendency to be concerned about adequacy of breasts.

**P** Obj. 1   Donna should demonstrate knowledge of the health hazards of adolescence.

Obj. 2   Donna should accept her changing body size and shape.

8,B   Learning and thought competency

**S** Mother states daughter is "A student." Is accepted into university of premedical curriculum.

**O** Is in formal operational period of intellectual development. Academic performance indirectly indicates mastery of concepts of relativity and use of systematic ways to solve problems.

**A** The young person develops a concept of relativity in the formal operations period through the application of hypotheses or propositional statements and with the use of implications. This is a necessary stage for the full development of intellectual thought as theorized by Piaget. Early in this stage there is a return to egocentrism in thinking. First relativity is applied indirectly, the child not realizing the application of the scientific method to thought. In academics this is formally applied as the young can take facts and principles as applied to present reality and hypothesis and predict outcomes of what could be as compared to what is. In this way the adolescent can move into logical thought, formulating ideas about the social and

**INITIAL PLAN—cont'd**

6/1/78    **No. 8    Child health maintenance—cont'd**

cosmic universe. This is necessary for the developmental task of developing intellectual and social sensitivities of a competent citizen. The adolescent needs academic success.

**P**    Obj. 1    Donna should demonstrate cognitive skills necessary for success in the university setting.

8,C    Social competency

**S**    Likes school and "enjoys the people" there. Active in clubs and activities at school. Especially likes "the guys." Mother and daughter like "to shop" together. Has her own car. Visits father frequently. Will live with him while attending college. Parents were divorced eight years ago. Recently mother and stepfather have also divorced. Mother is a university instructor. Expresses fondness for her 14-year-old brother. Babysits, has had part-time job after school and has full-time summer job arranged. Donna is the first-born child. Has expressed a chosen career of medicine. Looking forward to college and living with father.

**O**    Warm interchanges combined with touching between mother and daughter, teasing each other at home. Leaving her primary family unit soon. Feeling tones communicate fondness for her father. Good eye contact and open communication. Has sense of humor. Feels responsibility. No mention of mother's recent divorce.

**A**    Social competency of adolescence is partly dependent upon parental relationships and how the parents view the child. There is no longer the need for the adolescent to contribute financially to the family or for the family to teach vocational skills. Rapid changes in society leave gaps in skills, knowledge, and values of the generations. The young person is an important consumer and school gives a wide range of social interaction. All these things affect the developmental tasks of adolescence. Creation of adolescent behavior in U.S. culture includes expansion of life space due to cars, motorcycles, etc. Being neither a child or adult she/he may be treated ambivalently by those around him or her. The adolescent group may be viewed as a vehicle for movement out and away from the family unit and is a means of achieving goals of individuation. First achievements are recognized by the peer group and then the youth learns to identify personally meaningful goals for the future. Socially the adolescent must master the tasks of relating to a variety of people, achieving independence from parents while maintaining mature affection and interdependence upon them and selecting and preparing for an occupation providing for economic independence.

**P**    Obj. 1    Donna should achieve independence from the primary family unit.
Obj. 2    Donna should create a new group of friends at school.
Obj. 3    Donna should identify the family dynamics associated with divorce.

8,D    Inner competency

**S**    Dates. No steady boyfriend now but "likes the guys." Expresses herself through school, honor and social clubs. Expresses career plans for medicine. Expresses concern with body image. Wishes there was "more up front." States she "liked herself." Perceptions of herself as a student congruent with mother's comments. Mother allows her "independence." Parents were divorced in 1970.

**O**  Six years since onset of menarche. Body shape of a mature female figure. Seems at ease. Cooperative during interview and exams, questioned what was going on during exam. Demonstrates enthusiasm about career plans, school, and leaving home. Affectively is in identity formation vs. identity diffusion (Erikson).

Self-image seems congruent with others, has long-range plans for an occupation, actively seeks contacts with opposite sex, and peers are center of social interest. Does not smoke. Did not express "antagonism or being against" any conventional norm. Interview insufficient to discuss her working philosophy and values. Physical appearance and grooming are appropriate for her contemporary peer group (i.e., long straight hair, jeans). No mention of drug or alcohol use or experimentation. Mother mentioned no behaviors related to this.

**A**  Inner competency is central to all aspects of adolescence. The child who has a healthy self-concept performs appropriately physically and maintains physical appearance appropriate to contemporary standards. There is adequate learning and thought performance and her social behavior is appropriate. Behaviors are assessed and may be viewed as representing a serious social or inner impairment or a transient experimentation essential to identity formation. The central task of adolescence is to establish an identity formation. This is done by means of the adolescent clique. The adolescent's search for identity will depend on how well previous affective developmental crises were mastered. Self-identification should manifest as an accurate perception of self. The family and peer group should provide the positive regard and empathetic understanding for behavioral adaptability and growth. The ego becomes strengthened in adolescence and should facilitate reasoning, judgment, maintaining reality, subsuming contradictory values and attitudes, and maintaining unity and continuity of self.

**P**  Obj. 1  Donna should demonstrate mastery of tasks in identity formation.

**NURSING ORDERS**

6/1/78 **No. 1  Incomplete data base**                                         PERSONNEL

    Obj. 1  The client should plan for visit to clinic for further in-
           teraction and pelvic examination by clinical special-
           ist.
        A. Arrange for an appointment for 6/5/78 in clinic.   C.S.
        B. Share with client nurse's phone number. (6/1)   C.S.
        C. Arrange for preparatory time at clinic visit for   C.S.
           education about nature of procedure and sensa-
           tions occurring during exam. (6/5)
        D. Explore possibility of her bringing a friend with   C.S.
           her for the clinic visit should this make her more
           comfortable. (6/1)

6/1/78 **No. 7  Dysmenorrhea**

    Obj. 1  Donna should demonstrate relief from dysmenor-
           rhea.
        A. Ascertain a complete menstrual history including   C.S.
           beliefs about causes of discomfort, attitudes
           conveyed to her about menstruation. (6/5)
        B. Obtain menstrual history from mother and how   C.S.
           Donna was prepared for puberty and menstrua-
           tion. (6/5)
        C. After eliciting known information about the physi-   C.S.
           ology of the cycle from Donna, diagram the hor-
           monal and physical events in the cycle and re-
           late these to her symptoms. (6/5)
        D. After an orientation, perform a pelvic examina-   C.S.
           tion, perform Pap smear. (6/5)
        E. Share results of examination and Pap smear with   C.S.
           Donna and mother. (6/5)
        F. Determine how much over-the-counter analgesic   C.S.
           is being used for the pain. If excessive, refer to
           physician for prescription analgesic of sufficient
           strength to relieve pain. (6/5)
        G. Refer to physician should any structural or in-   C.S.
           flammatory alterations be identified in pelvic ex-
           am. (6/5)
        H. Explore the symptomatology further for signs re-   C.S.
           lated to vaginal irritation: bladder tenesmus, diar-
           rhea, vomiting, and fainting. (6/5)

**No. 8  Child health maintenance**

    8,A  Physical competency

    Obj. 1  Donna should demonstrate knowledge of the health
           hazards of adolescence.
        A. Elicit knowledge of basic four and of vitamins   C.S.
           and minerals from Donna. (6/14)
        B. Outline nutritional needs with her and allow her to   Donna
           choose foods to meet her deficiency. (6/14)   C.S.
        C. During clinic visit ascertain her knowledge of   C.S.
           sexual function, methods of contraception, and
           V.D. (6/5)

D. Using data from C plan an audiovisual presentation, giving information about sexual function methods of contraception and VD (6/14—in the clinic)  C.S.

E. After presentation, talk with her providing reinforcement and feedback asking how she may use this information to maintain her health. (6/14—clinic)  Donna C.S.

F. Have Donna list the methods of automobile safety she utilizes when in a car. (6/21)  Donna

G. Explore with her knowledge about drugs based on reading and/or any experimentation. Provide with pamphlet of facts about drugs. (6/21)  C.S.

H. Ask how she has coped with the drug scene and how she plans to deal with this when she is at the university (include alcohol in the discussion). (6/21)  C.S.

Obj. 2 Donna should accept her changing body and shape.

    A. Explore the seriousness of her concern about the adequacy of her breasts. (6/14—clinic)  C.S.

8,B Learning and thought competency

Obj. 1 Donna should demonstrate cognitive skills necessary for success in the university setting.

    A. Explore with Donna her study habits and how she plans to apply these in the college setting. (6/21)  C.S.

    B. Review with her the methods of viewing conceptually a problem or an idea. Work through an example. (6/21)  C.S.

    C. Encourage her to make use of counselors, teacher conferences in the academic setting. (6/21)  C.S.

    D. Have her outline strengths and weaknesses academically and how she will utilize them in her studies. (6/21)  C.S.

    E. Encourage her to share ideas and thoughts with her peers and professors. (6/21)  C.S.

8,C Social competency

Obj. 1 Donna should achieve independence from the primary family unit.

    A. Talk with mother about how she views her daughter as an individual and how she feels about her leaving the present unit. (6/21—home visit)  C.S.

    B. Explore how mother plans to cope with separation so as to foster interdependence between them. (6/21)  C.S.

    C. Have Donna role play through how she will cope with the effects of leaving mother and brother (i.e., "homesickness"). (6/21)  C.S.

    D. Explore her perception of how much independence she will have with her father and stepmother. (6/21)  C.S.

## NURSING ORDERS—cont'd

| 6/1/78 | **No. 8** | **Child health maintenance—cont'd** | PERSONNEL |

Obj. 2 Create a new group of friends at school.

    A. Encourage Donna to become a part of an orientation at school to initiate contacts for forming new relationships. (6/21) — C.S.

    B. Point out that living "off campus" will isolate her from much social interaction in the dormitory so that she may have to plan for opportunities to meet others. (6/21) — C.S.

Obj. 3 Identify the family dynamics associated with divorce.

    A. Ascertain feelings about her parents' divorce and how is this affecting her thinking about the forming of permanent relationships. (6/21) — C.S.

    B. Inquire how her mother's recent divorce is affecting her, Terry, and her mother. (6/21) — C.S.

    C. Refer for counseling should she desire or need information or intervention. — Psychologist C.S.

8,D Inner competency

Obj. 1 Donna should demonstrate mastery of tasks in identity formation.

    A. Further explore with Donna available help sources when she needs to share problems and doubts. — C.S.

    B. Encourage her to cultivate a confidant at school. — C.S.

    C. Teach mother about this developmental stage and how she can use this information to assess daughter's behavior. — Mother C.S.

    D. Collect more data from mother and Donna about nature of family life prior to divorce. — C.S.

    E. Teach Donna the tasks of identity formation and those of the forthcoming stage of intimacy vs. self-absorption. — C.S.

**REFERENCES**

Kugelmass, I. N.: Adolescent medicine; principles and practice, Springfield, Ill., 1975, Charles C Thomas, Publisher.

Murray, R., and Zentner, J.: Nursing assessment and health promotion through the life span, Englewood Cliffs, N.J., 1975, Prentice-Hall, Inc.

Thorn, G. W., Adams, R. D., Braunwald, E., and others, editors: Harrison's Principles of internal medicine, New York, 1977, McGraw-Hill Book Co.

Vaughn-Wrobel, B. C., and Henderson, B.: The problem oriented record in nursing practice, St. Louis, 1976, The C. V. Mosby Co.

# Serious health problems during childhood and adolescence

For some children, development incorporates a serious health problem. Severe acute illness, long-term illness, and handicapping conditions are special problems that confront health care professions and demand a large proportion of the resources offered by the health care system. Children who experience these kinds of problems are most often more like other children than they are unlike them. Development of adequate competencies can still be maintained and achieved in most areas in spite of a serious health problem. To accomplish these maintenance goals, the nature of the problem must be understood, and special skills must be utilized to help the family with multiple problems. This unit focuses upon the ways in which knowledge can be acquired relating to certain kinds of serious problems, and the means by which children and families can be assisted in achieving the basic goals of health.

The purposes of Chapter 16, "Hospitalization and Home Care," are (1) to discuss the known and hypothesized effects of hospitalization on a child and family, (2) to consider criteria for hospitalization and for home care of the child who experiences a serious health problem, (3) to discuss the basis of nursing assessment required when there is a serious health problem and the specific nursing diagnosis and management required in the face of a serious health problem, and (4) to discuss current trends in hospitalization of children that promote healthy child and family development.

Chapter 17, "Death and Dying During Childhood and Adoles-  **647** cence," concerns (1) attitudes toward death and the grieving process of children and parents who are faced with knowledge of a fatal illness and (2) a framework for acquisition of professional knowledge needed in administering care to the child and family.

Chapter 18, "Children and Youth with Long-Term Physical Problems," considers serious health problems that primarily affect or originate from physical competency. The purposes of this chapter are (1) to discuss the effect of physical problems on each area of competency development, (2) to present a framework for acquisition of knowledge related to particular physical problems, and (3) to discuss features of comprehensive health care required for the child and family when they face a serious physical problem.

Chapter 19, "The Child with Learning Problems," considers problems that primarily affect or originate from learning and thought competency. The purposes of this chapter are (1) to discuss the effect of learning problems on all areas of competency development, and the interactions that occur, (2) to define and describe the common learning problems that occur among children of all ages, and (3) to consider the means by which the family, teachers, and health care workers can mutually promote healthy development for these children.

Chapter 20, "The Child with Long-Term Social and Inner Problems," primarily concerns problems that affect or originate from social and inner competency development. The purposes of this chapter are (1) to discuss the effects of social and inner problems on other areas of competency development and the interactions between each of the areas of development, (2) to define and describe the common types of problems that occur in social and inner development, and (3) to discuss the health care needs that develop in the face of these long-term, serious problems.

# Hospitalization and home care

When children suffer long-term illness or handicapping conditions, hospitalization often becomes inevitable. In addition, some children must be hospitalized in relation to acute health problems. Although for most children experiences in the hospital comprise a very brief span of time compared with their total life experience, the encounter usually leaves a lasting impression on children and exerts a significant influence on their entire life. Because of the relatively high incidence of emotional problems related to hospitalization even for a brief period of time, much attention has been directed to ways in which this experience can be made less traumatic for children and families.[23,30,47,69]

Home care has been increasingly sought for children in all instances where this is feasible in order to avoid the trauma of hospitalization. In this chapter we will discuss primary care concerns that apply regardless of the setting in which care is given.

## EFFECTS OF HOSPITALIZATION

Long-term hospitalization in a setting that does not provide contact with other significant humans or that lacks environmental stimulation seriously affects the child's intellectual, physical, and emotional development.[17,68,74] In recent years, practice in hospitals and institutions has changed significantly to provide a healthier experience for the children confined. The child who experiences a brief hospitalization may react with problems in feeding or sleeping and with regressive behavior, aggressive behavior, irritability, or unreasonable fears.[30,49,74]

When hospitalization occurs for the first time, children are suddenly transferred into an environment that is totally new and unfamiliar. There is usually no past reference for many of the events that take place. The sounds are strange; the words people use are different. The smells of the air are different from anything before experienced. The food tastes different, and the lights and colors are different. The way their own parents act is also different, since their behavior is affected by the situation. In this situation the factors influencing growth and development become particularly significant. These factors determine the type of adjustment capacities the child possesses, and they influence the kind of experience that the hospitalization is to become for the child and the family. The more completely the child's past environment is understood by the hospital health care team, the more effectively they can plan and implement care that will promote the basic goal of health care—to motivate individuals to seek health and to use their own resources to attain, maintain, or regain optimal health and function (see Chapter 2). For the hospitalized child this goal demands attention not only to the restorative aspects of care but also to the child's need to con-

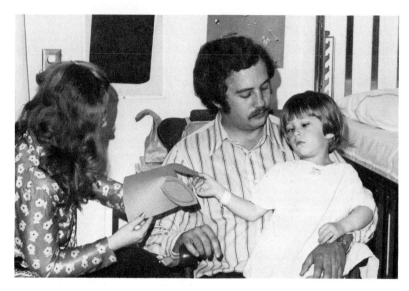

**Fig. 16-1.** Parents who maintain their previous mothering and fathering roles with minimal disruption are probably most facilitative in helping their child adjust and cope.

tinue development in each of the four competency areas with minimal disruption.[30,45,47,69]

There are several general factors of the child's home environment that are particularly significant in affecting adjustment to hospitalization and illness.

First, the attitudes of the parents toward the experience and toward the child influence the child's adjustment. This includes the particular roles assumed during the illness or hospitalization, as contrasted to the roles assumed by the parent before the event. Parents who maintain their previous mothering and fathering roles with minimal disruption probably help their child adjust and cope. If, on the other hand, they begin to assume the role of crusader, therapist, or expert-on-the-subject in relating to the child, they jeopardize the child's adjustment. Parents can and should participate as therapists, and they should become well acquainted with the child's illness, but these aspects of the parent's participation should not usurp the basic relationship between parent and child.[23,73]

Second, the duration and quality of the hospital or illness experience affect the child's adjustment. If the illness or disability is permanent, some adjustment must eventually be reached; if the illness is relatively temporary, the goal to restore the child to the former environment and optimal state of health should be implemented as early as possible. All efforts to bring the child's own familiar environment into the new and strange environment cannot substitute for actually being back home where things are totally familiar. The extent to which the hospital setting allows for familiarity and for help in coping with the stresses of unfamiliarity, fear, and pain defines the quality of the hospital or illness experience.

Third, the child's past experiences with hospitalization have a significant impact on the nature of each subsequent hospitalization. The child may appear to return to the hospital in a nonchalant manner or may require a new adjustment each time. Children who require repeated hospitalizations often suffer long-term illness with serious inner and social implications, and behavior problems during hospital experiences become a significant focus of nursing care. Such children may be expressing their frustration and anger, or their own approach to coping may interfere with social relationships with others and with the development of positive, healthy inner competency.

Finally, adequate preparation of children for a hospital experience or diagnostic procedure is considered to be an important factor in their adjustment to the experience. The exact timing and form that preparation takes depend upon the child's age, the illness, level of intelligence, and past history of coping with stress. When the hospitalization occurs as an emergency following a sudden accident, preparation is not possible, and adjustment begins abruptly upon entering the hospital. Young children who have not yet developed a concept of the future are prepared when the experience is just about to begin. Careful attention to the young children's initial responses and their ability to become acquainted are part of the preparation experience. The older children may have a period of several days of anticipation, which either positively or negatively prepare them for the actual experience.*

Four major risks have been identified with hospitalization of children:

1. Emotional and separation problems, particularly for children under 4 years of age, can be transient or permanent, but are significant for the child and the family.
2. The parents' confidence in their own ability to care for the child themselves may be undermined.
3. Exposure to infection is increased in the hospital setting.
4. The family and society sustain a significant economic cost, which for the family may constitute a lasting stress.[59]

## The hospital environment

Hospitalization clearly constitutes a crisis event for children and families.[5,25,31,76,82] The hospital environment itself can be a major source of unnecessary stress for children and families and should be designed to diminish such sources of stress as much as possible. The area of the hospital that is used for care of children needs to be carefully evaluated to determine the safety and suitability of the area for care of children, using the principles described below to determine if this area is conducive for providing sound, comprehensive care. When possible, children's rooms should be decorated in accord with the developmental needs of children and adolescents. For example, in an area

where infants and toddlers are placed, the rooms should provide age-appropriate stimulation such as wallpaper or wall hangings that portray storybook characters or familiar, favorite objects and toys. An area planned for the care of older children and adolescents, on the other hand, needs to be decorated at an age-appropriate level, using pictures and wall hangings that appeal to older children. The walls should be constructed in such a manner that hospitalized children can post their own drawings on the wall and hang objects they construct from the ceiling.[15,24,31,34]

Books, toys, and supplies for arts and crafts need to be readily available and planned for each age group of children. A special play area for group activities and group meals should be planned as a central part of the unit. Furnishings should be planned to facilitate active play and should be appropriate to a wide range of age groups and to planned therapeutic play activities. For example, a drawing easel permits drawing and painting on a large surface for the young child who needs a large area for drawing and painting. A punching bag provides a means for release of tension through large muscle activity. Ordinary hospital equipment provides play experiences in acting out therapeutic procedures. Objects and furnishings that are always out and available to children are selected for their value and safety in free, unsupervised play. Objects and furnishings that are used for planned, supervised play for therapeutic purposes are stored in an adjoining area where they can be obtained by nurses and other adults as they are required.[5,29,31]

Provision should be made for families and children to bring to the hospital environment their own clothing, toys, and objects that provide for familiarity. To whatever extent possible, children should dress in their own clothes during the day and be able to move about the hospital environment. Bathroom facilities should take into account the developmental needs of the children and young people who will be using them. Small toilets need to be available for young children who are just learning to use the toilet on their own, and older children need regular adult facilities. Bathrooms should provide for individual privacy, regardless of the

*References 2, 6, 12, 18, 30, 71, 72, 80.

**651**

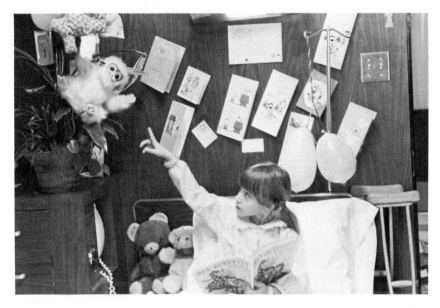

**Fig. 16-2.** The child's hospital room should be designed to encourage the child to hang cards, drawings, and toys on the wall and ceiling.

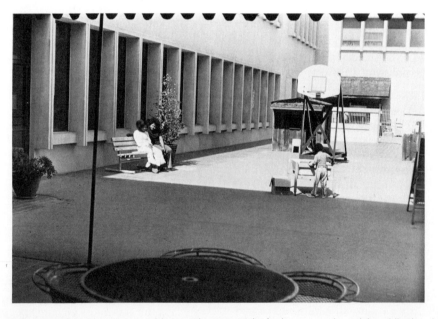

**Fig. 16-3.** An outdoor play area provides ample opportunity for large muscle activity while the child is hospitalized.

age of the child. Special attention needs to be given to provision of bathrooms for use by parents, and they need to be informed of the location of bathrooms for their use if these are separate from the facilities provided for their child.

The staff of a child care unit should be selected on the basis of their desire and ability to work with children of all age groups. The professional nursing staff needs to be qualified by their ability to relate to children, knowledge of developmental principles and ability to use this knowledge in planning nursing care, knowledge and application of therapeutic play techniques, skill in technical procedures used with children, ability to counsel with parents and integrate parents into the hospital environment, and ability to provide guidance and supervision for other health care workers, such as the technical nursing staff, nursing aides, and volunteer workers. Nurses who have a desire to work with children but who lack experience should be given the opportunity to work with more experienced nurses in order to receive guidance and counseling as they develop experience.[31,34]

The importance of planning for complete integration of parents and other primary caretakers into the hospital care of children cannot

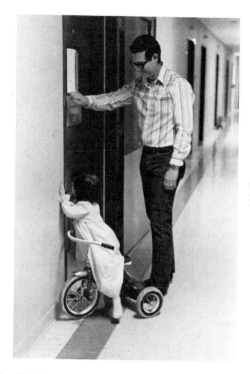

**Fig. 16-4.** The child and her father move freely about the hospital environment, providing for large muscle activity and achieving familiarity and mastery of the environment.

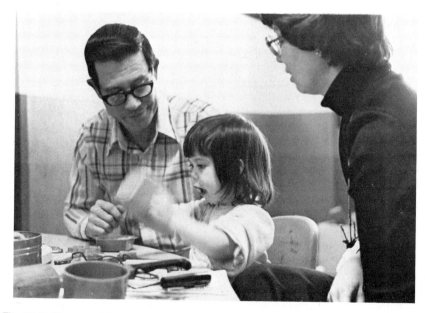

**Fig. 16-5.** Play materials are available for the child and her parents to use as they desire.

be overemphasized. Parents usually want to maintain intimate involvement with their children during this period of stress, and such involvement provides important learning that can improve the quality of health care for the child at home. A comprehensive plan that takes into account teaching of developmental principles, teaching and counseling related to the child's illness, teaching principles of regular health maintenance, and facilitating of optimal parent-child relationships can provide a great benefit in improving the health of children and families. The hospital environment should provide kitchen and laundry facilities for parents so that they have ready access to their use at any time during the day or night. Provision for sleeping and daytime relaxation in the child's room is provided by sofa beds, lounge chairs, or foldaway beds. Bathroom facilities suitable for adult use and convenient to the child's room should be provided. Early in the child's hospitalization, the parents are oriented to these provisions and counseled in regard to their own desire and ability. If the hospital serves groups who speak languages other than English, provision should be made for health care workers who can be available to work with the family in their own language and facilitate communication with English-speaking health care workers. Separate rooms for individual parent counseling, group meetings, and adult retreat from the child care area should be available.[10,31]

An emerging practice that facilitates parent involvement is complete access and sharing of information. Parents now have the legally protected right to complete access to the nursing and medical records, and the child health care team can facilitate their understanding of the material in these records by including the parents in team meetings involving their child's care. They should be considered, along with the child, as the primary members of the team, and all identification of problems and planning for intervention and evaluation of the effectiveness of care should center around their desires, goals, and perceptions. When differences of opinion or desire exist, the differences should be examined to determine the most desirable course of action. If the parents appear to be acting out of anger or denial, the counseling ap-

proach will be very different from a situation in which the parents are acting out of lack of understanding and accurate information. The health care team needs to be constantly aware of their own value system and together examine instances when they might be imposing their value system on a family unnecessarily.[30]

The hospital environment should be particularly sensitive to the needs of families who are disintegrated, in turmoil, experiencing serious external stress such as poverty, or who for some reason have not provided a healthy home environment for the child. Often the hospital environment is a welcome and relatively pleasant experience for the child who is unhappy at home. The parents may also be relieved to have the child removed from their responsibility at home, may be reluctant to be involved in hospital care, or may reject involvement. The health care team needs to plan for specific approaches during hospitalization that are directed toward identifying the real needs of the family, improving the child's physical and emotional health during the period of hospitalization, and providing for mobilization of a comprehensive health care team in the community that can begin to provide long-term intervention to assure optimal health for the child and family.[28,31]

### Emergency room care

It is estimated that approximately 86% of all hospitalizations of children under 5 years of age occur on an emergency basis. Emergency hospitalization for this age group intensifies the crisis and stress of hospitalization significantly. There is no opportunity for preparation of the child or the family for the experiences of hospitalization, they are thrown into a setting where the health care team is under the stress of the medical urgency of the child's problem, and their own anxiety level is likely to be extremely high.[37,51,52,56]

In spite of the high incidence of use of emergency room facilities by children of all age groups, very little attention has been directed to studying this experience and its effects on the health of children, and practically no attention has been given to the application of principles of child health care in emergency settings. Most health care workers in the emergency setting have little or no background preparation in working with children and families, and their approaches are seldom evaluated in terms of the developmental needs of children. Further, emergency room facilities are seldom, if ever, designed with the needs of parents and children taken into account. Little attention is given to adequate follow-through and long-term intervention, even though it is widely recognized that many children and families return to emergency rooms repeatedly with similar problems on each return or that they use the emergency room as a resource for some form of health supervision.[37,51,52]

Two studies describe the reactions of children, parents, and hospital health care workers during emergency care for children.[51,56] Children's reactions were often observed to be those that might be predicted, based on the child's developmental level and the nature of the trauma experienced. For example, preschool and middle-age children often expressed fear of body mutilation. Other fears expressed were fear of receiving an injection, fear of loss of support from parents, fear of losing control, and fear of pain. Children's questions were directed to clarifying the activities and procedures being conducted, concern about the immediate future, and as a diversionary tactic. Children asked for books, toys, food, water, or attention, apparently in an attempt to take their minds off the nature of the experience.

Parents' reactions in these two studies varied widely and reflected the wide range of circumstances that bring families to the emergency room for care. Many parents express concern, fear, guilt, and distress over the circumstances and are eager to comfort and quiet their child. In some instances the parents used the emergency room experience as a means of making the child feel guilty for what had happened, as a form of punishment, or as an opportunity to vent their anger toward someone not present who they identified as responsible for the child's emergency. Regression and withdrawal from the usual parenting role was observed in both groups of parents on occasion; the stress of the emergency exceeded their ability to cope on their own, much less provide parental support and comfort for their child. In some instances the parents were eager to have their child hospitalized in order to alleviate another external stress in the home.

The results of both of these studies confirm the lack of preparation of health care workers in caring for children and families in an emergency setting. Most of the health care workers had no concepts relevant to the preparation of children for a painful procedure or to communicating with children. Such procedures were simply administered, with no preparatory explanation or attempt to communicate with the child. There was no report of attempts made to provide counseling or guidance for the parents in relation to their parenting role in the emergency setting.

The need for further study of emergency care for children is sorely needed. Emergency care facilities need to be restructured and planned for integration of known principles of child health care, including improvement of emergency care itself and providing adequate follow-through care. Emergency rooms need to discard the blanket policy of asking all parents to remain in the waiting area while their child is treated. The psychologic care and attention to the parent and the child is probably as important as the actual physical care. Each parent-child relationship should be assessed, and the parents should be given support and guidance in providing a supportive parenting role for their child. If the parents seem unable or unwilling to remain with the child, their needs should be respected, and immediate attention turned to providing sound adult support for the child from the health care team. As soon as feasible, the adult's psychologic needs should be attended, and any need for long-term follow through planned as soon as possible.

Adequate facilities for parental counseling, including the provision of privacy, should be available. If the child's condition is grave, the health care staff needs to assist the family to identify and call friends and relatives who can offer support and assistance. Adequate facilities for food, refreshments, and bathrooms need to be available and identified for the family.

The child's need for play during emergency hospital experiences should be recognized, and materials and personnel prepared to provide for this experience. Books can provide an important source of diversion during the periods that waiting is required. Simple toys appropriate to each age group need to be available, particularly toys that are commonly used as sources of comfort and security. Most children arrive in an emergency setting without the security symbols that they might otherwise bring to a health care setting, and appropriate substitutes may be offered during this time of stress until their own objects can be made available. Blankets, dolls, and stuffed animals are recommended for this purpose. Drawing provides a very useful outlet for the child's fear and tension, as well as diversion. Often the child's drawing reveals fears that the child cannot express in words, such as fear of injections or fear of body mutilation. Puppets are often extremely useful in establishing communication and rapport with a child and provide another means through which the child can express fear and relieve tension. The emergency health care team who knows how to use puppets in relating to children can greatly enhance the effectiveness of their approaches to children and reduce the fear and anxiety that the emergency experience creates.[51,56]

## Ambulatory services in hospitals

Hospital ambulatory services have been established in recent years to meet the growing demand for health maintenance clinics, to decrease the need to hospitalize children, and to provide for continuity and coordination between hospital care and home care.[16,77,81] The hospital ambulatory clinic provides a setting where children can be initially evaluated for a serious health problem that exceeds the capability of the private physician, requiring the resources of the hospital diagnostic equipment and personnel. Using such a facility eliminates the need for an expensive and traumatic hospitalization. If the need for hospitalization becomes apparent, the clinic can serve as a setting for preparation, initial decision-making, planning, and orientation to the hospital setting. The ambulatory clinic provides an extremely valuable setting for children who have long-term illnesses requiring periodic hospitalizations. Sometimes the child can be served in the clinic rather than being rehospitalized, as for

periodic respiratory therapy for a child who has cystic fibrosis. The ambulatory clinic can also provide a setting for coordination and access among the various members of the health care team in the hospital and the community, and families. For example, a social worker and nutritionist may be available for regular consultations with parents who need their services and may participate in health team planning for comprehensive care.[1,5]

A hospital ambulatory service should include specific facilities for play, both for diversion and therapy. The waiting area can be used for this purpose and should include a variety of books and toys that appeal to each age group of children using the clinic. Specific play materials should be available for therapeutic use, such as puppets, hospital equipment, materials for drawing, and furnishings that encourage release of tension through large muscle activity.

Children who must experience repeated hospital admissions should be encouraged to maintain contact with the nursing staff in the hospital through the ambulatory clinic. Periodic visits should be planned as a part of the visits to the ambulatory clinic, and the child should be introduced to new nursing personnel and to children who are on the unit and should be encouraged to bring drawings and paintings that can be posted on the unit between periods of hospitalizations.[1,5]

## CRITERIA FOR HOSPITALIZATION

The decision to hospitalize a child has received careful attention in recent years as the physical and psychosocial risks of hospitalization have been recognized, as described previously in this chapter. When hospitalization is clearly required, these risks must be considered in terms of compensation during the hospitalization itself. When indications for hospitalization are less clear, they are weighed against the evidence for hospitalization and the ability of the family to care for the child at home. Thus it is helpful to consider carefully the criteria upon which a child should be hospitalized. While this decision is often a medical decision, all health care workers should be familiar with the criteria in order to contribute to gathering relevant information on which to base a decision, to facilitate optimal care, and to avoid delays in taking appropriate steps.

There are three classes of criteria for hospitalization of a child. These are (1) major emergencies, (2) potentially life-threatening or crippling illnesses, and (3) specific psychosocial indications for hospitalization.[59]

## Major emergencies

These are clear life-threatening circumstances such as shock, severe dehydration, coma, signs of major acute illness such as meningitis, respiratory distress, epiglottitis, renal failure, severe poisonings, life-threatening accidents, and surgical emergencies. The single criterion that applies universally is that the condition is life threatening.

## Potentially life-threatening or crippling illness

Criteria for these illnesses are less easily formulated, since accurate understanding of the extent of a problem may be difficult or impossible to delineate. Specific criteria for use by all members of the health care team should be developed to fit the preferences of the team members and the particular situation. The following guidelines are offered to assist in the development of more specific criteria for conditions commonly encountered in a given setting.

1. *Age and stage of development.* For infants there is a greater risk that physiologic imbalance will occur quickly and will threaten life. Hospitalization is necessary for such conditions as diarrhea, cellulitis, bleeding, respiratory infection (e.g., pneumonia), renal malfunction, or any suspicious condition that is not possible to fully describe without the specific resources of the hospital. An infant old enough to suffer separation anxiety (6 months or older) has enough of an advantage in maintaining physiologic balance that hospitalization might be delayed if the family can adequately care for the child at home. At this point the child's emotional response to hospitalization becomes a serious consideration, and hospitalization should be avoided if at all possible.

2. *Illness factors.* Illness that is not a major emergency, but which may become life threatening is difficult to differentiate from illness that

will not progress into a more serious condition. The guidelines developed for specific conditions may be somewhat arbitrary, and experience is needed in a particular setting to judge the adequacy of specified guidelines. The following are offered as examples:

*Burns:* The child who suffers (1) burns involving more than 10% to 15% of total body area (see Chapter 11), (2) burns involving the perineal area or hands, or (3) electrical burns should be hospitalized.

*Respiratory infections:* The child with an infection involving the respiratory tract that causes respiratory distress or potentially involves respiratory distress (e.g., diphtheria, pertussis), or who has complications such as hemoptysis, mastoiditis, anemia, or history of previous severe respiratory distress requires hospitalization.

*Head injury:* Children who suffer a head injury without apparent skull fracture and who are unconscious for longer than one minute, or who have persistent neurologic signs such as disorientation, irritability, decreased consciousness level, headaches, or who exhibit bleeding from any orifice of the head should be hospitalized.

*Febrile seizures:* If the seizure lasts for longer than five to ten minutes or if neurologic signs persist and consciousness level is decreased, the child should be hospitalized for the remainder of the febrile illness and for possible diagnostic investigation.

In addition, any child whose illness is managed at home and who does not begin to respond within two days of the onset of treatment should be considered for hospitalization.

3. *Diagnostic factors.* This criterion is particularly susceptible to misuse; in many cases a child's signs and symptoms are extremely elusive and, in a desire to fully delineate the nature of the problem, the child is hospitalized. This can be the preference of either the physician or the family, and while there are many instances that fully warrant such an approach, every effort should be made to avoid hospitalizing simply for diagnostic purposes. Diagnosis often can be accomplished through office and clinic facilities, but insurance policies held by many families do not provide for such diagnostic services.

Unless the family is suffering from undue financial strain, the child should not be hospitalized on insurance considerations alone.

Suspected illnesses that definitely warrant full diagnostic exploration within the hospital setting tend to meet specific guidelines. Such illnesses include those that are amenable to specific treatment if discovered early and if adequate treatment is begun promptly (such as pyelonephritis, thrombophlebitis, acute rheumatic fever, rheumatoid arthritis, osteomyelitis, lead poisoning, and failure to thrive). In addition, a condition may require that specific tests be done that can only be performed in the hospital. Hospitalization may be necessary because of special preparation for the tests, because observation of the recovery after the tests is necessary, or because a surgical procedure is required.

## Specific psychosocial indications

These indications arise primarily from a community's limitations in offering health care services during specific crisis situations. As resources of the community expand to help families with specific health care problems, the need for hospitalization decreases. The following guidelines should be used in developing criteria for specific conditions, and the community resources should be considered as alternatives to hospitalization as they are available.

### Parent factors

When a child has a health problem of any proportion and the criteria for home care cannot be met (see following section), hospitalization is required. Such problems include suspected or confirmed child abuse or neglect, severe economic deprivation, parental physical exhaustion, emotional incapacitation of one or both parents, or intellectually limited parents.

### Child factors

When a child has a problem that is not manageable at home or that arises from the home situation, hospitalization may be indicated. Emotional incapacitation of the child, emotional disturbance or crisis such as a suicide attempt, or socially dangerous or unduly disruptive behavior may indicate hospitalization until the crisis passes, therapy has been instituted, or some alternative plan to returning to the home can be implemented.

### Illness factors

There are three conditions that commonly lead to hospitalization even though none of the other criteria are met. These include:

*Initial diagnosis of an illness requiring a complex treatment regimen.* Even though the treatment is conducted at home throughout the remainder of the illness or the child's life, initial teaching and supervision may require the full concentration of the health care team in the hospital setting. For example, juvenile onset diabetes mellitus requires a careful, deliberate organized child and family-centered program of teaching and support in learning to carry out the administration of insulin and to balance all other aspects of life. Some communities have developed centers for provision of such teaching and guidance programs as alternatives to hospitalization. Such a program offers the advantage of more closely resembling the home setting and providing daily activities that simulate those experienced in everyday living. In addition, specialized health care workers are available who center upon the specific health problem of the individual.

*Initial diagnosis of a fatal illness.* Such a diagnosis may require hospitalization for psychosocial reasons alone. The family and the child may require the extra support and assistance found within the hospital as they work through the initial impact of the diagnosis (see Chapter 17).

*Terminal care of the dying child.* Hospitalization may be required if the family needs the support of the hospital health care team during this phase of illness, or if they prefer that the child not die at home. Further, while it is usually possible to care for the dying child in the home, the stress of physical care added to the burden of the emotional situation is more than some families can bear.

## CRITERIA FOR HOME CARE

When criteria for hospitalization are not clearly met, the criteria for home care should be fully explored by the health care worker and the family.

## Personal resources of the parents

For a child to remain in the home during an illness, there must be an adult present in the home who can give the physical and emotional care required. Further, there should be resources for obtaining relief from the physical burden of care, so that each adult involved in care has the opportunity for sleep and rest and for some diversion, particularly if the illness is prolonged. Adults caring for the child should have the capacity to understand the nature of the illness and the care and treatment regimen needed. They should demonstrate the needed skill in administering required treatment.[23,73]

## Physical environment of the home

The home should be reasonably conducive to the physical requirements of the child, including facilities for washing, elimination, food preparation, and reasonable diversion for the child; and it should be reasonably convenient for those who care for the child and maintain the household. There should be an indication that physical safety from injury or infection can be maintained throughout the illness or treatment period. For example, if humidification must be added to the room with an electrical device, the electrical facilities of the home should be safe, and there should be reasonable assurance of the family's capacity to use such a device safely.

## Social environment of the home

The presence of siblings or other relatives in the home may constitute an advantage or a disadvantage in home care of an ill child. If there are several young siblings who require a great deal of attention and care, the added burden of a sick child may not be reasonable to manage. On the other hand, if the other children can participate in certain aspects of the child's care, if they understand the child's needs for rest, treatment, or extra attention, and if there is no threat to the health of the siblings, they may contribute to the total care of the child. Adult relatives in the home may provide needed help in the physical and emotional burdens of caring for the ill child, or they may present a barrier to providing adequate care.

The interpersonal atmosphere should be reasonably harmonious and congruent with the goals of healthy living. A family that is ordinarily able to maintain its basic form and to cope with problems of everyday living or occasional extraordinary stress is ideally suited to caring for the ill child at home. Other families experience periodic stages of disorganization, have a borderline ability to cope with extraordinary stress, or seem to create stress among the members. Such families may respond favorably to the stress of a child's illness and gather together all of their positive resources to center on the needs of the child, or the illness may provide the stimulus that breaks the ties that have tenuously held the family unit together. When factors such as these are difficult to ascertain, a judgment must be made, together with the family, regarding whether to try to care for the child at home or turn to hospitalization from the outset. It must be acknowledged that hospitalization of the child may produce stress of a different kind, and the family must decide with which kind of stress they can most effectively cope.

## Supportive community resources

If the child's home meets the above requirements and any special health care needs can be met through resources in the community, home care is desirable. Special nursing services, nutrition teaching and consultation, and various forms of therapy and treatment may be available either through an out-patient clinic or in the home.[16]

Nursing services in the community are of vital importance in assuring the success of the family in caring for a child at home during a prolonged illness. The family often needs care and compassion from a qualified nurse in order to sustain the physical and emotional stress involved. Their efforts in providing continuing care need to be encouraged and reinforced, and attention must given to helping them work out suitable approaches that reduce the physical and emotional strain while assuring adequate care for the child. The nurse may give guidance and counseling in the family's arrangements for meeting the developmental needs of the child who is ill and in helping them to maintain healthy interpersonal and discipline relationships. The nurse must assess the needs of sib-

**659**

lings in the home and assist the family in achieving an adequate balance between the demands of the child who is ill and the demands of the siblings. Attention is particularly given to prevention of complications of the child's physical illness and complications of a social and emotional nature arising from the stress of the child's illness.[81]

## NURSING ASSESSMENT AND MANAGEMENT

Regardless of the setting in which care is given, the nurse uses the tools of the nursing assessment as a basis for formulating and implementing relevant nursing care. The nurse who cares for a child who is acutely ill in the hospital setting may need specific knowledge and skill related to the particular illness, but the approach and the tools of the nursing assessment remain the same. As experience, knowledge, and skill increase, the nurse becomes increasingly reliable in making sound, accurate observations and judgments and in giving effective care to the child. In this text we are concentrating on the development of a nursing approach to the attainment of the basic goals of health care of the child; specific knowledge relating to the illness and condition of a particular child will be developed through study of recent nursing and medical literature and through experience with children. The following sections present a discussion of the development of each competency area when a child suffers a major interruption in optimal health status.

## Competency development through illness experiences

Severe acute illness, long-term illness, and handicapping conditions exert a significant effect on competency development. In assessing the child and environment and in implementing relevant nursing care, each of the competencies is considered. The child may suffer a severe effect on previously mastered abilities, may be affected in one competency but not in others, or may be able to make great gains in development through the illness experience. Each child will have particular, unique strengths and other unique areas of vulnerability. Thus one child may suffer significant effects in areas of physical competency, while another with the same condition may handle the physical effects of the illness adequately but suffer severe effects in relation to social competency. Priorities of nursing care are, to a large extent, determined by the child's response to the experience.

There are few problems that affect only one area of competency; the condition or problem is identified in relation to the area that is primarily affected, and other areas of secondary effect are consequently identified by the nature of the child's unique response to the problem. For example, a child who is blind from the early months of life may be thought of as having a primary physical effect of blindness, in that the sensory nervous system that involves sight is damaged and the physical ability to see is not present. Each of the other competencies will be affected to some degree, but one blind child may be severely affected in learning and thought capacity, while another is seriously limited in social competency. Another blind child may be identified whose area of secondary problems is the development of adequate selfesteem.

### Physical competency

One aspect of the initial nursing assessment of the child during an illness episode (hospitalization, special care clinic, home) is to determine the level of physical competency that the child demonstrated prior to the onset of the present problem. If a professional team member was familiar with the child before the illness, firsthand knowledge of the prior circumstances is helpful for all health care team members involved. If this is not possible, the nursing and/ or medical history can begin to define these parameters. This information is then assessed in the context of what the child could reasonably be expected to achieve within the limitations of age, biologic endowments, and total environment. Physical development may have been appropriate or may have lagged behind what was reasonably expected. The expected influence of the current problem is then estimated, and the child's own strengths and weaknesses are evaluated to determine what can reasonably be expected during the illness experience. For example, a 3-year-old child may be estimated to have achieved most physical competencies appropriate for this age prior to a serious episode of meningitis. Many of the previously acquired tasks are lost during the acute phase of the illness, and ongoing reassessment indicates that the child may require several weeks to fully regain his former level of ability in bladder and bowel control, feeding skills, speech capacity, and fine motor control. Nursing problems are identified, and plans of management are implemented that will facilitate the restoration of former physical competencies and the acquisition of new abilities.

Another example might be a particular interruption of normal functioning of one or more of the child's physiologic systems. The respiratory system, for example, might be identified as functioning at a compromised level of efficiency during the acute phase of pneumonia, with impairment of oxygen transport to the tissues and impaired fluid and electrolyte balance. The related nursing problems identified include labored breathing, exhaustion, elevated body temperature, irritability, and anorexia. Nursing is directed toward intervention of each of these problems and toward support and restoration of normal homeostatic function.

Each of the physiologic systems is evaluated, with particular attention to the system or systems involved in the current illness. The ability to identify problems related to specific physiologic function or pathology depends upon thorough knowledge of both normal physiologic function of each of the systems at each period of life and the pathophysiology related to the illness or chronic condition.

Hospitalization often interrupts the progression of normal physical mastery and development during the early childhood years. Parents may need support and help in recognizing this regression as a necessary reaction to the stress of illness or hospitalization, and in finding ways to facilitate restoration of previously acquired skills. Equipped with an adequate understanding of the developmental capacities of the individual child, the nurse may use play, fantasy, stories, counseling, and guidance to help a child cope with stresses and begin to work out the inner feelings that lead to the need for physical or behavioral regression.

### Learning and thought competency

Assessment of the child's past and present capacity in learning and thinking may be more difficult than assessing physical competency. The young child's family may not be able to describe learning-related behaviors accurately, and the child's condition may interfere with efforts to evaluate the present capacity. Except in a condition of unconsciousness or coma or in the face of severe intellectual handicap, the child who is ill is experiencing the same kinds of learning that are described for the child who is healthy. Because of the stresses of the situation, the large proportion of new experiences, and the tendency to regress, the child may return to some of the earlier and more comfortable learning and thinking patterns. The illness and/or hospital situation is often a very discouraging learning environment; there is little positive reinforcement for adequate behavior, and negative or disagreeable events seem to predominate. The child has lost, at least temporarily, the many environmental factors that were associated with learning, such as associations with friends, play, mobility in and out of the school or preschool setting, and associations with the family that involve learning, thinking, problem-solving, or other forms of mental excursion.

Understanding and insight into the child's own perception of the illness and hospital situation can be significant additions to the nursing assessment. Children can be observed through play, art, writing, and interactions or verbal exchanges with other children or adults to expose their own interpretations and perceptions of the hospital or illness experience. Inaccuracies in thinking can thus be clarified, and nursing care can be planned on the basis of the existing level of understanding.*

Changes in behavior that occur over the period of illness represent some form of learning. If the behavior does not persist, the learning was relatively transient; on the other hand, a behavior may be learned that persists for months or years following the illness experience. For example, children may become increasingly manipulative of their environment in

*References 7, 12, 33, 47, 69.

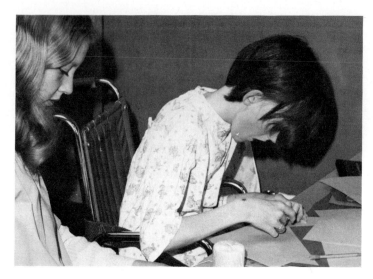

**Fig. 16-6.** Therapeutic play activities appropriate for the stage of development of the child provide understanding and insight into the child's own perceptions.

order to obtain needed attention. If the manipulation is rewarded by giving attention only in response to a manipulative effort, they may begin to use this approach as the most effective means of obtaining a desired end. If, on the other hand, they are not given the needed attention when manipulative efforts are made but are given significant attention at times when they are not attempting specific manipulation, they learn more acceptable means of reaching a goal and to forsake a socially undesirable behavior.

Academic learning may need to be pursued throughout an extended illness and/or hospitalization. This service is available through most school districts in the United States or through some cooperative effort by the schools and the health care institutions. Such programs can provide significant contributions to the total health care plan, because they promote the child's competency development in all areas.

### Social competency

Illness and hospitalization significantly interfere with social competency development at all ages of childhood. The hazard of separation anxiety, which is greatest between the ages of 6 months and 4 years, is one of several social disruptions that occur during illness. Disruption of associations with peers may be as traumatic for

the adolescent as the separation from mother is for the young child.

Nursing assessment of the previous social needs and capacities of children helps to identify the probable effect of the experience for the individual child. Their ability to draw upon previous social relationships to cope with the stress of illness is an indication of both past and present capacities. All children who have a severe illness or handicapping condition need to have and maintain relationships with significant adult members of the family. Children's expressions of dependency may predominate during the acute phase of an illness, and these should be predominantly directed toward those family members with whom they have formed attachments in the past. The inability to draw upon this attachment relationship signals a significant problem for the child.

Except during the most severe and acute phases of an illness, older children and adolescents should be observed to reestablish former patterns of relationships with peers, both newly acquired friends in the hospital and those friends with whom they had a relationship in the past. Such relationships can be important therapeutic tools for young people, and they should be encouraged and facilitated throughout the illness experience. As the older children progress from the most severe stages of their illness to a recuperative or restorative stage, they should progress away from dependency and intensified relationships with significant adults to the more usual pattern of peer group associations.

### Inner competency

As during periods of relative health and normal development, assessment of inner competency is indirect and often is derived from observations related to each of the other competencies. A child who does not perform physically appropriate skills, who demonstrates problems in learning and thought, or who is not able to establish expected social ties may be suffering from a primary problem in the area of inner competency. Illness is debilitating to the self; it degrades, demoralizes, and demeans. Even very young children are able to sense the loss of self-worth that can accompany severe illness. Attitudes of others around them toward their condition are often perceived by children as being directly applicable to them personally. For example, the child who suffers a distortion of the body through severe burns may elicit shock, disbelief, disdain, or pity from others. These reactions are perceived (perhaps accurately) by the child as being applicable to the self, to the person he or she is, and not just to the physical body which has been damaged.

The child's perceptions of the self through the illness experience may be observed through the skillful use of play, imitation, fantasy, or counseling. Even though accurate assessment of the child's inner experience may not be possible, these tools can be helpful in facilitating the child's use of his or her own resources for coping and adjusting to stress.[7,12,47,80]

## Nursing diagnoses

During the course of a serious illness experience, there are many nursing diagnoses made on the basis of the data collected in the nursing assessment. This process is used to continually adapt nursing care to the needs of the child and the family. We have previously cited a few examples of specific problems that might be identified relating to each competency area; we will now consider specific nursing problems which might be commonly identified during childhood illness.

Major areas of concern that involve specific nursing diagnoses are presented here. The reader is referred to the Appendix, pp. 884 to 895, Minnesota Nursing Problems Classification (MNPC), for review of specific labels that might be used in describing the specific nursing diagnosis that might be used for a particular child. As has been discussed in earlier chapters, a classification system such as the one presented here is useful in organizing data and evaluating the outcome of specific nursing intervention. Diagnostic labels that might be used in association with each of the general areas of concern are discussed in this chapter to assist the nurse in using this system in practice. Further discussion of specific diagnostic labels is found in the following chapters of this unit.

### Pain

The nursing diagnosis of pain in children is based upon subjective, indirect evidence. McCaffery[40,42] has identified six categories of response that can be observed in determining the presence of pain in children. These are:

1. Physiologic manifestation
2. Verbal statements
3. Vocalizations
4. Facial expressions
5. Body movements
6. Response to the surrounding environment

Often the most predominant and most reliable sign that a child is experiencing pain when the source of pain is not apparent to the nurse is irritability and a lowered frustration tolerance. Because children lack a background of experience with prolonged, chronic, or throbbing pain, they have no language with which to express their perception of pain. When such experiences of pain are suspected, the nurse can assist the child in describing the feelings experienced. A cardinal rule to remember in dealing with pain is that the child is the authority with regard to the experience of pain. Regardless of the source of the pain or adult interpretations of how the child "should" respond, the child's own experience is real and needs to be respected as such.[27,42,48]

Nursing intervention is directed toward de-

**663**

creasing or controlling the degree of pain that is anticipated and experienced by the child and toward decreasing the feelings of fear, anxiety, punishment, or abandonment that the child associates with the painful event. The approaches used in accomplishing these goals vary according to the child, the environment, and the nurse. People in the environment, particularly parents, are often in need of nursing intervention associated with a child's pain, because observing even a brief period of suffering in a child is an extremely difficult experience. Parents or other significant adults may be important participants in intervention, since their ability to comfort the child is usually greater than the professional worker's. Such participation is often therapeutic for the parent also. When the child in pain expresses a need for dependency, the adults who are significant need to be available and to understand this particular manifestation of pain.

The painful experience might be alleviated by a variety of physical interventions using the principles of heat and cold, elevation, movement or immobilization, and touch or massage. When a predictably painful episode is anticipated, the pain can be minimized by restraining the child appropriately, administering the painful procedure rapidly and efficiently, and giving appropriate emotional support throughout. When the pain is of longer duration or when prediction of pain is not possible, other means of decreasing both the anticipation and experience of pain, such as play, must be implemented.[40,41,42]

The nurse's relationship with the child and family provides the basis for effective pain relief for children. Pain often is augmented in a vicious cycle of the pain sensation, anxiety, and fear. This cycle leads to tension, and tension causes the pain to worsen. The relationship of caring and compassion provides a means of decreasing the fear and anxiety and a source of confidence that helps to alleviate anxiety and tension. In devoting time and attention to work with the child and family to achieve physical measures that help to relieve pain, the nurse builds a relationship that in itself is therapeutic.[42]

Distraction is a valuable means of alleviating

pain for children. Reading a book, listening to music, watching television, and playing games offer temporary distraction that diverts attention from the pain itself and decreases awareness of pain. Rhythmic breathing and rhythmic patting are useful forms of distraction when the child is experiencing a more acute, short-term type of pain, such as following a painful injection or during a painful procedure. The child can be taught to deep breathe in a rhythmic fashion or to imitate the rhythmic sound of a train by patting in order to divert attention from the source of the pain and to promote relaxation.[42]

Continuous stimulation of a painful area provides pain relief by stimulating large afferent fibers, thus exerting an inhibitory action on the central nervous system to reception of the pain stimuli. Such stimulation also provides distraction and comfort and promotes relaxation. Rubbing the painful area or other areas of the body or rhythmic patting are useful in this regard.

A nursing problem listed in the MNPC for nursing problems is "Preparation for Painful Procedures," Classification no. 351.6 (see Appendix). The objectives for the child when this diagnosis is made include desensitization toward the painful experience, learning about the pain experience, and knowing what pain relief measures will be taken. Desensitization to the pain experience occurs as a result of planned introduction of components of the experience that will involve pain on a gradual basis. A child who is to undergo a diagnostic procedure that will involve venipuncture (pain) is gradually introduced to the equipment that will be used, the people who will be present, and the means of being transported to the diagnostic area—all dimensions of the experience that will not produce pain but that could produce fear and anxiety if the child does not know from previous experience that these objects and events will not produce pain. Shortly before the experience itself, the child is informed of the actual painful event and is given honest and accurate information regarding what will happen, in detail and terminology appropriate for the stage of development. The child is reassured about what will not happen to prevent anxiety and fear of fantasized outcomes, such as loss of body parts or mutilation. The nurse practices with the child the techniques that will be used during and after the pain experience to reduce the pain itself, such as rhythmic breathing, patting, or singing a song. Specific measures to promote relaxation may be indicated for use during the procedure. The nurse practices these techniques with the child and gives positive feedback when relaxation of certain areas of the body is achieved. For example, the nurse instructs the child to tense his or her entire body for a few seconds, then let go. Subsequently, the child is instructed to relax completely the feet, then the lower portion of the leg, the thighs, and so forth. As the nurse gives these instructions in a slow, rhythmic tone of voice, the area of the body is palpated gently to determine achievement of relaxation, and positive feedback is given to let the child know that the goals of the relaxation exercise are being met.[42]

### Separation anxiety

Although the period of overwhelming separation anxiety occurs between the ages of 6 months and 4 years, older children undergoing the stress of hospitalization or illness can experience significant levels of separation anxiety and fear. The developmental level of the child, previous experiences with separation, the extent of previous social contacts outside of the family, preparation for the event, and the family's attitudes toward the separation are particularly important factors influencing the amount and kind of anxiety that the child feels. Before the age of 4 years and after attachment to mother occurs, young children are particularly vulnerable to anxiety and fears arising from separation from family members. Three stages have been identified in the separation process. The first stage involves *protest*, when children are restless, cry a great deal, and desperately attend all signals in the environment that suggest the arrival of family members or mother. The second stage involves *despair*, when children begin to ignore things and events in the environment, become apathetic, and rarely cry. They let things happen to them without resistance and do not participate actively. This stage is often mistaken as a positive sign of adjustment. When the final *denial* stage of separation anxiety be-

gins, children begin to show an interest in their surroundings and begin to enter into the activities around them with some degree of "adjustment." They may accept a parent's infrequent visit with some distress at the beginning of this stage, but eventually they allow the parent's departure without complaint. Close examination of the child-parent relationship often reveals impaired interactions, with subsequent difficulty in establishing a close relationship later in life as the period of separation and interruption of the parent-child relationship persists.[13,44,70,78]

Substitute mothering of children who are suffering the signs of separation anxiety cannot adequately compensate for the absence of a significant adult once children have established a strong attachment to their mother and other adults. Children may be supported and helped through their experience of inner suffering, and the adults of the family can be assisted with their own feelings and with reaching an understanding of the child's experience. Rather than stay away from the child because of the discomfort associated with leaving, they should understand that the child's expressions of grief help him or her to learn to cope adequately rather than to suppress frustration and inward feelings. The nurse can then offer the child some support in bearing the separation and can help the parents minimize separation during the stages when other sources of comfort are minimal. The older child can understand and talk about inner feelings, anticipate return, and can turn to games, adults, other children, books, television, or other activities. These activities help the child to develop more mature coping patterns.

The MNPC lists this problem as "enforced separation of child from parents or significant others," classification no. 351.4 (see Appendix).

When separation from parents must be repeated or prolonged, the hazards of the situation must be acknowledged. The complexities of the child's needs for human relationships and attachment are not well enough understood to definitively describe the nursing approach that will most reliably avoid the serious hazards of separation. Several recommendations for nursing intervention have been proposed by Wear[78] based on analysis of theories that deal with this phenomenon. The recommendations include:

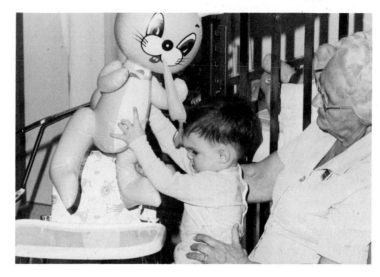

**Fig. 16-7.** A substitute "grandmother" is available to help the young child when separation from mother is necessary.

1. Provide continuous, individualized nursing care for the child by a limited number of individuals. These nurses should become familiar to the child and spend sufficient time with the child to build a relationship of confidence and a degree of attachment.

2. Support the child in coping with feelings and expressing these feelings. The child who has acquired receptive language abilities may find some comfort in hearing the nurse talk about the fears and anxieties, and if expressive language has developed, the child may be assisted in expressing these feelings. Play approaches, described below, are valuable in providing a nonverbal means of expressing feelings.

3. Nurture a sense of competence in the child. Provide positive reinforcement for positive coping skills and for the child's ability to do things independently.

4. Provide familiar clothing, food, toys, and rituals that help to decrease the sense of unfamiliarity with the environment.

5. Provide sights and sounds of the parents during their absence. The child can often maintain telephone contact with parents during periods of separation. Family members can provide photographs of themselves for the child, or instant-developed photographs may be taken of the child and parents together in the hospital setting and posted on the wall. Family members can be asked to tape record messages to the child that can be left with the child during periods of separation. If the child is accustomed to having a parent read a story at bedtime and he or she must be absent at this period of the day, the parent might be asked to read a favorite story to the child and tape record the story, capturing the parent's voice and the child's reactions and responses. This can then be played to the child at bedtime while a familiar nurse holds and rocks the child or otherwise provides companionship and comfort.[78] While these approaches have been proposed based on a sound analysis of theory, their usefulness in clinical practice needs to be investigated, and the practices refined for different developmental stages of development.

In managing the problem of separation anxiety, the factors that determine the child's reaction are important in determining the intervention that is provided. For example, if the child's attachment is very strongly formed to a single adult, this rather exclusive adult-child relationship should be guarded very carefully; the trauma of interruption added to the trauma of illness is rarely justifiable. Long-term goals with the family might be to help them gradually extend the child's relationships with other people,

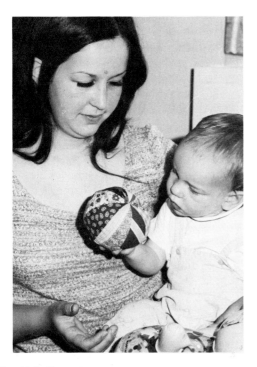

**Fig. 16-8.** When the child's attachment is very strongly formed with a single adult, this relationship should be guarded during the time of hospitalization.

but this kind of intervention is not possible or desirable under the stress of hospitalization and illness.

Even in the face of loud protest from children toward approaches made by adults in the strange environment of the hospital, infants or young children need the assurance that their needs are being met consistently by increasingly familiar individuals, and that this is one feature that they can count on.[60,78] By working at a "safe" distance, as defined by the child, a strange adult can be observed and watched by the child, and the child can assess whether or not this adult is acceptable. If children can see the adult interacting with other children, they begin to see what the adult might be like for them and will slowly accept more direct, personal approaches. In time, young children who have developed a sense of comfort related to a new adult will make the initial indication that they are ready for interaction and attention through some means of approach to the adult.

Play can be an important means of helping

children with separation anxiety. Games that involve the repeated appearance and disappearance of people and objects help the infant and toddler to experience active mastery of appearance and disappearance, thus relieving feelings of total helplessness in the situation. "Peek-a-boo," hide 'n seek, and variations of these simple games can be initiated by young children, parents, or another familiar adult to provide some means of mutual acknowledgement of the phenomenon. During early childhood and the school-age years, children can act out the situation with dolls, drawings, drama, or storybooks. In so doing they familiarize themselves with certain aspects of the situation, act out some of the feelings with which they associate, and experience some degree of active mastery of a situation that otherwise leaves them feeling helpless and distressed.[30,47]

### Control of body temperature

A problem frequently encountered in hospital or home care of a child with long-term illness is that of fever. The MNPC includes this nursing problem in major problem classification no. 31, nursing problems related to long-term illness or physical problems. Under each of the specific problems in this category, problem no. .3 provides for the identification of maintenance of body temperature (see Appendix, p. 888). Nursing management of fever as an acute, short-term problem is discussed in detail in Chapter 11. Each of the measures identified in that previous section is used in the nursing management of fever related to long-term problems. Intervention for fever includes specific intervention related to the predominant long-term problem and is integrated into the plan for care.

Special equipment may be available for management of fever in the hospital setting, such as cold water mattresses that provide for continuous circulation of cold water in a plastic mattress, which facilitates loss of body heat through conduction. Special equipment for use with a young infant who suffers from the inability to maintain a sufficient body temperature, such as radiant heat warmers, is discussed in Chapter 8.

When a child with a long-term illness suffers a fever, nursing and medical management must

**667**

be planned carefully to assure maximum intervention. When pharmacologic agents are used to reduce body temperature, the child needs to be observed carefully for various forms of drug incompatability. The antipyretic agent may interact adversely with another drug the child is taking, and each drug should be studied carefully in advance to reduce the chances of this occurring. In addition the antipyretic drug may interact with the child's system, causing an allergic reaction or other type of adverse reaction that compounds the problems the child is experiencing. For example, aspirin, which tends to produce gastrointestinal bleeding in normal children, may cause a serious bleeding problem for a child whose illness causes a tendency to bleed, as occurs in the child with leukemia.[9]

### Fluid and electrolyte disturbances

Monitoring, maintenance, and correction of fluid and electrolyte balance is a constant and unique concern for children. The physiology of fluids and electrolytes for children differs from that of adults, and children are more susceptible to severe, rapidly progressing states of imbalance. The MNPC includes the problem, "Marked disturbance of fluid and electrolytes," classification no. 350.2, which is used for children who have already suffered an imbalance in connection with vomiting, diarrhea, as a result of surgical procedures, or inadequate intake of fluids and electrolytes. Maintenance of fluids and electrolytes to prevent an imbalance is included in the physical maintenance problem for nursing problems related to long-term illness, classification no. 31 (see Appendix, p. 888).

Fig. 16-9 presents a diagrammatic representation of the shifts that occur in the body fluid compartments in hypertonic, isotonic, and hypotonic dehydration states. Body fluids are lost primarily through the urine, skin, and lungs, with a small proportion lost through the gastrointestinal tract. The first fluid compartment to lose fluids and solutes is the plasma, since it is this fluid that provides for exchange of solutes and transfer of water. When changes occur in the plasma fluid volume, the interstitial fluid volume reacts to maintain electroneutrality and balanced tonicity. Changes that occur in the in-

terstitial fluid volume mediate the fluid volume of the cells, which in turn responds to maintain electroneutrality and tonicity. When the net loss of water parallels the net loss of solutes, there is an isotonic body fluid dehydration, resulting in a simple decrease in both the extracellular and cellular fluid volumes. This is the most common form of dehydration in children and requires that fluids and solutes be replaced rapidly in a proportion equivalent to that of normal body fluids. (See discussion of fluids and electrolytes during infancy in Chapter 8.)

When the net loss of water is greater than the net loss of solutes, hypertonic extracellular fluid develops as a result of the high proportion of water lost from this compartment. The cellular water shifts from the cellular space to the extracellular space to achieve electroneutrality and equivalent tonicity, resulting in hypertonic dehydration with relatively decreased cellular fluid volume and relatively increased extracellular fluid volume. When the net loss of solutes is greater than the net loss of water, hypotonic extracellular fluid results, and there is an extracellular to cellular shift in fluid that results in hypotonic dehydration (see Fig. 16-9). These conditions occur less frequently than isotonic dehydration, but they present difficult problems in restoring a fluid and electrolyte balance. The young child has a particular risk for developing disorders of hydrogen ion metabolism, for the relatively immature compensating mechanisms of the system cannot keep up with the relatively rapid changes in the body fluid compartments. Immediate therapeutic correction is essential, and early recognition of signs of each form of dehydration can greatly enhance the therapeutic efforts and support of the child's own ability to compensate. Correction is achieved gradually over a period of about 24 hours, in order to decrease the risk of overhydration and allow the child's own compensatory mechanisms to achieve a balance.*

Table 16-1 presents a summary of the clinical signs that occur in children who have isotonic, hypertonic, and hypotonic dehydration. The clinical features that distinguish between hypotonic and hypertonic dehydration are related to

---

*References 20, 21, 36, 54, 55, 79.

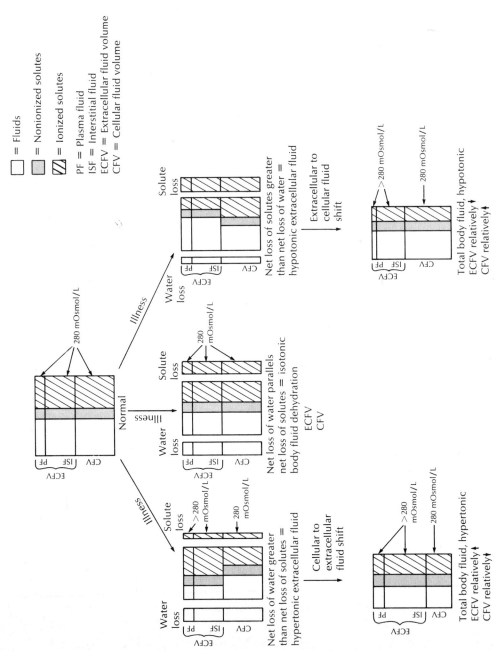

**Fig. 16-9.** Body fluid compartment changes occurring in hypertonic, isotonic, and hypotonic states. (Adapted from Hughes, J. G., editor: Synopsis of pediatrics, ed. 4, St. Louis, 1975, The C. V. Mosby Co., p. 143.)

**Table 16-1.** Signs of isotonic, hypertonic, and hypotonic dehydration*

| Area of assessment | Signs of dehydration | | |
|---|---|---|---|
| | **Isotonic** | **Hypertonic** | **Hypotonic** |
| Loss of body weight | Mild dehydration—up to 5% loss of body weight<br>Moderate dehydration—5% to 10% loss of body weight<br>Severe dehydration—over 10% loss of body weight | | |
| Behavior | Irritable and lethargic | Irritable when disturbed; lethargic | Lethargic to delirious; coma |
| Skin turgor | Decreased elasticity | Good turgor; foam rubber feel | Very poor turgor; clammy |
| Mucous membranes | Dry | Parched | Clammy |
| Eyeballs and fontanel | Sunken and soft | Sunken | Sunken and soft |
| Tearing and salivation | Absent or decreased | Absent or decreased | Absent or decreased |
| Thirst | Present | Marked | Present |
| Urine | Decreased output; SG elevated | Normal to decreased output; SG elevated or decreased | Decreased output; SG elevated |
| Body temperature | Subnormal to elevated | Elevated | Subnormal |
| Respiration | Rapid | Rapid | Rapid |
| Blood pressure | Normal to low | Normal to low | Very low |
| Pulse | Rapid | Rapid | Rapid |
| Blood chemistry | BUN increased<br>Na decreased<br>K normal or increased<br>Cl decreased<br>pH usually decreased | BUN increased<br>Na increased<br>K decreased<br>Cl low during correction<br>Ca decreased | BUN increased<br>Na decreased<br>K varies or increased<br>Cl decreased |

*Information from references 20, 21, 36.

**Table 16-2.** Solute composition and concentration of hydrating solutions*

| Solution | mEq/L | | | | | | | CHO g/L | ION mOsm/L† | CHO mOsm/L† | Total mOsm/L† |
|---|---|---|---|---|---|---|---|---|---|---|---|
| | **Na** | **K** | **Mg** | **Ca** | **HCO₃** | **Cl** | **HPO₄** | | | | |
| Sodium bicarbonate and chloride in 5% (or 2.5%) dextrose‡ | 75 | — | — | — | 50 | 25 | — | 50 | 150 | 278 (139) | 428 (289) |
| 0.33% NaCl (one-third physiologic strength) in 5% dextrose | 50 | — | — | — | — | 50 | — | 50 | 100 | 278 | 378 |
| 0.45% NaCl (one-half physiologic strength) in 5% dextrose | 77 | — | — | — | — | 77 | — | 50 | 154 | 278 | 432 |
| Half-strength lactated Ringer's solution in 5% dextrose | 65 | 2 | — | 1.5 | 14§ | 54.5 | — | 50 | 137 | 278 | 414 |

*From Etteldorf, J. N., and Sweeney, M. J.: Common fluid and electrolyte problems in pediatrics. In Hughes, J. G., editor: Synopsis of pediatrics, ed. 4, St. Louis, 1975, The C. V. Mosby Co., p. 152.
†Calculated.
‡Useful in metabolic acidosis.
§Lactate ion is replaced by metabolically generated HCO₃ ions in the body.

*Formula:* 7.5% sodium bicarbonate solution        56 ml
      Physiologic sodium chloride solution—2.5% or 5% dextrose    162 ml
      Dextrose (2.5% or 5%) in water    782 ml
                       1,000 ml

Sodium bicarbonate solution not to be heat sterilized.

**Table 16-3.** Solute composition and concentration of solutions for replacement and maintenance*†

| Solution | mEq/L | | | | | | | CHO g/L | ION mOsm/L§ | CHO mOsm/L§ | Total mOsm/L§ |
|---|---|---|---|---|---|---|---|---|---|---|---|
| | Na | K | Mg | Ca | HCO³‡ | Cl | HPO₄ | | | | |
| Butler-Talbot solution | 40 | 35 | — | — | 20 | 40 | 15 | 50 | 142.5 | 278 | 420.5 |
| Butler (modified) solution | 25 | 20 | 3 | — | 23 | 22 | 3 | 50 | 93 | 278 | 371 |
| Lactate-Ringer's solution (Hartmann's solution) | 130 | 4 | — | 3 | 28 | 109 | — | — | 272.5 | — | 272.5 |
| Half-strength lactate-Ringer's solution (Hartmann's solution) with 5% dextrose plus 30 mEq/L KCl | 65 | 32 | — | 1.5 | 14 | 84.5 | — | 50 | 196 | 278 | 474 |
| 5% dextrose in distilled water | — | — | — | — | — | — | — | 50 | — | 278 | 278 |
| 10% dextrose in distilled water | — | — | — | — | — | — | — | 100 | — | 556 | 556 |
| M/6 sodium r-lactate | 167 | — | — | — | 167 | — | — | — | 334 | — | 334 |
| 7.5% NaHCO₃ | 889 | — | — | — | 889 | — | — | — | 1,778 | — | 1,778 |

*From Etteldorf, J. N., and Sweeney, M. J.: Common fluid and electrolyte problems in pediatrics. In Hughes, J. G., editor: Synopsis of Pediatrics, ed. 4, St. Louis, 1975, The C. V. Mosby Co., p. 153.
†These solutions, or those of approximate solute concentration, are available commercially, or they may be prepared by dilution of available isotonic or near-isotonic solutions with 5% dextrose in water.
‡Except for the 7.5% NaHCO₃ solution, none of the solutions actually contains HCO₃ ion. Lactate ion is contained in most of the solutions and is replaced by metabolically generated HCO₃ ions in the body.
§Calculated.

**Table 16-4.** Initial hydrating solutions for use in treatment of dehydration and acid-base imbalance*†

| Mild to moderate dehydration | Severe dehydration | Hypertonic dehydration |
|---|---|---|
| **Dehydration with metabolic acidosis** | | |
| 1. Sodium bicarbonate and chloride in 2.5% or 5% dextrose | Sodium bicarbonate and chloride in 2.5% or 5% dextrose | Sodium bicarbonate and chloride in 2.5% or 5% dextrose |
| 2. 0.33% sodium chloride in 5% dextrose‡ | 0.33% sodium chloride in 5% dextrose‡ | 0.45% sodium chloride in 5% dextrose |
| 3. Half-strength lactated Ringer's solution in 5% dextrose | Half-strength lactated Ringer's solution in 5% dextrose | Half-strength lactated Ringer's solution in 5% dextrose |
| 4. 0.45% sodium chloride in 5% dextrose | 0.45% sodium chloride in 5% dextrose | 0.45% sodium chloride in 5% dextrose |
| **Dehydration with metabolic alkalosis** | | |
| 5. 0.33% sodium chloride in 5% dextrose | | |
| 6. 0.45% sodium chloride in 5% dextrose | 0.45% sodium chloride in 5% dextrose | 0.45% sodium chloride in 5% dextrose |

*From Etteldorf, J. N., and Sweeney, M. J.: Common fluid and electrolyte problems in pediatrics. In Hughes, J. G., editor: Synopsis of pediatrics, ed. 4, St. Louis, 1975, The C. V. Mosby Co., p. 154.
†See Table 16-2 for composition and concentration of initial hydrating solutions, and see Table 16-6 for quantities of solutions or mixtures of solutions to be used during treatment of fluid imbalances. If hypovolemic shock is present, rapidly administer whole blood, plasma, or other colloids (for example, Dextran) intravenously in a dose of 10 ml/kg (same dose for all age groups); then proceed with initial hydration therapy. Although any one of these hydrating solutions may be used as indicated in this table, we recommend no. 1 in the above table for acidemia, especially in small infants. For hypertonic dehydration the solutions listed under *Hypertonic dehydration* have not been associated with posthydration convulsions.
‡One-fourth or one-third strength physiologic solution of sodium chloride in 5% glucose and glucose in distilled water are to be avoided in the initial phase of hydration of patients with hypertonic dehydration.

**Table 16-5.** Solutions or mixtures of solutions used for maintenance and replacement in patients with dehydration and acid-base imbalance*†

**Dehydration with metabolic acidosis**
Butler-Talbot solution
Modified Butler's solution
Half-strength lactate-Ringer's solution with 5% dextrose + 30 mEq/L potassium chloride

**Protracted acidemia and acidosis**
7.5% sodium bicarbonate or less preferably, M/6 sodium lactate solution may be used, according to Table 16-6

**Dehydration with metabolic alkalosis**
Butler-Talbot solution
Physiologic sodium chloride solution with equal parts 10% glucose in water + 30 mEq/L potassium chloride
Half-strength lactate-Ringer's solution with 5% dextrose + 30 mEq/L potassium chloride

*From Etteldorf, J. N., and Sweeney, M. J.: Common fluid and electrolyte problems in pediatrics. In Hughes, J. G., editor: Synopsis of pediatrics, ed. 4, St. Louis, 1975, The C. V. Mosby Co., p. 155.
†See Table 16-6 for *quantities* of solutions to use during various phases of treatment of fluid imbalances. See Table 16-3 for composition of these fluids.

the relative volumes of extracellular fluid. In hypertonic dehydration, extracellular fluid volume is relatively increased, which results in relatively good tissue turgor, a foam rubber feel to the skin, fever, thirst, meningismus, irritability, delirium, and occasionally seizures. Hypotonic dehydration, on the other hand, involves a relative decrease in extracellular fluid volume, which causes poor tissue turgor, lethargy, and subnormal body temperature.[20,21,36]

Nursing management is directed to prevention of continued loss of fluids, monitoring of signs of reestablishing fluid and electrolyte balance, and provision of replacement and maintenance fluids and solutes. Nonpharmocologic nursing measures for control of vomiting and diarrhea are discussed in Chapter 11 and should be coordinated with medical provisions of pharmocologic measures for control of these sources of fluid loss. Insensible fluid loss may be minimized by provision of humidity in the air, which decreases evaporation of fluids from the lungs and the skin. Control of body tempera-

ture also minimizes insensible fluid loss from the lungs and skin.

Management of intravenous fluid administration requires particular attention and skill when working with children. The infusion equipment and site should be checked every half hour and recorded at least every hour to ensure as constant a rate of flow as possible. Microdrops are used for children in order to deliver smaller volumes of fluid at a regular rate over a period of time. The infusion rate should never be increased to make up deficits in volume administration; rather the fluid flow should be carefully regulated within a designated range. A child's IV should never be irrigated if the flow stops. The tubing may be aspirated to determine if an occluding clot can be removed; otherwise provisions should be made for changing the IV site of administration. Tables 16-2 to 16-6 present a summary of solutions used in achieving fluid and electrolyte balance in children and the appropriate rates of infusion.

Young children often need to have their limbs partially restrained in order to protect the infusion site. If restraint is necessary, it should be provided in a manner that permits some movement and that does not restrict the child's ability to observe people and things in the environment. The restraints need to be removed at periodic intervals, and the child should be supervised for movement of each extremity. While the child is restrained, particular attention is given to providing play, diversional activities, companionship, and comfort in order to decrease the child's distress over having to be restrained.[36]

Oral fluid intake is restored as soon as possible, providing the child frequent, small quantities of juice or electrolyte solution. The child's intake and output are carefully monitored and recorded every hour. Each of the signs listed in Table 16-1 is monitored every hour, and changes are noted in detail.

### Inadequate exchange of gases

Inadequate exchange of gases can occur in relationship to a wide range of long-term and acute health problems, involving primarily the respiratory, circulatory, and hematologic systems. These nursing problems are classified in

**Table 16-6.** Quantities and rates of administration of solutions or mixtures* of solutions used in the treatment of metabolic acidosis with dehydration according to body weight† and surface area‡

| | Surface area | Body weight† |
|---|---|---|
| Initial hydration | 400 ml/m²/hr at 8 ml/m²/min; repeat once if no urination | 30 ml/kg/hr at 0.5 ml/kg/min; repeat once if no urination |
| Replacement and maintenance in mild to moderate dehydration | 2,400 ml/m²/24 hr; 100 ml/m²/hr in 24 hr or 200 ml/m²/hr in 12 hr | 140 ml/kg/24 hr; 6 ml/kg/hr in 24 hr or 12 ml/kg/hr in 12 hr |
| Replacement and maintenance in severe dehydration | 3,000 ml/m²/24 hr; 125 ml/m²/hr in 24 hr or 250 ml/m²/hr in 12 hr | 180 ml/kg/24 hr; 7.5 ml/kg/hr in 24 hr or 15 ml/kg/hr in 12 hr |
| Maintenance alone | 1,500 ml/m²/24 hr; 60 ml/m²/hr in 24 hr or 120 ml/m²/hr in 12 hr | 100 ml/kg/day; 4 ml/kg/hr in 24 hr or 8 ml/kg/hr in 12 hr |
| Protracted acidemia and acidosis | M/6 sodium r-lactate, 4 ml/kg, or 7.5% $NaHCO_3$, 0.75 ml/kg, elevates $HCO_3$ 1 mEq/L. Quantity of these solutions calculated to raise plasma bicarbonate 5 mEq/L over 1-2 hr period is usually well tolerated and safe. Total quantity of these solutions to be given in 24 hr to majority of patients with severe acidosis should not exceed amount calculated to elevate plasma bicarbonate concentration to 20 mEq/L. | |

*See Tables 16-2 to 16-5 for types of solutions and composition of mixtures.
†Body weight dosage as given is recommended for infants from birth through 18 mo and should be modified for older children as follows:

| | |
|---|---|
| 19-36 mo | 80% |
| 3-6 yr | 70% } of stated quantities |
| 7-12 yr | 60% |
| Older than 12 yr | 50% |

‡From Etteldorf, J. N., and Sweeney, M. J.: Common fluid and electrolyte problems in pediatrics. In Hughes, J. G., editor: Synopsis of pediatrics, ed. 4, St. Louis, 1975, The C. V. Mosby Co., p. 156.

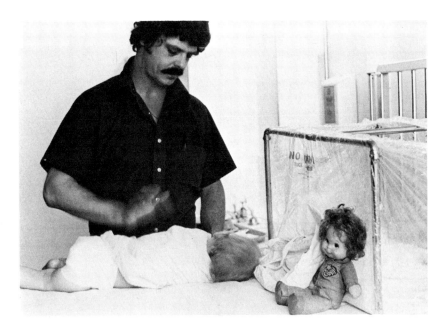

**Fig. 16-10.** This child is receiving respiratory therapy consisting of a mist tent and periodic percussion of the chest.

the MNPC as a component of physical care for long-term illness (see Appendix, p. 888). Inadequate gas exchange can occur with such nursing problems as inadequate food (MNPC no. 330.3) resulting in insufficient iron, which interferes with oxygen transport or upper respiratory infections (MNPC no. 350.5), resulting in inadequate filling and emptying of lung capacity or restriction of the airway.

Nursing measures include intervention directed primarily toward the correction of the underlying problem that is interfering with adequate gas exchange. Specific measures needed for specific problems, such as iron deficiency anemia, cystic fibrosis, bronchitis, and pneumonia, are discussed in other chapters.

When a child is hospitalized or attends an ambulatory clinic for regular respiratory therapy, specialized respiratory therapists may provide care and supervision of all respiratory therapy measures, including monitoring and care of the equipment. Often, however, it is desirable that a nurse who is consistently caring for a young child administer respiratory therapy and ultimately teach the child's parents to administer the therapy, particularly if the therapy is to be continued in the home. The most common approaches to respiratory therapy include provision of mist or oxygen or both, intermittent positive pressure breathing, and percussion of the chest. The technique of percussion is presented in Chapter 11. Intermittent positive pressure is administered by a machine that delivers measured portions of oxygen or air-oxygen mixture into the lungs at predetermined intervals. The child may initially be frightened by the machine, and often the child is too ill to respond to cognitive and psychologic preparation for the procedure. The parents or other adults who are with the child should be completely oriented to the procedure, and the nurse and parents together must decide how they might best assist the child in coping with the procedure. If the child is able to talk, it is recommended that a brief explanation and demonstration on a doll be offered before the first treatment. For very young children, a very brief, simple verbal explanation is given to the child as the child is placed in the nurse's lap, with the head positioned firmly against the

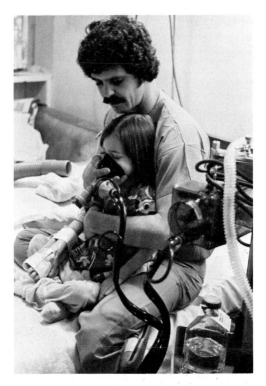

**Fig. 16-11.** Positioning of a young child for intermittent positive pressure breathing.

nurse's chest, one arm holding the child around the torso, and the other hand placing the mask firmly over the child's mouth and nose. A parent may need to help restrain the child's feet and legs and talk to the child to reassure him or her as the procedure begins. The young child is likely to object strenuously during the first few seconds of therapy but is likely to settle down after he or she becomes aware that no harm is going to result from the machine or the people. After the first treatment and as the child begins to feel better, play approaches should be used to assist the child in expressing and working through feelings of fear and anger toward the procedure.

Mist and oxygen or air-oxygen mixtures are delivered in a variety of ways in the hospital. The most common means of delivery is a mist tent that provides a high humidity ambient air without the use of tubes or masks. Intubation is required when there is a serious obstruction to the upper respiratory tract (see Chapter 11).

Inadequate exchange of gases can result in a

condition of respiratory acidosis. The child's pH falls below 7.3, and correction must be obtained immediately. The usual approach is administration of sodium bicarbonate intravenously. The dosage is calculated as follows:

$$\text{mEq bicarbonate needed} = \text{negative base excess} \times 0.3 \times \text{body weight in kg}$$

### Nutrition and feeding problems

Nutrition and feeding problems are very common for children who have a long-term illness. The MNPC system includes this category as a problem under each of the major categories of long-term illness, classification nos. 310 through 319, problem no. 1. (See Appendix, p. 888.) The specific problem of loss of appetite (MNPC no. 324.7) is frequent for hospitalized children, particularly in the younger age groups. Loss of appetite may stem from the physiologic illness, or it may be a somatic means of expressing despair arising from the separation from home and being in a strange environment.

Several of the hospital environment measures described earlier in this chapter are designed to promote healthy, positive eating experiences for children. Meals should be simple and planned in accord with the child's usual diet at home. Since most families feed young children simple, easily prepared meals, many of their meals can be prepared on the child care unit by the parents or the nurse. Familiar plates and cups, which may be an important part of meal-time ritual at home, should be brought to the hospital for use by the child. Children should be encouraged to eat out of bed at a table suited to their size, preferably with a group of children and supervising adults. The social experience provides an opportunity for the child to maintain a sense of personal autonomy and for adult encouragement and praise. Often, such a social environment provides a situation conducive to the child beginning to eat voluntarily. If children refuse to eat given optimal feeding settings, their refusal is accepted, the child distracted briefly, and the food offered again. Punishment and threats should not be used, and continued refusal should not be overattended. Both responses provide reinforcement for the noneating behavior. The child should be offered nutritious, appealing foods at frequent intervals, but efforts to entice eating should be limited to a simple statement that the food is available, encouragement to eat, integrating the child into a social situation, and offering the food again. When the child does take a bite or a drink, encouragement and praise is offered and the child is encouraged to eat and drink more, but not encouraged beyond limits of tolerance.[65]

### Adaptive/maladaptive behavior

Nursing care of hospitalized children or children who have long-term problems who remain at home involves frequent encounters with behavioral traits that are difficult for adults to understand and tolerate but that serve important adaptive or maladaptive functions for children. Maladaptive problems are included in the MNPC nos. 320 to 325 in the category of nursing problems related to behavior/emotions/learning (see Appendix, p. 890). The behaviors discussed in the following section are frequently exhibited in the hospital setting or in the home when a child is confined with a major illness and serve a useful function for the child. They need to be recognized as having potential for healthy adaptation, and specific health care should be planned to assist the child in progressively coping through mature and healthy behaviors. These behaviors cannot be assigned the label of adaptive or maladaptive but are assessed in light of the child's developmental stage, the needs the behavior is thought to reflect, and whether the behavior is instrumental in meeting that need. Each of these dimensions is discussed in interpreting the behaviors listed below.

**Regression.** Regression occurs when a child returns to a less mature behavior that had been abandoned. It tends to occur most frequently in children under 5 years of age but can occur in older children as well. An important dimension of the nursing assessment is determining if the behavior that appears immature for the child's developmental stage was truly abandoned. If the child has persisted in using an immature behavior or habit, the problem may be very different or there may not be a problem at all. For example, a 5-year-old who sucks a finger may have never abandoned the finger-sucking habit, and therefore using this habit in the hospital does not constitute regression.

Regression can be very frustrating for the parents, but it serves an important coping function for the child. Parents need assistance in understanding the way in which their child is temporarily behaving. Regression provides children a more comfortable, familiar pattern of behavior than recently acquired behaviors that are less familiar. The previous behaviors are more predictable to the child in attaining security, comfort, and mastery of an unknown situation. Regression also serves the purpose of providing less expenditure of emotional energy than that required in using more mature forms of coping, which are less familiar. This conservation of energy helps the child to regain energy needed for physical restoration.[3,67]

Children should be supported in using regressed behaviors for coping during the stress of acute illness, surgery, or brief hospitalization. If hospitalization lasts well into the recuperative period, the nurse and family need to plan together to encourage the child to begin to return to more mature behavior patterns and to reestablish previously accomplished developmental skills. If the child returns home for recuperation, the nurse needs to help the family to plan for and anticipate using a positive approach in helping their child regain developmental skills. For example, if the child had been able to use the toilet alone before hospitalization but needed to be diapered throughout hospitalization, the family may need to continue to use diapers until the child's recovery and readjustment at home is fully established and then begin to encourage the child to reestablish independent use of the toilet.

Regression becomes maladaptive when the child persists in using the regressed behavior well past the time of acute stress and crisis and has great difficulty in reestablishing the previously mastered developmental skills. The child should be able to return to the previously mastered skills with relative ease, and while the regressed behavior will continue to recur intermittently, it will gradually give way to the more mature behavior.

**Discharge of tension, fear, anxiety.** The most commonly used mechanism for discharge of tension, fear, and anxiety is crying. Unfortunately, many adults consider crying regressive and maladaptive behavior, failing to recognize the essential and healthy basis for crying. Often children cry most when their parents are present, indicating the need for relief of pent-up tension, fear and anxiety, and indicating that the child is continuing to relate to the parents as a source of comfort, support, and security. A common misinterpretation of this behavior is that the parent's presence is detrimental to the child and that he or she would be better off if they did not come. When parents react in this manner, they need to be assured of the healthy function of their child's behavior and of what it reveals about the nature of their relationship. They should be encouraged to actively foster this behavior and can also be assisted in finding means of helping their child to relieve tension, fear, and anxiety through means other than crying, but they also need to comfort and support the child when the need to cry occurs.

Other activities that provide for release of tension, fear, and anxiety are various forms of play and the use of large muscles. An organized program of exercise should be planned for the child as long as he or she is physically capable, and provisions should be made for the child to engage in this activity at will. Planned therapeutic play approaches, described in a following section of this chapter, provide for release of tension by acting out behaviors that are forbidden in reality and by expressing feelings that are not socially acceptable. For example, a child may act out through play a wish to attack and mutilate the physician or some other member of the health care team in retaliation for the perceived hurt which that person has inflicted on the child.[19]

**Direct expressions of anger.** As with crying behavior, direct expressions of anger are frequently misunderstood and misinterpreted. They are often thought to be regressive, immature, and even wrong or sinful, and may be punished as such. To the contrary, direct expressions of anger represent a child's direct and honest confrontation with real inner feelings, which are often quite justified from the child's point of view. Such feelings should be expected and anticipated in advance and provisions made for the child to express anger and hostility in a healthy, socially acceptable manner.[47] If a child's anger and hostility erupts into physical aggression, destruction of property, or self-punishment, the fact of the child's feelings needs to be openly acknowledged and accepted and a more positive alternative made immediately available for expression of angry feelings. One alternative that is almost always available is pounding on the mattress of the bed. The child can be told, "Your anger is an understandable feeling, and it needs to get out. The way to get it out is pounding on the bed, just as hard and long as you need to. You cannot (name the unacceptable behavior), but you can pound on the bed." Planning is then begun to facilitate the child's learning to express anger and hostility through means that allow for healthy release and to prevent building of pent-up anger that necessitates explosive outbursts. Angry feelings should be used in play and mentioned periodically by the nurse as acceptable feelings. The nurse uses play approaches in modeling healthy approaches to expressing anger. For example, the nurse might engage the child in puppet play, setting up a situation that will result in the nurse's puppet getting angry. The puppet then verbalizes the reasons for the anger and the felt inner feelings, confronts the person to whom the anger is directed, and then resolves the problem.

**Withdrawal.** Withdrawal is a common form of behavioral coping used by children of all ages and often is used by adolescents. As with other forms of behavior, such behavior is often misinterpreted in that the child who is withdrawn is viewed as behaving very well, being cooperative, quiet, causing little trouble, and making few demands. On the contrary the child is suffering serious inner misery, including feelings of despair, depression, homesickness, abandonment, fear, or separation anxiety. Reaching such a child may be very difficult for the nurse, and attempts to establish a relationship may appear to fail repeatedly. Particularly if the child has in reality been abandoned or is suffering enforced separation or loss of self-esteem, the child's withdrawal and depression needs professional intervention and planned team efforts to assist the child in coping. Caring and understanding need to be conveyed to the child consistently, regardless of the child's or teenager's repeated rejections of attempts to establish a relationship. When the child's withdrawal and depression is directed toward family members as well, they too need professional assistance in relating to their child and in handling their own feelings.

Whether the child or teenager expresses overt rejection or simply remains nonexpressive and withdrawn, the nurse can use several approaches in relating. The approaches used need to suit the nurse's own personality and natural abilities, but each of these approaches can be learned through planned role-play experience and practice in clinical situations. The play techniques described in the following section are often useful with a withdrawn child; they can respond to some form of play. If the child or teenager reads as a form of diversion and withdrawal, the nurse can suggest reading materials that are helpful in dealing with feelings that the young person might be experiencing. Fiction is particularly useful, in that it provides the child with a fantasized situation through which the emotions can be experienced, examined, and dealt with. The nurse can use fantasized or fictionalized stories to communicate to the child an understanding of how he or she might be feeling but through referral to an imagined or absent character.[57] For example, the nurse can talk about a person approximately the child's age and provide details of a story that are similar to the child's own situation, filling in the fictionalized child's feelings and frustrations. The child might relate to the story and begin to verbalize if the need is significant and the relationship with the nurse is sufficient to engender feelings of safety. The child may appear to ignore the story altogether and a reaction may not appear, or it may be delayed for several days. Or the child might strike out in anger and hostility toward the nurse, saying that the story is childish and stupid. This reaction is probably one of the most healthy and represents a major breakthrough, for the child feels secure enough to vent feelings of anger and hostility and come out of the withdrawal. The following dialogue is an example of how a nurse might respond to such an outburst of anger:

NURSE: Do you think that Susan was stupid?

CHILD: No, that whole story is just stupid, stupid, stupid.

NURSE: I think you have a point. It seems to not make any sense that people have to have such bad things happen to them, does it? (The nurse is acknowledging the child's right to think the story is stupid, and identifying, without focusing attention directly on the child, a possible source of frustration for the child.)

CHILD: You are darn right, I have a point. That is the most stupid story I have ever heard.

NURSE: What kind of story do you like? (The nurse is maintaining an indirect means of relating to the child until the child is clearly willing to relate and is willing to reveal something about herself.)

CHILD: I like stories where the people die.

The nurse has now clearly established sufficient rapport with the child to begin to probe more directly the child's feelings, but can still use the framework of stories to do so. The child has now revealed a probable preoccupation with death, which may involve wishing for death, wishing to have others who are hated to die, or an expression of fear that she herself will die. The nurse's continuing relationship and contact with the child make it imperative that dealing with feelings such as these is developed as an interpersonal skill and that the child is not automatically referred to a psychiatrist. Some children do need referral, and the skilled nurse will use regular consultation with specialists in psychiatry to assure continued development of sound therapeutic approaches.

**Manipulative behavior.** Manipulation is a relatively immature form of coping but serves the purpose of achieving mastery and control. It tends to be used by children who are faced with difficult facts of life over which they have no control and in situations where adults in the family are overwhelmed with their own problems and respond to their child with little or no parental control. The manipulative behavior, while reflecting a need for a sense of mastery and for attention from others, elicits intense feelings of resentment, anger, and alienation. Handling a negative form of behavior requires a coordinated team effort by everyone who contacts the child or young person. The team members need to acknowledge their feelings toward the child and may need to role play some typical

situations with the child in order to practice the desired responses so that when faced with the actual behavior and the feelings of anger toward the child, they will be able to respond in the desired, therapeutic fashion. The principles of positive behavior modification are applied with as much consistency as can be achieved, as described in the following section. The child is confronted directly with authentic responses to behaviors that are not desired. For example, if the child threatens not to eat dinner, the nurse openly acknowledges that the child's attitude is obnoxious or irritating. The fact of eating or not eating dinner is ignored, since this is a tool that the child has selected for manipulating, and this behavior is therefore not rewarded. When the child makes a real achievement or accomplishes a desired behavior, attention and praise is given. The long-term success of such behavioral modification is dependent upon the parents' ability to participate and follow through at home.[47]

## Special tools for child nursing intervention

The particular tools and approaches that are required for effective nursing care of children and families have been described throughout this text in relationship to particular problems and situations. The following section presents in further detail the techniques and approaches that are of particular concern in nursing care for hospitalized children and children at home with long-term illness.

### Therapeutic play

In the hospital the nurse is concerned with two basic types of play: diversional play, which is largely spontaneous and directed by the child with no specific therapeutic goals planned, and therapeutic play, which must draw on the child's spontaneity and the child's self-direction but which is planned to meet certain therapeutic goals related to the child's health. Diversional play facilities and materials are always available on a child care unit, and often the nurse will either observe the child's diversional play or participate with children at play in order to obtain information about the child or to establish rapport with the child. In planning facilities and materials for diversional play, all age groups need to be considered and space and toys made available for them. In addition, provision for diversional play needs to be made for children whose mobility is limited. Diversional play should include opportunities for fine and large muscle activity, for socialization with other children and adults, and for spontaneous expression of feelings. Toys should be selected for their value in learning, the safety of the toy, and the degree to which they stimulate spontaneity and creativity.[22]

In planning for participation in diversional and therapeutic play, the nurse needs to understand the meaning of children's play and gain experience in participation as an authentic "player." Play activities require an inner sense of spontaneity, creativity, and freedom. The person who is playing feels no restrictions or constraints in expressing the inner self. Thus, the child who is engaged in a play activity can, without fear or shame, act out an inner wish to mutilate an adult. If an adult who is interacting with a child persists in trying to teach the child what to do or to show the child how to work a toy, the child's ability and efforts at playing are totally thwarted. Play activities are totally absorbing and serious for the person who is playing. A person of any age who is engaged in a play activity finds such absorption and enjoyment and pleasure in the activity, for its own sake, that all else is forgotten and the person is totally absorbed in the activity of play. Any attempt by another person to disturb the individual who is playing is resisted in order to prolong the play. Play involves a sense of mastery and success, not in relationship to a product or an end result, but in the performing of the activity itself for its own sake, regardless of the outcome. This total concentration on the means, as described by Piaget,[50] is the key to interpreting the kind of mastery that is experienced through play. The quality or content is not judged in terms of mastery; the mastery lies solely in the feeling of total self-expression, in mastery of the self and not the external appearances of the play.[14,50]

In gaining expertise with play, the nurse needs first to feel comfortable with play, as a play participant. Roles of teacher, parent, coun-selor, and behavior officer need to be discarded and the nurse must become comfortable in the role of adult play participant. It is important to maintain the adult role and identity, for attempts to act as a child will appear stilted and false. Once comfort is achieved in being an adult play participant, the nurse can use play approaches for therapeutic purposes and alternately use the role of participant and observer, according to the needs of the child.[35]

There are three general categories of therapeutic goals that the nurse uses in planning play for hospitalized children. These are (1) expressions of inner feelings and perceptions, (2) mastery of a new perception or learning, and (3) release of emotions. Techniques that may be used to accomplish each of these goals are described below.

**Expression of inner feelings and perceptions.** Several play techniques can be used to stimulate expression of inner feelings and perceptions. The particular technique selected depends upon the child's developmental stage, background of social experience, and physical abilities. The most widely applicable technique for achieving this goal is drawing and other forms of art work. Most children, even in the face of severe physical or mental limitations, can participate in some form of art work or some form of drawing. The use of the self-portrait and family portrait have been described in Chapters 10 and 12. These portraits are extremely useful for the child who is hospitalized in expressing feelings of anxiety in maintaining self-control, fear of mutilation, death, and perceptions of body image. The self-portraits may be obtained over a period of time during a prolonged hospitalization to document changes that occur as the child works through changes in body image and self-perception. The family portrait may reveal traits of the child's feelings toward family members during the crisis period, and repeated portraits may document changes in family relationships that occur during the child's illness.

Shufer[61] has described a play-discussion group technique that encourages children to express, through group play, their own perceptions of hospitalization and illness. The children gather around a table equipped with doll and animal "patients" and a variety of hospital treat-

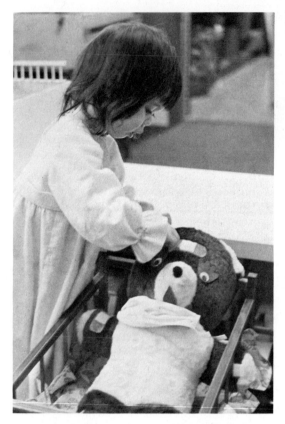

**Fig. 16-12.** The child achieves mastery of new experiences in the hospital by playing nurse for her patient and by "fixing" her patient's head with a bandage.

ment and diagnostic tools, such as stethoscopes, otoscopes, syringes with needles, IV bottles and tubing, and surgical caps and masks. The children may dress up in hospital costumes and then proceed to treat their selected patient. As the children treat their patient, the nurse stimulates discussion of what is happening and why. Misconceptions are uncovered and clarified, and accurate understanding is reinforced. At the conclusion of the play-discussion, each child is given the opportunity to tell the group about their patient, including why he or she came to the hospital and what kind of treatment was given. The children are given an opportunity to raise questions and discuss each child's report as they desire.

**Mastery of new perceptions or learnings.** There are many ways in which play is used for mastery of new perceptions and learning. The child often seeks such mastery of new perceptions through diversional play. In using play for therapeutic purposes, the nurse must first identify the nature of the new experience and the kind of mastery that is required of the child. One of the most common mastery experiences needed in the hospital is that involved in preparation for surgery and for postsurgical care. Initially the child is provided an opportunity to handle and become familiar with equipment and clothing that would otherwise be unfamiliar and frightening. Items that can be left in the child's room for diversional play are brought in, such as surgical caps and masks, green gown, and oxygen mask. At planned intervals, the nurse participates in play with the child, using equipment with which the child has become familiar. Gradually the child is introduced to new dimensions of the experience that are to come and is taken to the actual area of the hospital. The child can assume the role of a nurse or doctor as they walk a doll or animal "patient" through the experience. Equipment that will be surrounding the child when he or she comes out of surgery is, at some point, set up for the child to see, feel, and manipulate to gain familiarity. The child and the nurse again take care of their doll or animal "patient," who has now completed the surgery. Tubes and equipment are set up just as the child will experience them. The child is encouraged to move about, to get into an oxygen tent, try on a mask, and thoroughly gain familiarity with each piece of equipment. If the child will need to cooperate in postsurgical exercises, these are rehearsed during each play session.[35,47,58,66,75]

Books provide an important means of stimulating the child's inner thought and fantasy in gaining mastery of new perceptions and experiences. Books should be selected carefully for the accuracy of the content, appropriateness for the developmental stage of the child, and usefulness in helping the child master new perceptions.[26]

**Release of emotions.** The range and intensity of emotions generated by the stress and crisis of hospitalization and illness should never be discounted. Children and young people need the opportunity for expression and release of these feelings in as authentic a form as possible.

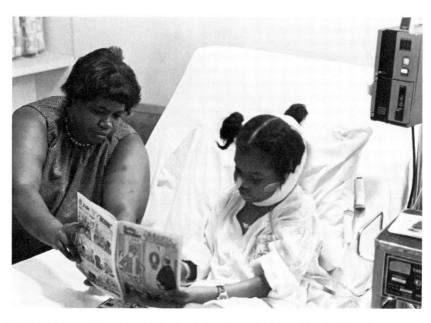

**Fig. 16-13.** Mother and daughter read a book together, which provides for diversion as well as for learning and a point of discussion between them.

Through play activities and planned nursing guidance, children and families learn coping skills that can be transferred and applied in the home setting.

Large muscle activity is important in the release of anger and hostility. A plastic clown that can be inflated and stands upright with a sandbag weight at the bottom makes a useful punching bag, and a child can fantasize striking out at adults and things toward which the anger is directed. The nurse encourages the child to punch as hard as possible and helps the child gain awareness of what he or she is accomplishing. Comments like "you are so angry, you just want to hit that old clown as hard as you can" provide guidance and encouragement for the activity, and convey the nurse's understanding of the child's plight. The nurse and the child discuss feelings of anger and the things the child feels angry toward, as well as the healthy ways, such as punching the clown, that the child can work out the anger.

Doll play provides a useful means for a child to act out inner emotions and the situations that stimulate those emotions. A doll family or group of dolls representing people in the hospital is made available for the child to select spontaneously. The child might have the alternates of clay, drawing, punching bag, or dolls, all of which provide an opportunity for expression of emotion. Children frequently select one doll to represent themselves and identify other figures as significant. The nurse observes and lets the child's play emerge spontaneously unless the child initiates interaction with the nurse as a participant or the nurse decides to ask a question that provides clarification of the meaning of the child's play for the child. For example, if the child develops a scene at home where mother and father are arguing, the nurse might ask the child to describe what the other dolls are feeling when that happens.

Clay provides a form of large muscle activity, particularly for children who have partial restriction of mobility. Clay can be punched, squeezed, pulled, and pounded. It also permits the child to use his or her own imaginative and creative skills in creating people and objects who can be used in a manner similar to the doll family. For example, the child might construct a doll figure and a rocket to go to the moon, which subsequently crashes with the doll on board.

**681**

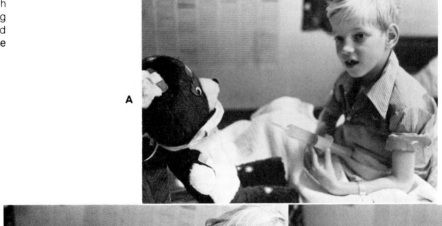

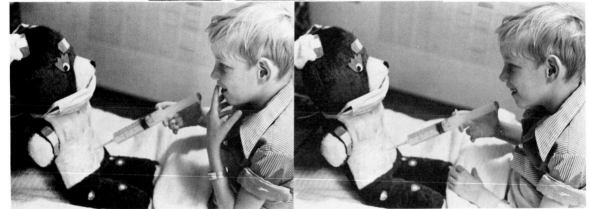

**Fig. 16-14.** This child was extremely fearful of shots, and a play experience was planned to provide for mastery of the problem and release of emotions. **A,** Upon being handed the syringe, he states, "I thought only nurses got to hold these." **B,** He inserts the needle with some apprehension. **C,** Begins to experience relief with the "job" done.

Such an enactment can have several interpretations, depending on the child's circumstance, but regardless of the interpretation it does, as an activity, provide for expression of emotions such as fear, anger, hostility.[35,64]

### Interview and dialogue with children

Many adults are uncomfortable and reluctant to enter into a dialogue with children, feeling as if they do not know what to say or how to relate to children. Observation of experienced nurses and child-care specialists provides an initial familiarity with ways in which people who are comfortable with children use their own personality and style in relating. While most adults who are effective with children are nat-

ural and talk and behave in a relaxed, confident manner, they easily make adjustments in their manner that is appropriate to the age group of the child. For example, in working with very young children, the adult gets on the child's eye level as much as possible by sitting on the floor, kneeling, or sitting down. Words and phrases are short and simple and direct, to enhance understanding and comprehension. A person relating to a child of school age, on the other hand, will relate in a manner similar to that used in relating to adults but will use teases and humor that are appropriate and popular with the child's peer group.

In interviewing and conducting an initial dialogue with young children, some form of play is often useful. Puppets provide almost instant response from children of the toddler age group through the lower grades in school. Children are comfortable and able to "talk" with a puppet more freely than a strange adult, and will eagerly enter into dialogue between the nurse's puppet and a puppet that they control. With or without puppets the nurse can engage the child in mutual story telling, which involves stimulating the child to fill in details of a story about a person or animal with whom the child can relate. If the nurse is interviewing a child to determine what his or her perceptions of hospitalization were before admission, the story might be initiated by the nurse telling about a fuzzy little puppy who had to go to the hospital, and when he found out he had to go, he thought . . . , and encouraging the child to pick up on the details of what the puppy thought about going to the hospital. The story-telling approach can be used with older children, providing a setting and story situation that is appropriate to their age group.[39,58,62,63]

### Positive modification of behavior

As was illustrated in the previous discussion of behavioral problems in this chapter, all behavior can be understood when it is viewed within the context of its occurrence. Techniques of behavior modification are based on the premise that behavior is regulated by environmental events; both antecedent stimuli and consequences or associated outcomes. (See discussion of behavior and personality development, Chapter 10.) Behavior of people of all ages can be successfully modified with the consistent and skilled use of behavior modification techniques, but young children are particularly responsive to this approach, as this type of learning constitutes a primary means through which daily learning occurs during this stage of growth. The following discussion presents a summary of the steps involved in design and implementation of a behavior modification program. Although these behavioral principles can be applied casually in nursing practice, thorough study and understanding of the behavioral change design and consistent, skilled application is required for the techniques to be effective in real modification of behavior. The reader is referred to the references for detailed study of this approach and is urged to use this technique initially with an experienced practitioner.[11,38,46]

The first consideration in designing a behavior modification program is identifying, with the child's mother or care-giver, the major trait or traits of behavior that are of concern. The behavior needs to be identified in explicit behavioral terms. For example, if the mother is concerned about her child being fussy and whiny, she needs to identify exactly what behavior occurs when the child is fussy. The precise behavior may be crying, or it may be verbal complaining in a specific tone of voice, or it may be clinging to mother in order to be held.[46]

The second step is to identify and assess the situations in which the behavior occurs. The mother or care-giver or nursing staff initially describes when, where, and with whom they have observed the undesirable behavior. This initial impression provides a starting point for direct observation and recording of behavior and the environmental events that immediately precede and immediately follow the undesired behavior. Systematic recording of the behavior and the related events needs to be done in as many situations as possible to estimate the range of environmental events that are related to the behavior and consistencies that exist from one situation to another.[46]

The child's developmental level is determined in order to interpret the meaning of the child's behavior and to select meaningful consequent events for reinforcing the behavior. The undesired behavior may be indicative of a normal developmental need that the child is expressing, and provision must be made to meet the child's needs in a positive manner while changing the behavior used to express the need. For example, if a child consistently expresses a need for interpersonal attention by crying during the second year of development and has begun to develop expressive verbal skills, the crying behavior is evaluated as being expressive of a real need, and positive interpersonal attention is planned for the child in response to more desirable behaviors, while the attention in response to crying is withheld.[46]

Next, the desired behavior that is to replace the undesired behavior is identified. The de-

**683**

sired behaviors must be observable, measurable activities that are repeatable and can be controlled by the child. An undesired behavior can be eliminated without specifying the alternate desired behavior, but if the desired behavior is specified and used in planning the behavior modification program, the problem behavior is extinguished through lack of opportunity for use and lack of reinforcement.[46]

The consequent events are selected for the known reinforcing value to the individual child. If a behavior is to increase, the events that follow the behavior must be rewarding and desirable to the child. If an undesirable behavior is not rewarded, the behavior will decrease. Reinforcers that are most often rewarding to young children are food, toys, and adult attention. These tend to also reinforce behaviors of older children, but special events and money are often important reinforcers as well. If the events that have been observed and documented to follow the undesired behavior appear to be consistently reinforcing to the child, that reinforcer might be used to increase the desired behavior. For example, if a child is picked up and held as a consequence of crying, the reinforcement is removed from the crying behavior and used instead in response to desired verbal behavior.[46]

The behavior change program is planned and discussed thoroughly with all persons involved in the child's care. The full cooperation of all adults in the setting is needed to assure maximum success. Once the behavior modification is underway, detailed recording of the child's behavior is documented in order to evaluate the effectiveness of the program. The frequency and/or duration of occurrence of the target behavior is observed and tallied or placed on a graph that depicts the rate of behavior change.[46]

### Care of the child who has surgery

Psychologic preparation of the child for surgery and complex diagnostic procedures has been discussed in relation to therapeutic play. Preparation of parents and other family members for the child's surgical and postsurgical experience is also of vital importance. Parents and family members can be included in many of the child's play experiences, can observe the nurse rehearsing postsurgical procedures and

exercises and become familiar with the use of equipment, and learn how to help the child with postsurgical experiences. Their listening and participation in the child's play experiences can serve as a point of discussion to initiate their expression of concerns, questions, and to explore their perceptions about what is going to happen to their child. Their questions need to be answered as directly and thoroughly as possible. Common misconceptions about the kind of surgery that their child is to experience should be raised by the nurse in order to help them establish a real base of understanding. Their presurgical expressions of desire or hesitancy to participate in the child's care after surgery are used as a basis for planning their involvement in care. If they appear to be eager to participate, but seem overwhelmed by the emotional impact of the experience when the time arrives, they need encouragement and support and can be urged to begin brief, limited participation.[8,32,43]

Physical preparation for surgery with children is similar to that for people of other age groups, as is standard postoperative care, with one major exception. That exception is in monitoring, regulating, and maintaining the delicate fluid and electrolyte balance of the child. Before surgery the child should be well hydrated and have adequate levels of hemoglobin, sodium, potassium, calcium, and other electrolytes. The preadmission and presurgical body weights are obtained to provide a basis for replacing lost fluids. The child's temperature, pulse, and respiration during the presurgical period serve as a basis for evaluating changes that might occur as a result of a fluid or electrolyte imbalance. Liquids should not be withheld from infants and small children longer than four to six hours before surgery; if a longer period of time is required, intravenous maintenance of fluids and electrolytes is required. During and after surgery, careful attention is given to replacement of fluid loss that occurs during surgery, and establishing normal intake and output patterns. In older children particularly, there may be an antidiuretic reaction to surgery due to release of ACTH, aldosterone, and ADH, which cause retention of sodium and water. Intake is carefully balanced with output, and all sources of fluid loss must be taken into account. Insensible loss from the skin and lungs, urinary loss, loss with feces, loss from gastric or nasopharyngeal suction, loss from bleeding, and loss from vomiting are all calculated and taken into account in planning for replacement and maintenance volumes. The child's state of hydration is carefully monitored, as described earlier in this chapter.[20,36]

### Counseling with parents and families

The degree to which the hospital and illness experience can be successfully weathered by the child and family depends to a great extent on the coping tolerance of the parents. Their emotional and cognitive needs are often overlooked, particularly if the family appears to be capable and intelligent. The parents' tendency to regress and to be unable to continue adequate parenting and supportive functions for the child must be recognized and specific early measures taken to plan for their continued support and to assist them in maintaining a parenting relationship with the child throughout the illness. The parents need to be fully informed and involved in early planning and preparation for hospitalization if at all possible. They need to be included from the beginning in care-taking activities and to know the hospital personnel and environment. Resources for special counseling and assistance are made available to them at the outset. When the parents are faced with uncertainties as to their child's illness or prognosis or when they are faced with difficult decisions regarding treatment and care, they need a great deal of ongoing counseling and understanding from all persons who work with them. Active listening, described in Chapter 2, is a valuable tool in helping them to think through and test the alternatives they face. When the family is faced with an ethical decision, they need to have full access to facts and information, assistance in understanding the meaning of the facts, and assistance in exploring their own ethical values and what each of the predicted consequences would mean to them if they were to come true. While health care workers cannot and should not impose their own values on a family, it is often helpful for the nurses and physicians involved to share with the family their real feelings and experiences rather than to avoid the personal dimensions of the problem. For example, if a family asks for advice about what they should do or what the nurse should do in a similar situation, the nurse might respond as follows: "I honestly do not know what I would do in your situation. It would be important to me to examine my own religion and my feelings about life and death. I do not have many family members who could help me with such a problem and my finances are limited, which would influence my own decision. I might have difficulty handling some alternatives that might seem best for you. As you think through the things that are important to you, I will share my own feelings with you to help you test and explore your own if that will be helpful."

If a nurse finds that the family's decision is difficult or impossible to cope with, the health care team needs to identify together those areas of care and counseling that need to be provided and identify ways in which each health care team member can best participate in order to meet the needs of the child and the family. For example, if a family decides that heroic measures to save a child's life are to be withdrawn and the nurse cannot cope with giving direct nursing care to the child under such a circumstance, other members of the nursing staff may be called upon to give care for the child, and the nurse might be able to continue to offer support and counseling for the parents as they await the outcome.

### STUDY QUESTIONS

1. Choose one of the criteria for hospitalization, and develop a statement of rationale for the criteria based on information in other chapters of this book and supplementary readings. For example, develop the rationale for hospitalization of an infant under 6 months of age with cellulitis (see Chapters 8 and 9). Expand the criteria to include consideration of the four major risks of hospitalization and criteria for the evaluation of family resources for home care. Discuss which factors would lead to the decision to hospitalize such a child and which would lead to the decision to encourage home care.
2. Participate in the hospital care of a child who is experiencing a separation anxiety. Describe in detail his or her reactions and behavior, identify the stage or stages of separation anxiety exhibited. Identify and plan nursing intervention with other health care team members and

give your impressions of the effectiveness of this intervention. What problems did you encounter in carrying out the plan? If possible, do this with several children in different stages of development, including the older age groups when the hazards of separation are thought to be not as great.

3. Interview one or more specialists who have particular skills in helping families and children with behavior problems, preferably one who has experience with hospitalized children. This person may be a nurse with advanced education and background or another health care team member. Identify the ways in which he or she assesses the behavior problem and the family's interrelationship with the child. Describe the approaches used and the ways in which he evaluates the success of their work.

4. Participate in the care of a child who is experiencing pain. Present a plan for care related to the pain experience, and the physiologic and psychologic principles that are related to the nursing intervention identified. Evaluate the effectiveness of your plan of care.

5. Describe a recent change or innovation in the hospital care of children in your local area. Determine the impact that this change has had on the experience of the family and the child and the ways in which professional health care workers in the setting have adjusted to the change. Describe the projections that are being made or could be made for further advances in this regard.

## REFERENCES

1. Alpert, J. J., and Feinbloom, R. I.: Advances in hospital ambulatory service for children, Pediatr. Clin. North Am. 21:263, May, 1974.
2. Amend, E. L.: Orientation for the short-time surgical patient. In Bergersen, B. S., and others, editors: Current concepts in clinical nursing, vol. 2, St. Louis, 1969, The C. V. Mosby Co., p. 230.
3. Audette, M. S.: The significance of regressive behavior for the hospitalized child, Matern. Child Nurs. J. 3:31, Spring, 1974.
4. Avey, M.: Primary care for handicapped children, Am. J. Nurs. 73:658, April, 1973.
5. Azarnoff, P.: Mediating the trauma of serious illness and hospitalization in childhood, Children Today 3:12, July-Aug., 1974.
6. Barnes, C. M., and others: Measurement in management of anxiety in children for open heart surgery, Pediatrics 49:250-259, Feb., 1972.
7. Barton, P. H.: Nursing assessment and intervention through plan. In Bergerson, B. S., and others, editors: Current concepts of clinical nursing, vol. 2, St. Louis, 1969, The C. V. Mosby Co.
8. Baxter, P.: Frustration felt by a mother and her child during the child's hospitalization, Matern. Child. Nurs. J. 1:159, May/June, 1976.
9. Beck, C., Johnson, M., and Silvest, M. L.: Nursing diagnosis of drug incompatibility; conceptual framework, process, and clinical evaluation, unpublished paper, Dallas, Texas, 1976, Texas Woman's University.
10. Beck, M.: Attitudes of parents of pediatric heart patients toward patient care units, Nurs. Res. 22:334, July-Aug., 1973.
11. Berni, R., and Fordyce, W. E.: Behavior modification and the nursing process, St. Louis, 1973, The C. V. Mosby Co.
12. Bothe, A., and Galdston, R.: The child's loss of consciousness; a psychiatric view of pediatric anesthesia, Pediatrics 50:252-263, Aug., 1972.
13. Bowlby, J., and others: Maternal care and mental health; deprivation of maternal care—a reassessment of its effect, ed. 2, New York, 1966, Schocken Books, Inc.
14. Caplan, F., and Caplan, T.: The power of play, New York, 1974, Anchor Press/Doubleday.
15. Characteristics of an in-patient unit for adolescents, Report of the Committee on In-patient Care for Adolescents of the Society for Adolescent Medicine, Clin. Pediatr. 12:17, Jan., 1973.
16. Condon, S. R.: Day-time hospital for children, Am. J. Nurs. 72:1431-1433, Aug., 1972.
17. Cooke, R. E.: The child in the hospital. In Cooke, R. E., editor: The biologic basis of pediatric practice, New York, 1968, McGraw-Hill Book Co., p. 1683.
18. Craford, C. F., and Palm, M. L.: Can I take my teddy bear? Am. J. Nurs. 73:286, Feb., 1973.
19. Dzik, M. A.: The use of motility by a preschool boy during hospitalization, Matern. Child Nurs. J. 3:169, Fall, 1974.
20. Etteldorf, J. N., and Sweeney, M. J.: Common fluid and electrolyte problems in pediatrics. In Hughes, J. G., editor: Synopsis of pediatrics, ed. 4, St. Louis, 1975, The C. V. Mosby Co., p. 139.
21. Finberg, L.: Water and electrolyte physiology. In Rudolf, A. M., editor: Pediatrics, ed. 16, New York, 1977, Appleton-Century-Crofts, p. 260.
22. Frank, D. J., and Drobish, M. L.: Toy safety in hospitals, Clin. Pediatr. 14:400, April, 1975.
23. Frieberg, K. H.: How parents react when their child is hospitalized, Am. J. Nurs. 72:1270-1272, July, 1972.
24. Friedberg, D. Z., and Caldart, L.: A center for pediatric cardiovascular patients, Am. J. Nurs. 75:1480, Sept., 1975.
25. Fujita, M. T.: The impact of illness or surgery on the body image of the child, Nurs. Clin. North Am. 7:641, Dec., 1972.
26. Galligan, A. C.: Books for the hospitalized child, Am. J. Nurs. 75:2164, Dec., 1975.
27. Gildea, J. H., and Quirk, T. R.: Assessing the pain experience in children, Nurs. Clin. North Am. 12:631, Dec., 1977.
28. Guerin, L. S.: Hospitalization as a positive experience for poverty children; observations on children from low-income multi-problem families, Clin. Pediatr. 16:509, June, 1977.
29. Haka-Ikse, K., and Van Leeuwen, J. V.: Care of the long-term hospitalized infant; a developmental approach, Clin. Pediatr. 15:585, July, 1976.
30. Hardgrove, C. B., and Dawson, R. B.: Parents and

children in the hospital; the family's role in pediatrics, Boston, 1972, Little, Brown and Co.

31. Hardgrove, C. B., and Dawson, R. B.: Ideas A to Z for personalizing pediatric units, Nursing '76, **6:**57, April, 1976.

32. Hardgrove, C., and Rutledge, A.: Parenting during hospitalization, Am. J. Nurs. **75:**836, May, 1975.

33. Hymovich, D. P.: Bobby . . . a very difficult little boy, Nursing '73 **3:**44, Feb., 1973.

34. Jackson, D. W.: The adolescent and the hospital, Pediatr. Clin. North Am. **20:**901, Nov., 1973.

35. Juenker, D.: Play as a tool for the nurse. In Steele, S., editor: Nursing care of the child with long-term illness, ed. 2, New York, 1977, Appleton-Century-Crofts, p. 31.

36. Kee, J. L., and Gregory, A. D.: The ABC's and mEq's of fluid imbalance in children, Nursing '74 **4:**28, June, 1974.

37. Lamb, G. A., and others: Emergency-room experience, Pediatrics **55:**266, Feb., 1975.

38. LeBow, M. D.: Behavior modification; a significant method in nursing practice, Englewood Cliffs, N.J., 1973, Prentice-Hall, Inc.

39. Luciano, K., and Shumsky, C. J.: Pediatric procedures—the explanation should always come first, Nursing '75 **5:**49, Jan., 1975.

40. McCaffery, M.: Brief episodes of pain in children. In Bergersen, B. S., and others, editors: Current concepts of clinical nursing, vol. 2, St. Louis, 1969, The C. V. Mosby Co., p. 178.

41. McCaffery, M.: Nursing management of the patient with pain, Philadelphia, 1972, J. B. Lippincott Co.

42. McCaffery, M.: Pain relief for the child; problem areas and selected non-pharmacological methods, Pediatr. Nurs. **4:**11, July/Aug., 1977.

43. Miller, J.: Cognitive dissonance in modifying families' perceptions, Am. J. Nurs. **74:**1468, Aug., 1974.

44. Neff, J. A.: Recapitulation of separation-individualization process in a toddler during hospitalization and home care, Matern. Child Nurs. J. **3:**87, Summer, 1974.

45. O'Grady, R. S.: Restraint and the hospitalized child. In Bergersen, B. S., and others, editors: Current concepts in clinical nursing, vol. 2, St. Louis, 1969, The C. V. Mosby Co., p. 192.

46. O'Neil, S. M., McLaughlin, B. N., and Knapp, M. B.: Behavioral approaches to children with developmental delays, St. Louis, 1977, The C. V. Mosby Co.

47. Petrillo, M., and Sanger, S.: Emotional care of hospitalized children; an environmental approach, Philadelphia, 1972, J. B. Lippincott Co.

48. Poznanski, E. O.: Children's reactions to pain; a psychiatrist's perceptive, Clin. Pediatr. **15:**1114, Dec., 1976.

49. Prugh, D. G., and others: A study of the emotional reaction of children and families to hospitalization and illness, Am. J. Orthopsychiatry **23:**70, 1973.

50. Pulaski, M. A.: Play symbolism in cognitive development. In Schaefer, C., editor: The therapeutic use of child's play, New York, 1976, Jason Aronson, Inc., p. 27.

51. Resnick, R., and Hergenroeder, E.: Children and the emergency room, Children Today **4:**5, Sept.-Oct., 1975.

52. Robbins, S. M., and Finklestein, J.: Reducing the emotional and economic costs of hospitalization of acutely ill asthmatics; description of an improved emergency room program, Clin. Pediatr. **12:**550, Sept., 1973.

53. Robertson, J.: Young children in hospitals, London, 1958, Tavistock Publications, Ltd.

54. Rose, B. D.: Clinical physiology of acid-base and electrolyte disorders, New York, 1977, McGraw-Hill Book Co.

55. Rosenfeld, W., and others: Improving the clinical management of hypernatremic dehydration, Clin. Pediatr. **16:**411, May, 1977.

56. Roskeis, E., and others: Emergency hospitalization of young children, Med. Care **13:**570, July, 1975.

57. Rothenberg, M. B.: Reactions of children to illness and hospitalization. In Smith, D., and Marshall, R., editors: Introduction to clinical pediatrics, Philadelphia, 1972, W. B. Saunders Co.

58. Rothenberg, M. B.: The unholy trinity—activity, authority, and magic, Clin. Pediatr. **13:**870, Oct., 1974.

59. Schmitt, B. D., and Duncan, B. R.: Ambulatory pediatrics. In Kempe, C. H., and others, editors: Current pediatric diagnosis and treatment, ed. 4, Los Altos, Calif., 1976, Lange Medical Publications, p. 133.

60. Sheil, E. P., and Rice, F.: Project perk-up, Am. J. Nurs. **73:**108, Jan., 1973.

61. Shufer, S.: Teaching via the play-discussion group, Am. J. Nurs. **77:**1960, Dec., 1977.

62. Smith, E. C.: Are you really communicating? Am. J. Nurs. **77:**1966, Dec., 1977.

63. Smith, J. C.: Spending time with the hospitalized child, Matern. Child Nurs. **1:**164, May/June, 1976.

64. Smith, L. F.: An experiment with play therapy, Am. J. Nurs. **77:**1963, Dec., 1977.

65. Snell, B., and McLellan, C. L.: Whetting hospitalized preschoolers' appetites, Am. J. Nurs. **76:**413, March, 1976.

66. Sopakar, B. A. B.: Trickery, white lies and deception in pediatrics, Nursing '74 **3:**11, March, 1974.

67. Spenner, D.: A preschool child copes with hospitalization, Matern. Child Nurs. J. **3:**41, Spring, 1974.

68. Spitz, R. A.: Hospitalism; a follow-up report. In Fenichel, O., and others, editors: The psychoanalytic study of the child, New York, 1946, International University Press.

69. Steele, S., editor: Nursing care of the child with long-term illness, ed. 2, New York, 1977, Appleton-Century-Crofts.

70. Stephens, K. S.: A toddler's separation anxiety, Am. J. Nurs. **73:**1553, Sept., 1973.

71. Tabler, M.: Preview of coming extractions, Nursing '73 **3:**40, Feb., 1973.

72. Tesler, M., and Hardgrove, C.: Cardiac catheterization; preparing the child, Am. J. Nurs. **73:**80, Jan., 1973.

73. Travelbee, J.: To find meaning in illness, Nursing '72 **2:**6, Dec., 1972.

74. Vernon, D. T., and others: The psychological responses of children to hospitalization and illness; a review of the literature, Springfield, Ill., 1965, Charles C Thomas, Publisher.

75. Visintainer, M. A., and Wolfer, J. A.: Psychological preparation for surgical pediatric patients, Pediatrics **56:**187, Aug., 1975.

76. Volicer, B. J.: Patients' perceptions of stressful events associated with hospitalization, Nurs. Res. **23:**235, May-June, 1974.

77. Wallace, H. M.: Survey of hospital care of children and youth in an urban-suburban area—Alameda County, California; implications for planning health care for children and youth, Clin. Pediatr. **16:**682, Aug., 1977.

78. Wear, E. T.: Separation anxiety reconsidered; nursing implications, Matern. Child Nurs. J. **3:**9, Spring, 1974.

79. Weil, W. B.: Acid-base phenomena and the hydrogen ion, J. Pediatr. **83:**359-371, Sept., 1973.

80. Whitson, B. J.: The puppet treatment in pediatrics, Am. J. Nurs. **72:**1612-1614, Sept., 1972.

81. Williams, C. D.: Health services in the home, Pediatrics **52:**773, Dec., 1973.

82. Williams, F.: The crisis of hospitalization, Nurs. Clin. North Am. **9:**37, March, 1974.

# Death and dying during childhood and adolescence

In modern technological societies illness has become a secondary cause of death in childhood, with accidents claiming more children's lives than any other single cause. Medical advances have gradually provided the means of prevention of previously fatal illnesses, and the prognostic outlook for many others has been changed. Thus in today's world a child may be stricken with an illness such as diabetes mellitus that might be expected to cause death eventually, but which can be controlled throughout a normal life span and may only secondarily contribute to the eventual cause of death. Other illnesses, such as cystic fibrosis or nephrotic syndrome, may significantly shorten life, but the possibility for controlling the illness into adulthood has become an increasing reality, and the prognosis is no longer definitely fatal. Such problems as these will be considered in the following chapter, since the focus of care for children with chronic illnesses is that of learning to live with the illness or disability as well as dealing with the face of impending death.

Cancer is the primary illness among children that is still considered fatal. All known forms of cancer can strike children of any age, but the incidence of types of cancer during childhood is unique: leukemia, 40%; brain tumors, 24.1%; kidney and lymph glands, 9.6%; bone cancers, 3.4%; endocrine system malignancy, 3.0%; digestive system malignancy, 1.7%; and all others 11.4%.[39] There are many other causes of death during childhood, including accidents, pneumonia, infectious diseases, and diseases and defects of the cardiovascular, respiratory, gastrointestinal, and nervous systems, but rarely is the anticipation of death such a reality as when the child is stricken with cancer. In many instances death is instantaneous, as with fatal accidents, or progression to death is rapid and not anticipated, such as occurs with fatal poisonings or some infectious diseases. The family is then thrown into immediate grieving, without involvement of the dying child. In other instances the child and family experience a prolonged period when death is anticipated and imminent. The time spent in the hospital with such illnesses has decreased in recent years, and professional medical and nursing care is provided increasingly through clinics and communities.[6] In this chapter we will consider aspects of grieving in relation to family members and the child or adolescent and nursing approaches that are needed for assessment and intervention when a child has died or is dying.

## GRIEF AND ATTITUDES TOWARD DEATH

Grief or mourning is an extremely complex emotion that is not completely understood. It is a difficult emotion to study, because few people have resolved their own inner anxieties regarding the phenomena that elicit mourning, such as death, severe disfigurement, and other human tragedies. We do not understand and cannot comprehend the full meaning of death and, therefore, suffer a great deal of anxiety when faced with it. We build various means of defending ourselves against this anxiety. Some responses are determined by the family and culture of which we are members; other features appear to be common human responses to tragedy.

### Parental grief

The phenomenon of adult mourning has been studied in American culture in recent years, and an increasing understanding is emerging. Emotions such as denial, despair, anger, fear, anxiety, and depression have been linked to the mourning process by various investigators and writers.[3,4,15,39] Many factors influence the response that a family experiences when they find out that their child will die. We will first explore the factors that are particularly important in relation to the mourning of parents and then consider some of the responses that appear to occur frequently among all parents in such a situation.

#### Factors influencing the grief reaction

The fact that a child in the family is dying has major significance for the mourning process. In American cultures, where the present is subordinated for future goals, youth and youthful vigor are admired and valued. When a child who has everything for which to live is found to have a fatal illness, the dreams and ideals of the future are suddenly destroyed. In addition the family may have a great deal of difficulty making optimal use of the time remaining with the child; many families in our culture have become so preoccupied with the future that they no longer appreciate the present for what it is. Finding richness and satisfaction in the experiences that are here and now may be difficult or impossible. The added stress of facing death rather than the anticipated pleasures of the future further inhibits the appreciation of the child as he or she is now. This sense of present orientation may, for some families, offer an important coping mechanism.

During the grieving process and after the death of the child, the family experiences many emotions that are intensified because a child, rather than an older person, has died. Guilt is compounded by feelings that the parent has somehow failed in providing a safe environment or adequate care for the child and that this parental failing is linked to the cause of death. There is a sense of unreality or disbelief that this can happen to a child. Each family member experiences and expresses grief in an individual manner, and their ability to help and support each other is often jeopardized by their own feelings of inner suffering. They cannot help other family members, and they cannot be helped in the intensely individual process of mourning. Rather, individual family members tend to view the grief responses of others in the family as inappropriate or not equal to their own experience of grief, and their anger toward the death is often directed to another family member who is perceived as not grieving or feeling sufficient sorrow. Family disruption frequently emerges, and divorce is common within the first year after the death of a child. The feeling of aloneness in grief is compounded by the fact that few other friends and acquaintances of the family have experienced the death of a child, and there is nobody who can share and understand the intense pain that the parents and family members feel. Other parents who have previously experienced the death of a child even years later are reluctant to reach out to the family because of fears of reactivating their own intense pain and sorrow.[20,22]

Societal avoidance and lack of support for families who experience the death of a child are evidenced by the relative lack of signs of bereavement for parents and the usual lack of emphasis on mourning ceremonies and rituals after a child's death. There is no word label that describes a parent or sibling who has lost a child, equivalent to widow or widower for one who has lost a spouse or orphan for a child who

CHAPTER 18

Children and
youth with
long-term
physical
problems

has lost a parent. Funeral ceremonies and services are often of the most simple type, and the work life of the parents and the school life of siblings and friends are usually expected to go on with little time or attention devoted to the memory of the dead child. Because most people are not able to reach out to assist the parents and siblings in their sorrow, the parents and siblings find themselves in the position of consoling their friends and neighbors by maintaining an external appearance of rapid reentry to a usual life-style, with little or no acknowledgment of their continuing grief.[12]

The nature of the attachment that the family has experienced with the dying child before the illness is an important factor influencing their response to the knowledge of death. Each individual in the family will have experienced a unique relationship with the dead or dying child, and their grief responses, including feelings of ambivalence, will be affected by the nature of their own previous relationship. The maternal relationship is the only attachment that has been studied in relationship to the grief response. The death of a child is a symbolic threat of death to the mother. Mothers report feeling as if they have lost a part of themselves in a way that does not exist for other losses. This may be particularly true for the mother of an infant or unborn child, when the mother has not yet identified the infant as separate from herself. This evidence is contrary to the popular belief that the loss of a fetus or infant is somehow eased by the fact that the family has not known the child as an individual. Resolution of grief for the mother often requires years and necessarily involves her coming to terms with her own mortality and ultimate death.[10,16,17,34,35]

If the child is very young or has been severely ill for a long period of time, the final knowledge that the child will die may bring a sense of relief and assurance that their mourning, which began at the child's birth, may soon be ended. Reinvestment in other interests may increase significantly as if the child were already dead. A similar reaction may be seen in a family that for some reason did not value this particular child. The child may have represented a great financial burden, or the personality and behavioral traits during illness may have been disagreeable

for one or both parents. The nature of this family's mourning will differ from the family who has intensely adored the dying child. Feelings of guilt are particularly significant for the parent who has had long-standing ambivalence toward the dying child.

The parents' previous experiences with death and dying are significant factors in their reaction. In addition the support that they have usually received in stressful situations becomes important in determining what they expect and need from others around them. If they have previously received little assistance from professional helpers during times of stress, they may not be able to easily accept and rely upon professional helpers. If the family is affiliated with a particular religion, a clergyman may be a valuable support during the mourning process.

The religion and beliefs of the family related to life after death also strongly influence their reaction to the death of a child. A family that relies heavily upon their religious beliefs during times of stress usually has straight-forward answers to which they can turn in trying to understand and cope with their sorrow. The parent who had strong religious training as a child and then forsook this background as an adult may have personal problems to resolve, particularly if a belief system has not been built to replace what was rejected. The feelings associated with the loss of childhood faith may stimulate the parent to turn back to that faith, to reject it more intensely, or to finally resolve some of the inner conflicts that have been waged over the years.

The cause of death, as well as the parents' past associations with this cause and their present level of understanding, influences their reaction to death. Cancer is viewed by many as a particularly dreaded disease and one that certainly cannot strike one's own family. It is often viewed as a disease of the elderly and, therefore, children are not expected to be stricken. Cancer is also viewed as an illness that causes a great deal of pain and suffering, and the anticipation of this aspect of the illness for the child is as frightening as the fact of death. Some parents may believe that cancer is contagious and that their other children or they themselves may already be afflicted or will become infected. They may view it as a disgrace, for things like this do not happen to "better" families. They may feel that if they had done their job in providing a healthy home, surely this would not have happened. Inherited disorders that lead to death create intense feelings of guilt. The parents may express feelings of regret for having brought the child into the world and feel that they deserve punishment for inflicting this on their child. Likewise, parents whose child dies as a result of an accident experience intense guilt for not having protected the child from the accident. The felt desire for punishment prolongs the grief and mourning, for the parent feels that their misery is deserved and it somehow pays recompense for the wrong that they have committed against the child.

The size of the family and the placement of the child within the family structure have some bearing on the parents' reactions to the death. The family's attitudes toward family size and the many factors that influenced the number of children in the family (including the planning or lack of planning that was used in structuring the family unit) influence the reaction to loss of a child. If the family values a large family that was not purposely planned, the loss of a single child within this unit may be viewed as another chapter in the family's destiny. If the culture places high values on such a family and they have not fulfilled this ideal either by chance or by choice, the loss of this child will have another meaning for them. If the family is oriented toward valuing each child as an individual regardless of the number of children in the family or the spacing of these children, the loss of the single child will be viewed in a manner different from the family who values the group more centrally. A family may turn their attention and affection to another child, who may yet be unborn, as a "replacement" for the child who is lost. This leads to an unsatisfactory resolution of grief and an inadequate parent-child relationship for the living child.[30]

The prior stability of the family as a unit affects the grieving process for the individuals involved. Parents who have recently experienced separation or divorce or for whom the marital relationship is less than satisfying, suddenly find their own relationship strained by another di-

mension. The illness and death of the child may bring them together, but it usually intensifies the conflict between them. Guilt for the unhappy state of affairs imposed in the dying child's home experiences may become overwhelming for one or both parents, and resolution of their despair may seem impossible. The adults may use the conflicts as a battle ground on which to express their anger and despair over the child's condition and further alienate both themselves and the child from important sources of comfort and support. They may find it difficult or impossible to support the child in the midst of their own suffering and conflict, and help is needed to bring the child's needs into focus for the present. If both parents cannot together provide for the dependency and support needs of the child, they may reach some agreement in providing separately for the needs of the child and thus lay aside some of their personal conflicts.

For any given family there may be other factors that are particularly significant for the child and the family, such as the presence of another adult relative in the family, financial resources, or the social status of the family. These may provide relatively positive or negative factors, depending on the nature of the influence.

### The grief reaction

When parents first learn that their child suffers from a fatal illness or has suddenly died, they initially respond with shock, disbelief, and bewilderment. They find that they cannot fully comprehend the fact for several days. They gradually begin to realize the reality of the facts, and to move gradually into a period of denial of the fact of death or of other aspects of the problem, such as the exact nature of the diagnosis or cause of death. Some degree of denial is probably necessary in the initial grieving process in order to allow the individual to face a reality that is otherwise unbearable. As adults begin to develop more acceptable and mature coping mechanisms for each aspect of the problem, they begin no longer to need denial of these aspects. Either concurrently with denial or as an outgrowth of this phase of mourning, the parents express anger and resentment and experience a period of seeking answers to the question "why did this happen to me?" They may strike out at the physician who has made the initial diagnosis, and as a means of expressing their denial they seek additional consultation and medical opinion in an effort to find out that the physician was mistaken. They may approach each member of the health care team seeking clarification and repeated reaffirmation of each detail of the child's condition. They may express unreasonable anger and resentment toward things that are said to them, and they may become very sensitive to the reactions and services of the professional staff. Some degree of this denial and anger must be respected and recognized for its functional nature.[3]

Most parents continue to express feelings of hope that something will happen to save their child even after they have ceased other forms of denial. They must still deny the inevitability of death, and for some parents this hope provides a significant coping mechanism. After the child's death, they may express the fact that they really knew that nothing could be done, but the hope that something might happen was always present. Other parents do not hope so desperately; they use other means of coping such as providing for the comfort and distraction of the child, withdrawing into a career, or becoming involved in religious activities. The individual parent tends to turn to those mechanisms for coping that have worked well in the past, and thus if the professional helper has some insight into the coping patterns of the parent under prior circumstances, a prediction can be made as to what might happen under the stress of grief. The parent who has turned to drugs or alcohol in the past will often do so again, possibly with greater intensity. If the family has demonstrated the ability to turn to one another in times of stress, they can be expected to be drawn closer together in supporting one another through the crisis. Predicting the responses of each individual in the situation would be a great asset to the professional person attempting to support the family that is coping with grief; potential problems and strengths might be understood and used in guiding the family. For example, one of the child's parents may have great needs to turn to another person for support and help in the grieving process. The other parent may cope by withdrawal into solitude or into the world of work. Because their means of coping are not suited to meeting one another's needs, the couple may experience mutual conflict and significant disruption of their individual capacities to cope. A great deal of professional assistance and understanding may be needed to help them help their child for whom they both mourn.

In the final stages of the mourning process, the parents may begin to come to some level of acceptance or resignation. They begin to reinvest their emotional energy toward another object or person, indicating that they are letting go of the object of their grief. Ideally, this reinvestment begins to some extent just before the death of the child but does not progress to the point of interfering with the parents' abilities to continue a close, supportive relationship with the child. When the child's illness is prolonged and difficult, this reinvestment may begin to occur long before the child dies, with the resulting withdrawal of the parent from the close contact needed by the child. The parents' energies are spent, and they have few resources left to continue to invest in the dying and grieving process. In some instances where the parent and child have experienced a very supportive and close relationship to this point, they may mutually "recognize" the termination of energy resources to give further, and the child begins to "help" the parents to stay away or to transfer their interest to other people and things. The child may find it too painful to watch the parents mourn, may bid the family goodbye too soon, and be left to die alone. If the family has not had a good relationship with the child, they may reinvest easily and quickly, with a minimum of grieving. If reinvestment does not begin to occur while the child lives, the family is faced with a sudden, acute need to reinvest when the child dies. If they cannot do this, they will be tied to the memory of the child, and emotional adjustment is impaired.[3]

When the child finally dies, the parents are faced with a reality that cannot be denied. They very often reexperience each of the components of mourning that they have gone through in the months since they learned of the child's condition. If they are left with very little energy and stamina or if their mourning has been relatively complete during the child's illness, their final reaction to the death of the child may be brief and one of relief. Regardless of the circumstances, their major task becomes one of reinvesting in a future that must exist for those who live and of making a healthy adjustment to a life that has suffered tragedy.[3,21,30]

## Childhood responses to death

While efforts have been made to describe childhood perceptions of death, these remain incompletely understood. We may be able to describe various aspects of the child's experience, but we are not able to know the child's own perceptions completely, because the child remains relatively inept in articulating inner experience. We will examine factors that seem to influence the child's experience and common features of children's responses based on present levels of understanding.

### Factors influencing children's responses

Early life experiences that contribute to the formation of concepts of life and death have not been thoroughly identified, although the literature reports several speculative points of view as to how children develop these highly abstract concepts. The infant may experience "pre-ideas" of death with the sensory experiences of waking and sleeping. The ability to play the game of peekaboo (a term stemming from Old English words meaning "alive or dead") reflects a sense of temporary loss of an object and regaining the object. The experiences of the infant and young child with separation from family members are thought to be a significant influence on the concepts of death that are developed later in childhood.[2,8,12,23] As the child acquires language and is exposed to experiences of death as portrayed on television or through the death of pets or family members, these early experiences contribute to the more conscious awareness of death and a development of a sense of the meaning of life and death.[28]

A child's stage of development in relation to the development of concepts of life and death are important factors influencing responses to his or her own death. Table 17-1 presents a summary of Piaget's[29] description of the development of the concept of life and of Nagy's[26] description of the development of the concept of death.

Each of the factors that were considered as important influences on the parents' grief reaction probably influence the child also. Parental distress is usually conveyed to children, and regardless of whether they are told directly of their condition, they sense the parents' reactions. Each of the stresses that the parents are feeling is likely to either directly or indirectly influence the child. Even if children are too young to comprehend or understand some of the problems involved, they are able to sense the despair and distress of their parents.

Whether or not children are told of their condition remains a significant factor in childrens' response to illness. Their own bodies continually give them clues that something is wrong, and repeated encounters with clinics and hospitals convey a sense of uncertainty and dread. Children's responses to their own impending death depend on their perception of what death is. Ideally, the decision to tell children about their own death should depend primarily on their prior perceptions.[37,38]

Evidence gathered from a projective technique of story-telling by children 6 to 10 years of age suggests that this age group does indeed have a conception of their own impending death, even when they have been carefully protected from knowledge of the diagnosis. These children are not able to express their inner distress and suffering as effectively as the older child, and thus they may use reactions to procedures as a means of coping with their fears of death.[41] Children under 9 or 10 years of age do not have a well-defined concept of death as a final biologic event. It seems evident that knowledge of impending death is not an absolute fact that is either known or not known, but rather that children have differing degrees of awareness and levels of perception of death. By the end of early childhood, most children have had a direct encounter with death, either through the loss of a friend or relative or a household pet. It is conceivable that during early childhood the child could be totally unaware of the phenomenon of death and that his or her concern is centered on physical illness

**Table 17-1.** Summary of the development of concepts of life (Piaget) and the development of concepts of death (Nagy)*

| Age (years) | Concepts of life (Piaget) | Age (years) | Concepts of death (Nagy) |
|---|---|---|---|
| 4-6 | Everything that moves is regarded as alive. | 3-5 | Death is temporary and reversible; death is equated with immobility. |
| 6-7 | Consciousness is attributed to things that move. | | |
| 8-10 | Makes distinction between objects that move of their own accord, which are viewed as conscious (sun, people), and objects that receive movement from another source, which are viewed as not conscious. | 5-9 | Personification of death occurs; death is perceived as inevitable for all people but is equated with old age and with other people. |
| Over 11 | Life and consciousness are regarded as the property of plants and animals, including humans, or to animals and humans alone. | 9-12 | Death is viewed as a cessation of body function, as an experience that is universal and final, and one to which the child is subject. |

*Adapted from Shuler, S. N.: Death during childhood; reactions in parents and children. In Brandt, P. A., and others, editors: Current practice in pediatric nursing, vol. 2, St. Louis, 1978, The C. V. Mosby Co., p. 109.

and the separation that is imposed as a result of the illness.

Related to children's perception of their own impending death is the degree to which they are able to express their fears and anxieties. Contrary to the common assumption that discussion with children of their own condition leads to further anxiety and distress, such discussion has been demonstrated to decrease insecurity related to loneliness, isolation, alienation, concern regarding the intent and purpose of therapeutic efforts, guilt related to the origin of the illness, and fear that life may end as a punishment for misdeeds.[41] Such discussions may be difficult or impossible for parents to participate in at first, but some provision must be made for these inner needs of the child. If parents are not able to face a discussion with the child involving impending death, they may be able to find some way to help their child concerning loneliness, alienation, guilt, or other factors that may be easier to approach than the fact of death. As they gain confidence in their own ability to provide help for their child and to cope with their own inner grief, they may be able to respond to the child's direct concerns with death.

The amount and extent of pain that children must endure influence their reaction. They may not be totally able to translate an extensive experience with pain as a bad prognostic sign, but the fact that they are suffering elicits fears and distress and demoralizes the young child's spirit. Other important factors are the child's previous coping capacities, religious education, and the nature of relationship with parents before the illness.

### Features of childhood responses

The more closely the child's perception of death approximates that of most adults in the culture, the more like the adult reaction is his or her own. Most adolescents understand death as a biologic reality, and they attach various religious meanings according to their cultural inheritance. Thus the adolescent most often progresses through a course of several interrelating reactions that might closely approximate that of the parents.[1,18,25,39,41]

During the later childhood years the reactions to impending death are more varied, since children's understanding of the problem varies greatly. The predominant reaction of the fatally ill child between the ages of 6 and 10 years has been identified by some investigators as being protest and fear of diagnostic and treatment procedures. The child of this age usually knows about death but often regards it as a person. It seems clear that most children in this age group are not able to express their own fears and distress as directly as the older child or adolescent, and they are only able to express fear of death through indirect means of play, reaction to procedures, and other behavioral changes.[39,41] Be-

**695**

havioral changes may have been the first clue that something was wrong, and these changes may be identified by adults as being related to the discomfort of the physical illness rather than as an expression of inner emotional suffering and fear.

Children under the age of 6 years react predominantly to the fear of separation. They deny death or view it as a condition that is not permanent. This reaction, as we have noted, is not unusual for children in this age group, and thus it is difficult to determine the child's specific reaction to death or to knowledge of impending death. Because their ability to conceptualize death is just beginning to develop, they probably react primarily to physical pain and to the clues they sense within their own bodies that all is not well. Their need for dependency and attachment to significant adults is heightened as their well-being is threatened, and indeed may be more intense than the same reaction experience in a child who is not fatally ill. The child may regress in expressing dependency and separation fears.[25,39,41,43]

### The professional helper

Becoming involved in a relationship with parents and children who are experiencing impending death is probably one of the most difficult aspects of child nursing. Most of us are uncertain of our own ability to relate to people who are suffering this human tragedy, and because of the intense feelings that we experience, we prefer to concentrate our attention and efforts on other areas of child health care. Nurses have not, in the past, been generally successful in helping families of dying children, and we need to consider carefully ways in which we might increase our ability to form a meaningful helping relationship in such a situation.[13]

#### Responses of the health care worker

The first consideration for professional health care workers to acknowledge is that most of the factors that typically influence the parent are important factors influencing their own reaction to the dying child and death. Simply being a professionally prepared health care worker does not make one immune to the effects of past training and learned attitudes toward death. We

tend to have specific reactions to the nature of certain illnesses, and we regard death from some conditions as more dreaded than others. We have inner reactions of mourning in the face of death, even though the dying child is not our own. Our own religious preferences influence our reaction to people who are involved in the dying process, as do other culturally determined attitudes. In addition, our past experiences with death and dying children greatly influence the reaction we experience. If we are facing our first experience with a dying child, we may react much as the parents in facing the child's death. We then begin either to develop defenses against the pain and discomfort felt upon that first encounter, along with increasing skill and talent in working with these families, or to develop defenses that inhibit our effectiveness. Thus it is important to consider one's own inner reactions and beliefs and to seek to resolve some of the inner anxieties regarding death.

Health care workers, like parents, tend to turn to their previous manner of coping with unusual stress when coping with dying children and their families.[3,39] If the professional person usually becomes increasingly compulsive under stress, this reaction will become more intense. The person who tends to become aloof and withdrawn will do so in relation to dying children and families. The individual who tends to intellectualize will do so increasingly as death nears. If our individual stress reactions tend to interfere with effective helping during the dying process, some measures must be taken to understand our own personality dynamics and to find ways to overcome the reaction or to recognize the signals that we are no longer able to carry out a helping relationship with the family.[7,31,40]

Experiences with each family will vary, and professional helpers may be able to cope adequately with inner stress with one family and not with another. In other situations they may be able to work effectively with a family for a period of time and then become unable to provide the needed helping relationship. A nurse, for example, may find that establishing a helping relationship with several families has been a rewarding and meaningful experience. Coping with inner stresses was possible, and the families expressed gratitude for and satisfaction with the help received. On one occasion, however, the fatally ill child may be one with whom the nurse identifies. The stress of working with this child may be too great, and the realization that this child could be her own may be overwhelming. Another member of the health care team must then become the primary helper for the family, and the nurse must maintain a rather distant, but interested, concern for the family and child. For the nurse, attention should be centered upon understanding the meaning of the experience for her own personal growth.

### Developing professional and personal coping skills

The most valuable therapeutic tool in working with families experiencing the death of a child is the self of the helper. However, in order to be able to use the self effectively in helping grieving families, the nurse and the health care team must be aware of their own needs for growth, for outlets for expression of their own sorrow experienced with the family and child, and for a network of interpersonal support. Without carefully planned provisions for these needs, the health care team will respond to repeated encounters with death in a manner similar to that of many families with repressed feelings—hostility toward one another, disruption within the group, and ineffectiveness in providing care.[13,14]

First, the health care team needs to determine their own philosophy, which will guide their actions and decisions in dealing with the emotional and physical needs of families and dying children. The underlying problems of the basic right of the child to know the facts and seriousness of the illness, the ethical problems inherent in prolonging life, and the responsibility of parents and health care workers in making life and death decisions need to be fully explored and discussed by every member of a health care team. In many settings where children are cared for who are dying, the additional problems of human experimentation with drugs and other life-saving measures are encountered daily, and the health care team must determine their own values and priorities in relation to human values and the advancement of science,

particularly when a conflict exists between these two areas of concern. The goal of mutual discussion is to achieve respect for each individual's point of view and establish a means of working within a mutually accepted group philosophy at the same time. For example, a health care team may develop a philosophy that favors discontinuing heroic measures for prolonging a child's life in the face of inevitable death and uses this philosophy to guide parents in making decisions related to the medical choices for treatment. If an individual working with this team favors, for herself, the use of heroic measures because of the inherent value of human life and the ultimate difficulty in defining a situation of "inevitable" death, the team can openly discuss the possible conflicts that might arise for the individual and support her when such a conflict arises.

Another concern that needs to be worked out by the health care team is that of individual reactions and response to personal grief. Each person's manner of responding needs to be respected and understood, and provisions made for expression of sorrow, anger, guilt, and fear. Some professional helpers need to talk freely and openly to ventilate their own feelings. Others need privacy and retreat, and others need to unload their feelings in "explosions" of words or tears. The health care team members need to apply all of their understanding of the varied reactions to grief in understanding one another and in providing mutual support for resolving these feelings. When a member of a health care team has reached his or her emotional limits in dealing with repeated death experiences, the individual needs support from the team in taking a period of time away from the situation in order to maintain a sense of emotional balance.[7,13,33,42]

## NURSING ASSESSMENT AND DIAGNOSIS
### Assessment tools

Comprehensive assessment of the child, the family, and the child's usual social environment is essential in planning adequate care for the child and each member of the family. Equipped with objective evidence regarding a particular child's life space and inner perceptions and the problems inherent to the child's illness, the nurse can plan for meeting the real needs of the child and the family.

The essential components of the nursing assessment are unchanged for the child and family experiencing impending death, but obtaining insight and accurate interpretation requires particular skill and experience with the family over an extended period of time. Children who suffer a fatal illness are in many respects more like their healthy peers than unlike them and continue to grow and develop in each competency area, even though the physical illness may take a toll in each area of function. While health care cannot provide an indefinite life span, the basic goals to attain, regain, and maintain a state of health may be possible for the periods of life remaining and for the entire family, who will live on. The quality of life remaining depends to a great extent on the ability of the child to maintain a healthy inner sense of self and satisfying relationships with significant people in the family and friendship circle. These factors also significantly influence the family's ability to reconstruct their own lives after the child's death. If they can finish unfinished business in their relationship with the child and achieve a sense of having provided for the child's care and comfort during the process of dying, their accomplishment of these tasks contributes to their ability to resolve feelings of guilt, anger, and sorrow when the fact of death arrives.[36] One of the hazards that exists for a family who experiences the sudden death of a child is the lack of an opportunity to finish unfinished business and to assure the child of their care, love, and support before the moment of permanent separation.

The following approaches in the early assessment are essential in obtaining accurate information upon which to plan care:

1. Careful observation of the child and family behaviors and detection of verbal cues is essential. Because they are fearful, disbelieving, and often in shock, the parents' ability to verbalize openly is often jeopardized, and the overt content of verbal responses to interview questions may present an overly optimistic or overly pessimistic interpretation of their coping powers.

2. Early assessment encounters should provide an opportunity to approach fears and areas of concern that frequently occur for families in order to assist them in bringing their own feelings to the surface.

3. A third-person style of interview is often helpful, not only for the child or adolescent but for parents as well. For example, the nurse might state, "Another mother I know had great difficulty in deciding how she was going to tell her parents about her child's illness. Is this a problem for you?" The fictitious third person's circumstances can be explored in more detail if the parents seem to respond favorably and are more easily able to talk about someone other than themselves.

4. Maintain frequent availability and interaction with the child and family, whether the child is treated in the hospital or at home. Frequent contact involving ordinary daily activities or centering on other concerns facilitates developing a sense of trust and confidence, which in turn makes it possible for the family to reveal more accurately the nature of their inner experience of the situation.

5. Doll play, puppet play, and drawing are important tools for assessment of the child. These approaches are described in previous chapters in relation to assessment of social and inner competencies. Themes that the child might express through these forms of play are fear of body mutilation, fear of separation, fear of abandonment, perceptions of death, and feelings of guilt and punishment for wrong-doing. Through play the child may also reveal the coping mechanisms that are being used in relation to the experiences that the child feels.

### Nursing diagnoses

In addition to the nursing diagnoses that are made in relation to the child's physical illness (see Chapter 18), the nurse will identify problems and diagnoses related to the psychosocial needs of the child in dealing with the illness and impending death (MNPC no. 4 in category no. 31). The assessment data that support the identification of each of these problems are variable and unique to each individual child, although further clinical investigation may reveal general patterns of response that can ultimately be described and formulated as criteria for diagnosis. Problems that are often identified for the child, parents, siblings, and other significant persons include:

1. Fear of body mutilation or pain
2. Fear of separation or abandonment
3. Premature separation between child and family
4. Repressed fear, anger, guilt or sorrow; depression
5. Loss of hope; despair
6. Excessive denial
7. Family disintegration related to stress of impending death
8. Psychosocial isolation and lack of support from significant others
9. Financial depletion related to illness
10. Neglect of siblings
11. Decision-making stress related to prolonging life
12. Spiritual/religious crisis
13. Inappropriate reinvestment object; child substitute
14. Need for knowledge and understanding of illness and responses to illness
15. Inappropriate feelings of guilt and self-punishment

## NURSING INTERVENTION

Some of the approaches recommended during the experience of death are not adequately understood and are subject to further investigation. The following discussion summarizes approaches that have been identified as particularly important for families and children.

### Informing child of illness and death

It appears clear that children need to have some understanding of their own illness in order to express and work out their own inner fears and anxieties.[39,41] They may or may not be told the exact diagnosis, but they need to have the reassurance that someone understands the distress they feel inside. The family and the professional members of the health care team usually come to some decision regarding what and how to tell a child about the illness. Factors to be considered include the family's preference, the age and stage of development of the child, the ways in which the child previously coped with stress, and the child's direct or indirect request for information. It seems evident that

most children over the age of 5 or 6 years have some comprehension of the seriousness of their illness even though they are not told the diagnosis. Adjustment to the problem appears to be more satisfactory if they are told certain important aspects of the problem. Older children and adolescents with leukemia, for example, need to have some understanding that they may experience repeated hospitalization, blood transfusion, drugs that may make them feel sick, and repeated physical signs of illness. They need the advantage of developing coping mechanisms for these experiences in advance, and they need the opportunity to express fears and anxieties before and as they happen.[13,27,39,41]

### Providing a network of support

Ample availability of health care workers seems essential in working with families of dying children.[7,13,33,39,42] Parents may find that it is exceedingly difficult to approach subjects of concern. They may need prolonged contact and interaction with a professional worker while attention is centered on peripheral concerns before they are able to approach a very sensitive concern. Prolonged, frequent contact with a family during such activities as physical care, treatment procedures, feeding, or play is made available. The sense of availability is enhanced when the nurse is unhurried and takes time to pursue casual conversation with the child and the family even though the time spent with them may not be optimal. Ways of approaching topics of common concern should be developed by the nurse to provide a means for assistance and support. For example, after the parents have learned of their child's condition, some member of the health care team should approach the topic of how the parents can relate to and help their child. Most parents are frightened and anxious in anticipating these first encounters, particularly when they have decided to tell the child the seriousness of the illness. The health care worker may be able to offer the parents suggestions on how to talk with their child the first time and to explore with them whether they would like help during their first conversations with their child. They may prefer to have the health care worker begin the conversation with the child and to remain with them as they enter into the interaction. Other families prefer to be alone but would like someone near to support them and the child once this first encounter has ended. Knowing that someone is near who can offer comfort and support after a difficult experience may make the difference in the parents being able to approach the experience. Whether these approaches are planned or not, the skillful helper is always aware of the needs of the people involved and provides real guidance and help as appropriate to the situation.

Another area of concern for the health care team is that of providing consistent information to the child and the family during the course of the illness. Most parents go through a period when they are desperate to have more information and to explore all of the possibilities for error. When they receive conflicting information during this time or at any other point during the grieving process, conflict and distress are likely to result.[39,41]

Even when they are given accurate information, there may be conflicting interpretations from various members of the health care team. Every effort should be made to have mutual understanding of what is being shared with the family at each point of the child's illness. For example, one health care worker may believe in promoting and supporting the family's feelings of hope throughout the course of the child's illness. This health care worker will tend to interpret new symptoms and events as temporary conditions that can be treated and overcome with medication. Another health care worker may feel that an attitude of realism should be fostered and will interpret the new symptoms as ominous signs that the child's condition is worsening. Such conflicting attitudes and approaches should be acknowledged by the health care team working together, and some unity should be developed when working with a particular family. This does not mean that individual workers need to discard their personal attitudes and beliefs, but they should consider the family's needs as a first priority and put aside their own feelings when necessary. One family may be identified by the team as becoming completely immobilized and ineffective in helping their child if they cannot continue to have hope

for the outcome of the illness. Another family may be identified as being paralyzed in the denial phase of their mourning experience when hope is emphasized. They continue, at great expense, to shop intently for new cures and miracles, and they neglect the reality of the child's distress.

## Support for siblings and playmates

Another aspect of the helping relationship involves other children who know the dying child. The child's siblings, playmates, and other children in a hospital setting need help in understanding the things that are happening to the child who is dying.[5,9,39] Children who are near the dying child in age or close in relationships tend to develop anxiety and fear on their own behalf; they are afraid that they will become ill or die. Their own concept of death and dying is greatly affected by the death of the child, and they need a great deal of help in working through their own confusing perceptions. Parents may be able to cope with this aspect well at first, but at the time of death they may not be able to help the other children for several days, and professional help may be particularly indicated. During the time that parents are beginning to reinvest their interest away from the dying child before the actual death, they may turn their attention and physical contact to siblings or to other children in the hospital. This diversion and reinvestment may be necessary and healthy for the parent and may be important for the children receiving attention. The dying child's needs must continue to be considered, however, and some balance should be maintained.

## Principles of counseling

In counseling children who are dying, their families, and families of a child who has died, several different counseling approaches may be needed. Active listening, described in Chapter 2, is one of the most important therapeutic approaches when a child or family needs to ventilate feelings of anger, fear, anxiety, guilt, despair, or sorrow. Skilled use of touch is an important means of communicating understanding and care. When a person is expressing anger, touch is usually not appropriate, and the person is likely to reject it. If feelings of anger are being repressed and touch elicits rejection or an outburst of anger directed toward the person who has touched, the response indicates the underlying feelings that need expression.

When a child or family ask questions about the illness, cause of death, or impending death, their questions should be answered truthfully, simply, and directly. The health care team needs to determine in advance how they will respond to usual questions posed by dying children and assist the parents in preparation for responding to these questions. For example, a young child, older child, or adolescent often asks the question, "Am I going to die?" The parents and health care team need to be prepared to respond simply with "Yes, you are going to die," and then wait to respond to any other questions the child might ask or to feelings that are expressed, rather than proceed with a lengthy and detailed explanation or discussion of other factors. Responses such as "Everybody dies" or "I don't know" are obvious evasions of the child's own needs and constitute for the child a rejection of his or her own experience and feeling. Likewise, asking if the child thinks he or she is going to die or using a question to explore the child's feelings is inappropriate in response to a direct question.[2,15]

## Decision-making related to prolonging life

One final consideration to be made in relation to modern treatment and care during terminal illness is the ethical and moral issue of when and how to prolong life and when to let the natural effects of illness intervene and let death occur. In some instances the wishes of the child and the family become very intense and they urge the physician to cease all efforts to prolong life, or they urge that all efforts necessary to prolong the child's life be taken. In other instances a medical decision is made to advise the family to take one course or the other. Professional health care workers' own attitudes toward medical and nursing intervention to either prolong life or to allow death vary considerably and involve great internal conflict. Most professional people find these decisions difficult or impossible to resolve. Legal considerations are great, but at present there are no universal guidelines, whether legal, moral, or ethical, that will help in making a decision. The decision may be made by a child and the family that intervention to prolong life be discontinued, but honoring this wish may be difficult or impossible for the health care worker who strongly opposes allowing death when life can be prolonged. Another professional person may feel that the cost of living is too great in a certain instance, and that death should be allowed to come naturally. Formulas to fit each occasion are not possible to outline, since each situation will be different from all others. The health care team may need help from other resources in the hospital or community as they face these difficult decisions, and they must live with the actions required to carry them out.*

## STUDY QUESTIONS

1. Identify a professional person who has had a great deal of experience in helping dying children and their families. Determine his or her philosophy toward the dying child and the family, and how he or she approaches these situations. Describe this person's recommendations for someone who is interested in developing skills that would be helpful to the child and family.

2. Investigate and contrast the major religious points of view toward death. Describe how these attitudes and beliefs would affect the grieving responses of both the child and the parents. Identify how a professional helper could enlist religious assistance for a given family who might desire this and what the nature of involvement with clergymen tends to be within the various major religions.

3. Choose a fatal illness in which there is a period of time between the knowledge of the prognosis and the actual death. Describe the illness or condition and identify the medical treatment and nursing care that might be indicated. Also indicate specific involvement of other health care team members that might be specifically required.

4. Explore either on your own or in cooperation with a classmate your own responses to the dying child. If possible, spend some time caring for a child who is dying either in the home or in the hospital and explore how your responses affected your encounter with the child and the family. Discuss your feelings and experience with your colleagues and explore ways in which various reactions of the group might either help or hinder a helping relationship with a family whose child is dying. An experienced professional helper might be enlisted as resource during your discussion.

*References 11, 19, 24, 32, 33, 42.

**REFERENCES**

1. Brandt, P. A.: The nurse and the adolescent face death. In Kalafatich, A. J., editor: Approaches to the care of adolescents, New York, 1975, Appleton-Century-Crofts, p. 221.
2. Crase, D.: Death and the young child; some practical suggestions on support and counseling, Clin. Pediatr. **14**:747, Aug., 1975.
3. Easson, W. M.: The family of the dying child, Pediatr. Clin. North Am. **19**:1157, Nov., 1972.
4. Engel, G. L.: Grief and grieving, Am. J. Nurs. **64**:93, Sept., 1964.
5. Everson, S.: Sibling counseling, Am. J. Nurs. **77**:644, April, 1977.
6. Fernbach, D. J., Henrich, W. L., and Starling, K. A.: Acute leukemia in children; time spent in hospitalization, Pediatrics **49**:765, May, 1972.
7. Gould, R. K., and Rothenberg, M. B.: The chronically ill child facing death—how can the pediatrician help? Clin. Pediatr. **12**:447, July, 1973.
8. Grollman, E. A.: Explaining death to children, Boston, 1967, Beacon Press.
9. Gyulay, J.: The forgotten grievers, Am. J. Nurs. **75**:1476, Sept., 1975.
10. Hagan, J. M.: Infant death; nursing interaction and intervention with grieving families, Nurs. Forum **13**:371, 1974.
11. Heffron, W. A., Bommelaere, K., and Masters, R.: Group discussions with the parents of leukemic children, Pediatrics **52**:831, Dec., 1973.
12. Kastenbaum, R. J.: Death, society, and human experience, St. Louis, 1977, The C. V. Mosby Co.
13. Kavanaugh, R. E.: Dealing naturally with dying, Nursing '76 **6**:22, Oct., 1976.
14. Kirkpatrick, J., Hoffman, I., and Futterman, E. H.: Dilemma of trust; relationship between medical care givers and parents of fatally ill children, Pediatrics **54**:169, Aug., 1974.
15. Kubler-Ross, E.: On death and dying, New York, 1969, Macmillan Publishing Co., Inc.
16. Kübler-Ross, E.: Questions and answers on death and dying, New York, 1974, Macmillan Publishing Co., Inc.
17. Kübler-Ross, E., editor: Death: The final stage of growth, Englewood Cliffs, N.J., 1975, Prentice-Hall, Inc.
18. Lacasse, C. M.: A dying adolescent, Am. J. Nurs. **75**:433, March, 1975.
19. Lascari, A. D., and Stehbens, J. A.: The reactions of families to childhood leukemia; an evaluation of a program of emotional management, Clin. Pediatr. **12**:210, April, 1973.
20. MacIver, R.: Death of a child, San Francisco Sunday Examiner and Chronicle, May 9, 1976.
21. Mann, S. A.: Coping with a child's fatal illness; a parent's dilemma, Nurs. Clin. North Am. **9**:81, March, 1974.
22. Marks, M. J. B.: The grieving patient and family, Am. J. Nurs. **76**:1488, Sept., 1976.
23. Maurer, A.: Maturation of concepts of death, Br. J. Med. Psychol. **39**:35, 1966.
24. Morison, R. S.: Dying, Sci. Am. **229**:54, Sept., 1973.
25. Morrisey, J. R.: Death anxiety in children with a fatal illness. In Parod, H., editor: Crisis intervention, New York, 1965, Family Service Association of America.
26. Nagy, M. H.: The child's theory concerning death, J. Genet. Psychol. **73**:3, 1948.
27. Northrup, F. C.: The dying child, Am. J. Nurs. **74**:1066, June, 1974.
28. Parness, E.: Effects of experiences with loss and death among preschool children, Children Today **4**:2, Nov.-Dec., 1975.
29. Piaget, J.: Six psychological studies, New York, 1968, Random House, Inc.
30. Poznanski, E. O.: The "replacement child"; a saga of unresolved parental grief, J. Pediatr. **81**:1190, Dec., 1972.
31. Schneiderman, G., Lowden, J. A., and Rae-Grant, Q.: Family reactions, physician responses and management issues in fatal lipid storage diseases, Clin. Pediatr. **15**:887, Oct., 1976.
32. Schowalter, J. E., Ferholt, J. B., and Mann, N. M.: The adolescent patient's decision to die, Pediatrics **51**:97, Jan., 1973.
33. Schulman, J.: Coping with tragedy—successfully facing the problem of a seriously-ill child, Chicago, 1976, Follett Publishing Co.
34. Seitz, P., and Warrick, L. H.: Perinatal death; the grieving mother, Am. J. Nurs. **74**:2028, Nov., 1974.
35. Shuler, S. N.: Death during childhood; reactions in parents and children. In Brandt, P. A., and others, editors: Current practice in pediatric nursing, vol. 2, St. Louis, 1978, The C. V. Mosby Co., p. 109.
36. Singher, L. J.: The slowly dying child, Clin. Pediatr. **13**:861, Oct., 1974.
37. Spinetta, J. J., and Maloney, L. J.: Death anxiety in the outpatient leukemic child, Pediatrics **56**:1034, Dec., 1975.
38. Spinetta, J. J., Rigler, D., and Karon, M.: Anxiety in the dying child, Pediatrics **52**:841, Dec., 1973.
39. Steele, S.: Nursing care of the child with a fatal prognosis. In Steele, S., editor: Nursing care of the child with long-term illness, ed. 2, New York, 1977, Appleton-Century-Crofts.
40. Tietz, W., and Powars, D.: The pediatrician and the dying child, Clin. Pediatr. **14**:585, June, 1975.
41. Waechter, E. H.: The responses of children to fatal illness. In Duffey, M., and others, editors: Current concepts in clinical nursing, vol. 3, St. Louis, 1971, The C. V. Mosby Co., p. 115.
42. Wessel, M. A.: The dilemma of dying, Clin. Pediatr. **16**:1093, Dec., 1977.
43. Yakulis, I. M.: Changing concepts of death in a child with sickle cell disease, Matern. Child Nurs. J. **4**:117, Summer, 1975.

# Children and youth with long-term physical problems

Children and youth who have long-term physical problems present a special challenge to the health care worker. Such problems may vary in severity, but the essential feature of a long-term problem is the need to continuously take the problem into account when giving health care. The condition may be severe to the extent that the child's life is periodically threatened, or it may be a minor problem that seldom needs direct attention. For example, children with cystic fibrosis, diabetes mellitus, or a central nervous system birth defect have daily concerns and problems with which to contend, including the possibility of acute phases of illness or death. Other children may have problems such as chronic allergies, asthma, permanent eye muscle imbalances, or permanent injury to a limb, which present relatively minor adjustment problems and usually are controlled and treated by medical or surgical means or by environmental control.

In this chapter we will consider factors common to problems that tend to last and continually affect the child's health and health care. Description of specific conditions is given, and the reader is referred to comprehensive literature for thorough understanding of these and other less common conditions.

Several problems of a long-term or chronic nature are discussed in other chapters of this text because of their relationship with specific age groups or because of the episodic nature of the course of illness. The pathophysiologic basis of allergy and the medical considerations related to asthma are presented in Chapter 13. Other allergic conditions are considered in Chapters 11 and 13. Other respiratory problems that sometimes develop into a long-term problem in early childhood, such as otitis media and tonsillitis, are presented in Chapter 11. Long-term sensory problems and learning problems are discussed in Chapter 19.

## COMPETENCY DEVELOPMENT AND LONG-TERM PHYSICAL PROBLEMS

A long-term physical problem inevitably is a factor to be considered in defining appropriate competency development for individual children. Their physical problem may impose a serious limiting factor in the development of competencies, or it may simply serve as a factor to shape and influence the unique way in which the child develops. In addition, a single competency is rarely affected alone. The primary effect of most physical problems is on the child's physical competency, but as the child grows and develops the effects on thinking, social, or inner competencies may be more significant. **703**

## Physical competency

Most long-term physical problems exert some influence on the child's physical competency. Nursing assessment provides (1) a continuing evaluation of the child's level of physical competency, (2) judgment regarding the optimal level of functioning, and (3) the basis upon which to plan and implement care to maintain and promote optimal health. Skill in making appropriate judgments may require that the health care worker initially focus upon a specific long-term problem, such as children with birth defects. This facilitates both development of a thorough knowledge base in this area and acquisition of experience in application of relevant knowledge in formulating health care decisions.

In some instances the effect of the problem may be relatively stable, in that the child's limitations or the adjustments required are usually predictable and rarely vary. For example, children who have a permanent orthopedic handicap may have permanent, unchangeable orthopedic limitations that require similar kinds of physical adjustments throughout life. They will probably go through periods when their coping capacity is greater or lesser than at other times, and their sensitivity to social limitations and interactions changes through the years, causing their physical adjustment to vary somewhat. However, the actual physical limitation and adjustment, as unaffected by other areas of adjustment, remain quite stable.

In some instances the child may begin with limitations and adjustments that are great in magnitude, and as the initial treatment, learning, and adjustment evolve, the effect may lessen. Such an instance might be the experience of children who suffer severe, extensive burns. The initial physical problems are great, and life may be threatened by the extent of the burns. Physical limitations are great and remain significant for several weeks or months. As the tissues heal and corrective surgery is undertaken, some degree of function is restored. Physical therapy further restores the physical capacity and helps them to gain new competencies that are appropriate for their stage of development. Some limitations and adjustments are permanent, but they gradually are able to improve and increase their capacity.

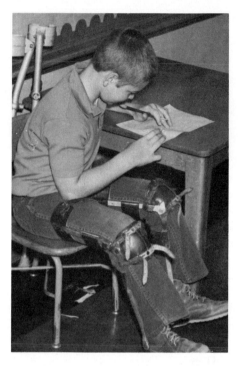

**Fig. 18-1.** The child who has a physical problem is often able to perform similarly to his peers in the areas of learning and thought.

Some children have a physical problem that tends to deteriorate or worsen over the years, with a decline in performance expected. Such circumstances are illustrated by children who are born with a central nervous system defect that leads to impairment of function at or below the level of the thoracic vertebrae. The physiologic function of the renal system may be expected to deteriorate over several months or years, with increasing demands for medical and surgical treatment and intervention in order to maintain optimal function.

Environmental factors often provide significant considerations in determining children's physical competency. If children are confined to wheel chairs, the problems of mobility that they face in an area where there are long winters with heavy snowfalls are significantly different from the mobility problems faced by children who live in a tropical area. The family's ability to adjust to the problem is a significant determinant in the kind of physical adjustments that are possible. The age at which children first encounter the long-term problem, the way in which their problem is viewed by others in society, whether they are boys or a girls, and their natural or acquired talents and capacities in other areas of functioning are all factors that influence their unique reaction and ongoing attainment of physical competency.

## Learning and thought competency

Learning and thought competency may or may not be affected by a long-term physical problem. In some instances, such as with a central nervous system defect, learning and thought competency deficits may be part of the child's total problem. In many instances, however, children with physical problems may be expected to function similarly to their peers in the area of learning and thought. Indirect influences on children's capacity often do occur. Children who have hemophilia may be gifted in learning and thought capacities and, indeed, may develop intense superior performance stimulated by the need to excel in at least one area.

In addition to the nursing assessment of cognitive and learning skills as described in Chapters 9, 10, 12, and 14, children's perceptions of their own physical problem and related treatment or management should be assessed. As their cognitive capacity increases, so should their understanding of the physical problem and of all aspects related to treatment. Their growing ability to participate in management or treatment should be encouraged as they demonstrate readiness to understand and comprehend essential information and concepts. For example, diabetic children who can comprehend essential facts about their condition and can perform motor and cognitive tasks essential to administration of insulin, diet, and exercise management should learn to assume these aspects of their care.[48]

## Social competency

Children's social competency depends primarily upon their relationship with parents. Parental attitudes toward their illness or disability and their ability to maintain appropriate parent-child relationships influence the ability to relate to all persons. If the nature of the parent-child relationship changes when a physical problem arises, the change is confusing and distressing to children. As children are able to maintain and experience satisfying social relationships, they are able to view themselves as competent and productive individuals.

The effect of long-term physical problems on social competency during later childhood depends significantly upon the visibility of the problem, the family's reaction to the problem, and the dynamics between each of the competencies and other aspects of the environment. If children have physical problems that are highly visible to other people and that set them apart as someone who is different, deformed, or unintelligent, they are likely to have increasingly difficult social adjustments to make as they grow older. Children and youth with cerebral palsy, for example, may have extreme difficulty in communicating and in performing ordinary motor tasks and may appear unattractive according to society's standards. Most people are afraid of interaction or contact with individuals who are so afflicted, or they avoid contact because they do not know what to do or say to the individual. Uncomfortable feelings of pity, sorrow, or inner conflict are aroused, and it is easier to remain distant from social contact with persons who have such physical problems. Thus these children are placed in a socially isolated position, and the problems of entering the social world of peers are so great that they or their family prefer to perpetuate comfortable isolation rather than to continually face social frustrations of the larger world. Most physically handicapped children have personal strengths that can be developed and cultivated in order to help them achieve satisfying social relationships, but these may be hidden from view by the reactions and feelings of the professional health care worker, the family, or children themselves.

At the times of life when peer relationships are vitally important to healthy social development, young physically handicapped person may find it almost unbearable to be so different. It may be advantageous to children to have a number of peers who have problems similar to their own in order to have social experiences that are not clouded with the reaction to being different. By sharing mutual problems, the children may help one another find and develop reasonable personal resources with which to cope in the larger world of peers. When children have been a member of a group of children without physical handicaps from early stages of development, they may not find this feeling of being different quite so distressing. Helping the family to find and promote satisfying social relationships early in life and to continue to seek these opportunities for the child throughout childhood can promote development in this area of competency.

When physical problems are not readily visible but impose some limitations on social participation, children have specific kinds of social adjustments to make. Children who have hemophilia, for example, may be limited in participation in physical contact sports. Having to sit on the sidelines sets them apart from other children, and they are faced with the need to continually make an explanation for their limitations. This kind of social isolation can be a significant deterrent to healthy social competency development, and the child may need special counseling and guidance through some of the years when peer relationships are particularly important.[18,34,76]

## Inner competency

As with each of the other competency areas, physical problems have variable effects on inner competency development. Because inner competency depends intimately on development in each of the other areas, children who have some difficulty or problem in other areas may be expected to be affected in relation to inner competency. Indirect clues that indicate that children are having some particular inner distress or struggle may lead to the decision to obtain professional evaluation of inner competency and to provide help for the child and family in finding ways to promote healthy inner development.

In addition to demonstrating well-adapted behavior at home, in school, and with peers, evaluation of certain aspects specifically related to the stress of long-term problems helps to identify the adequacy of children's inner adjustment. Understanding of their condition and ac-

ceptance of limitations, along with their ability to participate in their own care, indicates the nature of their adjustment. Most children with long-term physical problems use their problem occasionally as a vehicle for conflict between themselves and parents, peers, or teachers. They may refuse to cooperate with required care, or they use the problem as a means of escaping some unpleasant situation, such as a test or disciplinary action. These behaviors are not significantly different from those used by other children in attempting to control their environment. When the family is able to react to the behavior in the same realistic fashion that they would were the physical problem not involved, the child is able to develop adequate inner discipline and a self-concept that is not overly solicitous of the physical problem.

Well-adjusted children have an accurate sense of reality, without inappropriate use of defenses, denial, dependence, or independence. When children encounter stress, they can use effective means of coping that are appropriate for their stage of development. This may involve denial, dependence, hope, appropriate control and release of emotions, or rationalizations. For example, many children with long-term physical problems use denial as a means of coping with an uncertain future. They maintain hope for recovery during times of crisis, for more effective medical care that will relieve some of their suffering or will effect a cure, and for a relatively normal, productive adult life. These children also are able to use compensatory physical and/or cognitive activities to make up for certain physical limitations. They tend to subordinate their physical limitations in preference for factors over which they have more control. They are able to express their sadness, impatience, anger, or anxiety when they are having particular difficulty with their physical problem.

Children who have not made an adequate inner adjustment to a physical problem exhibit behavior and forms of adjustment that are not typical of a child with healthy inner adjustment. Children with physical problems may become dependent, confined to their home and family with no outside interest, inactive, and fearful of new experiences. Other children become exces-

**CHAPTER 18**

Children and
youth with
long-term
physical
problems

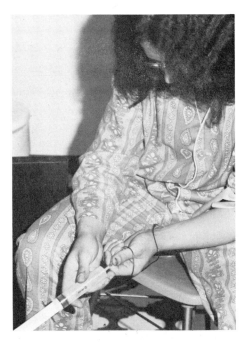

**Fig. 18-2.** The young person with hemophilia is supported and encouraged in taking over much of his own personal care and participation in health and medical treatment.

sively independent, demonstrate rebellious behavior, and appear to engage excessively in denial as a means of coping with real dangers and fears. During adolescence they become particularly defiant and rebellious, particularly against a parent who has been overly solicitous throughout earlier childhood. Very often children's symptoms of poor adjustment reflect family attitudes and poor patterns of parental adjustment. Children, modeling parental attitudes, may begin to resent other children who do not have similar physical problems; they may adopt the attitude that these more normal children owe them something for their suffering. They may emphasize their own limitations and handicaps, and tend to use them in gaining favors and acceptance from others.*

## FAMILY DYNAMICS

The vital role of the family in relation to children's adjustment and physical care has been

*References 18, 30, 69, 76, 78, 87, 114, 130, 137, 139.

implied in previous discussions. Without their family's support, care, and adjustment to the problem, children who have long-term physical problems cannot adjust or care for themselves. Thus the health care team must continually be concerned with the family's evolving situation and the dynamics that are intimately influencing the child. The reactions and adjustments that might be observed among families are as varied as the families themselves. Often the reaction is similar to that experienced by parents of the dying child, discussed in Chapter 17. Particularly when knowledge of the child's problem is sudden and unexpected, the reaction is often one of shock, disbelief, and inability to comprehend. When children are born with a serious birth defect, the family may mourn as if the hoped-for normal child had died, and then they begin a sad process of recognizing and accepting the living child as their own. In other instances awareness of the problem comes more gradually, and although there may be similarities in the reaction to a fatal illness, other dynamics operate. A sequence of reactions leading to acceptance of children who are mentally retarded has been described; it applies also to the reaction shared by parents of children with physical problems.[76,107] Some of the features described may be more or less prominent for an individual family, but consideration of the task faced by the family contributes to the health care worker's ability to assess the family's adjustment.

### Awareness of the problem

Awareness that something may be wrong with the child physically may come very gradually, even if the initial impact of the fact is sudden, as with a severe injury or a birth defect. With a sudden onset, the parents may only gradually begin to absorb the reality of the fact that this thing has happened. In other cases, where the problem actually develops gradually, the family may have become increasingly aware of physical symptoms, such as those that might occur with a child who has diabetes. This growing awareness of a problem stimulates the family to eventually seek evaluation and advice from professionals within the health care system.[8,76,107]

## Recognition of the problem

When the family can no longer avoid the problem and awareness has finally evolved, they must begin to face the problem for what it actually is. During this time the family may demonstrate denial mechanisms similar to those of the parents of the dying child. They express hopes that the diagnosis is incorrect or that someone somewhere knows of a cure for the condition. They may express anger toward those who have made the diagnosis and toward health care workers who are involved initially in the care and treatment. Most parents need some time to experience this phase of denial in order to accumulate needed resources to cope more adequately.[18,76,107]

## The search for a cause

At some point in the process of achieving some degree of acceptance, most parents of children with long-term physical problems seek some cause that can be identified. The search may consist of blaming environmental circumstances, but more often there is a self-accusing search that involves the gradual examination of all possible personal blame. When the condition is known to be inherited, there is often a search through both sides of the family to identify the source of the inherited trait. When the child has suffered accidental trauma, the parent replays the circumstances repeatedly to identify sources of blame or to mourn the neglected action that might have spared the child. If the parents are not able to master their resentment and self-accusatory feelings over having caused in some way their child's problem, they remain highly guilt-laden and tend to cope with their own emotional distress by overprotecting and pampering the child and being overly solicitous.[76,107]

## The search for a cure

Since medical advances have occurred so rapidly and miraculously in recent years, many parents engage in some search for a cure of the child's condition. Even if the child's condition is relatively easy to control and does not present a serious problem to the child or family, parents may make some effort to follow a clue they have read or heard that suggests a cure may hover on the horizon. Indeed, there are periodic claims from various sources in our society that allude to miraculous cures for conditions that have never before been curable, and some parents pursue these claims regardless of advice or evaluation from professional health care workers. For example, claims have been made in recent years regarding the curative power of vitamin E for diabetes. Even when the claim is implied rather than stated, an unsuspecting parent eagerly pursues the glimmer of hope.[18,76,107]

## Acceptance of the child

Acceptance of a child with a long-term physical problem has different meanings for different families. Parental acceptance does not often equate with acceptance as professionally defined for the parent of the healthy child. Rather, it implies healthy adjustment and adaptation to the child's problem and development of adequate coping mechanisms to deal with the continual stress imposed by the problem. The family that has adapted well to the child's physical problem imposes only necessary and realistic restrictions and does not impose unrealistic, overprotective limitations. The child is disciplined in accordance to the standards of behavior that apply to other children in the family and is encouraged to participate in all aspects of family and peer activities that are appropriate. The child is supported and encouraged to take over as much of his or her own personal care as possible, including responsibilities related to medical and health care requirements.

Well-adjusted parents develop coping mechanisms to handle the monotonous stress of living with the physical problem and to handle an occasional crisis. They tend to deny and isolate their anxiety and helplessness during a period of crisis, and as a result they may experience a period of depression and irritability once the danger is over and they can begin to more safely experience some of the denied fear.

Many parents develop attitudes of superiority over health specialists, using their own well-developed knowledge of their child's condition to criticize the care that is given. In so doing the parents are able to further deny some of their own inner helplessness and to project anger, resentment, and hostility about the child's condition onto the professional health care team. Various types of rationalizations about the child's condition are commonly heard. These include the attitude that the child has brought unusual joy and enrichment to the family, or that the experiences have brought an unusual sense of understanding for other people's problems. Although these statements may represent the family's reality, they also represent a relatively mature means of coping with sadness and monotony involved in living with a lasting burden. For some parents the intellectual processes mustered in mastering knowledge of all aspects of the child's problem provide the needed mastery over their continuing anxieties related to the child's condition.

Finally, association with other parents of children with similar conditions is often a healthy means of adjusting. Parents find that they can share their feelings, and that some of the feelings that have been too painful to express are felt by others also. The sharing somehow makes recognition more bearable, and they can mutually learn to adapt with more accepting, relaxed attitudes. A group can have destructive effects on some parents, particularly if they have problems requiring professional therapy. Groups should be encouraged for most parents, but individual assistance for special problems should be provided as well.*

## SCIENTIFIC BASES FOR UNDERSTANDING LONG-TERM PHYSICAL PROBLEMS

When working with a child who has a long-term physical problem, it is essential to understand the scientific bases for the physical problem and for the social dynamics that it creates. Equipped with such knowledge, the nurse is able to accurately assess the child and his or her competency development and environment and subsequently to make sound judgments in implementing care.

### Classification

For the purposes of this chapter, classification of long-term physical problems is accomplished according to the physiologic system that is primarily affected. This means of classification is consistent with the usual approach in conceptualizing the medical diagnosis, and the nursing problem classification system presented in the Appendix, p. 884, is arranged in this manner. Following sections of this chapter will present the definition, pathophysiology, incidence, etiology, essentials of medical diagnosis, essential features of the problem, special stress factors, medical treatment, and the prognosis related to common medical diagnoses for each physiologic system. The nursing problems that commonly occur with these groups of illness will be discussed, as classified in the MNPC (see Appendix, p. 888).

Because of the great scope of problems that are long-term during childhood, it is also helpful to review a means of classifying the disorders according to common factors such as etiology or pathology.

1. Conditions caused by chromosomal abnormalities include a wide range of problems, not all of which are physical in nature. Examples include Down's syndrome, Klinefelter's syndrome, and Turner's syndrome.

2. Conditions that result from abnormal hereditary traits usually are expressed as specific physical problems in the individual's phenotype. Identification of the hereditary factor may or may not be possible, and multiple causation is very often demonstrated or suspected. Evidence regarding the hereditary nature of most of these disorders is convincing, however, and they are considered inherited in most instances. Such problems include sickle cell anemia, hemophilia, cystic fibrosis, muscular dystrophy, osteogenesis imperfecta, diabetes mellitus, inborn errors of metabolism, club foot, cleft lip, cleft palate, dislocation of the hip, congenital blindness, and deafness.

3. Conditions caused by harmful intrauterine conditions may be the same or similar to those caused by hereditary factors. For example, rubella contracted by the mother during the first trimester of pregnancy can result in such problems as deafness, blindness, and congenital heart defects. Other intrauterine conditions that might result in physical damage include maternal infection, drug ingestion, radiation, pre-

*References 18, 29, 34, 49, 76, 107.

natal hypoxia, and blood incompatabilities (see Chapter 4).

4. Conditions that result from trauma or infection during labor, delivery and the immediate newborn period most often include damage to the central nervous system and/or motor capacity. Cerebral palsy and blindness caused by perinatal gonorrheal infection are examples of this type of condition.

5. Conditions that result from serious postnatal and childhood infections, trauma, neoplasms, and other factors constitute the remaining group of long-term physical problems in childhood. Such problems as meningitis, encephalitis, tuberculosis, rheumatic fever, chronic renal disease, physical injuries, and convulsive disorders may be permanent conditions, or they may result in permanent physical damage.[76]

## Definition and pathophysiology

To provide effective health care to a child with a long-term physical problem the nurse must thoroughly understand what the problem is and the basic pathophysiology involved. It is not sufficient, for example, to know that the child has a chronic kidney problem. The medical problem must be further delineated and differentiated as recurrent pyelonephritis, acute glomerulonephritis, nephrosis, renal failure, etc. For each condition the description factors are different, the medical treatment differs somewhat, and the pathologic effect on the renal system varies.[13,38,61] Thus a basic understanding of normal renal function and structure is essential. Since continuing investigation is needed to fully describe the pathology involved in many long-term physical problems, the clinician who is involved in care of an afflicted child must remain informed of the most recent advances and trends in relation to a given problem.

## Incidence

The incidence of all chronic illnesses of primary physical origin has been estimated variably as from 7% to 10% for all children.[42] The most common physical conditions are asthma, affecting about 2% of all children under 18 years of age; epilepsy, 1%; cardiac conditions, 0.5%;

and diabetes mellitus, 0.1%.[76] Incidence may also be related to a particular ethnic group, since some conditions occur with significant frequency among certain groups of people but are relatively rare among others. For example, sickle cell disease afflicts from 8% to 12% of all black Americans.[59]

## Etiology

The classification of long-term physical problems outlined earlier is based primarily on the etiology of a problem. However, for an individual child it is not always possible to define the specific etiology of a long-term problem. The nephrotic syndrome, for example, can be attributed to ingestion of drugs, concurrent renal or systemic disease, or an immunologic process.[23] Such a condition might be classified in the fifth etiologic category presented earlier because of the age of onset and the fact that it cannot be traced to a genetic or a prenatal etiology. But the specific etiology of most instances of the nephrotic syndrome remains unknown.[23] On the other hand, some long-term physical problems have a clearly defined etiology. Such a condition is hemophilia, which is a sex-linked inheritable disorder of the blood-clotting mechanism.[96,118] In other instances the etiology of a problem is specific to the circumstances of the individual child, as when severe trauma leads to permanent handicap.[132]

## Essentials of medical diagnosis

The medical diagnosis of long-term physical problems rests upon defined features or criteria. Some problems, such as injury or trauma, are clearly defined by the etiology or other self-evident fact. Other problems are less clearly described and diagnosis remains relatively difficult and inexact, as with some forms of allergy. Defining the essential features upon which the medical diagnosis rests provides a useful reference for members of the health care team in understanding the nature of a specific physical problem and in making relevant, reliable judgments regarding assessment findings. If a nurse is caring for a child who is known to suffer recurrent attacks of bronchial asthma, steps can be taken to facilitate the medical diagnosis and to obtain immediate medical consultation and

CHAPTER 18

Children and
youth with
long-term
physical
problems

referral as soon as signs and symptoms of the active condition are observed.

## Essential features of the problem

In addition to the definition and pathophysiology that identify a problem and the essential features that confirm a given medical diagnosis, there are other features of the condition that specify all known possible effects of the condition, the expected course of the illness or disabling condition, and the eventual outcome for most children with the problem. The primary features of the illness include those clinical signs and symptoms that usually occur when the problem is first identified. The typical course of the illness includes the expected changes that may be expected to occur over the child's developmental periods and into adulthood. Secondary effects include those pathologic changes that may occur in other physical systems as a result of the primary condition. For example, the primary disorder of the exocrine glands in cystic fibrosis leads to pathologic changes in the lungs and gastrointestinal tract, which in turn leads to failure to thrive and diminished physical stature.

## Medical treatment

When the initial medical diagnosis of a long-term physical problem has been made, the child and family may become involved in a long program of medical treatment. The medical objective of controlling the effects of the physical problem remains a central aspect of health care for these children and their families. Thus it is essential that each aspect of medical care be understood by the family and each professional worker. Ideally, the family should eventually become the central coordinating members of the team, identifying those aspects of care that they can reasonably assume and those services that are needed from individual health care workers. When the family is beginning to learn to cope with the problem or when their resources to manage are restricted, they may be able to assume only a portion of this ideal role. As children grow older and increasingly responsible, they can assume the family's participation role on their own behalf and thus learn to provide for themselves the basic goals of health care. Medical approaches to the treatment of many long-term conditions may vary according to a physician's own background and preference, but the basic features of management are usually similar. Thus various recommendations for treatment will be encountered, and the professional worker must exercise informed judgment in identifying the basic principles and goals toward which a particular approach applies and the rationale for choosing one method of treatment over another.

## Special stress factors

Most long-term physical problems impose particular physical, emotional, social, and economic stress factors upon most similarly affected children and families. The stresses that the particular problem creates should be understood by all members of the health care team, and early prevention and intervention should be planned with the family in order to minimize the stress involved. Long-term problems that require careful, constant attention in order to control the disease or prevent serious complications create a certain degree of emotional tension within the family. Diabetes, cystic fibrosis, convulsive disorders, bleeding disorders, and heart diseases, for example, require consistent care and attention by the family in order to control the problem or to prevent relapses, complications, or mishaps. There is often a significant fear associated with not following through adequately with the prescribed care regimen. The family and child with diabetes fear imbalances that might occur with hyperinsulinism or hyperglycemia. The child with a seizure disorder lives in fear of having a seizure at an unexpected time when friends are near or when there is no one to help. Children with respiratory problems such as those accompanying cystic fibrosis may fear suffocation, drowning, or death during sleep. In addition, the child with cystic fibrosis feels embarrassment because of flatulence, foul-smelling stools, and special needs for physical care. The family of a child with a congenital heart defect often lives in fear and anticipation of new complications and repeated surgical procedures. The child's disposition and behavior are often difficult to live with, and activity restrictions may be severe. The emotional distress of a physical problem may contribute to the occurrence of physical symptoms and signs. For example, some children with bleeding disorders have been observed to bleed spontaneously without apparent trauma in the face of emotional distress.[8,76,83,105]

## Prognosis

The prognosis of the condition should be understood. For some conditions, such as cancer, cystic fibrosis, and certain birth defects, the prognosis is very poor, and only in recent years has the outlook begun to change from certain early fatality to the possibility of prolonged life with adequate treatment. In other instances, as with certain allergic conditions, children may be expected to improve as they reach young adulthood.

## NURSING ASSESSMENT AND CARE

When skill, knowledge, understanding, and experience have been developed in management of a particular physical condition, maximal nursing participation in the medical plan which is coordinated with particular aspects of nursing care, can be assumed. In addition, all professional contacts with children include screening for long-term problems that may lead to early diagnosis and treatment of a gradually developing condition.

## Screening tools

The nursing assessment offers a valuable tool for identifying a number of long-term physical problems that might be developing gradually. When an unexpected change is noted in some aspect of the assessment from previous findings, the clue should stimulate further investigation either by the nurse or some other specialist on the health care team.

Specialized screening tools for particular conditions should be used for children who are particularly at risk for a certain condition. For example, black and Puerto Rican children are particularly at risk for sickle cell disease, and screening tests of blood samples should be used for newborns of these ethnic groups.[59,97] Older children should be screened if they have not been screened as infants, and screening for the heterozygous sickle cell trait can be conducted

in order to provide counseling and education for persons who carry the trait.[59,97] Regular screening of the urine and blood for increased glucose levels should be conducted for all children, particularly those with a known family history of diabetes.

Screening during infancy for the genetically inherited condition of phenylketonuria is now required in many states because of the dramatic results that can be achieved through early detection and treatment of this relatively rare condition. Because affected children become severely handicapped physically and mentally as the condition progresses, the economic impact of a single child upon the family and the community is severe enough to warrant screening of all infants in order to provide treatment for the few infants who are identified. Through effective treatment, the child can grow and develop into productive childhood and adulthood.[82]

## Prevention

Prevention of many long-term physical problems is possible through adequate accident prevention, including home, school, and automobile safety. Helping and encouraging the family to repeatedly take special notice of the hazards in and around the home and to practice adequate accident prevention in their daily living can prevent many tragic problems. Retrospective recognition of a danger once a serious burn, orthopedic injury, or poisoning has occurred emphasizes the many steps that might be taken by a family to increase the safety of their home, but this does not spare the child. A family cannot realistically remove all dangers from their child's life, but they can take significant steps to increase the safety of the environment.

## Comprehensive assessment

Assessment of the child who has a long-term physical problem includes each of the aspects of assessment appropriate for the age of the child (see Chapters 9, 10, 12, and 14). Additional attention and evaluation are directed toward the physiologic system or systems affected by the condition and toward each of the competencies affected by the physical problem. For example, diabetic children would be particularly assessed for the physiologic control of the effects of lack of insulin, including glucose tolerance, ketones in the urine, serum pH, or signs of tissue breakdown in any area of the body, particularly in the retina, kidney, skin, and cardiovascular system. Their adaptation to the condition and their ability to manage daily insulin and dietary requirements are assessed, as are the family's capacity in each of these areas.

## Nursing problems and plans

When the assessment provides data that supports the identification of a particular nursing problem, a plan is formulated in consultation with the family. For example, diabetic children may be identified who have developed to the point of being able to administer their own insulin, and thus a plan is formulated to teach them how to test their own urine, determine the appropriate amount of insulin to give, and how to inject the insulin. Such a plan requires a significant investment of professional and family time and effort, and the clinician's initial judgment in regard to the child's readiness to assume this responsibility is crucial to the success of the plan.

## Facilitating competency development

Facilitation of competency development for children with long-term physical problems presents a special challenge to the nurse. The special needs of each child are defined through evaluation of each competency and through environmental factors that affect development. Social and inner competencies are of particular significance for most children with a long-term health problem, and the role of the family in the ultimate adaptation of the child is a vitally important environmental factor. As the family's adaptation and understanding of the special needs and problems of the child become increasingly adequate, the potential for the child's development increases.

## Interdisciplinary role of other health care team members

Experience suggests that a comprehensive care program utilizing the specialized skills of several health care professionals facilitates adjustment and satisfactory progress of children and families with long-term problems.[10,98,129]

Rather than lead to fragmentation, the coordinated efforts of specialists with particular skills provide resources to the family far beyond what a single worker could offer.

A social worker may offer particular help for a family who has economic and social problems. Knowledge of community resources and of the ways in which a family might obtain needed resources are particular skills of a social worker. These professional workers are equipped with counseling and guidance skills, and they may have particular expertise in working with families as a group. Their understanding of health problems and health resources is usually such that they can recognize problems and refer the family to appropriate sources of help.[6]

Nutritionists and dietitians have vital resources to offer children and families with many long-term physical problems. A child with nutrition-related disorders, such as diabetes, cystic fibrosis, or allergies, may particularly benefit from the services and support of the nutritionist. In addition, they serve as important resource people for other team members who encounter nutrition-related problems.

Therapists who are able to provide special kinds of rehabilitational and physical therapy are important resources for children who have suffered the loss of some physical capacity or who have physical limitations that must be overcome in gaining physical skills. The therapists' particular understanding of the mechanisms of the nervous, skeletal, and muscle systems, related inner motivation to master a physical task, and means of promoting the restoration of function to damaged tissue may be vitally important for a child with extensive burns, orthopedic birth defects, or accidental injuries.

Counselors, psychologists, and psychiatrists have unique skills in helping children and families adjust, adapt, and cope with the stress of a long-term physical problem. While some families may need long-term counseling assistance, most families need such help at particular crisis points during the child's life. Recognizing the need for such help may come from the family, or they may feel reluctant to obtain outside assistance for problems they feel they should handle alone. The social stigma of obtaining professional help with emotional problems may be great, but acceptance of the child's problem may not be possible until some source of professional help is obtained. The family cannot be forced to receive help that they do not seek or desire, and health care workers may need to develop skill in helping families to reach the point of recognizing a need and accepting this particular kind of professional help.[99]

Counselors and mental health professionals can also offer the professional members of the health care team particular support and assistance in working with families and children. The health care worker may need to validate an observation, evaluation, or therapeutic approach used with a particular child or may need assistance in formulating alternative approaches to a particular problem. In addition the health care worker may experience personal stress related to working with a child and family and may need a resource for personal support and help.

Genetic counseling is often needed by parents who have an infant or young child with an inherited disorder and by adolescents who have an inherited disorder or whose sibling has such a problem. While basic and general principles of genetic inheritance may be discussed by all members of a health care team, specific counseling and recommendations should be given only by a specialist who has thoroughly studied the family's genetic history and endowment. The family may need long-term support and counseling related to family planning decisions.[138]

Finally, special educators may be available to help a child who has a particularly physical problem. While the special educator is most often viewed as working with children who primarily have learning and thought problems, many of the children whom they serve have primary physical problems that may or may not involve learning handicaps. Children who have neuromuscular handicaps or who have sensory handicaps such as blindness or deafness often need special educational provisions.[102] These problems are considered in Chapter 19.

## LONG-TERM MUSCULOSKELETAL PROBLEMS (MNPC no. 310)

Long-term physical problems that exert a major effect on musculoskeletal development and function are considered in this section. The etiology may be infectious, congenital, or prenatal, or may be acquired as a secondary problem of another physical system, often the nervous system. These problems usually cause visible physical deformity or disability, and even in instances where medical correction or cure is possible, the child and family often need long-term nursing care to maintain and restore full function in each of the areas of competency.

### Medical diagnoses and treatment
#### Rheumatoid arthritis

**Definition.** Juvenile rheumatoid arthritis is defined as a continuous inflammation of one or more joints of more than three months' duration. It is also known as Still's arthritis.[3,7,50]

**Incidence.** Approximately 250,000 children develop juvenile rheumatoid arthritis each year in the United States. This represents an estimated 1 in 1,000 to 1,500 school-age children each year. The female-to-male ratio estimates vary from 1.5:1 to 3:1. There are two peaks for age of onset: one peak occurs between 2 and 5 years of age; the second peak occurs between 9 and 12 years of age.[44]

**Etiology.** The etiology of juvenile rheumatoid arthritis is not known. Although there may be a predisposition to develop the disease, hereditary factors are not etiologic. Triggering events may include trauma, viral infections, climatic changes and psychologic stress, but there is no evidence that supports these factors as a cause, other than the possibility that a slow viral infection or viral alterations of tissues may be a cause. Immunologic pathogenesis is the most accepted etiologic theory, based on evidence that frequently demonstrates immune complexes of IgG in the joint fluid and phagocytic cells.[3,7,50]

**Pathophysiology.** The destructive changes of rheumatoid joint disease are thought to be caused by hydrolases discharged from lysosomal granules and increased amounts of fibrinogen. These substances are produced by an unidentified initiating factor that triggers the local synthesis of IgG and rheumatoid factor (IgM anti-IgG) by plasma cells within the joint. The antigen-antibody aggregates then activate the complement sequence, which is followed by a depletion of hemolytic complement activity in the synovial fluid while serum levels of complement remain normal. The activation of complement leads to generation of materials that attract polymorphonuclear leukocytes into the joint that phagocytize the immune complexes, thus leading to the formation of the rheumatoid arthritis (RA) cells. The phagocytized cells discharge the enzymes thought to be responsible for the degenerative changes that occur in the joint.[3]

**Essentials of medical diagnosis.** The essential features upon which a medical diagnosis rests are:

1. Nonmigratory joint inflammation involving one or more joints and lasting more than three months, with a tendency to involve large joints or proximal interphalangeal joints.

2. Systemic manifestations with fever, erythematous rash, nodules, and leukocytosis. Occasionally symptoms and signs of iridocyclitis, pleuritis, pericarditis, hepatitis, and nephritis will be present.

The nonmigratory nature of the arthritis is the primary feature that differentiates juvenile rheumatoid arthritis from the arthritis of rheumatic fever and infections of *Haemophilus influenzae* and gonorrhea, which involve a migratory pattern. If a single joint is involved, a differential diagnosis must be made considering the possibility of leukemia, neuroblastoma, rhabdomyosarcoma, or infection. X-ray examination and examination of the blood usually identify the possibility of malignancy, and the presence of a bacterial pathogen, an elevated white count, and low glucose in the synovial fluid suggests an infection. Systemic lupus erythematosus and inflammatory bowel disease often involve a presenting complaint of arthritis, but other systemic signs and symptoms of these problems will also be present.[50]

**Essential features of the illness.** There are three forms of juvenile rheumatoid arthritis. Each differs somewhat from the adult form of the illness, but it is not clear whether the differences arise from host factors or from illness factors. The acute febrile form is most common in children under the age of 4 years and is characterized by the presence of an evanescent salmon-pink macular rash, arthritis, hepato-

splenomegaly, leukocytosis, and polyserositis. The illness is episodic and usually resolves within a year of onset. Complications involving the eyes do not occur with this form of the illness.

A polyarticular form of juvenile rheumatoid arthritis resembles the adult disease, with chronic pain and swelling of many joints. The arthritis occurs in a symmetrical pattern, with both large and small joints usually involved. Systemic symptoms are not prominent, although low-grade fever, fatigue, rheumatoid nodules, and anemia may occur. This form of the illness tends to last indefinitely, although the symptoms may periodically lessen in intensity. Complications of the eyes occur occasionally.

The pauciarticular form of juvenile rheumatoid arthritis involves only a few joints, usually fewer than four. Usually these are the large weight-bearing joints in an asymmetric distribution. Inflammation of the joint may be painless, and few systemic symptoms occur. However, 30% of the children with this form of arthritis develop insidious, asymptomatic iridocyclitis, which frequently causes blindness. The development of eye disease does not occur with the joint symptoms and may occur months or years after the onset of joint symptoms. Ophthalmologic screening must be performed every six months until puberty to detect early signs of eye involvement and to institute early treatment for the prevention of blindness.[50]

**Special stress factors.** The impact of the diagnosis of juvenile rheumatoid arthritis and the many stress factors that accompany the course of chronic illness depend to a large extent on the severity of the child's illness. If the illness is severe, physical deformity often results, and the frequent exacerbations of illness, limitations in physical ability to conduct daily activities, and isolation from peers results in a serious interference with learning and thought, social, and inner competency development. Children with serious forms of illness often withdraw from activities outside of the family and become dependent on the family for assistance with daily activities and social interaction. Often children with severe forms of illness develop passive hostility, uncommunicativeness, and manipulative personality traits. Parents often have great difficulty in coping with the uncertainties inherent in predicting the degree of deformity that might develop, the problems that may result from the long-term use of drugs, and the social limitations that the child's illness presents in the conduct of daily living.[7]

**Medical treatment.** The primary objectives of medical treatment are to restore function of the joint, relieve pain, and maintain joint function. Drugs that reduce joint inflammation and relieve pain are the primary medical means of accomplishing these goals. Aspirin, 75 to 100 mg/kg/day in four doses often provides sufficient relief of pain and inflammation and makes it possible for the child to accomplish physical therapy and exercise to maintain joint function. If aspirin does not provide sufficient relief, prednisone in doses of less than 5 mg daily may be used without altering the child's growth pattern. Corticosteroids may be used temporarily when the symptoms have flared, when there is acute systemic illness, or for treatment of iridocyclitis. Gold salts may also be used for acute episodes. They are administered intramuscularly at a dose of 1 mg/kg/week, and the dose is gradually decreased as the symptoms subside. Drugs that are used for the adult form of the disease, such as cyclophosphamide (Cytoxan) and azathoeprine (Imuran) are not used for children because of the dangers of bone marrow depression and infertility.

Physical therapy, with complete range of motion and muscle-strengthening exercises, is an important component of the child's treatment. The child and parents are taught a specific program of planned active and passive exercises and are assisted in establishing a regular pattern of exercise in the home.[50] If the illness is mild, regular patterns of daily activities and play may be sufficient to meet the exercise requirements. Active play is frequently used as a means of accomplishing the exercise requirements, for it offers the advantage of diversion to offset the pain and discomfort the child may experience. During the acute phases of illness, hot water immersion baths are helpful to relieve discomfort during range of motion exercise. After acute inflammation subsides, active exercise such as tricycle or bicycle riding, running, and swimming are encouraged, with the only

limiting factor being the avoidance of physical contact sports, which increase the dangers of joint trauma.[7,44]

Splinting may be required to prevent deformities or to correct deformities. Surgical relief of contractures may be needed, and surgical stabilization of joints may be required after full growth has been achieved.[7]

**Prognosis.** For 95% of children who primarily exhibit joint symptoms without symptoms of systemic illness, the disease gradually decreases in severity and ceases altogether by puberty. If signs of the illness persist after puberty, the illness is likely to persist into adulthood. Children who have signs and symptoms that are difficult to control with drugs or who have hip involvement or positive rheumatoid factor tests are most likely to suffer permanent deformity and handicap. Death may occur as a complication of persistent carditis or renal amyloidosis.[50]

### Scoliosis

**Definition.** Idiopathic scoliosis is a curvature of the vertebral column in the lateral plane. Such a curvature can be a sign of congenital or acquired osteopathic, neuropathic, or myopathic conditions, but such underlying causes are rare, and the most predominant problem is a curvature that is apparently not related to underlying pathology of these related systems.[84,123]

**Incidence.** Idiopathic scoliosis in girls between 10 to 14 years of age comprises approximately 80% to 85% of all cases of scoliosis. Girls are affected seven to ten times more frequently than boys.[84]

**Etiology.** The cause of idiopathic scoliosis is not known. Factors that have been suggested as possible causes include congenital malformations of the vertebral column or other related structures, such as the femur or rib cage, or a clinically inapparent nervous system infection. Scoliosis may be related to poor posture in some instances.[123]

**Essential features.** Scoliosis is asymptomatic except for the appearance of deformity, which may not be detected while the child is sitting or standing. Careful observation of the curvature of the spine and the level of the hips and shoulders when the young person bends to touch the toes often reveals an early condition of scoliosis. The curvatures are usually limber during early stages but eventually become rigid and fixed. X-ray examination is essential to determine the extent of the problem. A single C-shaped curve is the most common form of scoliosis; occasionally there is an S-shaped curve with compensatory curves above and below. Rotation of the vertebral bodies may be present with some degree of deformity of the rib cage.[84]

**Special stress factors.** The age at which scoliosis usually develops is a primary stress factor. The majority of girls who develop this problem are entering puberty or just past puberty, when there is a normal developmental focus on body image and a need to achieve and maintain a body figure that is considered ideal by the peer group. The development of a postural deformity is a physical and inner developmental risk, as is the orthopedic treatment required to correct the problem.[87]

**Medical treatment.** Orthopedic evaluation and treatment is needed for all young people who develop idiopathic scoliosis. The severity and extent of the problem determine the type of orthopedic correction that is used and the length of time that is required. Correction sometimes involves a spinal fusion, followed by six months of immobilization in a body cast and another six months of treatment with a Milwaukee brace. Curves of less than 30 degrees can sometimes be treated by exercise alone. Curves between 30 to 60 degrees usually require treatment with a Milwaukee brace or body cast. Orthopedic management includes frequent evaluation of the progress and response of the curve to treatment and monitoring the degree of fixation that may occur. Regardless of the type of treatment needed, the length of time that is required for full correction of the condition is usually extended beyond a year and involves frequent monitoring and adjustment.[84,104]

**Prognosis.** Early intervention for compensated and slowly progressing curves usually results in full correction of the curvature. If the curve becomes fixed or if it involves a marked rotation of the vertebral bodies or pelvic obliquity, the possibility of lasting deformity is increased.[84]

**Table 18-1.** Summary of necrotic lesions of epiphyseal centers during childhood

| Epiphyseal center | Eponym | Typical age at appearance of symptoms |
|---|---|---|
| Capital femoral | Legg-Calvé-Perthes disease | 3-10 years |
| Tibial tuberosity | Osgood-Schlatter disease | 10-15 years |
| Tarsal navicular | Köhler's disease | 3-8 years |

*Osteochondroses*

**Definition.** The osteochondroses are avascular, aseptic necrosing lesions of epiphyseal centers. Table 18-1 indicates the location of epiphyseal centers that are typically affected during childhood and adolescence.

**Incidence.** The osteochondroses occur with undetermined frequency, but the incidence of the various types follows a typical pattern of age at appearance. This pattern is indicated in Table 18-1. Boys are affected more frequently than girls, at a ratio of about 6:1.[84,124]

**Pathophysiology.** The pathologic process involved in the osteochondroses involves an interruption of the vascular supply to the epiphyseal ossification centers, resulting in necrosis of bone tissue at the site of ossification. Unlike other tissues of the body, bone tissue removes the necrotic tissue and gradually replaces it with living bone in a process known as "creeping substitution." This process, which is similar to the normal process of growth in living bone, has a typical microscopic and radiologic appearance.[84,124]

**Etiology.** The etiology of the pathologic process is not known, but in many instances trauma is regarded as an etiologic factor. Infections have also been suspected but have not been documented as a cause. Idiopathic lesions appear to develop in relation to periods of rapid growth of the epiphyses and their ossification centers, which accounts for the unique age-related appearance of these conditions.[84,124]

**Essentials of medical diagnosis.** Serial x-ray examination is the basis for definitive medical diagnosis. Inflammatory and infectious lesions must be ruled out. During the early stages of

illness the radiographic findings may appear
normal, but because of the dangers of delay in
treatment resulting in permanent deformity,
medical treatment is usually instituted with the
appearance of clinical signs and symptoms, and
serial radiographic examination is obtained to
confirm the gradual changes that occur with the
osteochondroses.[84,119,124]

**Essential features.** The signs and symptoms
of osteochondroses are mild local tenderness,
pain, swelling, and motor disability. Legg-
Calvé-Perthes disease (coxa plana), which is the
most common and the most serious of the osteochondroses, may be manifested only by a mild
limp that is intermittent and by mild local pain
that is referred to the medial side of the ipsilat-
eral knee. A young boy may be observed during
assessment to have difficulty balancing on the
affected leg, or the leg may collapse while the
child attempts to balance. On questioning, he
may report the presence of mild signs of pain in
the hip and knee. The active phase of necrosis
usually lasts about 18 months, followed by a
quiescent phase of about 12 months and then
another 18 months of remineralization of the
epiphysis.[84]

**Special stress factors.** The length of time involved in the illness and the required immobilization for treatment are major stress factors for
a young person in an active stage of development. Further, the youngster does not experience pain or discomfort that interferes with the
desire to continue normal activity. The immobility that is required seriously interferes with
peer interaction and development of important
active skills, such as sports.

**Medical treatment.** Medical treatment consists of protection of the lesion. If the joint involved is a weight-bearing joint, the child must
not bear weight on the joint for an extended
period of time. During the early stages, traction
may be used, followed by plaster casting or the
use of a brace to keep the joint immobilized and
to allow the child to ambulate without bearing
weight on the joint. If a deformity of a weight-
bearing joint results, surgical intervention is
required to restore the joint to full function.[84,124]

**Prognosis.** The prognosis for spontaneous replacement of normal bone tissue is excellent,
but imperfect replacement may occur, which

results in derangement of joint function. The
prognosis is also related to the effectiveness of
early protection and continuous protection of
the affected joint. The younger the child at the
time of appearance of symptoms, the better the
prognosis.[84]

### Congenital deformities of the foot and ankle

**Definition.** Congenital deformities of the foot
and ankle are a variety of alterations in the normal bone, tendon, and ligament structures that
result in variations in normal alignment of the
foot. Fig. 18-3 shows the most common types of
variations that occur and the labels used for the
deformities, which are descriptive of the structures involved as well as the type of positional
deviation that occurs.[46]

**Etiology.** The most common etiology is a
positional deviation that occurs during intrauterine life. Positional deviations result in relatively mild forms of deformities that can usually
be passively corrected. If the foot cannot be
brought into correct alignment by passive rotation, the deformity probably arises from a congenital absence of muscles or bones or fusion of
bones. This is often the cause of severe forms of
congenital clubfoot, or talipes equinovarus.

**Essentials of medical diagnosis.** The response
of the foot to passive movement and radiologic
examination confirms the precise diagnosis.

**Medical treatment.** If the foot deformity is
caused by intrauterine positional inadequacy,
correction is accomplished by the use of simple
passive exercises and orthopedic shoes or
braces. Many deformities that arise from congenital deformities of the bones or muscles can
also be corrected by casts, wedgings, or Denis
Browne splints. Surgical lengthening of the heel
cord may be required after forefoot wedging for
severe forms of clubfoot.[46,66]

**Special stress factors.** Since congenital deformities of the foot are immediately apparent at
the time of birth, parents experience a great
deal of anxiety associated with the appearance of
birth defects. The uncertainty of the outcome of
treatment for severe deformities and the length
of treatment required present an emotional and
financial stress for young families.

**Prognosis.** The prognosis for correction of

**CHAPTER 18**

Children and
youth with
long-term
physical
problems

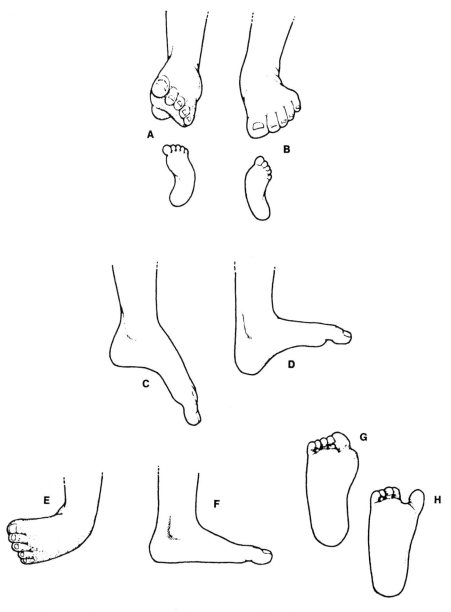

**Fig. 18-3.** Common foot and ankle deformities seen in children. **A,** Talipes varus. **B,** Talipes valgus. **C,** Talipes equinus. **D,** Talipes calcaneus. **E,** Clubfoot. **F,** Flatfoot. **G,** Metatarsus adductus. **H,** Metatarsus varus. (From Hilt, N. E., and Schmitt, E. W., Jr., Pediatric orthopedic nursing, St. Louis, 1975, The C. V. Mosby Co., p. 25.)

positional and bone or muscle defects is very good. Unless the child's deformity is associated with extensive deformities of other structures of the body, the outcome is usually complete correction of the deformity within the first year or two of life.[46,66]

### Congenital dysplasia of the hip

**Definition.** Congenital dysplasia of the hip is an abnormal development of the hip joint, the acetabulum, femoral head, capsule, and other soft tissues. Congenital subluxation of the hip is a partial dislocation of the head of the femur from the shallow acetabulum, while congenital dislocation of the hip is a complete dislocation of the femur head.[66]

**Incidence.** Black infants are rarely affected by congenital dysplasias of the hip, but in other populations the incidence is estimated to be 1.5 in 1,000 live births. These deformities are six to seven times more frequent in girls than in boys, and the left hip is affected more frequently than the right. Local variations in incidence occur, and where there is a relatively high local incidence there appears to be a familial tendency for hip dysplasias.[125]

**Etiology.** The etiology is not known, but fetal position, genetic inheritance, and abnormal relaxation of the capsule and ligaments of the joint by hormonal factors have been suggested as etiologic possibilities.[66,125] When there is a serious malformation of the structures of the hip related to the dysplasia, a teratogenic etiology that occurs during early intrauterine life is assumed to be responsible for the deformity.[125]

**Pathophysiology.** The pathology of teratogenic agents is discussed in Chapter 5. One theory suggests that development of the infant's enzyme systems, which are necessary for the degradation of transplacentally transmitted maternal hormones, particularly the hormone relaxin, is delayed. This theory has received some attention but has not been confirmed as a cause for dysplasias that do not involve abnormal structures of the hip. According to this theory, the maternal hormones are not degraded and cause an abnormal ligamentous laxity; the femoral heads are able to freely exit and enter the acetabular cavities, causing the clicks of Ortalani's maneuver. If the lower extremities are in a position favoring dislocation and the ligamentous resistance becomes normal when the enzyme system begins to degrade maternal hormones after the first week of life, the dislocation becomes relatively fixed, and secondary atrophy of the acetabular fossa develops.[125]

**Essentials of medical diagnosis.** Radiologic examination is required to confirm congenital malformations of the bony structures of the hips. A serious dislocation is usually evident by shortening of the affected leg, limitation in abduction, and asymmetry of the creases of the buttocks. A less evident dysplasia and subluxation of the hip are less apparent at birth and require careful observation during the first four months of life. Limitation in abduction may not develop until the third to fourth week of life. The criteria for medical diagnosis of congenital dysplasia of the hip are:[66]

1. The presence of Ortalani's sign
2. An acetabular angle above 40 degrees as confirmed by radiologic evidence
3. Lateral displacement of the upper end of the femur, confirmed by radiologic evidence
4. Persistent limitation of abduction of the flexed hip

**Essential features.** During the first month of life the essential features are those described for diagnosis. Once the child begins to bear weight on the hip and the condition has not been detected, a Trendelenburg gait develops, and there is a marked limitation of range of motion of the hip.

**Special stress factors.** The limitation of mobility required for treatment and the length of treatment constitute stress factors for the infant and the family. Depending on the severity of the deformity, financial stress exists as a result of long and complicated treatment. If a congenital deformity of bone structures exists, there may be a degree of permanent disability, depending upon the ability to achieve surgical replacement or correction.

**Medical treatment.** Orthopedic evaluation and diagnosis during the first month of life are essential to obtain full restoration of normal joint function. If medical treatment is delayed, treatment becomes more difficult and the outcome is jeopardized. Early treatment consists

CHAPTER 18

Children and
youth with
long-term
physical
problems

of external devices to maintain hip flexion and abduction, which are essential for reduction of the hip. For very mild subluxation of the hip, double diapers may suffice to achieve early correction. For more severe forms of subluxation, a Frejka abduction splint is used after 3 months of age to maintain the hip flexion and abduction until radiologic evidence confirms ossification of the acetabular roof and a stable hip joint. Skin and skeletal traction and surgery may be required as the child approaches a year of age, followed by plaster immobilization with a hip spica cast.[46,66,125]

**Prognosis.** Early diagnosis and treatment are essential for achieving full restoration of normal hip function. If treatment is delayed beyond the first year of life, surgical intervention is usually necessary to correct the dysplasia, and full function may not be possible.[66]

### Muscular dystrophies

**Definition.** Muscular dystrophy is a primary degenerative inherited disease of skeletal muscles characterized by muscular degeneration and weakness. Several different types have been identified and described, each of which is distinct in terms of clinical manifestation and genetic inheritance. Three major groups are discussed here: the pseudohypertrophic, or Duchenne's muscular dystrophy; facioscapulohumeral or Landouzy-Déjerine muscular dystrophy; and limb-girdle muscular dystrophy.[85]

**Incidence.** The most common of the muscular dystrophies is pseudohypertrophic muscular dystrophy, with an incidence of about 0.14 per 1,000 children. Boys are more commonly affected than girls.[57]

**Etiology.** The exact cause is not known, but the genetic pattern of inheritance has been described and can often be identified for children who develop symptoms. Pseudohypertrophic dystrophy is transmitted as a sex-linked recessive trait, although a rare instance of autosomal recessive inheritance is identified. Of all children who are diagnosed with this type of dystrophy, 30% to 50% have no family history.

Facioscapulohumeral dystrophy is usually transmitted by a autosomal dominant gene and rarely by an autosomal recessive gene. Limbgirdle muscular dystrophy is transmitted by an autosomal recessive gene in 60% of identified cases.[85,89]

**Pathophysiology.** The pathologic changes of muscle include a marked variation of muscle fiber size, internal migration of muscle nuclei, and varying degrees of necrosis and phagocytosis with replacement by fibrosis and fat. While these changes occur primarily in skeletal muscle, cardiac muscle is affected in pseudohypertrophic dystrophy. Electromyogram changes are reflected by rapid, low-voltage motor unit potentials, often with an increased number of short polyphasic potentials. Urinary creatine is increased, and creatinine is decreased as a result of muscle wasting. Elevated serum aldolase, creatine phosphokinase, and other enzymes are thought to result from a passive "leak" of normal muscle enzymes from abnormal fibers into the circulation.[27]

**Essentials of medical diagnosis.** Medical diagnosis is established by measurement of serum enzymes, electromyography, and muscle biopsy. Each of these measures confirms the pathologic changes described in the preceding section. A diagnosis of muscular dystrophy can be established at birth by an elevated creatine phosphokinase, and 60% to 80% of known carriers have a mild-to-moderate elevation of serum creatine phosphokinase, although no symptoms of the disease are present.[57]

**Essential features and prognosis.** Pseudohypertrophic dystrophy is a rapidly progressive disease that usually begins in early childhood between the ages of 2 and 6 years. The child often has a history of delayed sitting and walking and begins to exhibit clumsiness and a tendency to fall frequently. The child has difficulty in climbing stairs and develops a waddling gait and lordosis. The child develops a typical means of rising from a supine position—"climbing up the legs," which is known as Gower's sign. The child tends to walk on the toes, and the foot assumes a talipes equinovarus position due to the weakness of the anterior tibial and peroneal muscles. The muscles of the lower portion of the body are involved first, followed by the shoulder girdle within three to five years. The deep tendon reflexes are usually depressed or absent. There may be deformities of the skeleton that develop as a result of muscle wasting and contracture, and obesity is common due to the progressive lack of activity. A moderate degree of mental retardation is not uncommon. Fifty percent of all affected children eventually have involvement of the cardiac muscle, which occasionally is the cause of sudden death. The most common cause of death is pneumonia, which occurs as a result of immobility. Survival beyond the age of 20 years is unusual.

Facioscapulohumeral dystrophy is a slowly progressing form of this group of diseases that begins during late childhood or adolescence. Affected children have a normal life expectancy. The first muscles to be involved are the facial muscles and then the shoulder girdle, with occasional spread to the hips or distal legs. An inability to close the eyes may be the first sign, and pouting of the lips and immobility of facial expression are typical. The first symptoms are often noted when the child develops difficulty in lifting the arms above the shoulders. This form of the disease may become arrested for long periods of time, and progression to the lower limbs may not occur for 20 or 30 years, if at all.

Limb-girdle muscular dystrophy may develop at any age between early childhood to early adulthood. It is a mildly progressive form; life expectancy is from mid to late adulthood. In instances in which the shoulder girdle is affected first, the dystrophy is classified as juvenile scapulohumeral muscular dystrophy of Erb. In other instances the pelvic girdle and thigh muscles are first affected, and the dystrophy is classified as pelvifemoral dystrophy of Leyden and Moebius. Even though the course of the disease is slower than that of pseudohypertrophic dystrophy, it results in serious disability and progressive immobility.[57,85,89,140]

**Special stress factors.** The nature of genetic inheritance of muscular dystrophies presents a concern for the family members and for the child who has a form of the illness that progresses into adulthood. The emotional stress of dealing with the knowledge of a serious inheritable disease and the stresses of living with a progressively debilitating condition are major considerations in working with the child and the family. Psychologic counseling and support may be required for periods of crisis or over an extended period of time. Genetic counseling may be indicated or desired by the family.

**Medical treatment.** There is no specific treatment that can alter or alleviate the effects of the disease. Medical treatment is therefore aimed at preserving residual function of muscles as long as possible. The child is encouraged to engage in as many usual childhood activities as possible and remain mobile and involved in regular school programs as long as possible. Physical therapy and prescribed exercises may be used to maintain function. Braces may be used to prolong independent ambulation. When the child becomes unable to ambulate, a wheelchair may be used and the child may continue to participate in many school and community activities.[85,89,140]

### Osteomyelitis

**Definition.** Osteomyelitis is an infection of the bone. The infection may affect any part of the bone in any area of the body, but the most commonly affected sites are the distal end of the femur and the proximal end of the tibia and humerus.[84,131]

**Incidence.** The incidence of osteomyelitis is more common during infancy and in children 8 to 12 years of age but can occur at any time during childhood or adolescence.[131]

**Etiology.** Osteomyelitis develops from either of two sources of infection. One is from a penetrating wound or fracture, and related bone structure is infected as a result of inadequate care of the wound or fracture. The second type is infection by way of the bloodstream that gains access through furuncles or abrasions of the skin, impetigo, infections of the upper respiratory tract, acute otitis media, abscessed teeth, pyelonephritis, or infected burns. Children who are in poor physical condition are often more susceptible to developing osteomyelitis secondary to such infections.

The most common causative organism is *Staphylococcus aureus*, which is isolated in approximately 80% of all cases. A wide variety of other organisms may be involved, including streptococci, *Haemophilus influenzae*, *Escherichia coli*, *Salmonella*, and *Aerobacter aerogenes*. Children who have sickle cell disease have a predilection for salmonella osteomyelitis,

CHAPTER 18

Children and
youth with
long-term
physical
problems

and teenage drug abusers who fail to use adequate sterile technique tend to develop osteomyelitis caused by unusual organisms.[126,131]

**Pathophysiology.** The infection enters the bone by way of its nutrient artery. It spreads rapidly into the spongy cancellous marrow, destroying bone and producing necrosis through thrombosis of the vessels. It also spreads by way of the haversian canals through the cortex, forming an abscess that lifts the periosteum and spreads beneath it. In infants and very young children the periosteum ruptures easily and early in the course of the infection, causing a soft tissue abscess. In older children the periosteum resists rupture and contains the infection, causing intraosseous pressure and necrosis. Usually the epiphyseal plate is resistant to infection and protects the epiphysis unless the adjacent joint is also involved. The exception is the hip joint, since the neck of the femur is intracapsular and does not offer this protection. Sequestra, or necrotic cortical fragments, are formed by the death of large portions of the cortex and cannot be absorbed but become separated from the remainder of the bone and act as a foreign body that harbors the infection. The periosteum begins to produce new bone, known as the involucrum, surrounding the necrotic areas. This formation may be irregular with gaps that allow drainage of pus and sequestrum. In some instances, there is only a small walled-off area of osteomyelitis, known as Brodie's abscess. A chronic nonsuppurative sclerosing infection that produces an increased density of the cortex is known as Garré's osteomyelitis.[126]

**Essentials of medical diagnosis.** Medical diagnosis is made on the basis of blood findings, blood culture, culture and smears of aspirated pus, and radiographic evidence. Polymorphonuclear leukocytes in the blood are markedly increased, and the blood culture is usually positive early in the course of the illness. Smears of aspirated pus may indicate cocci or rods. Culture of aspirated pus is essential for identification of the organism and determination of antibiotic sensitivity. Radiographic findings may not indicate bony changes during the first 10 to 14 days but may indicate soft tissue swelling. If antibiotic treatment is rapidly effective in treating the infection, radiographic changes may not occur. However, it is more common for one or more areas of rarefaction of the cortex to appear on radiographic examination after the first 10 to 14 days. When the infection is severe or chronic, sequestra and involucrum are evident on the x-ray film. Acute osteomyelitis may exhibit similar signs and symptoms to such problems as acute pyogenic arthritis, cellulitis, rheumatic fever, and various malignant lesions and must be differentiated from these. In instances where osteomyelitis occurs as a complication of another severe disease or the child is in extremely poor physical condition, osteomyelitis may not be suspected.[84,131]

**Essential features.** Signs and symptoms of osteomyelitis typically begin abruptly and increase to maximum intensity within the first few days of illness. Initially, the child appears ill with a high fever, rapid pulse, severe and constant pain over the end of the shaft of affected bones, and limitation of joint motion. Often, local inflammatory signs may be absent in the first few days of illness, but later localized erythema, warmth, tenderness, and swelling over the site of infection appears. Rupture of the periosteum over the site of a subperiosteal abscess results in sudden decrease in pain and the appearance of local swelling, redness, and a temporary relief of systemic symptoms.[84,131]

**Special stress factors.** Because osteomyelitis is frequently a complication or sequelae of other problems and/or previous infection or trauma, it is an additional stress in an already stressful situation. The prolonged treatment and possibility of permanent damage to the bony structure may be a source of anxiety for the child and the family.

**Medical treatment.** Initial treatment with antibiotics is essential to interrupt the process of bone destruction and can be a life-saving measure. Until the results of blood and bone aspirate cultures have been obtained, the child is usually given intravenous penicillin G or methicillin in large doses. After culture results are available, antibiotic therapy may need to be altered. Strict bed rest is instituted, as well as measures for maintenance of adequate hydration and nutrition and symptomatic measures to relieve pain and fever. Blood transfusions may be required for children who develop anemia rapidly. The affected extremity is immobilized and elevated, and warm packs are used to promote circulation. Surgical drainage may be required, and polyethylene tubes may be inserted to allow the administration of an appropriate antibiotic directly into the affected area. Orthopedic evaluation and treatment may be required if bone destruction is extensive and if the child does not respond rapidly to treatment. Aggressive treatment is continued until all signs of active infection have subsided. Oral antibiotic treatment is continued for a period of 6 to 12 weeks after initial recovery from the infection, depending on the severity of the infection.[84,131]

**Prognosis.** The death rate from osteomyelitis remains approximately 2% for all confirmed cases. The chances for full recovery and restoration of normal bone structure are excellent with prompt, early, sustained, and effective treatment. When the condition is recognized and treated early, the extent of bone destruction is minimal and complete restoration is possible. However, if the infection is discovered later in the course of illness, inappropriate antibiotic therapy is used, antibiotic therapy is discontinued prematurely, or drainage is inadequate, permanent disability may result.[84,131]

### Nursing problems and intervention

The following section presents a discussion of nursing problems related to long-term musculoskeletal problems. Children and youth who have a medical diagnosis of a long-term problem may have health needs and other health problems that are not referred to in this section; the complete assessment of the child and family provides a basis for identification of the unique health status for each individual child.

#### Ambulation and exercise (MNPC no. 310.0)

Many long-term musculoskeletal problems involve extended periods of complete or partial immobilization, or the child's condition limits the full capacity for motion in parts of the body, as may occur with rheumatoid arthritis. However, it is important to determine the parts of the body that require specific types of exercise and plan for maintaining maximum function, strength, and endurance. Ambulation and exer-

cise planned to stimulate the child's maximum capacity throughout the illness also contribute to the child's independence and sense of inner competence, as well as providing diversion to combat boredom and discomfort.

Play approaches designed for the developmental level of the child are most useful in stimulating the child to participate in planned exercise programs. Once the health care team has determined the exercise needs of the child, specific play activities can be identified that stimulate the type of exercise needed and can provide variety in accomplishing the exercise program. Parents can be taught the essential purposes of planned exercise and play and can participate in the program in the hospital and continue the program independently at home.

The exercise program should aim to provide full range of motion for all of the child's joints unless they have been immobilized for treatment or are restricted by the disease process. For extremities that have been immobilized, muscle function can be improved and maintained by exercises that stimulate muscle contraction of the affected limb. Breathing exercises are essential to maintain optimal endurance and adequate function of the cardiovascular and respiratory systems. Breathing exercises should be designed to stimulate use of the diaphragm and abdominal muscles. Play exercises that can be used for this purpose include blowing soap bubbles, blowing balloons or windmill toys, or making the sounds of animals.

Passive exercises are indicated when the child has no active strength or is not alert enough to respond. When passive exercises are required because of the child's inability to participate in active exercise, each joint is passively moved through its full range of motion for several rotations at least twice a day. These exercises will maintain the range of function of the joint but will not contribute to strength or endurance of the muscle.

Active assistance exercises are used when the child is able to actively participate in the motion but does not have the ability to move freely through the full range of motion. These exercises may be used with a child who has rheumatoid arthritis or who is beginning to regain full function of a joint after a period of immobiliza-

**CHAPTER 18**

Children and
youth with
long-term
physical
problems

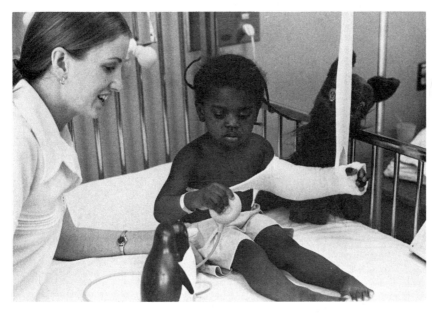

**Fig. 18-4.** This child's arm and cast are in suspension after application of a new cast. Exercise for the other arm and hand is accomplished using a squeeze toy.

tion. The child is encouraged to move the part through the range of motion that is possible, and some form of assistance is given to complete the motion. The assistance can be given by the nurse or parent, or in some instances the child can provide his or her own assistance. For example, the child may be able to use one hand to assist the other arm and hand to accomplish full range of motion. Another form of assistance is accomplished for the shoulder by having the child "climb" the wall with the fingers in order to assist the shoulders to extend the arms above the head.

Active exercises are used when the child has sufficient strength to move through the full range of motion but cannot move against resistance. These exercises maintain function and strength of muscles and contribute to maintaining minimal endurance. They are used after surgery or after a period of immobilization. For example, if the knee has been immobilized and the ankle and foot are free to move, active exercises of the foot are planned to maintain full function of the ankle and foot and contribute to maintaining strength of the leg muscles. A face can be drawn on the child's foot to provide di-

version and stimulate participation in planned exercises.

Resistive exercises are used when the child has sufficient strength to move against resistance. These exercises maintain function, strength, and endurance, and they may be accomplished isometrically. Isometric exercises are useful for a limb that is immobilized for long periods of time. A wide variety of play activities can be planned to accomplish active resistive exercise, both for the child in bed and for an ambulatory child. A child in a spica cast, for example, achieves active resistive exercise of the upper extremities, including the neck, by moving about independently on a spica "bug" or a platform set on ball-bearing casters. Playing with clay provides another type of active resistive exercise for the hands. Hitting a balloon suspended over the bed with a foot is another form of exercise that requires resistance against the weight of the leg.

Coordination exercises are planned when a child has difficulty performing coordinated functional movements. These are often needed after a long period of immobilization and can be stimulated through daily and play activities.[46]

Ambulation of some form should be accomplished for all children with musculoskeletal problems unless they are seriously ill. Provision should be made to move the child from the immediate surroundings of the hospital room or room at home and to make use of the child's own capacity to ambulate to the extent possible. If a child is able to use a wheel chair or spica "bug," space should be planned and designated for the child to move about freely. If the child cannot use a wheel chair, a wagon or the bed may be used to move the child about and provide regular changes in environment and stimulation. Regularly planned excursions beyond the confines of the hospital or home are also desirable if at all possible.

### Nutrition (MNPC no. 310.1)

Optimal nutrition is essential for the child with long-term musculoskeletal problems, with particular focus on the need for providing adequate protein and minerals needed for healing and reconstruction of damaged tissue. Another major concern is restoring nutritional deficits that may have contributed to the child's condition, as might occur when a child who develops osteomyelitis in the face of a debilitated physical condition. Weight gain presents a special problem for a child who is completely immobilized in a body cast, as following a spinal fusion for correction of scoliosis.[104]

Fruits and vegetables and adequate fluid intake are important for a child in a cast or one who is immobilized for periods of time. These dietary components promote adequate function of the bowels and the kidneys, which may be jeopardized as a result of relative inactivity.[46]

### Skin care (MNPC no. 310.2)

Skin care is a primary concern for a child who is immobilized or who is in traction or a cast. Provision must be made for regular changes in position to relieve points of pressure. If a child is in traction and cannot be freely repositioned, the skin should be rubbed with 70% isopropyl alcohol at least every four hours, particularly areas that are subject to pressure. Alcohol is also used around the edges of a cast to toughen the skin and decrease irritation around the cast edges. Powders, lotions, and oils should not be

used, as they soften the skin and increase the skin's vulnerability to breakdown. Cast edges should be petaled with adhesive tape or another material that will provide a smooth edge to minimize irritation to the skin at the edge of the cast and under the cast from dislodged cast particles and help to protect the edge of the cast from damage from the child picking on it or wetting it. Cast edges that are susceptible to soiling, particularly around the perineal area, can be lined with plastic wrap tucked under the edges to protect the cast from becoming wet and soiled, for wetting and soiling of the cast can lead to breakdown and irritation of the skin under the cast as well as damage the effectiveness of the cast.[46]

### Maintenance of body temperature, and other physical care (MNPC no. 310.3)

Measures described in Chapter 11 for maintenance of body temperature are used for children who have an elevated body temperature due to the acute stage of an illness or during postoperative periods. Of particular concern is maintainance of adequate ventilatory function, which is accomplished by using deep breathing exercises described in the section on ambulation and exercise above.

### Psychosocial and intellectual stimulation (MNPC no. 310.4)

The child with long-term musculoskeletal problems has particular needs with regard to self-esteem and body image. Periodic assessment of inner competency, as described in previous chapters for each stage of development, is important to determine how the child's physical problem has affected self-esteem and body image and to determine the effects of therapeutic measures to strengthen the child's inner competency.[77]

Family dynamics that emerge as a result of the child's illness need to be assessed, and specific supportive intervention planned and implemented. The family needs to be fully involved in identifying the nature of stress that they experience and their own needs and goals for coping with the demands created by the circumstances of the child's illness.

Stimulation and learning needs for the child

**CHAPTER 18**

Children and
youth with
long-term
physical
problems

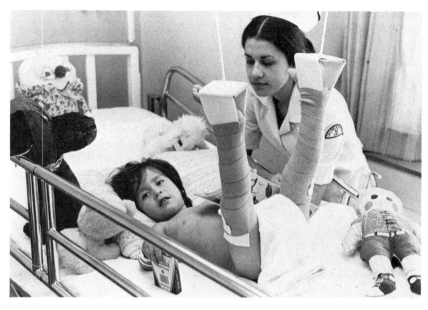

**Fig. 18-5.** This child, who is in Bryant's traction for a fractured pelvis and femur, is getting ready to draw with crayons for nursing assessment of inner competency.

should be provided in accord with the child's stage of development. The long-term isolation and immobilization that often occurs with long-term musculoskeletal problems usually requires that special provisions be made to meet the child's needs for learning and thought either in the hospital or at home.

### Environmental dangers (MNPC no. 310.5)

Protection of the child who is immobilized or disabled in some respect is an important aspect of nursing care. Adequate restraint and precaution to protect the child from falls are especially important when the child is in a cast or when mobility is limited by disability. Teaching is planned to help the child learn to ambulate, use a wheel chair or crutches, and conduct activities of daily living with safety.[46]

### Elimination (MNPC no. 310.6)

Dietary factors related to elimination were mentioned in the section above on nutrition. Special provisions may need to be made for elimination for a child who is immobilized in traction or in a cast.

### Follow-through (MNPC no. 310.7)

Preparation for optimal follow-through care begins early in the child's course of illness through teaching and counseling with the child and parents. During hospitalization the parent or other person who will provide primary care for the child at home should gradually participate in every aspect of care that will be required in the home and demonstrate competence and confidence in the ability to provide care for the child. A home visit is often needed before the child's arrival to assist the family in setting up the home environment to provide care for the child that will be needed. Telephone contact with the health care team in the hospital is often helpful during the first few days after the child arrives at home to assure the family of a resource for answering questions, ventilating feelings, and obtaining support for management of care at home. If long-term use of drugs is needed, the family needs to have periodic assistance in assessing the efficacy of the drugs used. They may also need assistance with any problems that might have emerged for the child.[104]

# LONG-TERM GASTROINTESTINAL AND ENDOCRINE PROBLEMS (MNPC no. 314)

Long-term physical problems that exert a major effect on gastrointestinal and endocrine function are considered in this section. The etiology of these problems often has a genetic basis, but the age at which the problem is expressed is highly variable. While there is usually not a visible physical deformity, many of these problems result in some form of interference with physical growth and development.

## Medical diagnoses and treatment

### Celiac disease (gluten-induced enteropathy)

**Definition.** Celiac disease is a specific defect of gluten metabolism resulting in malabsorption in the jejunal mucosa. This disease is one of several intestinal malabsorption problems that are generally classified as the celiac syndrome. The symptoms of these various problems are similar to those of celiac disease, but the malabsorption deficiency and treatment varies. Gluten-induced enteropathy is the most common of these disorders and is illustrative of the diagnostic and treatment approaches used.[111]

**Incidence.** Celiac disease is the second most common cause of malabsorption in children, with cystic fibrosis being the most common malabsorption disorder. The most frequent age of onset is during the second year of life, although onset can begin at any age, including adulthood. Black and Asian children are rarely affected, and the disease occurs more frequently in Europe than in the United States.[111]

**Etiology.** Celiac disease is generally accepted to be an inborn error of metabolism that is triggered by a variety of mechanisms, including the ingestion of gluten, dietary deficiencies, and emotional stress. The basic defect is thought to be an absence of peptidase in intestinal mucosal cells, resulting in an inability to metabolize the peptides of gliadin, a component of gluten. The toxic factor that initiates the disease is thought to be contained in gliaden.[19,53]

**Pathophysiology.** The ingestion of wheat, oat, or rye gluten is responsible for the underlying pathology of this disease, which results in loss of mucosal villi, obliteration of intervillous spaces, and loss of the brush borders of the epithelial cells. These intestinal changes result in a fundamental malabsorption of fat, predominantly long-chain saturated fatty acids. Hypoproteinemia and nutritional edema sometimes result from diversion of essential amino acids to abnormal metabolic pathways by the atrophied intestinal mucosa.[19]

**Essentials of medical diagnosis.** Medical diagnosis is confirmed by small bowel biopsy that reveals villous atrophy and by improvement of symptoms when the child is placed on a gluten-free diet. The typical symptoms of steatorrhea, failure to thrive, and abdominal distension are often present and suggest the presence of celiac disease; however the bowel biopsy and response to a gluten-free diet are essential to differentiate this disease from other forms of celiac syndrome and other causes of chronic diarrhea. Occasionally, a child does not exhibit diarrhea but may have symptoms of abdominal obstruction.[111]

**Essential features.** Typically, the child has a history of repeated digestive disturbances throughout infancy and early childhood, often thought to be associated with a minor infectious illness. Celiac disease is considered when the child develops continuous diarrhea characterized by voluminous, bulky, pale, frothy, greasy, floating, and offensive-smelling stool. When this pattern of stool develops, the child often exhibits loss of appetite, failure to gain weight, and increased irritability. The loss of weight usually occurs in the limbs and buttocks, while the face remains filled out and the abdomen becomes distended secondary to poor musculature and the accumulation of gas and fluid in the intestinal tract. Anemia and deficiency of fat-soluble vitamins are common, resulting in secondary rickets, osteomalacia, and pathologic fractures. Hypoprothrombinemia and severe intestinal hemorrhage may develop.

Impaired carbohydrate metabolism, hypoalbuminemia, increased fat content of the stool, and evidence of abnormal intestinal function on barium enema examination are common laboratory findings. Hypoalbuminemia is thought to be responsible for the celiac crisis, which is an acute episode of precipitous weight loss and dehydration stimulated by an acute digestive upset, such as a gastrointestinal viral infection that would cause only a minor disturbance in most children.[9,19,111]

**Special stress factors.** The degree of stress created by celiac disease depends upon the severity of the problem, which can vary from very mild and almost imperceptible to very severe with marked failure to thrive. If strict dietary restrictions are required to control the disease, this factor and the persistent threat of celiac crisis place major stress on the family and child.

**Medical treatment.** Dietary gluten restriction is the primary therapy used for celiac disease. Improvement of signs and symptoms occurs within a week of instituting a gluten-free diet, and histologic repair of intestinal atrophy is complete after three months. The gluten-restricted diet must be maintained for life, although in some instances a child may develop a greater tolerance for gluten after several years of therapy. The degree of gluten restriction that must be maintained is dependent upon the severity of the disease for an individual child. In addition to gluten restriction, the diet should provide about 25% more calories than would otherwise be required for the child's weight and at least 6 to 8 g of protein per kilogram of body weight per day. Restriction of fat intake is not necessary.

A gluten-free diet eliminates from the diet the following foods, which contain sources of wheat, rye, and oat gluten:

All breads, rolls, crackers, cakes, and cookies made from wheat, rye, or oats
All wheat, oat, and rye cereals, spaghetti, macaroni, and noodles
All canned soups except clear broth
Commercial ice cream
Prepared mixes and puddings
Postum, Ovaltine, and some instant coffees
Beer and ale
Commercial candies containing cereal products

Corticosteroids may be used for a child who has a celiac crisis or for a child who continues to fail to thrive despite enforcement of a strict gluten-free diet. Corticosteroid therapy produces dramatic remission of the disease and can be withdrawn after a remission has been established.[111]

**Prognosis.** Most children who receive adequate dietary therapy gradually improve and have a complete remission of clinical signs and symptoms. However, intermittent exacerbations of the symptoms may occur frequently, and severe responses to digestive tract infections may continue. Death due to celiac disease is unusual.[111]

### Juvenile-onset diabetes mellitus

**Definition.** Diabetes mellitus is a disturbance of carbohydrate metabolism usually associated with a deficiency of insulin, which begins during childhood or adolescence. It is differentiated from adult-onset diabetes only because of the unique, abrupt onset of the condition and the greater difficulty in controlling the symptoms than typically occurs with adult onset.[91]

**Incidence.** The incidence of diabetes mellitus in children under the age of 15 years in the United States is estimated to be 40 cases per 100,000 children. Approximately 10,000 children are newly diagnosed with diabetes mellitus each year.[136]

**Etiology.** A number of causes have been explored for the phenomena of diabetes mellitus, and it appears that there are probably several different causes resulting in multiple distinct entities with differences observed in symptom severity, age of onset, and genetic heterogeneity. It is generally agreed that there is a genetic predisposition that contributes to the clinical onset of diabetes mellitus but that specific environmental factors such as infection, diet, and life stress may trigger the onset of symptoms. It is now clear that the etiology does not simply rest in a deficiency of insulin production and that the underlying lesion may be in extrapancreatic body tissues, the pancreas, or both. One possible explanation is the presence of a primary insensitivity to insulin action in the peripheral muscle and adipose tissue that might initially stimulate elevated insulin secretion for maintenance of normoglycemia, resulting in the ultimate exhaustion of pancreatic beta cell secretory capacity. Another explanation that has received attention is the possibility of peripheral factors that set limits on the pancreatic ability to respond to increased demands for insulin secretion. Serum antagonists or specific antibodies that reduce the effectiveness of circulating insulin have also been considered as a possible cause of diabetic symptoms. An autoimmune reaction to the islet of Langerhans cells has also been postulated, with some evidence of support in some children.[136]

**Pathophysiology.** As is true concerning etiologic factors, the altered metabolic state of diabetes mellitus is complex and is not yet understood entirely. Once the etiologic pathology has occurred, a deficiency of endogenous insulin results and glucose utilization by body tissues is impaired, with a resulting hyperglycemia. Glycogen synthesis in the liver is decreased, and reserves of glycogen are depleted. The major physiologic effect of this state is as follows:

First, there is decreased utilization of glucose by the body cells for essential metabolic and energy requirements. This results in a significant increase in blood glucose level to as high as 300 to 1,200 mg/100 ml. Glucose is lost in the urine, causing an obligatory diuretic effect because of the osmotic pressure in the renal tubules. Both water and electrolytes are lost in the urine. This extracellular water loss in turn causes compensatory dehydration of the intracellular fluid.

Second, since glucose cannot be used for cellular metabolism, there is significant mobilization of fats from the fat storage areas, along with abnormal fat metabolism in the cells. There is a resulting accumulation of keto acids in the body fluids, with a resulting acidosis. The concentration of keto acids in the extracellular fluids contributes further to progressive acidosis through obligatory loss of sodium, which occurs in the renal excretion of a proportion of the keto acids.

Third, the lack of glucose available for metabolic purposes also stimulates the utilization of protein for cellular metabolism, with a resulting diminished deposition of protein in the tissues of the body. This effect is also partially caused by the loss of the direct effect of insulin in promoting protein anabolism, which to some degree accounts for the diabetic individual's lack of energy, tendency to develop skin lesions that will not heal, and degeneration of various organs of the body.[26,41]

**Essentials of medical diagnosis.** The essential features of medical diagnosis are[45]:
1. Hyperglycemia and glycosuria with or without ketonuria
2. Weight loss, polyuria, polydipsia, and abdominal or leg cramps
3. Enuresis, mild appetite loss, emotional disturbances, and lassitude
4. Diminished glucose tolerance

**Essential features.** The onset of juvenile diabetes mellitus is rapid, with progression to severe ketoacidosis and coma in a matter of hours or days. Twenty percent of all children diagnosed with diabetes mellitus are first seen in a coma or near coma.[45] During the early or prediabetic phase, there is an excess of insulin circulating in the blood. Atrophy of the cells of the islets of Langerhans occurs later, and a complete diabetic state results within five to ten years after onset. Usually within three months after the initiation of insulin therapy, there is a temporary remission of the diabetic state, referred to as the "honeymoon" period. The diabetic state then progresses over a period of four to five years with increasingly less frequent remissions, until there is complete insulin insufficiency. Oral hypoglycemic agents are usually ineffective, and insulin replacement is required. Management of an appropriate insulin dosage is difficult to attain, for variations in response to insulin occur with significant swings from hypoglycemia to hyperglycemia. If insulin replacement is not provided, ketoacidosis develops rapidly. Exercise has a significant effect on lowering blood glucose levels, which contributes to the difficulty in regulating insulin dosage. Emotional responses of the child and the parents are great, and these reactions affect the stability of management of insulin administration and diet and exercise management. Complications occur frequently in juvenile diabetes, with most children suffering some type of complication within 20 years of the onset of symptoms.[26,117]

Etteldorf and Burghen[26] suggest the following guidelines for classification of a child's condition according to the degree of hyperglycemia and disturbance in acid-base balance:

**Stage I**
Glycosuria without ketonuria; minimal dehydration
Blood glucose < 350 mg/100 ml

$HCO_3^- > 15$ mEq/L
Blood pH—normal range
Not acidotic clinically

**Stage II**

Glycosuria and ketonuria without significant acidosis
Blood glucose > 350 mg/100 ml
$HCO_3^- > 15$ mEq/L
Blood pH—normal range

**Stage III**

Glycosuria, ketonuria, and significant acidosis (Kussmaul respiration, dehydrated skin, and subcutaneous tissue, lethargy)
Blood glucose usually > 500 mg/100 ml
$HCO_3^- < 15$ mEq/L
Blood pH 7.1 to 7.35

**Stage IV**

Glycosuria, ketonuria, with severe acidosis and impending coma or coma
Blood glucose 500 to 750 mg/100 ml or higher
$HCO_3^- < 10$ mEq/L
Blood pH < 7.1

**Special stress factors.** Special stresses created by the diabetic condition are related to the monotonous task of daily attention to insulin administration, diet, and exercise. The child and the family are tied to constant consideration of the special needs imposed by the diabetic condition and the necessity to continually adjust and take this into account. For example, when diabetic children go to parties with friends, they must consider what they eat when faced with high carbohydrate party foods. Depending on the severity of the problem and the success they have achieving insulin control, they may

**Table 18-2.** Specific treatment during first 24 hours according to stage of severity

| Dosage of regular insulin | Diet and parenteral fluids and electrolytes |
|---|---|
| **Stage I** | |
| First dose, give insulin according to the sliding scale (Table 18-3)<br>Repeat insulin administration according to sliding scale before each meal and at bedtime snack | Parenteral fluids usually necessary<br>ADA diet: 1,500 Cal/m² or 1,000 Cal + 100 Cal/year of age to be started promptly; 30%-30%-30% of calories with major meals and 10% as bedtime snack |
| **Stage II** | |
| First dose, give 1 unit/kg subcutaneously; not to exceed 35 units;<br>After 4-6 hr give ½ unit/kg every 4-6 hr until urine 1+ or negative for sugar, then start sliding scale every 6 hr<br>Note: Add 1 unit crystalline insulin for each 2 g of glucose in parenteral fluids | Oral fluids: in absence of nausea and vomiting, give 2-4 oz of orange juice or skim milk and water as tolerated every 4 hr<br>If unable to take oral fluids, give intravenous fluids, 2,400 ml/m²/24 hr electrolyte solution No. 75 (Table 18-5)<br>No initial hydrating fluid required if plasma $K^+$ is normal and patient voiding; added $HCO_3^-$ usually not indicated |
| **Stage III** | |
| First dose, give 2 units/kg subcutaneously<br>Subsequent doses as in stage II<br>Note: Add 1 unit crystalline insulin for 2 g glucose in intravenous fluids | Initial hydrating fluid: 400 ml/m² (Table 18-4) and infuse over 1-2 hr period<br>Repeat hydrating fluids without glucose if patient has not voided<br>Then start replacement and maintenance, 3,000 ml/m²/24 hr electrolyte solution No. 75 (Table 18-5) |
| **Stage IV** | |
| First dose, give 3 units/kg crystalline insulin if blood glucose 500-750 mg/100 ml or 4 units/kg if blood glucose > 750 mg/100 ml<br>If after 6 hr blood glucose > 500 mg/100 ml, give 1-2 units/kg insulin<br>Subsequent doses same as in stage II<br>Note: Add insulin to intravenous fluids as in stages II and III | Initial hydrating fluid: same as in stage III<br>Replacement and maintenance, 3,600 ml/m²/24 hr electrolyte solution No. 75 (Table 18-5) |

From Etteldorf, J. N., and Burghen, G. A.: Juvenile diabetes. In Hughes, J. G., editor: Synopsis of pediatrics, ed. 4, St. Louis, 1975, The C. V. Mosby Co., p. 620.

**Table 18-3.** Regular insulin by sliding scale

| | Weight (kg) | | | |
|---|---|---|---|---|
| | **70** | **35** | **15** | **10** |
| 4+ glycosuria | 20 U | 10 U | 8 U | 5 U |
| 3+ glycosuria | 15 U | 8 U | 5 U | 3 U |
| 2+ glycosuria | 10 U | 5 U | ±3 U | 0 U |

When a fractionally collected urine specimen is negative or 1+ with an ADA diet, calculate the insulin dosage on the basis of 1:20 insulin:glucose (in the diet) ratio; ADA diet contains 140 g available carbohydrate/1,000 Cal.

**Table 18-4.** Composition of initial hydrating fluid

Formula*
| | |
|---|---|
| $Na^+$ | 75 mEq/L |
| $HCO_3^-$ | 50 mEq/L |
| $Cl^-$ | 25 mEq/L |
| Glucose | 5 g/100 ml if blood glucose < 250 mg/100 ml |
| | 2.5 g/100 ml if blood glucose > 250 mg/100 ml |
| | No glucose if blood glucose > 600 mg/100 ml |

This solution may be prepared as follows*:
| | |
|---|---|
| 7.5% $NaHCO_3$ solution | 56 ml |
| Physiologic NaCl solution | 162 ml in 2.5% or 5% dextrose |
| Dextrose in water (2.5% or 5%) | 782 ml |

One-half strength physiologic saline with appropriate concentration of glucose may be used*

*Omit dextrose when not desired.

**Table 18-5.** Composition of replacement and maintenance fluid–electrolyte solution No. 75 or Inosol T

| Formula | Concentration |
|---|---|
| $Na^+$ | 40 mEq/L |
| $K^+$ | 35 mEq/L |
| Lactate | 20 mEq/L |
| $Cl^-$ | 40 mEq/L |
| $PO_4^-$ | 15 mEq/L |
| Glucose | 5 g/100 ml |

From Etteldorf, J. N., and Burghen, G. A.: Juvenile diabetes. In Hughes, J. G., editor: Synopsis of pediatrics, ed. 4, St. Louis, 1975, The C. V. Mosby Co., p. 621.

have to decline some of the delectable goodies enjoyed by their peers. They live with constant awareness of the possibility of insulin shock or diabetic coma. The adolescent is faced with the problems of the effect that the diabetic condition will have in adult life, particularly in establishing intimate adult relationships and childbearing.[5,26,39,40,108]

**Medical treatment.** Table 18-2 summarizes initial medical treatment that is essential during the first 24 hours of the onset of symptoms or when a child has an imbalance crisis. Table 18-3 gives a sliding scale for the calculation of insulin dosage. Tables 18-4 and 18-5 present the composition of fluids for hydration and replacement of fluid and electrolytes. After the first 24 hours, children in stages I and II will gradually tolerate a full diet, which is based on the American Diabetic Association recommendations. Insulin requirements may be calculated according to the sliding scale in Table 18-3. Crystalline insulin, administered 20 minutes before meals and bedtime snack, is used for the first few days, after which the child may begin to use an intermediate-acting insulin such as isophane (NPH). Table 18-6 shows the types of insulin that are commonly used and describes features of their action.

Children who are initially in stages III and IV require parenteral therapy and intensive insulin therapy for several hours beyond the first 24 hours. Oral fluids of orange juice, skim milk, and water are given as tolerated. When oral fluids are well tolerated, the child can be gradually managed with diet and insulin therapy.

After the initial crisis, a prolonged period of time is required to achieve control using insulin therapy, balanced with diet and exercise management. In addition the child and family must learn about the diabetic condition and begin to acquire the ability to plan and manage the diet and regulate insulin requirements.

Several different models for dietary management are used; however the diet of the American Diabetic Association is the most widely recognized. This diet provides 20% of the calories as protein, 40% of the calories as carbohydrate, and 40% of the calories as fat. It supplies 140 g of available glucose and 50 g of protein/1,000 calories. Instructions for using the diet

CHAPTER 18

Children and
youth with
long-term
physical
problems

**Table 18-6.** Types of insulin and their action

| Type of insulin | Time of administration | Onset of action | Peak effect | Duration of action | Probable glycosuria | Probable hypo-glycemia | Remarks |
|---|---|---|---|---|---|---|---|
| Crystalline or regular | 20 min before meals, subcutaneously, intra-muscularly, or intra-venously | Within 1 hr | 2 hr | 6-8 hr | Night | 10 AM-12 NOON | |
| Isophane (NPH) | 45-60 min before† breakfast, subcutane-ously | 2 hr | 8-12 hr | 18-24 hr | 10 AM-12 NOON; before break-fast | 3 to 6 PM | |
| Globin | 45-60 min before* break-fast, subcutaneously | 2 hr | 8-12 hr | 18-24 hr | 10 AM-12 NOON; before break-fast | 3 to 6 PM | Similar to NPH |
| Lente | 45-60 min before* break-fast, subcutaneously | 2 hr | 8-12 hr | 20-26 hr | 10 AM-12 NOON | 3 to 6 PM | Contains no prota-mine or globin; useful in insulin allergy |

*From Etteldorf, J. N., and Burghen, G. A.: Juvenile diabetes. In Hughes, J. G., editor: Synopsis of pediatrics, ed. 4, St. Louis, 1975, The C. V. Mosby Co., p. 623.
†When mixed with crystalline insulin, the mixture should be given 20-30 min before breakfast.

include an exchange system that allows for a wide range of selection of foods. Calories must be distributed throughout the day and balanced with activity requirements. Each of three major meals during the day usually contains 30% of the total daily caloric intake, with another 10% taken at bedtime. An 8-ounce glass of milk is often recommended in addition to the regular diet for every one to two hours of active exercise. Twenty-four-hour calorie requirements may be calculated by age or by body surface area as follows:

**Age**
1,000 calories for the first year of life plus 100 calories for each additional year.

**Body surface area**
1,500 Cal/m²

The maximum daily calorie intake ranges from 1,800 to 2,000 calories per day for girls and from 1,800 to 2,400 calories per day for boys. During strenuous activity, such as work or sports, an additional 200 calories every one or two hours is recommended rather than a decrease in insulin dosage.

As soon as possible the child is switched to intermediate-acting insulin. The initial 24-hour dose of intermediate-acting insulin is 80% of the previously established 24-hour regular in-sulin dose. If the dose for 24 hours does not exceed 20 units, a single morning dose may suffice, but control is usually more effective if the dose is given in two divided doses. Two thirds of the total 24-hour dose is usually given 45 to 60 minutes before breakfast, and the remaining portion of the dose 12 hours later. Regular insulin may be combined with the morning dose of intermediate-acting insulin if the child consistently exhibits glycosuria before or after breakfast. The dose of regular insulin is calculated according to the sliding scale in Table 18-3.

Strict control of juvenile diabetes is impractical and leads to emotional and behavioral problems. Temporary mild hyperglycemia and glycosuria may be tolerated, and the child and family can be taught to recognize moderate or severe hyperglycemia and ketosis and to take appropriate action to prevent repeated episodes. Insulin-induced hypoglycemia is characterized by weakness, pallor, diplopia, sweating, and twitching and is treated with glucagon, 1 mg, administered subcutaneously or intramuscularly. The child and family need to learn to recognize an impending insulin reaction and to use oral sugar, orange juice, milk, or sweetened beverages to prevent it.

Long-term education is essential for the

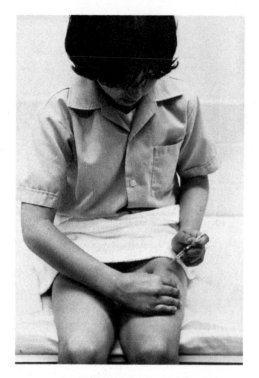

**Fig. 18-6.** The child is learning to administer his own insulin injection.

child, and new learning needs emerge with each developmental stage. The child needs to acquire an ability in maintaining good body hygiene, protection from infection, insulin administration and regulation, diet management, and exercise management. Temporary live-in programs for the child and family have been designed to bring several families together where they can learn to manage the requirements of diabetic control with a comfortable and active life-style. Summer camps have been particularly effective in bringing groups of diabetic children together for periods of time where they can learn independence in managing their daily living and diabetic control measures, as well as share their experiences and feelings with peers.*

**Prognosis.** The prognosis for diabetic children and youth achieving a productive adult life is optimistic. Children who have juvenile-onset diabetes tend to develop complications such as retinal, renal, and cardiac disease, with accompanying disability or shortening of the life span. The factors leading to complications are not clearly understood, and existing evidence suggests that these developments are not related to the degree of control maintained or the age of onset. Future research and clinical investigation are needed to more adequately define aspects of treatment that might affect the eventual prognosis for individual children.[136]

### Cleft lip and cleft palate

**Definition.** Cleft lip and cleft palate result from failure of the maxillary and premaxillary processes to fuse at about the fifth week of intrauterine development. The resulting defect runs from the vermillion border of the lip to the inferior surface of the nostril and may be bilateral or unilateral, and partial or complete.[2]

**Incidence.** Cleft lip and cleft palate are the most common anomalies of the face and mouth. It is estimated that this problem occurs in 1 of every 800 live births.[116]

**Etiology.** Cleft lip and cleft palate defects are thought to be caused by a multifactorial inheritance combined with toxic environmental factors that interfere with normal development in intrauterine life. An embryo who has an inherited susceptibility for the development of this defect will manifest the defect if, at a critical period of development, a toxic factor interferes with the movement of the palatal shelves from a vertical position alongside the tongue to a horizontal position above the tongue. When this shift is delayed beyond the critical period of development (about the fifth week of gestation), development of the structures is arrested and fusion of the structures does not occur.[106]

**Pathophysiology.** Once the defect has developed in the gestational period, no further interference with development and function occurs during intrauterine life. However, after birth, the infant experiences varying degrees of interference with gastrointestinal and otolaryngeal function arising from the defect. The infant is unable to suck effectively and experiences nasal regurgitation and episodes of coughing and choking. Insufficient intake of calories accounts for a lack of weight gain in the first few months

*References 4, 26, 63, 64, 91, 101, 115, 136.

**CHAPTER 18**

Children and
youth with
long-term
physical
problems

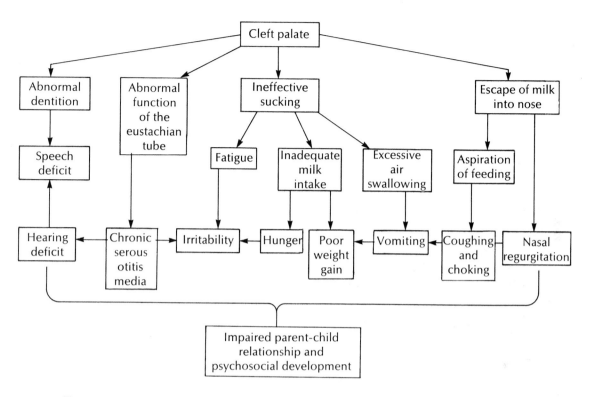

**Fig. 18-7.** Interrelationship of problems for a child with cleft palate. (Adapted from Pradise, J. L., and McWilliams, B. J.: Simplified feeder for infants with cleft palate, Pediatrics **53**:567, April, 1974.)

of life. Middle ear disease is almost invariably present at birth or soon thereafter for infants with cleft palate. It is thought that middle ear disease arises from impairment of the opening mechanism of the eustachian tube, which results in functional obstruction and abnormal compliance of the tubal wall.[94]

**Essentials of medical diagnosis.** A cleft lip deformity is readily apparent at birth and suggests the presence of a cleft palate. Cleft palate deformities without the presence of a cleft lip may not be apparent until the infant has difficulty feeding, which is usually accompanied by nasal regurgitation. A cleft that involves only the uvula or soft palate may only be detected by palpation of the palate.[116]

**Essential features.** Fig. 18-7 represents diagrammatically the multiple problems that result from a cleft palate deformity. The severity of the deformity is related to the severity of the sequelae, which are outlined in Fig. 18-7. Cleft palate severity is classified into four types, as follows:[25]

TYPE I: Cleft confined to the soft palate
TYPE II: Unilateral cleft of the entire soft and hard palate
TYPE III: Unilateral cleft of the entire soft and hard palate and the alveolar ridge
TYPE IV: Bilateral cleft of the entire palate and the alveolar ridge

A cleft lip that exists without a cleft palate may not lead to multiple physiologic problems for the infant but may create a strong emotional response in the parents, leading to a risk of impaired early parent-child relationships.

**Special stress factors.** In addition to the stress involved in giving birth to a child with a visible deformity, the family faces a long period of therapeutic intervention, including surgery, medical care, speech and hearing therapy, dental and orthodontic treatment. Feeding and caring for the infant is difficult and often leads to frustration rather than being a mutually satisfying experience. Speech and hearing deficits ultimately lead to impaired social relationships for the child and to difficulty in learning and school performance, even though surgical repair of the palate and/or lip may have been accomplished.

**Medical treatment.** Feeding the infant is the first major problem. A variety of methods is used to assist the infant in obtaining sufficient volume of intake, and the mother needs teaching and assistance in acquiring skill in using the method chosen. Prosthetic feeding devices that obturate the palatal cleft, "Ducky" or lambs' nipples, have been used with varying success. The simplest and often preferred method of feeding is the use of a device that permits manual expression of milk into the infant's mouth. The Beniflex Cleft Lip/Palate Nurser (Mead Johnson Laboratories) is one such device that is available and is usually effective, but the cost of using these disposable appliances for each feeding is a problem for many families. A disposable Playtex nurser that is readily available on the market may be modified by enlarging the vertical slit along the side of the plastic bottle-holder to allow space for the mother to gently compress the milk bag as the infant sucks. Vomiting and choking can be minimized by holding the infant in a relatively upright position during feeding and regulating the expression of milk with signs of the infant's readiness to swallow.[95]

Surgical repair of a cleft lip is usually planned for the first few months of infancy or by the time the infant reaches about 12 pounds of body weight. An incomplete or complete unilateral cleft lip can usually be repaired with little residual deformity. A bilateral cleft lip often has some residual deformity because of the anterior displacement of the premaxillary process and the absence or marked shortening of the columella of the nose. Repair of a cleft palate is usually planned for approximately 14 to 18 months of age or when the child reaches about 20 pounds in body weight. Speech therapy is begun at the time of the cleft palate repair and is continued for at least four to five years. If the gingival margin is involved in the cleft, deformed or supernumerary teeth must be re-

moved as they erupt, and dental prosthetic devices built. Orthodontic treatment is usually instituted at about 5 years of age.[2]

Treatment for chronic serous otitis media includes providing middle ear aeration by myringotomy, aspiration of middle ear fluid, and insertion of tympanotomy tubes. This procedure is repeated as necessary to maintain adequate aeration of the middle ear and prevent acoustic damage. Marked improvement in the child's otolaryngeal problems occurs after the palate is repaired.[93,94]

**Prognosis.** The child's long-term prognosis depends on the severity of the deformity, the degree of hearing loss and speech deficit that develops, and the response of the child and family to the stresses of the problem and treatment.

## Nursing problems and intervention

The following section presents a discussion of the nursing problems and intervention that are particularly important in relation to long-term gastrointestinal and endocrine problems. The complete nursing assessment will reveal the exact nature of these problems for the individual child, as well as health maintenance needs and other types of health problems.

### Elimination (MNPC no. 314.0)

As reflected in the previous discussion of medical diagnoses, elimination is often a particular problem for the child with long-term gastrointestinal and endocrine problems. Dietary measures to control elimination problems are designed in accord with the particular needs of the child, based on the nature of the underlying illness. For example, a child with celiac disease must limit or exclude the intake of gluten to control elimination problems, while the child with diabetes must balance the dietary sources of calories. The nursing focus in providing care is teaching the child and family the features of the illness of the child and how the diet affects their elimination and facts regarding foods and dietary supplements. Assistance in planning for the dietary needs of the child and recognizing signs of dietary effectiveness or failure is often needed. Often the nurse is able to help the family recognize the effect that other problems might have on their ability to achieve control of elimination problems, such as might occur if the child uses the illness to gain manipulative control of the environment or if the mental health of the parents is such that they cannot cope with the effective management of the diet.

### Nutrition (MNPC no. 314.1)

In addition to the particular requirements of the diet in achieving control of problems such as elimination, the child's nutrition needs to be maintained at an optimal level in order to maintain optimal physical health and growth. The total intake needs to be evaluated periodically for its adequacy in meeting the minimum daily requirements, and changes in dietary requirements must be assessed as the child grows. Feeding problems are not uncommon for children who must adhere to special dietary requirements and arise as an expression of the emotional stress of the illness and the social stress that it creates. For example, a diabetic child might refuse to eat as a behavioral attempt to control and manipulate the family. Other types of feeding problems that occur are the feeding difficulty encountered with a child who has a cleft palate or loss of appetite. Nursing teaching and counseling are focused on helping the family provide optimal nutrition for the child within any dietary restrictions that must be considered and achieve compatible mealtime arrangements for the entire family.

### Skin care (MNPC no. 314.2)

Body hygiene and prevention of infection are the major concerns for a child who has long-term gastrointestinal or endocrine problems. This is a particular concern for the diabetic child who is prone to complications of the integumentary system and for children whose illness creates a debilitated state. As the child grows into the school-age and adolescent periods of development and assumes personal responsibility for body hygiene and prevention of infection, teaching and counseling with the child focuses on this problem area.

### Psychosocial needs (MNPC no. 314.4)

Regardless of the extent to which the child's illness is visibly apparent, children with long-term gastrointestinal and endocrine problems have difficulty in establishing a healthy self-concept and body image. Young children often perceive some wrong-doing that might have caused their physical problems and have greatly distorted perceptions of their body and its internal function. Children who can "hide" their illness, such as a diabetic child or a child with celiac disease, may exert much attention and energy toward keeping their problem from peers or may widely publicize their problem in order to gain attention from peers, which may result in inadequate peer relationships.

The life-long, day-to-day demands of managing illnesses like diabetes make problems particularly stressful for families. Families vary in their ability to cope over a long period of time, and all families experience periodic crises when the child's condition worsens or when another type of stress event, which may not otherwise be considered stressful, occurs but which the family perceives as "the last straw." Health care workers need to be sensitive to the stress experiences of the family and make provisions for crisis intervention or counseling and psychotherapy in accord with the family's needs.

### Environmental dangers (MNPC no. 314.5)

The increased risk of infection for many children with long-term gastrointestinal and endocrine problems is a particular concern. Measures to increase the child's resistance to infection may suffice for most children; however in some instances measures to decrease environmental sources of infection may be needed. If the hygienic condition of the home is poor, the family may need assistance in learning to provide an environment that will decrease sources of infection. Some families, such as a family with a severely affected child with a cleft palate and chronic otitis media, may need to alter their social contacts in the home, forego travel, or make other alterations in their life-style in order to protect the child from infection.

### Rest, recreation, and exercise (MNPC no. 314.6)

The child's condition and nature of the illness are assessed to determine the optimal balance needed between rest and exercise. The family life-style is assessed to determine the extent to which their usual pattern of rest and activity will tend to promote an optimal balance or if alterations are needed to meet the child's needs. For example, a family who is accustomed to a sedentary life-style may need to alter their life-style to provide planned activity on a regular basis for a diabetic child. If a life-style change is needed, this change presents a particular stress on each member of the family, and their individual needs must be taken into account in helping them work out a suitable plan that is beneficial for the child but that respects their own life-style preferences.

### Follow-through (MNPC no. 314.7)

Adequate follow-through for children with long-term gastrointestinal and endocrine problems is an aspect of care that should be carefully planned by the entire health care team working with the family. Often the family is served by several different health care workers, and fragmentation of care and inadequate follow-through for particular aspects of care can easily develop. The nurse who is providing primary health care and teaching needs to periodically assist the family in reviewing the health care services they are receiving and determine their needs for follow-through and priorities for each area of care.

## CENTRAL NERVOUS SYSTEM PROBLEMS (MNPC no. 315)

This section presents a discussion of long-term disorders of the central nervous system. A discussion of seizure disorders is presented in Chapter 13; hyperkinetic problems are discussed in Chapters 13 and 19.

### Medical diagnoses and treatment
#### Cerebral palsy

**Definition.** Cerebral palsy is a term used to denote a group of diverse nonprogressive impairments of neurologic function caused by brain injury or deficient structure, growth or development of the central nervous system. The term is usually limited to disorders that are presumed to have developed before birth, during the birth process, or within the first year of life.[73,89]

**Incidence.** The incidence of cerebral palsy is estimated to be between 1 to 5/1,000 live births.[89]

**Etiology.** Cerebral palsy is usually considered to be an acquired problem of the prenatal, perinatal, or early infancy periods of development, although genetic factors may contribute to the development of the impairment. During the early gestational period, faulty implantation of the ovum or diseases of the mother may be responsible for the neurologic impairment. Maternal conditions that are sometimes associated with early neurologic impairment include extreme nutritional deficiency, infection, injuries, toxins, and radiation. These factors are thought to injure the developing fetal brain and lead to permanent motor defects. Prematurity and low birth weight are the most commonly associated problems, with 20% to 25% of children with cerebral palsy having a birth weight of less than 2,500 g. Asphyxiation, cerebral hemorrhage, and meningitis are the most frequent perinatal conditions leading to brain damage and permanent neurologic impairment for both preterm and full-term infants.[73]

**Pathology.** About one third of cerebral palsy children have gross malformations of the brain, regardless of the etiology. The changes in the remaining two thirds of the children are often microscopic changes and usually involve the cortical or subcortical tissues. Cortical lesions are characterized by laminar degeneration, fallout of neurons, and cortical atrophy with narrowing of gyri and widening of sulci. Subcortical lesions are characterized by atrophy of white matter and gliosis of the deep central structures. Symmetric demyelination of the globus pallidus and the subthalamic nucleus is found in children who have an athetoid type of palsy resulting from kernicterus.[73]

**Essentials of medical diagnosis.** The essentials of medical diagnosis are:[89]
1. Impairment of neurologic function, particularly voluntary motor activity
2. Nonprogressive condition
3. Condition apparent at birth or during early infancy

**Essential features.** Table 18-7 presents a classification of cerebral palsy disorders based on anatomic site and clinical manifestations.

CHAPTER 18

Children and
youth with
long-term
physical
problems

**Table 18-7.** Clinical, anatomic classification of neuromotor disorders

| Anatomic site | Clinical manifestations | Topographic manifestations |
|---|---|---|
| Pyramidal tracts | Spastic paralysis | Paraparesis—legs only; diplegia—legs more than arms; quadriparesis—all four extremities; hemiparesis—half the body; monoparesis—usually one extremity |
| Extrapyramidal tracts | Athetosis, choreiform movements, dystonia, tremor, rigidity | Arms, legs, neck, trunk |
| Cerebellum and/or connections | Ataxia | Arms, legs, trunk |

From Jabbour, J. T., Duenas, D. A., and Gilmartin, R. C.: Diseases of the nervous system. In Hughes, J. G., editor: Synopsis of pediatrics, ed. 4, St. Louis, 1975, The C. V. Mosby Co., p. 852.

Spasticity is the most common type of manifestation, with about 65% of children with cerebral palsy exhibiting spasticity in some part of the body; 40% have spastic hemiparesis and 22% have spastic quadriparesis. Spasticity consists of hyperreflexia, clasp-knife phenomena, hypertonia, and an extensor toe sign.

Extrapyramidal impairment results in several different types of faulty motor movements. About 22% of children with cerebral palsy have these types of disorders. Athetosis consists of a slow, writhing, twisting movement of the limbs, which is in contrast to the quick, jerky, purposeless limb and face movements of choreiform movements. Mixed movements, termed choreoathetosis, may occur and are often accompanied by intermittent plastic or cog-wheel rigidity.

About 10% to 15% of children with cerebral palsy have ataxia, hypotonia, or mixed disorders. These children exhibit incoordination, dysmetria, an inability to perform rapid and alternating movements, and hypotonia. Hypotonia types of disorders may only be manifested at birth by general muscle hypotonia, which lasts for six to eight months. Gradually, over a period of one to two years, the child develops hypertonia, hyperreflexia, and spasticity. Delayed developmental milestones may become apparent by 3 years of age, and strabismus and behavior problems occur during the preschool and school-age period.

About 50% of children with cerebral palsy have some degree of mental retardation. Visual problems, such as refractive errors, astigmatism, and squints, are present in about half of all affected children. Other sensory defects, such as proprioceptive and spatial orientation disturbances, occur in about 30% of affected children. Language and learning disorders are present in about 30% of children with cerebral palsy.[58]

**Special stress factors.** Regardless of the severity of neurologic impairment, the family faces the life-long problems of living with a disabled child. Initially, most families assume that their child is mentally retarded, and even if this proves not to be the case, they are faced with the inevitable response of society to their child, which labels the individual with cerebral palsy as mentally deficient in some manner. Their response to the child and their ability to achieve a reality-based attitude toward their child as an individual are of paramount importance in helping the child achieve maximum potential for physical, learning, and social and inner development. If the child is severely disabled, the family is faced with life-long custodial care for the child, either in the home or through placing the child in a custodial care facility outside of the home. If the child has normal or near-normal intellectual capacity and can achieve independence in mobility and most daily activities, the family needs to facilitate maximal independent function and integration into society, which presents new stresses each time the child enters into a different stage of development.

**Medical treatment.** Control of seizures is achieved with drug therapy as described in Chapter 13, p. 512. Dextroamphetamine may be used to control hyperactivity to some extent. The dose used is 2.5 to 15 mg orally in the morning and at noon, depending on the size, age, and degree of hyperactivity in the child. Other psychotropic drugs, such as methylphenidate, chlorpromazine, or chlordiazepoxide may also be effective in controlling hyperactivity. Spasticity may be controlled to some extent with diazepam, 2 to 5 mg orally two to four times a day, or by dantrolene, 3 to 12 mg/kg/day in three to four divided doses. Dantrolene may cause hepatotoxicity, and the safety of the drug for children under 5 years has not been established.[89]

Physical therapy and orthopedic treatment are essential for many children to achieve and maintain maximal function. Physical therapy exercises are used to achieve and maintain maximum range of motion and prevent contractures. Orthopedic bracing and splinting are used to prevent and correct deformities of spastic disorders. Rigid bracing and rigid night splinting are used to maintain the limbs in a position of maximal extension. Reconstructive orthopedic surgery may be used for some children, including tenotomies, muscle and tendon transfers, joint arthrodeses, and denervations. Surgical intervention is subject to dispute, for the benefits are often disappointing and do not yield substantial functional improvement. Children with athetoid disorders are not benefited by braces, and neurosurgical procedures may be the only approach that offers improvement in the condition.[84]

Special education may be needed for the child and is planned according to the needs of the child and the desires of the family. Special programs for children with cerebral palsy often include facilities for physical therapy and assistance with managing the activities of daily living as an integral part of the educational program.

**Prognosis.** Severely affected children with mental retardation and seizures that are difficult to control usually die during childhood, due to intercurrent infections and complications arising from the neurologic disability. Children who can achieve a degree of mobility and independence have a better prognosis for survival. If the child has normal or near-normal intellectual capacity, it is usually possible for him or her to experience productive and satisfying adult living.[89]

*Hydrocephalus*

**Definition.** Hydrocephalus is a condition of increased volume of cerebrospinal fluid that either has been or is under pressure and that accumulates in the ventricular system of the brain as a result of distal obstruction to normal cerebrospinal fluid circulation. If the condition develops before closure of the sutures of the skull, enlargement of the head occurs. If the condition occurs after the closure of the sutures, signs of intracranial pressure occur.[103]

**Incidence.** The incidence of congenital hydrocephalus varies in different populations, with a range reported of 0.2 per 1,000 births to 4 per 1,000 births. The incidence of other types of hydrocephalus is estimated as just under 1 per 1,000.[56]

**Etiology.** There are three major causes of hydrocephalus: neoplasms, congenital malformations, and posttraumatic or postinflammatory obstruction. Neoplasms seldom occur during early infancy but may occur at any time during development. The most common neoplasms that occur during infancy and childhood that are associated with hydrocephalus are gliomas located in either the third ventricle, the periaqueductal region, or the fourth ventricle and cerebellum. Several congenital anomalies can produce hydrocephalus. These include aqueductal stenosis or atresia, absence or atresia of the foramens of Luschka and Magendie (Dandy-Walker syndrome), elongation of the lower brain stem and caudal displacement of the fourth ventricle in the upper cervical canal (Arnold-Chiari syndrome, frequently associated with myelomeningocele), arteriovenous malformation of the great vein of Galen compressing the aqueduct of Sylvius, and blockage of the interventricular foramens of Monro. The most frequent cause of hydrocephalus is postinflammatory or posttraumatic obstruction of the basilar cisterns and associated subarachnoid pathways, particularly in the tentorium region.[89,103]

**Pathophysiology.** The three mechanisms by which hydrocephalus develops are: (1) obstruction of circulation of cerebrospinal fluid with the ventricular system or in the subarachnoid pathways with secondary dilatation of the channels proximal to the site of obstruction, (2)

CHAPTER 18

Children and
youth with
long-term
physical
problems

defective absorption of cerebrospinal fluid through the arachnoid villi, associated with progressive fibrosis of the arachnoidal pathways as a sequela of trauma or infection, and (3) overproduction of cerebrospinal fluid due to a choroid plexus tumor.

Secondary changes occur in the brain as a result of increased volume of cerebrospinal fluid. Pressure from the ventricles leads to progressive thinning of brain tissue and demyelination and loss of white matter. Rupture of the septum pellucidum may occur with marked ventricular dilatation, and there may be areas of cortical rupture into the subarachnoid space that form external cerebrospinal fluid fistulas. In less severe cases, there is only flattening of the convolutions of the brain, and atrophic changes in ganglion cells may occur. When hydrocephalus occurs before closure of cranial sutures, the head bones are often thinned, the fontanels enlarged, and suture margins separated.[103]

**Essentials of medical diagnosis.** Abnormal enlargement of the cerebral ventricles due to an increased pressure gradient between the intraventricular fluid and the brain is the primary criteria for diagnosis of hydrocephalus. Evidence of ventricular enlargement is obtained by air encephalography, computerized axial tomography, or both. Air encephalography is accomplished by injecting air into a ventricle (ventriculography) or by the lumbar route (pneumoencephalography), and subsequent x rays are taken to observe the size of the ventricles and locate the site of obstruction or presence of a tumor. Computerized axial tomography is a noninvasive technique that provides a picture of the entire ventricular system and from which the etiology may be inferred.[89]

**Essential features.** The signs and symptoms of hydrocephalus vary with the age of onset, the underlying cause, and the rapidity with which hydrocephalus develops. In infants with a severe, rapidly progressing hydrocephalus that develops before birth, death often occurs in utero or the infant's head is enlarged to the extent that a caesarean section is required for delivery. The infant has a large head, frontal bossing, thinning of the skull and skin over the head, translucent skin with visible veins over the head, and a "setting sun" appearance of the

eyes, in which the eyes appear to be depressed and more sclera than normal shows above the iris. An infant who has a rapidly developing condition may develop these signs and symptoms within a few weeks. For the majority of infants, no apparent malformation is present at birth, and there is a gradual increase in head size with the head circumference exceeding the percentile measurement present at birth and exceeding the percentile of growth in height and weight. The fontanel measurement reflects a gradual increase, rather than the expected gradual decrease. Neurologic signs are often normal, with the exception that the infant may have a delayed ability to hold up the head and demonstrate other developmental delays. Spasticity or ataxic phenomena may be present at any age. If an acute obstruction is present, the infant or child may have vomiting, irritability or listlessness, and difficulty with vision and gait. In the older infant or child, signs and symptoms include Macewen's cracked pot sign of sprung sutures, papilledema or other eye findings, disturbances of muscle tone and reflexes, and incoordination.

A markedly elevated cerebrospinal fluid protein is often present with a choroid plexus tumor and occasionally after a central nervous system infection or hemorrhage. Low cerebrospinal fluid glucose is present in hydrocephalus that results from a previous infection. Obstructive hydrocephalus results in an increased 5-hydroxyindoleacetic acid in the cerebrospinal fluid.[89,103]

**Medical treatment.** Occasionally, hydrocephalus arrests spontaneously, but usually surgical intervention is needed to assure survival and adequate intellectual development. Isosorbide, an osmotic agent capable of reducing the formation of cerebrospinal fluid without inducing significant diuresis, is sometimes used to delay or prevent the need for surgical intervention.[72]

Surgical intervention consists of shunting to drain excessive cerebrospinal fluid from the lateral ventricles into the great veins and into the heart. Occasionally the fluid is shunted into the peritoneal cavity as a temporary measure, and the shunt is later revised to a vascular shunt. Inert plastic tubing with a Silicone valve allowing unidirectional flow is placed from the cerebral ventricle into the right atrium by way of the jugular vein. After placement of the shunt, serial head and chest roentgenograms are taken to confirm proper placement of the shunt, and manometric testing of ventricular pressure and ventriculography with $CO_2$ are used to confirm the success of the surgery. The shunt is usually replaced periodically to prevent complications from infection and assure continued proper placement as the child grows. Complications from the shunt include a sudden rise in intracranial pressure due to blockage or other malfunction; displacement of the shunt mechanism, particularly at the distal end with growth; infections (most frequently a coagulase-positive *Staphylococcus albus*) with septicemia, meningitis and ventriculitis; electrolyte imbalances; and subdural hematoma following abrupt collapse of enlarged ventricles. Periodic evaluation of the function of the shunt is necessary to detect early signs of complications and to intervene with a revision of the shunt before a serious complication arises.[89,103]

**Prognosis.** If hydrocephalus can be arrested with shunting procedures, the prognosis for survival and functioning is improved considerably, with other handicaps that might be present having a major determining role in predicting the prognosis. For children who do not receive shunting control of the condition, the survival rate at 10 years of age is only about 25%, with only about 5% being able to continue to function and carry out activities of daily living. For children who receive shunting intervention, the survival rate at 10 years of age is about 60%, with many of these children able to function and care for themselves. About 25% of these survivors have normal or higher than normal intelligence. Follow-up evidence indicates that of children who survive the first one or two years after shunting, spontaneous arrests of the condition occur in 40% to 50%, which may be a result of the ependymal surface growing sufficiently large to absorb excessive amounts of cerebrospinal fluid.[89,103]

### Spina bifida

**Definition.** Spina bifida is a midline closure defect of the vertebral column. Spina bifida occulta is the most frequent form of this type of defect, but it is rarely symptomatic and often goes undetected. It is a failure of closure of the bony vertebral column, and the spinal cord beneath the vertebral column remains intact. This deformity usually occurs in the fifth lumbar and first sacral vertebral segments. Cystic forms of spina bifida involve some degree of malformation of the spinal cord. Meningocele is a cystic lesion in the midline of the back that contains only meninges or perhaps meninges and nerve roots and is well covered with skin. There is no neurologic impairment associated with the spinal defect, although hydrocephalus may develop. These lesions occur with similar frequency in the cervical, thoracic, and lumbar spines. Meningomyelocele is a cystic lesion in which the nerve roots have failed to separate from the epithelium, resulting in a sac that contains cerebrospinal fluid, incompletely formed meninges, and malformed spinal cord. There is neurologic impairment below the level of the defect, which most frequently occurs in the lumbosacral region.[120]

**Incidence.** Spina bifida occulta is estimated to be present in about 25% of young children, with the majority of the defects not detected, and eventual fusion of the posterior vertebral arches occurs. An estimated 5% of these defects are estimated to persist into adult development. Cystic forms of spina bifida occur in about 2 per 1,000 births, with meningomyelocele occurring in about 1 per 800 births.[89]

**Etiology.** The etiology of these defects is not known, but genetic factors appear to be present in that a history of other affected family members is present for about 8% of all affected children. Environmental causes, such as viral or irradiation injury to the embryo, have been suggested as possible etiologic factors.

**Essentials of medical diagnosis.** Radiographic evidence of spina bifida occulta confirms a defect of the vertebral column that is not apparent otherwise. A meningocele may not be recognized immediately if there is a sufficient skin covering and if the sac does not contain sufficient cerebrospinal fluid to protrude visibly. Radiographic evidence of the defect confirms failure of closure of the bony vertebrae, and surgical intervention confirms a differentiation of the lesion from meningomyelocele in that no abnormalities of the spinal cord tissue are found. Meningomyelocele is readily recognized because of the lack of skin covering the sac and neurologic impairment.[120]

**Essential features.** A few children with spina bifida occulta will develop neurologic difficulty during periods of rapid growth. Signs and symptoms include muscle weakness resulting in gait disorders, trophic ulcers that develop as a result of sensory loss, or incontinence due to loss of sphincter control.

Signs and symptoms of cystic forms of spina bifida are often extensive, and associated malformations and complications are common. Hydrocephalus develops in 65% of children who have a meningomyelocele and in 10% of children with meningocele. Hydrocephalus is usually associated with an Arnold-Chiari malformation (see discussion of hydrocephalus, above) or as a sequela of meningitis that occurs from infection of a leaking sac or after surgical repair of the spinal defect. Congenital deformities of the feet or legs and congenital dislocation of the hips are not uncommon. Children with meningomylocele have neurologic deficits in the limbs and pelvis below the level of the deficit. The lower extremities may be normal with lesions in the sacral region, but there is loss of sphincter control and sensory loss in the sacral area. A child with a lesion in the lumbosacral region often has fairly good movement of the hips and knees, but the ankles are paralyzed and the feet are inverted in an equinovarus position. A child with a lesion in the thoracolumbar region has flaccid paralysis of the legs, poor development of the abdominal musculature, congenitally dislocated hips, and loss of sphincter control. Meningitis and urinary tract disease are common complications of meningomyelocele. Meningeal infections are commonly caused by *Escherichia coli, Pseudomonas aeruginosa,* or *Staphylococcus epidermidis.* Urinary tract diseases that develop include urinary tract infections, bladder atony, vesicoureteral reflux, hydronephrosis, and eventual renal failure.[120]

**Special stress factors.** The readily apparent spinal defect and related neurologic impairment cause a major traumatic impact for the parents at birth. The family is faced with coping with uncertain outcomes of surgery, uncertain development of the child, the possibility of many serious complications, and the life-long stress of daily coping with the complex needs of the child. As with other types of serious congenital problems, the child requires intensive therapy from many different specialists on the health care team, including neurosurgeon, orthopedist, urologist, physical therapist, and nurse. The financial burden of care for the child is usually such that financial assistance is needed. If the child is born with multiple problems and has a poor prognosis, the family is faced with making decisions between proceeding with life-saving intervention or providing supportive care only. A less severely affected child who has a good prognosis for survival and improved function with adequate intervention is faced with life-long disability of varying degrees and the possibility of major complications, repeated surgical procedures, and extensive therapy to achieve maximal function.

**Medical treatment.** Surgical intervention for spina bifida occulta is not indicated unless the child develops symptoms that indicate the need for surgical correction of the defect. Surgical repair of a meningocele defect is usually delayed until after the child reaches 3 months of age. If the child with a meningocele is destined to develop hydrocephalus, evidence of this complication will emerge by the third month, and surgical shunting for the hydrocephalus is often performed before correction of the spinal defect.

A meningomyelocele that ruptures and leaks before delivery or during the neonatal period must be repaired as soon as possible to decrease the dangers of ascending meningitis. The only contraindication to immediate surgical repair is when the child has many related congenital and birth problems with a poor prognosis, in which case the health care team and the family may elect to provide only supportive care for the infant. If a meningomyelocele is intact and appears to present no threat of rupture, delay of surgical repair may be desirable until after 3 months of age. If surgical repair is delayed, the sac must be protected with a "doughnut" of foam rubber covered by plastic, raised sufficiently above the level of the sac to prevent contact. The sac may be treated with silver nitrate to encourage epithelialization and prevent subsequent rupture or leakage.

Orthopedic surgery to correct congenital deformities of the feet, legs, and hips is indicated to enhance the child's ability to ambulate. Urologic medical and surgical intervention is essential, and the child's urologic status must be carefully assessed at frequent intervals. The incidence of renal complications is decreased by suprapubic manual expression of urine from the bladder, the use of in-dwelling catheters, and ultimately a surgical ureteroileostomy. Urinary tract infections must be recognized early and treated with appropriate antibiotic therapy. Mandelamine or cranberry juice in the diet acidifies the urine and may reduce the frequency of urinary tract infections. Fecal incontinence may be reduced by the use of constipating foods and drugs. A colostomy may be indicated for an older child who is able to function but who is inhibited by fecal incontinence. Skin care of the perineal area, around abdominal ostomies, and at pressure areas is essential.[71,89,120]

**Prognosis.** The prognosis for children with repaired spina bifida occulta and meningocele is the same as that of the complications that may occur with these conditions. About 30% of children with meningomyelocele achieve long-term functional capability with normal mental ability, although they may be multiply handicapped due to neurologic and orthopedic deficits. The predominant long-term threat to life and health is impairment of renal function. About 10% of infants who are born with a meningomyelocele die within the first six weeks of life, and another 5% to 10% die within the first year. The most common causes of early death are meningitis and hydrocephalus. These complications and renal failure account for death during later childhood.[89]

### Bacterial meningitis

**Definition.** Bacterial meningitis is an inflammation of the meninges following invasions of the spinal fluid by any of a wide range of organisms. This problem is included in this chapter because of the frequency with which it occurs in infants and young children and the high risk of long-term neurologic sequelae.[54] Discus-

sion of the unique characteristics of bacterial meningitis in the newborn and early infancy period of development is presented in Chapter 8.

**Etiology and epidemiology.** *Haemophilus influenzae* type B, pneumococcus, and meningococcus are the most common causative organisms of bacterial meningitis in infancy and early childhood. However, a wide variety of organisms can be isolated as the causative organism, and the predominant organisms involved vary geographically and from year to year. Bacterial meningitis occurs predominantly in infancy and childhood, and the relationship between the illness and age is presumed to be due to the young child's lack of acquired resistance to the invading organisms. Meningococcal infections cause epidemic outbreaks. *H. influenzae* infections occur most frequently between 3 months and 3 years of age, while pneumococcal and meningococcal infections occur most frequently in the first year of life. During the newborn period, the most common organisms involved are *E. coli* and other gram-negative organisms.[24,54]

**Pathophysiology.** Usually meningitis is the result of bacteremia from an upper respiratory infection. Direct extension of an infection of the paranasal sinuses, mastoid, or abscesses contiguous to the meninges may occur. Entry from penetrating wounds, spinal puncture, or neurosurgical operative procedures also occurs. The infection causes hyperemia and edema in the brain. An exudate composed of fibrin, pus cells, red cells, and the infectious organism collects in the subarachnoid space. Blockage may occur in the foramens of Luschka and Magendie, the aqueduct of Sylvius, or the foramen of Monro. The cerebral cortex may suffer destructive changes, and thromboses may form in the meningeal veins or venous sinuses. Deafness, blindness, or facial weakness may result from infection and exudate about the cranial nerves. Serious lesions in other areas of the body may occur as a result of a meningococcal infection, including petechiae from septic thrombi in the vessels of the skin, purulent lesions in the peritoneum, pericardium, and pleura, and hemorrhage into the adrenal gland.[24,54]

**Essentials of diagnosis.** The medical diagnosis is based on the following features:

1. Fever, headache, vomiting, and convulsions, and tense fontanel
2. Petechial rash of skin and mucous membranes (specifically with a meningococcal infection)
3. Stiff neck
4. Flexion at the hip, knee, or ankle in response to flexion of the neck (Brudzinski's sign)
5. Inability to extend the leg with the hip flexed (Kernig's sign)
6. Cultures of blood and cerebrospinal fluid to determine the invading organism

It is estimated that in about 15% of patients admitted to hospitals with meningitis, culture evidence cannot be obtained because of antibiotic therapy previously administered for treatment of an upper respiratory infection, which masks the early symptoms of meningitis and makes it impossible to grow the organism in culture.[24,54]

**Essential features.** Signs and symptoms of meningitis vary initially because of the varying symptoms that emerge with different age groups, the nature of the invading organism, the duration of the illness, the type and duration of previous therapy for a previous infection, and whether the meningitis is a complication of another severe illness or exists as a single illness. Older children react similarly to adults in that the onset is likely to be abrupt and there are clear classic signs of meningeal irritation. Initially the child has fever, headache, and vomiting, which may be accompanied by or is shortly followed by changes in levels of consciousness. The child is extremely irritable and may become delirious, alternating with periods of extreme drowsiness. Later, the child becomes comatose. Convulsions may occur at any stage of the illness. The young child or infant often does not exhibit symptoms of meningeal irritation and serious illness until the infection is well advanced. Early signs and symptoms may be loss of appetite, irritability, and persistent fever. The only signs of central nervous system irritability may be irritability alternating with drowsiness, a high-pitched cry, and a transient vacant stare as if the infant or child is disconnected with the environment. Tension of the fontanel is the most important sign of central nervous system involvement. When the child or infant already has another illness, the signs and symptoms of meningeal irritation may be very difficult to detect, and the major clue might be that the child appears to be more seriously ill than might be expected from the present illness.

The cerebrospinal fluid pressure may be increased, and the appearance is usually cloudy, although in the earliest stages of the infection the fluid may be clear. The blood cell count is elevated, and protein is elevated. The cerebrospinal fluid glucose level is low, and when compared to the blood glucose level, the cerebrospinal glucose level is less than two-thirds that of the blood glucose level. Cultures of the blood and cerebrospinal fluid must be obtained before administering antibiotic therapy and reveal the invading organism. Gram-stained smears of scrapings from petechiae lesions may be used to detect meningococci.[54]

**Medical treatment.** Early detection and treatment of bacterial meningitis is imperative to prevent long-term neurologic damage or death. The child is isolated as soon as a diagnosis of meningitis is suspected and remains in isolation until at least 24 hours of therapy with a known effective antibiotic has been accomplished. Until the etiologic organism is identified, the child is treated with ampicillin administered parenterally. Chloramphenicol is used for children with a documented sensitivity to penicillin. Supportive care and symptomatic management that must be instituted include maintenance of adequate hydration, maintenance of ventilation, management of bacterial shock, reduction of intracranial pressure, control of seizures, control of extremes in body temperature, and correction of anemia. Initially, the child's hydration level may be depleted, and the fluids and electrolyte balance must be corrected. Thereafter, a low maintenance level of fluid intake is maintained to minimize cerebral edema. Signs of increased intracranial pressure must be carefully monitored. These include an irregular respiratory rate, increase in systolic blood pressure, bradycardia, and persistent seizure activity. Reduction of increased intracranial pressure may be accomplished by the use of a hypertonic solution such as mannitol administered as a 20% solution of mannitol in distilled water (1.5 to 2.0 g/kg). A 30% to 60% reduction in cerebrospinal fluid pressure lasting for from two to four hours may be expected with this type of hypertonic solution. Hydrocortisone, 25 to 50 mg/kg/day in four divided doses, may be used when the inflammatory response is maximal to reduce intracranial pressure and to treat bacterial shock. Signs of bacterial shock include initially a mild change in sensorium, diminution in urinary output, and alteration in blood pressure and cardiac output, followed by rapid deterioration. Blood volume must be restored and acid-base balance corrected immediately, and the child may need digitalization and the administration of heparin for associated disseminated intravascular coagulopathy.

Subdural effusions develop in almost half of the infants and young children with meningitis, with about 10% developing a condition requiring treatment. This complication is most commonly associated with *H. influenzae* and pneumococcal infections. The signs and symptoms of a serious subdural effusion include (1) persistence of fever or a return of fever after the child has been afebrile, (2) persistence of abnormal neurologic signs or the return of abnormal neurologic signs after they have disappeared, (3) persistence of a full fontanel, (4) persistence of pathogenic organisms in the cerebrospinal fluid, (5) an increase in head circumference, and (6) persistent vomiting. When these signs are present, bilateral subdural taps are performed; the presence of more than 2 ml of fluid confirms the presence of a subdural effusion. Daily tapping is used to remove the fluid until it ceases forming, which usually occurs within a few days in children whose condition is diagnosed early. If fluid continues to form after two weeks of daily tapping, a neurologic procedure of stripping the membranes may be performed in an effort to treat the condition and prevent permanent neurologic handicaps, such as convulsive seizure disorders.

The Waterhouse-Friderichsen syndrome is an extremely serious complication caused by bilateral adrenal hemorrhage. It is usually associated with meningococcal meningitis, but it can occur with any type of infection. The survival rate is extremely poor. The child develops

signs and symptoms including profound shock, petechial and ecchymotic lesions that spread rapidly, and vomiting and prostration. Symptomatic treatment of shock is the primary means of therapy and includes replacement of blood, fluids for maintenance of electrolyte balance, and drugs to elevate the blood pressure. Corticoid therapy may be used and may improve the child's chances for survival.

Young children in the family and other children who have been exposed to the child should be evaluated for signs of a similar infection. No prophylactic treatment is used for persons exposed to *H. influenzae* or pneumococcal infection, but because of the epidemic nature of meningococcal infections, family members may be given prophylactic antibacterial therapy in an effort to prevent their contracting the infection.

The child who has recovered from bacterial meningitis must be periodically evaluated at intervals of three to four months for at least a year following recovery. Neurologic sequelae may not be immediately apparent, and early detection of residual damage is needed to provide appropriate intervention for the child and to plan for special considerations that may be needed for learning.*

**Prognosis.** The prognosis for the child depends upon early detection of the illness, the age of the child, and the nature of the invading organism. The overall fatality rate for meningitis is 10% to 15%, with another 15% exhibiting long-term neurologic sequelae. The lowest fatality rate is reported for children over a year of age with *H. influenzae* meningitis; the fatality rate associated with this infection for infants and children combined is 8%, but an estimated 35% of these infants and children are incapacitated for life or have permanent sensory or neuromotor impairment. In pneumococcal infections, the death rate exceeds 25% in infants under 1 year of age. The Waterhouse-Friderichsen syndrome is responsible for 20% of the fatalities associated with meningococcal meningitis.

Neurologic impairments following meningitis include cerebral damage, hydrocephalus, motor deficits, spastic hemiplegia, visual or auditory

---

*References 12, 15, 32, 54, 60, 86, 128.

**CHAPTER 18**

Children and
youth with
long-term
physical
problems

impairment, vestibular damage, seizure states, mental retardation, hyperactivity, and specific learning disabilities.[24]

## Nursing problems and intervention

The following section sumarizes health problems that are particularly associated with central nervous system disorders. The comprehensive nursing assessment and intervention includes identification of health maintenance needs appropriate to the age and stage of development of the child in addition to the problems discussed in this section.

### Ambulation and exercise (MNPC no. 315.0)

Many disorders of the central nervous system result in some type of interference with full ambulation capacity. When such an impairment is present, nursing care is focused on assisting the child to achieve the maximum degree of locomotion possible and includes teaching the child and family to use braces, crutches, or wheelchair devices for self-locomotion. Careful and consistent nursing care must be given to maintaining the integrity of the skin in areas that are subject to pressure or friction and to maintain maximum range of motion of all joints. Practice and exercise are important in developing self-locomotion skill, as is nurturing an inner motivation on the part of the child and the family. Specific exercises are used to prevent secondary deformities as well as to maintain maximal motion capacity.

Besides specific exercises designed for therapeutic purposes, the level of activity that the child engages in is an important component of maintaining health. If the child uses self-locomotion capacities, achieves independence in most activities of daily living, and has opportunity for social involvement that promotes activity, the child's activity level is probably sufficient to promote an optimal state of health.

### Nutrition problems (MNPC no. 315.1)

One of the predominant problems for many children with central nervous system impairment is feeding. A severely affected child with cerebral palsy, for example, may require several months of planned teaching and assistance in order to gain the ability to manipulate feeding utensils. Specially designed feeding utensils may be needed to make it possible for the child to grasp a spoon and hold it in a position whereby food can be delivered to the mouth. The patience and effort required to develop this capacity are considerable, but the resulting satisfaction makes the effort worthwhile.

Dietary planning is important in working with a child who has bladder or bowel incontinence or who has an ostomy, as often occurs with a child who has a meningomyelocele. Regular mealtimes and foods that promote optimal bowel function are important considerations for the child with bowel incontinence or a colostomy. Adequate fluid intake is essential to maintain optimal renal function for a child who has bladder impairment and renal impairment.

### Skin care (MNPC no. 315.2)

Meticulous skin care is essential for a child who has limited functional mobility or who has bowel or bladder incontinence or an ostomy. Areas of pressure from lying or sitting or from the use of crutches or braces must be carefully observed daily, and attention must be given to periodically relieving the pressure by repositioning the child. Ostomy care or care of the perineum must be thorough and frequent in order to maintain adequate skin integrity where urine or feces come in contact with the skin.

### Maintenance of body temperature and other physical care (MNPC no. 315.3)

Maintenance of body temperature is most often associated with acute episodes of illness to which the child is prone or to acute conditions that cause increased intracranial pressure, such as meningitis. Measures to prevent infection are of vital importance for children who have central nervous system disorders.

Provision of ventilation and adequate pulmonary function is a consideration for children whose neurologic impairment involves the thorax or whose level of activity is limited. Specific measures to exercise and to expand the lungs may be needed on a daily basis.

### Psychosocial needs

A child with permanent neurologic impairment has many unique psychosocial needs, for the limitations of the condition interfere greatly with the development of social and inner competencies. The social experiences and stimulation experiences that a nonhandicapped child of a comparable stage of development may be used as a guideline to plan for the needs of the handicapped child. During childhood and adolescence, peer group experiences are of great importance, and the family may need assistance in finding a way to meet this need for the child. Often there are provisions for the handicapped child in school groups that primarily serve nonhandicapped children and facilities that serve handicapped children only. Both types of peer group experiences are desirable for most handicapped youngsters, but a multitude of problems interfere with providing such experiences for the child. Transportation for the handicapped child may be difficult to obtain, or an appropriate facility may be located a distance away from the child's home. Special provisions for ambulation, feeding, toileting, and other physical care must be provided for many handicapped children, which limits the numbers of settings that can accommodate a handicapped child in a social group experience. A child's limited ability to communicate, as often occurs with cerebral palsy, presents a major psychosocial handicap. The nursing focus in working with children with these types of problems is to assist the family in identifying their needs, the experiences that would be optimal for the child, and the provisions that can realistically be made in providing these experiences.

### Follow-through (MNPC no. 315.7)

Adequate follow-through is imperative for children with neurologic problems. Several specific follow-through needs have been described for the medical diagnoses in this section. In addition to the particular concerns related to the child's medical problems, the nurse should periodically evaluate the child's developmental level and identify emerging needs based on developmental changes. A child may have developmental delays in some areas of competency, while in other areas the child's development may be congruent with age-standardized norms. Stimulation of optimal development in each competency area needs to be planned for each

stage of development and periodically reviewed to determine the child's developmental progress.

## CARDIOVASCULAR PROBLEMS (MNPC no. 316)

Congenital heart defects are the most common cause of cardiovascular problems during childhood. The most common of these are discussed in the following section. A discussion of rheumatic fever and hypertension, both of which may have long-term cardiovascular problems associated, is presented in Chapter 13.

### Medical diagnosis and treatment of congenital heart disease
#### General considerations

**Definition.** Congenital heart disease is any functional disturbance in cardiovascular function that arises from a structural defect present at birth. The functional disturbance is often apparent at birth but may first appear during childhood or even adulthood.

**Incidence.** Congenital heart diseases occur in about 1% of all children. Table 18-8 presents the incidence of the most common types of defects among children who have congenital heart defects and the risk of recurrence of the defect in subsequent siblings.[47]

**Etiology.** Approximately 2% to 3% of all congenital heart defects are caused by a single mutant autosomal or sex-linked gene. The cardiac defect is one of several abnormalities. The most common of these conditions is Noonan's syndrome (Turner phenotype), which usually involves pulmonic stenosis. Another 4% to 5% of all congenital heart defects are associated with chromosomal abnormalities, with the cardiac defect being one of several other abnormalities. The most common of these types of defects are those associated with trisomies. Trisomy 21 (Down's syndrome) has a 50% incidence of cardiac defects, trisomy 18 has a 99% incidence of cardiac defects, and trisomy 13 has a 90% incidence of cardiac defects. The remaining 92% to 94% of all congenital heart defects are probably caused by multifactorial inheritance, in which there is a polygenetic predisposition interacting with environmental triggers. The environmental triggers that are most often

CHAPTER 18

Children and
youth with
long-term
physical
problems

**Table 18-8.** Incidence and risk of recurrence of congenital heart defects (CHD)*†

| Lesion | Incidence/100 children with CHD | Recurrence risk (%) |
|---|---|---|
| Ventricular septal defect | 35-50 | 6-7‡ |
| Patent ductus arteriosus | 10-15 | 3-4 |
| Atrial septal defect (secundum) | 5-10 | 2.5-3 |
| Endocardial cushion defects | 5-10 | 2.5-3 |
| Coarctation of the aorta | 6-8 | 2.5-3 |
| Aortic stenosis | 6-8 | 2.5-3 |
| Pulmonic stenosis | 6-8 | 2.5-3 |
| Tetralogy of Fallot | 4-6 | 2-2.5 |
| Transposition of great arteries | 4-6 | 2-2.5 |
| Pulmonary atresia | 1-2 | 1-1.5 |
| Tricuspid atresia | 1-2 | 1-5 |
| Truncus arteriosus | 1-2 | 1-1.5 |
| Total anomalous pulmonary venous connection | 1-2 | 1-1.5 |

*From Hoffman, J. I. E.: Congenital heart disease; introduction. In Rudolf, A. M., editor: Pediatrics, ed. 16, New York, 1977, Appleton-Century-Crofts, p. 1404.

†This table does not include bicuspid aortic valves, which occur in about 2% to 3% of live-born children.

‡This is theoretical and higher than the 4.5% to 5% actually observed, because the latter does not take into account people whose defects closed spontaneously.

associated with congenital heart defects are drugs, viruses, environmental toxins, and maternal conditions that affect embryonic development during the first trimester of development. Infants of diabetic women have an increased risk of congenital heart defects, and about 50% of infants of alcoholic women have heart defects.[47,90]

**Pathophysiology.** There are two major factors that determine the nature and magnitude of the hemodynamic alterations produced by congenital heart defects. These two factors are the presence of abnormal pathways of flow of blood and resistance opposing blood flow through a portion of the circulation. The volume of blood flow through any pathway in the cardiovascular system is defined by the following relation:[134]

$$\text{Flow} = \text{Pressure/resistance}$$

In fetal circulation the pulmonic and systemic vascular beds are parallel to one another; with birth these two pathways change in series with one another. This change is created by the elimination of the pathways of flow provided in fetal circulation by the foramen ovale, the ductus arteriosus, the ductus venosus, and the placenta. In addition the resistance to flow changes in the two vascular beds. In fetal circulation, pulmonary vascular resistance is higher than systemic vascular resistance. At birth, pulmonary vascular resistance decreases dramatically due to the reduction of vasomotor tone in the pathway with the first inspiration and gradually because of reduction of medial muscle in the small muscular pulmonary arteries. Systemic vascular resistance, on the other hand, increases because of the elimination of the low resistance pathway of flow in the placenta. Because of these changes the right ventricle is able to perfuse the pulmonary vascular bed at a much lower pressure than is true of the systemic circulation. If an anatomic communication between the two pathways of flow persists after fetal life, such as occurs with a ventricular septal defect or a patent ductus arteriosus, the direction of blood flow is determined by two factors: the pressure relationship between the two chambers or vessels connected by the defect and the relationship between the resistance in the two vascular beds that are connected. Specific anatomic and functional relationships will be presented for each defect in the following section, which describes several common defects in more detail.

Congenital heart defects that produce cyanosis are characterized by an anatomic abnormality that produces obligatory shunting of blood that is relatively unsaturated with oxygen from the systemic circulation back into the systemic circulation, without passing through the pulmonary pathway. The pathophysiologic features of these defects can be categorized as follows:

1. Conditions in which there is almost complete mixing of the systemic and pulmonary venous streams in an atrium, ventricle, or the great vessels because of an anatomic pathway of flow that brings the two streams together. Examples of this type of defect are the tricuspid atresia, total anomalous venous return, hypoplastic left ventricle syndrome (conditions that result in atrial mixing), a single ventricle (resulting in ventricular mixing), and truncus arteriosus (resulting in arterial mixing).

2. Lesions with reduced pulmonary flow result in significant arterial hypoxemia. The ventricular pressures are usually identical, and pulmonary artery pressure is low. The major hemodynamic stress on the myocardium is the increased pressure work that is required of the right ventricle. An example of this type of lesion is tetralogy of Fallot.

3. Lesions in which the systemic and the pulmonary circulations remain separate and do not connect serially either through direct channels or through a capillary bed result in no mixing between the two major pathways. An example of this type of lesion is transposition of the great arteries. For the patient to survive, an associated defect that permits mixing between the two systems must be present, such as an arterial septal defect, a ventricular septal defect, or a patent ductus arteriosus.

While these categories are useful in conceptualizing the hemodynamic alterations that create cyanosis, they are arbitrary. Overlap between the groups frequently occurs. Furthermore, the severity of the defects influences the extent to which hemodynamic function is altered.[134]

**Essentials of diagnosis.** Medical diagnosis is based on complex evaluation and description of several dimensions, which make possible the differentiation of the type of defect that exists and provide a basis for medical intervention. The areas of diagnostic study include:[90]

1. Auscultation of heart sounds. Of particular importance in the diagnosis of congenital heart defects is the second heart sound. The intensity and manner of splitting provide important diagnostic clues. Murmurs, which occur innocently in most young children, require expert evaluation in relation to the characteristics of the murmur, the persistence of the murmur with changes of position and manipulation, and the child's overall state of health and other physical findings.

2. Evaluation of femoral and arterial pulses, arterial blood pressure, and venous pressure and pulse. The quality and amplitude of the pulses in each pulse site, as well as the rate and the rhythm of the pulse, are evaluated for variations from expected normal findings.

3. Electrocardiogram findings. The electrocardiogram is essential for diagnosis of cardiac defects. Although some defects yield no changes in the electrocardiogram, changes that do occur are important in diagnosis of the defect. The electrocardiogram shows age-related variations in that the rate gradually decreases and intervals generally increase with age. Ventricular dominance progresses from right ventricular dominance in young infants to left ventricular dominance in the older infant and child. A persistence of an infantile pattern is a clue to possible defects. Abnormalities in the propagation of electrical force are manifested as alterations in the direction and duration of force or as increased or decreased electrical force (e.g., amplitude of the QRS complex). Fig. 18-8 defines the events that are recorded on the electrocardiogram. A general description of each event that is usually recorded and upon which an interruption of the electrocardiogram is based follows:[90]

a. Rate. The paper speed at which the electrocardiogram is usually recorded is 25 mm/sec. Each small square is 1 mm and represents 0.04 second, and each large square is 5 mm and represents 0.2 second. Five large squares extend for 25 mm and represent 1 second. To estimate the ventricular rate, the number of large squares between two QRS complexes is counted. If two large squares appear between QRS complexes, the ventricular rate is estimated to be 150 per minute.

b. Rhythm. Interpretation of rhythm is very

**CHAPTER 18**

Children and
youth with
long-term
physical
problems

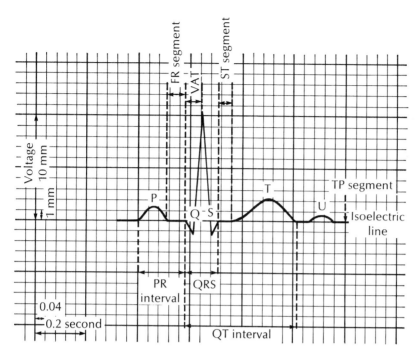

**Fig. 18-8.** Complexes and intervals of the electrocardiogram.

complex, but a general guideline for a normal rhythm is a normal P wave followed by a normal P-R interval and a normal QRS complex.

c. P wave. The P wave represents atrial depolarization and in the child is normally not taller than 2.5 mm and not longer than 0.08 second in duration.

d. P-R interval. The P-R interval is measured from the beginning of the P wave to the beginning of the QRS complex. It ranges from a minimum of 0.11 in infants to a maximum of 0.18 in older children with slow rates.

e. QRS complex. The QRS complex represents ventricular depolarization, and the interpretation of this complex is one of the most important aspects of diagnosis. The amplitude and direction of force of the QRS complex reveal the relative size of viable ventricular mass and abnormal ventricular conduction.

f. Q-T interval. The Q-T interval is measured from the beginning of the QRS com-

plex to the end of the T wave. The normal duration is rate-related and is affected by drugs such as digitalis and electrolyte imbalances such as hypocalcemia and hypokalemia.

g. ST segment. This segment is measured from the end of the QRS complex and the beginning of the T wave and is affected by drugs and electrolyte imbalances. It reflects myocardial injury.

h. T wave. The T wave represents myocardial repolarization. It is altered by electrolytes, myocardial hypertrophy, and ischemia.

4. Chest roentgenogram. The chest roentgenogram may be useful in revealing enlargement of chambers of the heart, great vessels of the heart, and vascular markings of the lungs. X-ray studies for congenital heart defect diagnosis include posteroanterior, lateral, and right and left oblique views with barium swallow.

5. Echocardiography. Echocardiography is an important noninvasive technique that reveals information regarding chamber size, anatomic

relationships of great vessels and valves, valve motion, wall and septal thickness, and myocardial performance.

6. Cardiac catheterization. Cardiac catheterization performed by a qualified pediatric cardiologist is usually a low-risk procedure and is essential for a definitive diagnosis of the anatomic and physiologic characteristics of a defect. Cardiac catheterization reveals oxygen content and saturation (expressed in percent) and pressure (expressed in mm Hg) in the cardiac chambers and the great arteries, pulmonary and systemic blood flow (cardiac output), and pulmonary and systemic vascular resistance.

**Essential features.** Signs and symptoms that appear vary with the type and severity of the defect. This section presents a discussion of the common signs and symptoms that appear and that may provide the first clue that some form of congenital heart defect is present.

There is often a family history of cardiovascular disease or defect. Poor feeding, often related to easy fatigability, is sometimes the first complaint recognized by the mother. The infant may take an hour to feed and appears to be too tired to suck. Older children may exhibit easy fatigability, growth retardation, sweating, orthopnea, dyspnea, or squatting as signals of cardiac defects. Repeated upper respiratory infections and pneumonia are not uncommon. Tachypnea and hypoxemic spells may be present with varying degrees of severity. Tachypnea is a sign that is frequently recognized by mothers and is a cardinal sign of left-sided heart failure. Hypoxemic spells begin with tachypnea. The infant or child becomes progressively more gray or blue and cries as if in severe pain. The attack may progress to unconsciousness, paresis, or death.[90]

Cyanosis and congestive heart failure are the two most important signs of serious cardiovascular disease in children. Cyanosis is sometimes difficult to detect unless it is severe, and its detectability is influenced by skin coloring, hemoglobin level, lighting conditions, and the experience of the observer. During the newborn period, extracardiac factors cause cyanosis; these are described in Chapters 7 and 8. In the older infant and child, cyanosis is almost invariably caused by a cardiac problem and is usu-

ally related to a defect with a right-to-left shunt. Persistent cardiac-related cyanosis implies a reduction of approximately 5 g/100 ml hemoglobin in the systemic arterial circuit and is apparent in the nail beds, skin, and oral mucosa and is not significantly improved with the administration of oxygen. A "precyanotic state" may exist, which is characterized by an outstanding reddish appearance of the highly vascularized areas such as the ends of the fingers, earlobes, and mucous membranes. It is related to the polycythemia of mild arterial unsaturation. The observable degree of cyanosis is often not related to the true degree of oxygen saturation of the blood, and arterial or arterialized capillary blood gases must be obtained to determine the presence and degree of arterial unsaturation.

Congestive heart failure occurs when cardiac output is not adequate to meet the metabolic demands of the body, and accumulation of excessive blood volume results in the pulmonary and/or the systemic circulation. Heart failure occurs in about 20% of all children with congenital heart disease, with the majority of these children being under 1 year of age. The signs of heart failure in the infant are usually subtle and are related to left ventricular failure. Right heart failure usually develops later; when it develops early it is usually associated with defects such as pulmonary valve stenosis with intact ventricular septum, congenital tricuspid insufficiency, Ebstein's malformation of the tricuspid valve, and congenital absence of the pulmonary valve.

The cardinal sign of congestive heart failure is enlargement of the chambers of the heart, which is the result of a homeostatic mechanism to maintain adequate cardiac output by enlarging the capacity of the pump (Starling's law of the heart). Tachypnea is considered to be a cardinal sign of left-sided failure and may be present for a short time before hepatomegaly and right-sided failure occur. Hepatomegaly develops with right-sided failure and occurs as a result of trapping of relatively large amounts of edema in the liver. This trapping of fluid in the liver occurs in the infant before peripheral edema, common in older children and adults, is apparent.

CHAPTER 18

Children and
youth with
long-term
physical
problems

Other signs and symptoms of congestive heart failure include feeding difficulty, dyspnea, restlessness, easy fatigability, weak pulses, pallor, rales, weight gain from fluid accumulation, tachycardia, sweating, pneumonia, orthopnea, and growth retardation.[31,47,90,134]

**Special stress factors.** Parents of children with congenital heart defects often have severe guilt feelings associated with their search for a cause of the defect. Empathic counseling, sometimes for a prolonged period of time, is needed to assist their resolution of these feelings. The prognosis associated with their child's defect and the ability and prognosis for medical or surgical intervention are important factors in determining the counseling approach that is needed. Parents are often concerned about the chances for reoccurrence of the defect in future children, and some form of genetic counseling may be indicated to assist them in family-planning decisions.

As the child grows older, temporary or permanent restriction of strenuous activity may be indicated. In the young child, spontaneous restriction of activity usually occurs, with the child responding to his or her own levels of energy and fatigue. For the older child and adolescent, motivation to participate in peer group activities and sports may be present even though the physical energy and capacity to participate is limited. Nursing intervention for the child who has surgery, particularly in relation to preparation for surgery and postoperative care, is discussed in Chapter 16.

**Medical and surgical intervention.** Medical and surgical techniques used to treat specific defects are presented with the description of common defects in the following section. Medical management of common symptoms must be maintained for a child whose defect has not yet been repaired or whose defect can be only partially alleviated by surgical intervention. Congestive heart failure is treated primarily with the use of oxygen, digoxin, and diuretics. The child is placed in oxygen in an upright, semi-reclining position. The initial digitalizing dose of oral digoxin is 0.08 mg/kg for infants, and 0.06 mg/kg for children over 2 years of age, given in three divided doses daily. The parenteral dose is three-fourths the oral dose and is also given in three divided doses daily. The daily maintenance dose is one-quarter to one-third of the initial digitalizing dose and is given in two equal portions 12 hours apart. For rapid diuresis, intravenous ethacrynic acid or furosemide (1 mg/kg) is given as a single dose. For maintenance therapy, oral thiazides are alternated every other day with oral spironolactone. The dose for chlorothiazide suspension (250 mg/tsp) is 20 mg/kg/day. The dose for hydrochlorothiazide tablets is 2 mg/kg/day. The dose for spironolactone is 2 to 4 mg/kg/day in two divided doses. Serum electrolytes must be monitored periodically while a child is receiving diuretics.

A child with decompensated congestive heart failure in mild distress requires rest; a severely distressed infant or child also requires sedation. Parenteral morphine, 0.1 mg/kg, sedates the child and also helps to relieve acute pulmonary edema. Positive pressure breathing may be used to raise the alveolar pressure above pulmonary capillary pressure. Peritoneal dialysis with a hypertonic solution may be indicated for children who have not responded to diuretics, when fluid retention and electrolyte imbalance require heroic correction, and in the early postoperative period for an infant who has transient renal failure with fluid retention and hyperkalemia.

Hypoxemic spells can be life threatening, and must be treated immediately. The objective of treatment is to increase pulmonary blood flow and enhance peripheral oxygenation. The child is placed in oxygen in a knee-chest position. Morphine sulfate is administered intravenously to reduce anxiety and diminish spasm of the right ventricular outflow tract. Propanolol (Inderal), which is a beta-adrenergic blocking agent, is also effective in reducing spastic obstruction to pulmonary blood flow.

Supraventricular tachycardia is a frequent problem in young infants and can result in congestive heart failure. Digitalization, as described above, is the major therapeutic approach.[31,90,110,134]

**Prognosis.** The prognosis for a child with congenital heart disease depends upon early detection of signs and symptoms, accurate medical diagnosis, and the ability to correct the defect surgically and provide long-term medical treat-

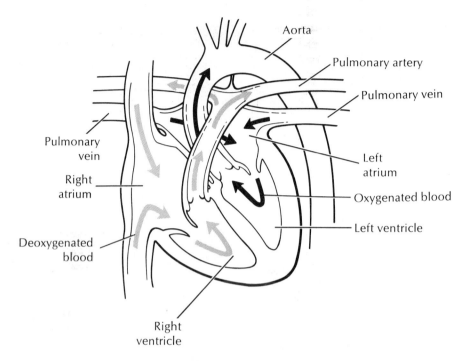

**Fig. 18-9.** Normal heart.

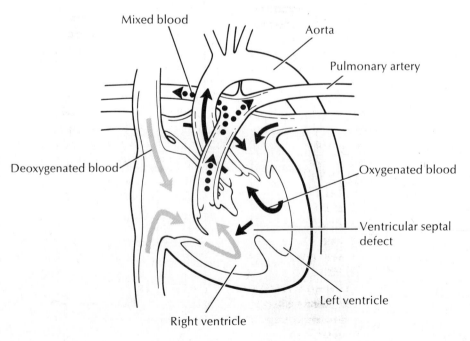

**Fig. 18-10.** Ventricular septal defect.

**CHAPTER 18**

Children and
youth with
long-term
physical
problems

ment if needed. Without adequate diagnosis and intervention, over half of all children with congenital heart disease die before reaching 1 year of age. However, 90% of the congenital heart defects can now be accurately diagnosed, and palliative or corrective surgery can be used to dramatically improve the prognosis for these infants and children.[90,134]

### Description of common congenital heart defects

**Ventricular septal defect.** A ventricular septal defect is an opening in the septum between the ventricles that can be as small as a pinpoint or so large that the septum is essentially absent (Fig. 18-10). The higher pressure in the left ventricle causes blood to be shunted from the left to the right ventricle. The effect on the lungs of the increased volume of blood in the right ventricle depends upon the size of the defect and its proximity to the pulmonary artery. The child with a small defect is often asymptomatic except for a murmur that is heard along the middle and lower left sternal margin, which is usually a harsh, pansystolic murmur. It may be accompanied by a thrill. Because of an increased risk for endocarditis, the child is given prophylactic antibiotic therapy for invasive procedures such as dental work or genitourinary procedures. The child is periodically evaluated until the murmur disappears. When the defect is larger, the young infant may be asymptomatic at birth and remain so until there is a sufficient pressure gradient established in the ventricles to cause the left-to-right shunt. This usually occurs within the first three weeks of life. If the infant has an unusually rapid decline in pulmonary vascular resistance within the first one or two weeks of life, congestive heart failure may develop rapidly within this period. However, more commonly, the pulmonary vascular resistance declines slowly, and signs of congestive heart failure emerge between the third and sixth weeks of life. Medical management for congestive heart failure is the initial course of treatment. If surgical intervention is deemed appropriate, the defect is repaired by direct closure or with a patch graft. Spontaneous closure is estimated to occur in 20% to 50% of all affected children, even for some infants who ini-

tially exhibit congestive heart failure. Spontaneous closure is most likely to occur by the third year of life, although some closures occur later. It is thought to be accomplished by muscular or fibrous encroachment or by adherence of the septal leaflet of the tricuspid valve. Partial spontaneous closure of a large defect improves the prognosis for a severely affected child.[110,113,134]

**Patent ductus arteriosus.** A patent ductus arteriosus results from persistence of the fetal channel between the pulmonary artery and the descending aorta (Fig. 18-11). With the onset of extrauterine circulation and failure of the ductus to contract, blood from the high pressure systemic circulation flows into the pulmonary circulation, causing an increased volume of blood to the lungs and a subsequent burden on the left side of the heart. In most instances the defect is small and the child is asymptomatic except for a murmur that is heard maximally at the upper left sternal border and under the left clavicle. The murmur is usually a faint late systolic crescendo murmur of high frequency, with or without a diastolic component. The second heart sound is normal, and pulses are not bounding. Mild symptoms include some growth retardation, easy fatigability, and increased incidence of upper respiratory infections.

Premature infants are particularly prone to persistence of the ductus arteriosis, presumably because of a more poorly developed muscular wall and decreased responsiveness to the stimuli that normally induce constriction. These infants are more likely to have a serious defect and develop congestive heart failure. Symptoms of a severe defect with a large left-to-right shunt are typical of left ventricular failure. Cyanosis is absent, and peripheral pulses are bounding. A systolic thrill may be palpable at the upper left sternal margin and in the suprasternal notch. The first heart sound is normal, but the second sound is narrowly split or obscured. A continuous murmur, grade 3 or greater, is heard at the upper left sternal border. It has an uneven rasping or clanging character, which is known as "machinery" quality. A late complication of a large patent ductus arteriosus is a true reversal of the shunt due to severe elevation of pulmonary vascular resistance. Pulmonary blood flow is then decreased, and there is no longer a vol-

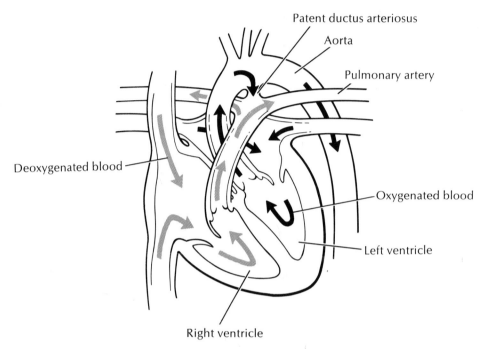

**Fig. 18-11.** Patent ductus arteriosus.

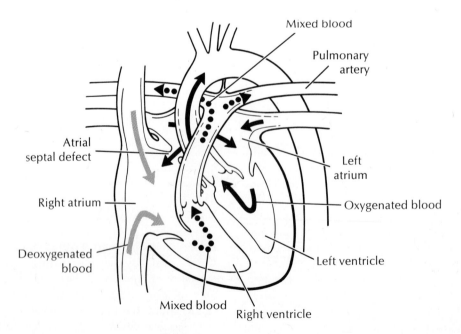

**Fig. 18-12.** Atrial septal defect.

**CHAPTER 18**

Children and
youth with
long-term
physical
problems

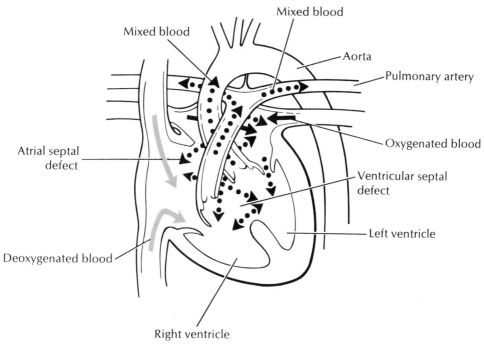

Mixed blood

Mixed blood

Aorta

Pulmonary artery

Oxygenated blood

Atrial septal
defect

Ventricular septal
defect

Left ventricle

Deoxygenated blood

Right ventricle

**Fig. 18-13.** Endocardial cushion defect.

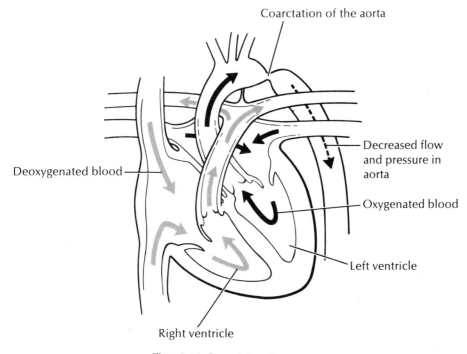

Coarctation of the aorta

Decreased flow
and pressure in
aorta

Deoxygenated blood

Oxygenated blood

Left ventricle

Right ventricle

**Fig. 18-14.** Coarctation of the aorta.

757

ume overload of the left heart chambers. The right ventricle, however, hypertrophies because of the increased pressure required by the reversal of the shunt.

The electrocardiogram of asymptomatic children may show no evidence of the defect. Symptomatic children may exhibit left ventricular dominance or hypertrophy on the electrocardiogram. Complete surgical repair is possible by ligation of the ductus. Since spontaneous closure of the ductus may occur up till 6 months of age, an infant may be observed for this period of time and surgery delayed.[110,113,134]

**Atrial septal defect.** Atrial septal defects are usually of sufficient size to allow unrestricted flow of blood between the atria (Fig. 18-12). There is a left-to-right shunt due to the higher pressure in the left atrium, creating a volume overload of the right ventricle and the pulmonary vascular beds. Often there are coexisting right-to-left shunts because of transient dominance of right atrial pressure during certain phases of the cardiac cycle or because of streaming from the inferior or superior vena cava when the defect is close to those structures. Defects in the latter location are often associated with anomalous pulmonary venous return and are termed sinus venosus defects. If the defect is located at the lower end of the septum, it is termed an ostium primum defect; if it is in the center of the septum, it is called an ostium secundum. Most children with atrial septal defects are asymptomatic. Infants may develop congestive heart failure, and older children may experience easy fatigability, dyspnea, and recurrent upper respiratory tract infections. A murmur is detected at the second left intercostal space. It is a systolic ejection type murmur, with wide splitting of the second heart sound without phasic variation (fixed splitting). The electrocardiogram reveals right ventricular hypertrophy. Often the defect is well tolerated, and surgical intervention is not indicated. If there is a significant left-to-right shunt, surgical correction by direct closure of the defect or patch grafting is indicated.[110,113,134]

**Endocardial cushion defect.** Endocardial cushion defects result from failure of fusion of the structures that divide the heart into four chambers and involve the atrial and ventricular septa, as well as the atrioventricular valves (Fig. 18-13). Pulmonary stenosis is a commonly associated lesion. The hemodynamic abnormalities that result from an endocardial cushion defect are those associated with the underlying lesions of the septa and the valves, with the pathways of flow being determined by the level of pulmonary and systemic resistances, left and right ventricular pressures, and the compliances of each chamber. Pulmonary hypertension is common.

The evident murmurs are variable and depend on the nature of the defect. They are usually associated with the ventricular septal defect or mitral regurgitation. Congestive heart failure is a chronic condition, growth is retarded, and respiratory infections are frequent. Complete surgical correction for the defects involved is possible before the child develops pulmonary vascular obstruction, but the risk of surgery is higher than that associated with simpler defects of the atrial or ventricular septum alone. Surgical repair involves direct or patch closure of the septal defects, and simultaneous repair of the atrioventricular valve abnormalities. Mitral valve replacement may be needed. The prognosis for children whose defect is repaired is good.[110,113,134]

**Coarctation of the aorta.** Coarctation of the aorta is a narrowing of the aortic lumen, usually near the point of attachment of the ductus arteriosus (Fig. 18-14). Associated defects are frequent, including patent ductus arteriosus, ventricular septal defect, and tubular hypoplasia of the aortic arch. Three compensatory mechanisms develop to maintain adequate distal aortic blood pressure and flow. These include (1) peripheral vasoconstriction to maintain a higher level of diastolic pressure in the aorta, (2) an increase in blood pressure in the proximal aortic compartment, and (3) the development of extensive collateral arterial pathways to bypass the site of the obstruction. The collateral pathways include the intercostal arteries, branches of the subclavian arteries, and anterior spinal arteries. The left ventricle must work against the increased resistance created by the obstruction, which may be complicated by a left ventricular volume overload in children with left-to-right shunts. The obstruction to flow and the circu-

CHAPTER 18

Children and
youth with
long-term
physical
problems

itous collateral pathway result in damping of the peak systolic pressure in the distal aortic segment, with a narrow pulse pressure and weak delayed pulses in the lower extremities. The femoral pulse may be weak or absent. The blood pressure in the upper extremities is increased in the upper extremities and decreased in the lower extremities.

Some children remain asymptomatic during infancy, but later the defect becomes apparent because of the associated murmur and hypertension. The hypertension is not an absolute hypertension but instead is a relative disparity between the pressures of the upper and lower extremities. It develops with increasing frequency as the child grows older. If the condition is not corrected, complications including hypertension, cerebral aneurysm formation and hemorrhage, rupture of the aorta, bacterial endocarditis, and congestive heart failure develop. The life expectancy for a child with an uncorrected coarctation of the aorta is about 35 years.

If symptoms develop during infancy, the first sign of the defect may be congestive heart failure that develops by the end of the first month of life, or the infant may exhibit tachypnea, dyspnea, poor feeding, and slow growth rate. The most significant sign is weak or absent femoral pulses and a significant disparity between the blood pressure of the upper and lower extremities.

Murmurs associated with coarctation of the aorta arise from turbulence at the site of the lesion and flow through arterial collateral pathways, or they may be associated with other defects. The electrocardiograph changes are variable. In infants under 6 months of age the electrocardiograph often reveals right or combined ventricular hypertrophy, while in older children left ventricular hypertrophy may be revealed.

Surgical correction of an uncomplicated coarctation involves end-to-end anastomosis and is usually done between 4 and 6 years of age. Surgical correction may be needed during infancy if the child does not respond to medical treatment. Surgical intervention may also be influenced by the nature of complicating defects that may be present.[110,113,134]

**Aortic stenosis.** Lesions resulting in left ventricular outflow obstruction may be supravalvular, valvular, or subvalvular (Fig. 18-15). The most common congenital aortic stenosis is valvular. Regardless of the site of the lesion, a systolic pressure gradient exists between the left ventricle and the ascending aorta, and the left ventricle is stressed by the increased pressure work that results. Associated anomalies such as patent ductus arteriosus and coarctation of the aorta are common. A congenital valvular stenosis may be asymptomatic and insignificant in early life but leads to significant stenosis with calcification in adult life because of the trauma of abnormal flow dynamics and atherosclerotic changes. The young infant with a critical stenosis may be asymptomatic at birth but develops early congestive heart failure due to severe obstruction. The symptomatic infant exhibits tachypnea, dyspnea, and has a dusky pallor characteristic of the low output of the left ventricle. Left ventricular or combined ventricular enlargement is present. An audible murmur may be heard at the mid-left sternal border or the apex. If the valve is mobile, the murmur is associated with a constant apical systolic ejection click. The electrocardiogram typically reveals abnormal left ventricular forces and may also reveal combined or right ventricular hypertrophy if pulmonary hypertension due to elevated pulmonary venous pressure is present.

An infant who exhibits symptoms of congenital aortic stenosis requires early surgical correction, for medical treatment of symptoms provides only temporary improvement. Aortic commissurotomy is the surgical procedure usually performed.

A child who has been asymptomatic with an aortic stenosis is usually identified by the presence of a murmur. The child may be easily fatigued and show exertional dyspnea and, with a more severe obstruction, may experience angina, exertional dizziness or syncope, or frank left heart failure. Sudden death is a potential hazard, probably due to myocardial ischemia and dysrhythmia, and the child must refrain from strenuous exercise and participation in sports. Cardiac catheterization is needed to determine the extent of stenosis by obtaining the relative pressure gradients across the

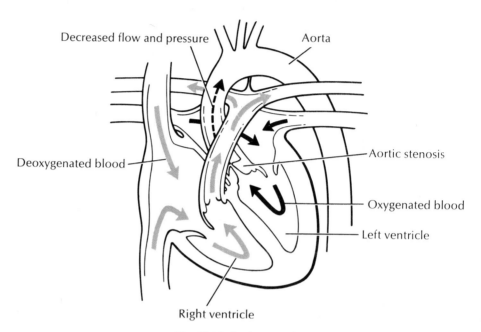

**Fig. 18-15.** Aortic stenosis.

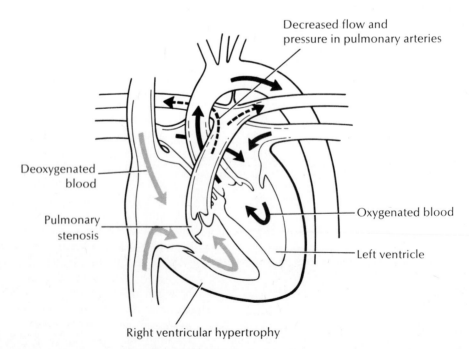

**Fig. 18-16.** Pulmonary stenosis.

**CHAPTER 18**

Children and
youth with
long-term
physical
problems

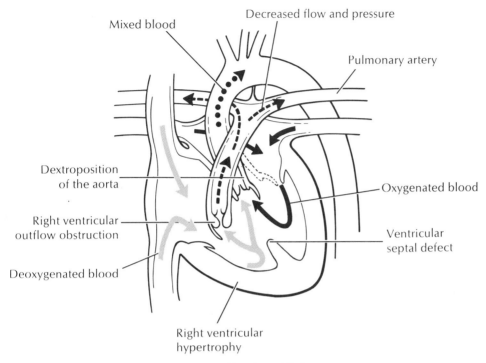

Mixed blood

Decreased flow and pressure

Pulmonary artery

Dextroposition
of the aorta

Oxygenated blood

Right ventricular
outflow obstruction

Ventricular
septal defect

Deoxygenated blood

Right ventricular
hypertrophy

**Fig. 18-17.** Tetralogy of Fallot.

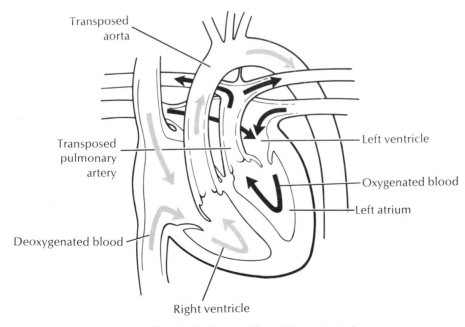

Transposed
aorta

Transposed
pulmonary
artery

Left ventricle

Oxygenated blood

Left atrium

Deoxygenated blood

Right ventricle

**Fig. 18-18.** Transposition of the great arteries.

aortic valve. Commissurotomy is the procedure of choice, but since this procedure does not produce a functionally normal valve, the child is treated postoperatively as a child with untreated aortic stenosis, and careful periodic evaluation is needed to detect complications. Eventual aortic valve replacement is anticipated for most children with aortic stenosis.[110,113,134]

**Pulmonary stenosis.** Pulmonary stenosis is an obstruction to the right ventricular outflow that may be valvular, subvalvular, or supravalvular (Fig. 18-16). The most common congenital condition is a valvular lesion with commissural fusion and thickened leaflets that result in a membranelike obstruction. Pulmonary stenosis is often associated with other lesions such as a patent foramen ovale or atrial defect. The lesion produces an increase in the pressure of the right ventricle, with a resulting right ventricular hypertrophy. As a result, right atrial pressure may rise, with hypertrophy of the right atrium.

Children with mild stenosis are asymptomatic and are likely to remain asymptomatic. If there is a significant obstruction, the child usually develops symptoms after 2 or 3 years of age. Fatigue on exertion and dyspnea are the most common complaints, but chest pain, exertional dizziness, or syncope may be present. Cyanosis and clubbing are present in about one third of all persons with pulmonary stenosis, but squatting is not characteristic. Cyanosis usually develops from venoarterial right-to-left shunting at the atrial level but may be of peripheral origin in children with low cardiac output. Growth and development are usually normal. A systolic thrill is usually present in the pulmonic area and frequently at the suprasternal notch. There is a widely split second sound, a diminished pulmonic component, and a prominent systolic ejection click of variable intensity that is louder with expiration. There is a harsh systolic ejection murmur at the pulmonary area.

Commissurotomy is the preferred surgical intervention. Extremely stenosed valves may need complete valve excision, and widening of the valve annulus by a patch may be required. Associated defects are also repaired at the time of surgical correction of the valve.[110,113,134]

**Tetralogy of Fallot.** Tetralogy of Fallot is a classic cyanotic defect consisting of four anatomic abnormalities: (1) ventricular septal defect, (2) pulmonic stenosis, (3) overriding aorta, and (4) hypertrophy of the right ventricle (Fig. 18-17). The pulmonic stenosis creates hypertrophy and increased pressure in the right ventricle, which causes a right-to-left shunt through the large ventricular septal defect. This results in mixing of unsaturated blood from the right ventricle with saturated blood from the left ventricle, which is pumped into the systemic circulation by way of the overriding aorta.

Cyanosis may be present at birth with a severe defect or may appear first during infancy or childhood. It usually becomes progressively severe, with clubbing of the fingers and toes. Squatting is a common symptom, and hypoxemic spells may develop. A severely cyanotic infant requires immediate palliative surgery. Based on the findings of cardiac catheterization, the decision may be made to support the child with medical intervention or to use palliative surgery until the child is larger. Full corrective surgery is possible for most infants and children, but when a palliative procedure is indicated, the aim is to relieve hypoxemia by increasing pulmonary blood flow. The Blalock-Taussig procedure provides anastomosis of the right pulmonary artery to the right subclavian artery. The Potts procedure is the anastomosis of the left pulmonary artery to the descending aorta. The Waterston procedure is an anastomosis of the right pulmonary artery to the ascending aorta. If a child is maintained with medical treatment in order to delay surgical intervention, the primary objectives are to maintain an optimum hemoglobin level, prevent bacterial endocarditis, intervention for acute hypoxemic spells, and observation for signs of increasing hypoxemia.[31,110,113,134]

**Transposition of the great arteries.** This is a cyanotic defect characterized by the aorta arising from the right ventricle and the pulmonary artery from the left ventricle, producing two parallel and separate circulatory systems (Fig. 18-18). If coexisting lesions such as a patent ductus arteriosus or a ventricular septal defect permit mixing of venous and arterial blood, the infant can survive the first few days of life. If marked cyanosis is immediately apparent at

CHAPTER 18

Children and
youth with
long-term
physical
problems

birth, there is probably no mixing, and immediate palliative surgery is done to create a channel for mixing. One such procedure is the Rashkind balloon septostomy, in which a balloon catheter is passed through the foramen ovale, inflated, and withdrawn to rupture the atrial septum. Functional surgical correction of transposition of the great arteries is performed using the Mustard technique, which redirects venous input by means of a baffle inserted within the atria so that pulmonary venous blood is directed across the tricuspid valve to the right ventricle and aorta, and systemic venous blood is directed to the mitral valve, left ventricle, and pulmonary artery. If a ventricular septal defect or pulmonary stenosis is also present, the outcome of corrective surgery is not as promising as that for simple transposition of the arteries.[31,110,113,134]

## Nursing problems and intervention

Health maintenance needs are important to optimal physical and emotional development of the child who has a congenital heart defect. Young children with congenital heart defects are prone to frequent upper respiratory infection; identification and management of these conditions are discussed in Chapter 11. The following section presents nursing problems related to the long-term problem of cardiovascular defects.

### Ambulation and exercise (MNPC no. 316.0)

The previous discussion of cardiovascular defects has presented instances when a child's exercise must be restricted. Most young children with cardiovascular defects spontaneously regulate their level of exercise to that which is compatible with their tolerance. As the child grows older, there may be a desire to become more active than can be tolerated, or the child may become overly cautious and fearful of exercise. Nursing assessment of the actual activity level of the child, compared with the expected tolerance that is usually predicted for the child's condition, can identify an appropriate activity level.

Ambulation and exercise after cardiac diagnostic procedures and cardiac surgery are planned in accord with the nature of the child's condition and the nature of the procedure that has been performed. In most instances of corrective surgery and in many instances of palliative surgery, the child may gradually resume full activity levels typical of other children at a similar stage of development.

### Nutrition (MNPC no. 316.1)

Optimal nutrition for children with cardiovascular disease is of major importance, particularly when hemoglobin level is compromised and growth retardation is present. Children who have chronic congestive heart failure or who are prone to develop congestive heart failure may be placed on a diet that restricts salt intake or that assures optimal intake of fluids and electrolytes. If the child is hospitalized, nursing assessment and management of dietary intake, including fluid and electrolyte intake, is a central concern. If the child is cared for at home, nursing care must focus on teaching the parents and the child about optimal nutrition and special dietary requirements for the child, as well as periodic evaluation of the child's nutritional status.

### Physical care (MNPC no. 316.3)

A child hospitalized for congestive heart failure, diagnostic procedures, or cardiovascular surgery requires expert nursing care for maintenance of ventilation and provision of adequate gas exchange, particularly during acute periods of congestive heart failure and during the postoperative period. Nursing measures related to these problems are discussed in detail in Chapter 16, as well as in the above discussion related to congestive heart failure.

### Psychosocial needs (MNPC no. 316.4)

Teaching and counseling for the family when the child is first recognized to have a congenital heart defect are of great importance. The fact that the parents can often not see visible evidence of the child's problem makes it difficult for them to understand and comprehend the nature of the problem, and it is particularly difficult for them to understand the need for drastic surgical procedures or to deal with the uncertain prognosis that is often inherent with a mild or moderately severe defect. For example, the initial course of treatment may be to pro-

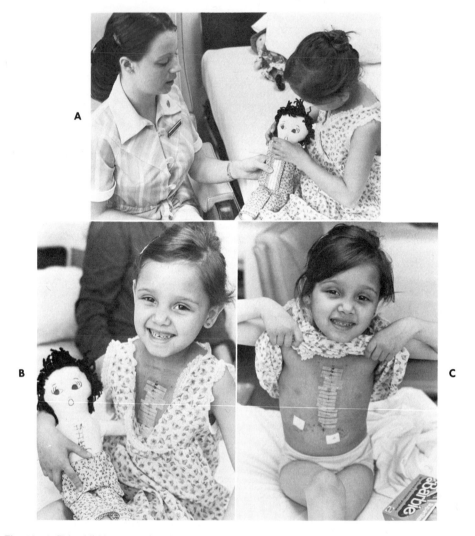

**Fig. 18-19.** This child has completed a surgical procedure for correction of a congenital heart defect. **A,** She shows a nurse her doll, which she "operated on" before her own surgery. **B,** She shows their matching scars and, **C,** her own complete incision.

vide the child with medical support and wait to observe the extent to which a defect will resolve spontaneously. Families may assume an attitude of extremes in the face of uncertainty in that they are unable to comprehend the full extent of the problem and deny or ignore the possible implications of the child's condition, or they become very attentive of the child's condition and be overly protective and cautious, anticipating the worst possible outcome. Nursing guidance and counseling are aimed toward

helping them comprehend the nature of the problem, understand the medical and surgical approaches that may become necessary, and develop a realistic attitude toward the child that promotes full development of each competency.

The child's response to the extensive diagnostic procedures necessary, particularly cardiac catheterization, should be assessed, and nursing intervention should be planned to prepare the child for each diagnostic encounter and to follow the procedures with therapeutic mea-

CHAPTER 18

Children and
youth with
long-term
physical
problems

sures to help the child work through feelings of anger, fear, or anxiety. A detailed discussion of play approaches for preparation for diagnostic procedures and surgery is presented in Chapter 16. Assessment of inner competency at periodic intervals is important in determining the nature of response that the child has in relation to these procedures.[1,65]

### Follow-through (MNPC no. 316.6)

Long-term follow-through is required for most children who have a congenital cardiac disease. If palliative or corrective surgery is not used and the child's condition is observed in anticipation of possible spontaneous resolution of the defect, long-term follow-through and evaluation of the child's progress is needed. If the child has undergone palliative or corrective surgery, long-term observation of the child to evaluate continued optimal functioning is essential to detect the development of complications and to provide adequate care.[110]

## LONG-TERM GENITOURINARY PROBLEMS (MNPC no. 317)

Urinary tract infections, which are discussed in Chapter 13, are often associated with congenital malformations of the genitourinary tract. Such infections can become chronic, leading to pyelonephritis, scar formation in the affected kidney, growth retardation, and ultimate renal failure. The following section presents a discussion of two conditions that affect the renal glomeruli during childhood: poststreptococcal acute glomerulonephritis and the idiopathic nephrotic syndrome of childhood.

### Medical diagnoses and treatment

#### Poststreptococcal acute glomerulonephritis

**Definition.** Poststreptococcal acute glomerulonephritis is a renal parenchymal disease that follows an infection with a nephritogenic strain of group A beta hemolytic streptococci. Glomerulonephritis is a term used for a number of diseases of the kidney that affect primarily the glomeruli and exhibit similar clinical courses and histologic changes. While it is recognized that there are many diverse causes for these disorders, the specific etiologies are not fully understood, nor is the pathologic relationship among these disorders clear. For purposes of clarity, only the poststreptococcal form of the disorder is presented here and may be used as a basis for understanding other related glomerulonephritic illnesses.[22,112]

**Incidence.** Poststreptococcal acute glomerulonephritis is the most common form of renal parenchymal disease in childhood. The actual incidence of occurrence is not known because of differences that exist in diagnostic criteria and in labeling the related disorders and the fact that undetected cases are not uncommon. Seventy percent of all cases occur in children between 2 and 8 years of age, with the peak age of occurrence being 7 years. It is rarely observed during infancy.[112]

**Etiology.** While the theory that poststreptococcal acute glomerulonephritis is an immune complex disease has not been confirmed, evidence strongly supports the role of an antigen-antibody reaction in the etiology of the disease. The renal disease is preceded by a nephritogenic strain of group A beta hemolytic streptococci infection of the tonsils, pharynx, sinuses, middle ear, or skin in 70% to 80% of cases. Several immune complex reactions are apparently involved, including specific antibody, complement, and polymorphonuclear leukocytes that are apparently capable of producing the altered tissue reaction and damage to the glomeruli. Discrete irregular granular deposits of circulating, nonglomerular antigen-antibody complexes plus complement accumulate along the epithelial side of the glomerular basement membrane.[13,22,112]

**Pathophysiology.** As a result of the immune complex reactions, the capillary tufts are swollen, and the mesangial and endothelial cells of the glomeruli are increased in number. All glomeruli are involved. Early in the course of the disease, neutrophils and eosinophils are present. The capillary lumina are obliterated by the cell proliferation, but the capillary walls remain normal. Bowman's capsule is usually obliterated by the swollen capillary tuft. Tubular changes are minimal. When there is a decrease in inflammatory and endothelial cells, capillary patency is restored, and there is improved glomerular perfusion.

Decreased effective filtration pressure is

caused by the occlusion of the capillary lumina and by vasospasm of the afferent arteriole. The decrease in normal filtration persists even though renal plasma flow is normal or increased. Hematuria is caused by glomerular damage, while proteinuria is caused by both glomerular and tubular damage. Tubular reabsorption of filtered sodium occurs with the decreased amount of glomerular filtrate, leading to salt and water retention. Edema and an expansion of the extracellular fluid volume results, producing in some cases cardiac decompensation and encephalopathy. Hypertension results from the expanded vascular fluid volume and vascular spasm, which also contributes to the development of encephalopathy.[22,112]

**Essentials of medical diagnosis.** Medical diagnosis is based upon the following traits:[81,112]

1. History of group A beta-hemolytic streptococcal infection seven to ten days previously, which can often be confirmed by positive culture of the site of the infection at the time of renal involvement or by increased antistreptolysin (ASO) titer (greater than 250 Todd units).
2. General malaise, headache, vomiting, fever, loss of appetite, and occasional abdominal pain
3. Negligible or moderate hypertension, which is sometimes of rapid onset and may produce sudden seizures or cardiac failure
4. Proteinuria and hematuria with hyalin, granular, and red cell casts in the urine
5. Oliguria, anuria, or acute renal failure
6. Transient mild-to-moderate elevation of BUN, low C3 complement level, high erythrocyte sedimentation rate, cryoglobulinemia, hypergammaglobulinemia

**Essential features.** The diagnostic criteria above reflect the range of signs and symptoms that can exist. If the onset is mild, the child may have few symptoms, such as hematuria, malaise, anorexia, nausea, vomiting, and abdominal pain. Edema, usually limited to periorbital puffiness, may be present. Hypertension may or may not be present initially but appears abruptly at any time during the initial phase of the disease. If severely affected, the child may exhibit cardiovascular and cerebral symptoms. Tachypnea may be associated with hyper-

tension; cardiac decompensation is reflected by tachypnea, dyspnea, arrhythmia, gallop rhythm, venous enlargement, hepatomegaly, and/or cardiomegaly. Symptoms of encephalopathy include nausea, vomiting, severe headache, changes in visual acuity, diplopia, focal or generalized seizures, or coma.[22,81,112]

**Medical treatment.** There is no therapy specific for the immune complex reactions that damage the glomeruli, and therefore medical treatment consists of supportive care and early recognition and treatment of complications such as hypertension, cardiac decompensation, and encephalopathy. Monitoring of vital signs, body weight, and fluid balance is essential for the early recognition of complications. If there is severe impairment of renal function, long-term hospitalization and treatment related to renal function are necessary.

Bed rest is maintained during the acute phase of the illness and continued until renal function has significantly improved. For children who suffer renal impairment, activity is limited until renal function returns to normal or plateaus at a level compatible with increased activity. When the child first resumes activity, a rebound of transient increase in BUN, hematuria, and/or proteinuria may occur, but usually it is not necessary to resume bed rest.

If the child's illness is mild and uncomplicated, a regular diet is maintained. While there are symptoms of edema, hypertension, or cardiac or renal failure, salt restriction is indicated. Protein intake is restricted if the child has oliguria or anuria. Fluid intake is restricted while the child has edema and in some instances during the acute phase of the illness even if edema is not present. The recommended fluid intake is 500 ml/m²/24 hours plus a volume equal to urinary output.

If there is culture evidence of a persisting streptococcal infection, antibiotic therapy is used for a full ten-day course. Cultures should be taken from sibling contacts for evidence of a streptococcal infection, and urinalysis should be performed to detect the presence of a subacute glomerulonephritis, which occurs in about 20% of all sibling contacts.[22,70,81,112]

**Prognosis.** The long-term outcome for most children with poststreptococcal acute glomerulonephritis is more favorable than the projected outcome of glomerulonephritis from other causes. Current evidence indicates that renal lesions are fully resolved in 80% of affected children within five years from the date of onset of the disease and that these and the remaining children with persistent renal lesions are asymptomatic within five years. Occasionally a child progresses rapidly to acute renal failure, but death from this and other complications has been almost eliminated with effective intervention, including peritoneal dialysis, hemodialysis, and early effective treatment of cardiac and cerebral complications.[22,81,112]

### Idiopathic nephrotic syndrome of childhood

**Definition.** The idiopathic nephrotic syndrome of childhood is a group of disorders associated with abnormal permeability of the glomerular basement membrane that are characterized by proteinuria, hypoalbuminemia, hypercholesterolemia, and edema. The idiopathic nephrotic syndrome occurs in the absence of any associated systemic disease or precipitating factor in about 80% of all children who develop a nephrotic syndrome. The relationship between the associated disease and the nephrotic syndrome that occurs in the remaining 20% of affected children is not known. Associated problems can include other glomerulopathies, congenital syphilis, lupus erythematosus, sickle cell disease, cyanotic congenital heart disease, diabetes mellitus, and drug toxicity. A rare form of congenital nephrotic syndrome is present at birth and is generally fatal.[23,81,112]

**Incidence.** The incidence has been estimated to be 1.9/100,000 white children and 2.8/100,000 nonwhite children below the age of 16 years. The peak age of onset is 2 to 3 years, with more than half of the children below age 4 and three-quarters of the children below age 7 years. About 60% to 65% of affected children are male.[23]

**Etiology.** The etiology of the idiopathic syndrome is not known, and the relationship between associated illnesses and the nephrotic syndrome is not known. Immunologic mechanisms have been explored, but the evidence supporting these theories has not been substantial enough to confirm this possible etiology.[23,81,112]

**Pathophysiology.** The basic disturbance of the idiopathic nephrotic syndrome is increased glomerular permeability to protein, with the metabolism of lipids, electrolytes, and water also affected. Several different types of histologic lesions appear on renal biopsy, with the most common type classified as minimal change disease. In minimal change disease there are only minor changes from normal glomerular structure, including mild degrees of stalk hypercellularity, slight leukocytosis, and focal mesangial thickening. Electron microscopy reveals fusion of the foot processes of glomerular epithelial cells. Tubular abnormalities may also be present. There are usually no abnormalities in the glomerular basement membranes. This type of idiopathic nephrotic syndrome occurs in 80% of affected children. Other less common forms of the syndrome reveal such changes as sclerosis and hyalinosis of the glomerular tufts or abnormalities in the basement membrane.

Increased permeability of the glomerular basement membrane to normal plasma protein accounts for the proteinuria of the syndrome. Proteinuria is a major factor that causes hypoproteinemia, but there is also an increased rate of catabolism of protein. The cause of a marked elevation of serum lipids (hyperlipemia) and occasional elevation of serum cholesterol is not known. The basis for edema formation and electrolyte imbalance is complex. One factor is the loss of protein from the urine that exceeds the synthetic capacity of the liver, reducing the oncotic pressure of the plasma and causing a shift of fluid from the vascular compartment to the interstitial tissues. This shift also causes a contraction of vascular fluid volume, which stimulates the kidney to increase the reabsorption of filtered sodium and water. This response of the kidney is mediated by an increase in aldosterone, antidiuretic hormone, and other mechanisms that influence renal hemodynamics. While the net retention of water and sodium preserves the vascular fluid volume, the hypoproteinemia allows a considerable portion of this additional fluid to shift into the interstitial space, furthering the development of edema. While this physiologic process is thought to account for the major mechanisms that create edema, other factors may exist and are as yet incompletely understood.[23,112]

**Essentials of medical diagnosis.** Medical diagnosis is confirmed by biopsy and examination of renal tissue, which reveals the typical histologic patterns of the syndrome. The clinical characteristics upon which diagnosis is based include proteinemia (greater than 40 mg/m²/hour), hypoalbuminemia (less than 2.5 g/100 ml), hypercholesterolemia, and edema.[112]

**Essential features.** The typical onset of symptoms is characterized by a gradual appearance of periorbital edema that is present upon arising in the morning and subsides during the day, persisting for several days or weeks before it is noticed by the child's family or before other symptoms emerge. Proteinuria may have been present but is not detected until the family seeks medical care, usually because they have noticed the progressive edema. Generalized malaise and abdominal pain may also have been noticed. There may be a gradual or a rapid increase in generalized edema, with abdominal ascites, labial and scrotal edema, and respiratory embarrassment from pleural effusion. Extreme skin pallor is usually present, and diarrhea is frequently present, probably due to edema of the intestinal mucosa. Intravascular volume depletion may result in symptoms of shock. Hypertension is rarely present.[23,112]

**Special stress factors.** The uncertainty of the prognosis and long-term course of the disease present major problems for the child and the family. The lack of definitive knowledge about the causes of the disease leaves the family further perplexed and uncertain, and they may question the competence of the health care workers who have participated in the early diagnosis and care of the child. A great deal of counseling and support and efforts to build and maintain a relationship of trust are often needed to help the family cope with the child's illness.[23]

**Medical treatment.** Adrenocorticosteroid therapy is used to control the edema, and it appears to alter the underlying disease process and the ultimate outcome, particularly for minimal change disease. The specific drug and dosage vary, but the aim of therapy is to maintain the child free of proteinuria on the minimum possible dosage. Daily determination of urinary protein, which can be performed at home using Albustix with the first morning urine specimen, is used to regulate the dose of steroid drug. One recommended approach to steroid therapy is initial treatment with prednisone orally for 28 days in a dosage of approximately 60 mg/m²/day in three divided doses, up to a maximum dose of 80 mg/day. Diuresis and lowering of urinary protein to less than 50 mg/m²/12-hour night specimen are achieved within 7 to 21 days for the majority of children. Following completion of the initial course of therapy and remission of symptoms, the child is given a daily dose of 40 mg/m² for three consecutive days out of each week for a period of four weeks. If the child remains asymptomatic, no further treatment is given. If improvement is not sustained, the child may be changed to another drug or the initial drug may be continued for a period of time. If the condition recurs, the child is treated as in the initial regimen. Tapering of the steroid after many months of therapy may result in symptoms of headache, lethargy, weakness, anorexia, and vomiting. The child is then maintained on minimal dosages needed to alleviate the symptoms for two- to three-month periods until therapy can be gradually and completely withdrawn. The serious side effects of high doses of steroid therapy include growth retardation, Cushing's syndrome, and vertebral compression fractures. When side effects become apparent, the child may be placed on immunosuppressant drugs such as cyclophosphamide or chlorambucil in combination with a reduced dosage of the steroid drug.

Dietary intake of sodium is moderately restricted while the child exhibits edema. Foods are not salted during cooking, no salt is added at the table, and high-sodium-content foods are avoided. Diuretic agents are not usually given initially, since most children respond adequately to steroid therapy. If the child is extremely edematous or does not respond to steroid therapy within two to three weeks, diuretics may be used to provide symptomatic relief. Hydrochlorothiazide may be used in a dose of 2 to 4 mg/kg/day.

Because of the threat of serious intercurrent infection, particular caution is given to prevention of infection and to prompt treatment of signs of infection in the child. Prophylactic antibiotics are not usually given on a routine basis but may be used if the child has been exposed to a known infection. While the activity of the child is not restricted except for self-imposed restriction that occurs during periods of edema, the child's contacts with large groups of children or with children known to have an infectious illness are avoided to the extent possible. Most children can remain at home for the full course of treatment and can continue to attend preschool and school classes except during periods of acute illness, when they may remain at home or may need hospitalization.[14,23,81,112,122]

**Prognosis.** Before the advent of antibiotic therapy, most children died as a result of an intercurrent infection. Before the use of steroid therapy, the usual course of the disease was a prolonged illness with gradual improvement and recovery for about half of affected children, the remainder dying during active stages of the disease or developing chronic renal insufficiency and dying at an early age. With steroid therapy, 95% or more of children with minimal change disease are fully recovered or have infrequent relapses during the first five years after onset. A few have frequent relapses for many years but ultimately stabilize or recover. For a few children with minimal change disease and for those with other types of idiopathic nephrotic syndrome the prognosis is not as favorable, and ultimate renal failure and early death occurs. If a child remains asymptomatic after two to three years without steroid therapy, permanent recovery is assumed to have occurred.[23,81,112]

## Nursing problems and intervention
### Ambulation and exercise (MNPC no. 317.0)

The level of activity for a child with long-term genitourinary problems must be planned in accord with the nature of the condition of the child and the stage of development. If periods of bed rest or restricted activity are required, as occurs with glomerulonephritis, measures to help the child tolerate restriction of activity and not suffer residual physical and emotional effects of the restriction must be planned and implemented. Play activities involving a level of activity that is appropriate for the child are useful to provide diversion as well as to provide for therapeutic expression of feelings.

### Nutrition (MNPC no. 317.1)

Optimal intake of nutrients, fluids, and electrolytes is essential for the child whose renal metabolism is altered. Conditions under which fluid or salt intake is restricted are described in the above section. When the child is cared for at home over a long period of time, the family may need assistance in understanding the nutritional and dietary requirements for the child. During periods of hospitalization the nurse carries primary responsibility for careful monitoring of intake and output and for managing the intake requirements of the child as required for medical treatment. The parents need to begin to learn about these requirements and gradually participate in monitoring intake and output.

### Elimination and other physical care (MNPC no. 317.3)

If a child is catheterized during periods of hospitalization, proper techniques for insertion and management of the catheter are used, with particular attention to maintaining sterile technique and prevention of infection. Daily urinary testing may be required either in the hospital or at home to provide monitoring of the child's progress and to guide medical therapy decisions. The nurse gradually includes the parents in assuming responsibility for these procedures in the hospital and provides assistance as needed at home.

### Psychosocial needs (MNPC no. 317.4)

The uncertain prognosis for most children with long-term genitourinary problems is especially stressful. Many children who develop urinary problems early in childhood experience several years of therapy during which there are alternating periods of extreme optimism and extreme pessimism. If the child progresses to renal failure, repeated dialysis, and possible renal transplant, the ultimate possibility of early death creates a major impact on the child's development as well as on the family.[17,88]

*Follow-through (MNPC no. 317.7)*

Teaching and guidance in relation to administering drugs at home, dietary management, activity level, protection of the child from infection, and the nature of the child's illness and its effect on development are planned and implemented according to the needs of the family and the child. Periodic reevaluation of the child's development and of the family as a unit are needed to provide for changes that occur over a period of time.

## MULTIPLE AND/OR SYSTEMIC PROBLEMS (MNPC no. 318)
### Medical diagnoses and treatment

A multitude of medical disorders may be associated with this group of nursing problems. Three such problems are presented in this section: cystic fibrosis, sickle cell disease, and leukemia, which is representative of cancer in childhood.

### Cystic fibrosis

**Definition.** Cystic fibrosis is an autosomal-recessive inherited disorder of the exocrine glands, which leads to disturbed functioning, in varying degrees, of the lungs, gastrointestinal tract, and sweat glands. Mucous secretions are increased and thickened in all of these structures, and fluid and electrolyte exchange is impaired, leading to secondary destruction and change in function of the organs.[16,55,135]

**Incidence.** In the general population the incidence of cystic fibrosis is approximately 1:1,500, with a carrier rate of about 5% of the general population. The disorder occurs less frequently in the black population than in other groups. There is a 25% risk of the disease being present in any child of an affected family.[55]

**Etiology.** The genetic inheritance of cystic fibrosis is well documented as a Mendelian recessive trait. Both parents must be carriers (heterozygotes), and the child must inherit the recessive trait from each parent in order to exhibit traits of the disease. The basic defect consists of the production of abnormally viscid secretions by various glands of the body.

**Pathophysiology.** The most commonly affected organs are the pancreas and the lungs. Instead of producing a watery secretion that flows freely through the ducts to transport digestive enzymes to the duodenum, the pancreas produces an inspissated secretion of abnormal mucoprotein material, which blocks the ducts and leads to cystic dilatations of the acini. The acini become distended and degenerate. Subsequently a mild inflammatory reaction occurs about the acini, and progressive, diffuse pancreatic fibrosis develops. The islands of Langerhans are usually not affected, but glucose intolerance may develop in advanced stages of the disease due to reduction in islet numbers.

In the lungs, mucus occludes the lumen of the bronchioles, leading to an expiratory bronchiolar obstruction and hyperinflation of the lungs. Mucus stasis and air trapping in the lungs promote infection in the lungs, which produces bronchiolitis, bronchitis, and destructive changes in the bronchial walls and ultimate fibrosis. The frequency and persistence of lung infections arise from the impairment of three important defenses against infection: (1) free-flowing mucus, (2) ciliary activity, and (3) the ability to rid the lung of secretions by coughing. The most frequent invading organisms in children with cystic fibrosis are *Staphylococcus aureus* and *Pseudomonas aeruginosa*.[55,135] Table 18-9 summarizes the secretory dysfunction, clinical manifestations, and complications that develop in the pancreas and lungs and other organs that may be involved in the pathologic process.

**Essentials of medical diagnosis.** The criteria upon which medical diagnosis is based include:[16,135]

1. Sodium in sweat elevated above 70 mEq/liter
2. Absent or decreased pancreatic exocrine function
3. Recurrent infections of the lung
4. Characteristic changes in the chest roentgenogram
5. Frequent bulky stools
6. Failure to thrive

**Essential features.** Signs and symptoms vary greatly in severity and degree of involvement. If the disease is apparent in the newborn period, it is likely to develop into a severe form; if signs and symptoms appear later in childhood or adolescence the individual is likely to exhibit a

CHAPTER 18

Children and
youth with
long-term
physical
problems

**Table 18-9.** Pathophysiology, clinical manifestations, and complications in various organs involved in cystic fibrosis

| Organ involved | Secretory dysfunction | Clinical manifestations | Complications |
|---|---|---|---|
| Sweat glands | Elevated concentration of sodium and chloride in sweat | Hyponatremia, hypochloremia | Heat prostration shock |
| Intestine | | | |
| Newborn | Viscid meconium | Meconium ileus with intestinal obstruction | Meconium peritonitis |
| Older child and adults | Inspissated mucofecal masses (intestinal sludging) | Partial intestinal obstruction with severe cramping pains | Intestinal obstruction Intussusception |
| Pancreas | Inspissation and precipitation of pancreatic secretions causing obstruction of pancreatic ducts | Absence of pancreatic enzymes causing malabsorption of food and fatty, bulky stools | Hypoproteinemia, iron deficiency anemia, vitamin K deficiency and rectal prolapse, and/or insulin deficiency |
| Liver | Insulin deficiency | Glucose intolerance | Diabetes mellitus |
| | Inspissation and precipitation of bile in biliary system | Focal biliary cirrhosis; shrunken "hob-nail" liver | Portal hypertension with esophageal varices and hematemesis |
| Salivary glands | Inspissation and precipitation of secretions in small ducts of submaxillary and sublingual salivary glands | Mild patchy fibrosis of salivary glands | None |
| Paranasal | Viscid mucus | Retention of mucus. Clouding on sinus roentgenograms | Mucopyoceles wtih nasal deformity or orbital cavity extension |
| Nose | Nasal polyps | Obstruction to nasal airflow | None |
| Lungs | Viscid mucus in bronchioles and bronchi | Obstruction of bronchioles causing bronchiolectasis, bronchiectasis, and chronic suppurative lung infection | Hemoptysis, pneumothorax, cor pulmonale |
| Reproductive tract | | | |
| Males | Viscid genital tract secretions during embryologic development, causing failure of formation of normal wolffian duct structures | Sterility | None |
| Females | Distension of the endocervical epithelial cells with cytoplasmic mucin | None proved; ? decreased fertility | Polypoid cervicitis while taking oral contraceptives |

From Tooley, W. H., and Lipow, H. W.: Specific diseases causing obstruction. In Rudolf, A. M., editor: Pediatrics, ed. 16, New York, 1977, Appleton-Century-Crofts, p. 1564.

mild form of the disease. Approximately 15% of affected children exhibit only pulmonary signs and symptoms, while another 10% to 15% exhibit only gastrointestinal signs and symptoms.

In a severely affected infant the first sign of illness is meconium ileus, causing intestinal obstruction, usually in the distal ileum near the ileocecal valve. Abdominal distention, vomiting, failure to pass stools, and rapid onset of dehydration and electrolyte imbalance signal the presence of intestinal obstruction. Approximately 10% of affected infants exhibit early meconium ileus as the first sign of the disease.

Beyond the newborn period, infants and children who exhibit signs of intestinal effects fail to gain weight appropriate for their stage of development. Despite an enormous appetite, the child gains weight very slowly due to an enormous degree of wastage of ingested food. Carbohydrate absorption is only slightly impaired, but about half of the ingested fat and protein passes through the intestine unabsorbed due to the reduction or absence of pancreatic enzymes in the duodenum. The weight of the stool is as

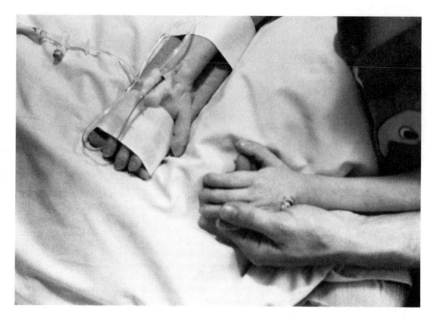

**Fig. 18-20.** Severe impairment of ventilation due to respiratory involvement of cystic fibrosis results in clubbing of fingers and cyanosis.

much as three times the normal weight. Initially, the bulky nature of the stool may pass unnoticed, but gradually the stools become clearly abnormal in that they are loose and passed with normal frequency or unformed and passed with increased frequency. The addition of starches and cereals to the diet of an infant usually causes the stool to become frothy and foul smelling. The onset of a pulmonary infection may stimulate diarrhea, failing appetite, and progressive weight loss and malnourishment.

Signs and symptoms in the lungs are initially obstructive with superimposed infection. Wheezing respiration and hacking cough are often the first symptoms. The cough may become paroxysmal, simulating that of pertussis. Mucopurulent sputum may be present with infection. Dyspnea is caused by generalized obstructive emphysema and may appear gradually or suddenly. Cyanosis and clubbing of fingers and toes may develop if ventilation is sufficiently impaired.[55,67,133]

**Special stress factors.** The stress factors that arise when a child is diagnosed with cystic fibrosis are multiple. The constant care and spe-

cial provisions that must be made in the home for the child's physical care are complicated, time consuming, and exhausting, as well as expensive. The genetic implications for the parents and siblings, as well as the child, are serious and result in the need for genetic evaluation and counseling. The nature of the illness results in a major alteration of life-style for the family and a long-term emotional process of dealing with chronic illness and the possibility of early death for the child. Adequate care for the child requires the involvement of a large number of health care workers, repeated hospitalization, and constant care for the child by an adult family member.[92,135]

**Medical treatment.** The major challenge of medical treatment is the relief of obstruction of the bronchioles and combating persistent infection in the lungs. Postural drainage, percussion of the chest, and mist therapy are essential components of therapy. An ultrasonic nebulizer and mist tent are used during sleep to loosen tenacious secretions. Percussion and postural drainage are required as often as four times a day, preceded by inhalation of mist and the use of a bronchodilator aerosol. In addition to a reg-

CHAPTER 18

Children and
youth with
long-term
physical
problems

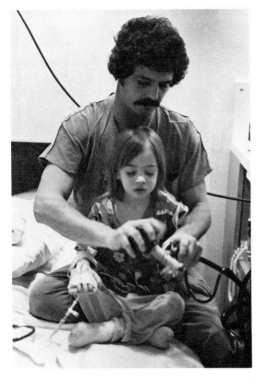

**Fig. 18-21.** The father's involvement in care of the child can contribute to the child's sense of worth and assist the father in dealing with his own feelings about the child's illness and early death.

ular home program, periodic hospitalization for intensive respiratory therapy may be required. Hospitalization is also indicated when the child develops a serious lung infection that cannot be adequately controlled and treated at home.

Controversy exists over the best approach to use in administering antibiotics to combat the almost continual pulmonary infections of severely affected children. If antibiotics are used continuously on a prophylactic basis or over an extended period of time to attempt to eradicate a well-established infection, the antibiotics are rotated over several weeks at a time to prevent developing drug sensitivity in the child and resistance of organisms to the drugs. Antibiotics should be selected on the basis of cultures from the sputum, which are usually obtained during postural drainage. Sensitivity studies of the organisms that are cultured guides the selection

of the most effective antibiotic for a selected period of time.

Pancreatic insufficiency is treated with replacement of lipase, trypsin, and amylase (Cotazym, Viokase) taken just before meals. The child's diet should be high in proteins and carbohydrates; sometimes a low-fat diet is recommended. Vitamin supplements are also given.

Surgery is required for neonatal meconium ileus, refractory intussusception in an older child, removal of airway obstruction of nasal polyps, persistent atelectasis, pneumothorax, and empyema, which may develop as complications of cystic fibrosis.*

**Prognosis.** The prognosis for children with cystic fibrosis remains poor, despite improved management of respiratory complications in recent years. Most affected children die in their teens or during young adulthood, with the primary cause of death being respiratory complications.[16,135]

### Sickle cell disease

**Definition.** Sickle cell disease is a condition in which sickling of the red cells results in a significant and chronic clinical disorder. The most common forms of the disease are sickle cell anemia, sickle beta-thalassemia, and sickle–hemoglobin C disease. The sickle cell trait is the heterozygous carrier state.[33,74]

**Incidence.** Sickle cell anemia is estimated to occur in 1 out of every 600 black newborns. Sickle cell–hemoglobin C disease occurs in about 1 out of every 800 black newborns, and sickle beta-thalassemia occurs in 1 out of every 1,700 black newborns in the United States. The incidence in Africa among blacks is much higher than that reported for the United States.[21,74]

**Etiology.** Sickle cell disease is transmitted as a dominant autosomal gene for the particular structural abnormalities of the hemoglobin molecule that are characteristic of each form of the disease and that result in the abnormal sickle shape of the red blood cells. In the sickle cell trait, a heterozygous genotype results when both normal cells and abnormal sickled cells are present.[74]

**Pathophysiology.** Sickled cells are trans-

---

*References 16, 55, 92, 109, 121, 135.

formed to a normal unsickled shape upon oxygenation. As the hemoglobin loses oxygen to body tissues, the abnormal, sickled shape returns. The rigid, deformed cells are readily damaged by mechanical stresses of passage through the vasculature, which creates a chronic hemolytic anemia. If the individual is subjected to conditions that suppress red blood cell production, such as infection, the anemic state worsens. Sickled cells are also subject to entanglement and sequestration in areas where blood flow is slow, and they also increase the viscosity of the blood, thus compromising blood flow. These conditions produce observable local ischemia, thrombosis, and/or infarction, resulting in a vaso-occlusive crisis.[74]

**Essentials of medical diagnosis.** Medical diagnosis is based on the following traits:

1. Anemia, elevated reticulocyte count, jaundice
2. Positive sickling test
3. Pains in the legs and abdomen
4. Splenomegaly in early childhood, with later disappearance
5. Hemolytic crises

Differentiation between the various forms of sickle cell disease is sometimes difficult but can be accomplished by studies of family members and of the blood, including hemoglobin electrophoresis, studies of fetal hemoglobin, and the sickling test.[33]

**Essential features.** The child with sickle cell trait (heterozygous carrier state) usually remains asymptomatic throughout life, but occasionally hematuria, with progressive impairment of the ability of the kidneys to concentrate urine, occurs. Infarcts in the spleen and lungs may occur in the presence of low oxygen tension or at high altitudes.

The child with sickle cell disease usually develops symptoms between 9 and 12 months of age. Anemia is moderately severe (usually between 7 and 10 g/100 ml), and mild scleral jaundice is usually present. Physical growth may be delayed, and the child begins to experience frequent crises. The two major types of crises that occur are anemic and vaso-occlusive, with multiple signs and symptoms of each. Anemic crisis usually occurs as a result of a transient condition that interferes with red blood cell production in the bone marrow, often a bacterial or viral infection. The reticulocyte count drops, and severe anemia occurs. Anemic crises can also be caused by an increased rate of destruction of red cells. The most common type of crisis is the vaso-occlusive crisis, which can involve any organ system and leads to permanent occlusive damage. In young children the most common site is the hands and feet, which results in painful swelling, and in the abdominal organs, which results in abdominal pain and gastrointestinal spasms. In older children and adults, crises occur in the low back, abdomen, and long bones as well. The crises may last a few hours or several days and are not predictable in onset or duration.

Death from sickle cell disease is often associated with bacterial septicemia or splenic sequestration. Children who live beyond the first decade often have growth retardation and delay in puberty and in the development of secondary sex characteristics, although ultimately adult size and development is attained. Signs and symptoms of the disease vary markedly but can include leg ulcers, failure of the heart, kidneys, or liver, infarction of the retina causing visual disturbance and blindness, and neurologic problems such as hemiplegia, coma, convulsions, and visual disturbances.[33,74,79,80]

**Special stress factors.** Unpredictable crises pose a major physical and emotional stress on the child and family and interfere with daily activities, school, and later work. The child often develops excessive dependency on family members and impaired social relationships with peers because of limitations on regular participation in school activities.

Genetic counseling is essential for all family members and provides the major approach to prevention. Individuals with the sickle cell trait or disease are faced with difficult family planning decisions based on the probability of giving birth to an affected child.[45,74]

**Medical treatment.** Medical management is directed to crises intervention and regular evaluation of the child's condition to determine the extent of organ damage that may have occurred. Rest, analgesics, and sedatives may be sufficient to manage a mild crisis. When the crisis is severe, the child is given blood transfusions with whole blood or packed cells. Oxygen may be indicated, and hydration and electrolyte balance must be corrected and maintained. Prevention of infection is of great importance, and the onset of infections needs to be recognized early and treated promptly.[33,74]

**Prognosis.** Although a few children with sickle cell disease die during childhood, most individuals die during young adulthood. The most common causes of death during adulthood are renal and cardiac failure. Individuals with sickle cell trait, and a few with mild symptoms of sickle cell disease, have a normal life expectancy.[33,74]

### Leukemia

**Definition.** Leukemia is a group of disorders of the blood system characterized by hyperplasia of the sites of leukopoiesis and by abnormal proliferation of leukocytes. Increased numbers of leukocytes and their precursors, or immature leukocyte cells, enter the peripheral circulation and invade many of the internal organs.[52,127]

**Incidence.** Acute leukemia is second only to accidents as a cause of death during the childhood years. The annual incidence in the United States is about 4 per 100,000 children under 15 years of age, or about 4,000 new cases each year. The peak age group for the occurrence of acute leukemia is 2 to 6 years of age, although it can occur at any age. The incidence is somewhat higher for boys than for girls, with a ratio of 1.3 to 1. White children are affected twice as frequently as nonwhite children.[52]

**Etiology.** The etiology is unknown, although several important factors appear to be related to the incidence of the disease. Viruses or viruslike particles have been isolated in some types of leukemia, particularly in animal research, but the exact role of the agents in the development of the leukemic condition is not clearly understood. It appears that there is a close relationship between the presence of a virus and the nature of the chromosomal division of cells, and there is a great deal of ongoing research investigating these phenomena.[43]

Other factors have been identified as related to the illness, but the nature of their relationship to leukemia is not known. Socioeconomic factors seem to bear some relationship, with the incidence of leukemia being greatest where there are few physicians in large urban areas. This raises a question as to whether the relationship is more a factor of rate of diagnosis than of actual incidence.

There is an unusually high incidence of leukemia occurring in children with other forms of cancer, in children with Down's syndrome, and in children who have a family history of leukemia or other types of cancer. However, the role of inheritance in the etiology of cancer is still not completely understood.

Environmental influences, such as radiation and air, water and food pollution, have come under recent investigation to determine a possible relationship. Tumors and other forms of cancer have been demonstrated to be induced by radiation experimentally in laboratory animals, but this etiology is uncertain for humans.[43]

**Essentials of diagnosis.** Medical diagnosis is established by the following factors:

1. Pallor, petechiae, fatigue, fever, and bone pain
2. Lymph node enlargement and enlargement of the liver and spleen
3. Thrombocytopenia with low, normal, or elevated white blood count and normal or low hemoglobin
4. Confirmation of the suspected diagnosis by bone marrow aspiration, showing differential features of the type of leukemia that is present

Usually there is a predominance of blastocytes, or immature-appearing mononuclear cells with pale-staining nuclei and little or no clumping of nuclear chromatin. Frequently the cells lack differentiation. There is often marked decrease in megakaryocytes, erythroid cells, and granulocytes.

Diagnosis of the type of leukemia is important in order to determine the type of treatment that is needed. Recent methods of differential treatment have led to improvement in obtaining a long-lasting remission and possible cure of some types of leukemia. The likelihood of accurate diagnosis is increased through the use of tissue culture techniques, special stains, biochemical studies, and electron microscopy.

Acute leukemia can be divided into two basic classes depending upon the morphology of the abnormal blastocytes present in a sample of bone marrow. These are acute lymphoblastic leukemia (ALL) and acute myelogenous leukemia (AML). About 80% of all childhood leukemia is acute lymphoblastic leukemia. There are several subclasses of acute myelogenous leukemia: myeloblastic, myelomonoblastic, monoblastic, promyelocytic, and erythroleukemia.[52,127]

**Pathophysiology.** When leukemia occurs, leukemic blast cells in the bone marrow divide, apparently without the control that normally regulates the number of stem cells that divide and differentiate. The blast cells produced in large numbers fail to mature and therefore accumulate. In the marrow, leukemic proliferation interferes with the production of normal erythrocytes, granulocytes, and platelets, which results in anemia, infection, and hemorrhage. The leukemic cells infiltrate body organs and cause enlargement and dysfunction. The most commonly involved organs are the liver, spleen, and lymph nodes. The kidneys, gonads, meninges, and intestine are commonly involved and rarely the eyes, endocrine glands, heart, and lungs.[127]

**Essential features.** The essential features of illness are common to all types of leukemia. These include a low-grade fever, irritability, easy fatigue, pallor, and weight loss. The child may have skin manifestations and signs, including petechiae, purpura, bruising of the skin, excessive bleeding from mucous membranes, and skin lesions that do not readily heal. The child commonly experiences nausea and vomiting, anorexia, and vague, generalized aches and pains or pain associated with bones and joints. Palpable glands and lymph nodes are often enlarged. As the illness progresses or worsens, many of these signs and symptoms increase in severity, and other signs and symptoms arise from specific organ involvement. For example, with central nervous system involvement, the child may begin to exhibit papilledema, increased intracranial pressure, headache, vomiting, or cranial nerve palsy.[36,43,52,127]

**Special stress factors.** The uncertainty of remission, repeated trials with drugs that produce toxic side effects, and the probability of impending death are exceedingly stressful for the child and the family. During periods of remission the child may continue to participate in usual activities and school, but behavioral and personality changes may occur, and peer relationships may be altered (see Chapter 17).

**Medical treatment.** The objective of medical treatment is to prolong the useful life of the child and remission of the disease. Some centers have developed treatment regimens that provide for increasing remission periods, and cure appears to have been accomplished in a few cases. Children with acute lymphoblastic leukemia respond more completely to chemotherapy than do children with acute myelogenous leukemia, and the drugs of choice for each type of leukemia differ. Children who have begun to exhibit signs of advanced stages of the disease, with exceedingly high white blood counts, massive liver and spleen enlargement, and central nervous system involvement tend not to respond to drug therapy. Children who begin to demonstrate symptoms before the end of the first year or during adolescence have a poorer prognosis than children from 1 to 10 years of age.

Medical therapy includes supportive measures to counteract the effects of the disease and establishment of control of abnormally proliferating cells by the use of specific antileukemic drugs and radiation. The most commonly used supportive medical measures are: (1) correction of anemia and thrombocytopenia by use of blood transfusions with fresh whole blood, sedimented erythrocytes, or concentrated platelets; (2) appropriate prevention and treatment of infection; (3) symptomatic treatment of pain and discomfort; and (4) maintenance of appropriate fluid and electrolyte balance.[52,127]

Remission is obtained by the use of various combinations of drugs and radiation therapy. Remission is defined as a 5% or less abnormal blast content in the marrow and 40% or less lymphocytes plus blasts in the marrow. The child must also be free of symptoms and physical findings that could be attributable to the disease, and the complete blood count must be within normal limits.[52,68,127]

Table 18-10 summarizes the drugs used for

**Table 18-10.** Chemotherapeutic agents commonly used for acute leukemia

| Agent<br>Common dose | Type | Most effective use | Marrow toxicity | Immuno-suppression | Other toxic effects |
|---|---|---|---|---|---|
| Prednisone<br>40 mg/m²/day | Corticosteroid<br>? Membrane effect | Remission induction-ALL | No | Yes | Salt and water retention, increased appetite, hypertension, hyperglycemia, protein catabolism, osteoporosis |
| Vincristine<br>1.5 mg/m²/wk | Periwinkle alkaloid<br>Inhibits mitosis by preventing spindle formation | Remission induction-ALL | Little | Yes | Peripheral neuropathy, constipation, jaw pain, hair loss |
| Methotrexate<br>20-40 mg/m²/wk | Folate antagonist<br>Blocks folic acid reductase, inhibits purine synthesis | Remission maintenance-ALL<br>Intrathecal therapy | Yes | Yes | Mucosal ulceration, hepatic cirrhosis, encephalopathy, megaloblastosis |
| Mercaptopurine and thioguanine<br>50-100 mg/m²/day | Purine analogues<br>Block purine synthesis | Remission maintenance-ALL<br>Remission induction and maintenance-AML | Yes | Yes | Mucosal ulceration, hepatic dysfunction |
| Cyclophosphamide<br>200-300 mg/m²/wk | Alkylating agent<br>Cross-links DNA, inhibits replication | Remission maintenance-ALL<br>Remission induction and maintenance-AML<br>Limited efficacy in both | Yes | Yes | Nausea, vomiting, hair loss, hemorrhagic cystitis |
| Cytosine arabinoside<br>50-300 mg/m²/wk | Pyrimidine analogues<br>Inhibits DNA polymerase | Remission induction and maintenance-AML<br>Less effective for ALL | Yes | Yes | Nausea, vomiting, mucosal ulceration, hepatic dysfunction |
| Asparaginase<br>10,000-50,000 units/m²/wk | Enzyme<br>Deprives cell of asparagine | Remission induction-ALL | Little | Yes | Allergic reactions, anaphylaxis, hepatitis, pancreatitis, hypofibrinogenemia |
| Daunorubicin and adriamycin<br>20-50 mg/m²/wk | Anthracycline antibiotics<br>Bind DNA, prevent transcription | Remission induction-AML and ALL | Yes | Yes | Mucosal ulceration, hair loss, myocardial damage |

From Simone, J.: Leukemia. In Rudolf, A. M., editor: Pediatrics, ed. 16, New York, 1977, Appleton-Century-Crofts, p. 1187.

induction and maintenance of remission, the doses used, and side effects. These drugs are used sequentially and/or cyclically to produce resmissions and maintain them as long as possible. A combination of prednisone and vincristine is most commonly used to induce initial remission, and the child's response is then used as a guideline for further therapy. Since response decreases with prolonged use of the drugs, some physicians prefer to use cyclic therapy, alternating the drugs used to avoid decreased effectiveness of a single drug.

With the increased remission spans that are being accomplished with chemotherapy, there has been an increased incidence of invasion of the central nervous system by the leukemic cells, because the antileukemic agents do not cross the blood-brain barrier. Radiation therapy as prophylaxis against the development of central nervous system involvement is administered by some physicians at the time that the initial remission is achieved. Once involvement of the central nervous system develops, intrathecal administration of antileukemic agents and intensive radiation therapy are required.[28,52,68,100,127]

## Nursing problems and intervention

Even though many children with multiple and systemic problems have a guarded prognosis and are faced with imminent death, the goal of nursing intervention is to assist the child and family to attain maximal development in each area of competency throughout the remaining life span and to provide for their needs in crises. Health maintenance needs continue to be important in maintaining the optimal state of health that is possible for the child. Approaches for dealing with the dying child have been discussed in Chapter 17. The following section presents a discussion of the problems that are likely to emerge for these children that are directly related to their illness.

### Ambulation and exercise (MNPC no. 318.0)

Fatigue and transient intolerance for exercise occurs with children who have systemic problems. Often they will regulate their own activity level in accord with their tolerance for activity. When limitation of activity and exercise is either necessary or desirable, nursing intervention to help the child cope with the limitation may be needed. Activities that are in accord with the child's limits of tolerance yet promote learning and thought, social, or inner competency development are very important to continued development of the child as a person.[35,51]

### Nutrition (MNPC no. 318.1)

Loss of appetite may interfere with optimal nutrition of a child who has a systemic illness or who is on drugs that cause extensive side effects. Nursing assessment of the nutritional status of the child may be difficult because of the signs and symptoms of the child's illness; evaluation of the dietary intake and assistance in providing foods that appeal to the child and provide optimal nutrition are often the primary means of approaching nutrition problems.

### Skin care (MNPC no. 318.2)

Prevention of breakdown of the skin is an important aspect of nursing care for the child whose systemic disease affects the skin and causes difficulty in healing of skin lesions. If a skin lesion occurs, meticulous care is given to prevent infection, alleviate irritation of the area, and promote healing with aeration, light, and warmth.

### Maintenance of body temperature and physical care (MNPC no. 318.3)

Prevention of pulmonary infections and provision of optimal ventilation of the lungs are a major concern for children with systemic problems because of their increased risk for infection and complications of respiratory infection. The child's contact with other children who have a known infection should be limited. Optimal nutrition and exercise help maintain the child's own defenses against infection. Teaching the family to prevent infection and recognize its early signs is important in providing for protection of the child and in achieving early diagnosis and treatment when an infection occurs.

### Psychosocial and intellectual stimulation (MNPC no. 318.4)

Support and counseling for the child and family are one of the most critical areas of health care and yet the most difficult to achieve in the face of systemic problems that have a grave outlook. Maintaining trust and communication between the family and the health care team is essential if the team is to be able to recognize the real needs of the family and to make provisions for the type of support that is needed by the family at various stages in the child's illness. Approaches for working with the family and the dying child are discussed in Chapter 17. Periodic family assessment, as described in Chapter 3, provides information as to how the family is coping or not coping with the stress of the illness. Assessment of the child's inner competency at various stages of illness provides an evaluation of the child's means of coping or not coping, and approaches can be identified that might assist the child and family in a meaningful way.[62]

Continued attention to learning and thought, social, and inner competencies throughout the course of the child's illness is one means of helping the child and family cope with their stress. If the child can continue to develop an

CHAPTER 18

Children and
youth with
long-term
physical
problems

inner sense of worth and of success, the inner resources for dealing with the reality of the physical illness is greatly enhanced. If the family can experience a meaningful relationship with their child during the months and years of illness and direct their energy during these months toward using their time and experience with the child in a positive manner, their own resolution of the sorrow and grief related to the child's illness and possible early death is altered in a positive manner.[11,35,37,75]

### Follow-through (MNPC no. 318.7)

The child with systemic problems usually requires life-long follow-through, often with continuing and increasing medical care. Particular attention is given to complications and recurrences of problems related to the systemic illness and to early identification and treatment of these conditions that can alter the course of the illness.

## STUDY QUESTIONS

1. Present a case study of a child with whom you work who has a long-term physical problem. Describe the problem as outlined in this chapter. Discuss the medical treatment being used and the nursing problems and intervention that are being implemented. Discuss the child's level of competency development and ways in which the health care team is facilitating this development.
2. Identify groups active in your community that are composed of parents whose children have particular long-term health problems. If possible, attend one of their meetings or interview one of the active parents. Identify the services that the organization offers to parents and how the group serves to help families and children.
3. Identify resources in your community that offer financial assistance to families who have long-term financial burdens with children afflicted with a physical problem. Include resources available to people of all socioeconomic levels; for example, insurance, public assistance, special foundations and funds, and government agencies. If a specialized clinic serves children with a particular problem, such as congenital heart defects, determine the source of financial support for the clinic and the cost to the family.

## REFERENCES

1. Aisenberg, R. B., and others: Psychological impact of cardiac catheterization, Pediatrics **51**:1051, June, 1973.
2. Allen, R. G., and Wrenn, E. L., Jr.: Pediatric surgery. In Hughes, J. G., editor: Synopsis of pediatrics, ed. 4, St. Louis, 1975, The C. V. Mosby Co., p. 899.
3. Ammann, A. J., and Wara, D. W.: Collagen vascular diseases (rheumatic diseases). In Rudolf, A. M., editor: Pediatrics, ed. 16, New York, 1977, Appleton-Century-Crofts, p. 373.
4. Backscheider, J. E.: Self-care requirements, self-care capabilities, and nursing systems in the diabetic nurse management clinic, Am. J. Public Health **64**:1138, Dec., 1974.
5. Benoliel, J. Q.: Childhood diabetes; the commonplace in living becomes uncommon. In Strauss, A. L.: Chronic illness and the quality of life, St. Louis, 1975, The C. V. Mosby Co., p. 89.
6. Bezzeg, E. D., and others: The role of the child care worker in the treatment of severely burned children, Pediatrics **50**:617, Oct., 1972.
7. Boone, J. E., Baldwin, J., and Levine, C.: Juvenile rheumatoid arthritis, Pediatr. Clin. North Am. **21**:885, Nov., 1974.
8. Bowden, M. L., and Feller, I.: Family reaction to a severe burn, Am. J. Nurs. **73**:317, Feb., 1973.
9. Brown, M. R. and Lillibridge, C. B.: When to think of celiac disease. The classical features of gluten sensitive enteropathy are often absent, Clin. Pediatr. **14**:76, Jan., 1975.
10. Burke, C.: Working with parents of children with hemophilia, Nurs. Clin. North Am. **7**:787, Dec., 1972.
11. Burnette, B. A. S.: Family adjustment to cystic fibrosis Am. J. Nurs. **75**:1986, Nov., 1975.
12. Butler, I. J., and Johnson, R. T.: Central nervous system infections, Pediatr. Clin. North Am. **21**:649, Aug., 1974.
13. Chan, J. C. M.: Perspectives in pediatric nephrology, Clin. Pediatr. **15**:990, Nov., 1976.
14. Chiu, J., and others: A controlled prospective study of cyclophosphamide in relapsing corticosteroid-responsive, minimal-lesion nephrotic syndrome in childhood, J. Pediatr. **82**:607, April, 1973.
15. Conway, B. L.: Pediatric neurologic nursing, St. Louis, 1977, The C. V. Mosby Co.
16. Cotton, E. K., and Parry, W. H.: Respiratory tract and mediastinum. In Kempe, C. H., Silver, H. K., and O'Brien, D., editors: Current pediatric diagnosis and treatment, ed. 4, Los Altos, Calif. 1976, Lange Medical Publications, p. 266.
17. Crittenden, M. R., Waechter, E., and Mikklesen, C. A.: Taking it day by day; when children undergo hemodialysis and renal transplantation, Children Today **6**:6, May-June, 1977.
18. Cytryn, L.: Factors in psychosocial adjustment of children with chronic illness and handicaps, Clin. Proc. Child. Hosp. **27**:200, July-Aug., 1971.
19. Davidson, M.: Diarrhea. In Rudolf, A. M., editor: Pediatrics, ed. 16, New York, 1977, Appleton-Century-Crofts, p. 990.
20. Dees, S. C.: Some unsolved problems in clinical allergy; observations on milk and egg hemagglutinating antibody titers in allergic children, Pediatrics **50**:420-428, Sept., 1972.
21. De Lamerens, S. A., and Simone, J. V.: Pediatric hematology. In Hughes, J. G., editor: Synopsis of

pediatrics, ed. 4, St. Louis, 1975, The C. V. Mosby
Co., p. 464.

22. Edelmann, C. M., Jr.: Acute glomerulonephritis. In
Rudolf, A. M., editor: Pediatrics, ed. 16, New York,
1977, Appleton-Century-Crofts, p. 1266.

23. Edelmann, C. M., Jr.: Idiopathic nephrotic syndrome
of childhood. In Rudolf, A. M., editor: Pediatrics, ed.
16, New York, 1977, Appleton-Century-Crofts, p.
1280.

24. Einhorn, A. H.: Bacterial meningitis. In Rudolf, A.
M., editor: Pediatrics, ed. 16, New York, 1977, Appleton-Century-Crofts, p. 418.

25. Einhorn, A. H.: The mouth. In Rudolf, A. M., editor:
Pediatrics, ed. 16, New York, 1977, Appleton-Century-Crofts, p. 911.

26. Etteldorf, J. N., and Burghen, G. A.: Juvenile diabetes. In Hughes, J. G., editor: Synopsis of pediatrics,
ed. 4, St. Louis, 1975, The C. V. Mosby Co., p. 616.

27. Feldman, D. J., Chambers, D. C., and Altrocchi, P.:
Developmental and acquired disorders of muscle. In
Cooke, R. E., editor: The biologic basis of pediatric
practice, New York, 1968, McGraw-Hill Book Co., p.
243.

28. Foley, G., and McCarthy, A. M.: The child with leukemia; the disease and its treatment, Am. J. Nurs. 76:
1108, July, 1976.

29. Fostel, C.: Chronic illness and handicapping conditions; coping patterns of the child and the family. In
Brandt, P. A., and others, editors: Current practice
in pediatric nursing, vol. 2, St. Louis, 1978, The C. V.
Mosby Co., p. 53.

30. Freeman, R. D.: Emotional reactions of handicapped
children. In Chess, S., and Thomas, A., editors: Annual progress in child psychiatry and child development, New York, 1968, Brunner/Mazel, Inc., p. 379.

31. Friedberg, D. Z., and Litwin, B.: The medical and
surgical management of patients with congenital heart
disease, a survey of current knowledge and practices,
Clin. Pediatr. 15:324, April, 1976.

32. Gardner, P., Breton, S., and Carles, D. G.: Hospital
isolation and precaution guidelines, Pediatrics 53:663,
May, 1974.

33. Githens, J. H., and Hathaway, W.: Hematologic disorders. In Kempe, C. H., Silver, H. K., and O'Brien,
D., editors: Current pediatric diagnosis and treatment, ed. 4, Los Altos, Calif., 1976, Lange Medical
Publications, p. 358.

34. Gracely, K. A.: Parental attachment to a child with
congenital defect, Pediatr. Nurs. 3:15, Sept.-Oct.,
1977.

35. Greene, P.: The child with leukemia in the classroom,
Am. J. Nurs. 75:86, Jan., 1975.

36. Greene, P.: Acute leukemia in children, Am. J. Nurs.
75:1709, Oct., 1975.

37. Grossman, M. L.: The psychosocial approach to the
medical management of patients with cystic fibrosis,
Clin. Pediatr. 14:830, Sept., 1975.

38. Grupe, W. E.: Chlorambucil in steroid-dependent
nephrotic syndrome, J. Pediatr. 82:598, April, 1973.

39. Guthrie, D. W.: Diabetic children; special needs,
diets, drugs, and difficulties, Nursing '73 3:10, March,
1973.

40. Guthrie, D. W., and Guthrie, R. A.: Diabetes in adolescence, Am. J. Nurs. 75:1740, Oct., 1975.

41. Guyton, A. C.: Textbook of medical physiology, ed. 5,
Philadelphia, 1976, W. B. Saunders Co.

42. Haggerty, R. J., and Greene, M.: Illnesses and prob-
lems. In Green, M., and Haggerty, R. J., editors:
Ambulatory pediatrics, II, Philadelphia, 1977, W. B.
Saunders Co., p. 13.

43. Hammond, G. D.: Leukemia, lymphoma, and the
reticuloendothelioses. In Cooke, R. E., editor: The
biologic basis of pediatric practice, New York, 1968,
McGraw-Hill Book Co., p. 462.

44. Hanissian, A. S.: Arthritis in childhood. In Hughes,
J. G., editor: Synopsis of pediatrics, ed. 4, St. Louis,
1975, The C. V. Mosby Co., p. 441.

45. Headings, V., and Fielding, J.: Guidelines for counseling young adults with sickle cell trait, Am. J. Public
Health 65:819, Aug., 1975.

46. Hilt, N. E., and Schmitt, E. W., Jr.: Pediatric orthopedic nursing, St. Louis, 1975, The C. V. Mosby Co.

47. Hoffman, J. I. E.: Congenital heart diseases. In Rudolf, A. M., editor: Pediatrics, ed. 16, New York,
1977, Appleton-Century-Crofts, p. 1403.

48. Holaday, B. J.: Achievement behavior in chronically
ill children, Nurs. Res. 23:25, Jan.-Feb., 1974.

49. Holaday, B. J.: Parenting the chronically-ill child. In
Brandt, P. A., and others, editors: Current practice
in pediatric nursing, vol. 2, St. Louis, 1978, The C. V.
Mosby Co., p. 68.

50. Hollister, R., and O'Brien, D.: Immune complex diseases. In Kempe, C. H., Silver, H. K., and O'Brien,
D., editors: Current pediatric diagnosis and treatment, ed. 4, Los Altos, Calif., 1976, Lange Medical
Publications, p. 520.

51. Holmes, H. A., and Holmes, F. F.: After ten years,
what are the handicaps and life styles of children
treated for cancer? Clin. Pediatr. 14:819, Sept., 1975.

52. Holt, C. P.: Neoplastic diseases. In Kemps, C. H.,
Silver, H. K., and O'Brien, D., editors: Current pediatric diagnosis and treatment, ed. 4, Los Altos, Calif.,
1976, Lange Medical Publications, p. 848.

53. Hughes, J. G.: Digestive system. In Hughes, J. G.,
editor: Synopsis of pediatrics, ed. 4, St. Louis, 1975,
The C. V. Mosby Co., p. 286.

54. Hughes, J. G.: Infectious diseases. In Hughes, J. G.,
editor: Synopsis of pediatrics, ed. 4, St. Louis, 1975,
The C. V. Mosby Co., p. 694.

55. Hughes, J. G., and Hanissian, A. S.: Cystic fibrosis
of the pancreas (fibrocystic disease of the pancreas;
mucoviscidosis). In Hughes, J. G., editor: Synopsis of
pediatrics, ed. 4, St. Louis, 1975, The C. V. Mosby
Co., p. 320.

56. Huttenlocher, P. R.: Diseases of the nervous system.
In Vaughan, V. C., III, and McKay, R. J., editors:
Nelson's Textbook of pediatrics, ed. 10, Philadelphia,
1975, W. B. Saunders Co., p. 1411.

57. Huttenlocher, P. R.: Neuropathies and muscular disorders. In Vaughan, V. C., III, and McKay, R. J.,

editors: Nelson's Textbook of pediatrics, ed. 10, Philadelphia, 1975, W. B. Saunders Co., p. 1457.

58. Jabbour, J. T., Duenas, D. A., and Gilmartin, R. C.: Diseases of the nervous system. In Hughes, J. G., editor: Synopsis of pediatrics, ed. 4, St. Louis, 1975, The C. V. Mosby Co., p. 811.

59. Jackson, D. E.: Sickle cell disease; meeting a need, Nurs. Clin. North Am. 7:727, Dec., 1972.

60. Johnsen, S. D.: Some important pitfalls in the diagnosis and treatment of bacterial meningitis in children, Clin. Pediatr. 14:191, Feb., 1975.

61. Kallen, R. J., and Lewis, E. J.: "Immunosuppressive" treatment of "chronic glomerulonephritis," J. Pediatr. 82:335, Feb., 1973.

62. Kartha, M., and Ertel, I. J.: Short-term therapy for mothers of leukemic children, Clin. Pediatr. 15:803, Sept., 1976.

63. Kaufmann, S. J.: In diabetic diets, realism gets results, Nursing '76 6:74, Nov., 1976.

64. Kohler, D.: Diabetic day; setting goals for a child-directed ambulatory program, Clin. Pediatr. 17:24, Jan., 1978.

65. Kupst, M. J., and others: Improving physician-parent communication; some lessons learned from parents concerned about their child's congenital heart defect, Clin. Pediatr. 15:27, Jan., 1976.

66. Lachman, J.: Pediatric orthopedics. In Vaughan, V. C., III, and McKay, R. J., editors: Nelson's Textbook of pediatrics, ed. 10, Philadelphia, 1975, W. B. Saunders Co., p. 1491.

67. Lamarre, A.: Early detection of pulmonary function abnormalities in cystic fibrosis, Pediatrics 50:291-298, Aug., 1972.

68. Lampkin, B. C., McWilliams, N. B., and Mauer, A. M.: Treatment of acute leukemia, Pediatr. Clin. North Am. 19:1123, Nov., 1972.

69. Lazarus, R. S.: Psychological stress and the coping process, New York, 1966, McGraw-Hill Book Co.

70. Linshaw, M. A., and Gruskin, A. B.: Management of the nephrotic syndrome; a summary of progress in the use of immunosuppressive therapy, Clin. Pediatr. 13:45, Jan., 1974.

71. Lorber, J.: Selective treatment of myelomeningocele; to treat or not to treat? Pediatrics 53:307, March, 1974.

72. Lorber, J.: Isosorbide in the treatment of infantile hydrocephalus, observations with a new drug, Clin. Pediatr. 14:916, Oct., 1975.

73. Low, N. L.: Cerebral palsy. In Rudolf, A. M., editor: Pediatrics, ed. 16, New York, 1977, Appleton-Century-Crofts, p. 1779.

74. Lubin, B. H., and Mentzer, W. C.: Sickle cell disease. In Rudolf, A. M., editor: Pediatrics, ed. 16, New York, 1977, Appleton-Century-Crofts, p. 1149.

75. Martinson, I. S.: The child with leukemia; Parents help each other, Am. J. Nurs. 76:1120, July, 1976.

76. Mattson, A.: Long-term physical illness in childhood; a challenge to psychosocial adaptation, Pediatrics 50:801, Nov., 1972.

77. McAnarney, E. R., and others: Psychological problems of children with chronic juvenile arthritis, Pediatrics 53:523, April, 1974.

78. McDermott, J. F., and Akina, E.: Understanding and improving the personality development of children with physical handicaps, Clin. Pediatr. 11:130, March, 1972.

79. McFarlane, J. M.: The child with sickle cell anemia, Nursing '75 5:29, May, 1975.

80. McFarlane, J. M.: Sickle cell disorders, Am. J. Nurs. 77:1948, Dec., 1977.

81. McIntosh, R. M., and O'Brien, D.: Kidney and urinary tract. In Kempe, C. H., Silver, H. K., and O'Brien, D., editors: Current pediatric diagnosis and treatment, ed. 4, Los Altos, Calif., 1976, Lange Medical Publications, p. 470.

82. Menkes, J. H.: Metabolic disorders. In Cooke, R. E., editor: The biologic basis of pediatric practice, New York, 1968, McGraw-Hill Book Co., p. 1234.

83. Meyers, R. D., and others: The social and economic impact of hemophilia—a survey of 70 cases of Vermont and New Hampshire Am. J. Nurs. 62:530-535, April, 1972.

84. Miles, J. S., and Solomons, C. C.: Orthopedics. In Kempe, C. H., Silver, H. K., and O'Brien, D., editors: Current pediatric diagnosis and treatment, ed. 4, Los Altos, Calif., 1976, Lange Medical Publications, p. 520.

85. Millichap, J. G.: Diseases of the muscles. In Rudolf, A. M., editor: Pediatrics, ed. 16, New York, 1977, Appleton-Century-Crofts, p. 1881.

86. Murray, M. D., and others: The continuing problem of purulent meningitis in infants and children, Pediatr. Clin. North Am. 21:967, Nov., 1974.

87. Myers, B. A., Friedman, S. B., and Weiner, I. B.: Coping with a chronic disability; psychosocial observations of girls with scoliosis treated with the Milwaukee brace, Am. J. Dis. Chil 120:175, 1970.

88. Neff, J. A.: Autonomy concerns of a child on dialysis, Matern. Child Nurs. J. 4:101, Summer, 1975.

89. Nellhaus, G.: Neurologic and muscular disorders. In Kempe, C. H., Silver, H. K., and O'Brien, D., editors: Current pediatric diagnosis and treatment, ed. 4, Los Altos, Calif., 1976, Lange Medical Publications, p. 526.

90. Nora, J. J., and Wolfe, R. R.: Cardiovascular diseases. In Kempe, C. H., Silver, M. H., and O'Brien, D., editors: Current pediatric diagnosis and treatment, ed. 4, Los Altos, Calif., 1976, Lange Medical Publications, p. 301.

91. O'Brien, D.: Diabetes mellitus. In Kempe, C. H., Silver, H. K., and O'Brien, D., editors: Current pediatric diagnosis and treatment, ed. 4, Los Altos, Calif., 1976, Lange Medical Publications, p. 673.

92. O'Hara, M. N.: Nursing care of the child with respiratory problems. In Steele, S., editor: Nursing care of the child with long-term illness, ed. 2, New York, 1977, Appleton-Century-Crofts, p. 285.

93. Paradise, J. L., and others: Pediatric and otologic aspects of clinical research in cleft palate, Clin. Pediatr. 13:587, July, 1974.

**781**

94. Paradise, J. L., and Bluestone, C. D.: Early treatment of the universal otitis media of infants with cleft palate, Pediatrics 53:48, Jan., 1974.

95. Paradise, J. L., and McWilliams, B. J.: Simplified feeder for infants with cleft palate, Pediatrics 53:566, April, 1974.

96. Patterson, P. C.: Hemophilia; the new look, Nurs. Clin. North Am. 7:777, Dec., 1972.

97. Pearson, H. A., and O'Brien, R. T.: Sickle cell testing programs, J. Pediatr. 81:1201-1204, Dec., 1972.

98. Perrin, J. C. S., and others: Evaluation of a ten-year experience in a comprehensive care program for handicapped children, Pediatrics 50:793, Nov., 1972.

99. Pless, I. B., and Satterwhite, B.: Chronic illness in childhood; selection, activities and evaluation of nonprofessional family counselors, Clin. Pediatr. 11:403, July, 1972.

100. Pocheldy, C.: Management of CNS leukemia in childhood; an outline of current concepts, Clin. Pediatr. 11:503, Sept., 1972.

101. Prater, B. M., Denton, N. J., and Fisher, K.: Food and you; nutrition in diabetes, Salt Lake City, Utah, 1970, Intermountain Regional Medical Program.

102. Rafael, B.: Early education for multihandicapped children, Children Today 2:22, Jan.-Feb., 1973.

103. Ransohoff, J., and Epstein, F.: Hydrocephalus, In Rudolf, A. M., editor: Pediatrics, ed. 16, New York, 1977, Appleton-Century-Crofts, p. 1753.

104. Raynolds, N.: When children go home after surgery for scoliosis, Am. J. Nurs. 74:1090, June, 1974.

105. Roberts, F. B.: The child with heart disease, Am. J. Nurs. 72:1080-1084, June, 1972.

106. Robinson, A., Goodman, S. I., and O'Brien, D.: Genetic and chromosomal disorders, including inborn errors of metabolism. In Kempe, C. H., Silver, H. K., and O'Brien, D., editors: Current pediatric diagnosis and treatment, ed. 4, Los Altos, Calif., 1976, Lange Medical Publications, p. 885.

107. Robinson, H. B., and Robinson, N. M.: The mentally retarded child; a psychological approach, New York, 1965, McGraw-Hill Book Co.

108. Romm, K. M., McArthur, R. G., and Leahey, M. D.: Psychologic management of children with diabetes mellitus, Clin. Pediatr. 16:1151, Dec., 1977.

109. Rosenlund, M. L.: Cystic fibrosis—survival could depend on you, Clin. Pediatr. 11:667, Dec., 1972.

110. Rowe, R. D., Kidd, B. S. L., Fowler, R. S., Olley, P. M., Isukawa, T., Rose, B., and Trusler, S. A.: Long-term management of heart defects, Pediatr. Clin. North Am. 21:841, Nov., 1974.

111. Roy, C. C., Silverman, A., and Dubois, R. S.: Gastrointestinal tract. In Kempe, C. H., Silver, H. K., and O'Brien, D., editors: Current pediatric diagnosis and treatment, ed. 4, Los Altos, Calif., 1976, Lange Medical Publications, p. 414.

112. Roy, S., III, and Arant, B. S., Jr.: Nephrology. In Hughes, J. G., editor: Synopsis of pediatrics, ed. 4, St. Louis, 1975, The C. V. Mosby Co., p. 502.

113. Sacksteder, S., Gildea, J. H., and Dassy, C.: Common congenital cardiac defects, Am. J. Nurs. 78:266, Feb., 1978.

114. Samaniego, L., and others: Exploring the physically ill child's self-perceptions and the mother's perceptions of her child's needs, Clin. Pediatr. 16:154, Feb., 1977.

115. Schmitt, B. D.: An argument for the unmeasured diet in juvenile diabetes mellitus; the physical and emotional risks of the measured diet, Clin. Pediatr. 14: 68, Jan., 1975.

116. Schmitt, B. D.: Ear, nose and throat. In Kempe, C. H., Silver, H. K., and O'Brien, D., editors: Current pediatric diagnosis and treatment, ed. 4, Los Altos, Calif., 1976, Lange Medical Publications, p. 240.

117. Schumann, D.: Assessing the diabetic, Nursing '76 6:62, March, 1976.

118. Sergis, E., and Hilgartner, M. W.: Hemophilia, Am. J. Nurs. 72:2011, Nov., 1972.

119. Shands, A. R., Jr., MacEwen, G. D., and Cowell, H. R.: Pediatric orthopaedics. In Shirkey, H. C., editor: Pediatric therapy, ed. 5, St. Louis, 1975, The C. V. Mosby Co., p. 1150.

120. Shulman, K., and Shapiro, K.: Closure defects of neural plate. In Rudolf, A. M., editor: Pediatrics, ed. 16, New York, 1977, Appleton-Century-Crofts, p. 1757.

121. Shwachman, H., Khaw, K. T., and Kowalski, S. M.: The management of cystic fibrosis, Clin. Pediatr. 14: 1115, Dec., 1975.

122. Siegel, N. J., and others: Long-term follow-up of children with steroid-responsive nephrotic syndrome, J. Pediatr. 81:251-258, Aug., 1972.

123. Silverman, F. N.: Axial skeleton. In Rudolf, A. M., editor: Pediatrics, ed. 16, New York, 1977, Appleton-Century-Crofts, p. 1994.

124. Silverman, F. N.: Systemic affections of the skeleton. In Rudolf, A. M., editor, Pediatrics, ed. 16, New York, 1977, Appleton-Century-Crofts, p. 2003.

125. Silverman, F. N., and Kleiman, M. B.: Joints. In Rudolf, A. M., editor: Pediatrics, ed. 16, New York, 1977, Appleton-Century-Crofts, p. 2026.

126. Silverman, F. N., and Kleiman, M. B.: Osteomyelitis. In Rudolf, A. M., editor: Pediatrics, ed. 16, New York, 1977, Appleton-Century-Crofts, p. 1999.

127. Silmone, J.: Leukemia. In Rudolf, A. M., editor: Pediatrics, ed. 16, New York, 1977, Appleton-Century-Crofts, p. 1183.

128. Smith, D. H., and others: Bacterial meningitis; a symposium, Pediatrics 52:586, Oct., 1973.

129. Smith, M.: A community approach to meeting the needs of diabetic youths and their families, Children Today 3:28, Jan.-Feb., 1974.

130. Steinhauer, P. D., Mushin, D. N., and Rae-Grant, Q.: Psychological aspects of chronic illness, Pediatr. Clin. North Am. 21:825, Nov., 1974.

131. Stewart, M. J.: Pediatric orthopedics. In Hughes, J. G., editor: Synopsis of pediatrics, ed. 4, St. Louis, 1975, The C. V. Mosby Co., p. 937.

132. Syme, S. L.: Behavioral factors associated with the etiology of disease; a social epidemiological approach, Am. J. Public Health 64:1043, Nov., 1974.

133. Taussig, L. M.: A new prognostic score and clinical

**CHAPTER 18**

Children and
youth with
long-term
physical
problems

evaluation system for cystic fibrosis, J. Pediatr. **82:** 380, March, 1973.

134. Tierney, R. C., Fitch, C. W., and Anthony, C. L., Jr.: Pediatric cardiology. In Hughes, J. G., editor: Synopsis of pediatrics, ed. 4, St. Louis, 1975, The C. V. Mosby Co., p. 382.

135. Tooley, W. H., and Lipow, H. W.: Specific diseases causing obstruction. In Rudolf, A. M., editor: Pediatrics, ed. 16, New York, 1977, Appleton-Century-Crofts, p. 1554.

136. Weil, W. B., Jr., and Kohrman, A. F.: Diabetes mellitus. In Rudolf, A. M., editor: Pediatrics, ed. 16, New York, 1977, Appleton-Century-Crofts, p. 694.

137. Wolfish, M. G., and McLean, J. A.: Chronic illness in adolescents, Pediatr. Clin. North Am. **21:**1043, Nov., 1974.

138. Wood, J. W.: The pediatrician as genetic counselor, Pediatr. Clin. North Am. **21:**401, May, 1974.

139. Wright, B. A.: Physical disability—a psychological approach, New York, 1960, Harper and Brothers.

140. Ziter, F. A., and Allsop, K. G.: The diagnosis and management of childhood muscular dystrophy; clinicians must provide the best care and support possible. Clin. Pediatr. **15:**140, June, 1976.

# The child with learning problems

Co-authored with Philip C. Chinn, Ed.D.

Children with learning handicaps present a unique challenge to professional workers involved in primary health care. These children have many problems similar to those of children with long-term physical problems, and a few children have primary problems in both areas. There are, however, special concerns related to the area of learning handicaps, and these will be the focus of attention for this chapter. In addition to a basic understanding of learning problems the child health care worker needs to be aware of measures that can be taken to prevent the development of learning handicaps or to minimize the problems encountered by the child and family.

## LEARNING HANDICAPS AND COMPETENCY DEVELOPMENT

Conditions or problems that primarily interfere with learning and thought competency development can originate from the environment or from the child. Environmental factors such as malnutrition, lack of stimulation, or disturbing interpersonal relationships can result in measurable deficiencies in the child's learning processes, which appear very similar to conditions originating as physical or organic problems. Mental retardation, learning disabilities, and certain physical handicaps such as blindness and deafness are the specific problems considered in this chapter. As with physical problems, there is rarely an effect on only one competency area; children with a primary learning problem may also have significant problems and concerns in other areas of development. They may be limited by biologic endowment in terms of intellectual capacity or have average or above average intellectual capacity. Yet children with learning problems do not perform in a learning situation in accordance with cultural and societal expectations. Societal stigma related to learning problems have changed, but the family usually remains significantly affected by these problems.

Since the child's problem is primarily one of learning difficulty, considerations for the child's educational experience are paramount. Promotion of optimal competency development becomes an effort jointly shared by those in health care and professional people in education who have special skills in serving these children and their families. These children's physical capacity may be limited by their intellectual capacity, or the condition causing the learning handicap may also result in a physical problem. Such conditions as cerebral palsy, blindness, and deafness involve limitations in physical competency and in many instances contribute to deficits in learning and thought capacity. In other instances children afflicted with these conditions are able to perform adequately in learning and thought, but they need special educational provisions in order to achieve their maximal level of performance. Children with Down's syndrome invariably have limitations in both physical and learning competencies.

Children with learning problems are at a particular risk for developing significant social and inner problems. They may have difficulty adjusting to their environment, and those around them may have problems adjusting to them. The level of satisfactory adjustment made by the family and child is a significant factor in determining the child's social and inner competency. Only rarely does a child with learning problems suffer from social and inner problems that are directly a function of the handicapping condition; but often there is a complex interrelationship among environmental factors and all areas of competency development.[31,40]

## DEFINITION AND SCOPE OF LEARNING PROBLEMS

Numerous attempts have been made to determine the prevalence of handicapping conditions that interfere with learning. Estimates have lacked consistency for two major reasons. First, each survey tends to utilize its own unique criteria for defining a handicapping condition. Second, where multiple handicaps exist,

**Table 19-1.** Estimate of percentages of handicapped children, ages 5 to 19 years, requiring special educational provisions*

| Condition | Percent affected |
|---|---|
| Speech impaired | 3.5 |
| Mentally retarded | 2.3 |
| Emotionally disturbed | 2.0 |
| Learning disabled | 1.0 |
| Hard of hearing | 0.5 |
| Deaf | 0.075 |
| Crippled and other health impaired | 0.5 |
| Visually impaired | 0.1 |
| Multiple handicapped | 0.06 |
| TOTAL | 10.035 |

*From United States Office of Education, Bureau of Education for the Handicapped, 1970.

the individual may be reported in each category in one survey and in only one category in another survey.

In a report, the Bureau of Education for the Handicapped of the United States Office of Education estimated that slightly more than 10% of children between the ages of 5 and 19 years suffer from handicapping conditions sufficiently pronounced to require some special educational provisions in order for these children to reach their maximum educational potential.[7] The bureau's categorical estimate of percentages of school-age handicapped children is presented in Table 19-1.

### Mental retardation

Mental retardation has often been simply defined as a low intelligence quotient (IQ). Most states use IQ score levels of 70 or below to legally qualify a child for special educational classes for the intellectually handicapped. One of the most widely utilized definitions of mental retardation is that of the American Association of Mental Deficiency (AAMD), which is included in the organization's *A Manual on Terminology and Classification in Mental Retardation:*[16] "Mental retardation refers to significantly subaverage general intellectual capacity existing concurrently with deficits in adaptive behavior, and manifested during the developmental period."

Chinn, Drew, and Logan[9] state that "Mental retardation as defined denotes a level of behavioral performance without reference to etiology. Thus it does not distinguish between retardation associated with psychosocial or polygenic influences and retardation associated with biological deficit. Mental retardation is descriptive of current behavior and does not imply prognosis. Prognosis is related to such factors as associated conditions, motivation, treatment, and training opportunities rather than to the mental retardation itself."

The AAMD definition thus implies that there are three major criteria for an individual to be considered mentally retarded: (1) The child must demonstrate significantly subaverage intellectual functioning, which is usually defined as two or more standard deviations below the mean IQ score. The two most commonly used

**785**

individual tests of intelligence are the Stanford Binet and the Weschler. On these two scales, significantly subaverage performance is represented by IQ scores of 67 and 69, respectively. (2) The upper age limit of the developmental period is 18 years and distinguishes mental retardation from other disorders of human behavior. (3) Adaptive behavior is defined as effectiveness or the degree with which the individual meets the cultural standards of personal independence and social responsibility expected at a particular developmental level. Deficits in adaptive behavior are manifested in learning, maturation, and social adjustment.

Among professional and parent groups serving mentally retarded and handicapped children, there is a growing trend toward the inclusion of concepts of mental retardation within a broad classification of developmental disabilities.[2,3,34,35] Developmental disabilities include children who are mentally retarded, autistic, cerebral palsied, physically handicapped, and those with learning disabilities and tend to focus on the child's actual behavioral capacity in relation to developmental norms for behavior rather than on intellectual capacity. Traits of specific disabilities related to learning and thought competency are presented in this chapter; disabilities related to social and inner competency are presented in Chapter 20.

Mentally retarded children are usually classified by symptom etiology, symptom severity, or by clinical types. Clinicians in the health sciences are often interested in all three systems of classification. Clinicians in the behavioral sciences and education tend to place a greater emphasis on symptom severity, since their primary service is to provide programs to meet the individual needs of each child regardless of etiology or clinical type.

### Symptom etiology

Classification based on symptom etiology is provided by the AAMD manual on terminology and classification.[16] Briefly summarized, the eight categories are:

I. Mental retardation associated with diseases and conditions caused by infection (e.g., congenital rubella, postnatal encephalitis, syphilis).

II. Mental retardation associated with diseases and conditions caused by intoxication (e.g., Rh incompatibility causing bilirubin encephalopathy, congenital maternal intoxications, such as toxemia of pregnancy).

III. Mental retardation associated with diseases and conditions caused by trauma or physical agents (e.g., prenatal, perinatal, or postnatal physical injuries, anoxia at birth).

IV. Mental retardation associated with diseases and conditions caused by disorders of metabolism, growth, or nutrition (e.g., phenylketonuria).

V. Mental retardation associated with diseases and conditions caused by new growths (e.g., neurofibromatosis).

VI. Mental retardation associated with diseases and conditions caused by unknown prenatal influence (e.g., hydrocephalus, Down's syndrome).

VII. Mental retardation associated with diseases and conditions of unknown cause with central nervous system deviation present (e.g., spinal sclerosis).

VIII. Mental retardation of uncertain or presumed psychologic cause with functional or behavioral reactions alone expressed (e.g., cultural-familial retardation).

As many as 75% to 85% of all retarded children may be classified in category VIII. The remaining percentage of children would be distributed by etiology in categories I through VII.

### Symptom severity

Symptom severity is most commonly expressed in either educational terms or under the AAMD classification system. While most school systems continue to use the traditional educational classification system for the mentally retarded, the advent of Public Law 94-142, the Education of Handicapped Children Act of 1975, has prompted some schools to use the AAMD classification system. Public Law 94-142 is a right to education act that ensures the right of severely and profoundly handicapped children to an appropriate public education. Prior to the advent of this act, many schools refused services to those children considered difficult to

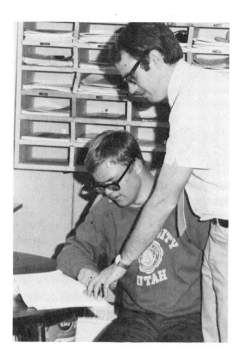

**Fig. 19-1.** Limited academic skills are achieved by the trainable mentally retarded child.

handle in the usual school program. Previously, schools only provided services for those retarded children whose IQ score was above 25 or 30. With the more severely handicapped now able to receive public education, school programs are being expanded to make provisions for the special needs of these children, and families are relieved of great financial and personal stresses associated with making private arrangements for their child's needs.

Using the educational classification by symptom severity, retarded children are most frequently identified according to their capacity to adapt to the requirements of standard education.

Educable—IQ score approximately 50 to 70
Trainable—IQ score approximately 30 to 49
Custodial—IQ score below 30

Educable children can generally respond to traditional education in reading, writing, and arithmetic. Academic expectations range from about the second to the fifth grade levels of achievement in the United States educational system. Preschool development in speech and/or motor skills usually proceeds with a notice-

able lag in rate, although sequence of development is like other children. In most instances educable children possess few if any physical characteristics that would distinguish them from their intellectually average peers.[9,24] Although educable retarded individuals tend to be limited in the kinds of vocational choices that they can make, they are capable of competitive employment and often become an integral part of their community by gaining productive employment.[8]

Preschool development for trainable mentally retarded children proceeds with a noticeable rate lag in all competencies. They can be expected to learn academic subjects only on a very limited basis during later childhood and adolescence. Although some school programs are now encouraging academics for these children, emphasis in classes for trainable children is usually placed on social and self-help skills. Trainable children may have noticeable physical and sensory deviations. A great number of children with clinical syndromes, such as Down's syndrome, function at trainable levels of achievement.[8] If trainable individuals are employed, they are usually limited to sheltered workshops or other situations where they are closely supervised. The majority of these individuals will require some sort of supervision in personal matters throughout life.

Custodial children are those who seldom, if ever, are capable of responding to traditional education. While custodial children are frequently kept at home or are institutionalized, the advent of Public Law 94-142 has resulted in larger numbers of these children being served in public school classroom settings.

Another type of classification is based on symptom severity and is provided by the AAMD using standard deviations (SD) of IQ scores.[16] These are as follows:

*Mildly mentally retarded:* SD $-2$ to $-3$; Stanford Binet scores 67 to 52. These children correspond approximately to the educational classification of educable.

*Moderately mentally retarded:* SD $-3$ to $-4$; Stanford Binet scores 51 to 36. These children correspond closely to the educational classification of trainable.

*Severely mentally retarded:* SD $-4$ to $-5$;

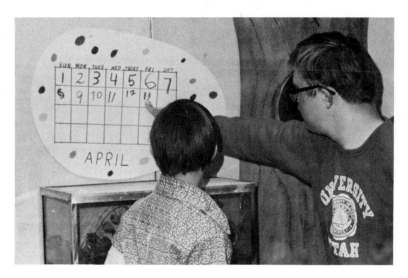

**Fig. 19-2.** Socialization and independence are gained by mentally retarded children in the school setting through experiences similar to those of all other children.

Stanford Binet scores 35 to 20. A few of these children at the upper level of this group correspond with the trainable. The remainder of the group corresponds with educational classification of custodial.

*Profoundly mentally retarded:* SD −5 or below; Stanford Binet scores below 20. All of these children correspond with the educational classification of custodial.

It is estimated that approximately 2.6% of the total population is mildly retarded. Moderately retarded children are estimated to comprise 0.3% of the population, and severe and profoundly retarded individuals combined are estimated to comprise 0.1% of the population.[9]

### Clinical types

A third approach to classification is according to clinical types. Certain retarded children possess anatomic, physiognomic, or pathologic characteristics sufficiently pronounced to allow them to be placed in particular clinical groupings. Examples of some of the more commonly mentioned clinical types of retardation include Down's syndrome, hydrocephaly, microcephaly, cretinism, Marfan's syndrome, neurofibromatosis, and Klinefelter's syndrome.

## Learning disabilities
### Definition

For years, educators have found it administratively convenient to categorize children with specific handicapping conditions in order to describe and implement programs that take into account the child's limitations. However, it has become increasingly apparent that many children who do not respond well to traditional academic requirements do not have defined characteristics of handicapped children, such as blindness, hearing loss, mental retardation, or emotional disturbance. This group of children has become recognized in recent years as having specific learning disabilities. Because the problems observed among these children are extremely diverse, a simple definition of the problem is seemingly elusive. A broad definition indicates that a learning disability is "a specific retardation or disorder in one or more of the processes of speech, language, perception, behavior, reading, spelling, writing, or arithmetic."[23]

Recognizing the confusion that exists in relation to learning disabilities, a National Advisory Committee on Handicapped Children formulated a tentative statement as follows:

Children with special learning disabilities exhibit a disorder in one or more of the basic psychological processes involved in understanding or in using spoken or written languages. These may be manifested in disorders of listening, thinking, talking, reading, writing, spelling, or arithmetic. They include conditions which have been referred to as perceptual handicaps, brain injury, minimal brain dysfunction, dyslexia, developmental phasia, etc. They do not include learning problems which are due primarily to visual, hearing, or motor handicaps, to mental retardation, emotional disturbance, or to environmental disadvantage.[39]

Children with learning disabilities, as implied by this definition, have three basic characteristics in common. First, their intellectual functioning is average or above average. Second, they have adequate sensory acuity. Third, their academic achievement is below what would be expected by the composite of their IQ score, age, educational opportunity, health, and cultural opportunities.[15]

The Bureau of Education for the Handicapped estimates that about 1.0% of all school-age children are learning disabled. However, until more adequate criteria and procedures for identification are established, statements identifying the prevalence of such conditions among children will tend to be based on rough estimates rather than on reliable scientific data.[24]

### Educational approaches

Most children with learning disabilities are not identified until they begin to fail academically in school. The most common failure is in reading, and the school often requests evaluation from several sources to determine the exact nature of the problem. A health evaluation is often required to rule out physical impairment that might be subject to medical intervention. However, a child who has a learning disability is specifically identified and the nature of the problem is diagnosed through psychoeducational diagnostic procedures. This process of diagnosis leads to a program of educational remediation for the specific problem.

The first step in educational diagnosis is determination of whether the problem is general or specific. If the failure is related to general inadequacy in functioning, the child will most likely be identified as having some type of retardation. If the problem is specific, the child will be identified as having difficulty in performing skills related to an isolated area of performance, such as reading. All other indications of capacity, such as IQ score, estimated mental age, or capacities in other academic skills, will be consistently more advanced and near the average range that would be expected for the child.

Next, the child's specific area of difficulty is further evaluated to determine the exact nature of the problem. The diagnostician determines the nature of the child's reading habits, what kinds of symbols he expresses verbally, what confusions he has in relation to printed symbols, and how he makes use of phonics. Such evaluation requires skilled observations and evaluation of various specific performances.[5,9,24,25] A few tools, such as the Illinois Test of Psycholinguistic Abilities (ITPA), have been developed to aid in the description of specific disabilities. The ITPA is one of the most widely used tools in evaluating various aspects of the process of communication, including memory, cognitive, associative, and expressive abilities. It is designed to assess the abilities of children between 3 and 10 years of age in five major areas[25]:

1. The ability to receive and understand what is seen and heard
2. The ability to make associations and understand interrelationships of what is seen and heard
3. The ability to express oneself by verbal and motor responses
4. The ability to automatically grasp the whole of a visual pattern or verbal expression when only a part of its is presented
5. The ability to remember and repeat visual and auditory sequences of material.[12]

The physical, environmental, and psychologic factors that might be associated with the child's disability are explored and described. Physical factors include visual deficits, auditory deficits, confused spatial orientation, hyperactivity, poor body image, and undernourishment. Environmental factors considered include such things as traumatic experiences in the family or community, conditioned avoidance reactions, bilingualism, sensory deprivation, or lack of school experiences. Psychologic factors that might be associated with a child's problem in achieve-

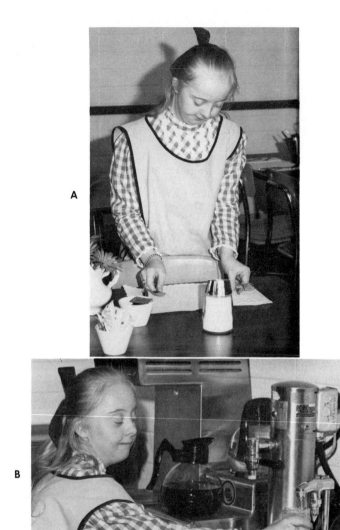

**Fig. 19-3.** In a sheltered workshop setting the trainable mentally retarded child can gain skills that enable her to make a meaningful contribution and limited earnings. Skills are acquired in waiting on tables, including **A,** setting the table, **B,** obtaining ordered items from the kitchen, **C,** serving the customer, and **D,** receiving payment for services rendered.

ment include poor sensory discrimination, slow perception and interpretation of concepts, inability to express concepts vocally or manually, and defective short-term memory capacity.

The diagnostician then formulates an inference based on the behavior that has been identified and the associated factors that have been explored. This inference, or hypothesis, specifies the nature of relevant variables that seem to have contributed to the child's problem and the specific disabilities toward which the remediation program must be directed. The appropriate program is then organized and implemented.[17,39]

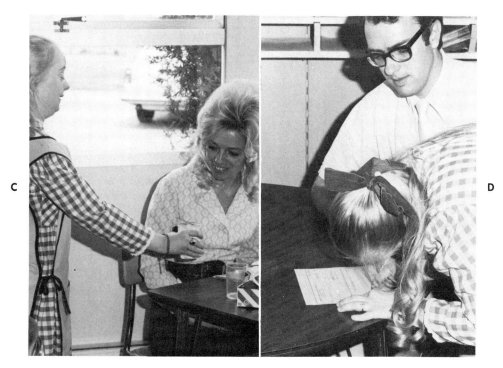

**Fig, 19-3, cont'd.** For legend see opposite page.

## Sensory handicaps with special implications for learning competency

There are several reasons why children with visual and auditory sensory handicaps tend to have unique learning problems. First, they often are dependent on individuals with normal sensory capacity for much of their day-to-day existence. Second, they are often readily identifiable. Third, the general public is culturally expected to demonstrate a sympathetic and at times patronizing attitude toward people with these handicaps.

There are several psychologic implications related to these factors. Many people view blindness as the worst handicap that an individual could have; however, many blind people tend to consider deafness as the most devastating of all handicaps. For many years the blind have received special privileges that have not been accorded to other handicapped individuals. For example, they are permitted double income tax exemptions; until recently they were the only handicapped group entitled to the free use of talking book equipment and to free mail service for their talking books.

Old wives' tales, such as blind individuals being able to place the "evil eye" on someone, still may influence the reaction of rational people to blind individuals. From a semantic standpoint, blindness is often used as a term synonymous with ignorance. For example, in speaking of cognitive understanding of a difficult problem, we often use the expression, "I was just too blind to see."

Physically handicapped individuals (crippled as well as deaf and blind) may feel the subtle pressures of a society that places great emphasis on the body beautiful/body whole concept, as does the typical American society. It is not uncommon for physically handicapped individuals to suffer from feelings of social, occupational, academic and/or sexual inadequacy because their handicap may psychologically preclude the possibility of forming satisfying relationships and personal achievements.

There are many variables that affect the learning and thought competency of the sensory-impaired child. The health care specialist who is aware of these variables can curtail or minimize the negative implications that often result.

The range and variety of experiences may be unduly limited for sensory-impaired children. They suffer from sensory deprivation effects that are not necessarily imposed by their handicap. Families may assume that because they are blind or deaf they cannot fully appreciate objects or events as normal children do. They may not provide their children special encouragement to "see" with their hands and ears or to "hear" with their eyes and sense of touch. They may be confined to a playpen as protection rather than allowed to explore. They can learn to experience their environment safely as long as appropriate provisions are made to guard against predictable dangers. In the home they can learn to experience, appreciate, predict, and control their environment, as do children with full sensory capacity. Provision should also be made for these children to have experiences outside the home appropriate to their stage of development; they should not be "protected" from the hazards of the greater world. They can enjoy a circus, trips to the zoo, or picnics; they can participate in preschool programs, and can play with neighborhood children.

Well-adjusted children who have a sensory handicap attain a balance of control with their environment. Children who are completely dependent upon the "normal" members of their family may develop the attitude of helplessness and a loss of self-identity. The other extreme is equally insidious. Blind or deaf children who completely dominate and control their environment by overwhelming their overly patronizing family with unreasonable demands fail to make an acceptable adjustment. Children's learning in relation to their own capacity to participate as a successful, loved member of the family is transferred into the educational situation and into peer group and other social contacts later in life.

The suddenness of onset of the handicap may be an important factor in the adjustment of a sensory handicapped child. If children suffer a sudden trauma, their adjustment may be different from that of children who gradually lost their capacity. The kind of learning that is required when loss of sensory function is sudden is also different from that required of children who gradually lose capacity.

The age of onset is an extremely important variable in adjustment and learning. If the condition is congenital and there is total absence of sensory capacity from birth, children do not have memory associated with the missing sensory capacity. They have never experienced perceptions involving these capacities, and thus they have not had the opportunity to build concepts utilizing these sensory modalities. The congenitally blind child, for example, cannot formulate the same concept of "green" grass as is possible for the child who loses sight after experiencing the perception of "green." Concepts such as deep, up, down, over, or wide may be difficult concepts to develop for a child who has never experienced related visual clues. While educational deficits can occur for blind children, the overall academic achievement of blind children with special educational provisions tends to be similar to seeing children of similar age and intellectual capacity.[1] Hearing loss tends to result in more severe effects on learning and is estimated to cause academic achievement lags of two to five years. When children become deaf or significantly hard of hearing after 6 years of age, they have formed notably more subtle concepts and advanced language and speech capacities than those of children who lose hearing capacity at 2 or 3 years of age or earlier. Thus the effect on academic achievement is closely related to the age when the loss occurred.[32]

Another variable that may significantly affect the capacity and adjustment of the sensory handicapped child is the amount of residual sensory acuity. Within the definitions involving visual and acoustic impairments, there is a wide variation in functioning abilities. For example, two children may be declared legally blind. One child may have 20/200 vision with correction and will have few, if any, pedestrian mobility problems. Another child may have only poor light perception and will have to rely on other individuals, a guide dog, or a long cane for pedestrian mobility.

The prognosis of the child's condition is also important in education and counseling. A child with glaucoma whose condition is progressively deteriorating needs to be prepared gradually for the emotional and educational problems that will occur when complete loss of vision becomes a reality.

### Visually impaired children

Visually impaired children are usually placed into one of two categories based on symptom severity. These are (1) blind and (2) partially seeing. To be considered legally blind, the child must meet the criteria of corrected vision of 20/200 or worse in the better eye, or peripheral vision where the visual field subtends an angle no greater than 20 degrees. Children whose corrected vision is between 20/200 and 20/70 are considered partially seeing and eligible for special classes in most public schools.[38]

The prevalence of visually impaired children of school age is estimated at 0.1%. The incidence of visual impairment in the general population is considerably higher since many visual problems relate directly to advanced age.

The National Society for the Prevention of Blindness has estimated that prenatal factors such as rubella and hereditary factors cause 47.7% of legal blindness in children. Poisonings (e.g., retrolental fibroplasia from oxygen toxicity) account for 33.3% of all blindness in children. Infectious disease, tumors, and accidental injuries account for most of the remaining percentage.[33]

### Acoustically impaired children

Acoustically impaired children have problems that transcend the reduction of hearing sensitivity, because impaired hearing tends to impair speech. Thus with both auditory and verbal communication skills affected, the child with a hearing loss is affected in language skills vital for both academic and social purposes.

The major types of hearing loss are conductive, sensorineural, and central impairment. Conductive losses result when there is any dysfunction of the outer or middle ear. The primary effect of this type of loss is a loss of loudness. As loudness is increased, perception of sound is restored. Hearing aids are often helpful, and there may be surgical means of restoring some of the loss.

Sensorineural, or nerve impairment, loss results from a dysfunction of the inner ear. The degree of hearing loss may be variable, and

**Table 19-2.** Scale of hearing impairment

| Classification of hearing loss | Hearing level decibels* loss (1964 International Standards Organization Reference) |
|---|---|
| None | 26 db or less |
| Slight | 27-24 db |
| Mild | 41-55 db |
| Marked | 56-70 db |
| Severe | 71-90 db |
| Extreme | 91 db or more |

*Average of hearing level loss are decibels at 500, 1,000, and 2,000 cycles per second. Decibel means a ratio by which one level of sound is greater or lesser than another.

there is presently no satisfactory way to restore hearing loss. The use of hearing aid may be helpful, but early identification and education are of prime importance in helping the child achieve maximal use of any sensory function that the child may retain.

Central impairment results from a dysfunction along the pathways of the brain from the brain stem through the cerebral cortex. This type of impairment frequently involves the symbolic processes of the mind in terms of receptive and expressive language.[37]

Table 19-2 indicates an example of a classification system for hearing loss based on audiometric measurement of hearing levels. Children who have a slight hearing loss have difficulty hearing faint sounds in their environment. They experience little interference in school and have no defective speech as a result of the loss. They may benefit from favorable seating in a group of children, and they may favor hearing from one ear over the other.

Children with mild hearing loss are able to understand conversational speech at a distance of 3 to 5 feet when facing the other person. They may miss as much as half of a class discussion if voices are faint or if they are not directly facing the person who is speaking. They may have a limited vocabulary and some speech problems if their loss is in the higher frequencies of sound. This child often benefits from the use of a hearing aid, and some supplementary educational assistance with speech and language development may be necessary.

Children who have a marked loss require

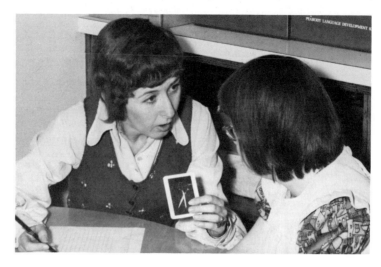

**Fig. 19-4.** Speech therapy is essential in helping a child with a hearing loss to attain optimal capacity in speech and language.

amplified levels of conversation in order to hear. They may misunderstand most of a conversation, and frequently have some speech impairment. Most often these children benefit from a hearing aid, and they need special assistance in voice, speech, and language development. They may need special class assignment for a portion of their educational experience.

Children who have a severe hearing loss hear voices only when the source is a few inches from their ear. Loud noises may be heard at some distance. Speech and language do not develop spontaneously, and special education is required very early in life. A child with this level of impairment who has had a rich background of experience with special auditory training, family enrichment, and contacts with normal peers may be successful in pursuing education integrated into a regular classroom.

Children who have an extreme hearing loss may hear a shout 1 inch away from the ear. They respond to tactile vibrations rather than to sounds. Speech and language are significantly impaired, and they rely on vision rather than hearing for communication. The quality of the voice is affected, and integration into a regular classroom situation is not possible for most of these children. They have very special needs for continuing special education, particularly in re-

lation to communication skills. Constant association with hearing peers and family members is important for optimal adjustment of these children.

The causes of hearing loss during childhood include prenatal factors, childhood illnesses, tumors, noise damage, entry of foreign bodies into the ear canal, and other forms of accidental injury. The major prenatal factor leading to hearing loss is maternal infection such as rubella. Childhood illnesses such as meningitis can also lead to hearing loss. Otitis media is a particular concern in causing hearing loss during the early childhood period. The Bureau of Education for the Handicapped estimated that 0.5% of all school-age children have some hearing loss which interferes with education and learning. Totally deaf children comprise about 0.075% of all school-age children.[7]

## THE FAMILY, EDUCATION, AND HEALTH CARE
### The family and the child with learning handicaps

American society tends to place a great emphasis on the body beautiful/body whole concept. Equally valued are traits that suggest bright mental function. The girl who looks as if she has just stepped off the cover of a fashion magazine or the all-around athletic boy is often the focus of attention. Most parents view their children as an extension of themselves, with desires for all of society's valued traits to be seen in their children. When the child is less than is hope for, there is often a feeling of personal loss and inadequacy on the part of the parent. Their own self-concept suffers as a result of having a child who does not meet their own and society's expectations. The degree of acceptance or rejection of the child is related to the perceptions that the parents have of the child's problem and the social and personal implications that it carries. Thus a child with a moderate hearing loss may be more easily accepted by a given family than a child who is educably retarded, even though the academic achievement of the two children may be quite similar.

Parental acceptance may depend upon the type and severity of the condition. Families of mentally retarded children often use denial in relation to the severity of their child's problem and refer to the child as having a learning disability rather than mental retardation. When a severely retarded child is in the family, family integration and development are often arrested, and acceptance of the child cannot develop.[9]

The presence of a handicapped child in the family may have varying effects on siblings. In some instances the siblings appear extremely well adjusted and have a great sense of understanding for the child with a learning handicap, along with a sense of tolerance for individuality. Often the placement of the handicapped child within the sequence of siblings affects the adjustment made by each member of the family. When a child with a learning handicap is first-born, acceptance by the parents may be more difficult, although younger siblings may adjust more adequately.[20]

In counseling with the families of handicapped children, the facts, alternative choices, and possible consequences of each alternative should be made available. Because families of children with learning handicaps tend to experience many of the same reactions in adjustment as those whose child has a physical problem, coordination among each professional worker who is helping the family is extremely important (see Chapter 18). The family who is search-ing for causes and cures may repeatedly seek advice and information from people in education and in the health care system. Each of these professional workers should work collaboratively with the family and find ways to provide coordinated assistance for the family. Conflicting information can confuse rather than help the family reach some level of acceptance of the child. Uncoordinated efforts to help the family may inhibit movement toward working out the inner and social problems involved. The family must continually deal with new information and advice, and they can remain in a state of denial and false hope about the child's actual condition for many years.

The ultimate decisions regarding the education and care of the child must be made by the family. The more completely they have been able to work through their own feelings and reactions, the more sound their decision is likely to be and the more likely they will be able to accept and live with the decision they make. The most difficult decisions for many families are whether to place the child with a learning handicap in a residential care facility and whether to have additional children after a handicapped child is born. The severity of the child's condition is often a factor to consider, but for any one family another factor may be equally important.[11]

Through genetic counseling the family can obtain information regarding the statistics of occurrence and reoccurrence of a given handicapping condition. For some conditions, such as Down's syndrome, the family can obtain information as to whether their child's problem is inherited or is the result of an isolated chromosomal defect. In subsequent pregnancies the family can obtain genetic evaluation of the amniotic fluid to determine the condition of the embryo.[36]

The moral, ethical, and emotional problems for the family in making decisions based upon genetic information may be exceedingly difficult. For example, if they are told that there is a 25% chance of a condition occurring for another child in their family, they need to realize that it will be either an all-win or an all-lose proposition. The child who is born is either normal or handicapped. They must, therefore, reach a decision in advance regarding the full implications of having another handicapped child in the family, rather than decide to have another child in the hope that this child will be normal.[11]

## Education of the child with learning handicaps

Through the years, many different kinds of programs have emerged to provide educational services for children with learning handicaps. It appears that individual children differ in their response to different approaches, and the needs of the child must be determined in making an educational decision. While the preference of the family and the school may be an important factor in the decision that is made, the child's own needs and response should be the central basis for the decision.

### Residential schools

Residential state-supported and private schools are among the earliest provisions made for children with learning handicaps. These schools have been and continue to be widely used in providing for the needs of mentally retarded, blind, or deaf children. They are most frequently utilized for children who are more severely handicapped and for whom there are no suitable community resources. At times the family situation is such that residential placement of the child is justified regardless of the severity of the child's condition or the availability of community resources. In addition, small, isolated communities are not able to provide special services for the very few children who might have learning problems, and these children need to be placed in a residential school in order to obtain educational provisions.[28]

### Special schools

Special schools are provided in some communities for children who might profit from a segregated, special school setting but who can live in their own home. A residential school may serve as a daytime special school for children who live in a nearby community. Such schools for trainable retarded, blind, and deaf children are usually available in larger cities in the United States.

### Special self-contained classrooms

The self-contained classroom has been one of the most popular provisions for educating children with learning problems. The classes are located in neighborhood schools, and the children are assigned to special education teachers who work with them throughout the day. In such a setting the child is not expected to compete against the academic standards of peers with average intellectual capacity, and they are able to reach educational goals designed for their expected level of achievement. Integration with other children is provided on a limited basis.

### Special resource programs

In recent years special educators have recognized the need to provide specific experiences for individual children that are not ordinarily available in self-contained classrooms or special schools. While these approaches are administratively convenient and they provide many of the special educational considerations needed by handicapped children, they tend to remove them from the mainstream of social and educational experience, and they emphasize the stigma associated with learning handicaps.

Alternatives to the special classroom have developed in order to maximize integration of the child with a learning handicap into the regular school experience. Emphasis is placed on providing the child with the least restrictive alternative or the type of program that will place the child in as much of the mainstream of regular education as his or her abilities will permit. Approaches that have been implemented include the following:

1. *Resource rooms* provide selected educational support for individual children. The child with a learning handicap is assigned to a regular classroom but goes to the resource room for special attention to his or her needs. This type of program reflects a philosophy of shared responsibility involving both the regular classroom teacher and the specially prepared teacher.

2. *Cooperative programs* are similar to the resource room concept, but the child is assigned primarily to the special classroom teacher and is integrated into regular classes whenever feasible. Children with more pervasive handicaps,

such as blind or deaf children or mentally retarded children with orthopedic limitations,
might achieve greater benefit from this type of
program, which utilizes special resources more
centrally.

3. *Itinerate resource personnel* are specially
prepared teachers who provide assistance for
the regular classroom teacher who has full educational responsibility for a child with a learning problem. Many children with learning
handicaps can respond well to the regular classroom situation on a full-time basis if the teacher
is assisted in identifying the special needs of
the child and in planning and implementing
special provisions for the child. Many children
with specific learning disabilities, as well as children with mild retardation, marginal hearing
loss, or visual impairment respond well with
such programs.

These trends in special education have provided a more child-centered approach to meeting the needs of children with learning problems. Children are not assigned a label or a
diagnostic category; rather their learning problem is identified, and special provision is made
to help them overcome their problem with optimal performance in the affected area. At the
same time, they are encouraged to maintain
and develop skills in each area of performance
that is not necessarily affected by the learning
handicap. Thus children who have limited intellectual function are encouraged to develop
social competencies appropriate for their stage
of development.[9,19]

## Health care of the child with learning handicaps

### Mentally retarded children

One of the major concerns of child health
maintenance is the evaluation of learning and
thought competency. Although health care
workers are seldom skilled in the evaluation of
IQ scores, several means of screening learning
and thought competency can reveal objective
observations regarding the adequacy of the
child's level of intellectual functioning and adaptive behavior. Tools such as the Denver Developmental Screening Test and the Preschool
Readiness Experimental Screening Scale have
been discussed, which provide screening of the

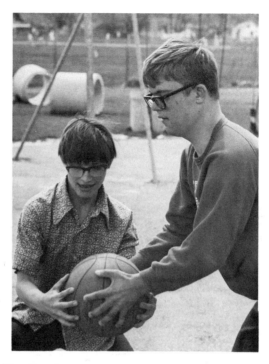

**Fig. 19-5.** Retarded children can achieve physical and
social skills similar to those acquired by other children.
In so doing they can gain healthy inner competency and a
satisfying relationship with peers.

child's mental and adaptive behavior (see Chapter 10). The neurologic and motor evaluation
and the assessment of speech and language development provide important indications of the
child's development in learning competency.

When a child has some form of mental retardation, health care for the child often becomes a
central concern. Many retarded children have
special related health problems. Special provisions must often be made for meeting daily
health care needs and for teaching the child to
assume some of his or her own health care. In
addition, the child develops physiologically as a
mature adult, and some understanding of the
growing and changing body becomes a health
concern just as it does for the mentally average
individual. Thus the health care worker may
become involved in both care and education of
mentally retarded children.[13,26,43]

In teaching health care concepts to mentally
retarded children, it is helpful to apply a few
basic principles that take into account their

special learning limitations. First, retarded children generally respond more adequately to concrete ideas and objects rather than to abstractions. For example, if the nurse is trying to help children understand the need for bathing, it is difficult for them to respond to abstract explanations of what to do and how it should be done. Success will be enhanced if the nurse instructs the child through the actual bathing experience, using demonstrations and return demonstrations from the child. The seemingly simple concept of rinsing shampoo out of the hair may need to be transferred several times to the actual experience in a teaching situation in order for the child to learn the behavior.

Second, retarded children usually respond better to distributed practice as opposed to massed practice.[27] The behavior that is being taught needs to be practiced in brief, frequent intervals rather than in one longer learning session. This may require a great deal of time and effort, and there must be cooperation from the child's family to achieve the type of practice that the child needs. For example, if the child is learning to prepare a meal, he or she may need many practice experiences with a small aspect of meal preparation spaced over an extended period of time. If they can obtain this practice in the school setting and again at home, their opportunities for brief, frequent practice are increased and learning is enhanced.

In addition, the health care worker who is able to offer the family help and guidance in teaching the child has a vital role in assisting the family through ongoing adaptations and adjustments. Regardless of past experience, no family is prepared to cope with either the realization or the adaptation required when a child is mentally retarded. Stimulation approaches described in Chapter 9 provide valuable benefits for the infant and child in promoting development, and they also promote the family's physical and emotional interaction with the child. Supportive counseling may be beneficial in relation to health care of the child and in promoting the continuing development of all aspects of family life and competency development.*

*References 3, 13, 14, 22, 30, 34.

### The child with learning disabilities

Professional health care workers are often confronted with the need to evaluate a child who is not performing adequately in school in spite of indications that he could do better. Although this type of discrepancy in performance may be related to several other health or social problems, awareness of the common manifestations of a learning disability may enhance the assessment of the child. Gearheart[15] has identified several characteristics, one or more of which might be exhibited in the behavior of children with learning disabilities. Although these characteristics do not provide either a diagnosis of learning disabilities or delineation of the specific nature of the problem, they do provide a basis upon which referral can be made for psychoeducational diagnosis.

**Hyperactivity.** Increased levels of inappropriate activity tend to be present when a child has a particular brain injury. These children may be inappropriately restless, fidgety, nervous, unable to sit still, and so on. Their noticeably different rate of movement is annoying to others and interferes with their ability to focus attention on anything long enough to learn effectively.

**Hypoactivity.** Although decreased activity levels are less common among children with learning disabilities, this does occur. Rather than being active and fidgety, these children are consistently tired, unable to participate in ordinary activities, and require a great deal of rest and sleep. This problem points out the error in equating learning disabilities with hyperactivity, or hyperkinesis.

**Lack of motivation.** This problem may be caused by children's specific learning disability and the continual frustration that they have already encountered in the academic setting. It is often listed as a symptom, however, and should alert the clinician to observe for other characteristics typical of the learning disabled child.

**Inattention.** Regardless of the typical activity level of the child, some learning-disabled children have a specific problem in focusing attention on any one activity or problem for an extended length of time. They may be described as flighty, unable to concentrate, or unable to listen and follow directions.

**Overattention.** In contrast to the child who cannot concentrate, the child with overattention tends to fixate attention on one particular object and has great difficulty in changing attention to something else. This problem relates to figure-ground problems, in which the child is unable to focus attention on the significant aspect of a total setting because he or she fixates attention on a less significant aspect of the background.

**Perceptual disorders.** Disorders of visual, auditory, tactile, kinesthetic, olfactory, and gustatory perception have been identified. Those that appear to create the greatest academic interference are disorders in visual and auditory perception. These children may be observed to consistently copy letters and figures incorrectly, with the letters reversed or mirrored typical of those produced by the preschool child. They may be unable to differentiate auditory sound such as the ring of the telephone and the door bell. Sensory acuity is within normal limitations, but perceptual function is deviated.[29]

**Lack of coordination.** Many learning-disabled children, regardless of activity level, are described as clumsy or slow to develop the motor skills used in playing, such as throwing or catching a ball, skipping, or running.

**Perseveration.** Children who exhibit perseveration are similar to the children who are identified as overattending. They are not able to switch concepts or tasks easily, and they tend to repeat persistently in any behavioral area. Perseveration may refer to a specific repetitive behavior in writing or in speaking, rather than to the general behavioral trait of overattention.

**Memory disorders.** The phenomena of memory are not clearly understood, and memory disorders without impairment of general intellectual function are particularly puzzling. Children with this sort of problem may not be able to remember the placement of furniture in a room, demonstrating a visual memory disorder, or they may not be able to repeat a simple sequence of three or four numbers, demonstrating an auditory memory disorder.[7]

For children with learning disabilities the potential is great for serious effect on social and inner competency. The repeated failure experienced by these children leads to progressive deterioration of social relationships with peers and the associated inner feelings of inadequacy and incompetency.[42] Intervention that is directed to remediation of their learning disability is of primary importance, but health care workers can assist the family and school in finding ways to provide success experiences for the child.[4]

Once the child has obtained effective educational assistance directed toward remediation of the problem, his or her competency in all adversely affected areas tends to increase. Some children with learning disabilities associated with hyperactivity are placed on behavior-modifying drugs; the health care implications of this treatment are discussed in Chapter 13.[10,21]

### Sensory-impaired children

Many problems of sensory function may be identified through the health care assessment. Several cues are particularly important in assessing sensory function, and they provide a basis for special attention to evaluation of particular sensory capacities.

1. The child's parents or teacher may express concern regarding the adequacy of the child's vision or hearing. Even in the face of suggestive inadequacies in the parent-child or teacher-child relationship, such concerns should be investigated thoroughly with actual sensory acuity determined as accurately as possible.

2. The child may exhibit behaviors that are unusual and tend to draw attention. Excessive blinking, squinting, tilting of the head in an extra effort to see or to hear, holding reading material unusually near, or consistently asking people to repeat conversation may indicate a loss of sensory function.

3. Physical signs and symptoms may be observed that suggest sensory problems. Headaches, dizziness, sensitivity to light, clumsiness in mobility and fine motor control, recurrent signs of infection in the eyes or ears, and muscular imbalance of the eyes indicate special attention to sensory acuity.

Further, several approaches to the screening of visual and hearing acuity appropriate for the child's developmental stage have been reviewed in Chapters 9 and 10. Children of all ages should be screened periodically with the most reliable means available.

Particular skill in working with children who have sensory impairment may be developed by acquiring special communication skills appropriate for the child. Family members may be vital in interpreting the child's means of communication to the health care worker and in offering suggestions as to how the child relates to others in ways that compensate for sensory loss. Since individual children tend to develop and learn different ways of adjustment and of compensation, knowledge of the individual child may be needed before a successful relationship can be developed.

Health care workers should be particularly aware of the child's need to have realistic expectations set for behavior, without undue pressure to perform beyond actual capacity. Equally devastating, however, is the tendency of people to be overly solicitous and to praise and reward the child for every accomplishment that is considered by the sensory normal adult as truly remarkable. The blind child who learns to perform tasks that sighted individuals think of as dependent upon sight does so with a feeling of great inner satisfaction, just as a seeing child would when the initial accomplishment is made. Once this accomplishment is mastered, however, it is demeaning to the child to continually receive benevolent praise for usual activities. A realistic approach to the child with sensory deficits can help in establishing a relationship of rapport similar to that achieved with any other child.[6,14,41]

## STUDY QUESTIONS

1. Identify a child who has a learning problem such as those discussed in this chapter. Investigate the etiology of the condition, and describe the features of the handicap. Obtain a complete health history, perform a nursing assessment, and indicate your impression of health care needs. If possible, also investigate the educational provisions that are being made for the child and describe these.
2. Visit a residential or special school in your community that provides special educational services for retarded children. Describe the educational programs conducted in this facility. Describe the health care program that is available to the children while they are in school or in relation to their school experience. Determine the role of the health care system in the children's diagnosis and continuing care.
3. Investigate further the means of communication that might be used by a child who has a sensory impairment.

If possible, interview a person who is involved in teaching sensory impaired children, and observe the activities that are conducted. If possible, plan an experience with a selected child who has a sensory impairment, and describe how you made provisions for establishing a relationship with the child.

## REFERENCES

1. Ascroft, S. C.: The blind and partially seeing, Rev. Educ. Res. **29**:519, 1959.
2. Barnard, K.: Developmental disabilities, Am. J. Nurs. **75**:1700, Oct., 1975.
3. Barnard, K. E., and Erickson, M. L.: Teaching children with developmental problems; a family care approach. ed. 2, St. Louis, 1976, The C. V. Mosby Co.
4. Bierbauer, E.: Tips for parents of a neurologically handicapped child, Am. J. Nurs. **72**:1872, Oct., 1972.
5. Bishop, J. S.: An investigation of the efficacy of the Frostig program for the development of visual perception, Pediatrics **50**:154, July, 1972.
6. Boone, D. R., and Hartman, B. H.: The benevolent overreaction; a well-intentioned but malignant influence on the handicapped child, Clin. Pediatr. **11**:268, May, 1972.
7. Bureau of Education for the Handicapped: Better education for the handicapped, Annual Report FR 1969, Washington, D.C., 1970.
8. Capute, A. J., and Biehl, R. F.: Functional developmental evaluation; prerequisite to habilitation, Pediatr. Clin. North Am. **20**:3, Feb., 1973.
9. Chinn, P. C., Drew, C. J., and Logan, D. R.: Mental retardation; a life cycle approach, St. Louis, 1975, The C. V. Mosby Co.
10. Cline, F. W.: The nurse practitioner and learning disorders, Nurse Practitioner **2**:31, Sept.-Oct., 1977.
11. Crocker, A. C., and Crushna, B.: Pediatric decisions in children with serious mental retardation, Pediatr. Clin. North Am. **19**:413, May, 1972.
12. Durbin, L.: New horizons for the mentally handicapped, Child. Today **2**:17, Jan.-Feb., 1973.
13. Etters, L. E.: Adolescent retardates in a therapy group, Am. J. Nurs. **75**:1174, July, 1975.
14. Fleming, J. W.: Care and management of exceptional children, New York, 1973, Appleton-Century-Crofts.
15. Gearheart, B. R.: Learning disabilities: Educational strategies, St. Louis, 1973, The C. V. Mosby Co.
16. Grossman, H. J., editor: Manual on terminology and classification in mental retardation, Washington, D.C., 1977, American Association on Mental Deficiency.
17. Guthrie, J. T.: Educational assessment of the handicapped child, Pediatr. Clin. North Am. **20**:89, Feb., 1973.
18. Hersey, W. J., Jr., and Lapidus, K. R.: Restoring the balance, Pediatr. Clin. North Am. **20**:221, Feb., 1973.
19. Hewett, F. M.: Strategies in special education, Pediatr. Clin. North Am. **20**:695, Aug., 1973.
20. Howell, S. E.: Psychiatric aspects of habilitation, Pediatr. Clin. North Am. **20**:203, Feb., 1973.
21. Johnson, C. F., and Prinz, R.: Hyperactivity is in the eyes of the beholder; an evaluation of how teachers

view the hyperactive child, Clin. Pediatr. **15**:222, March, 1976.

22. Kanthor, H., Pless, B., Satterwhite, B., and Myers, G.: Areas of responsibility in the health care of multiply handicapped children, Pediatrics **54**:779, Dec., 1974.

23. Kirk, S. A.: The Illinois Test of Psycholinguistic Abilities; its origin and implications. In Hellmuth, J., editor: Learning disorders, vol. 3, Seattle, Wash., 1968, Special Child Publications.

24. Kirk, S. A.: Educating exceptional children, ed. 2, Boston, 1972, Houghton Mifflin.

25. Kirk, S. A., McCarthy, J. J., and Kirk, W. D.: The Illinois Test of Psycholinguistic Abilities, rev. ed., Urbana, Ill., 1968, University of Illinois Press.

26. Levine, M. S., and others: Adolescents with developmental disabilities; a survey of their problems and their management, Clin. Pediatr. **14**:25, Jan., 1975.

27. Madsen, M. C.: Distribution of practice and level of intelligence, Psychol. Resp. **13**:39, 1963.

28. Magnus, R. A.: Teaching parents to parent; parent involvement in residential treatment programs, Child. Today **3**:25, Jan.-Feb., 1974.

29. Mencher, G. T., and Stick, S. L.: Auditory perceptual disorders, Clin. Pediatr. **13**:977, Nov., 1974.

30. Murphy, A., and others: Meeting with brothers and sisters of children with Down's syndrome, Child. Today **5**:20, March-April, 1976.

31. Myers, P. A., and Warkany, S. F.: Working with parents of children with profound developmental retardation; a group approach, Clin. Pediatr. **16**:367, April, 1977.

32. Mykelbust, H. R.: The psychology of deafness, New York, 1960, Grune & Stratton, Inc.

33. National Society for the Prevention of Blindness: Fact book; estimated statistics of blindness and visual problems, New York, 1966, The Society.

34. O'Neil, S. M., McLaughlin, B. N., and Knapp, M. B.: Behavioral approaches to children with developmental delays, St. Louis, 1977, The C. V. Mosby Co.

35. Paris, S. G., and Haywood, H. C.: Mental retardation as a learning disorder, Pediatr. Clin. North Am. **20**:641, Aug., 1973.

36. Reisman, L. E., and Matheny, A. P.: Genetics and counseling in medical practice, St. Louis, 1969, The C. V. Mosby Co.

37. Rushford, G.: Glossary of terms relating to children with hearing problems, Vota Rev. **66**:750, Dec., 1964.

38. Scholl, G. T.: The education of children with visual impairments. In Cruickshank, W. M., and Johnson, G. D., editors: Education of exceptional children and youth, ed. 2, Englewood Cliffs, N.J., 1967, Prentice-Hall, Inc.

39. Special Education for Handicapped Children: First Annual Report of the National Advisory Committee on Handicapped Children, Washington, D.C., 1968, Office of Education, Department of Health, Education and Welfare.

40. Taichert, L. C.: Parental denial as a factor in the management of severely retarded child, Clin. Pediatr. **14**:666, July, 1975.

41. Ulrich, S.: Elizabeth, Ann Arbor, 1972, The University of Michigan Press.

42. Wender, P. G.: Minimal brain dysfunction in children, New York, 1971, John Wiley & Sons, Inc.

43. Wilson, R. R., and Baldwin, B. A.: A pilot sexuality training workshop for staff at an institution for the mentally retarded, Am. J. Public Health **66**:77, Jan., 1976.

# The child with long-term social and inner problems

Co-authored with Philip C. Chinn, Ed.D.

Long-term social and inner problems of childhood are a particular concern for society and families. When a child develops a serious problem in either social or inner competency, the effect upon all aspects of development is great. It may be impossible, in fact, to determine the source of the problem or to identify which competency area is primarily involved. Interference with development is so pervasive that the child's development in each of the other competencies becomes as disturbed as that of the inner self-concept. Physical competency is often the least affected competency, but some effect on physical function is usually present. In this chapter we will consider the primary features of serious, long-term social and inner problems, but the interrelationship between these two disturbances is so great that in many instances they cannot be clearly delineated.

## SOCIAL IMPLICATIONS OF HANDICAPPING CONDITIONS

Nearly all handicapping conditions preclude total social interaction to some degree, and they interfere with totally adequate inner development. For example, deaf and speech-impaired children lack communication skills. The visually impaired and physically handicapped are often limited in their mobility. As discussed in Chapter 19, the general public has developed an accepting and sometimes patronizing attitude toward some conditions, such as blindness, deafness, and physical handicaps. Solicitors for public contributions to help people with these conditions seldom find resistance.

Mental retardation, learning disabilities, and speech impairment have in the past carried varying degrees of stigma. While they interfere with the individual's social competency, the child and parents can often find some social acceptability and satisfaction in today's societies. Society has reached a point where it does not overtly hold the child or parents accountable and responsible for these conditions or for their failure to develop completely as average individuals in all competencies. There is increasing recognition that these handicaps can occur to anyone regardless of the family's adequacy, behavior, or socioeconomic status.

Emotionally disturbed and socially maladjusted children and their families, however, continue to be plagued with great social stigma and personal blame. The behavior patterns of these children significantly affect adequate func-

CHAPTER 20

The child with
long-term social
and inner
problems

tion of the family as a unit as well as all social contacts beyond the family. The behavior exhibited by these children is invariably negative, and the response to this outward manifestation of the problem is usually rejection. Because the behavior may grossly affect the well-being of society, the child and parents are often held accountable for their actions in a criminal sense, even if these actions are, in reality, beyond their willful control.[4]

## DEFINITIONS, SCOPE, AND INTERVENTION
### Defining the problems

While emotionally disturbed and socially maladjusted children are frequently treated as having synonymous problems, two separate conditions, which occasionally overlap in their symptoms, can be identified. Emotionally disturbed children are described as mentally ill, and their behavior patterns range from aggressive destruction to morbid withdrawal. Because of their psychologic stress, they are unable to produce work or to be integrated into a social group typical of those of their peers. They cannot achieve academic goals and often do not fit well into the family unit.

Socially maladjusted children, on the other hand, may be described as chronic social offenders who disregard the values and rules of society and substitute the rules and value system of their particular peer group. These children differ from emotionally disturbed children in that they do identify with a group, even though the group shares the maladjustment in relation to acceptable social standards. These children may participate as members of delinquent gangs that defy authority and the recognized standards of socially adjusted children. These children are frequently from families who have many social problems that closely interact with emotional difficulties. In many instances it is impossible to identify the primary, or etiologic, problems; the interrelationship of all factors becomes a vicious cycle that is self-perpetuating.

It is recognized that some socially maladjusted children are also emotionally disturbed, but it is believed that the majority are not.[21] Gang membership requires a certain degree of conformity, which few emotionally disturbed children can attain. It requires its own unique type of social skill and purposefulness, which can rarely be achieved by emotionally disturbed children.

There is little doubt that emotionally disturbed children often exhibit behavior that is indicative of serious social maladjustment, including violation of legal, moral, and ethical standards, and nonconformity to generally accepted behavior. However, these social deviations are often isolated and spontaneous, and they usually do not involve the deliberate challenge of authority planned by the socially maladjusted child. It has been estimated that emotionally disturbed children are responsible for roughly 25% of all the delinquent acts committed.[19]

### Scope

Determining the scope of any problem depends upon adequate definition of the problem being investigated. Since definitive description and definition of social and inner problems have not been possible, there is uncertainty as to the prevalence of these problems. Further, even when consistent definitions are used in attempting to identify the prevalence of a specific problem, it is not possible to determine the accuracy of diagnosis. In addition, there may be many affected children who have not been identified or who are "hidden" in the community and family.

Because of the lack of consensus regarding definition of the problems and the lack of standardized methods of obtaining data, estimates of the prevalence of emotional and social disturbance among children vary. Shultz and associates[30] found prevalence estimates ranging from 0.05% to 15% nationally in the United States. The United States Office of Education[34] estimated a prevalence of 2% in 1975. Bower suggested that an estimated 10% of school-age children in the United States need special attention due to behavioral difficulties.[6]

Estimates of the prevalence of socially maladjusted children likewise vary considerably, and some overlap between the categories of social maladjustment and emotional disturbance leads to further confusion. Crime rates among children and youth are used to estimate the prevalence of social maladjustment. A more definitive description of the exact problem being studied might yield somewhat different statistics, but this parameter has provided some interesting information. Crime rates appear to decline steadily with movement from inner urban zones to outer city zones. It is estimated that crime rates among children and youth are three times higher in metropolitan areas than in rural areas. It has been estimated that about 1.5% of all young people from 10 to 16 years of age living in urban areas are so socially maladjusted that they require special educational provisions. It appears that environmental circumstances of the urban area contribute significantly to the development of social maladjustment.[28] Granbard[11] found that more aggressive, acting-out behavior problems are generally reported in lower-class than in middle-class or upper-class children. Boys are more often considered behavior problems than are girls.[25,31]

Prevalence figures are confusing, because the criteria and definitions used are inconsistent. However, it seems apparent that a great number of children suffer from emotional problems and social maladjustment. The loss of these individuals as useful, functional, integral members of society represents one of the most significant losses to humanity. Although older individuals suffering from these handicapping conditions may be rehabilitated for more satisfying functions, the obvious emphasis should be on prevention, early detection, and remediation during childhood. The cost of financing diagnosis and rehabilitation is great, but the economic worth is obvious if early treatment results in more rapid recovery and an increased number of productive years of life for the individual. The lack of adequate economic support for prevention of these problems and for early detection and remediation programs is a continuing source of frustration for health care specialists.

### Inner disturbance
#### Description of the problem

Emotional disturbance may be generally described as a reaction to life situations that is so personally unrewarding and so inappropriate as to be unacceptable to peers and adults in the child's life. The child experiences great deficits in inner development, and observable indications of an adequate self-concept are lacking. These children may isolate themselves from all contact with others, in which case it is not possible to describe the nature of their inner perceptions except by inference. If they are able to reveal some of their perceptions, they are most often found to have consistent and lasting inadequacies in relation to the structure, function, and quality of their self-concept (see Chapter 1). Their conversation and behavior reflect such structural traits as rigidity, simplicity, narrowness, and incongruence. For example, such children may focus on one aspect of themselves as being the significant factor that characterizes them as persons, such as seeing themselves as "bad." They see themselves reflected in this frame of reference always and are not able to recognize the incongruence that may exist between this perception of the self and environmental clues that would indicate otherwise. This self-concept serves negative functions for the child, and leads to predictions of failure and participation in behavior that leads to social rejection and disapproval (see Chapter 1).

#### Psychologic evaluation

When children are identified as having a possible emotional problem, they should undergo psychologic evaluation. The initial identification may come from several sources, including the health care worker, the family, the school, or the child.

Group tests for identification and initial description of an individual child's problem are limited and not widely used. However, the Junior Eysenck Personality Inventory and the California Test of Personality may be used for elementary level school-age children in groups as a psychologic screening device. The Minnesota Multiphasic Personality Inventory can be used for middle adolescents and young adults; the California Psychological Inventory is useful for older adolescents and adults. Interpretation of group test results must be made by a specialist who understands the test and its particular qualities and limitations.

When a child is referred for psychologic evaluation because of a suspected serious emotional

CHAPTER 20

The child with
long-term social
and inner
problems

disturbance, projective tests are frequently utilized. The basic objective of these tools is to have the child project feelings or inner emotions and perceptions into what he or she sees. Among the more commonly used projective tests are the ink blot tests, such as the Rorschach and the Holtzman. In these tests the child is shown a standardized ink blot and is asked what he or she sees in the design. The answer may reflect a story based in reality or in fantasy, but the content that is chosen and the themes developed through the testing serve as indications of inner experiences and feelings.

Another commonly used projective test is the Thematic Apperception Test. In this test the individual is shown a set of pictures in which the subjects, actions, and objects portrayed are clearly definable. In this test the child is asked to tell a story about the picture. The story may include conditions leading to the situation portrayed, what is happening at the time, and/or what future outcomes will be. Again, the content of the stories and the themes that are developed give indications of the child's inner experiences. A children's version, the Children's Apperception Test, is used for younger children, incorporating pictures appropriate to the age level of the child.

Psychologic standardization procedures used in developing the projective techniques have led to the identification of certain expected, or "normal," patterns of response. Themes that are not typical of the emotionally healthy individual have been identified and described, such as those expressing excessive conflict, anger, anxiety, self-destructive tendencies, or death wishes.[5,15]

### Specific disorders

Emotional disturbance may be viewed as a general problem that incorporates five major psychiatric disorders. The reader may wish to pursue more detailed investigation and study of the basic concept in abnormal personality development.[16] We will briefly consider the essential features that have been associated with these five major types of disorders, and some of the implications for health care and competency development.

*Transient stress disorders* are acute reactions to catastrophic psychologic pressures. The death of a loved one, divorce of parents, and some of the problems of adolescence discussed in Chapters 14 and 15 may bring about temporary but serious disturbance that results in abrupt changes in emotional behavior. Although the disturbance may be temporary, the effect on the child's personality development is often lasting. The importance of such trauma to the child should never be minimized with the view that another child has been known to handle such a stress without a severe emotional reaction. For example, one child may demonstrate a severe reaction to the divorce of parents while a sibling appears to adjust more adequately. The child who has trouble is often blamed or one or both parents are held accountable for the fact that one child is not "strong" enough to make an adequate adjustment. The disturbed child's suffering is minimized because of the expectation that he or she will make an adjustment similar to the sibling, and further pressure is brought to bear on the child to conform to these expectations. It is often overlooked that emotional events in the lives of children are relative to their unique reactions and abilities to cope and not to the performances of other children.

An event that an adult may view as relatively unimportant may be extremely important to a child, leading to an emotional reaction that seems inappropriate from the adult's perspective. The arrival of a new baby in the family may be a joyful experience for the parents, and they may feel that their other children should share their enthusiasm. Yet this arrival may provoke a transient stress disorder for a young child who views the new infant as a distinct threat to security.[24]

*Personality disorders* make up a broad category of chronic problems described as inadequacies in personality development and behavior patterns, which present a serious problem to the family and society. These children may be extremely shy or excessively outgoing, or they may express excessive conflicts and hostilities typical of paranoia. Children who exhibit these types of problems are characteristically unconcerned about their problem because they do not feel that their behavior is unusual, and thus help is not ordinarily sought voluntarily.

The list of specific personality disorders that have been described is extensive and beyond the scope of this text. Among the more commonly identified disorders are paranoid reactions, sociopathic personalities, sexual deviations such as exhibitionism, and drug addiction. There is controversy regarding the appropriate classification of some of these problems, and the literature is inconsistent in this respect. For example, homosexuality has been identified as an emotional disturbance partly because of the social aversion to this pattern of sexual behavior. Whether or not personality, or emotional, disturbance is always associated with homosexuality remains an issue of controversy. Likewise, drug addiction may not be considered by some as always involving personality disorders. Such disorders may be identified for some users, but the universality of a personality problem that typifies the drug addict has not been clearly delineated.[16]

*Psychoneurotic disorders* are among the most common of all types of personality disorganizations. Prevalence is high compared to other types of emotional disturbances, and these problems are considered relatively mild, although some types of psychoneuroses are disabling. Many psychoneurotic conditions respond very favorably to treatment. These children seldom need institutionalization but may need prolonged psychiatric treatment.

These problems are characterized by anxiety expressed in either a direct or indirect manner. Often it is difficult to describe the exact nature of a child's reaction, and diagnosis requires skilled psychiatric evaluation. Phobic reactions can occur at any time during childhood, and include specific, excessive fears of such objects or circumstances as animals, darkness, high places, or enclosed areas. During early childhood most children experience fear that appears to adults as unreasonable, but the emotionally healthy child is able to respond to supportive measures offered by adults and siblings, and gradually overcomes the fear within a few months. Phobic reactions may grow out of this phase of development, with the child continuing to experience excessive fear of a specific circumstance, or it can occur later as an event that is seemingly unrelated to earlier childhood fears.

Anxiety reactions may occur during childhood. One of the most prevalent is a later childhood reaction to school, commonly referred to as "school phobia." These children do not experience a phobia, or fear, in the accurate sense of the term, but rather they develop an acute anxiety reaction associated with going to school and separating from a significant adult. Most healthy children experience periods when school is more distasteful than pleasant. They may express the desire to remain at home and become disturbed over having to go to school. This may be quite distressing to the parents. However, emotionally healthy children are able to respond to supportive measures offered by their parents, to acknowledge a specific problem that they may be having in school, and to resolve the issue of going to school and contributing to the solution of any specific problem. Children who are experiencing an anxiety reaction associated with going to school, on the other hand, are not able to respond to measures that would ordinarily help a child over a momentary difficulty. Their complaints about the school situation are usually vague and inconsistent, and they may complain repeatedly of nonspecific, vague physical symptoms in order to avoid going to school.

Anxiety reactions are manifested in a great variety of ways among children, and it is impossible to describe a single definitive syndrome. The reactions stem from difficulties experienced with the transition between dependency and independency during early childhood. When parents are insensitive to the needs of children for dependency and independency as they gain autonomy and initiative, the child experiences inner conflict toward the breakdown of the mutual regulation interaction that needs to occur during the transition. The parent is often overcontrolling and overprotective or overly permissive, either of which denies a balanced regulation of behavior. As children grow older, they experience inner anxiety associated with these lasting conflicts, and their behavior reflects such traits as aggressiveness, withholding of feelings, inordinate shyness, or rebelliousness.

Obsessive-compulsive reactions are manifested in repeated, ritualistic behaviors and pre-

The child with
long-term social
and inner
problems

occupation with a certain behavior or activity. During childhood, compulsive masturbation or exhibitionism, for example, may become an expression of this neurotic type of reaction. Masturbation, which is typical of the normal developmental task of learning about one's own body during early childhood and of dealing with sexual tensions during adolescence, becomes an expression of an emotional disturbance only when the child demonstrates the compulsive urge to excessively engage in the behavior and a preoccupation with thoughts surrounding the activity.

*Conversion reactions* involve unconscious anxiety that is converted into a physical symptom. This type of reaction tends to be dramatic and severe, and involves expression through the central nervous system. It is observed during early and later childhood and adolescence, and the kinds of physical symptoms that commonly occur include tics, or excessive facial grimacing, stuttering, and certain types of enuresis. Because the physical symptoms are not socially tolerable, they usually attract much attention from the family and other adults, and they may be mistaken for behaviors over which the child has purposeful control. "Normal" stuttering, which tends to occur in ordinary patterns of speech during the first two years after the child begins to use sentences, may be mistaken for the type of stuttering that is symptomatic of a disturbance. When the child continues to stutter and is not able to gradually and naturally evolve more mature patterns of speech, the possibility of an emotional neurotic disorder should be explored (see Chapter 10).

The fine balance that exists between normal development and psychoneurotic disturbance may be exceedingly delicate for some children. Some children appear to be quite resistant to great external stress, while others appear vulnerable and sensitive to minimal stress. Assessment of behaviors that appear to have traits in common with the psychoneurotic disorders requires well-developed skill and knowledge on the part of the health care worker. Thorough judgment and evaluation are made by the specialist, but the professional health care worker who is dealing with child health may develop some skills in determining the potential seriousness of a problem. As has been implied in the above discussions, the child's stage of development and age are important factors in distinguishing between behavior that is acceptable for healthy children and behavior that is indicative of a serious problem. During early childhood some children experience episodes of enuresis, fears of objects and animals, various fantasies, or periods of extreme shyness or aggressiveness that are more severe than occur for other children of the same age. However, the behavior or "disturbance" is resolved within a few weeks or months, and healthy children are able to gradually utilize more mature means of coping. They respond to the support and encouragement they receive from significant people in their lives. The child who is suffering from a psychoneurotic disturbance, on the other hand, demonstrates behavior that is extreme in character, with accompanying signs of disturbance, or the behavior persists beyond the developmental stage in which it originated.[36]

*Psychophysiologic disorders* are emotional disturbances resulting in physical malfunctioning but without observable, overt anxiety on the part of the person affected. The effects of psychophysiologic disorders are not unlike that of the conversion reaction neurosis, but they are thought to be mediated through the autonomic nervous system. Among the many conditions that may be related to psychophysiologic disorders are peptic ulcers, respiratory reactions such as bronchial asthma, skin reactions, and headaches. Although these reactions may be psychogenic, the health care specialist must be aware of multiple etiologic factors that should be considered. The symptoms themselves are real, regardless of whether the basis for the problem is organic or psychologic. In many instances the specific etiology does not appreciably alter the symptomatic relief measures that are indicated during an acute attack; however, the etiology does make a difference in relation to the long-term effectiveness of treatment, since symptomatic relief does not alleviate the cause of the condition. When the cause is recognized, appropriate medical, psychiatric, or surgical intervention can be attempted in treatment.[10]

*Psychosis* is the most severe and debilitating

of the psychiatric disturbances. One of the most well-known psychotic conditions of childhood is autism, which usually is recognized in the first or second year of life. This condition is sometimes referred to as childhood schizophrenia; however, in other instances the conditions are clearly differentiated, with autism being a condition present from birth and childhood schizophrenia following a period of relatively normal development. Kanner[14] provided a classic description of autism in childhood, which incorporates the following features:

1. The child is unable to relate to other people and situations from the very beginning of life.
2. The child maintains extreme aloneness and isolation.
3. The child fails to develop language or the use of language for the purpose of communication with other people. Verbalizations may exist but they are not directed toward interpersonal communications.
4. The child's behavior may be described as anxiously obsessive in a desire to maintain sameness.
5. There is a tendency to engage in stereotypic preoccupation with certain inanimate objects.

Since the time of this early description, there have been many efforts to determine the etiology of the condition and to more completely describe the underlying neurophysiology and associated metabolic problems. Although basic issues and controversy regarding etiology have not been resolved, it appears that there are associated abnormalities of central nervous system function and metabolism that underlie a particular vulnerability to the autistic syndrome.[8,9,17,35]

Neurotic children manage to hang onto the real world in which they live, but psychotic children lose contact with reality. They suffer from disorientation, delusions, hallucinations, and disordered verbal and nonverbal communication. Their pervasive problem interferes with every aspect of development. These children present a serious challenge to health care workers who attempt to work with them and their families in maintaining other aspects of health.[3,8,23]

## Social maladjustment
### Description

Social maladjustment is behavior that is offensive to most members of society and that fails to meet minimum standards of conduct required by society. Behavior patterns of socially maladjusted children include intimidation and harassment of peers who do not participate in their particular group and violation of the codes of conduct accepted by adults or by socially adjusted peers. The failure of these children to adjust to accepted societal norms for behavior often leads to exclusion from regular school programs.

### Related factors

In addition to the relationship between urban residence and social maladjustment that was discussed earlier, there are several significantly related factors that have provided some understanding of the problems involved, and have stimulated additional investigation regarding the complex issues that remain to be resolved. Problems with social maladjustment in childhood tend to be related to lower socioeconomic circumstances, including being supported on public welfare, living in low-rent housing, and membership in minority groups who tend to be caught in the low-income and poverty cycles.[28]

There is a higher incidence of social maladjustment among boys than among girls. The estimated ratios range from about 5 to 1 to about 8 to 1.[33] It is also interesting to note that grade retention rates are disproportionately high among boys. It is speculated that retention may be related to social maladjustment problems among boys, because intellectual and cognitive capacity differences between boys and girls do not exist.[2]

There is speculation regarding the reasons for the relationships among several of these social factors and social maladjustment during childhood. In some instances it is thought that the children are rebelling against social standards that are different from those of their own minority or disadvantaged group. In other instances the resentment and rebellion seem to be directed toward their own social and economic system, such as the maladjustment problems observed among children and youth in middle-

The child with
long-term social
and inner
problems

class and higher socioeconomic groups.[7,21]

A group of related theories involving a legitimate-illegitimate theme has been developed, which concentrates upon the discrepancies between the goals that society indicates an individual should have and the legitimate structure that society provides for individuals to reach those goals.[20-22,28,29] As most American children begin to enter the social world beyond the family, they observe environmental settings different from their own. They experience to some extent a desire to perform the tasks of daily living and achievement in surroundings that provide legitimacy, ease, flexibility, individuality, personal safety, challenge, and opportunity for self-improvement. Their own surroundings begin to be judged in relation to the degree to which they offer the particular opportunities that become important to the individual child. At some point during development, the children also begin to incorporate societal expectations for achievement and behavior. When these norms are relatively lacking, children tend to formulate aspirations and goals that are not realistic or attainable. Disillusioned by the circumstances that have led to unrealistic goals and by the inability of the surroundings to provide a means of attaining their goals, these children begin to develop social alienation and maladjustment. For example, children or young people from low-income, disadvantaged groups are very often confronted with the set of circumstances described below:

1. The family and culture do not provide behavioral and achievement norms.

2. There are few legitimate means available for achieving the goals that they recognize to exist for other members of the society.

3. They may formulate early unlimited aspirations and conceptions of what should happen in life, with limited perception of the real means of achieving these goals. Economically disadvantaged children, for example, may recognize that some people have unlimited resources of money. They form a dream of someday having so much money that they could not spend it all. Their concept of how to achieve the dream may simply be that it will automatically happen because they wish it to happen.

4. When children realize that their unlimited aspirations will not come to pass automatically, they feel disillusioned and disappointed in their circumstances and society, and they then begin to seek illegitimate means of achieving whatever they can salvage of their dream.[20-22,28,29]

These theoretical notions might be equally applicable to socially maladjusted children of another socioeconomic group. If children from financially established families do not, for some reason, incorporate appropriate behavior and achievement norms and instead formulate unlimited aspirations, a similar set of circumstances might evolve. For example, children might reject the goal of becoming a professional person, because they find it too constricting and limiting. In the absence of other equally desirable norms for behavior, they formulate unrealistic aspirations; for example, they may decide to enter the performing arts despite their lack of talent. Finding themselves deprived of legitimate means of achieving their unrealistic goal in the form of financial support and encouragement from family and friends, they become frustrated and resentful and turn to socially unacceptable approaches in living. There may be some legitimate ways in which such a young person could, in fact, enter a career related to the performing arts (such as stage management and design, film editing, etc.) and develop their interest and real talents, but they fail to recognize these legitimate opportunities because they are not incorporated into their unlimited aspirations to actually perform.

The many factors involved in social maladjustment are complex and not clearly understood. It appears that illegitimate means of attaining goals is usually a last-resort measure, which occurs only after the individuals have exhausted all known legitimate means available to them. The fewer the legitimate opportunities offered by society, the sooner they will resort to socially unacceptable behavior. If this theory is accurate, then the availability of illegitimate opportunities is less important than the availability of legitimate opportunities for behavior and goal achievements.[21]

Another important factor appears to be the means by which goals for behavior and achievement are formulated by young people. The effects of various kinds of societal expectations and norms for behavior are not clearly understood. For example, clearly delineated, highly specific expectations (e.g., high academic achievement) and the relative absence of any expectation for achievement appear to differentially affect social adjustment in different children, but the outcome for a given child cannot presently be predicted. Apparently an important interaction exists between the child's unique personality and the environment, the precise nature of which remains speculative.[1]

## Approaches to intervention

Intervention involves both accurate identification of social and inner problems among children and remediation and rehabilitation when a problem has been detected. Of primary concern for the health care worker is the detection of real problems. The mental health specialist is most adequately prepared to provide definitive evaluation, diagnosis, remediation, and rehabilitation. Often the nature of the specialist's participation in individual treatment programs depends upon his or her particular background and level of expertise.

### Detection and screening

The health care worker can contribute a vitally important role in accurate detection and screening for social and inner problems. While the definitive diagnosis must be made by a competent psychologist or psychiatrist, the child is usually referred to these specialists because of observations made by other members of the health care team, family, or teachers who identify the child as having a possible social or inner disturbance.

Criteria for identification of possible inner disturbances are described below, one or more of which would indicate the need for special evaluation.[32]

1. Behavior tends to be excessive in a particular direction, or is not typical of the child's stage of development.
2. The child fails to develop language competency.
3. The child exhibits excessive nervous behavior such as the biting of nails, thumbsucking, hyperactivity, stuttering, extreme restlessness, muscle twitching,

hair twisting, picking of the skin, scratching, frequent sighing, or bed-wetting.
4. The child imposes isolation and aloneness upon himself or herself.
5. The child is actively excluded by other children of his or her own age or equivalent developmental stage.
6. The child appears consistently inattentive and indifferent, unable to concentrate on activities at home or on school work and needs constant prodding to complete assignments.
7. The child appears to be excessively jealous and overly competitive.
8. The child conveys verbal and behavioral cues indicating an inordinate degree of dissatisfaction and unhappiness with the self and the environment.
9. The child expresses an apparent dislike for school beyond what might be expected; he or she is frequently tardy or absent and complains of illness frequently.
10. Academic achievement is at a level that is lower than the child's known capacity, although he or she is not failing.
11. The child is failing in school work with no immediately apparent reason.

Criteria for the identification and screening for social problems may likewise be described. It should be noted that circumstances such as those listed do not invariably lead to disturbances in social development, but they are associated with a higher incidence of problems and thus place the child in a position of risk. One set of criteria for further evaluation may be formulated as follows:

1. The child's home is characterized by consistent instability.
2. The family provides inconsistent and erratic discipline.
3. The home is lacking in understanding, affection, and individual interaction among the members of the family.
4. There is a lack of methodologic approaches to problems that might be expected for the stage of development and a tendency toward direct and concrete expressions rather than symbolic representations.
5. The child demonstrates behavior that indicates disregard for legitimate authority.

CHAPTER 20

The child with
long-term social
and inner
problems

6. The child's temperament is typically restless, destructive, overtly extroverted, and aggressive.
7. The child demonstrates behavior that reflects attitudes of hostility, defiance, resentfulness of others, nonconformity, social assertiveness, and stubbornness.

A comprehensive assessment of the child and the environment facilitates the total psychiatric evaluation of the child. This might involve several members of the health care team, but the more comprehensive the information regarding the child's environment, the more accurately the multiple factors influencing development will be perceived by the person who is seeking to fully describe the unique nature of the child's problem.

### Remediation and rehabilitation

Emotionally disturbed and socially maladjusted children have long been considered the problems of psychiatric-medical therapists. A limited number of children have been treated by psychologists, social workers, psychiatrists, nurse therapists, and specially prepared mental health care workers, but the needs of children who demonstrate disturbances far exceed the available resources for therapy. The fact that most children who have these problems are in public school settings has led to a recognition of the ways in which the school can provide certain kinds of therapy. The schools can aid in recognition of problems, provide for special needs, and design special group programs that can enhance the child's adjustment. These programs may be offered either as an alternative to services from other sources or in conjunction with medical and psychiatric treatment. Teachers who specialize in working with emotionally and socially disturbed children can bring about effective change for some children, and can become important agents in mental health care.

Clinicians working with handicapped children usually attempt to provide a plan of treatment for each child that is particularly suited to his or her needs. Several kinds of approaches that are commonly employed in medical and educational treatment programs will be described. Each approach has been successful, but the exact basis for success of one approach over another with a given child has not been determined. An important factor seems to be the personality of the therapist; it appears that some therapists gain consistent success when using one type of approach, while others experience success with an entirely different approach.

*Psychodynamic strategy* is a model based primarily upon psychoanalytic concepts and theory of personality development. Maladaptive behavior is viewed as a function of intrapsychic conflict involving the id, ego, and superego. Treatment emphasizes removal of the underlying cause rather than just the symptom. Removal of the symptom and not the cause only results in the substitution of another symptom.

The underlying causes are believed to originate during childhood through traumatic experiences that are repressed. The treatment is based upon psychotherapy that focuses attention on the analysis of the unconscious. This strategy is seldom used outside of psychiatric hospitals and treatment centers because long-term treatment is required, there are too few professional persons prepared in this mode of therapy, and the treatment is expensive. It most often requires an individual relationship with a child, but some of the principles can be applied in working with groups of children.

The *behavior modification strategy* does not involve reconstruction of the past traumatic or etiologic events in order to accomplish therapeutic results. Behavior is viewed as learned, and the objective of the therapy is to extinguish maladaptive behavior through learning techniques and to provide for learning of adaptive behavior. The behavior that is unacceptable must first be identified and the replacement behavior described. The therapist then implements skillfully planned reinforcements, or associated events, that are designed to perpetuate the occurrence of the desired behavior. Individual diagnosis of the child's problem is required, and it is necessary to identify, on an individual basis, what might serve as a reinforcement. Once the diagnosis and plan have been established, therapeutic intervention can be maintained within a group setting, and parents, teachers, and specially prepared assistants can participate in the therapeutic plan.

**811**

*Developmental strategies* are similar to behavior modification, but the learning process involves seven defined developmental sequences. For children to learn, they must complete these developmental tasks in order. They must (1) pay attention to a stimulus for learning, (2) respond to the stimulus, (3) follow directions, (4) freely and accurately explore the environment, (5) function appropriately in relation to others, (6) master the learning task, and (7) achieve a feeling of success in their accomplishment. This approach to therapy has been engineered in detail for application in groups of school-age children; it achieves therapeutic behavior change by not providing, or removing, the opportunity for the child to engage in maladaptive behavior. As soon as the therapist or teacher observes signs of maladaptive behavior, these children are distracted to another activity that requires a behavior change in the positive direction. Children then experience repeated success rather than the negative reinforcement that occurs when they are able to pursue maladaptive means of achieving goals. For example, a boy in a specially engineered classroom setting begins to work on a project, and he gradually becomes disruptive to those around him. At the first sign of the disturbance, the teacher moves him from the original activity to one that has been predetermined to preclude, for this child, the possibility of behaving in a disruptive manner. He has been identified as being able to respond positively to a communication learning center, for instance, and he gradually builds the capacity to perpetuate his ability to control his behavior in a socially acceptable manner, while at the same time incorporating the basic developmental learning skills that are designed into the total strategy.

*Learning disabilities remediation,* discussed in Chapter 19, often provides therapy for the child who is disturbed and frustrated with repeated failure in school. Frustration and maladaptive behavior lead to varying degrees of social and inner disturbance. Remediation of the specific learning disability and provision of success are valuable emotional therapeutic approaches for many children.

*Psychoeducational approaches* are eclectic in that features of behavior modification, psycho-dynamics, and learning disabilities strategies are incorporated in a therapeutic program. The basic principle of the program is acceptance of the child regardless of his or her behavior. Each child is viewed as possessing innate biologic potentials that are combined with early experiences. This combination determines the self-concept and behavior patterns. When children enter school they are expected to possess certain skills and behaviors. If they fail to meet the imposed standards, they will suffer from frustration and anxiety, which may lead to maladaptive behavior. The psychoeducational approach begins by attempting to understand the child's perception of the situation, including the past experiences that have led to the current problem. Modification is aimed at changing the child's perceptions of the problems, and thereby changing behavior.

*Ecologic strategy* is a model that focuses on the environment as well as the child in identifying desired therapy and outcomes of therapy. Proponents of this approach reject the idea that the child alone must change; rather, they work from the premise that the undesired behavior is a function of a misfit between the child and the environment, and the interactions between these two elements must be altered in order to achieve therapeutic results. Psychotherapy is used in working with the child, but efforts are made simultaneously to prepare the child's environment to accommodate him or her and the existing problems.

## EFFECTS OF LONG-TERM SOCIAL AND INNER PROBLEMS ON COMPETENCY DEVELOPMENT AND HEALTH CARE

Emotional and social disturbances lead to varying degrees of interference with expected growth and development patterns. They can provide minimal stress that interferes periodically with competency in a specific area of development, or they can provide pervasive stress leading to total incapacitation. The basis for a child's particular reaction to stressors in the environment is not clearly understood. It is thought that there may be genetically determined biologic factors involved in the complex reactions observed in these dynamics, and that biologic determinants of the reaction to stress

CHAPTER 20

The child with
long-term social
and inner
problems

may be significant factors. Children seem to vary in their tolerance and vulnerability to stressful stimuli, and their reactions are unique, ranging from great flexibility and resilience to rigidity and delicate maintenance of balance. While it is not presently possible to predict one child's response to emotional and social stress, these kinds of events can affect each area of competency development.

Emotional disturbance can be expressed in disturbances in physical competency, or it can cause deficits in this area of development. As we have discussed, the child may develop physical symptoms mediated through the central and autonomic nervous systems in response to neurotic and psychotic disorders. A severe emotional disturbance of any type can result in failure to thrive, associated with a life-threatening loss of appetite and/or metabolic responses that interfere with the utilization of food taken.

Learning and thought competency is often affected in some way by either social or inner disturbances. In fact, as demonstrated in the above discussion, failure to progress according to expected levels of development in learning and thought is often one of the first objective observations that lead to the evaluation of a possible social or inner disturbance.

Finally, we have seen that social and inner indices of adequate development are so closely intertwined that it is often impossible to clearly distinguish one from another. The child who has a disturbance in one area of function is invariably affected in the other. Some of the approaches to treatment, in fact, depend upon this close interrelationship. For example, the child who is identified as having a basic inner disturbance may be helped if provided with opportunities for satisfying social achievements. Another child who has a basic problem in social adjustment may find therapeutic help through intensive therapy aimed toward accurate inner concepts and goals related to the self.

The family is a special concern for the health care worker who is helping the child with a social or inner disturbance. The severe implications for the family who has a child with serious problems in these areas of development often lead to avoidance in dealing with the family's problems. Even though the family may contrib-ute significantly to the child's problem and may be limited in being able to help themselves or their child, there must be some attempt to explore the resources that the family does offer. In some instances the family will be able to respond to therapy as a group and thus help their child. In other instances, the family's contribution to the problem may be minimal, as when a single traumatic event creates long-term disturbance for a particularly vulnerable child. The guilt and self-incrimination that the parents may experience may lead to the initial impression that their contribution to the creation of the problem is greater than it actually is, and their actual strengths and resources are not recognized either by themselves or by health care workers. In other instances the family may be almost totally incapable of contributing toward therapy, and the child must be placed in an environment more conducive to recovery. Professional decisions and judgments of this nature require great skill and experience, and the family must be fully involved. A family may be unable to provide environmental help for their own child, but they often desire some sort of help. They can acknowledge the alternatives available and the predicted benefits and risks involved for each alternative that may be available. [12,13,26,27]

Because many families bring problems having a social or inner basis to the initial attention of those in the health care system, it is vitally important for clinicians to be aware of the ways in which a possible problem can be identified. The types of social and emotional problems and their behavioral clues have been discussed. Health care workers must remember that emotional problems can affect any of the body systems, and a child who is seemingly healthy on initial inspection may have bothersome symptoms of nonspecific disorders, which would suggest the need to consider emotional problems as the cause. A description of the child's total environment can be helpful in identifying children at risk for special stress factors that tend to lead to social and emotional disturbance. Conversation with the child is often revealing of inner thinking, perception, and feelings. [10] During early childhood various types of play and fantasy can be useful in helping the child express feelings.

School-age children enjoy conversation and will often openly discuss impressions, feelings, and concerns with an interested health care worker. They may respond to a game or a fantasy situation, such as naming three wishes they might make if they could wish for anything they wanted. Their thoughts and fantasies provide information as to the adequacy of their perceptions of themselves and the environment. Young adolescents may be best able to express themselves in the presence of peers who share their innermost feelings of distress. They may be able to respond to fantasy and play appropriate for their age, and yet they are gaining capacities to reason and deliberate and to become self-directed agents in using their own resources in maintaining health.[18]

## STUDY QUESTIONS

1. Investigate a therapeutic approach being used in your community directed toward remediation of some emotional or social problem during childhood. Describe the kinds of problems that are involved and details of the underlying principles upon which the therapeutic approach is based. Describe your observations of the application of therapy and the results that are being achieved by the children.
2. Observe an emotionally disturbed child for a period of time. What behaviors does this child demonstrate that are considered normal for his or her age; what behaviors might be expected for a child of another age or developmental stage? What behaviors are atypical and inappropriate?
3. After observing the emotionally disturbed child, find a child who is emotionally healthy but whose developmental stage might enable you to see some of the same behaviors you saw exhibited by the emotionally disturbed child (e.g., immature speech patterns, dependency, shyness). Can you detect a difference in quality of the same behavior between the two children? Describe and discuss your impressions.
4. Select a physical problem that can evolve as the result of either physical illness or emotional disturbances. Pursue further in-depth study of the literature available on this problem from the points of view of a physical and an emotional etiology. What criteria might be described for delineating between the etiologies involved, and what kinds of therapies are employed for each kind of problem?

## REFERENCES

1. Anderson, L. S.: The aggressive child, Child. Today **7:** 11, Jan.-Feb., 1978.
2. Arrington, J. W.: A study of retention in the Ogden, Utah, school district. Unpublished master's thesis, University of Utah, 1973.
3. Aug, R., and Ables, B. S.: A clinician's guide to childhood psychosis, Pediatrics **47:**327, 1971.
4. Bentz, W. K., and Davis, A.: Perceptions of emotional disorders among children as viewed by leaders, teachers, and the general public, Am. J. Public Health **65:** 129, Feb., 1975.
5. Berry, K. K: Effectively using the psychologic evaluation with children; some guidelines to assist the pediatrician on making referrals for psychologic evaluation, Clin. Pediatr. **12:**174, March, 1973.
6. Bower, E. M.: Early identification of emotionally handicapped in school, ed. 2, Springfield, Ill., 1969, Charles C Thomas, Publisher.
7. Cohen, A. K.: Delinquent boys; the culture of the gang, Glencoe, Ill., 1955, The Free Press.
8. Cohen, D. J.: The medical care of autistic children, Pediatrics **51:**278, Feb., 1973.
9. Cohen, D. J., and Caparulo, B.: Childhood autism, Child. Today **4:**2, July-Aug., 1975.
10. Goodall, J.: Clinical clues to emotional disturbance in children; how to suspect and treat disturbances due to nonorganic causes, Clin. Pediatr. **12:**178, March, 1973.
11. Granbard, P. S.: Children with behavioral disabilities. In Dunn, L. M., editor: Exceptional children in the schools, ed. 2, New York, 1973, Holt, Rinehart, and Winston.
12. Hartman, K., and Bush, M.: Action-oriented family therapy, Am. J. Nurs. **75:**1184, July, 1975.
13. Hazzard, M. E., and Scheuerman, A.: Family therapy—new ways to help families in trouble, Nursing '76, **6:**22, July, 1976.
14. Kanner, L.: Autistic disturbances of affective contact, Nervous Child **2:**217, 1943.
15. Kirk, S. A.: Educating exceptional children, ed. 2, Boston, 1972, Houghton Mifflin Co.
16. Kisker, G. W.: The disorganized personality, New York, 1964, McGraw-Hill Book Co.
17. Knobloch, H., and Pasamanick, B.: Infantile autism and psychosis, Pediatrics **55:**182, Feb., 1975.
18. Kosidlak, J. G.: Improving health care for troubled youths, Am. J. Nurs. **76:**95, Jan., 1976.
19. Kvaraceus, W. B., and Miller, W. B.: Delinquency and behavior; culture and the individual, Washington, D.C., 1969, NEA Juvenile Delinquency Project.
20. Landis, J. R., and Scarpitti, F. R.: Perceptions regarding value orientations and legitimate opportunity; delinquents and non-delinquents, Social Forces **44:**83, 1965.
21. McCandless, B. R.: Adolescents; behavior and development, Hinsdale, Ill., 1970, The Dryden Press.
22. Merton, R. K.: Social theory and social structure, New York, 1961, Free Press of Glencoe.
23. Ostendorf, M.: Dan is schizophrenic; possible causes, probable course, Am. J. Nurs. **76:**944, June, 1976.
24. Pederson, W. M.: A case study of neurosis secondary to trauma in an eight-year-old girl; comments on the tendency for psychogenic illness to become chronic, Clin. Pediatr. **15:**859, Sept., 1975.

25. Quay, N. C.: Patterns of aggression, withdrawal and immaturity. In Quay, H. C., and Werry, J. S., editors: Psychopathological disorders of childhood, New York, 1972, John Wiley & Sons.
26. Salerno, E. M.: A family in crisis, Am. J. Nurs. **73:**100, Jan., 1973.
27. Shaw, D., and others: Multiple impact therapy, Am. J. Nurs. **77:**246, Feb., 1977.
28. Short, J. F., Jr.: Juvenile delinquency; the sociocultural context. In Hoffman, L. W., and Hoffman, M. L., editors: Review of child development research, vol. 2, New York, 1966, Russell Sage Foundation, p. 423.
29. Short, J. F., Jr., Rivera, R., and Tennyson, R. A.: Perceived opportunities, gang membership, and delinquency, Am. Soc. Rev. **30:**56, 1965.
30. Shultz, E. W., Hirshoren, A., Manton, A. B., and Henderson, R. A.: Special education for the emotionally disturbed, Except. Child. **38:**313, May, 1971.
31. Shultz, E. W., Salvia, J. A., and Feinn, J.: Prevalence of behavioral symptoms in rural elementary school children, J. Abnormal Child Psychol. **2:**17, Jan., 1974.
32. Stocking, M., and others: Psychopathology in the pediatric hospital—implications for community health, Am. J. Public Health **62:**551, April, 1972.
33. United Nations Comparative Survey of Juvenile Delinquency. I. North America, New York, 1958, Department of Economic and Social Affairs, United Nations.
34. United States Office of Education: Estimated number of handicapped children in the United States, 1974-1975. Washington, D.C., 1975, U.S. Office of Education.
35. Wing, L., and Wing, J.: Multiple impairments in early childhood autism, J. Autism Child. Schiz. **1:**256, 1971.
36. Wright, L., and Walker, C. E.: Treatment of the child with psychogenic encopresis; an effective program of therapy, Clin. Pediatr. **16:**1042, Nov., 1977.

The child with long-term social and inner problems

# Jerry—CYSTIC FIBROSIS
# Randy G.—ACUTE LYMPHOBLASTIC LEUKEMIA

Cheryl Hundley

## HEALTH STATUS LIST—Jerry

| Onset | Date | No. | Active | Date | Inactive/resolved |
|---|---|---|---|---|---|
| | | 1 | Incomplete data base | | |
| 9/10/74 | 6/15/78 | 2 | | 10/26/74 | Malabsorption 2° to cystic fibrosis |
| 9/10/74 | 6/15/78 | 3 | Child health maintenance | | (See problem 3,A) |
| | | 3,A | Physical competency—cystic fibrosis | | 3,A Inactive physical problems: |
| | | | | 4/74 | Ear infection |
| | | | | 6/75 | Ear infection |
| | | | | 8/77 | "Virus" |
| | | | | 2/78 | "Cold in eyes" |
| 9/10/74 | 6/15/78 | 3,B | Learning and thought competency | | |
| | | 3,C | Social competency | | |
| | | 3,D | Inner competency | | |
| | | 4 | Need for knowledge and guidance in the care of the child with long-term illness | | |
| | | 4,A | Child entering preschool | | |
| | | 4,B | Management of child's illness | | |
| | | 4,C | Coping with family problems produced by chronically ill child | | |
| | | 4,D | Provision of safety needs of preschooler | | |

Client **Jerry**  Sex M  Age 3½  B.D. 9/10/74
Date 6/15/78  Race C

**Information sources:** Parents
Records

**Reason health care worker sought client**

To assist parents with Jerry's transition into a day-school setting. Jerry has cystic fibrosis and has never been away from his parents for long.

**Reason for seeking health care (mother's and child's comments)**

We feel Jerry should be as normal as possible, and we want him to learn to function with kids his age.

**What events led up to the situation?**

Child has been wanting group activities and friends. Physicians concur that physiologically he is stable and believe he needs socialization also.

### When did this situation occur?

Just last week after visiting the cystic fibrosis clinic, parents and specialist concurred that since the life span of CF children is increasing, the child needs to have as many normal experiences as possible, even though it may mean an occasional URI.

### Describe the situation and/or how you are feeling. What made you decide to seek health care?

Both parents discuss the problem and try to form a mutual decision. In this case they believe child needs more than what they can give him at home, where they fear he may become "isolated" and "overprotected." Has gone to one day of school.

### How is this affecting you and your family at the present time?

Nervous about how son will get along with others and worry about him getting sick being around kids with colds and viruses.

### MOTHER PROFILE
HEALTH HISTORY

Sharon, age 26, is tall and slim and vivacious. Has high school education with "some college."

### Present health status

She believes she is in "good health" except for recent bout with "flu."

### Previous medical-surgical events

No other surgeries except for caesarian section for delivery of Jerry. No past serious illnesses.

PRENATAL HISTORY WITH THIS CHILD

Gravida i Para i. Child was a planned pregnancy.

### Medical supervision

Medical supervision throughout.

### Nutrition, diet

Ate anything she wanted to eat. Had morning sickness for three months. Gained 15 pounds during the pregnancy.

### Illness, infections, complications

Pregnancy complicated with bleeding in the seventh and ninth months. Stayed in bed for a week during the ninth month.

### Treatments, procedures

Was x-rayed during labor, and pelvic outlet was "too small" for vaginal delivery of Jerry.

### Anesthesia

General anesthesia for a C-section. Remembers no drugs or IV.

### Course of labor and delivery

Labored 18 hours. Used breathing techniques from natural childbirth classes.

### Availability in home

Always at home. Tried working when Jerry was a baby but he got sick too much staying at the baby-sitter's.

### Number of people in the home

Five—Jerry, Sharon (mother), and J. D. (father), Sharon's mother and father.

### Employment/work environment

Not employed since Jerry was 9 months old. Enrolled in real estate course at local college.

### Date of last menstrual period

May 28, 1978. Taking oral contraceptive.

## FATHER PROFILE

J. D., age 34, is congenial and very enthusiastic about his son. Has smiling countenance, is slim, and moves quickly. Has high school education and dropped out of college before finishing a degree in architecture (expressed much remorse over this event).

### Present health status

"Good." No problems except for "flu" a few months ago.

### Previous medical-surgical events

Positive family history of cystic fibrosis on father's side. Had severe "whooping cough" as a child and had much "bronchitis" until puberty with few URIs after that.

### Number of people he supports

Sharon and Jerry. Two daughters by a previous marriage.

### Availability in home/work habits

Presently home most of the time as he quit his job last week.

### Employment/work environment

Until recently was employed selling new homes. Is enrolled in a real estate course. Has plans to become a builder and wants to do real estate as a sideline.

### Range of income

$1,000 per month. Financially have been "strapped" due to monthly child support payment and wife not working.

### Insurance

Hospitalization for wife and husband. Policy did not cover Jerry as he is considered uninsurable. He gets "insurance" from the Crippled Children's Society.

LIFE CHANGE EVENTS (dates)

Two LCEs in past year.

Death (family, close friend) __No__  New baby __No__

Divorce __No__  Marital separation __No__  Return to school __No__

Injury, illness __No__  Job loss __5/78__

Change of residence __Moved in with her parents two months ago__  Retirement __No__

**Pedigree (include chronic, inherited conditions, allergies, causes of death, illness in siblings)**

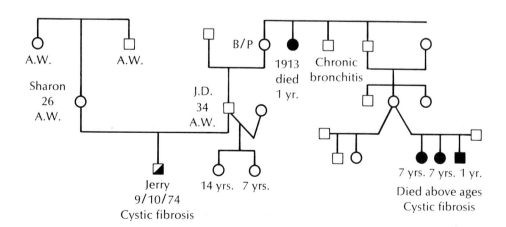

### Does your family see itself as a healthy family or as a sick family?

Believes they are basically a healthy family.

## CHILD PROFILE
### Neonatal status (risk, Apgar, congenital abnormalities)

Birth weight 7 lbs. 5½ oz. Breast-fed for three weeks. Began spitting up and vomiting after each feeding. Stools were "yellow and slimy." Infrequently retained a whole meal.

### Postnatal course

Switched to Similac with iron at age 3 weeks. At fourth-week visit weighed 7 lbs. 2 oz. Calories increased to 32 calories per ounce for three days without weight gain. 10/26/74 Malabsorption ruled out with positive sweat chloride test.

### Previous illnesses (dates)

10/26/74 Admitted for malabsorption, diagnosed with CF.
4/17/75 Ear infection
6/75 Ear infection
8/77 Virus (four-five days' duration)

### Medications

Cotazym, ½ packet after each feeding, but is varied according to how much he eats. Aerosol b.i.d. with Aralone in normal saline.

### Accidents and injuries (dates)

None either parent can remember.

### Nutrition history (example of a 24-hour intake)

"Watch" his diet and do not allow him too many eggs or whole milk. Is tolerating more foods as he gets older. Loves pancakes. Bread causes stomach aches, so he doesn't eat this much.

| BREAKFAST | LUNCH | SUPPER | SNACKS |
|-----------|-------|--------|--------|
| Toast and jelly | Milk | Meat | "Pringles" |
| Skim milk | Chicken | Potatoes | Cheese (lite-line) |
|  | Rice | Green beans | Bologna |
|  | Broccoli | Milk |  |
|  | Peaches |  |  |

### Food groups

Meats (2) $\underline{2}$   Veg. (4) $\underline{3}$   Fruit $\underline{2}$   Breads/cereals (4) $\underline{2}$   Milk/products (3) $\underline{3}$

### Formula: type/amt.

Breast milk 0 to 3 weeks. Similac with iron 3 weeks to 5 weeks. Progestamil until solid foods.

### Compare weight/height/age ratio

3 years, 9 months, weight = 32 lbs. (25%); height = 38 inches (25%)

### Identify developmental milestones

11/21/75   Sleeps all night, reaches for mobile on bed, lots of hand and feet movement.
4/17/75   Pulling up in crib, cutting teeth.
7/10/75   Junior foods.
9/75   Said several words. "Talked early."

### Sleep patterns/disturbances

Sleeping from 8 P.M. to 7 A.M. in the morning. May awaken about once a night. Many times may have "stomach trouble." Sleeps better after full day of activity. Takes afternoon nap of about one hour duration.

### Allergies

None known.

### Immunizations

DPT and TOPV ×4. Record "packed away." Had MMR. Can't remember how old he was—they will check.

PSYCHOLOGIC PROFILE (data here to be obtained during interactions, inquiry, observation, DDST)

### COGNITION
**CONCRETE OPERATIONS; PRECONCEPTUAL THOUGHT**
**(2-4 YEARS)**

_Yes_ Believes everyone views world as he does

_Yes_ Play is chief activity; assigns elements of reality to toys, objects

_Yes_ Centering: can identify only one quality of an object

_No_ Imitates parental model

_Yes_ Events judged by outward appearance

_No_ Unable to perform a completed process in reverse (reversibility)

### EGO
**INITIATIVE VS. GUILT**
**(3-6 YEARS)**

_Yes_ Cares for own body, toys, pets

_Yes_ Observes differences between men and women

_Yes_ Interacts more with parents and peers

_Yes_ Intrusive behavior; questioning, noisy

_Yes_ Rivals with older siblings; _solitary play_ or group play with peers; play out feelings

_No_ Identifies with parent of the same sex

### Comments

Does not understand other points of view. Played all through interview. Changed hats—played fire fighter most of the time using fire hat. Could only identify that the girl doll was "a girl, just because she was a girl." Did not see him imitate a parental model. During exam judged events by outward appearance. After using reflex hammer on nurse, decided the hammer wouldn't hurt him. Did not observe or test for reversibility.

Can dress himself. Grouped dolls into boys and girls. Loves school and talks about his friends. Behavior is noisy, attention-getting, but minds his parents. Engaged in solitary play without interruption for 30 minutes.

#### SCHOOL PROGRESS

Just enrolled in "special" day school run by local school district.

**What would you like to tell me about school?**

I like the kids.

**What do you like or dislike most about school?**

Dislikes the nap. Likes playing with kids and liked finger painting.

**Talk with parent or teacher about memory.**

Child recited accurately the sequence of a story in a short book. Parents say he "never forgets anything."

**Tell me: What kind of a student do you think you are?**

Not applicable.

#### PERCEPTION OF SELF
**Self-evaluation**

(Describe yourself to me.)
"I'm a little boy."

**Tell me things you like about yourself; dislike.**

No response.

**Let's pretend you could change something about yourself. Would you change anything?**

No response.

**Describe how you feel about what's happening to you now.**

Just wanted to talk about his "new school" and his "friends."

SOCIAL PROFILE
**Personal-social (DDST)**

3/9 Plan for second home visit.

Cases

**Father/mother–child interaction**

Both parents come with child to clinic visit. May take him to the park.

Eye contact   Good contact with both parents and with nurse during conversations.

Touching   Father and mother held son's hand as they walked in and out. Mother dressed son. Jerry did not pull away from examining physician and nurse.

Tone of voice of parent   Mother's tone is vivacious with soft quick speech. Father has a quiet low voice when speaking to son.

Child-parent activities   Plan lots of play activities in and around the house (mother and son). Mother, father, and grandparents read books to him daily.

Ease of separation   Never been separated from his parents or has been with a sitter on a consistent basis. Parents dreaded how he would react to separation, but he "got along well" the first day.

**Position of child in family**

First and only child in this primary unit.

**Describe life-style**

Presently living with her parents in their moderately spacious suburban home. All seem content with this temporary arrangement.

Is there more than one language spoken in the home? No

ENVIRONMENTAL PROFILE

**Pollutants**

Determine from city agencies.

**Population density**

Check with local agencies.

**Infestations**

Investigate during next home visit.

**Fire hazards**

None seen.

**Safety features in home and environment**

No obvious hazards seen. Fireplace well screened. No stairs in house.

**Medications/poisons**

When painting trim outside house, father turned back and thought Jerry drank paint thinner. After the trip to ER discovered he didn't. Since then keeps all potential poisons up and lids secured on containers. Will confirm this next home visit.

**Crime**

Will check local statistics.

**Availability of transportation**

Have two cars.

REVIEW OF SYSTEMS

Jerry, age 3½, diagnosed with cystic fibrosis at 6 weeks of age.

**General**

Active child with brown eyes and brown hair. Eyes sparkle, but expression is more somber. Seemed acclimated to the clinic environs and is very comfortable at home.

**Hair and scalp (dandruff, lice, cradle cap, itchiness, hair loss)**

Cradle cap (11/74), otherwise negative history.

### Skin (infections, scaling, burns, allergies)

10/24/74 Sweat chlorides (163) confirmed diagnosis of CF.

### Hematopoietic (anemias, bleeding, bruising)

10/24/74 Prothrombin time WNL. No history of anemias, bleeding, bruising. Hgb range (10.9 g to 12.3 g). Hct range (31.3 to 34.4) 8/77 RBCs 4.5 cu/mm.

### Eyes (infections, blurred vision, squinting, color blindness)

Has recently had "cold" in his eyes successfully treated with ophthalmic antibiotic; otherwise history is negative.

### Ears (infection, discharge, eardrum perforation, foreign objects, wax removals, decreased hearing)

Ear infections 4/75 and 6/75 resolved with ampicillin injections. No recurrences since then. Otherwise history is negative.

### Nose, throat, sinuses (runny nose, colds, decreased smell, foreign body, broken nose, tonsillitis)

Sometimes may have a runny nose, but parents avoid places and people to avert "a cold." Otherwise negative history.

### Mouth and dentition (dental caries, gingivitis, malocclusion, cleft lip and/or palate)

Has never been to dentist but brushes teeth regularly with parental assistance. History otherwise negative.

### Respiratory (bronchitis, pneumonia, whooping cough, histoplasmosis, tuberculosis, cough)

Respiratory distress when admitted for malabsorption 10/74. RR then was 30 per minute. Chest clear to auscultation 10/74. 1/75 had "raspy breathing" at clinic visit with negative chest film. Since 7/75 AP chest diameter ranged from 11 cm to 14 cm (8/77). Lateral diameter ranged from 15 cm (7/75) to 17 cm (8/77). 8/77 Chest x ray showed increased markings in the RML. Receives aerosol with Aralone twice daily. Gets tired of the treatments. Sleeps with vaporizer at night.

Parents were instructed about respiratory care, medication, postural drainage at time of child's diagnosis.

### Cardiovascular (heart murmurs, cyanosis)

Negative history for murmurs. No documented episodes of cyanosis. Mother denies any cyanotic episodes. Records negative for clubbing.

### Gastrointestinal (nausea/vomiting, diarrhea, constipation, jaundice, pain, colic, gas, hernias, anorexia)

(See neonatal and postnatal course.) By 1/23/75, after enzymes and Progestamil, was having three "mushy" BMs daily. Since then well-controlled digestion and elimination. Mother claims appetite "is good." Has occasional "stomach aches" at night, which awaken him. Will get stomach ache if "he gorges himself," which they try not to let him do. Stools alter in consistency if diet and Cotazym are not balanced. Usually has a daily BM.

### Genitourinary (frequency, urgency, burning, toilet training, bedwetting, odor, stream)

Toilet trained by 29 months without any regular bedwetting. Has had no frequency or urgency to their knowledge.

### Reproductive (irritations/rashes, deviations, secondary sexual characteristics)

Negative history. Circumcised at birth. Parents have received genetic counseling. (10/74)

### Neuromuscular (convulsions, headache, imbalance, incoordination, muscle weakness, numbness, tremors, tics)

Negative history. Father thinks child is "very coordinated."

### Psychologic (thumb sucking, fears, masturbation)

Does not suck thumb. History negative.

Cases

PHYSICAL PROFILE

## Measurements

Head <u>20 inches</u> (50 percentile)    Chest <u>22 inches</u>    Ht. <u>38 inches</u>    Wt. <u>32 lbs.</u>

## Vital signs

B/P _____    H.R. <u>90/min (after exercise)</u>    R.R. <u>22/min</u>    Temp. <u>98.4° F oral</u>

## Neuromuscular system

Runs during play. Relaxed coordinated gait. Posture is straight. Has good muscle development in arms and legs.

## Present status

Normal neuromuscular status.

## Social affect

Eyes are bright and alert. Has many smiling and inquisitive expressions. Intrusive behavior observed with all adults.

## Speech development

Speech is articulate. Six- and seven-word sentences. Told mother she "was being difficult."

## Reflexes

Biceps <u>2+</u> } Equal bilaterally
Triceps <u>2+</u>
Brachioradialis <u>2+</u>
Patellar <u>Unable to relax leg</u>    Achilles <u>Unable to relax leg</u>
Babinski <u>Negative</u>    Eye <u>Good blink</u>

## Cranial nerves

I (olfactory): Intact. Identified smell of alcohol as "medicine smell."
II (optic): Gross vision intact. Next visit plan to do DEST.
III, IV, and VI (oculomotor, trochlear, abducens): Intact. EOMs intact, peripheral vision at 90 degrees. Good convergence. Symmetrical blink. No ptosis of lids.
V (trigeminal): Intact. Detects light touch of cotton swab in mandibular and maxillary areas. Bit is bilaterally equal in strength.
VIII (acoustic): Intact. Gross hearing tested—heard examiner's finger rubbing together in front of ears.
IX, X (glossopharyngeal and vagus): Intact. Gags, uvula in midline, coordinated swallow. Tongue in midline when protruded. Buccal cavity is moist with saliva.
XI (accessory): Intact. Equal shoulder strength.
XII (hypoglossal): Intact. Can move tongue from side to side and equally apply pressure to both cheeks with tongue.

## Cerebellar function (Rhomberg, walk heel-toe, run in place, touch tip of nose, copy hand movements, pincer grasp, draw and copy geometric shapes)

Walked heel-to-toe smoothly. Able to touch top of nose, ran in place, and copied hand movements. Drew a picture of himself.

## Parietal lobe (object identification)

Intact. Tactilely identified a rubberband, a key, and a safety pin.

## Proprioception (positional sense of toe)

Unable to cooperate with this maneuver.

## Tactile capacity (cold, two-point discrimination, pin prick)

Discriminates between hot and cold. Feels pin prick on forearms and thighs.

### Skin (scars, lesions, turgor, bruises, moles)

No scars or lesions seen. Turgor reflects hydration.

### Head (circumference, fontanel measurement, palpation, transillumination)

Circumference 20 inches (6/15/78). No bulges seen or masses felt. Fontanels closed.

### Face (expression, palpebral fissures, placement of ears, percussion of sinuses, symmetry)

Face and structures bilaterally equal and symmetrical. Ears in line with outer canthus. Sinuses nontender. Relaxed expression.

### Hair, scalp (hairline, hygiene, distribution)

Thick brown hair with normal distribution. Hair is clean with fine texture and pliant. Normal hairline. No flaking or accumulation on scalp.

### Eyes (infection, conjunctival, red reflex, strabismus)

No strabismus, amblyopia. Conjunctivae pink, moist, and without exudates. No periorbital edema. PERRLA.

### Nose (patency, discharge, smell)

Nose in midline of face. Clear loose mucus in nose. Nares patent.

### Mouth and throat (teeth, gums, pharynx, tongue, palates, swallowing, tonsils)

Mucosa pink and moist without inflammation. No caries of primary dentition. Tonsils enlarged without inflammations or exudates. Tongue not coated. Palates without clefts or arch deviations.

### Ears (landmarks, structure, hearing)

Ears clean, canals patent. Bony landmarks visualized through some scarring of tympanums. Cone of light visualized 4-5 o'clock on L, 6-7 o'clock on R. No inflammation of canal or bulging of tympanum.

### Neck (nodules, masses, bruits, ROM)

Neck supple and without masses. No lymphadenopathy or bruits. Full ROM. Unable to palpate thyroid. No openings seen.

### Chest (symmetry, excursion, nodes, nipples)

Bilaterally equal symmetry and excursion. Nipples in apposition. No masses palpated. No lymphadenopathy. Enlargement of A-P diameter is slight. No cough.

### Heart (size, position, PMI, sounds)

No visible impulses on chest wall. No thrills. PMI at 4th interspace 1-2 cm L of MCL. $S_1$ loudest at mitral area, $S_2$ loudest at pulmonic with physiologic splitting of $S_2$. No murmurs, $S_3$ sound. Sinus arrhythmia. Rate 90/minute and regular with breath holding. Pulses equal bilaterally.

### Lungs (breath sounds, fremitus, percussion, duration of inspiration, expiration, rate)

Chest clear to percussion and auscultation and tests for fremitus and egophony negative. Inspiration to expiration 2:1. Rate is 22 per min. Breathes deeply. No clubbing of toes or fingers. No cyanosis.

### Abdomen (size, contour, bowel sounds, umbilicus, liver, spleen, femorals)

Abdomen protuberant with pale thin skin with prominent vasculature. Flared costal margins. Bowel sounds present, umbilicus inverted and clean. Unable to palpate liver and spleen. Abdomen nontender and without masses.

### Back and spine (structure, symmetry, column curvature)

Straight spine, straight posture. Bilateral symmetry of scapulas. No defects of column palpated. No openings in sacral area. Fine dark downy hair between shoulders. Buttocks have little adipose tissue.

### Extremities (palmar creases, ROM, hip abduction)

Normal palmar creases. Warm perfused extremities. Full active ROM and passive ROM without joint crepitus.

Cases

**Urinary (position of meatus, charae of voiding, appearance of urine)**

Urethra normally placed. Voids clear yellow urine. No recent urinalysis.

**Genitalia (structure, secondary sexual characteristics)**

Normal circumcised male with descended testes.

**Anus (structure, function)**

Patent. No fissures or prolapse.

## INITIAL PLAN

6/15/78 **No. 1 Incomplete data base**

**S** Parents talked much about their life since Jerry's birth—their "ups and downs."

**O** Home visit did not allow enough time for testing of Jerry. Seem eager about the visits.

**A** Need ongoing data collection for accurate problem identification.

**P** Obj. 1 The family should assist in planning for another home visit.
Obj. 2 The family should identify purpose of clinical specialists' interventions.

6/15/78 **No. 3 Child health maintenance**

3,A Physical competency—cystic fibrosis

**S** After neonatal feeding and growth problems, Jerry's parents were told he "probably had cystic fibrosis." After referral to major medical center as an in-patient a definite diagnosis was made on 10/26/74. Parents state they have carefully complied with his therapy, and he has been "fairly healthy" all along. Ear infections were resolved after mother quit work and elected to stay home all the time. They feel he was not cared for properly by the babysitter. They feel fortunate Jerry was diagnosed early as parents stated "the life span is longer and they are less sick" when this happens. Father and mother believe child is bright and is active and well coordinated. Jerry appears younger than 3½, looking about 2½ years of age as to size and weight. No obvious barreling of the chest with clothes on. Brushes teeth with parental assistance. Has bowel movement daily consistently and odor controlled by Cotazym. Immunizations are "up-to-date." Aerosol treatments provide medication and nebulization twice a day. Gets Cotazym after eating. Visits CF clinic two to three times yearly. Diet history reveals balanced diet.

**O** Physical exam revealed Jerry physiologically stable. Sensory and motor systems are intact. Weight is 32 pounds (twenty-fifth percentile) and height is 38 inches (twenty-fifth percentile), verifying the visual impression of being small for his chronological age. He is active, movements are coordinated. Respiratory excursion is equal bilaterally. No obvious increase in the A-P diameter of the chest. Rate is 22/minute, auscultation negative for adventitious sounds. Abdomen is protuberant with obvious vasculature. Buttocks lacking adipose tissue. No cough or expectorations during exam. No dental caries of the deciduous dentition. Need to assess further vision, hearing, and speech development and DTRs. Mother will check on age Jerry was given MMR. Clinic records reveal near-normal chest films and pulmonary function. No objective data to confirm adequacy of diet.

**A** Cystic fibrosis is an inherited autosomal recessive disorder of infancy and childhood. The pancreatic acini are replaced by fibrous tissue, and eventually fat replaces the fibrous tissue. Clinical manifestations of the consequent pancreatic deficiency are malnutrition and steatorrhea. In the newborn, viscous intestinal mucous secretions may cause meconium ileus. Later the child may develop fecal impaction, rectal prolapse, and intussusception. In a few cases the smaller hepatic biliary channels are plugged, with subsequent cirrhosis and portal hypertension developing The sweat contains very high concentration of chloride and sodium so

**827**

## INITIAL PLAN—cont'd

6/15/78    **No. 3   Child health maintenance—cont'd**

in hot weather this abnormality can cause acute dehydration and cardio-vascular collapse. The most devastating obstructive pathologic changes affect the lungs, in which an overabundance of thick mucus starts a cycle of obstruction of air passages, infection, and inflammation leading to chronic pulmonary disease. The pulmonary disease varies from mild to severe. If the child is diagnosed early and medical care and a health team are available for supervision and management, the outlook is brighter. Dietary management includes high protein, high caloric snacks, and moderate restriction of fatty foods. The child usually has a voracious appetite. Cotazym is a pancreatic enzyme preparation that aids in absorption of nutrients from the GI tract, the dosage dependent on appearance of the stools. Prognosis for CF child is better since advent of reliable sweat tests, use of antibiotics, and use of chest physical therapy and pulmonary function studies. Indicators of a bacterial infection in the lungs are increased cough, increased sputum production, and weight loss with or without fever. Usual pathogens are *Staphylococcus* and *Pseudomonas* and *Hemophilus*. Since CF literally affects every system in the body, the concept of maintenance of the physical competency of the child is vital to his optimum health and longevity of life.

**P**    Obj. 1   Jerry should demonstrate growth parameters proportional to baseline data.

Obj. 2   Jerry should begin to identify foods therapeutically excluded from his diet.

Obj. 3   Jerry should demonstrate adequate gaseous exchange at the alveolar level.

Obj. 4   Jerry should continue to increase his skills in caring for his body.

3,B    Learning and thought competency

**S**    Parents believe child is "very bright." Parents have spent lots of time reading to him. Likes to play. Has started to preschool.

**O**    Is by age in phase of preconceptual thought. He plays continually. He changed characters as he changed hats, but played fire fighter most of the time, assigning an element of reality to play. Could only center on idea that girl doll was a girl but unable to distinguish several features making her different (i.e., hair, dress). Judges events by outward appearances by realizing if reflex hammer didn't hurt nurse it wouldn't hurt him. Recited the sequence of events in a story book. He has no gross sensory or motor deficits that might interfere with learning.

**A**    In this phase the child believes that everyone views the world as he does. The child uses assimilation and accommodation to conceptualize his sensory perceptions. At this age he may begin magical thinking. Play is the medium for learning, for expression of creativity and joy, a way of testing and dealing with reality, building self-esteem, and learning social roles. It is also a medium through which the child can express a sense of power and exploration. A preschooler's play has elements of reality, and he plays with an earnest attitude. He should have a beginning concept of time in hours but not an understanding of the future. Development of a strong learning and thought competency in a chronically ill child may contribute later to strengthening his inner competency when his illness limits his activity or alters his body image.

**P**    Obj. 1   Jerry should demonstrate continuing cognitive development.

3,C    Social competency

**S**    Parents fear child may become "isolated" and "overprotected" and believe preschool will give him a normal social outlet. They state child desires friends his own age. Child hasn't been separated from them for any length of time. After one day in school Jerry liked the "kids." Parents play with child daily.

**O**    Both parents speak in soft voices to child and he comes to them occasionally to be held or touched on a brief moment. Child has good eye contact with the parents. Interacts with adults in a relaxed manner.

**A**    The social competency of the chronically ill child depends primarily on how the parents relate to him. Their attitudes toward illness or disability will determine if the child can maintain an appropriate role. When a child who is chronically ill or disabled has been a member of a peer group from early stages, he may not find "being different" so distressing. There is a necessity to assess the adequacy of the environment to assist in promoting social adaptation. Children with cystic fibrosis are living to be young adults with increasing frequency, so their needs must be met to facilitate normal development. Developmentally, he needs to learn to communicate with an increasing number of others and to conform to others' expectations and to become a participating member in the family. Is starting interactive play and can cooperate briefly. In preschool years the peer group is becoming important as the child must learn to understand limits the group places on the individual. The time the preschooler spends away from his parents should increase in length and frequency.

**P**    Obj. 1   Jerry should be able to separate easily from his parents.
       Obj. 2   Jerry should form relationships with his peer group.

3,D    Inner competency

**S**    Behavior appears to be well adapted to his home. Mother states child sometimes tires of aerosol treatments. Parents believe he is "spoiled."

**O**    Chronologically is in initiative vs. guilt stage of affective development. Behavior is intrusive, is able to dress himself, asks questions and observes differences in men and women dolls. Played without interruption for 30 minutes. Did not observe child imitating a parental model. Seemed eager and enthusiastic in school and was not clinging to parents during interview.

**A**    A child with a chronic illness may be expected at some point to have some difficulty with self-esteem. He can best cope by understanding his condition and his limitations. Parents that react to behavior of the child in a realistic fashion (not allowing presence of a physical problem to override) allow the child to develop adequate inner discipline and a self-concept that is not oversolicitous of his physical problem. The child's perception of himself in illness may be observed through skilled use of play. Gender identity is a part of total task of identification and should occur during this developmental period. This identity is necessary for emotional stability and ego development. Inadequate self-esteem may produce very dependent behavior, excessive fear of new experiments, and manipulative use of his handicap.

**P**    Obj. 1   Jerry should demonstrate a positive sense of self.

**829**

**INITIAL PLAN—cont'd**

6/15/78 **No. 4  Need for knowledge and guidance in the care of the child with a long-term illness**

4,A    Child entering preschool

**S**    Mother is anxious that no one in school will care for him as she does. Both parents believe this will cause some adjustments to be made by all three. They want son to have as normal a social life as possible. They are nervous about how he will get along with other kids and how he will fare being exposed to colds and viruses. Child has had one uneventful day at school.

**O**    This situation has caused tension and discomfort, both parents expressing ambivalent feelings about how he will get along in school. This appears to be a mild crisis for them. They are still a little anxious even though he's had one good day at school.

**A**    The person experiencing a stressful event can move into a state of disequilibrium where regular coping mechanisms and problem-solving techniques fail to meet the needs of the situation. This couple see school for child as good but fraught with health hazards and are frightened as to how it will affect Jerry's health. They seem to have a realistic perception of the event but need some support as they carry through this endeavor. The question of whether or not it was a "good idea" to send Jerry to school may possibly be more realistically discussed after he has had a URI from school. At this time they can more realistically view the situation and think about how they plan to handle preschool on a long-term basis.

**P**    Obj. 1  The parents should develop coping mechanisms for handling problems related to the child's entry into preschool.

4,B    Management of child's illness

**S**    Mother quit work to care for child as he was sick a lot while at the babysitter's. Since then child has been well most of the time and she feels the financial sacrifice "is worth it." At medical center they learned how to give respiratory care and medications, how to do postural drainage, and received genetic counseling. Child wakes almost every night.

**O**    Conversation reflects knowledge of CF, i.e., early diagnosis means a longer life span. Both parents seem involved with child's care. Did not observe them doing pulmonary hygiene with Jerry. Did not find out the exact routine and how this affects their home life.

**A**    Problems of managing a child with CF are numerous for the family. The treatments and postural drainage require a great deal of time and energy and learning of skills. They must have a place for special equipment and know how to maintain it. Sleep may be disturbed as parents may listen for a cough or sleep lightly if the child calls. The threat of infection by visitors in the home may curtail visits by relatives, neighbors, peers. It is imperative that the parents understand the special needs and problems, as this increases the child's potential for growth and development.

**P**    Obj. 1  The parents should be able to identify the pathophysiology of cystic fibrosis as a basis for their management.
       Obj. 2  The parents should be able to do a respiratory assessment on Jerry using physical exam techniques.

**830**    4,C    Coping with family problems produced by chronically ill child

**S**    Parents "are strapped" financially due to his child support payments and mother not working. Parents' medical insurance company considers Jerry uninsurable, so his medical costs relating to CF are not covered. Should child need care or hospitalization they would assume cost. Father is presently unemployed. They are temporarily living with her parents. Sharon has stayed home with child for last three years. Babysitter did not properly care for infant when she tried to work. Enrolling in real estate courses.

**O**    Life seems centered around care for child. Are having financial problems as mother does not think she should work while Jerry is home as they did not want to hassle with babysitters and URIs.

**A**    Sleeping arrangements, child's therapy routine, social isolation from friends and organization, complicated family outings or vacations, problems finding a babysitter are everyday problems that confront the family of the CF child. The cost of care will eventually strain a family budget, and financial assistance may be necessary. The local Cystic Fibrosis Research Foundation chapter can help in finding services and assistance. There is also the problem of the genetic transmission of the disease as in any pregnancy there is a 1:4 chance that child will have cystic fibrosis. In a child-bearing family this may severely alter plans for a certain size family. The family needs basic strategies for coping with key problems and thus needs family organizational arrangements.

**P**    Obj. 1   The family should develop basic strategies for coping with problems produced by their chronically ill child.

4,D    Provision for safety needs of the preschooler

**S**    Want child to be as normal as possible and not be "overprotected." Parents and grandparents read to and play with child. Father once careless with paint thinner and thought Jerry drank it.

**O**    No overt physical safety hazards. Fireplace screen covered entire fireplace. No staircases in house. No mention of child's developmental needs or how they discipline child.

**A**    Providing for optimal health includes knowledge and provisions about physical safety hazards and developmental hazards of the child—immediate and forthcoming tasks. Jerry is cognitively in preconceptual phase of development and affectively is in stage of initiative vs. guilt in which the major task is gender identity with parent of same sex. The most common cause of death at this age is accidents: motor vehicle–related accidents, burns, drowning, poisoning, and falls. Preschooler needs clear-cut safety rules and needs to start learning to protect himself. Parents need knowledge of play as this is the medium through which the child experiences the world through the sensory modes.

**P**    Obj. 1   The parents should utilize knowledge of developmental tasks to direct child's behavior.

        Obj. 2   The parents should provide injury control and safety for Jerry.

**NURSING ORDERS**

6/15/78   **No. 1  Incomplete data base**           **PERSONNEL**

Obj. 1  The family should assist in planning for another home visit.
- A. Arrange time on 6/20/78 for next visit at 3 PM.     Family C.S.

Obj. 2  The family should identify purpose of clinical specialist's interventions.
- A. Have family identify what they perceive as their health needs. (6/20)     C.S.
- B. Using their identified needs, explain nurse's role in assisting family with stated needs. (6/20)     C.S.
- C. Solicit suggestions from them as to how nurse can be better utilized in working with CF families (ongoing).     C.S.

6/15/78   **No. 3  Child health maintenance**

3,A   Physical competency—cystic fibrosis

Obj. 1  Jerry should demonstrate growth parameters proportional to baseline data.
- A. Graph height, weight, head and chest circumferences since birth using clinic records. (6/18)     C.S.
- B. Evaluate diet and absorption deficiencies should growth and size not increase proportionately (ongoing).     C.S.
- C. Share the need for keeping records of this data with the parents. (6/20)     C.S.

Obj. 2  Jerry should begin to identify foods that are therapeutically excluded from his diet
- A. Ascertain from talking with Jerry if he has any knowledge of types of foods by using pictures and puzzles of types of food. (6/20)     C.S.
- B. Plan a simple program whereby he will be able to identify foods with fat. (6/20)     C.S.
- C. Talk with preschool teacher about assisting him in this exercise at mealtime at school. (6/21)     C.S.

Obj. 3  Jerry should demonstrate adequate gaseous exchange at the alveolar level
- A. Review clinical records and record data of pulmonary function tests to determine inspiratory and expiratory volumes for baseline data. (6/18)     C.S.
- B. Monitor chest circumference and A-P chest diameters and record on each exam (ongoing).     C.S.
- C. Respiratory assessment each visit.     C.S.
- D. Teach parents techniques of percussion and auscultation of the chest and abdomen. (Start on 6/27)     C.S.
- E. Encourage exercise and play as this promotes deeper breathing and facilitates ciliary activity and coughing up of secretions (ongoing).     C.S.

|  |  |  |
|---|---|---|
| F. Teach parents clinical symptoms of respiratory infections. (6/20) | C.S. | Cases |
| G. Instruct teacher as to the nature of Jerry's illness. (6/21) | C.S. | |

Obj. 4   Jerry should continue to increase his skills in caring for his body

|  |  |
|---|---|
| A. Encourage parents to allow independence in dressing and oral hygiene. (6/20) | C.S. |
| B. Teach Jerry about caring for his teeth and mouth. (6/20 or 6/27) | C.S. |
| C. Talk with teacher to determine if hygiene teaching is part of the daily activities. (6/21) | C.S. |

6/15/78   3,B   Learning and thought competency

Obj. 1   Jerry should demonstrate continuing cognitive development

|  |  |
|---|---|
| A. Next visit inventory play items and determine play activities he and parents do. (6/20) | C.S. |
| B. Encourage parents to stimulate Jerry as much as possible as he may need this strength for a future sense of well-being (ongoing). | Parents C.S. |
| C. Briefly explain Jerry's cognitive abilities as outlined by the preconceptual period. (6/20) | C.S. |
| D. Ascertain types of learning activities at school and encourage parents to follow through with these at home. (6/21) | Teacher Parents C.S. |

3,C   Social competency

Obj. 1   Jerry should be able to separate easily from his parents

|  |  |
|---|---|
| A. Have parents relate child's separation behaviors for past week and their response. | C.S. |
| B. Encourage them to look for additional social outlets for the child in the near future (church groups, Bible school). | Parents C.S. |
| C. Have parents communicate with teacher as to Jerry's behavior upon their leaving. | Parents C.S. |

Obj. 2   Jerry should form relationship with his peer group.

|  |  |
|---|---|
| A. Assess Jerry with DDST for personal social interactions. | C.S. |
| B. Have parents work with teacher to foster his play within the group. | Parents C.S. |
| C. Encourage parents to make Jerry share. | C.S. |
| D. Encourage mother to invite a playmate regularly to the home. | Mother C.S. |

6/15/78   3,D   Inner competency

Obj. 1   Jerry should demonstrate a positive sense of self.

|  |  |
|---|---|
| A. Next visit plan a play session with a "sick doll" and record roles he takes or comments. (6/20) | C.S. |

## NURSING ORDERS—cont'd

6/15/78   **No. 3   Child health maintenance—cont'd**

B. Have Jerry draw a picture of himself. Repeat this at intervals for comparison. (6/20)    C.S.

C. Teach parents behaviors that indicate inadequate sense of self. (6/20)    C.S.

D. Talk with teacher at preschool as to how Jerry is integrating. (6/21)    Parents

E. Ask teacher to play down anything that might set Jerry apart from the other children. (6/21)    Parents

6/15/78   **No. 4   Need for knowledge and guidance in the care of the child with a long-term illness**

4,A   Child entering preschool

Obj. 1   The parents should develop coping mechanisms for handling problems related to child's entry into preschool.

A. Have parents identify on a sheet of paper all the pros and cons of son going to school. (6/20)    Parents   C.S.

B. Discuss with them how they will handle their feelings should Jerry become ill, i.e., will they feel guilty? (6/27)    C.S.

C. Encourage them to have a conference with the teacher, listing for her all the safety precautions Jerry must observe to maintain health. (6/21)    Parents   C.S.

D. Explore Sharon's feelings now that child is away from her six hours daily. (6/20)    C.S.

E. Suggest to Sharon that she explore an outside interest in her free time, i.e., part-time work, hobby. (6/20)    C.S.

F. Have them keep a log of events during first week of school as a reference for discussion of how they have coped. (6/27)    Parents   C.S.

4,B   Management of child's illness

Obj. 1   The parents should be able to identify the pathophysiology of cystic fibrosis as a basis for their management.

A. Ascertain parental knowledge of cystic fibrosis.    C.S.

B. Discuss with them what they would like to learn further.    C.S.

C. Have them identify basic pathologic mechanisms and relate it to care they give son.    Parents   C.S.

Obj. 2   The parents should be able to do a respiratory assessment on Jerry using physical exam techniques.

A. Explore with them verbally their knowledge of use of stethoscope, percussion, and the types of breath sounds.    C.S.

B. Discuss with them the feasibility of learning the above to monitor son's pulmonary status.    Parents   C.S.

C. Provide pamphlet "Living with Fibrosis."    C.S.

**834**

4,C   Coping with family problems produced by chronically ill child

Obj. 1   The family should develop basic strategies for coping with problems produced by their chronically ill child.

A. Perform a family assessment delving into meaning of illness to the parents, financial resources. (6/27)

C.S.

B. Refer the father to an employment service should he desire. (6/20)

C.S.

C. Investigate further sources of insurance and aid for the family.

C.S.

D. After family assessment analyze family as open or closed system and assess for degree of social isolation and support persons.

C.S.

E. Explore with them verbally what they consider key problems in coping with long-term illness.

Parents
C.S.

F. Subsequently assist them as they formulate or revise strategies used to manage the illness and normalize their lives.

Parents
C.S.

4,D   Provision for safety needs of the preschooler

Obj. 1   The parents should utilize knowledge of developmental tasks to direct child's behavior.

A. In family assessment have them identify expected developmental events of forthcoming year. (6/27)

Parents
C.S.

B. Provide literature giving developmental tasks in the cognitive and affective realms.

C.S.

C. In writing, have them name toys, sensory experiences, materials they would use to stimulate development of these tasks.

Parents
C.S.

D. List methods of guidance.

Parents

Obj. 2   The parents should provide injury control and safety for Jerry.

A. See if they use a car seat and a seat belt for Jerry when in motor vehicle.

C.S.

B. Plan to collect specific data about safety hazards and location of poisons on next home visit.

C.S.

C. Have parents give clear-cut safety rules to Jerry and repeat them consistently.

C.S.

D. Have them praise child when he takes responsibility for his own safety.

Parents

E. Teach child full name, his address and phone number, and how to utilize police and fire fighters.

Parents

F. Never allow child to play in driveways or near water.

Parents

## PROGRESS NOTES

6/20/78    **No. 1    Incomplete data base**

**S**    Home visit cancelled due to illness of nurse. In the phone call Sharon stated she had gotten a bookkeeping job with the Dairy Owen Corporation and J. D. had gotten a job as construction superintendent. Jerry had developed an ear infection. Ears were "bright red." Was going to pediatrician for medicine. Child "loves" school. Stated they were pleased with his adjustment.

**O**    Arranged visit for 6/27 at 3 PM.

**A**    Family actively solving problems as to unemployment and financial difficulties. Will use next visit to collect additional data and implement scheduled nursing orders.

**P**    Continue with present overall plan until further collection of data.

## NURSING ORDERS

### No. 1    Incomplete data base

Obj. 1    The family should assist in planning in another home visit.
A.  Arrange a visit for 6/27 at 3 PM.

## PROGRESS NOTES

6/27/78    **No. 1    Incomplete data base**

**S**    Sharon called to say that grandfather suddenly became ill and that they would be gone during scheduled visit. Reported they both liked their jobs and that Jerry's ear infection was resolving and that she was worried that school might be going to cause child increase in his frequency of ear infections.

**O**    Another home visit planned for 6/31.

**A**    Since both parents are busier with work and Jerry is in school the time available for planning visits is limited. Sharon is considerate and responsible for calling to cancel the scheduled visit.

**P**    Continue with stated plan until opportunity to reassess family's progress and ongoing needs.

## NURSING ORDERS

### No. 1    Incomplete data base

Obj. 1    The family should assist in planning in another home visit.
A.  Arrange another visit on 6/31 at 3 PM.

## PROGRESS NOTES

6/31/78    **No. 1    Incomplete data base**

**S**    Sharon reviewed the outline of identified needs and the plan for Jerry and stated she believed these were areas for need. She stated she believed these interventions to be helpful.

**O**    Explained to family my role and that any need they had at any time could be added to the present plan. Parents seem to accept nurse's purpose and interventions as helpful.

**A**    There is always need for ongoing problem identification and reassessment and evaluation of the original plan. Family is identifying what they see as health needs and accepting interventions by the nurse as helpful. Family does cooperate in planning visits and can identify nurse's purposes thus objectives 1 and 2 have been met.

**P**  Revise Obj. 1 of nursing orders to read:
Obj. 1  The family will assist in the process of data collection and problem identification on an ongoing basis.

### No. 3  Child health maintenance

3,A  Physical competency—cystic fibrosis

**S**  Sharon reported that Jerry's ear infection was resolved and mentioned that the pediatrician said that he might need "tubes" in his ears. Stated Jerry now weighed 35 pounds and that he took his lunch to school as he wasn't liking what was in school lunches. Child knows he must take Cotazym or "my stomach will hurt." Mother doesn't know if he can identify actively foods he shouldn't eat. Appetite has "picked up" since getting antibiotic for ears. Mother had a conference with the teacher, giving her a list of foods that he could not tolerate. Mother also gave teacher the pamphlet, "A Teacher's Guide to Cystic Fibrosis," which gives an overview of CF, explains the therapy, and child's adjustment needs.

**O**  Jerry's respiratory rate is 23/minute. Lungs are clear to auscultation. No retractions of the chest wall or suprasternal notch. Color is good; conjunctivae are pink. No cyanosis of nail beds. Extremities are warm. Outer ears are nontender. Unable to visualize tympanums as examiner did not have an otoscope. Child was able to name pictures of food in a book. Could not identify any food with fat, i.e., butter, cheese. Child weighed 35 pounds on the family's scales. Parents agreed that they would like to learn proper auscultation of Jerry's lungs to assess his respiratory status and the adequacy of his treatments.

**A**  Jerry's respiratory status is stable; he is gaining weight. He cannot identify foods that are excluded from his diet by food group. Does know his medication is necessary to avoid stomach aches. Mother has instructed teacher about dietary restrictions. Child takes his lunch now, which eliminates the necessity for him to actively identify foods he can't eat, although he must learn to do this eventually. Parents seem eager to want accurate techniques for assessing child's respiratory status and will plan this for the next visit. Mother has conference with teacher about his special physical needs in relationship to cystic fibrosis. Need to continue with dietary teaching for the child. Jerry may be viewed as a system whose subsystems are affected by his illness. A system is known as a set of elements standing in interaction. Jerry may also be viewed as a subsystem of the family system. The client and his family may be thought as fully functioning if they are able to carry out all processes of which they are capable. Certainly long-term goals are those that will allow for full function of a system. A living system is an open one that maintains a steady state within a narrow range of variables. Negative feedback allows the organism to adapt, thus maintaining the steady state. Therefore, how Jerry's illness affects his system and subsystems and how Jerry as a subsystem is maintained physically within his family system should be identified.

**P**  Continue with present plan but omit 2,C, and 3,G, from the nursing orders and notate them as done in nursing order section. Add long-range objectives.
Obj. 5  Jerry should demonstrate the ability to share responsibility for regulating his therapy with his parents.

**837**

**PROGRESS NOTES—cont'd**

**No. 3   Child health maintenance—cont'd**

> Obj. 6 Jerry should eventually demonstrate the ability to regulate his therapy for maintenance of his physical competency.

4/14/78   3,B   Learning and thought competency

**S**   Mother states child "loves" school. Was tested for an intelligence quotient "with a score around 130." He brings home finished projects from school —drawings, finger paintings.

**O**   Discussed with the mother the need to strengthen his learning and thought abilities as a safeguard for a future sense of well-being. *Inventory of Home Stimulation: Three to Six* was done as a general assessment of the child's environment. Percentile scores ranged from 83-100 on indicating that the child's environment is adequate in the following areas: provision of stimulation through equipment and toys, stimulation of mature behavior, provision of stimulating physical and language environment, avoidance of restriction and punishment, stimulation of pride, affection, and thoughtfulness, masculine stimulation, and independence from parental control. Sharon showed nurse Jerry's art work and projects from school. Jerry is able to center or see the striking characteristic of an object.

**A**   The "Home" tool is based on the hypothesis that characteristics of an environment could predict a child's developmental outcome. The tool evaluates subtle aspects of the young child's environment likely to influence the child's development. It obtains samples of the quantity and quality of cognitive, social, and emotional support available to the child in his home. Feedback can be used to help parents meet their own needs for assuring their child an appropriate environment. Did not have an opportunity to outline the cognitive tasks of the preconceptual period. Inventory reveals that parents are providing an environment for cognitive stimulation. The task in teaching Jerry is to break through his egocentric thinking. Centering is the beginning for sorting and classifying.

**P**   Continue with present plan but notate Obj. 1,A as done and add Obj. 2 to nursing orders.
Obj. 2   Jerry will demonstrate ability for intellectual thought.

3,C   Social competency

**S**   Parents state child does not cry when he goes to school and was only slightly fearful the first day and did not cry then. Mother states child frequently plays with a nearby cousin. Teacher told parents that Jerry is well adjusted to the school routine. Jerry describes play activities at school and states "it's fun." Child has not missed a day of school. Parents are pleased with the way school has worked out for them.

**O**   None.

**A**   Jerry seems to be separating easily from his parents. Parents have been communicating with the teacher about Jerry's behavior in school. School adjustment presently is adequate. Subjective data reveals child does have a cousin for a frequent playmate. Time did not allow for administering of the DDST. Jerry, by becoming involved in preschool, is being influenced by the environment and by his peers, which causes change in the structure of his life space. For Lewin changes in the structure of the

**838**

life space are accomplished by need satisfaction and tension reduction. The life space consists of the person and his psychologic environment. Cells of the personality function comprising the life space should develop progressively and differentiate as the individual grows and matures. Behavior then may be interpreted in terms of the total life space. In expanding his life space the parents are allowing the child to come to a state of social equilibrium appropriate to his developmental needs.

**P**  Note Obj. 1 as met and orders A, B, C as completed. Continue with remainder of plan adding immediate and long-range goals.

Obj. 3 Jerry will demonstrate ability to master age-appropriate social tasks.

Obj. 4 Jerry will demonstrate ability to function responsibly in society.

3,D  Inner competency

**S**  Mother reports that child was tested at school and that he refused to draw a picture of a man or himself. States that teacher reports he at times will not join in activities "if he doesn't like how he's talked to." Mother, after conference with the teacher, believes child is integrated with the other children at school. Mother reports Jerry seems more satisfied and content since child goes to school.

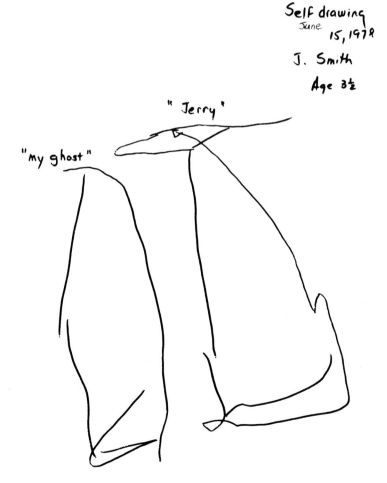

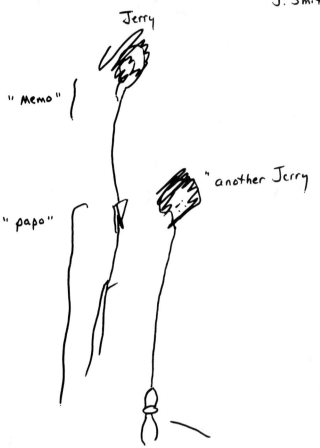

*June 31, 1978*

*Self drawing
J. Smith*

*Jerry*

*"Memo"*

*"another Jerry"*

*"papo"*

## PROGRESS NOTES—cont'd

### No. 3 Child health maintenance—cont'd

**O** HOME data revealed that child does have masculine stimulation: spends time each evening with father, eats breakfast with father, and has toys that provide large muscle development and riding toys. Child drew a picture of himself, and to the right side he drew a similar picture stating this was "his ghost." Child did not discuss the self-portrait any more. Dependent behavior, excessive fear of new experiments, and manipulative use of his handicap were explained as signs of inadequate self-esteem. Both parents actively talk with the child and touch him at frequent intervals.

**A** Child's picture of himself indicates not enough body parts for his chronological age according to Goodenough's Draw-A-Man Data. The presence of "my ghost" may represent a fear or fears that he has. Since he is also entering into an era of magical thinking and imaginary playmates this may explain "my ghost." The concept of a child's self is reflected in the way he talks, draws pictures, and plays. Usually the 3-year-old draws a man consisting of a circle, sometimes with an appendage, a crude representation of the face, and no differentiation of the body parts. Jerry's

**840**

drawing of himself much reflects the latter. To ascertain the significance of the ghost figure serial drawings may identify whether the ghost figure is significant. According to Murphy, coping for the child should lead to adaptation. If the child's first efforts at coping fail, the child may develop defensive rigidity resulting in continued frustration, further anxiety, and defensive attitudes. Therefore, coping should be viewed with focus on the purpose, the function, and the result of the behavior for the child. Defense mechanisms used for coping are projection, rationalization, and denial. These are manipulations of reality that make reality bearable. It is possible that the ghost figure is a symbolic representation of fears about his illness or threat of the illness to his body. Children need to learn to express their emotions but how they communicate is a function of parental imitation. Parents need to give examples of affective language like "I feel happy today" or "I feel sad today because you're sick." Parents need to clarify expressions of sadness, anger, joy, or confusion by asking child "You seem sad today, are you worried?" In this way the young child can learn to recognize and identify how he feels and later verbalize his inner feelings.

**P** Revise objectives of nursing orders.

Obj. 1 Jerry should demonstrate the ability to play or draw as mediums for expressing inner needs.

Obj. 2 Jerry will demonstrate coping mechanisms that provide for a positive sense of self.

### No. 4 Need for knowledge and guidance in the care of the child with a chronic illness

4,A Child entering preschool

**S** Parents believe child is adjusted to school setting, and that this is meeting his need for expanding his social contacts and their need for child to have normal childhood experiences. The advent of the ear infection worries mother. She states she fears school might cause these to increase. Grandmother is the school secretary where child attends school. Mother is now working. Sharon states she enjoys work and having some time away from the child. Grandmother checks on child while he is in school and communicates with the teacher any special needs Jerry may have. Sharon stated that teacher said she would call her if any of the children had colds or "flu" so Jerry could stay home.

**O** Mother still seems worried about how school environment will affect child's health, although the signs of this being a crisis event are not evident.

**A** To parents of chronically ill children contacts such as a nursery school, outside playmates may be a source of intense worry. Parents need to control overprotective impulses by giving guidance to the school personnel about special vulnerabilities. Parents need support for themselves by sharing their concerns with a supportive individual. Parents should know that all parents wish to protect their children and that this is a normal impulse. Parents appear to be coping with worrisome aspects of child's schooling. They have identified fears and given guidance to teacher about child's special vulnerabilities.

**P** Revise Obj. 1 of nursing orders.

Obj. 1 The parents should develop coping mechanisms for handling problems related to child's presence in preschool.

**PROGRESS NOTES—cont'd**

### No. 4 Need for knowledge and guidance in the care of the child with a chronic illness—cont'd

Continue with present plan. Omit D and E as Sharon is enjoying her free time with work.

4,B    Management of child's illness

**S**    Jerry gets aerosol treatments twice a day using compressor with nebulized normal saline. Not using a bronchodilator now. Also gets clapping and postural drainage following aerosol. Child is sleeping better since going to school. Mother keeps an active file of pamphlets and articles about disease process of CF and management techniques. Parents are able to detect changes in child's lungs with a stethoscope. Are using tape recordings of normal and abnormal breath sounds.

**O**    Teaching plan for use of the stethoscope and auscultatory techniques of the lungs implemented by parents meeting stated learning objectives. Parents demonstrated proper auscultation of child's lungs. Parents verbally identified rationale of their intervention based on the disease process. Parents want more information about abnormal breath sounds you would expect to hear if Jerry were to have increasing lung changes.

**A**    Parents have a basic understanding of the pathophysiology of cystic fibrosis and are able to relate their interventions to this. They have correct beginning skills in the use of the stethoscope and auscultatory techniques and can identify normal breath sounds. They have written information about cystic fibrosis.

**P**    Discontinue Obj. 1 and orders A-C as implementation of interventions have met the objective. Continue with Obj. 2. Revise orders A-C. Add Obj. 3 to nursing orders.

Obj. 3    Parents will identify verbally their feelings that may affect management of the child's illness.

4,C    Coping with family problems produced by chronically ill child

**S**    Sharon has gotten a job working M-F at a local business. J. D. has gotten a position as construction superintendent. Father is pleased as the pay is good and he is to learn about construction business in order to eventually become a builder. Jerry will soon have insurance for his regular pediatric needs by coverage from Sharon's group policy hospitalization, a benefit of her job. They have enrolled in college real estate courses. They expressed that father's child support payments and one income have really caused them much stress because of "tight finances." They are feeling relief from this now with increased income. They are presently living with her parents and express gratitude for their support emotionally and materially during the last few months. They are making plans to eventually try to build a "small home" as soon as possible.

Sharon stated she reacted to Jerry's illness with "why us?" Stated that husband's parents were not supportive at this time, but her parents were and encouraged them to seek support by getting to know other families with children with CF. She said she cried and mourned for about three months and finally as a couple, they decided that Jerry was given to them because they could best care for him. A former teacher helped her to work through her feelings during the crisis. J. D. was disillusioned because his parents had never told him of his cousins' deaths from CF. They had only planned one child since R. L. has two other children that he supports and they both care for and see frequently. They believe they have accepted the child's illness and that they are committed to providing the best possible family life working within the child's needs. Sharon stated it still bothers her when she thinks that Jerry will not live or be disabled or not have children. They were active in the local CF chapter of which R. L. was president. Every time a child died she stated they reexperienced the crisis of Jerry's illness and the fear of his death. They are not active presently due to disagreements about how organization was being run. Parents have a daily routine for child's care and this has become an accepted part of their life.

Social work consultant in 1975 felt parents had minimal acceptance of the illness. Sharon stated she still has problems with grief but tries not to think about negative outcomes of CF. Parents confirmed that despite the stresses of child's illness and the resulting financial difficulties that both are committed to each other and to providing for Jerry.

**O** Child's physical competency is stable, which reflects the success of the preventive and rehabilitative interventions. Family assessment not performed. No need for services to assist in seeking employment. Sharon's parents do provide a support system. Anger about child's illness may have been displaced onto CF organization with subsequent rejection of that support system. Parents have progressed through denial and depression to the outcome of crisis solution as evidenced by accepting illness and limitations realistically.

**A** Parents of a chronically ill child use denial throughout to some degree, particularly when the child is stable. The family has reacted to chronic illness with reintegration and has realistically accepted the illness and limitations imposed upon them. Since the child has not had any severe remission since diagnosis, the family has not had to adapt to a more mature stage of crisis solution in which they can adapt successfully to their feelings. Family unit appears stable, with no evidence of family disintegration.

**P** Continue with present plan. Delete orders B and C.

6/31/74    No. 4,D    Provision for safety needs of the preschooler

**S** Parents do not have literature giving age-appropriate developmental needs. Parents stated they would like this information. Parents believe school is assisting to meet Jerry's growth and development needs and their desire for him to reach his full potential physically, socially, and psychologically. They believe the child is bright and that they have stimulated him with play materials, books, records, and tapes. Expressed concern because he will not use his car seat. Child is not allowed to play in the driveway.

**O** Cleaning fluids and chemicals are on high shelves. There are no deep drainage ditches or bodies of water near the house. The house is situated close to a busy street with no fence in the front yard. The child can open and close doors. His toys, swing are located in the chain-linked fenced back yard. The *Home* data reveals all scores above 83 percentile indicating that the parents provide a safe environment for development of social, cognitive, and emotional competencies. The home is physically safe for the child. Parents could not identify specifically expected developmental tasks for the forthcoming year.

**843**

**PROGRESS NOTES—cont'd**

### No. 4  Need for knowledge and guidance in the care of the child with a chronic illness—cont'd

**A**  Provision for the child's physical and developmental safety needs will allow the child to grow so he can function responsibly in society, develop a healthy ego, and develop the capacity for intellectual thought. Differentiation of the personality is viewed by Lewin as expanding the cells or life spaces in the child's perceptual motor areas produced by internal drives and psychologic tension reduction. Cognitive development can be stimulated with knowledge of Piaget's stages of epigenesis of thought. Affectively the child must master the stages of Erikson's affective development for healthy ego function and adaptive living. Need to share with the parents data that validates their provision of a developmentally safe environment. Parents seem to view Jerry as having the same needs as a well child, which allows parenting that is not oversolicitous of child's illness. Will provide parents with written material to reinforce information about his cognitive, emotional, social, and physical needs.

**P**  Continue with present plan. Add long-range goals.
Obj. 3  Jerry will progress into stage of industry vs. inferiority.
Obj. 4  Jerry will demonstrate ability to master age-appropriate social tasks.
Obj. 5  Parents stimulate cognitive development leading to intellectual thought.

## NURSING ORDERS

6/31/78    **No. 1   Incomplete data base**        **PERSONNEL**

Obj. 1   The family will assist the nurse in the process of data collection and problem identification on an ongoing basis.

     A.   Continue at each visit to elicit new data about Jerry and the family (ongoing).     C.S.

     B.   Plan regular home visits convenient for the family (ongoing).     Family C.S.

6/31/78    **No. 3   Child health maintenance**

3,A   Child with chronic illness affecting the physical competency.

Obj. 5   Jerry should demonstrate the ability to share responsibility for regulating his therapy with his parents.

     A.   Teach parents to give Jerry reasons for the pulmonary therapy, drugs, and dietary treatment. (7/6)     C.S. Parents

     B.   Instruct Jerry to describe why he believes he receives treatments and drugs. (7/7)     C.S. Parents

     C.   Teach parents to use puppets or dolls to build connections between therapeutic procedures and his illness. (7/7)     C.S. Parents

Obj. 6   Jerry should eventually demonstrate the ability to regulate his therapy for maintenance of his physical competency.

     A.   Discuss with the parents that this must be the long-term goal for the child. (7/7)     C.S. Parents

     B.   Elicit their ideas for this preparation. (6/7)     C.S. Parents

3,B   Provision of optimum learning and thought competency for a chronically ill child

Obj. 1   Continue orders B-D.

Obj. 2   Jerry will demonstrate ability for intellectual thought.

     A.   Identify for the parents the definition of intellectual thought as the highest level of cognitive development. (7/7)     C.S.

     B.   Discuss with them how mastery of the basic concepts of each cognitive stage will allow Jerry full cognitive development.     C.S.

3,C   Expansion of life spaces related to maintaining social competency of the chronically ill child

Obj. 1   Completed. Orders A, B, C completed.

Obj. 2   Continue orders A-D as stated.

Obj. 3   Jerry will demonstrate ability to master age-appropriate social tasks.

     A.   Continue to follow his school progress (ongoing).     C.S.

**845**

**NURSING ORDERS—cont'd**

6/31/78 **No. 3   Child health maintenance—cont'd**

B. Arrange a time when child can be observed interacting with peers. (7/7)   C.S.

C. Explore other methods of which the parents have thought to expand his social competency. (7/7)   Parents C.S.

Obj. 4   Jerry will demonstrate ability to function responsibly in society.

A. Educate parents as to this long-term goal as the product of appropriate mastery of social tasks. (7/7)   C.S.

B. Elicit from them how they envision Jerry functioning as an adult. (7/7)   Parents C.S.

3,D   Inner competency needs related to child with chronic illness

Obj. 1   Jerry should demonstrate a positive sense of self.
A. Orders B-E notated as implemented.
B. Revise Obj. 1 and place A under revised objective.

Obj. 1   (Revised.) Jerry should demonstrate the ability to play or draw as a medium for expressing inner needs.

A. Have Jerry repeat drawing a picture of himself (ongoing).   Jerry C.S.

B. Plan a play session with a "sick doll" and record roles and comments. (7/7)   C.S.

C. Teach parents to use observations and play to assist in identifying fears or needs. (7/7)   Parents C.S.

Obj. 2   Jerry will demonstrate coping mechanisms that will provide for a positive sense of self.

A. Educate parents to behaviors that indicate defense mechanisms used in coping. (7/7)   C.S.

B. Teach parents to verbalize affective or feeling tones and to clarify Jerry's nonverbal expressions with expressed verbal counterparts by questioning. (7/7)   C.S. Parents

6/31/78 **No. 4   Need for knowledge and guidance in the care of the child with a chronic illness**

4,A   Child entering preschool

Obj. 1   The parents should develop coping mechanisms for handling problems related to child's presence in preschool.
Continue orders A-C and G.   C.S.

4,B   Management of child's illness

Obj. 1   Orders A-C discontinued.

Obj. 2   The parents should be able to perform a respiratory assessment on Jerry using physical exam techniques.
Revise A-C to read:

    A. Have parents assess child's respiratory status using auscultatory techniques before and after treatments. (7/7)     Parents C.S.

    B. Provide literature and a tape recording of abnormal breath sounds. (7/7)     C.S.

    C. Monitor their auscultation at the home visit. (7/7)     C.S.

    D. Teach parents other aspects of respiratory assessment:     C.S. Parents

      1. Behavioral signs of respiratory distress

      2. Retractions of chest wall and suprasternal notch

      3. Elevation of heart rate

      4. Color of conjunctivae and mucosas

      5. Degree of clubbing (7/7)

Obj. 3   Parents will identify verbally their feelings (anxiety, guilt, and fear) that may affect management of the child's illness.

    A. Explore with parents feelings associated with care for the child. (7/7)     Parents C.S.

4,C   Coping with family problems produced by chronically ill child

Obj. 1   The family should develop basic strategies for coping with problems produced by their chronically ill child.
Continue A, D-F.     C.S.
Omit B and C.     C.S.

4,D   Provision for safety needs of the preschooler.

Continue with present orders. Add Obj. 3-5 to nursing orders.     C.S.

Obj. 3   Jerry will progress into the stage of industry vs. inferiority.

    A. Provide parents with literature about ego development and methods by which the child can resolve the present tasks in initiative vs. guilt. (7/7)     C.S.

Obj. 4   Jerry will demonstrate the ability to master age-appropriate social tasks.

    A. Elicit from parents what future socialization experiences they can provide. (7/7)     Parents C.S.

Obj. 5   Parents will be able to stimulate cognitive development leading to intellectual thought.     Parents

    A. Outline the major cognitive tasks of each stage and ways of stimulating the mastery of cognitive concepts. (7/7)     C.S. Parents

## Jerry's thoracic dimensions*

|  | Lateral | Norm* | Anteroposterior | Norm* |
|---|---|---|---|---|
| 2 mos. | 13 | 13 | 10 | 10.2 |
| 4 mos. | 14 | 13.8 | 11 | 11.2 |
| 10 mos. | 15 | 15.4 | 11 | 12.0 |
| 1 year | 15 | 16.1 | 13 | 13 |
| 2 years | 16 | 16.7 | 12 | 13.1 |
| 3 years | 18 | 16.9 | 14 | 12.6 |
| 3½ years | 17 | 17.1 | 13 | 12.7 |

*Data from Meredith, H. V.: The rhythm of physical growth, vol. 2, no. 3, Iowa City, 1935, University of Iowa.

### Pulmonary function studies

None done yet. No available data.

## HEALTH STATUS LIST—Randy

| Onset | Date | No. | Active | Date | Inactive/resolved |
|---|---|---|---|---|---|
|  |  | 1 | Incomplete data base |  |  |
| ? | ? | 2 |  | 3/13/78 | Ear infections |
| 12/74 | 6/13/78 | 3 | Acute lymphoblastic leukemia |  |  |
| 12/74 | 6/13/78 | 4 |  |  | Relapses of ALL |
|  |  |  |  | 12/74 | a. C.N.S. |
|  |  |  |  | 9/75 | b. Testicular |
|  |  |  |  | 12/76 | c. Bone marrow |
|  |  |  |  | 2/78 | d. Viral effusions of lungs |
| 9/21/69 | 6/13/78 | 5 | Child health maintenance |  |  |
|  |  | 5,A | Physical competency |  |  |
|  |  | 5,B | Learning and thought competency |  |  |
|  |  | 5,C | Social competency |  |  |
|  |  | 5,D | Inner competency |  |  |
| 9/21/69 | 6/13/78 | 6 | Provision of safe home environment |  |  |
| ? | 6/13/78 | 7 | Preservation of family stability |  |  |

Client **Randy G.**  Sex M  Age 8  B.D. 9/21/69
Date 3/13/78  Race Cauc.

**Information sources:** Randy
Parents
Record

### Reason health care worker sought client

Randy is seen almost weekly in clinic. He is in terminal stages of acute lymphoblastic leukemia. Family may need support during the child's final treatment phases.

### Reason for seeking health care (mother's and child's comments)

Last month child was hospitalized for chest pain diagnosed as viral pleuritic effusion. Had bone marrow and transfusions last week. Vincristine and prednisone not effective so a new experimental drug, vindesine, is being used to maintain remission. It is not known if the drug will work with Randy. Parents may need some support and nursing interventions during this period.

### What events led up to the situation?

In 1974 was diagnosed with acute lymphoblastic leukemia and has had "many" exacerbations. Has been in a hematology management program; sometimes seen weekly for tests and medications.

### When did this situation occur?

Randy has had "the flu" and has not been feeling well since last week's treatments in the clinic. Has returned today for a bone marrow and IV medication.

**Describe the situation and/or how you are feeling. What made you decide to seek health care?**

Mother states she is relieved that Randy is feeling better since last week and he is beginning to play again. Child wishes to return to school. Nurse sought out this family as they may need intervention to support them should present therapy not be effective.

**What do you and your family do when something like this happens?**

Family attempts to make Randy as comfortable as possible. Mother's father, who lives nearby, helps her with Randy and comes with them to each clinic visit. He is involved in Randy's case. Five-year-old sister is beginning to be more sympathetic with Randy when he is not feeling well.

**How is this affecting you and your family at the present time?**

Mother states home life is geared to allowing Randy to function as best he can: limiting visitors to prevent him catching something, homebound teachers for school. Family has become accustomed to this life-style.

## MOTHER PROFILE
HEALTH HISTORY

Marcia, age 37. Stays at home with children. Is college graduate. Taught speech and drama for seven years before Randy's birth. Seems energetic and talks freely.

**Present health status**

No present problems; believes she is in "good health."

**Previous medical-surgical events**

Has history of sinusitis.

PRENATAL HISTORY WITH THIS CHILD (RANDY)

Regular prenatal care and no complications of pregnancy (Gr i Para i $AB_0$)

**Medical supervision**

Regular obstetrical visits.

**Nutrition, diet**

Weight gain—she can't remember. Ate most anything she desired. Transient morning sickness in early pregnancy.

**Illness, infections, complications**

None during pregnancy.

**Treatments, procedures**

None she can remember.

**Anesthesia**

Saddle block, she thinks. Remembers no drugs.

**Course of labor and delivery**

Labor was complicated by abruptio placenta. Labor began prematurely with gestation estimated at 33 weeks.

**Availability in home**

Stays at home. Helps operate a family photography business located in the home—in "what used to be their garage."

**Number of people in the home**

Father—Jack, age 41; mother—Marcia, age 37; Randy—age 8; Melissa—age 5. Maternal grandparents live nearby.

**Employment/work environment**

Assists in the family business when time allows.

Cases
**Date of last menstrual period**
3/1/78.

**FATHER PROFILE**
Currently a college professor. Teaches physics. Was formerly an engineer.

**Present health status**
"Good."

**Previous medical-surgical events**
Has in past had "colitis."

**Number of people he supports**
His own nuclear family—five persons.

**Availability in home/work habits**
Available most evenings after work. Works in photography shop at home.

**Employment/work environment**
College professor, teaches several levels of physics. Drives 20 minutes to work.

**Range of income**
$20,000 yearly. Own their home in the suburbs.

**Insurance**
Two types of hospitalization: a private and a group plan that pays most of their medical costs. Have car, home, and life insurance.

LIFE CHANGE EVENTS (dates)
No recent life change events. Son has been ill since 1974.
Death (family, close friend) No   New baby No
Divorce No   Marital separation No   Return to school No
Injury, illness Son since 1974   Job loss No
Change of residence No   Retirement No
**Pedigree (include chronic, inherited conditions, allergies, causes of death, illness in siblings):**

A.W. = Alive and well
O = Female
□ = Male
? = Unknown

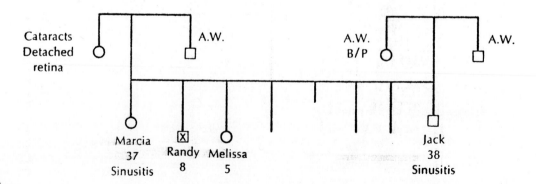

Cataracts Detached retina

A.W.

A.W. B/P

A.W.

Marcia 37 Sinusitis    Randy 8    Melissa 5    Jack 38 Sinusitis

**Does your family see itself as a healthy family or as a sick family?**

They believe they are generally a healthy family.

## CHILD PROFILE
HEALTH HISTORY
**Neonatal status (risk, Apgar, congenital abnormalities)**

Born at 33 weeks' gestation weighing 3 lbs. and 2 ounces. No congenital abnormalities noted. No data as to Apgar. By gestational age was high risk.

**Postnatal course**

Stayed in hospital for five weeks after birth. Mother knows little of his hospital course.

**Previous illnesses (dates)**

Diagnosed with ALL 4/74
Numerous ear infections as baby (dates?)
CNS relapse 12/74. Testicular relapse 9/75.
Bone marrow relapse 12/76.
Hospitalized for viral pleuritic effusion of lungs 2/78.
2/78 had thoracentesis and bone marrow during hospitalization.
3/1/78 contracted "flu bug."
Over the years had mouth ulcerations from Methotrexate.

**Medications**

Until recently received weekly IV Vincristine and Cytoxan in clinic. Experimental drug vindestine has been started now. Tylenol with codeine every six hours for pain.

**Accidents and injuries (dates)**

Mother can remember none.

**Nutrition history (example of 24-hour intake)**

During virus two weeks ago, lost his appetite. Now is eating good.

| BREAKFAST | LUNCH | SUPPER | SNACKS |
|---|---|---|---|
| Cereal with milk | Peanut butter and | Roast beef | Fruits |
| Toast/butter | jelly sandwich | Green beans | Cheeses |
| Hot chocolate | Banana | Potatoes | Chips |
| | French fries | Twinkies | |
| | Milk | Milk | |

**Food groups**

Meats (2) _2_  Veg. (4) _3_  Fruit _2_  Breads/cereals (4) _4_  Milk/products (3) _3_

**Formula: type/amt.**

Similac with iron until he began baby foods.

**Compare weight/height/age ratio**

8 yrs., weight = 23.1 kg (10%); height = 120.5 cm (10%)

**Identify developmental milestones**

After neonatal period gained weight rapidly. Walked at 8 months, babbled at 5-6 months.

**Sleep patterns/disturbances**

Mother states he sleeps until he has pain, and she will get up about once a night to give Tylenol when he's hurting.

**Allergies**

No medication allergies, but mother believes he may have some environmental allergies.

**Immunizations**

No immunizations since 3½. Has had DPT and TOPV X4 and has had MMR (record confirms).

**851**

Cases    PSYCHOLOGIC PROFILE (data here to be obtained during interactions, inquiry, observation, DDST)

| **COGNITION** | **EGO** |
| CONCRETE OPERATIONS: OPERATIONAL THOUGHT | INDUSTRY VS. INFERIORITY |
| (8-11 YEARS) | (6-13 YEARS) |

_Yes_ Operational thought: mentally orders and relates the experience to an organized whole

_Yes_ Sees events from different perspectives

_Not seen_ Able to return to starting point of an operation (reversibility)

_Not seen_ Deduction from simple experiences

_Not seen_ Concentrates on communication with peers

_Not known_ Activities segregated by sex

_Limited by illness_ Competitive activities

_Yes_ Participated eagerly in learning activities

_Yes_ Play: relives real-life situation

_Yes_ Identifies with an adult other than a parent

**Comments**

Played uninterrupted with hospital toy that had people, beds, equipment he could move from room to room. He assumed different roles (patient, doctor, father) depending on the figure he was using. He interchanged the nurse doll and mother of the patient and he made adult play partner (female) assume these roles and voice. Patient had "flu" bug. He related all the phantasized situation to the patient's situation in which the doctor, nurse, and mother were getting him some ice cream. Changing roles evidenced that he can see events from different perspectives. Child is able to play guitar and banjo. Makes B's in school.

Had much difficulty in first grade as mother reported that children started to see Randy as "different and clumsy" because "of comments and behavior of teacher." Since then he had to have a homebound teacher since this problem in classroom couldn't be resolved. These were same children he was with in kindergarten. Mother believes this very negatively has affected his self-esteem.

He does not have any peers that live nearby to play with. He tires of playing with sister who "drives me crazy" sometimes. Play indicates he reenacts real life situations, i.e., his recent hospitalization. Identifies with his grandfather and his teacher. Working through this affective phase of ego development as he relives real-life situations in play and is eager about learning.

**SCHOOL PROGRESS**
**What would you like to tell me about school?**
I want to go back to school as soon as I can.

**What do you like or dislike most about school?**
Likes being "with the kids and learning stuff." Sometimes lunches aren't good.

**Talk with parent or teacher about memory.**
Mother says Randy is bright and has a good vocabulary and remembers most everything he experiences, especially in relationship to his treatment.

**Tell me, What kind of a student do you think you are?**
"I make B's most of the time."

**PERCEPTION OF SELF**
**Self-evaluation (Describe yourself to me.)**
I'm 8 years old and have brown hair and eyes.

**Tell me things you like about yourself; dislike.**
Can't ride a bicycle very well, but I can play the banjo "O.K."

**Let's pretend you could change something about yourself. Would you change anything?**
I'd like to be able to play better.

**Describe how you feel about what's happening to you now.**

I'm at the clinic for tests and medicine.

SOCIAL PROFILE
**Personal-social**

Was busy playing, and there was no interaction observed between mother and child.

**Mother/child interaction**

He turned to tell her he was going to another part of the clinic.
Eye contact: There was eye contact during this exchange.
Touching: No touching seen.
Tone of voice of parent: Mother had medium-pitched tone of voice and addresses Randy in same tone as she did her father.
Child-parent activities: Need to explore this further.
Ease of separation: Child when hurting does not want his mother to be away from him. They are rarely separated.

**Position of child in family**

First child.

**Describe life-style**

According to data live a comfortable suburban existence geared to accommodate having a chronically ill child.
Is there more than one language spoken in the home? No

ENVIRONMENTAL PROFILE
**Pollutants**
**Population density**
**Infestations**         } Obtain this information in a home visit
**Fire hazards**
**Medications/poisons**
**Crime**

**Availability of transportation**

Mother has a car.

REVIEW OF SYSTEMS
**General**

Thin, pale 8-year-old boy, who is dressed in overalls and a plaid shirt and sneakers. Has a wide stiff gait. Eyes sparkle, and he smiles as he plays and jokes with playmate.

**Hair and scalp (dandruff, lice, cradle cap, itchiness, hair loss)**

Hair loss associated with antineoplastic medications. Last time this occurred was last year.

**Skin (infections, scaling, burns, allergies)**

Last year had eczema around mouth, which cleared up.

**Hematopoietic (anemias, bleeding, bruising)**

Hgb and Hct have been kept within normal range and medication administered to maintain WBC in 2,000-4,000 range. Has had no bleeding or bruising problems. Has had numerous bone marrow biopsies. After diagnosis received 2,250 rad's to skull and had five intrathecal injections of methotrexate. Has been on Vincristine and prednisone, methotrexate, 6-Mercaptopurine, Cytoxin at some time since his illness.

3/7/78 Hgb = 9.3 g, Hct. = 27.1, platelets 83,000 and WBC = 1,800 (1/25/78 Hgb = 12.2, Hct = 35.9, Platelets = 162,000, WBC = 12,000)

Now receives Vindesine 4 mg (per meter squared) IV weekly, which will be reduced to 3.7 mg IV weekly. Bone marrow on 2/20/78 during hospitalization revealed 83% blasts and prolymphocyte cells. No cells were seen on the cyto spin.

Remission induction was begun on third hospital day with Prednisone 40 mg/m² daily and allopurinal 200 mg/m²/day. Received on fourth hospital day IV. Vincristine 1.5 mg/m² and Adriamycin 50 mg/m². Concurrently he received large doses of analgesic (Demerol 35 mg every 3-4 hours).

### Eyes (infections, blurred vision, squinting, color blindness)

Prior exam noted L estrophia. Negative history for rest of above.

### Ears (infection, discharge, eardrum perforation, foreign objects, wax removals, decreased hearing)

Audiology exam reported mild bilateral conductive hearing loss in 1974. Has history of ear infections as a baby and toddler.

### Nose, throat, sinuses (runny nose, colds, decreased smell, foreign body, broken nose, tonsillitis)

Been under treatment for swelling of tissue in left maxillary region with reflex. Sometimes has a runny nose. No history of decreased smell, broken nose. Still has tonsils.

### Mouth and dentition (dental caries, gingivitis, malocclusion, cleft lip, and/or palate)

Negative history for the above. Occasionally medications have caused mucosal ulceration of mouth.

### Respiratory (bronchitis, pneumonia, whooping cough, histoplasmosis, tuberculosis, cough)

Chest films up to this point have shown clear lung fields and normal heart size but on 2/77 chest A-P and lateral showed small pleural effusions bilaterally. This is resolved now. Thoracentesis specimen did not show any malignant cells, WBC count was 6,700 with 13% segs, and 87% monohistoids.

### Cardiovascular (heart murmurs, cyanosis)

No history of cardiovascular problems. Sister has heart murmur and is followed in the cardiac clinic.

### Gastrointestinal (nausea/vomiting, diarrhea, constipation, jaundice, pain, colic, gas, hernias, anorexia)

Has had some nausea and vomiting and constipation associated with the drug therapy. Appetite is not as good in last few months but has improved since recent "flu" bug.

### Genitourinary (frequency, urgency, burning, toilet training, bedwetting, odor, stream)

Medications watched to avoid hemorrhagic cystitis of Cytoxan. Toilet trained at 28 months. No history of bedwetting, frequency.

### Reproductive (irritations, rashes, deviations, secondary sexual characteristics)

L testicle became enlarged and was treated—as leukemic testicular relapse. Negative history for deviations, rashes.

### Neuromuscular (convulsions, headache, imbalance, incoordination, muscle weakness, numbness, tremors, tics)

Has difficulty riding a bike in past and is not good at sports activities. Mother reports negative history of convulsions. Had CNS relapse 12/24. Has slow movements of arms and legs. Has been having leg pains and cramping in calves.

### Psychologic (thumb sucking, fears, masturbation)

Does not or did not suck thumb. Plan to discuss later with family and child his and their fears.

PHYSICAL PROFILE
**Measurements**

Head <u>21½ inches</u>  Chest <u>23½ inches</u>  Ht. <u>120.5 cm</u>  Wt. <u>23.1 kg</u>

**Vital signs**

B/P <u>100/60 R.A.</u>  H.R. <u>80/min—regular</u>  R.R. <u>24/min</u>  Temp. <u>36.4° C</u>

**Neuromuscular system**

Is oriented to time, date, and place. No gross abnormalities seen.

### Present status

Walk is wide stanced and stiff. Moves toy figures slowly and has slow grasp. Elevates head and neck slowly when he looks up to speak to a taller person.

### Social affect

Face expression is placid except when smiling. Communicates feelings, i.e., smiles when joking.

### Speech development

Speech is low but articulate, and vocabulary seems advanced.

### Reflexes

Biceps _____ 2+  
Triceps _____ 2+  
Brachioradialis ___ 1+  
Patellar _____ 1+  } Equal bilaterally  
Achilles _____ 1+  
Babinski __Negative__  
Eye __Good blink__

### Cranial nerves

I (olfactory): Intact. Identified smell of alcohol.

II (optic): Intact. Gross vision intact. Snellen to be done at a later time.

III, IV, and VI (oculomotor, trochlear, abducens): Intact. EOMs intact with L esotropia. Peripheral vision is at 90°. Slow but symmetrical blink.

V (trigeminal): Intact. Detects light touch in maxillary and mandibular areas. Equal bite bilaterally.

VII (facial): Intact. Able to mimic frown, smile, and eye squinting. Discriminates salt and sugar tastes.

VIII (acoustic): Intact. Gross hearing intact. Heard watch tick 3 inches from his ears. Need to do Weber and Rhinne (see hx).

IX, X (glossopharyngeal and vagus): Intact. Uvula in midline, gag, reflex present coordinated swallow, tongue in midline.

XI (accessory): Intact. Equal shoulder strength bilaterally.

XII (hypoglossal): Intact. Can stick tongue from side to side and equally apply pressure to cheeks.

### Cerebellar function (Rhomberg, walk heel-toe, run in place, touch tip of nose, copy hand movements, pincer grasp, draw and copy geometric shapes)

Can slowly walk heel-to-toe with difficulty. Touches tip of nose with eye closed. Slowly copies hand movements and can copy geometric shapes. Negative Rhomberg.

### Parietal lobe (object identification)

Able to tactilely identify key, paper clip, and rubber band.

### Proprioception (positional sense of toe)

Correctly identified up and down position of the big toe.

### Tactile capacity (cold, two-point discrimination, pin prick)

Feels hot and cold sensations and pin pricks on surfaces on arms and legs.

### Skin (scars, lesions, turgor, bruises, moles)

Cafe au lait spot 2 by 2 cm L forearm. Skin is pale. Rugor reflects hydrations. No bruising or petechiae seen.

### Head (circumference, fontanel measurement, palpation, transillumination)

Symmetry equal. No masses palpable on skull. Head circumference is 21½ inches (25 percentile).

### Face (expression, palpebral fissures, placement of ears, percussion of sinuses, symmetry)

Placid expression, ears in line with outer canthus of eye. No tenderness over the sinuses. Facial symmetry equal except for some L maxillary noninflammatory swelling of tissues.

Cases

### Hair, scalp (hairline, hygiene, distribution)

Hairline normal. Fine thinly distributed brown hair. Clean hair and scalp. Hair is fine and pliant.

### Eyes (strabismus, amblyopia, red reflex, conjunctiva)

Red reflex present. L. esotropia. Conjunctiva pale pink but moist and without exudates. PERRLA.

### Nose (patency, discharge, smell)

Nares patent, no septal deviations, no discharges.

### Mouth and throat (teeth, gums, pharynx, tongue, palates, swallowing, tonsils)

Tongue and mouth clean, no mucosal inflammation. Tonsils present but not enlarged. Palates intact. No caries, malocclusion. No gingival bleeding.

### Ears (landmarks, structure, hearing)

Ears close to head with supple structure. Ear canals clean and nontender. Bony landmarks visualized. Cone of light at 6-7 o'clock on the right and 4-5 o'clock on the left. No bulging or redness of tympanums. Some scarring of tympanums seen.

### Neck (nodes, masses, bruits, ROM)

No openings seen. Can slowly move through active ROM of neck. Some swelling of postcervical node on the left and slightly tender to palpation.

### Chest (symmetry, excursion, nodes, nipples)

Equal excursion bilaterally. Bilateral symmetry of thorax. No lymphadenopathy, no masses.

### Lungs (breath sounds, fremitus, percussion, duration of inspiration, expiration, rate)

Percussion symmetrically resonant; inspiration to expiration is $2:1$. Rate is 24/minute. Breath sounds negative for adventitious sounds. No flaring of nares at rest or retractions.

### Heart (size, position, PMI, sounds)

PMI is at fifth interspace at MCL. Rate is 80 per minute. $S_1$ loudest at mitral area. $S_2$ loudest at pulmonic with physiologic splitting. No M or $S_3$ or $S_4$. Pulses equal bilaterally. Extremities warm.

### Abdomen (size, contour, bowel sounds, umbilicus, liver, spleen, femorals)

Abdomen is flat. Bowel sounds are present. Liver is at right costal margin. Spleen is not palpable. No masses found on light or deep palpation. Umbilicus clean and dry. No respiratory movements of abdomen.

### Back and spine (structure, symmetry, column curvature)

Back is straight, but posture is slumped slightly at the shoulders. No kyphosis or vertebral defects. No openings in sacral area.

### Extremities (palmar creases, ROM, hip abduction)

Arms and legs thinly muscled but with equal bilateral strength. Full active and passive ROM without joint crepitus. Negative Ortalani's sign.

### Urinary (position of meatus, charae of voiding, appearance of urine)

Urinanalysis: SG = 1.023, pH = 6.5, dipstick = neg., micro = 0-2 WBCs, urine yellow and clear. Meatus normally placed.

### Genitalia (structure, secondary sexual characteristics)

Normal circumcised male with descended testes equal in size and nontender.

### Anus (structure, function)

No fissures or masses. Patent sphincter.

## INITIAL PLAN

3/13/78    **No. 1    Incomplete data base**

**S**    None.

**O**    First conversation with mother in a clinic waiting area. Mother curious about services nurse could provide and forthcoming home visit. Mother introduced her father, with whom nurse did not interact. Not enough time to thoroughly assess Randy. Nurse approached family believing they may need additional intervention from health care team.

**A**    Additional data is needed to clarify and further identify the health needs of Randy and his family. A home visit would be conducive for this purpose.

**P**    Obj. 1    The family should collaborate with nurse for planning a home visit.

6/13/74    **No. 3    Acute lymphoblastic leukemia**

**S**    Mother talked about Randy getting mouth ulcers from the medication and that he's had "many" exacerbations. Stated he's been in the hematology management program since his diagnosis. States he is coming weekly for IV medication and recently for bone marrows. Was hospitalized last month with pleural effusions determined not to be due to leukemia. Since then he has had flu compounded by starting a new drug. Randy's grandfather comes with Randy and his mother for the weekly clinic visits. Has been having cramps in his legs lately.

**O**    Diagnosed with ALL in 4/74. Has had relapses of CNS system after 12/74 after prophylactic radiation and intracathecal injections. Was in remission until 9/75 when he had L testicular swelling. Again was in remission until a relapse 12/76. Laboratory data from hospitalization of 2/20: bone marrow results 83% blasts and prolymphocyte cells; CBC-Hgb 10.1 g., Hct. 30.2, WBCs 4300, U-A normal and peripheral smear 10% blasts. Remission induction was begun 2/28/78 with prednisone and allopurinol. On 2/24 received IV vincristine and adriamycin. At this time, needed much pain medication. Was later discharged on prednisone 10 mg p.o. q.i.d. and Septra 2 teaspoons in AM and 1 teaspoon every PM. On 3/2 Hgb = 9.3 g, Hct = 27.1, platelets = 83,000, and WBCs = 1,800. Vindesine 4 mg/m$^2$ IV weekly was begun. Tylenol with codeine q 6 hours for pain ordered. Decreased DTFs upon examination. Child is very pale and has slow neuromuscular coordination. Height and weight are in the tenth percentile for his age. Cranial nerves are intact. Has adequate nutritional intake when feeling well.

**A**    Leukemia is a disease characterized by neoplastic proliferation of one of the blood-forming cells. Types of leukemia are classified according to the cell type involved and as acute or chronic depending on the state of maturity of the neoplastic cells and the expected duration of the disease. Acute leukemias are divided into two types: acute lymphoblastic (ALL) and acute nonlymphoblastic leukemia. The response to chemotherapy is much more favorable with ALL. The peak incidence of ALL occurs between the ages of 2 to 4 years. The etiology is unknown, although the following factors are thought to predispose to its development: ionizing radiation, chemical agents (chloramphenicol), hereditary factors (Down's syndrome), and viruses. It is firmly established that viruses may cause leukemia in birds, monkeys, cats, and rodents. Leukemia originates with the transformation of a single or a few hematopoietic cells. The critical

**857**

**INITIAL PLAN—cont'd**

6/13/74    **No. 3   Acute lymphoblastic leukemia—cont'd**

defect is intrinsic and inheritable by the cells' progeny. Diagnosis is confirmed and classed with bone marrow aspiration. Symptoms include pallor, petechiae, fever, bone pain, lymph node enlargement, and hepatosplenomegaly, thrombocytopenia with low, normal, or elevated WBCs and normal or low hemoglobin. Relapse after remission is caused by regrowth of residual surviving cells from the original leukemic population. Chemotherapy reduces the leukemic population so normal cells may proliferate and repopulate the bone marrow at a faster rate than the leukemic cells. If enough leukemic cells are destroyed, remission will result. Remission is defined as a 5% or less abnormal blast content in the marrow and 40% or less lymphocytes plus blasts in the marrow.

Vindesine is an investigational drug and has been used since 1975. One third of patients achieve remission in four weeks. It is given weekly intravenously and is similar to vincristine. Side effects include nausea. vomiting, abdominal pain, fever, hair loss, leukopenia, sodium and chloride imbalance. Mouth sores and skin rash rarely occur. May also produce constipation and tingling of hands and feet. Decrease DTRs in the lower legs. Other clinical manifestations include fever present in attempted remission, bleeding at any site, thrombophlebitis, local infections, bone and joint pains, and neurologic findings due to CNS infiltration. The most serious bleeding episodes develop when platelets are fewer than 20,000/mm³. Although prolonged and permanent second remissions have occurred, in general second and later remissions become progressively shorter and more difficult to maintain. Infection and bleeding and central nervous system involvement are the immediate causes of death in leukemia.

**P**    Obj. 1   Randy should demonstrate clinical manifestations of remission.

       Obj. 2   The parents should be able to verbally identify the side effects of Vindesine.

3/13/74    **No. 5   Child health maintenance**

5,A   Physical competency

**S**    Baby born at 33 weeks' gestation and was kept in nursery for five weeks. Weighed 3 lbs. and 3 ounces. Mother reports he quickly gained weight once home and proceeded through developmental milestone early, i.e., walked at 8 months. Was diagnosed with ALL 4/74. Immunized completely before diagnosed with leukemia. Mother reports child has had much leg pain recently. Randy appears small for his age. Presently is being treated to produce remission. Has difficulty riding a bike and is not good at sports activities. Mother reports son is more active since remission induction 17 days ago.

**O**    Growth charts reveal he is in tenth percentile on height and weight. B/P is 100/60, HR is 80/min and regular, and RR is 24/min. Temperature is 36.4° C. Has decreased DTRs. Walk is wide-stanced and stiff. Slowly elevates head and neck. Fine motor function of fingers is slow but precise. Speech is slow but articulate. Need to further test bone conduction hearing and vision (Snellen). Skin reflects turgor, is pale without petechiae and bruising. No bleeding in the oral cavity. Lab reveals leukopenia, thrombocytopenia, and anemia. Pleural effusion of 2/78 resolved. Lungs clear, no M, pulses equal bilaterally, L postcervical node enlarged. Good hygiene.

No dental caries. Sinuses nontender.

**A**     The essential components of assessing the well child are unchanged for the fatally ill child. Knowing the physical competency of the child allows for more pertinent intervention as this relates to his illness. In the physical realm the school-age child is learning finer neuromuscular skills for participation in work and in games. Randy has slow neuromotor functions, especially fine motor movements. This will affect the other competencies. The school-age child needs to accept the care for his own hygiene. Good dental hygiene for Randy would be important to maintain the integrity of his gums and to decrease possibility of respiratory infection from tooth decay and food accumulation. Randy is old enough to assess his own skin for bruising, nodes, or petechiae. Because of the leukopenia and thrombocytopenia, there is a great tendency to develop infections and bleeding.

**P**     Obj. 1   Randy should demonstrate the optimal physical competency for this phase of ALL.

5,B   Learning and thought competency

**S**     Mother and son state he is a B student. States he enjoys learning. Parents are college educated. Wants to go back to school. Memory is good according to mother. Child has learned to play the banjo and guitar.

**O**     In phase of concrete operations thought. Play revealed ability to see other points of view (played roles of health personnel) and that he can mentally order and relate an experience to an organized whole. Speech is articulate but slow. Sensory and motor systems are intact.

**A**     Cognitive phase of operational thought involves systematic reasoning about actual or imagined situations. Gradually hypotheses are extracted from concrete examples. The 8- or 9-year-old is realistic, reasonably self-motivated, and intellectually curious and energetic. He is busy and does not like to be interrupted. He is a good pupil and likes to plan in advance. He likes to classify, inventory, and identify. He learns by his own experience as well as from others. Randy seems to have cognitive development appropriate to his age.

**P**     Obj. 1   Randy should demonstrate cognitive abilities appropriate to his age.

5,C   Social competency

**S**     Due to problems with teacher Randy was removed from school and put on homebound program. Desires to return to school. No peer playmates nearby. Sister "drives him crazy." Parents are college educated. Mother states when child is hurting he wants her nearby. They are rarely separated. First child in the family. Live in the suburbs.

**O**     Good eye contact with nurse and mother in conversation. No touching was observed. Mother uses same tone of voice with Randy as she does with others. Records reflect mother and child were separated for five weeks after birth. No data on child-parent activities. No peer involvement.

**A**     At this age the child needs to be involved with peers, and in preadolescence the gang becomes important. A gang is a group whose membership is earned on the basis of skilled performance of some activity fre-

**859**

**INITIAL PLAN—cont'd**

3/13/74 **No. 5   Child health maintenance—cont'd**

quently physical in nature. The chum stage becomes apparent at the age of 9. A chum is a peer of same sex and age and may be the child's first love attachment outside of the home. The friend becomes an extension of the child's nonself. Randy is socially isolated except for trips to the clinic. Physical limitations do not allow for group activities of a physical nature at this time. He is missing opportunities to form important social relationships due to his illness.

**P**  Obj. 1   Randy should return to school when physically able.

Obj. 2   Randy should develop a skill that would safely allow him to become a member of a peer group.

Obj. 3   Randy should experience satisfying interactions with his family.

5,D   Inner competency

**S**  Mother related that children referred to Randy as "different and clumsy" and that the teacher allowed this situation to develop. Believes this still negatively affects his self-esteem. Dislikes being unable to ride a bicycle very well and desires to play better. No reference to word leukemia in his prognosis by mother.

**O**  Congruent image of himself academically and of his physical limitations. Refers to events of clinic when asked how he feels about what's happening to him. Affectively is in stage of industry vs. inferiority. No data about Randy's knowledge about his illness and its consequences. Expresses eagerness to learn and relives real life situations in play.

**A**  In industry vs. inferiority, the child must feel he can learn and solve problems so he can feel pride in doing something well. Parents need to have realistic expectations of the child to avoid his developing a sense of inferiority. The child under 9 or 10 years does not have a well-defined concept of final biologic death. Inner needs of the child may be met if parents discuss the illness with the child, but this may not occur until they have worked through their own grief. The predominant reaction of the fatally ill child at this age is protesting and fear of diagnostic treatments. Child of this age may regard death as a person. The child may be able to express his fears indirectly through play and behavioral changes. Parents must be careful to interpret behavioral changes and consider them an expression of inner suffering and fear rather than reactions to physical changes. Need objective evidence of the child's life space and inner perceptions to accurately give care to meet the child's inner needs.

**P**  Obj. 1   Randy should master tasks of industry for appropriate ego development

Obj. 2   Randy should be able to express fears and inner needs

3/13/78 **No. 6   Provision of a safe home environment**

**S**  Mother states home life is geared to allowing Randy to function as best he can. Aware that he has no peers with whom to play. Limit visitors in home to prevent him "catching something." Child is in school at home. Seem knowledgeable about drugs used in the past.

**O**  Child is progressing through a remission. Mother did not mention developmental needs of child. No data about environmental and safety hazards of the home.

**A** A safe home environment is provided when parents are aware of the potential physical and developmental hazards for the child. Parents need knowledge of safety precautions and of developmental tasks of child's age. Providing a safe home environment necessitates protecting the leukemic child from infection and hemorrhage and being aware of changes made in the child's care.

**P** Obj. 1  Parents should demonstrate ability to provide a safe home environment.

3/13/78 **No. 7  Preservation of family stability**

**S** Maternal grandparents are a support to the family as they live nearby. Mother believes daughter is more sympathetic toward Randy. Daughter is 5 years old. Father is home most evenings. Insurance provides for most of health expenses. Mother and Randy separated five weeks after his birth.

**O** No data about nature of parental attachment before child's illness or parents' previous reactions to experience with death or the stability of the family unit before the child's illness. Have 5-year-old daughter.

**A** Family assessment is needed to ascertain nature of the parental tie to child and degree of family stability before illness as this may influence parental response to grief and death. Most parents express feeling of hope even after they have ceased forms of denial. Predicting responses of each individual assists the professional person in support of these families as they cope. Children who are near the dying child in age or relationships tend to develop anxiety and fear on their own behalf. They may need help working through their perceptions of death. The goal of intervention of these families is to preserve the stability of the family unit from the disrupting effects of the fatal illness of the child. The extended family providing support aids in maintaining stability in most cases. Religious beliefs may strengthen the family unit. Interventions need to be aimed at providing support so parents can maintain control of child's situation and limiting uncertainty by preparing parents for complications that might occur. It is necessary that the nurse providing this kind of support be available to clients on an on-call basis when in between planned interactions. A common observation has been that parents' grief over the loss of their child is eased by the knowledge that they themselves have done everything possible to help their dying child.

**P** Obj. 1  The family should be able to function as a stable unit.

Cases

## NURSING ORDERS

| | | PERSONNEL |
|---|---|---|
| 3/13/78 | **No. 1  Incomplete data base** | |

Obj. 1  The family should collaborate with nurse for planning a home visit.

    A. Will call family 3/14 and arrange for a visit on 3/17 if agreeable.     **C.S.\***

    B. At that time, explain that after getting acquainted with Randy and them, I would like to assist them in any way possible during this time.     **C.S.**

3/13/78    **No. 3  Acute lymphoblastic leukemia**

Obj. 1  Randy should demonstrate manifestations of remission.

    A. Observe child in the home for increased tolerance to activity, increased appetite, and decrease of leg pain (ongoing).     **C.S.**

    B. Observe for initial signs of any local or general infection as WBC is 1,800 (start 3/17 ongoing).     **C.S.**

    C. At home visit reexamine child for any lymphadenopathy, hepatosplenomegaly, petechiae, bleeding, or bruising (start 3/17).     **C.S.**

    D. Teach child to assess his own skin for redness, swelling, or bruising. (3/17)     **Randy C.S.**

    E. Review CBC and bone marrow and platelet counts for clinical evidence of remission (start 3/14; ongoing).     **C.S.**

3/13/78    **No. 5  Child health maintenance**

5,A   Physical competency

Obj. 1  Randy should demonstrate the optimal physical competency for this phase of ALL.

    A. Identify the degree of endurance of physical activity through observation and talking with parents (start 3/17; ongoing).     **C.S.**

    B. Determine during home visit how much of his personal hygiene is his responsibility. (3/17)     **C.S.**

    C. Outline a program of oral hygiene (if indicated) with Randy explaining its importance. (3/21)

    D. Teach him to carefully care for and examine his skin for bruising, lymph nodes, or petechiae. (3/17)     **Randy C.S.**

    E. Assess play materials at home for purpose of searching with parents for indirect ways of working on fine motor activities. (3/17)     **C.S.**

    F. Complete sensory assessment—do Snellen, Rhinne, and Weber. (3/17)     **C.S.**

    G. Gather data about safety hazards. (3/17)     **C.S.**

Obj. 2  The parents should be able to verbally identify the side effects of Vindesine

    A. Ascertain how much information they have processed about the drug. (3/17)     **C.S.**

  *Clinical specialist.

B. Determine if they realize the implications of using one of the last drugs on the spectrum of chemotherapy. (3/17)    C.S.

C. Provide them with written information containing drug's action and side effects. (3/17)    C.S.

D. Review with them what they should observe for in Randy. (3/17)    C.S.

5,B   Learning and thought competency

Obj. 1   Randy should continue to demonstrate cognitive abilities appropriate to his age.

A. Encourage parents to take advantage of his enthusiasm to learn to develop intellectual abilities that may compensate for social loss (ongoing).    C.S.

B. Explain to parents that developmentally his ability to work alone uninterrupted is an advantage since he is a student in a home-bound program. (3/17)    C.S.

C. Talk to parents about how much Randy understands about the nature of his illness (ongoing).    C.S.

D. Talk with teacher about giving child projects that will give him a solid sense of academic achievement. (3/21)    C.S.

E. Explore with Randy other activities or games he would like to learn. (3/17)    C.S.

5,C   Social competency

Obj. 1   Randy should return to school when physically able.

A. Discuss with parents their thoughts about child returning to school. (3/23)    C.S.

B. Explain developmentally his great need to be with peers. (3/17)    C.S.

Obj. 2   Randy should develop a skill that would safely allow him to become a member of a peer group.

A. Collaborate with the home-bound teacher and Randy and choose a subject or skill his peer group at school would value (i.e., playing guitar). (3/21)    C.S.

Obj. 3   Randy should experience satisfactory interactions with his family.

A. Observe interactions of family members and communication patterns at next home visit. (3/17)    C.S.

B. Observe touching behaviors of family members as related to children. (3/17)    C.S.

C. Explore sibling relationship with parents next visit. (3/17)    C.S.

5,D   Inner competency

Obj. 1   Randy should master tasks of industry for appropriate ego development.

Cases **NURSING ORDERS—cont'd**
3/13/78 **No. 5 Child health maintenance—cont'd**

    A. Talk further with child about his school experi-   C.S.
       ence. (3/17)
    B. Have child draw a picture of himself. (3/17)   C.S.
    C. Talk with teacher to see if he could be a part of   C.S.
       competitive academic activities at home. (3/21)
    D. Encourage parents to stimulate play that relives   C.S.
       situations in reality (ongoing).

Obj. 2  Randy should be able to express fears and inner
    needs.
    A. Discuss with parents how they have dealt with   C.S.
       Randy's illness and if they have discussed ill-
       ness with Randy. (3/23)
    B. If they have not discussed illness, assess how   C.S.
       they are coping with their own grief. (3/23)
    C. Teach parents how child views death in terms of   C.S.
       his developmental level (ongoing).
    D. Establish a rapport with Randy and plan play   Parents
       sessions in which he may express fears and   C.S.
       anxieties (ongoing).
    E. Teach parents that behavioral changes and   C.S.
       protest of treatments and procedures are ways
       of expressing inner emotional suffering. (3/17)

3/13/78 **No. 6 Provision of a safe home environment**

Obj. 1  Parents should demonstrate ability to provide a
    safe home environment.
    A. Assess home environment for safety hazards.   C.S.
       (3/17)
    B. Assess parents' knowledge of their children's   C.S.
       developmental needs. (3/17)
    C. Further explore how they arrange the home en-   C.S.
       vironment to protect Randy from infection and
       bleeding (ongoing).

3/13/78 **No. 7 Preservation of family stability**

Obj. 1  The family should be able to function as a stable
    unit.
    A. Perform family assessment with all members   C.S.
       present. (3/23)
    B. Investigate with parents Melissa's reaction to
       Randy and his condition. (3/17)
    C. Document the nature of parental ties to Randy   C.S.
       before the illness and previous experiences
       with death. (3/23)
    D. Further assess support resources. (3/17)   C.S.
    E. Encourage parents to utilize nurse for questions   C.S.
       and to act as sounding board for fears and as a
       resource for aid at any time (ongoing).

## CONVERSION TABLES
### Metric system

The units of measurement in the metric system are:

**meter (m)** for length
**gram (g)** for weight
**liter** for capacity or volume
(Note: cubic centimeter [cc] also indicates volume.)

With these units the following prefixes are used:

| | |
|---|---|
| **micro** | 1/1,000,000 of a unit |
| **milli** | 0.001 (1/1000) of a unit |
| **centi** | 0.01 (1/100) of a unit |
| **deci** | 0.1 (1/10) of a unit |
| **deka** | 10 times the unit |
| **hekto** | 100 times the unit |
| **kilo** | 1,000 times the unit |
| **cubic** | the total area covered, measured in square lengths |

Thus:

1 kilogram (kg) = 1,000 grams (g)
1 gram (g) = 1,000 milligrams (mg)
1 milligram (mg) = 1,000 micrograms ($\mu$g)

### Avoirdupois and imperial systems
#### Weight

1 pound (lb) = 16 ounces (oz)
1 oz = 437.5 grains (gr)

#### Height

1 yard (yd) = 3 feet (ft)
1 foot (ft) = 12 inches (in)

#### Capacity

1 gallon = 4 quarts = 8 pints
1 quart = 2 pints
1 pint = 20 fluid ounces
1 fluid ounce = 8 drams (or drachm)
1 dram = 60 minims

## Conversion of pounds to kilograms for pediatric weights

| Pounds→ ↓ | 0 | 1 | 2 | 3 | 4 | 5 | 6 | 7 | 8 | 9 |
|---|---|---|---|---|---|---|---|---|---|---|
| 0 | 0.00 | 0.45 | 0.90 | 1.36 | 1.81 | 2.26 | 2.72 | 3.17 | 3.62 | 4.08 |
| 10 | 4.53 | 4.98 | 5.44 | 5.89 | 6.35 | 6.80 | 7.25 | 7.71 | 8.16 | 8.61 |
| 20 | 9.07 | 9.52 | 9.97 | 10.43 | 10.88 | 11.34 | 11.79 | 12.24 | 12.70 | 13.15 |
| 30 | 13.60 | 14.06 | 14.51 | 14.96 | 15.42 | 15.87 | 16.32 | 16.78 | 17.23 | 17.69 |
| 40 | 18.14 | 18.59 | 19.05 | 19.50 | 19.95 | 20.41 | 20.86 | 21.31 | 21.77 | 22.22 |
| 50 | 22.68 | 23.13 | 23.58 | 24.04 | 24.49 | 24.94 | 25.40 | 25.85 | 26.30 | 26.76 |
| 60 | 27.21 | 27.66 | 28.12 | 28.57 | 29.03 | 29.48 | 29.93 | 30.39 | 30.84 | 31.29 |
| 70 | 31.75 | 32.20 | 32.65 | 33.11 | 33.56 | 34.02 | 34.47 | 34.92 | 35.38 | 35.83 |
| 80 | 36.28 | 36.74 | 37.19 | 37.64 | 38.10 | 38.55 | 39.00 | 39.46 | 39.91 | 40.37 |
| 90 | 40.82 | 41.27 | 41.73 | 42.18 | 42.63 | 43.09 | 43.54 | 43.99 | 44.45 | 44.90 |
| 100 | 45.36 | 45.81 | 46.26 | 46.72 | 47.17 | 47.62 | 48.08 | 48.53 | 48.98 | 49.44 |
| 110 | 49.89 | 50.34 | 50.80 | 51.25 | 51.71 | 52.16 | 52.61 | 53.07 | 53.52 | 53.97 |
| 120 | 54.43 | 54.88 | 55.33 | 55.79 | 56.24 | 56.70 | 57.15 | 57.60 | 58.06 | 58.51 |
| 130 | 58.96 | 59.42 | 59.87 | 60.32 | 60.78 | 61.23 | 61.68 | 62.14 | 62.59 | 63.05 |
| 140 | 63.50 | 63.95 | 64.41 | 64.86 | 65.31 | 65.77 | 66.22 | 66.67 | 67.13 | 67.58 |
| 150 | 68.04 | 68.49 | 68.94 | 69.40 | 69.85 | 70.30 | 70.76 | 71.21 | 71.66 | 72.12 |
| 160 | 72.57 | 73.02 | 73.48 | 73.93 | 74.39 | 74.84 | 75.29 | 75.75 | 76.20 | 76.65 |
| 170 | 77.11 | 77.56 | 78.01 | 78.47 | 78.92 | 79.38 | 79.83 | 80.28 | 80.74 | 81.19 |
| 180 | 81.64 | 82.10 | 82.55 | 83.00 | 83.46 | 83.91 | 84.36 | 84.82 | 85.27 | 85.73 |
| 190 | 86.18 | 86.68 | 87.09 | 87.54 | 87.99 | 88.45 | 88.90 | 89.35 | 89.81 | 90.26 |
| 200 | 90.72 | 91.17 | 91.62 | 92.08 | 92.53 | 92.98 | 93.44 | 93.89 | 94.34 | 94.80 |

## Conversion of pounds and ounces to kilograms

| Pounds | Kilograms | Ounces | Kilograms | Pounds | Kilograms | Ounces | Kilograms |
|---|---|---|---|---|---|---|---|
| 1 | 0.454 | 1 | 0.028 | 9 | 4.082 | 9 | 0.255 |
| 2 | 0.907 | 2 | 0.057 | 10 | 4.536 | 10 | 0.283 |
| 3 | 1.361 | 3 | 0.085 | 11 | 4.990 | 11 | 0.312 |
| 4 | 1.814 | 4 | 0.113 | 12 | 5.443 | 12 | 0.340 |
| 5 | 2.268 | 5 | 0.142 | 13 | 5.897 | 13 | 0.369 |
| 6 | 2.722 | 6 | 0.170 | | | 14 | 0.397 |
| 7 | 3.175 | 7 | 0.198 | | | 15 | 0.425 |
| 8 | 3.629 | 8 | 0.227 | | | | |

# Conversion of pounds and ounces to grams

| Pounds | 0 | 1 | 2 | 3 | 4 | 5 | 6 | 7 | 8 | 9 | 10 | 11 | 12 | 13 | 14 | 15 |
|---|---|---|---|---|---|---|---|---|---|---|---|---|---|---|---|---|
| | | | | | | | | | | Ounces | | | | | | |
| 0 | — | 28 | 57 | 85 | 113 | 142 | 170 | 198 | 227 | 255 | 283 | 312 | 340 | 369 | 397 | 425 |
| 1 | 454 | 482 | 510 | 539 | 567 | 595 | 624 | 652 | 680 | 709 | 737 | 765 | 794 | 822 | 850 | 879 |
| 2 | 907 | 936 | 964 | 992 | 1021 | 1049 | 1077 | 1106 | 1134 | 1162 | 1191 | 1219 | 1247 | 1276 | 1304 | 1332 |
| 3 | 1361 | 1389 | 1417 | 1446 | 1474 | 1503 | 1531 | 1559 | 1588 | 1616 | 1644 | 1673 | 1701 | 1729 | 1758 | 1786 |
| 4 | 1814 | 1843 | 1871 | 1899 | 1928 | 1956 | 1984 | 2013 | 2041 | 2070 | 2098 | 2126 | 2155 | 2183 | 2211 | 2240 |
| 5 | 2268 | 2296 | 2325 | 2353 | 2381 | 2410 | 2438 | 2466 | 2495 | 2523 | 2551 | 2580 | 2608 | 2637 | 2665 | 2693 |
| 6 | 2722 | 2750 | 2778 | 2807 | 2835 | 2863 | 2892 | 2920 | 2948 | 2977 | 3005 | 3033 | 3062 | 3090 | 3118 | 3147 |
| 7 | 3175 | 3203 | 3232 | 3260 | 3289 | 3317 | 3345 | 3374 | 3402 | 3430 | 3459 | 3487 | 3515 | 3544 | 3572 | 3600 |
| 8 | 3629 | 3657 | 3685 | 3714 | 3742 | 3770 | 3799 | 3827 | 3856 | 3884 | 3912 | 3941 | 3969 | 3997 | 4026 | 4054 |
| 9 | 4082 | 4111 | 4139 | 4167 | 4196 | 4224 | 4252 | 4281 | 4309 | 4337 | 4366 | 4394 | 4423 | 4451 | 4479 | 4508 |
| 10 | 4536 | 4564 | 4593 | 4621 | 4649 | 4678 | 4706 | 4734 | 4763 | 4791 | 4819 | 4848 | 4876 | 4904 | 4933 | 4961 |
| 11 | 4990 | 5018 | 5046 | 5075 | 5103 | 5131 | 5160 | 5188 | 5216 | 5245 | 5273 | 5301 | 5330 | 5358 | 5386 | 5415 |
| 12 | 5443 | 5471 | 5500 | 5528 | 5557 | 5585 | 5613 | 5642 | 5670 | 5698 | 5727 | 5755 | 5783 | 5812 | 5840 | 5868 |
| 13 | 5897 | 5925 | 5953 | 5982 | 6010 | 6038 | 6067 | 6095 | 6123 | 6152 | 6180 | 6209 | 6237 | 6265 | 6294 | 6322 |
| 14 | 6350 | 6379 | 6407 | 6435 | 6464 | 6492 | 6520 | 6549 | 6577 | 6605 | 6634 | 6662 | 6690 | 6719 | 6747 | 6776 |
| 15 | 6804 | 6832 | 6860 | 6889 | 6917 | 6945 | 6973 | 7002 | 7030 | 7059 | 7087 | 7115 | 7144 | 7172 | 7201 | 7228 |
| 16 | 7257 | 7286 | 7313 | 7342 | 7371 | 7399 | 7427 | 7456 | 7484 | 7512 | 7541 | 7569 | 7597 | 7626 | 7654 | 7682 |
| 17 | 7711 | 7739 | 7768 | 7796 | 7824 | 7853 | 7881 | 7909 | 7938 | 7966 | 7994 | 8023 | 8051 | 8079 | 8108 | 8136 |
| 18 | 8165 | 8192 | 8221 | 8249 | 8278 | 8306 | 8335 | 8363 | 8391 | 8420 | 8448 | 8476 | 8504 | 8533 | 8561 | 8590 |
| 19 | 8618 | 8646 | 8675 | 8703 | 8731 | 8760 | 8788 | 8816 | 8845 | 8873 | 8902 | 8930 | 8958 | 8987 | 9015 | 9043 |
| 20 | 9072 | 9100 | 9128 | 9157 | 9185 | 9213 | 9242 | 9270 | 9298 | 9327 | 9355 | 9383 | 9412 | 9440 | 9469 | 9497 |
| 21 | 9525 | 9554 | 9582 | 9610 | 9639 | 9667 | 9695 | 9724 | 9752 | 9780 | 9809 | 9837 | 9865 | 9894 | 9922 | 9950 |
| 22 | 9979 | 10007 | 10036 | 10064 | 10092 | 10120 | 10149 | 10177 | 10206 | 10234 | 10262 | 10291 | 10319 | 10347 | 10376 | 10404 |

## Approximate metric and imperial equivalents

| Metric | Imperial | Metric | Imperial |
|--------|----------|--------|----------|
| 30 g | 1 oz | 30 mg | ½ gr |
| 15 g | ½ oz | 20 mg | ⅓ gr |
| 8 g | 120 gr | 15 mg | ¼ gr |
| 4 g | 60 gr | 10 mg | ⅙ gr |
| 2 g | 30 gr | 7.5 mg | ⅛ gr |
| 1 g | 15 gr | 6 mg | 1/10 gr |
| 600 mg | 10 gr | 3 mg | 1/20 gr |
| 450 mg | 7½ gr | 1 mg | 1/60 gr |
| 300 mg | 5 gr | (1,000 $\mu$g) | |
| 250 mg | 4 gr | 0.6 mg | 1/100 gr |
| 200 mg | 3 gr | 0.5 mg | 1/120 gr |
| 150 mg | 2½ gr | 0.3 mg | 1/200 gr |
| 100 mg | 1½ gr | 0.2 mg | 1/300 gr |
| 60 mg | 1 gr | 0.1 mg | 1/600 gr |
| 50 mg | ¾ gr | | |

Useful approximate metric and imperial equivalents:

| | |
|---|---|
| 1 cm = 0.39 inches | 1 in = 2.54 cm |
| 1 meter = 1.1 yards | 1 ft = 30.48 cm |

To convert centimeters to inches:
  Divide the length in centimeters by 2.54.
  EXAMPLE: The average newborn infant measures 50.8 cm:

$$\frac{50.8}{2.54} = 20 \text{ inches}$$

To convert inches to centimeters:
  Multiply the length in inches by 2.54.
  EXAMPLE: The average newborn infant measures 20 inches:

$$20 \times 2.54 = 50.8 \text{ cm}$$

## Approximate weight equivalents

| Apothecary | Metric | Apothecary | Metric |
|------------|--------|------------|--------|
| 1/320 gr | 0.2 mg | ½ gr | 32.0 mg |
| 1/210 gr | 0.3 mg | ¾ gr | 50.0 mg |
| 1/160 gr | 0.4 mg | 1 gr | 65.0 mg |
| 1/100 gr | 0.65 mg | 1½ gr | 0.1 g |
| 1/64 gr | 1.0 mg | 2 gr | 0.13 g |
| 1/32 gr | 2.0 mg | 2½ gr | 0.16 g |
| 1/16 gr | 4.0 mg | 3 gr | 0.2 g |
| 1/12 gr | 5.4 mg | 5 gr | 0.32 g |
| 1/10 gr | 6.5 mg | 7½ gr | 0.5 g |
| ⅛ gr | 8.0 mg | 10 gr | 0.65 g |
| ⅙ gr | 11.0 mg | 15 gr | 1.0 g |
| ¼ gr | 16.0 mg | 1 dr | 4.0 g |
| ⅓ gr | 22.0 mg | 1 oz | 30.0 g |
| ⅜ gr | 24.0 mg | | |

## Conversion of inches to centimeters

| Inches | Centimeters | Inches | Centimeters |
|--------|-------------|--------|-------------|
| 10 | 25.40 | 17½ | 44.45 |
| 10½ | 26.67 | 18 | 45.72 |
| 11 | 27.94 | 18½ | 46.99 |
| 11½ | 29.21 | 19 | 48.26 |
| 12 | 30.48 | 19½ | 49.58 |
| 12½ | 31.75 | 20 | 50.80 |
| 13 | 33.02 | 20½ | 52.07 |
| 13½ | 34.29 | 21 | 53.34 |
| 14 | 35.56 | 21½ | 54.61 |
| 14½ | 36.83 | 22 | 55.88 |
| 15 | 38.10 | 22½ | 57.15 |
| 15½ | 39.37 | 23 | 58.42 |
| 16 | 40.61 | 23½ | 56.69 |
| 16½ | 41.91 | 24 | 60.96 |
| 17 | 43.18 | | |

## Capacity (volume) equivalents

**Useful approximate metric and imperial equivalents**

| | |
|---|---|
| 1 liter | = 1.75 pints |
| 1 oz | = 30 ml |
| 1 pint | = 0.568 liters or 568 ml |
| 1 gallon | = 4.55 liters |

**Conversion table**

| Liters | | Pints |
|--------|---|-------|
| 0.28 | 0.5 | 0.88 |
| 0.57 | 1 | 1.75 |
| 1.14 | 2 | 3.50 |
| 1.70 | 3 | 5.28 |
| 1.28 | 4 | 7.04 |
| 2.85 | 5 | 8.80 |
| 3.42 | 6 | 10.50 |
| 3.99 | 7 | 12.30 |
| 4.55 | 8 | 14.08 |

To read the table:  3 liters = 5.28 pints
3 pints = 1.70 liters

## Household measurements

| | Apothecary | Metric |
|---|------------|--------|
| 1 teaspoon | 1 dram | 4 ml |
| 1 tablespoon | ½ fl oz | 15 ml |
| 1 teacup | 4 oz | 120 ml |
| 1 tumbler | 8 oz | 240 ml |

## Approximate volume equivalents

| Apothecary | Metric | Apothecary | Metric |
|---|---|---|---|
| 1 minim | 0.06 ml | 80 minims | 5.0 ml |
| 1⅝ minims | 0.1 ml | 2 fl dr | 7.5 ml |
| 3 minims | 0.18 ml | 2¾ fl dr | 10.0 ml |
| 5 minims | 0.3 ml | 4 fl dr | 15.0 ml |
| 8 minims | 0.5 ml | 5½ fl dr | 20.0 ml |
| 10 minims | 0.6 ml | 1 fl oz | 30.0 ml |
| 12 minims | 0.75 ml | 1⅔ fl oz | 50.0 ml |
| 15 minims | 0.9 ml | 2 fl oz | 60.0 ml |
| 16 minims | 1.0 ml | 3⅜ fl oz | 100.0 ml |
| 20 minims | 1.2 ml | 4 fl oz | 120.0 ml |
| 30 minims | 1.8 ml | 8 fl oz | 240.0 ml |
| 50 minims | 3.0 ml | 12 fl oz | 360.0 ml |
| 1 fl dr | 3.7 ml | 1 pt | 480.0 ml |
| 65 minims | 4.0 ml | | |

## Temperature equivalents

| Centigrade | Fahrenheit | Centigrade | Fahrenheit |
|---|---|---|---|
| 34.0 | 93.2 | 39.0 | 102.2 |
| 34.2 | 93.6 | 39.2 | 102.5 |
| 34.4 | 93.9 | 39.4 | 102.9 |
| 34.6 | 94.3 | 39.6 | 103.2 |
| 34.8 | 94.6 | 39.8 | 103.6 |
| 35.0 | 95.0 | 40.0 | 104.0 |
| 35.2 | 95.4 | 40.2 | 104.3 |
| 35.4 | 95.7 | 40.4 | 104.7 |
| 35.6 | 96.1 | 40.6 | 105.1 |
| 35.8 | 96.4 | 40.8 | 105.4 |
| 36.0 | 96.8 | 41.0 | 105.8 |
| 36.2 | 97.1 | 41.2 | 106.1 |
| 36.4 | 97.5 | 41.4 | 106.5 |
| 36.6 | 97.8 | 41.6 | 106.8 |
| 36.8 | 98.2 | 41.8 | 107.2 |
| 37.0 | 98.6 | 42.0 | 107.6 |
| 37.2 | 98.9 | 42.2 | 108.0 |
| 37.4 | 99.3 | 42.4 | 108.3 |
| 37.6 | 99.6 | 42.6 | 108.7 |
| 37.8 | 100.0 | 42.8 | 109.0 |
| 38.0 | 100.4 | 43.0 | 109.4 |
| 38.2 | 100.7 | | |
| 38.4 | 101.1 | | |
| 38.6 | 101.4 | | |
| 38.8 | 101.8 | | |

## Chest circumference for Negro children, in centimeters*

| | Chest circumference | | | |
|---|---|---|---|---|
| | Boys | | Girls | |
| Age | Mean | SD | Mean | SD |
| 3 months | 38.2 | 3.3 | 38.1 | 1.8 |
| 6 months | 41.7 | 1.9 | 40.2 | 2.4 |
| 9 months | 42.7 | 2.5 | 41.7 | 2.8 |
| 12 months | 43.7 | 2.4 | 43.6 | 1.8 |
| 15 months | 44.4 | 2.3 | 44.2 | 2.8 |
| 18 months | 46.2 | 2.9 | 45.3 | 2.6 |
| 21 months | 47.4 | 2.4 | 46.4 | 2.9 |
| 24 months | 48.6 | 3.4 | 47.0 | 3.3 |
| 2½ years | 49.6 | 3.3 | 47.6 | 3.1 |
| 3 years | 50.1 | 3.1 | 48.0 | 3.2 |
| 3½ years | 50.7 | 3.4 | 48.4 | 3.4 |
| 4 years | 50.8 | 4.0 | 48.9 | 3.1 |
| 4½ years | 51.4 | 2.4 | 49.8 | 3.1 |
| 5 years | 52.3 | 4.1 | 52.7 | 3.1 |
| 5½ years | 54.3 | 3.6 | 53.5 | 3.8 |
| 6 years | 56.5 | 3.8 | 54.7 | 3.8 |
| 7 years | 58.5 | 3.6 | 56.0 | 3.2 |
| 8 years | 60.8 | 3.0 | 58.2 | 4.6 |
| 9 years | 62.9 | 3.4 | 60.4 | 6.4 |
| 10 years | 64.5 | 4.5 | 62.0 | 5.2 |
| 11 years | 66.5 | 3.7 | 64.4 | 7.0 |
| 12 years | 70.3 | 5.4 | 66.1 | 4.0 |
| 13 years | 73.6 | 5.7 | 67.6 | 6.1 |
| 14 years | 76.8 | 5.9 | 68.0 | 4.2 |
| 15 years | 80.7 | 5.6 | 68.6 | 5.3 |
| 16 years | 83.8 | 4.5 | 70.2 | 3.8 |
| 17 years | 85.6 | 6.3 | 70.8 | 9.5 |

For conversion: 1 inch = 2.54 cm

*Derived from measurements obtained from 2,632 well children from low-income families in Washington, D.C. Abstracted from Verghese, K. P., Scott, R. B., Teixeira, G., and Ferguson, A. D.: Studies in growth and development. XII. Physical growth of North American Negro children, Pediatrics **44**:243, Aug., 1969. Graphs prepared from those of Freedmen's Hospital, Department of Pediatrics, Washington, D.C. Reprinted by permission of Roland B. Scott, M.D., Howard University College of Medicine, Washington, D.C.

To convert centigrade to Fahrenheit:
$$9/5 \times \text{temperature} + 32$$
EXAMPLE: To convert 40° centigrade to Fahrenheit

$$9/5 \times 40 - 72 + 32 = 104° \text{ Fahrenheit}$$

To convert Fahrenheit to centigrade:
$$(\text{Temperature} - 32) \times 5/9$$
EXAMPLE: To convert 98.6° Fahrenheit to centigrade

$$98.6 - 32 = 66.6 \times 5/9 = 37° \text{ centigrade}$$

## Chest circumference, boys and girls, birth to 5 years, in centimeters*

| Percentile (boys) | | | Chest circumference | Percentile (girls) | | |
|---|---|---|---|---|---|---|
| 10 | 50 | 90 | | 10 | 50 | 90 |
| 30.6 | 33.2 | 35.7 | Birth | 30.8 | 32.9 | 35.0 |
| 38.3 | 40.6 | 42.9 | 3 months | 37.6 | 39.8 | 42.0 |
| 41.6 | 43.7 | 46.3 | 6 months | 40.6 | 43.0 | 45.4 |
| 43.7 | 46.0 | 48.9 | 9 months | 42.7 | 45.4 | 47.9 |
| 45.1 | 47.6 | 50.7 | 12 months | 44.2 | 57.0 | 49.5 |
| 46.1 | 48.6 | 51.7 | 15 months | 45.1 | 47.9 | 50.5 |
| 47.0 | 49.5 | 52.6 | 18 months | 46.0 | 48.8 | 51.4 |
| 48.4 | 50.8 | 53.9 | 2 years | 47.4 | 50.1 | 53.0 |
| 49.3 | 51.7 | 54.9 | 2½ years | 48.4 | 51.2 | 54.3 |
| 49.9 | 52.4 | 55.8 | 3 years | 49.3 | 51.9 | 55.1 |
| 50.5 | 53.1 | 56.6 | 3½ years | 50.1 | 52.5 | 55.8 |
| 51.1 | 53.7 | 57.2 | 4 years | 50.7 | 53.1 | 56.5 |
| 51.7 | 54.4 | 58.0 | 4½ years | 51.3 | 53.7 | 57.3 |
| 52.3 | 55.0 | 58.8 | 5 years | 51.7 | 54.2 | 57.9 |

*From Nelson, W. E., Vaughan, V. C., III, and McKay, R. J., editors: Textbook of pediatrics, ed. 9, Philadelphia, 1969, W. B. Saunders Co. From Studies of Child Health and Development, Department of Maternal and Child Health, Harvard School of Public Health.

## Chest circumference, boys and girls, 5 to 18 years, in centimeters*

| Percentile (boys) | | | Chest circumference | Percentile (girls) | | |
|---|---|---|---|---|---|---|
| 10 | 50 | 90 | | 10 | 50 | 90 |
| 51.6 | 54.5 | 57.5 | 5 years | 50.2 | 52.9 | 56.5 |
| 52.4 | 55.3 | 58.5 | 5½ years | 50.9 | 53.7 | 57.4 |
| 53.2 | 56.1 | 59.5 | 6 years | 51.5 | 54.5 | 58.2 |
| 54.1 | 57.0 | 60.6 | 6½ years | 52.2 | 55.3 | 59.2 |
| 54.9 | 57.8 | 61.6 | 7 years | 52.8 | 56.1 | 60.1 |
| 55.8 | 58.8 | 62.9 | 7½ years | 53.5 | 57.0 | 61.2 |
| 56.7 | 59.8 | 64.1 | 8 years | 54.2 | 57.8 | 62.3 |
| 57.6 | 60.8 | 65.4 | 8½ years | 54.9 | 58.7 | 63.5 |
| 58.4 | 61.8 | 66.7 | 9 years | 55.5 | 59.6 | 64.7 |
| 59.3 | 62.9 | 68.1 | 9½ years | 56.2 | 60.5 | 66.1 |
| 60.1 | 63.9 | 69.4 | 10 years | 56.9 | 61.4 | 67.4 |
| 60.9 | 64.9 | 70.7 | 10½ years | 57.8 | 62.8 | 69.0 |
| 61.7 | 65.9 | 71.9 | 11 years | 58.6 | 64.2 | 70.5 |
| 62.5 | 66.9 | 73.1 | 11½ years | 59.6 | 65.5 | 72.2 |
| 63.3 | 67.8 | 74.2 | 12 years | 60.6 | 66.7 | 73.8 |
| 64.2 | 69.1 | 75.8 | 12½ years | 61.8 | 67.7 | 75.3 |
| 65.0 | 70.3 | 77.4 | 13 years | 62.9 | 68.6 | 76.7 |
| 66.3 | 72.4 | 79.4 | 13½ years | 63.8 | 69.3 | 77.7 |
| 67.6 | 74.5 | 81.4 | 14 years | 64.6 | 69.9 | 78.6 |
| 69.4 | 76.3 | 83.1 | 14½ years | 65.1 | 70.4 | 79.2 |
| 71.1 | 78.0 | 84.8 | 15 years | 65.5 | 70.9 | 79.8 |
| 72.8 | 79.4 | 86.3 | 15½ years | 65.8 | 71.3 | 80.2 |
| 74.4 | 80.7 | 87.8 | 16 years | 66.1 | 71.6 | 80.5 |
| 75.4 | 81.6 | 88.8 | 16½ years | 66.3 | 71.9 | 80.7 |
| 76.4 | 82.5 | 89.7 | 17 years | 66.4 | 72.1 | 80.9 |
| 77.0 | 83.0 | 90.2 | 17½ years | 66.5 | 72.2 | 81.0 |
| 77.5 | 83.4 | 90.7 | 18 years | 66.6 | 72.3 | 81.1 |

*From Nelson, W. E., Vaughan, V. C., III, and McKay, R. J., editors: Textbook of pediatrics, ed. 9, Philadelphia, 1969, W. B. Saunders Co. From Studies of Child Health and Development, Department of Maternal and Child Health, Harvard School of Public Health.

# Landmarks of visual development*

| Age | Characteristic development | | |
|---|---|---|---|
| Birth | Pupils react to light. Blink reflex in response to light stimulus. Corneal reflex in response to touch. Rudimentary fixation on objects with ability to follow to the midline. | 28 to 44 weeks —cont'd | Exhibits smooth visual pursuit of objects and sound in the vertical and horizontal planes. Visual acuity exceeds 20/200. |
| 2 to 4 weeks | Fixation ability advances; stares at light source. Follows to midline more reliably. Tear glands begin to function. | 44 weeks to 12 months | Transverse diameter of the cornea is 12 mm, the adult size. Amblyopia may develop with lack of binocularity. Fixates intently on facial expressions. Discriminates simple geometric forms. Visual acuity 20/100. Full binocular vision developed. |
| 4 to 12 weeks | Convergence appears. Binocular fixation is established. Follows moving objects with head and eye movements through 180 degrees. Fascinated by bright colors and lights. Tear glands display response to emotion. | 12 to 18 months | Able to identify forms. Associates with visual experiences. Displays an intent interest in pictures. Able to scribble on a paper. Convergence becomes well established. Depth perception remains crude. |
| 12 to 20 weeks | Begins to inspect own hands. Accommodation begins to develop. Able to fixate on objects more than 3 feet distant. Foveal pit becomes distinguishable as macula development proceeds. Pigmentation of fundus not developed; appearance of fundus is pale. Visual acuity 20/200. | 18 months to 2 years | Accommodation well developed. Visual acuity 20/40. |
| | | 2 to 3 years | Convergence smooth. Fixation on small objects or pictures should approach 50 seconds. Able to recall visual images. Visual acuity 20/30. |
| 20 to 28 weeks | Able to rescue a dropped block. Hand-eye coordination is developing. Binocular fixation becomes fully developed. Ultimate color of iris is established. Discrimination between simple geometric forms is beginning to develop. Color preference for reds and yellows develops. | 3 years to 4 years | Able to copy geometric figures. Reading readiness is present. Lacrimal glands are fully developed. |
| | | 5 years | Minimal potential for amblyopia to develop. Color recognition is well established. |
| 28 to 44 weeks | Depth perception begins to develop. Displays interest in tiny objects. Tilts head backward to see upward. | 6 years | Visual acuity approaches 20/20. Color shading may be differentiated. Astigmatism may develop at any point throughout life. Depth perception fully developed. |

*Adapted from Whipple, D. V.: Dynamics of development; euthenic pediatrics, New York, 1966, McGraw-Hill Book Co.; Liebman, S. D., and Gellis, S. S.: The pediatrician's ophthalmology, St. Louis, 1966, The C. V. Mosby Co.; Keeney, A. H.: Development of vision. In Falkner, F., editor: Human development, Philadelphia, 1966, W. B. Saunders Co.

## Landmarks of speech, language, and hearing ability*

| Chronological age | Receptive language | Expressive language | Related hearing ability |
|---|---|---|---|
| 3 months | | | Is startled by loud sounds and soothed by mother's voice. Lateral turning to the side of sound; turning in general direction but not looking directly at sound source. |
| 6 months | Responds by raising arms when mother says come here and reaches toward the child; responds appropriately to friendly or angry voices; moves or looks toward family member when named. | Repeats self-produced sounds; imitates sounds; vocalizes to persons; and uses 12 different phonemes. | Turns eyes and head to search for location of sound but does not necessarily find the sound source on the first attempt. Responds to mother's voice and own name, imitates own noises, and enjoys sound-making toys. |
| 8 months | | | Turns eyes and head in a sweeping motion to the sound source. Locates sound source. |
| 10 months | | | Looks directly, promptly, and predictably to the sound source. Responds to own name, telephone ringing, and someone's voice. |
| 12 months | Up to ten words, such as no, bye-bye, pat-a-cake, hot, own name; one simple direction such as sit down or give it to me; these commands are usually accompanied by gesture. | Up to 3 words besides mama and dada; may say such words as bye-bye, hi, baby, kitty, and puppy; uses up to 18 different phonemes. | Begins to show voluntary control over responses to sound; may or may not respond or may delay response. This selective response should not be interpreted as a hearing loss so long as it is intermittent and of recent origin. This might be representative of beginning of listening refinement. |
| 18 months | Up to 50 words; recognizes between 6 and 12 objects by name, such as dog, cat, bottle, ball; identifies 3 body parts such as eyes, nose, mouth; understands the concept "now," simple commands unaccompanied by gesture, such as give me the doll, open your mouth, stick out your tongue. | Up to 20 words and 21 different phonemes; jargon and echolalia are present; uses names of familiar objects and 1-word sentences such as go or eat; uses gestures; uses words such as no, mine, eat, good, bad, hot, cold, and expressions such as oh oh, what's that, all gone; the use of words may be quite inconsistent; 25% of speech is intelligible. | Has begun to develop gross discrimination by learning to distinguish between highly dissimilar noises such as doorbell and train, barking dog and auto horn, or mother's and father's voice. |

*Adapted from Weiss, C. E., and Lillywhite, H. S., Communicative disorders, St. Louis, 1976, The C. V. Mosby Co., pp. 51, 54-58, 65-66.

# Landmarks of speech, language, and hearing ability—cont'd

| Chronological age | Receptive language | Expressive language | Related hearing ability |
|---|---|---|---|
| 24 months | Up to 1,200 words; in, on, under; identifies dog, ball, engine, bed, doll, scissors, hair, mouth, feet, nose, cup, spoon, car, key; distinguishes between one and many, and formulates a negative judgment—a knife is not a fork; understands the concept "soon," simple stories; follows simple directions; is beginning to make distinctions between you and me. | Up to 270 words and 25 different phonemes; jargon and echolalia almost gone; averages 75 words per hour during free play; talks in words, phrases, and 2- to 3-word sentences; averages 2 words per response; first pronouns appear such as I, me, mine, it, who, that; adjectives and adverbs are just beginning to appear; names objects and common pictures; enjoys Mother Goose; refers to self by name such as Bobby go bye-bye; uses phrases such as I want, go bye-bye, want cookie, ball all gone. 60% of speech is intelligible. | Refinement of gross discriminative skills. |
| 30 months | Up to 2400 words; identifies action in pictures and objects by use; carries out 1- and 2-part commands such as pick up your shoe and give it to mommy; knows what we drink out of, what goes on our feet, what we can buy candy with; understands plurals, questions, difference between boy and girl, the concept "one," up, down, run, walk, throw, fast, more, my. | Up to 425 words and 27 phonemes; jargon and echolalia no longer exist; averages 140 words per hour; names words such as chair, can, box, key, door; repeats 2 digits from memory; average sentence length is about 2½ words; uses more adjectives and adverbs; demands repetition from others, such as do it again; almost always announces intentions before acting; begins to ask questions of adults; 75% of speech is intelligible. | |
| 36 months | Up to 3,600 words; understands both, two, not today, what we do when we are thirsty, hungry, sleepy, why we have stoves, wait, later, big, new, different, strong, today, another, and taking turns at play; carries out 2- and some 3-item commands such as give me the ball, pick up the doll, and sit down; identifies several colors, and is aware of past and future. | Up to 900 words in simple sentences averaging 3-4 words per sentence; averages 15,000 words per day and 170 words per hour; uses words such as when, time, today, not today, new, different, big, strong, surprise, secret; can repeat 3 digits, name 1 color, say name, give simple account of experiences, and tell stories that can be understood; begins to use more pronouns, adjectives, and adverbs; describes at least 1 element of a picture; is aware of past and future; uses commands such as you make it; also expressions such as I can't, I don't want to; verbalizes toilet needs, and expresses desire to take turns, communication includes criticisms, commands, requests, threats, questions, answers; 85% of speech is intelligible. | Starts to distinguish dissimilar speech sounds such as the difference between "ee" and "er," although there may be some difficulty with the concepts of "same" and "different." |

*Continued.*

## Landmarks of speech, language, and hearing ability—cont'd

| Chronological age | Receptive language | Expressive language | Related hearing ability |
|---|---|---|---|
| 42 months | Up to 4,200 words; knows words such as what, where, how, funny, we, surprise, secret; knows number concepts to 2, how to answer questions accurately, such as do you have a dog, which is the girl, what toys do you have. | Up to 1,200 words in mostly complete sentences averaging 4-5 words per sentence; uses all 50 phenomes; 7% of sentences are compound or complex; averages 203 words per hour; rate of speech is faster; relates experiences and tells about activities in sequential order; uses words such as what, where, how, see, little, funny, they, we, he, she, several; can say a nursery rhyme; asks permission; 95% of speech is intelligible. | |
| 48 months | Up to 5,600 words; carries out 3-item commands consistently; knows why we have houses, books, umbrella, key; knows nearly all the colors, words such as somebody, anybody, even, almost, now, something, like, bigger, too, full name, 1 or 2 songs, number concepts to 4; understands most preschool stories; can complete opposite analogies such as brother is a boy, sister is a _____; in daytime it is light, at night it is _____. | Up to 1,500 words in sentences averaging 5-6 words per sentence; averages 400 words per hour; counts to 3, repeats 4 digits, names 3 objects, and repeats 9-word sentences from memory; names the primary colors, some coins; relates fanciful tales; enjoys rhyming nonsense words and using exaggerations; demands reasons why and how; questioning is at a peak, up to 500 a day; passes judgment on own activity; can recite a poem from memory or sing a song; uses words such as even, almost, something, like, but; typical expressions might include I'm so tired, you almost hit me, now I'll make something else. | Begins to make find discriminations among similar speech sounds such as the difference between "f" and "th" or "f" and "s." The child has matured enough to be tested with an audiometer. At this age formal hearing testing can usually be carried out. Not only has hearing developed to its optimum level, but listening has also become considerably refined. |
| 54 months | Up to 6,500 words; knows what a house, window, chair, and dress are made of and what we do with our eyes and ears; understands differences in texture and composition, such as hard, soft, rough, smooth; begins to name or point to penny, nickel, dime; understands if, because, why, when. | Up to 1,800 words in sentences averaging 5-6 words; now averages only 230 words per hour—is satisfied with less verbalization; does little commanding or demanding; likes surprises; about 1 in 10 sentences is compound or complex, and only 8% of sentences are incomplete; can define 10 common words and count to 20; common expressions are I don't know, I said, tiny, funny, because; asks questions for information, and learns to manipulate and control persons and situations with language. | |

# Landmarks of speech, language, and hearing ability—cont'd

| Chronological age | Receptive language | Expressive language | Related hearing ability |
|---|---|---|---|
| 60 months | Up to 9,600 words; knows number concepts to 5; knows and names colors; defines words in terms of use such as a horse is to ride; also defines wind, ball, hat, stove; understands words such as if, because, when; knows what the following are for: horse, fork, legs; begins to understand right and left. | Up to 2,200 words in sentences averaging 6 words; can define ball, hat, stove, policeman, wind, horse, fork; can count 5 objects and repeat 4 or 5 digits; definitions are in terms of use; can single out a word and ask its meaning; makes serious inquiries —what is this for, how does this work, who made those, what does it mean; language is now essentially complete in structure and form; uses all types of sentences, clauses, and parts of speech; reads by way of pictures, and prints simple words. | |
| 66 months | Up to 13,500 words; knows number concepts to 7, right and left, most simple, compound, and complex sentences if not too long; knows functions of body parts—what are your eyes, ears, and so on, for; understands dependent clauses such as when I open the door, put the cat out. | Up to 2,300 words; sentence length varies from 6-7 words; grammatical errors continue to decrease as sentences and vocabulary become more sophisticated. | |
| 72 months | Up to 15,00 words; knows number concepts to 10, the meaning of morning, afternoon, night, summer, winter; can relate differences between objects, animals, and clothing; is beginning to answer a few similarities correctly, such in what way are _____ and _____ alike. | Up to 2,500 words in sentences averaging 7 words; relates fanciful tales; recites numbers to 30; asks meaning of words; repeats 5 digits from memory; can complete analogies such as a table is made of wood and a window of _____, a bird flies and a fish _____, an inch is short and a mile is _____. | |

## Suggested schedule for preventive child dental health care*

| Age | Developmental landmarks | Discussion and guidance | Procedures |
|---|---|---|---|
| Prenatal period | | Parent education to dental needs<br>Effect of drugs on developing dentition during pregnancy<br>Diet and proper dental habits | Brochures and pamphlets from American Dental Association; fluoridated drinking water |
| Newborn | Edentulous gum pads<br>Infantile swallowing pattern | Parent education to dental needs<br>Effect of drugs on developing dentition during pregnancy<br>Diet and proper dental habit<br>Congenital anomalies<br>Birth trauma | Thorough oral examination by obstetrician, pediatrician, etc. |
| Birth to 6 months | Neonatal teeth<br>Lower deciduous incisor eruption<br>Epstein pearls | Parent education to dental needs<br>Effect of drugs on developing dentition during pregnancy<br>Diet and proper dental habit<br>Congenital anomalies<br>Dental arch and dentitional development | Fluoridated drinking water |
| 6 to 30 months | Correct eruption sequence and time of eruption<br>Completion of deciduous dentition<br>Transitional period from infantile to mature swallow<br>Tongue, lip, finger habits<br>Learning and sleeping habits | Effect of drugs on developing dentition during pregnancy<br>Diet and proper dental habit<br>Dental arch and dentitional development<br>Traumatic injuries<br>Oral habit patterns | Oral hygiene<br>Oral habit control<br>Dietary regimen check |
| 30 months to 6 years | Complete deciduous dentition<br>Appearance of spaces between incisor teeth | Period of use of complete deciduous dentition and developmental preparation for permanent teeth<br>Routine periodic visits to the dentist<br>Oral manifestations of medication and drug therapy<br>Traumatic injuries more likely<br>Temporomandibular joint disturbances (bruxism, clenching, rheumatoid arthritis, etc.)<br>Dietary regimen | First visit to dentist<br>Supervision of dental occlusion and development (arch and jaw relationships and space control)<br>Control of abnormal pressure habits<br>Caries control procedures<br>Oral hygiene instruction |
| 6 to 12 years | Mixed dentition period<br>Eruption of eight permanent incisors and four permanent molars by 8½ years<br>Loss of deciduous molars, eruption of premolars by 10½ to 12 years | Periodic dental visits (at least twice a year)<br>Caries, soft tissue problems<br>Malocclusion<br>Oral manifestations of medication and drug therapy<br>Traumatic injuries more likely | Supervision of dental development (arch and jaw relationships and space control)<br>Optimal time for orthodontic consultation and guidance; possible interceptive procedures<br>Oral hygiene instruction |

*Joint statement prepared by a committee of representatives from the American Academy of Pedodontics, the American Society of Dentistry for Children, the American Association of Orthodontists, and the American Academy of Pediatrics, Sept. 1966. From Standards of child health care, Evanston, Ill., 1967, American Academy of Pediatrics, p. 115.

## Suggested schedule for preventive child dental health care—cont'd

| Age | Developmental landmarks | Discussion and guidance | Procedures |
|---|---|---|---|
| | Eruption of second molars (12 year molars) | Temporomandibular joint disturbances (bruxism, clenching, rheumatoid arthritis, etc.)<br>Dietary regimen<br>Oral effects of endocrine activity | Caries control<br>Soft tissue care |
| 12 to 19 years | Completion of permanent dentition<br>Possible third molar eruption (girls first) | Periodic dental visits (at least twice a year)<br>Caries, soft tissue problems<br>Malocclusion<br>Oral manifestations of medication and drug therapy<br>Traumatic injuries more likely<br>Temporomandibular joint disturbances (bruxism, clenching, rheumatoid arthritis, etc.)<br>Dietary regimen<br>Oral effects of endocrine activity | Supervision of dental development (arch and jaw relationships and space control)<br>Optimal time for orthodontic consultation and guidance; possible interceptive procedures<br>Oral hygiene instruction<br>Caries control<br>Soft tissue care<br>Active orthodontic therapy<br>Replacement of missing teeth<br>Esthetic and functional considerations |

## Pulse rates for boys and girls up to 18 years*†

| | Pulse rate per minute | | | | | |
|---|---|---|---|---|---|---|
| | Boys | | | Girls | | |
| Age in years | No. of tests | Mean $\pm\ \sigma_m$ | SD | No. of tests | Mean $\pm\ \sigma_m$ | SD |
| 0- 1 | 33 | 135 ± 3.1 | 18 | 56 | 126 ± 2.8 | 21 |
| 1- 2 | 82 | 105 ± 1.8 | 16 | 93 | 104 ± 1.8 | 17 |
| 2- 3 | 150 | 93 ± 1.0 | 12 | 177 | 93 ± 0.7 | 9 |
| 3- 4 | 157 | 87 ± 0.7 | 9 | 145 | 89 ± 0.7 | 9 |
| 4- 5 | 157 | 84 ± 0.7 | 8 | 137 | 84 ± 0.7 | 8 |
| 5- 6 | 150 | 79 ± 0.6 | 7 | 129 | 79 ± 0.6 | 7 |
| 6- 7 | 146 | 76 ± 0.6 | 8 | 122 | 77 ± 0.7 | 8 |
| 7- 8 | 140 | 75 ± 0.7 | 8 | 117 | 76 ± 0.8 | 8 |
| 8- 9 | 142 | 73 ± 0.7 | 9 | 114 | 73 ± 0.6 | 7 |
| 9-10 | 168 | 70 ± 0.6 | 7 | 106 | 70 ± 0.7 | 8 |
| 10-11 | 164 | 67 ± 0.6 | 7 | 98 | 69 ± 0.8 | 8 |
| 11-12 | 129 | 67 ± 0.6 | 7 | 84 | 69 ± 0.8 | 7 |
| 12-13 | 131 | 66 ± 0.6 | 7 | 72 | 69 ± 0.9 | 8 |
| 13-14 | 110 | 65 ± 0.8 | 8 | 68 | 68 ± 0.9 | 8 |
| 14-15 | 106 | 62 ± 0.7 | 7 | 57 | 66 ± 1.1 | 8 |
| 15-16 | 76 | 61 ± 0.9 | 8 | 47 | 65 ± 1.1 | 8 |
| 16-17 | 45 | 61 ± 0.9 | 6 | 30 | 66 ± 1.4 | 8 |
| 17-18 | 38 | 60 ± 1.4 | 8 | 20 | 65 ± 1.7 | 7 |

*Adapted from Iliff, A., and Lee, V. A.: Pulse rate, respiratory rate, and body temperature of children between 2 months and 18 years, Child Dev. **23**:237, 1952. By permission of the Society for Research in Child Development, Inc.
†Measurements were made following the basal metabolism determinations, and all those after 3 years were made in the morning.

## Respiratory rates for boys and girls up to 18 years*†

| Age in years | Respiratory rate per minute | | | | | |
|---|---|---|---|---|---|---|
| | Boys | | | Girls | | |
| | No. of tests | Mean ± $\sigma_m$ | SD | No. of tests | Mean ± $\sigma_m$ | SD |
| 0- 1 | 38 | 31 ± 1.3 | 8 | 55 | 30 ± 0.8 | 6 |
| 1- 2 | 69 | 26 ± 0.5 | 4 | 79 | 27 ± 0.5 | 4 |
| 2- 3 | 118 | 25 ± 0.4 | 4 | 134 | 25 ± 0.3 | 3 |
| 3- 4 | 131 | 24 ± 0.2 | 3 | 119 | 24 ± 0.2 | 3 |
| 4- 5 | 122 | 23 ± 0.2 | 2 | 113 | 22 ± 0.2 | 2 |
| 5- 6 | 110 | 22 ± 0.2 | 2 | 100 | 21 ± 0.2 | 2 |
| 6- 7 | 128 | 21 ± 0.2 | 3 | 97 | 21 ± 0.3 | 3 |
| 7- 8 | 119 | 20 ± 0.2 | 3 | 97 | 20 ± 0.2 | 2 |
| 8- 9 | 113 | 20 ± 0.2 | 2 | 101 | 20 ± 0.2 | 2 |
| 9-10 | 141 | 19 ± 0.2 | 2 | 98 | 19 ± 0.2 | 2 |
| 10-11 | 141 | 19 ± 0.2 | 2 | 90 | 19 ± 0.2 | 2 |
| 11-12 | 123 | 19 ± 0.2 | 3 | 82 | 19 ± 0.3 | 3 |
| 12-13 | 131 | 19 ± 0.2 | 3 | 72 | 19 ± 0.3 | 2 |
| 13-14 | 110 | 19 ± 0.2 | 2 | 68 | 18 ± 0.3 | 2 |
| 14-15 | 106 | 18 ± 0.2 | 2 | 57 | 18 ± 0.4 | 3 |
| 15-16 | 76 | 17 ± 0.3 | 3 | 47 | 18 ± 0.4 | 3 |
| 16-17 | 45 | 17 ± 0.4 | 2 | 30 | 17 ± 0.5 | 3 |
| 17-18 | 38 | 16 ± 0.5 | 3 | 20 | 17 ± 0.7 | 3 |

*Adapted from Iliff, A., and Lee, V. A.: Pulse rate, respiratory rate, and body temperature of children between 2 months and 18 years, Child Dev. **23**:237, 1952. By permission of the Society for Research in Child Development, Inc.
†Measurements were made at the time of the basal metabolism determinations, and all those after 3 years were made in the morning.

## Body temperatures for boys and girls up to 18 years*†

| Age in years | Body temperature (°F) | | | | | |
|---|---|---|---|---|---|---|
| | Boys | | | Girls | | |
| | No. of tests | Mean ± $\sigma_m$ | SD | No. of tests | Mean ± $\sigma_m$ | SD |
| 0- 1 | 38 | R 99.1 ± 0.12 | 0.7 | 57 | R 99.1 ± 0.05 | 0.4 |
| 1- 2 | 86 | R 99.1 ± 0.05 | 0.5 | 92 | R 98.9 ± 0.05 | 0.5 |
| 2- 3 | 145 | R 99.0 ± 0.03 | 0.4 | 167 | R 98.8 ± 0.03 | 0.4 |
| 3- 4 | 96 | R 98.9 ± 0.04 | 0.4 | 96 | R 98.8 ± 0.04 | 0.4 |
| 3- 4 | 59 | 98.7 ± 0.06 | 0.5 | 45 | 98.7 ± 0.08 | 0.5 |
| 4- 5 | 116 | 98.6 ± 0.04 | 0.5 | 98 | 98.5 ± 0.06 | 0.5 |
| 5- 6 | 141 | 98.5 ± 0.04 | 0.4 | 121 | 98.5 ± 0.04 | 0.4 |
| 6- 7 | 144 | 98.4 ± 0.04 | 0.4 | 120 | 98.5 ± 0.04 | 0.4 |
| 7- 8 | 141 | 98.3 ± 0.04 | 0.4 | 117 | 98.4 ± 0.04 | 0.4 |
| 8- 9 | 142 | 98.3 ± 0.04 | 0.4 | 113 | 98.3 ± 0.03 | 0.4 |
| 9-10 | 167 | 98.1 ± 0.04 | 0.5 | 106 | 98.2 ± 0.04 | 0.4 |
| 10-11 | 163 | 98.0 ± 0.04 | 0.5 | 98 | 98.1 ± 0.04 | 0.4 |
| 11-12 | 129 | 98.0 ± 0.03 | 0.4 | 84 | 98.0 ± 0.05 | 0.5 |
| 12-13 | 131 | 97.8 ± 0.04 | 0.4 | 71 | 97.9 ± 0.05 | 0.4 |
| 13-14 | 110 | 97.7 ± 0.04 | 0.4 | 68 | 97.9 ± 0.06 | 0.5 |
| 14-15 | 106 | 97.6 ± 0.04 | 0.4 | 57 | 97.9 ± 0.08 | 0.6 |
| 15-16 | 76 | 97.4 ± 0.05 | 0.4 | 47 | 97.9 ± 0.06 | 0.4 |
| 16-17 | 45 | 97.3 ± 0.07 | 0.5 | 30 | 97.8 ± 0.09 | 0.5 |
| 17-18 | 38 | 97.2 ± 0.06 | 0.4 | 20 | 97.9 ± 0.12 | 0.5 |

*Adapted from Iliff, A., and Lee, V. A.: Pulse rate, respiratory rate, and body temperature of children between 2 months and 18 years, Child Dev. **23**:237, 1952. By permission of the Society for Research in Child Development, Inc.
†Measurements were made following the basal metabolism determinations and all those after 3 years were made in the morning. Temperatures measured rectally are indicated by the letter "R"; other temperatures were taken orally.

## Normal blood pressure at various ages*

| Ages | Mean systolic ± 2 SD | Mean diastolic ± 2 SD |
|---|---|---|
| Newborn | 80 ± 16 | 46 ± 16 |
| 6-12 months | 89 ± 29 | 60 ± 10 |
| 1 year | 96 ± 30 | 66 ± 25 |
| 2 years | 99 ± 25 | 64 ± 25 |
| 3 years | 100 ± 25 | 67 ± 23 |
| 4 years | 99 ± 20 | 65 ± 20 |
| 5-6 years | 94 ± 14 | 55 ± 9 |
| 6-7 years | 100 ± 15 | 56 ± 9 |
| 7-8 years | 102 ± 15 | 56 ± 8 |
| 8-9 years | 105 ± 16 | 57 ± 9 |
| 9-10 years | 107 ± 16 | 57 ± 9 |
| 10-11 years | 111 ± 17 | 58 ± 10 |
| 11-12 years | 113 ± 18 | 59 ± 10 |
| 12-13 years | 115 ± 19 | 59 ± 10 |
| 13-14 years | 118 ± 19 | 60 ± 10 |

*From Haggerty, R. J., Maroney, M. W., and Nadas, A. S.: Essential hypertension in infancy and childhood, Am. J. Dis. Child. **92:**535, 1956. Copyright 1956, American Medical Association.

## Normal values for hematocrit and hemoglobin*

**Hematocrit**

| | |
|---|---|
| Birth | 44%-64% |
| 14-90 days | 35%-49% |
| 6 months-1 year | 30%-40% |
| 4-10 years | 31%-43% |

**Hemoglobin**

| | |
|---|---|
| Day 1 | 19 (14-24) g/100 ml |
| Day 2 | 19 (15-23) g/100 ml |
| Day 6 | 18 (13-23) g/100 ml |
| 2 weeks | 16.5 (15-20) g/100 ml |
| 1 month | 14 (11-17) g/100 ml |
| 2 months | 12 (11-14) g/100 ml |
| 3 months | 11 (10-13) g/100 ml |
| 6 months | 11.5 (10.5-14.5) g/100 ml |
| 1 year | 12 (11-15) g/100 ml |
| 2 years | 13 (12-15) g/100 ml |
| 5 years | 13.5 (12.5-15) g/100 ml |
| 8-13 years | 14 (13-15.5) g/100 ml |

*From Kempe, C. H., Silver, H. K., and O'Brien, D.: Current pediatric diagnosis and treatment, ed. 2, Los Altos, Calif., 1972, Lange Medical Publications, p. 978.

## Denver Articulation Screening Examination*
### For children 2½ to 6 years of age

Name: _____  Hosp. no.: _____

Address: _____

Date: _____ Child's age: _____ Examiner: _____ Raw score _____

Percentile: _____ Intelligibility: _____ Results: _____

**Instructions:** Have child repeat each word after you. Circle the underlined sounds that he pronounces correctly. Total correct sounds is the raw score. Use charts.

| | | | | |
|---|---|---|---|---|
| 1. table | 6. zipper | 11. sock | 16. wagon | 21. leaf |
| 2. shirt | 7. grapes | 12. vacuum | 17. gum | 22. carrot |
| 3. door | 8. flag | 13. yarn | 18. house | |
| 4. trunk | 9. thumb | 14. mother | 19. pencil | |
| 5. jumping | 10. toothbrush | 15. twinkle | 20. fish | |

**INTELLIGIBILITY** (CIRCLE ONE)

1. Easy to understand
2. Understandable ½ the time
3. Not understandable
4. Can't evaluate

**TEST RESULT**

1. **Normal** on DASE and Intelligibility = **normal.**
2. **Abnormal** on DASE and/or Intelligibility = **abnormal.**
   If abnormal on initial screening, rescreen within 2 weeks. If abnormal again, child should be referred for complete speech evaluation.

# Denver Articulation Screening Examination—cont'd

**COMMENTS**

*By Amelia B. Drumwright, University of Colorado Medical Center, 1971.

**TO SCORE INTELLIGIBILITY**

|  | Normal | Abnormal |
|---|---|---|
| **2½ years** | Understandable ½ the time, or "easy" | Not understandable |
| **3 years and older** | Easy to understand | Understandable ½ time<br>Not understandable |

To score DASE words: Note raw score for child's performance. Match raw score line (extreme left of chart) with column representing child's age (to the closest *previous* age group). Where raw score line and age column meet number in that square denotes percentile rank of child's performance when compared to other children that age. Percentiles above heavy line are **abnormal** percentiles, below heavy line are **normal.**

| Raw score | 2.5 yr | 3.0 | 3.5 | 4.0 | 4.5 | 5.0 | 5.5 | 6 years |
|---|---|---|---|---|---|---|---|---|
| | | | | Percentile rank | | | | |
| 2 | 1 | | | | | | | |
| 3 | 2 | | | | | | | |
| 4 | 5 | | | | | | | |
| 5 | 9 | | | | | | | |
| 6 | 16 | | | | | | | |
| 7 | 23 | | | | | | | |
| 8 | 31 | 2 | | | | | | |
| 9 | 37 | 4 | 1 | | | | | |
| 10 | 42 | 6 | 2 | | | | | |
| 11 | 48 | 7 | 4 | | | | | |
| 12 | 54 | 9 | 6 | 1 | 1 | | | |
| 13 | 58 | 12 | 9 | 2 | 3 | 1 | 1 | |
| 14 | 62 | 17 | 11 | 5 | 4 | 2 | 2 | |
| 15 | 68 | 23 | 15 | 9 | 5 | 3 | 2 | |
| 16 | 75 | 31 | 19 | 12 | 5 | 4 | 3 | |
| 17 | 79 | 38 | 25 | 15 | 6 | 6 | 4 | |
| 18 | 83 | 46 | 31 | 19 | 8 | 7 | 4 | |
| 19 | 86 | 51 | 38 | 24 | 10 | 9 | 5 | 1 |
| 20 | 89 | 58 | 45 | 30 | 12 | 11 | 7 | 3 |
| 21 | 92 | 65 | 52 | 36 | 15 | 15 | 9 | 4 |
| 22 | 94 | 72 | 58 | 43 | 18 | 19 | 12 | 5 |
| 23 | 96 | 77 | 63 | 50 | 22 | 24 | 15 | 7 |
| 24 | 97 | 82 | 70 | 58 | 29 | 29 | 20 | 15 |
| 25 | 99 | 87 | 78 | 66 | 36 | 34 | 26 | 17 |
| 26 | 99 | 91 | 84 | 75 | 46 | 43 | 34 | 24 |
| 27 | | 94 | 89 | 82 | 57 | 54 | 44 | 34 |
| 28 | | 96 | 94 | 88 | 70 | 68 | 59 | 47 |
| 29 | | 98 | 98 | 94 | 84 | 84 | 77 | 68 |
| 30 | | 100 | 100 | 100 | 100 | 100 | 100 | 100 |

# GUIDE TO GOOD EATING*

### A recommended daily pattern

The recommended daily pattern provides the foundation for a nutritious, healthful diet.

The recommended servings from the Four Food Groups for adults supply about 1,200 calories. The chart below gives recommendations for the number and size of servings for several categories of people.

| Food group | Recommended number of servings |
|---|---|
| **Milk**<br>1 cup milk, yogurt, OR<br>*Calcium equivalent:*<br>  1½ slices (1½ oz) cheddar<br>    cheese†<br>  1 cup pudding<br>  1¾ cups ice cream<br>  2 cups cottage cheese† | Child: 3<br>Teenager: 4<br>Adult: 2<br>Pregnant woman: 4<br>Lactating woman: 4 |
| **Meat**<br>2 ounces cooked, lean meat,<br>  fish, poultry, OR<br>*Protein equivalent:*<br>  2 eggs<br>  2 slices (2 oz) cheddar<br>    cheese†<br>  ½ cup cottage cheese†<br>  1 cup dried beans, peas<br>  4 tbsp peanut butter | Child: 2<br>Teenager: 2<br>Adult: 2<br>Pregnant woman: 3<br>Lactating woman: 2 |
| **Fruit-vegetable**<br>½ cup cooked or juice<br>1 cup raw<br>Portion commonly served<br>  such as a medium-size<br>  apple or banana | Child: 4<br>Teenager: 4<br>Adult: 4<br>Pregnant woman: 4<br>Lactating woman: 4 |
| **Grain, whole grain,<br>fortified, enriched**<br>1 slice bread<br>1 cup ready-to-eat cereal<br>½ cup cooked cereal,<br>  pasta, grits | Child: 4<br>Teenager: 4<br>Adult: 4<br>Pregnant woman: 4<br>Lactating woman: 4 |

*Courtesy National Dairy Council, ed. 4, copyright 1977.
†Count cheese as serving of milk OR meat, not both simultaneously.

**"Others"** complement but do not replace foods from the Four Food Groups. Amounts should be determined by individual caloric needs.

## Nutrients for health

| Nutrient | Important sources of nutrient |
|---|---|
| Protein | Meat, poultry, fish<br>Dried beans and peas<br>Egg<br>Cheese<br>Milk |
| Carbohydrate | Cereal<br>Potatoes<br>Dried beans<br>Corn<br>Bread<br>Sugar |
| Fat | Shortening, oil<br>Butter, margarine<br>Salad dressing<br>Sausages |
| Vitamin A (retinol) | Liver<br>Carrots<br>Sweet potatoes<br>Greens<br>Butter, margarine |
| Vitamin C (ascorbic acid) | Broccoli<br>Orange<br>Grapefruit<br>Papaya<br>Mango<br>Strawberries |
| Thiamin (B₁) | Lean pork<br>Nuts<br>Fortified cereal products |
| Riboflavin (B₂) | Liver<br>Milk<br>Yogurt<br>Cottage cheese |
| Niacin | Liver<br>Meat, poultry, fish<br>Peanuts<br>Fortified cereal products |
| Calcium | Milk, yogurt<br>Cheese<br>Sardines and salmon with bones<br>Collard, kale, mustard, and turnip<br>  greens |
| Iron | Enriched farina<br>Prune juice<br>Liver<br>Dried beans and peas<br>Red meat |

Nutrients are chemical substances obtained from foods during digestion. They are needed to build and maintain body cells, regulate body processes, and supply energy.

About 50 nutrients, including water, are needed daily for optimum health. If one obtains the proper amount of the 10 "leader" nutrients in the daily diet, the other 40 or so nutrients will likely be consumed in amounts sufficient to meet body needs.

One's diet should include a variety of foods because no *single* food supplies all the 50 nutrients, and because many nutrients work together.

When a nutrient is added or a nutritional claim is made, nutrition labeling regulations require listing the 10 leader nutrients on food packages. These nutrients appear in the chart below with food sources and some major physiologic functions.

| Some major physiologic functions | | |
|---|---|---|
| **Provide energy** | **Build and maintain body cells** | **Regulate body processes** |
| Supplies 4 calories per gram. | Constitutes part of the structure of every cell, such as muscle, blood, and bone; supports growth and maintains healthy body cells. | Constitutes part of enzymes, some hormones and body fluids, and antibodies that increase resistance to infection. |
| Supplies 4 calories per gram. Major source of energy for central nervous system. | Supplies energy so protein can be used for growth and maintenance of body cells. | Unrefined products supply fiber—complex carbohydrates in fruits, vegetables, and whole grains—for regular elimination. Assists in fat utilization. |
| Supplies 9 calories per gram. | Constitutes part of the structure of every cell. Supplies essential fatty acids. | Provides and carries fat-soluble vitamins (A, D, E, and K). |
| | Assists formation and maintenance of skin and mucous membranes that line body cavities and tracts, such as nasal passages and intestinal tract, thus increasing resistance to infection. | Functions in visual processes and forms visual purple, thus promoting healthy eye tissues and eye adaptation in dim light. |
| | Forms cementing substances, such as collagen, that hold body cells together, thus strengthening blood vessels, hastening healing of wounds and bones, and increasing resistance to infection. | Aids utilization of iron. |
| Aids in utilization of energy. | | Functions as part of a coenzyme to promote the utilization of carbohydrate. Promotes normal appetite. Contributes to normal functioning of nervous system. |
| Aids in utilization of energy. | | Functions as part of a coenzyme in the production of energy within body cells. Promotes healthy skin, eyes, and clear vision. |
| Aids in utilization of energy. | | Functions as part of a coenzyme in fat synthesis, tissue respiration, and utilization of carbohydrate. Promotes healthy skin, nerves, and digestive tract. Aids digestion and fosters normal appetite. |
| | Combines with other minerals within a protein framework to give structure and strength to bones and teeth. | Assists in blood clotting. Functions in normal muscle contraction and relaxation, and normal nerve transmission. |
| Aids in utilization of energy. | Combines with protein to form hemoglobin, the red substance in blood that carries oxygen to and carbon dioxide from the cells. Prevents nutritional anemia and its accompanying fatigue. Increases resistance to infection. | Functions as part of enzymes involved in tissue respiration. |

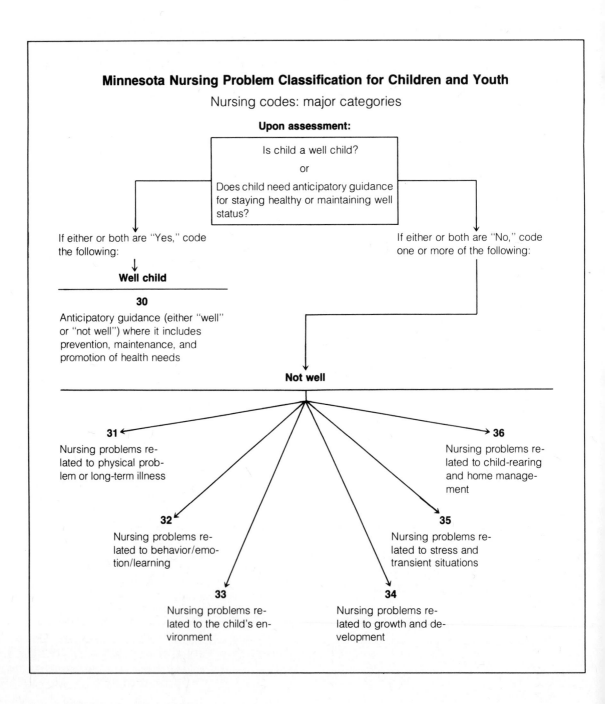

**Minnesota Nursing Problem Classification for Children and Youth**

Nursing codes: major categories

**Upon assessment:**

Is child a well child?

or

Does child need anticipatory guidance for staying healthy or maintaining well status?

If either or both are "Yes," code the following:

**Well child**

**30**

Anticipatory guidance (either "well" or "not well") where it includes prevention, maintenance, and promotion of health needs

If either or both are "No," code one or more of the following:

**Not well**

**31** Nursing problems related to physical problem or long-term illness

**32** Nursing problems related to behavior/emotion/learning

**33** Nursing problems related to the child's environment

**34** Nursing problems related to growth and development

**35** Nursing problems related to stress and transient situations

**36** Nursing problems related to child-rearing and home management

884

## MINNESOTA NURSING PROBLEM CLASSIFICATION FOR CHILDREN AND YOUTH*
### First position digit identifies the discipline or functional area

3-- Nursing
4-- Nutrition
5-- Social work
6-- Psychology

### Second position digit identifies the major categories (see chart)

30- Well child; anticipatory guidance for "well" and "not well" children, i.e., prevention, maintenance, and promotion of health needs
31- Nursing problems related to physical problem or long-term illness
32- Behavioral/emotional/learning problems of the child affecting nursing status
33- Environmental problems affecting nursing status
34- Nursing problems related to overt problems due to temporary deviations from normal growth and development
35- Nursing management problems related to stress and transient situations (short term)
36- Child-rearing and home management problems affecting health status

### Third position digit identifies the problem more specifically

The third position digits, --0 to --9 in the code structure, identify more specifically the nursing problems in each of the major categories. The third digit, --9, has been designated "Other" and is to be used consistently for the few of a kind problems not otherwise specified. The recorder should always state the problem when this third digit 009—Other is used. Users may wish to designate a separate code for a certain "other" problem group if that problem exists in their setting in sufficient numbers.

*Nursing problem classifications and codes for children and youth: Developed under DHEW Maternal and Child Health Training Grant No. MCT-001036-02. Minneapolis, 1975, Minnesota Systems Research, Inc. Revised October, 1977. Reprinted by permission of Minnesota Systems Research, Inc., 2412 University Ave. S.E., Minneapolis, Minn. 55414.

### Fourth position digit identifies the problem by name or very specifically

The fourth position digits, ---.0 to ---.9, in the code structure identify by name the exact problem assessed in the nursing area. The fourth digit, ---.9, has been designated "Other" and is to be used consistently for the few of a kind problems not otherwise specified. The recorder should always name the problem when this fourth digit ---.9—Other is used.

## AREAS OF SPECIAL NOTE WHEN ASSIGNING CODES
### Coding of well child status/anticipatory guidance

Category 30 includes a code for the well child who at the present time has no needs other than routine health promotion counseling—300.0. If, however, the nurse judges that the well child has a specific area of potential need, a code from 301-309 should be assigned which will specify that particular anticipated health need. When there are areas of anticipatory guidance covered routinely as part of the overall nursing program, it is not necessary to code this routine. Only when the nurse has particular concern or sees a special anticipatory guidance need does a specific code need to be assigned to the well child.

### Coding of anticipatory needs

In addition to applying the anticipatory guidance codes in 301-309 to a well child status, these codes may also be used in association with illness conditions or problems of not well children (310-399). If a child has a problem and needs related anticipatory counseling, code the problem(s) and also code any anticipatory or supportive counseling need(s).

### Problems of family or environment affecting child

As has been stated, this nomenclature and classification system is based on patient specific assessment and is limited to problems of a child and youth population. It includes sections for coding the child's community or household environment, as well as cultural and family practices which appear to impinge directly on the child's health status. However, these codes are not intended to describe fully the status or problems of those other persons or situations.

**885**

## Distinction in similar nomenclature used at third and fourth digit positions

In some cases the same or similar phrases are used to code conditions at both the third digit level and fourth digit level. The assignment of the appropriate code is dependent on the depth and thoroughness of the assessment/workup process, as well as the role and focus of the nursing program and practitioner. It may not be possible for the assessment/workup to be sufficiently in depth to name the specific condition. At that time a third level code should be used. The completeness with which the practitioner is able to define and describe the patient's overall health status may, therefore, dictate the level of code which can be assigned.

## Follow-up visits

When patients return for a follow-up visit for a previously identified problem, the recording system to which this coding applies must include some mechanism to assure that it is a *revisit* and not a new condition. Although the follow-up mechanism should be documented as part of a summary data system, it is beyond the scope of this tool. Comment is included here to be certain that multiple recording and reporting of the same condition does not occur in the uses for planning or estimating prevalence or incidence.

## Identification of problems, not intervention techniques

In utilizing this classification system, it is important to remember that the result of the assessment of a situation which exists or potentially exists as a problem or need is what is being classified, not an intervention technique or method. As a result of the assessment/workup process, one or more short descriptive statements or phrases are written which summarize the findings of that process, i.e., problems are described or "wellness" is documented and numerical codes are assigned to these statements. Following this assessment a plan of care should be developed which will include methods or techniques of intervention or treatment to resolve the problems or maintain the "wellness." It is not possible to classify these intervention techniques or methods using these

codes as presently developed, although this system would form the basic data set for any subsequent monitoring of intervention or evaluation of outcomes.

## 3--NURSING CLASSIFICATIONS AND CODES (TABULAR LISTING)

### 30-  Anticipatory guidance for well and not well children

**300  Well child**
300.0  Well child, only routine anticipatory guidance needed, no specific problem

**301  Need for general health information**
301.0  Health maintenance (hygiene, nutrition, importance of health supervision, immunizations, vision and hearing screening, pregnancy testing)
301.1  Home environment (garbage, rat-insect control, preservation of food)
301.2  Rest, recreation (socialization), exercise
301.3  Child spacing, birth control information
301.4  Utilization of community resources
301.5  Lead poisoning information
301.6  Genetic information and/or screening (PKU, sickle cell)
301.7  Communicable disease and other common illness
301.8
301.9  Other

**302  Need for motivation in carrying out preventive measures and health maintenance**
302.0  Immunization
302.1  Making and keeping appointments for routine health assessment and supervision, follow-through on screening procedures, Mantoux, audio, dental, etc.
302.2  Importance of taking prescribed prophylactic drugs
302.3  Illness recognition and management
302.4  Orientation to crisis care
302.5  Low priority of health care
302.6  Cultural/religious bias for health care (Christian Science, Jehovah's Witness, old wives' tales)
302.7
302.8
302.9  Other

**303  Need for knowledge and guidance in managing early infancy (0-3 months)**
303.0  Infant-mother-family emotional relationships (other caretakers)
303.1  Physical care (skin, cord, scalp, bathing)
303.2  Feeding (bottle, breast, solids)

303.3 Growth expectations
303.4 Development expectations (reflexes, responses, strength, movement, stimulation)
303.5 Behavior expectations (smiling, crying, etc.)
303.6 Safety (toys, positions, clothing, falls)
303.7 Social (extended family)
303.8
303.9 Other

**304 Need for knowledge and guidance in managing infancy (4-24 months)**

304.0 Emotional relationships: family and other caretakers (separation anxiety, sibling rivalry, attachment)
304.1 Physical care (skin, hair, teeth, skin rashes, cuts, bruises)
304.2 Feeding (weaning, solids, finger foods, messiness, amounts)
304.3 Growth (weight, height, teething)
304.4 Development (speech, fine motor, gross motor, adaptability, walking, toilet training, stimulation)
304.5 Behavior expectations (fears, autonomy, discipline versus punishment)
304.6 Safety (accident, poisoning, toys)
304.7 Social (parallel play, socialization, toys)
304.8
304.9 Other

**305 Need for knowledge and guidance in managing early childhood (2-4 years)**

305.0 Family emotional relationships (separation anxiety, sibling rivalry, babysitters)
305.1 Physical care (skin, grooming, dental)
305.2 Feeding (self, manners, messiness, decreased appetite)
305.3 Growth (physical size)
305.4 Development (intellectual stimulation, need to be self-sufficient, independent, speech patterns, toilet training)
305.5 Behavior expectations (fears, ritualism, rage, bad language, desires to please, temper tantrums, fighting)
305.6 Safety (poison, accident prevention, toys)
305.7 Social (peer relationships, cooperative play, socialization, toys, school entry)
305.8 Sexuality (identity, sexual play)
305.9 Other

**306 Need for knowledge and guidance in managing middle and late childhood (5-9 years)**

306.0 Emotional relationships (family and significant others, babysitters)
306.1 Physical care (skin, hygiene, grooming, dental)
306.2 Nutrition (periodic food fads)

306.3 Growth (periodic spurts with concurrent clumsiness)
306.4 Development (school entry and adjustment, initiative, industry, imagination, the gifted or slow child)
306.5 Behavior (ambivalence, fighting, independence)
306.6 Safety (accidents, poisonings, misuse of drugs and other chemical agents, smoking, fires, water safety)
306.7 Social (peer relationships, teachers, clubs, gangs, play and recreation, school entry)
306.8 Sexuality (sex education, identity, sexual play)
306.9 Other

**307 Need for knowledge and guidance in preadolescence and puberty (10-13 years)**

307.0 Emotional relationships (family and parents, authority figures, generation gap, best friend of same sex, attraction for opposite sex)
307.1 Physical care (hygiene, grooming, acne, oily hair, dental)
307.2 Nutrition (eating habits, fads, growth spurt needs)
307.3 Growth (prepubertal and pubertal changes, growth spurts, wide ranges are normal)
307.4 Development (identity, self-image, self-criticism, intellectual)
307.5 Behavior (rebellion, mood swings)
307.6 Safety (vehicle and sport accidents, misuse of drugs and other chemical agents, street safety, smoking)
307.7 Social (gangs, cliques, recreational outlets, sports, parties)
307.8 Sexuality (education, birth control, experimentation, identity)
307.9 Other

**308 Need for knowledge and guidance in adolescence (14-17 years)**

308.0 Emotional relationships (family, generation gap, best friends of same and opposite sex)
308.1 Physical care (hygiene, grooming, acne, exercise needs, dental)
308.2 Nutrition (eating habits, fads, weight maintenance)
308.3 Growth (pubertal changes, growth, adjustment to personal appearance)
308.4 Development (identity, self-image, high school and preparation for college or specialized training for career planning)
308.5 Behavior (mood and emotional changes, independence, responsibility for own health, other responsibilities)

308.6 Safety (vehicle and sport accidents, misuse of drugs, tobacco, alcohol, street safety)

308.7 Social (group identification and selection, recreational outlets)

308.8 Sexuality (identity, education, birth control, V.D. control, planning for parenthood)

308.9 Other

**309 Need for knowledge and guidance in late adolescence (18-21 years)**

309.0 Emotional relationships (family, mate selection, proposed or realized parenthood)

309.1 Physical care (hygiene, grooming, exercise needs, dental)

309.2 Nutrition (to maintain fitness, preparation for childbearing in female, weight maintenance)

309.3 Growth (end of height growth, adjustment to personal appearance)

309.4 Development (self-image and acceptance, advanced training or college, career choices and selection)

309.5 Behavior (responsibility for self and others, independence, responsibility for own health maintenance)

309.6 Safety (accidents, misuse of drugs, tobacco and alcohol)

309.7 Social (group selection, recreational outlets)

309.8 Sexuality (identity, birth control, V.D. control)

309.0 Other

**31- Nursing problems related to long-term illness or physical problems**

**310 Long-term musculoskeletal problems (post polio, muscular dystrophy, congenital hip, post fracture complications, scoliosis, paraplegia, cleft palate)**

310.0 Ambulation and exercise (self-locomotion, transferring techniques, maintenance of movement and posture, ROM, crutch walking, wheelchair, special appliances)

310.1 Nutrition (difficulty in swallowing, feeding problems)

310.2 Skin care (positioning, posture, prevention of infection)

310.3 Maintenance of body temperature and other physical care (maintenance of breathing, correct ventilation, pulmonary infections)

310.4 Psychosocial (self-image problems with deformity, family understanding, support, independence) and intellectual stimulation (schooling, group activities)

310.5 Environmental dangers (avoid self-injury, burns, falls)

310.6 Elimination (catheter care, perineal hygiene)

310.7 Follow-through (appointments, taking medication, treatments)

310.8 At risk (patient returned to maximum functioning but subject to disruption without appropriate ongoing care and health supervision)

310.9 Other

**311 Sensory modifiable problems (hearing loss, strabismus, refractory errors, recurrent otitis media)**

311.0 Ambulation and exercise (self-locomotion, transferring techniques, maintenance of movement and posture, ROM, crutch walking, wheelchair)

311.1 Nutrition (difficulty in swallowing, feeding problems)

311.2 Skin care (positioning, posture, prevention of infection)

311.3 Other physical care

311.4 Psychosocial (self-image problems with deformity, family understanding, support, independence)

311.5 Environmental dangers (avoiding self-injury, burns, falls)

311.6 Use of appliance (glasses, hearing aid)

311.7 Follow-through (keeping appointments, medications, treatments)

311.8 At risk (condition returned to maximum functioning but subject to disruption without appropriate ongoing care and health supervision)

311.9 Other

**312 Sensory nonmodifiable problems (loss of speech, blind, totally deaf, equilibrium problems, etc.)**

312.0 Exercise (activity level)

312.1 Nutrition (difficulty in swallowing, feeding problems)

312.2 Skin care (positioning, posture, prevention of infection)

312.3 Other physical care

312.4 Psychosocial (self-image problems with deformity, family understanding, support, independence)

312.5 Environmental dangers (avoiding self-injury, burns, falls)

312.6 Communication (learning to talk, write, anxiety about speech and learning)

312.7 Follow-through (keeping appointments, medications, treatments)

312.8 At risk (condition returned to maximum functioning but subject to disruption without appropriate ongoing care and health supervision)

312.9 Other

**313 Allergy and respiratory problems (allergies, asthma, recurrent URI, recurrent bronchitis, recurrent pneumonia, TB, croup, allergic dermatitis)**

313.0 Acute exacerbation or episode

313.1 Nutrition (feeding problems, special diets)

313.2 Skin care (cleanliness, prevention of infection)

313.3 Respiratory maintenance, ventilation, body temperature (exercises, special equipment)

313.4 Psychosocial (self-image, support, understanding, acceptance of problem, family guidance counseling, anxiety about problem)

313.5 Environmental dangers (source of allergy)

313.6 Rest, recreation, exercise (activity level)

313.7 Follow-through (appointments, taking medications, treatments)

313.8 At risk (patient returned to maximum functioning but subject to disruption without appropriate ongoing care and health supervision)

313.9 Other

**314 Gastrointestinal and endocrine problems (chronic diarrhea, constipation, obesity, dental caries, nutritional anemias, ulcerative colitis, diabetes, CF)**

314.0 Elimination (bowel or bladder problems)

314.1 Nutrition (feeding problems, acceptable diet, diet supplements)

314.2 Skin care (cleanliness, prevention of infection)

314.3 Other physical care

314.4 Psychosocial (self-image, support, family guidance, understanding, acceptance of problems, counseling)

314.5 Acute exacerbation or episode

314.6 Rest, recreation, exercise

314.7 Follow-through (appointments, taking medications, treatments)

314.8 At risk (patient returned to maximum functioning but subject to disruption without appropriate ongoing care and health supervision)

314.9 Other

**315 Central nervous system problems (CP, mental retardation, Down's, PKU, hydrocephalus, seizure disorders)**

315.0 Ambulation and exercise (self-locomotion, transferring techniques, maintenance of movement and posture, ROM, crutch walking, wheelchair)

315.1 Nutrition (feeding problems)

315.2 Skin care (cleanliness, prevention of infection)

315.3 Maintenance of body temperature and other physical care including elimination (maintenance of breathing, correct ventilation, prevention of pulmonary infection)

315.4 Psychosocial (self-image, support, understanding, acceptance of problem, family guidance, counseling, day care, independence, communication) rest and recreation

315.5 Environmental dangers

315.6 Genetic counseling

315.7 Follow-through (appointments, taking medications, treatments)

315.8 At risk (patient returned to maximum functioning, but subject to disruption without appropriate ongoing care and health supervision)

315.9 Other

**316 Cardiovascular problems (congenital heart conditions, rheumatic heart disease)**

316.0 Ambulation and exercise (activity level)

316.1 Nutrition (special diet, feeding problem)

316.2 Skin care (cleanliness, prevention of infection)

316.3 Physical care (maintenance of breathing, body temperature, correct ventilation, prevention of pulmonary infections)

316.4 Psychosocial (support, understanding, acceptance and understanding of problem, family guidance, counseling, independence)

316.5 Environmental dangers

316.6 Rest and recreation

316.7 Follow-through (appointments, taking medications, treatments)

316.8 At risk (patient returned to maximum functioning but subject to disruption without appropriate ongoing care and health supervision)

316.9 Other

**317 Genitourinary problems (menstrual problems, GU infections, congenital anomalies)**

317.0 Ambulation and exercise (self-locomotion, maintenance of movement and posture, ROM, wheelchair)

317.1 Nutrition (special diet, feeding problem)

317.2 Skin care (cleanliness, prevention of disease)

317.3 Elimination (catheter care) and other physical care

317.4 Psychosocial (self-image, support, family guidance, understanding of problem)

317.5   Acute exacerbation or episode
317.6
317.7   Follow-through (appointments, taking medication, treatments)
317.8   At risk (patient returned to maximum functioning but subject to disruption without appropriate ongoing care and health supervision)
317.9   Other

318   **Multiple and/or systemic problems (tumors, leukemia, Hodgkin's disease, collagen disease, sickle cell anemia, hemophilia, lead poisoning)**
318.0   Ambulation and exercise (self-locomotion, activity level, maintenance of movement and posture, ROM, crutch walking, wheelchair)
318.1   Nutrition (special diet, feeding problems)
318.2   Skin care (cleanliness, prevention of disease)
318.3   Maintenance of body temperature and physical care (maintenance of breathing, correct ventilation, pulmonary infections)
318.4   Psychosocial (self-image, support, family guidance, understanding of problem, independence) intellectual stimulation, rest and recreation
318.5   Examination of environmental dangers
318.6   Genetic counseling
318.7   Follow-through (appointments, taking medications, treatments)
318.8   At risk (patient returned to maximum functioning but subject to disruption without appropriate ongoing care and health supervision)
318.9   Other

319   **Miscellaneous chronic problems (worms, infestation, impetigo, acne, cellulitis, other skin conditions**
319.0   Ambulation and exercise (self-locomotion, transferring techniques, maintenance of movement and posture, ROM, crutch walking, wheelchair)
319.1   Nutrition (special diet, feeding problems)
319.2   Skin care (cleanliness, prevention of further infection)
319.3   Other physical care
319.4   Psychosocial (self-image, support, family guidance, understanding or problem, independence)
319.5   Environmental hygiene (reinfection of self or others)
319.6   Acute exacerbation or episode
319.7   Follow-through (appointments, taking medication, treatments)
319.8   At risk (patient returned to maximum functioning but subject to disruption without appropriate ongoing care and health supervision)
319.9   Other

32-   **Nursing problems related to behavior/emotions/learning**
320   **Aggressive behaviors**
320.0   Physically assaultive to people (fighting, sexual attack)
320.1   Destructive of property (fire setting, vandalism, stealing)
320.2   Abusive to animals
320.3   Verbally abusive
320.4   Explosive temper (tantrums)
320.5   Exhibitionism (excessive)
320.6   Running away/truancy
320.7   Rebellious
320.8   Overactive
320.9   Other

321   **Passive behaviors**
321.0   Withdrawn (very quiet, isolative, seclusive, sleeps excessively)
321.1   Unable to express anger
321.2   Unwilling or unable to compete (intellectually or physically)
321.3   Relates to animals rather than people
321.4   Lack of assertiveness
321.5   Overly dependent (conforming, compliant)
321.6   Excessive daydreaming and fantasizing
321.7
321.8
321.9   Other

322   **Self-abusive behaviors**
322.0   Masochistic behaviors (scratching, burning, cutting, picking)
322.1   Accident prone
322.2   Alcohol abuse/addiction
322.3   Drug abuse/addiction (hard drugs, glue, volatiles)
322.4   Suicide attempt
322.5   Verbal degradation, excessive self-criticism
322.6   Refuses to eat
322.7
322.8
322.9   Other

323   **Emotional problems**
323.0   Feelings of inadequacy, poor self-image
323.1   Feelings of guilt
323.2   Insecure
323.3   Overly fearful of people, situations, things
323.4   Compulsive
323.5   Depressed (lethargic, excessive crying, suicidal, etc.)

323.6 Phobic
323.7 Out of touch with reality (hallucinates, paranoid, delusional, autistic, schizophrenic)
323.8
323.9 Other

## 324 Physical symptoms/behaviors associated with emotional problems
324.0 Bowel and bladder incontinence or retention
324.1 Abdominal problems (pain, nausea, etc.)
324.2 Skin reactions (hives, rashes, etc.)
324.3 Respiratory symptoms (hyperventilation, wheezing, holding breath)
324.4 Headaches, stiff neck
324.5 Tics, twitches, stuttering
324.6 Habit disturbances (finger sucking, pulling, hand movements, etc.)
324.7 Loss of appetite
324.8 Unable to sleep
324.9 Other

## 325 Relationship problems
325.0 Unable to relate to children the same age (no friends, relates to older or younger persons)
325.1 Unable to relate to parents
325.2 Unable to relate to authority figures (teachers, police, etc.)
325.3 Relates predominantly to animals
325.4 Afraid to be alone
325.5 Symbiotic relationships with parent, sibling
325.6 Feelings easily hurt (feels rejected, sensitive)
325.7 Bullies others, domineering
325.8
325.9 Other

## 326 Learning problems (school age)
326.0 Underachiever
326.1 Vision, hearing, speech problem
326.2 Hyperactive (short attention span, distractible, distracting, etc.)
326.3 Poor reader
326.4 Special learning disabilities
326.5 Slow learner (intellectually slow)
326.6 Mentally retarded
326.7 Gifted
326.8
326.9 Other

## 327 Currently unused, open for future use and expansion
327.0
327.1
327.2
327.3
327.4
327.5
327.6
327.7
327.8
327.9

## 328 Currently unused, open for future use and expansion
328.0
328.1
328.2
328.3
328.4
328.5
328.6
328.7
328.8
328.9

## 329 Currently unused, open for future use and expansion
329.0
329.1
329.2
329.3
329.4
329.5
329.6
329.7
329.8
329.9

## 33- Nursing problems related to child's environment

## 330 Physical environmental problems (home)
330.0 Difficulty securing adequate housing
330.1 Inadequate physical facilities
330.2 Overcrowding/lack of privacy/sleeping arrangements
330.3 Inadequate food (amount and nutrition)
330.4 Inadequate clothing
330.5 Inadequate basic furnishings
330.6 Faulty and/or inadequate heating facilities
330.7 Lack of transportation
330.8
330.9 Other

## 331 Physical safety problems
331.0 Fire hazard
331.1 Paint peeling, plaster cracking
331.2 Rats or rodent infestation
331.3 Inadequate security
331.4 Inadequate sanitation
331.5 Accident hazards apparent
331.6 Inadequate safe play facilities
331.7 Poisons or other toxic substances available (bleach, ammonia, glue, medicine, etc.)

331.8
331.9  Other

**332  Social environmental problems**
332.0  School adjustment problems
332.1  Extreme mobility of family
332.2  Conflict in relationships between family and social institutions, community and/or significant others
332.3  Conflict of relationships within family
332.4  Parental responsibilities given to child (excessive cooking, housekeeping, babysitting, etc.)
332.5  Insufficient income
332.6
332.7
332.8
332.9  Other

**333  Cultural environmental problems**
333.0  Traditional patterns differ
333.1  Foods—nutritional deficiencies
333.2  Food—inappropriate substitution or inclusion
333.3  Cultural isolation
333.4  Health beliefs
333.5  Language barriers
333.6
333.7
333.8
333.9  Other

**334  Currently unused, open for future use and expansion**
334.0
334.1
334.2
334.3
334.4
334.5
334.6
334.7
334.8
334.9

**335  Currently unused, open for future use and expansion**
335.0
335.1
335.2
335.3
335.4
335.5
335.6
335.7
335.8
335.9

**336  Currently unused, open for future use and expansion**
336.0
336.1
336.2
336.3
336.4
336.5
336.6
336.7
336.8
336.9

**337  Currently unused, open for future use and expansion**
337.0
337.1
337.2
337.3
337.4
337.5
337.6
337.7
337.8
337.9

**338  Currently unused, open for future use and expansion**
338.0
338.1
338.2
338.3
338.4
338.5
338.6
338.7
338.8
338.9

**339  Currently unused, open for future use and expansion**
339.0
339.1
339.2
339.3
339.4
339.5
339.6
339.7
339.8
339.9

**34-  Nursing problems related to growth and development**

**340  Growth and development—lags in development**

340.0  Delayed speech or language development
340.1  Delayed gross motor development
340.2  Delayed fine motor development
340.3  Delayed social development
340.4  Delayed physical development (slow weight gain, small size of head)
340.5
340.6
340.7
340.8
340.9  Other

**341  Prematurity**
341.0  Emotional relationships (infant-mother-family)
341.1  Physical care (hygiene, skin care, nails)
341.2  Nutritional care (bottle, breast, solids)
341.3  Growth and development
341.4  Behavioral expectations
341.5  Safety (positioning, clothing, falls, toys)
341.6  Social needs (extended family, babysitters)
341.7  Illness prevention, recognition, and management
341.8  Follow-through (appointments, planned care)
341.9  Other

**342  Failure to thrive**
342.0  Emotional relationships and needs
342.1  Physical care
342.2  Nutritional care
342.3  Growth and development
342.4  Behavioral expectations
342.5  Safety
342.6  Social needs
342.7  Illness prevention, recognition and management
342.8  Follow-through (appointments, planned care)
342.9  Other

**343  Currently unused, open for future use and expansion**
343.0
343.1
343.2
343.3
343.4
343.5
343.6
343.7
343.8
343.9

**344  Currently unused, open for future use and expansion**
344.0
344.1
344.2
344.3
344.4
344.5
344.6
344.7
344.8
344.9

**345  Currently unused, open for future use and expansion**
345.0
345.1
345.2
345.3
345.4
345.5
345.6
345.7
345.8
345.9

**346  Currently unused, open for future use and expansion**
346.0
346.1
346.2
346.3
346.4
346.5
346.6
346.7
346.8
346.9

**347  Currently unused, open for future use and expansion**
347.0
347.1
347.2
347.3
347.4
347.5
347.6
347.7
347.8
347.9

**348  Currently unused, open for future use and expansion**
348.0
348.1
348.2
348.3
348.4
348.5
348.6

348.7
348.8
348.9

**349　Currently unused, open for future use and expansion**
349.0
349.1
349.2
349.3
349.4
349.5
349.6
349.7
349.8
349.9

**35-　Nursing problems related to transient, stress, or crisis situations**

**350　Acute physical illness management**
350.0　Acute febrile states
350.1　Shock, collapse, hemorrhage
350.2　Disturbance of fluid and electrolytes (dehydration, fluid retention)
350.3　Wound, injury, skin problems, localized burn, or infection
350.4　Acute GI problems
350.5　URI or other respiratory infection
350.6　Venereal disease
350.7　Other communicable disease
350.8　Acute GU problems
350.9　Other

**351　Psychosocial stress (crisis) management**
351.0　Adjustment crisis
351.1　School crisis
351.2　Identity crisis
351.3　Drug crisis
351.4　Enforced separation of child from parents or significant other (through death, moving, divorce, absence, desertion)
351.5　Preparation for hospitalization
351.6　Preparation for painful procedures
351.7　Rape, assault
351.8　Enuresis, encopresis
351.9　Other

**352　Environmental stress (crisis) management**
352.0　Loss of employment leading to financial crisis
352.1　Moving into new community
352.2　Fire, flood, destruction of home
352.3　Eviction
352.4　Immediate financial need
352.5　Neighborhood crisis (riot, violence)
352.6
352.7

352.8
352.9　Other

**353　Crisis in facing child's terminal illness or death**
353.0　Child's physical comfort
353.1　Child's emotional security
353.2　Family's emotional support
353.3　Teaching the family
353.4　Family and child communication
353.5　Family and child interaction (social interaction)
353.6　Child's mental/physical activity
353.7　Family's behavioral expectations
353.8　Disease complications
353.9　Coordination of family, professional, and community resources

**354　Teenage pregnancy**
354.0　Emotional (with parents, father of infant)
354.1　Physical (hygiene and personal care)
354.2　Nutritional (need to control weight, need for diet modification and supplement, inappropriate inclusion of nonnutritive substances)
354.3　Physical growth changes of pregnancy
354.4　Development—understanding developing fetus
354.5　Behavior—norms for age group with stresses of pregnancy
354.6　Safety (accidents, drugs and alcohol, medications)
354.7　Social group identification (recreation outlets, peer and social group)
354.8　Sexuality (identity, education, birth control after pregnancy, VD control)
354.9　Acceptancy—denial conflict of pregnancy by teenager

**355　Teenage pregnancy (continued)**
355.0　Conflict with significant others over pregnancy
355.1　Options—abortion, marriage, adoption, keeping the child, foster care
355.2　Education options—career, school
355.3　Physical care, preparation for infant
355.4　Emotional care, preparation for infant
355.5　Follow-through (appointments, following recommendations)
355.6　Physical complication of pregnancy (anemia, spontaneous abortion, induced abortion)
355.7　No special problems
355.8
355.9　Other

**356　Currently unused, open for future use and expansion**
356.0

356.1
356.2
356.3
356.4
356.5
356.6
356.7
356.8
356.9

**357 Currently unused, open for future use and expansion**

357.0
357.1
357.2
357.3
357.4
357.5
357.6
357.7
357.8
357.9

**358 Currently unused, open for future use and expansion**

358.0
358.1
358.2
358.3
358.4
358.5
358.6
358.7
358.8
358.9

**359 Currently unused, open for future use and expansion**

359.0
359.1
359.2
359.3
359.4
359.5
359.6
359.7
359.8
359.9

## 36- Nursing problems related to child rearing and home management

**360 Child-rearing problems (parental functioning)**
360.0  Physical care
360.1  Feeding (weaning, nutrient amounts)

360.2  Nurturing or parenting (parent-child relationship)
360.3  Stimulation
360.4  Supervision
360.5  Child discipline
360.6  Physical or mental abuse
360.7  Day care
360.8
360.9  Other

**361 Infancy and early childhood problems (child's functioning)**
361.0  Eating (poor eater, constipation)
361.1  Sleeping
361.2  Toileting
361.3  Crying
361.4  Teething
361.5  Pica
361.6  Bedwetting
361.7
361.8
361.9  Other

**362 Home management problems**
362.0  Planning the day
362.1  Coping with numerous children
362.2  Budgeting
362.3  Food shopping
362.4  Cleanliness, sanitation, nutrition
362.5  Lack of stamina or energy
362.6  Use of money
362.7
362.8
362.9  Other

**363 Parental problems**
363.0  Physical illness of parent
363.1  Mental or emotional problems of parent
363.2  Drug and/or alcohol abuse in parent
363.3  Mentally retarded parent
363.4  Marital discord or conflict
363.5  Parent(s) without support system
363.6
363.7
363.8
363.9  Other

**364** ⎤
 ⎟ **Currently unused, open for future use and expansion**
**369** ⎦

**37-**
**38-** ⎤ **Currently unused, open for future use and expansion**
**39-** ⎦

## CASE AUDIT GUIDE

Instructions: After review of this case, answer the following questions and cite the evidence that is found in the record.

### I. Application of the framework of child competencies
  A. Does the record contain assessment data related to physical, learning and thought, social, and inner competencies?
  B. Does the assessment data support the conclusions made regarding the child's stage of development?
  C. What additional information is needed for each competency?
  D. Does the plan provide for future acquisition of needed data?

### II. Achievement of the nursing process
  A. 1. Are the values of the child/adult client and of the nurse acknowledged in relation to the needs of the client?
  2. Is the child/adult client involved in identification of problems and planning for care?
  3. Is the nurse an advocate for the child/adult client?
  B. 1. Is the structure needed for goal attainment identified, including personnel, monetary resources, and physical facilities?
  2. Is the process, or the actions needed to achieve health care goals, identified?
  3. Are the outcomes, or goals of health care, described in measurable or observable terms?
  C. 1. Is baseline date, or initial health status, reported in relation to each health care goal?
  2. Is progress toward goal attainment reported?
  D. 1. Is the data obtained interpreted in relation to developmental norms?
  2. Is the data obtained interpreted in relation to cultural values of the family?
  3. Is the interpretation of health needs, health problems, and nursing diagnoses supported by the available data?
  E. 1. Does the record reflect consideration of alternative actions and involvement of the child/adult client in selecting the desired action?
  2. Do the actions selected appear to be defensible based on the available data, or would other alternatives be indicated?
  F. 1. Do the actions selected reflect sound professional judgment?
  2. Are the actions selected in accord with the values of the child/adult client?
  G. Does the recrod reflect realistic implementation of actions, accounting for the structure, process, and outcomes needed to achieve health care goals?

### III. Use of the problem-oriented record
  A. Does the data base support the health needs and problems listed on the health status list?
  B. Does the data base include:
  1. initial statement of the client's reason for seeking health care
  2. profile of the child/adult client
  3. past history of the child, parents and family
  4. review of physiological systems
  5. physical assessment data
  6. psychosocial assessment data
  7. results of testing or laboratory data
  8. summary of the child's stage of development and health status
  C. Does the initial plan include, for each problem on the health status list, the following:
  1. Subjective data
  2. Objective data
  3. Assessment

4. Plan
D. Are nursing orders included for each client objective?
E. Do the progress notes reflect implementation of the plan and nursing orders?

## IV. Quality of care as determined by nursing care standards

Using the Maternal and Child Health Standards of Nursing Practice on pp. 47-51, determine the following:
A. Which assessment factors are demonstrated in this record?
B. Which assessment factors have not been demonstrated that could have been demonstrated in this record?
C. Based on this evaluation, what recommendations would you make for improvement of this nurse's practice?

### REFERENCES

Eshleman, R. J.: The family, Boston, 1974, Allyn & Bacon, Inc.

Murray, R., and Zentner, J.: Nursing assessment and health promotion through the life span, Englewood Cliffs, N.J., 1975, Prentice-Hall, Inc.

Satir, V., Stachowaick, J., and Taschman, H.: Helping families to change, New York, 1976, Jason Aronson, Inc.

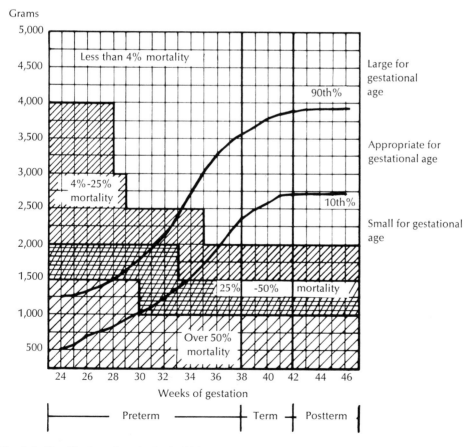

**Fig. A-1.** Classification of newborns by birth weight and gestational age. (After Battaglia, F. C., and Lubchenco, L. O.: J. Pediatr. **71:**161, 1967.)

## Growth Charts for U.S. Girls

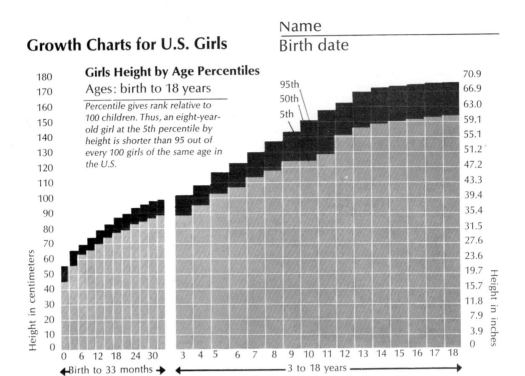

**Girls Height by Age Percentiles**

Ages: birth to 18 years

*Percentile gives rank relative to 100 children. Thus, an eight-year-old girl at the 5th percentile by height is shorter than 95 out of every 100 girls of the same age in the U.S.*

Height in centimeters

Height in inches

95th
50th
5th

0  6  12  18  24  30     3  4  5  6  7  8  9  10  11  12  13  14  15  16  17  18

◄Birth to 33 months ►     ◄—————— 3 to 18 years ——————►

**Fig. A-2.**

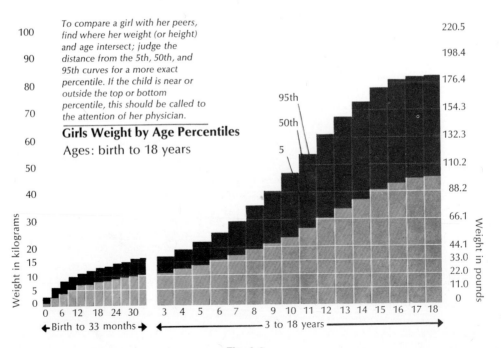

*To compare a girl with her peers, find where her weight (or height) and age intersect; judge the distance from the 5th, 50th, and 95th curves for a more exact percentile. If the child is near or outside the top or bottom percentile, this should be called to the attention of her physician.*

**Girls Weight by Age Percentiles**

Ages: birth to 18 years

Weight in kilograms

Weight in pounds

95th
50th
5

0  6  12  18  24  30     3  4  5  6  7  8  9  10  11  12  13  14  15  16  17  18

◄Birth to 33 months ►     ◄—————— 3 to 18 years ——————►

**898**

**Fig. A-3.**

# Growth Charts for U.S. Boys

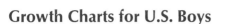

## Boys Height by Age Percentiles
### Ages: birth to 18 years

*Percentile gives rank relative to 100 children. An 11-year-old boy at the 50th percentile by height is taller than 50 out of every 100 11-year-old boys in the U.S. and shorter than the other 50.*

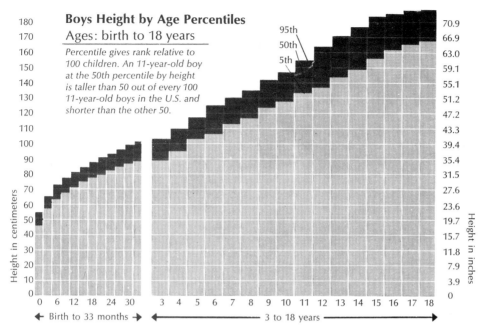

**Fig. A-4.**

*To compare a boy with his peers, find where his weight (or height) and age intersect; judge the distance from the 5th, 50th, and 95th curves for a more exact percentile. If the child is near or outside the top or bottom percentile, this should be called to the attention of his physician.*

## Boys Weight by Age Percentiles
### Ages: birth to 18 years

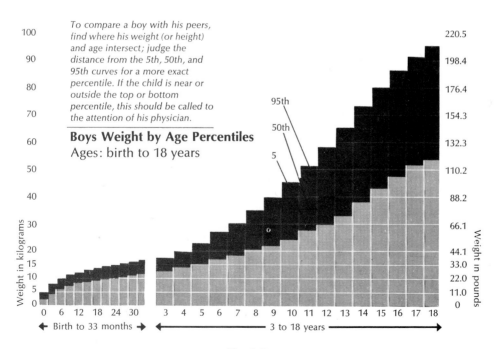

**Fig. A-5.**

Girls from birth to 36 months

Head circumference for age

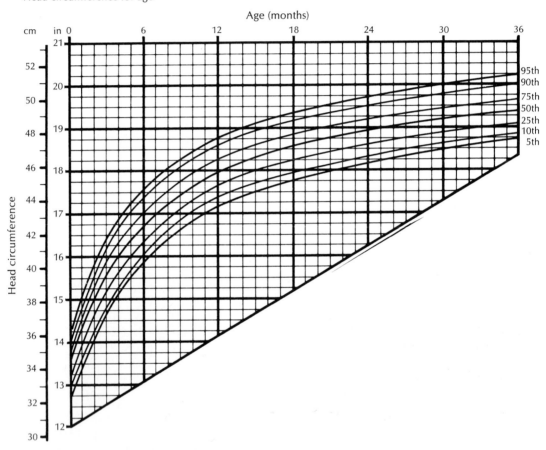

**Fig. A-6.** Head circumference chart for girls. (Courtesy Department of Health, Education and Welfare, Public Health Service Center for Disease Control.)

Boys from birth to 36 months

Head circumference for age

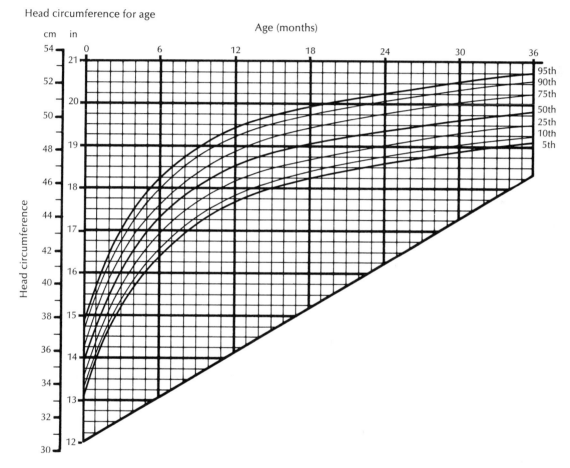

**Fig. A-7.** Head circumference chart for boys. (Courtesy Department of Health, Education and Welfare, Public Health Service Center for Disease Control.)

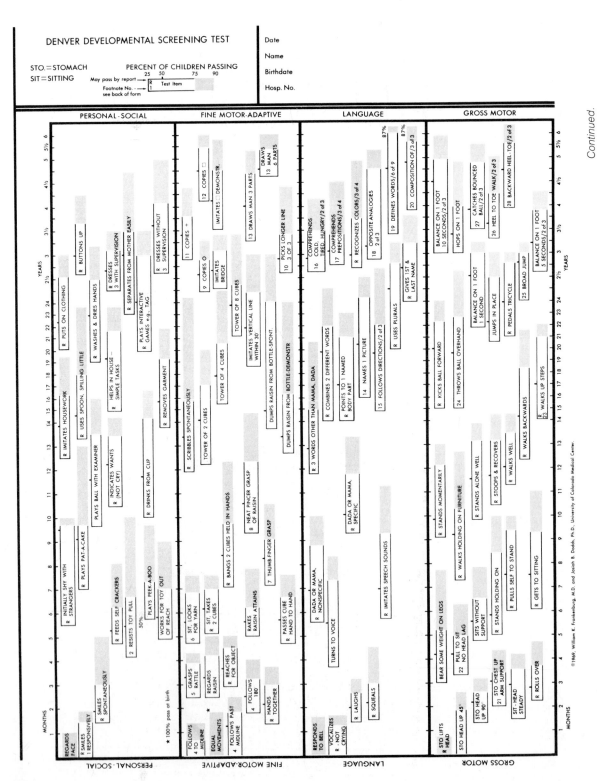

**Fig. A-8.** Denver Developmental Screening Test. (Courtesy William K. Frankenburg, M.D., University of Colorado Medical Center, Denver, Colorado.)

902

1. Try to get child to smile by smiling, talking or waving to him. Do not touch him.
2. When child is playing with toy, pull it away from him. Pass if he resists.
3. Child does not have to be able to tie shoes or button in the back.
4. Move yarn slowly in an arc from one side to the other, about 6" above child's face. Pass if eyes follow 90° to midline. (Past midline; 180°)
5. Pass if child grasps rattle when it is touched to the backs or tips of fingers.
6. Pass if child continues to look where yarn disappeared or tries to see where it went. Yarn should be dropped quickly from sight from tester's hand without arm movement.
7. Pass if child picks up raisin with any part of thumb and a finger.
8. Pass if child picks up raisin with the ends of thumb and index finger using an over hand approach.

9. Pass any enclosed form. Fail continuous round motions.
10. Which line is longer? (Not bigger.) Turn paper upside down and repeat. (3/3 or 5/6)
11. Pass any crossing lines.
12. Have child copy first. If failed, demonstrate

When giving items 9, 11 and 12, do not name the forms. Do not demonstrate 9 and 11.
13. When scoring, each pair (2 arms, 2 legs, etc.) counts as one part.
14. Point to picture and have child name it. (No credit is given for sounds only.)

  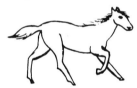 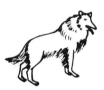 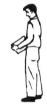

15. Tell child to: Give block to Mommie; put block on table; put block on floor. Pass 2 of 3. (Do not help child by pointing, moving head or eyes.)
16. Ask child: What do you do when you are cold? ..hungry? ..tired? Pass 2 of 3.
17. Tell child to: Put block on table; under table; in front of chair, behind chair. Pass 3 of 4. (Do not help child by pointing, moving head or eyes.)
18. Ask child: If fire is hot, ice is ?; Mother is a woman, Dad is a ?; a horse is big, a mouse is ?. Pass 2 of 3.
19. Ask child: What is a ball? ..lake? ..desk? ..house? ..banana? ..curtain? ..ceiling? ..hedge? ..pavement? Pass if defined in terms of use, shape, what it is made of or general category (such as banana is fruit, not just yellow). Pass 6 of 9.
20. Ask child: What is a spoon made of? ..a shoe made of? ..a door made of? (No other objects may be substituted.) Pass 3 of 3.
21. When placed on stomach, child lifts chest off table with support of forearms and/or hands.
22. When child is on back, grasp his hands and pull him to sitting. Pass if head does not hang back.
23. Child may use wall or rail only, not person. May not crawl.
24. Child must throw ball overhand 3 feet to within arm's reach of tester.
25. Child must perform standing broad jump over width of test sheet. (8-1/2 inches)
26. Tell child to walk forward, ⬭⬭⬭➝ heel within 1 inch of toe. Tester may demonstrate. Child must walk 4 consecutive steps, 2 out of 3 trials.
27. Bounce ball to child who should stand 3 feet away from tester. Child must catch ball with hands, not arms, 2 out of 3 trials.
28. Tell child to walk backward, ⬅⬭⬭⬭ toe within 1 inch of heel. Tester may demonstrate. Child must walk 4 consecutive steps, 2 out of 3 trials.

DATE AND BEHAVIORAL OBSERVATIONS (how child feels at time of test, relation to tester, attention span, verbal behavior, self-confidence, etc,):

**Fig. A-8, cont'd.** For legend see opposite page.

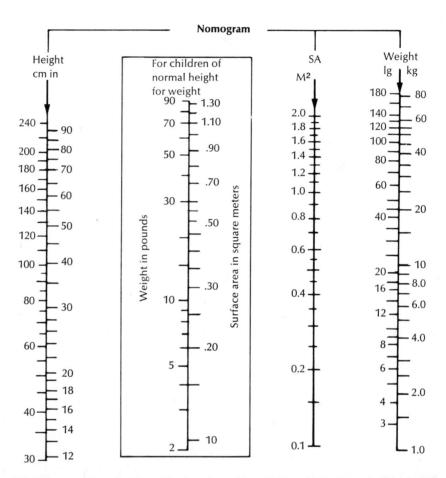

**Fig. A-9.** Nomogram for estimation of body surface. (From Shirkey, H. D.: Drug therapy. In Nelson, W. E., Vaughan, V. C. III, and McKay, R. J., editors: Textbook of pediatrics, ed. 9, Philadelphia, 1969, W. B. Saunders Co.)

# Index

**905**

932